MANUAL OF ENDOCRINOLOGY AND METABOLISM

Fourth Edition

MANUAL OF ENDOCRINOLOGY AND METABOLISM

Fourth Edition

Editor

Norman Lavin, M.D., Ph.D., F.A.A.P., F.A.C.E.

Clinical Professor of Endocrinology and Pediatrics
Director of Clinical Education in Endocrinology
UCLA School of Medicine
Los Angeles, California

Editor-in-Chief: *Growth, Growth Hormone, IGF-1, and Metabolism*
London, England

Director of the Diabetes Care Center
Director of Medical Education
Providence Tarzana Regional Medical Center
Tarzana, California

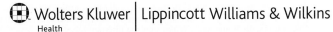

Wolters Kluwer | Lippincott Williams & Wilkins
Health

Philadelphia · Baltimore · New York · London
Buenos Aires · Hong Kong · Sydney · Tokyo

Publisher: Charles W. Mitchell
Managing Editor: Sirkka E. Howes
Senior Marketing Manager: Angela Panetta
Associate Production Manager: Kevin P. Johnson
Designer: Teresa Mallon
Compositor: Aptara, Inc.

351 West Camden Street   530 Walnut Street
Baltimore, MD 21201   Philadelphia, PA 19106

Printed in China

9 8 7 6 5 4 3 2

Library of Congress Cataloging-in-Publication Data

Manual of endocrinology and metabolism / editor, Norman Lavin. – 4th ed.
   p. ; cm.
  Includes bibliographical references and index.
  ISBN 978-0-7817-6886-3 (alk. paper)
  1. Endocrinology–Handbooks, manuals, etc. 2. Endocrine glands–
Diseases–Handbooks, manuals, etc. 3. Metabolism–Disorders–
Handbooks, manuals, etc.   I. Lavin, Norman.
  [DNLM: 1. Endocrine System Diseases–Handbooks. 2. Metabolic
Diseases–Handbooks.   WK 39 M294 2009]
  RC648.M365 2009
  616.4–dc22

                         2008049705

DISCLAIMER

This book is dedicated to:

To my **mother** and **father,** and my **brother, Sheldon:** One day, we will all be together again.

To my **sister, Barbara**—I cherish our continuing close friendship. Thank you for always "holding my hand." We all love you.

To my **sons, Arye and Jonah**—who continue to be on a reflective journey towards spiritual, intellectual, and emotional enlightenment, and are teaming with great promise and fresh starts. One day, you will locate your coordinates on the arc of history. You are both full of tender wisdom, brawling insight, and sharp-edged humor as you explore the tricky journey to adulthood with honesty and generosity. You have woven a radiant tapestry that illuminates the experience of adolescence. As you approach adulthood, you will explore its complexities, feel its ambivalences, struggle with its choices, and live imaginatively its moral life.

You make me laugh, cry, and cherish every moment, but mostly you make me aware of joy—the wild, clattering joy of being alive. From both of you, I have learned about the power of love, the enduring strength of family, and the possibilities of life.

Thank you. I love both of you dearly.

To my **wife, Michele,** a woman of extreme caring and giving, who propels the shifting tides of love and need into something close to majesty. Every day, every year, your arms stretch farther and farther to encompass more people, more life.

Your spirit is generous and embracing and your triumph is the breathing, shimmering world you create around our family and friends. Your beauty, intelligence, kindness, easy charm, and steadfast individuality make me cherish every moment of our lives together.

Michele—you are the pulsing emotional center of my life. I love you now and forever.

N.L.

CONTENTS

VI: THYROID DISORDERS

VII: METABOLIC DISORDERS

VIII: INBORN ERRORS OF METABOLISM

IX: DIABETES MELLITUS

X: SPECIAL TOPICS IN CLINICAL ENDOCRINOLOGY

APPENDICES

$\int$n this fourth current edition, we present significantly updated information regarding recent developments in the field of endocrinology as well as an introduction to risk assessment and screening. Results of recent clinical trials and their implications for future treatment modalities and prevention are highlighted. We also provide in a summary form recently released guidelines from the Endocrine Society and the American Academy of Clinical Endocrinology for prevention and management of many endocrine disorders including diabetes, growth hormone deficiency, dysmetabolic syndrome, dyslipidemia, and obesity.

The fourth edition of *The Manual of Endocrinology and Metabolism* blends three primary subdivisions—namely, Adult, Pediatric and Reproductive—into a text that closely examines genetic and environmental factors that contribute to endocrine diseases in every age group. Because of our new understanding of endocrine disorder causation, a primary focus of this text is to develop interventional programs to reverse these factors and/or prevent their transmission. Cardiovascular disease in adults, for example, often begins in childhood and in some cases has been traced back to fetal life. Thus, an underlying theme of this book is to present evaluation, pathophysiology, management and treatment at every age of life with short and long term goals of reversibility and prevention. By providing succinct chapters on pathogenesis, evaluation, and ample therapeutic options for both prevention and treatment, our interventional programs not only eliminate or reverse the disease process but also help prevent contributing etiologic factors.

This manual allows the reader to quickly identify and understand topics of interest, which translates into very practical treatment planning. Our authors, who are pioneers in the field of endocrinology, present relevant pathophysiology with practical protocols for evaluation and treatment.

The target audience continues to be any health professional who desires a rapid answer to any challenging question in Endocrinology including endocrinologists, diabetologists, endocrine surgeons, fellows, house officers, nurses, and medical students.

All chapters have been updated with a focus on new technologies and laboratory assessment as well as new treatment options. Some chapters have been eliminated and others have been added to parallel the evolution of modern medicine. With the global epidemic of obesity and type 2 diabetes mellitus in children, new chapters focus on comorbidities (e.g., dyslipidemia, and essential hypertension). Newer drugs for both type 1 and 2 are presented with a target goal of optimal glucose control as well as an attempt at retention of beta cell function.

The book again is divided into ten sections arranging closely related subjects into clusters. Basic Sciences in Part I provides the underlying theme of endocrinology, but it is kept to a minimum with chapters on genetics, molecular biology and the molecular endocrine laboratory. Hypothalamus and pituitary disorders are described in Part II, with a new chapter on the use of growth hormone in adults. Part III addresses adrenal gland disorders, focusing on the molecular basis for evaluation and clearly outlined treatments.

Pubertal and reproductive endocrinology is highlighted in Part IV, while Part V encompasses the most recent understanding of calcium metabolism emphasizing prevention as well as immediate and long-term treatment.

Thyroid disorders ranging in age from the fetus to the elderly are covered in Part VI with separate chapters on thyroid function tests, hypothyroidism and hyperthyroidism and thyroid cancer in children and adults. Part VII incorporates important metabolic diseases including obesity, dyslipidemia, insulin resistance syndrome, and hypoglycemia, while Part VIII highlights common inborn errors of metabolism.

The global epidemic of type 2 diabetes mellitus in adults, and now in children, necessitates a thorough examination of the prevention, evaluation and treatment of this challenging problem found in Part IX. Once again, Nobel Laureate Andrew Schally presents his recent research on hormone-dependent cancers in Part X. Other chapters in this section include Aging and Hormones, Pregnancy and Surgical Correction of Hormone Related Tumors.

It is therefore with great pleasure that I have the distinct honor to be the editor of the fourth edition of *The Manual of Endocrinology and Metabolism* written by distinguished scholars, scientists, endocrinologists, researchers and clinicians as well as the 1983 Nobel Laureate in Medicine.

Norman Lavin, M.D.

Omar Ali, M.D.
Assistant Professor of Pediatric
  Endocrinology
Medical College of Wisconsin
Attending Physician
Childrens Hospital of Wisconsin
Milwaukee, Wisconsin

Marie U. Beall, M.D.
Professor
Director of Maternal Fetal
  Medicine Fellowship
Department of Obstetrics and
  Gynecology
Harbor UCLA Medical Center
Torrance, California

Asif Bhutto, M.D.
Assistant Professor of Internal Medicine
Division of Geriatric Medicine
Saint Louis University
Saint Louis University Hospital
Saint Louis, Missouri

Norman L. Block, M.D., F.A.C.S.
Weeks Professor of Urology/Oncology
University of Miami
Miller School of Medicine
Attending Physician
Jackson Memorial Hospital
Miami, Florida

**George A. Bray, M.D., M.A.C.P.,
M.A.C.E.**
Boyd Professor
Chief of Clinical Obesity
Pennington Center at LSU System
Baton Rouge, Louisiana

Stuart J. Brink, M.D.
Associate Clinical Professor of Pediatrics
Tufts University School of Medicine
Boston, Massachusetts
Senior Endocrinologist
New England Diabetes and Endocrinology
  Center (NEDEC)
Waltham, Massachusetts

Harold E. Carlson, M.D.
Professor of Medicine
Head of Division of Endocrinology
Stony Brook University
Attending Physician
University Hospital-Stony Brook
Stony Brook, New York

Stephen D. Cederbaum, M.D.
Professor of Psychiatry
Pediatrics, and Human Genetics
University of California
Los Angeles
Attending Physician
Department of Pediatrics
UCLA Medical Center
Los Angeles, California

Charles H. Choe, M.D.
Assistant Clinical Professor of Medicine
Department of Endocrinology
Diabetes and Metabolism
University of California
San Diego
Staff Physician
San Diego VA Healthcare System
San Diego, California

Orlo H. Clark, M.D., F.A.C.S.
Professor of Surgery
University of California
San Francisco
Mount Zion Medical Center
San Francisco, California

Pinchas Cohen, M.D.
Professor of Pediatrics
David Geffen School of Medicine at UCLA
Chief of Pediatric Endocrinology
Mattel Children's Hospital at UCLA
Los Angeles, California

Alfred M. Dashe, M.D., F.A.C.P.
Clinical Professor
Department of Medicine
Endocrinology
Geffen School of Medicine at UCLA
Los Angeles, California

Mayer B. Davidson, M.D.
Professor of Medicine
UCLA School of Medicine
Director
Clinical Center of Research Excellence
Charles R. Drew University
Los Angeles, California

Alan H. DeCherney, M.D.
Chief
Reproductive Biology and Medicine
   Branch
Head
Program in Adult and Reproductive
   Endocrinology
Eunice Kennedy Shriver National Institute
   of Child Health and Human Development
National Institutes of Health
Bethesda, Maryland

Michael A. Dedekian, M.D.
Fellow in Endocrinology
Department of Medicine
Division of Endocrinology
Harvard Medical School
Children's Hospital Boston
Boston, Massachusetts

Cem S. Demirci, M.D.
Fellow
PGY-6
Department of Pediatric Endocrinology
Diabetes and Metabolism
UPMC University of Pittsburgh Medical
   Center
Children's Hospital of Pittsburgh UPMC
Pittsburgh, Pennsylvania

Richard A. Dickey, M.D.
Clinical Assistant Professor
Department of Internal Medicine/
   Endocrinology
Wake Forest University School
   of Medicine
Winston-Salem, North Carolina

Andrew Jay Drexler, M.D.
Clinical Professor of Medicine
Division of Endocrinology
UCLA David Geffen School
   of Medicine
Los Angeles, California

Nicole Ducharme, D.O.
Endocrinology Fellow
Saint Louis University
Saint Louis, Missouri

Steven V. Edelman, M.D.
Professor of Medicine
Department of Endocrinology
Diabetes, and Metabolism
University of California
San Diego
Staff Physician
San Diego VA Healthcare System
San Diego, California

George S. Eisenbarth, M.D., Ph.D.
Director
Barbara Davis Center for Childhood
   Diabetes
Colorado University, Denver
Aurora, Colorado

Calvin Ezrin, M.D.
Clinical Professor
Department of Medicine
University of California, Los Angeles
Attending Physician
Encino-Tarzana Medical Center
Tarzana, California

Rena Ellen Falk, M.D.
Professor
Department of Pediatrics
David Geffen School of Medicine at UCLA
Associate Medical Director
Cytogenetics Laboratory
Co-Director
Prenatal Diagnosis Center
Clinical Pathology and Laboratory
   Medicine and Medical Genetics Institute
Cedars-Sinai Medical Center
Los Angeles, California

Benjamin Fass, M.D.
Assistant Clinical Professor of Pediatrics
University of California
Los Angeles
School of Medicine
Staff Pediatrician/Pediatric Endocrinology
Southern California Kaiser Permanente
   Medical Group
Los Angeles, California

Mitchell E. Geffner, M.D.
Professor of Pediatrics
USC Keck School of Medicine
Director of Fellowship Training
Division of Endocrinology
Diabetes, and Metabolism
Saban Research Institute of Childrens
   Hospital Los Angeles
Los Angeles, California

Guido Lastra Gonzalez, M.D.
Department of Internal Medicine
Endocrinology
University of Missouri-Columbia
Columbia, Missouri

Wayne W. Grody, M.D., Ph.D.
Professor
Departments of Pathology & Laboratory
  Medicine
Pediatrics, and Human Genetics
UCLA School of Medicine
Director
Diagnostic Molecular Pathology
  Laboratory
Attending Physician
Division of Medical Genetics
UCLA Medical Center
Los Angeles, California

Theodore J. Hahn, M.D.
Professor of Medicine and Director
Osteoporosis and Bone Disorders Program
Department of Medicine
University of California, Los Angeles
Director
Geriatric Research
Education, and Clinical Center
VA Greater Los Angeles Healthcare System
Los Angeles, California

Jerome M. Hershman, M.D., M.S.
Distinguished Professor of Medicine
David Geffen School of Medicine at UCLA
Associate Chief
Endocrinology and Diabetes Division
Greater Los Angeles Healthcare System
Los Angeles, California

Christopher P. Houk, M.D.
Associate Professor of Pediatrics
Medical College of Georgia
Pediatric Endocrinologist
Medical College of Georgia
Augusta, Georgia

Stanley H. Hsia, M.D.
Assistant Professor of Medicine
Division of Endocrinology
Metabolism, and Molecular Medicine
Charles R. Drew University of Medicine
  and Science
Consultant Physician
Division of Endocrinology
Metabolism, and Molecular Medicine
Department of Internal Medicine
Martin Luther King Jr.
Multi-Service Ambulatory Care Center
Los Angeles, California

Stephen Albert Huang, M.D.
Assistant Professor of Pediatrics
Harvard Medical School
Director, Thyroid Program
Children's Hospital Boston
Endocrine Division
Boston, Massachusetts

Naomi Horowitz James
Pediatrics Assistant
Mount Sinai School of Medicine
New York, New York

John L. Kitzmiller, M.D.
Division of Maternal-Fetal
  Medicine
Santa Clara Valley Medical Center
San Jose, California

Siri L. Kjos, M.D., M.S.Ed.
Professor
Chief of Obstetrics
Department of Obstetrics and
  Gynecology
Program Director
OB/GYN Residency
Harbor-UCLA Medical Center
Torrance, California

Stephen H. LaFranchi, M.D.
Professor of Pediatrics
Oregon Health & Science
  University
Staff Physician
Pediatrics—Endocrinology
Doernbecher Children's Hospital
Portland, Oregon

Adrian Langleben, M.D.
Associate Professor
Department of Oncology
McGill University
Attending Physician
Departments of Oncology and
  Medicine
Jewish General Hospital
Montreal
Quebec, Canada

**Norman Lavin, M.D., Ph.D., F.A.A.P.,
  F.A.C.E.**
Clinical Professor of Endocrinology
  and Pediatrics
Director of Clinical Education in
  Endocrinology
UCLA School of Medicine
Los Angeles, California

Kuk-Wha Lee, M.D., Ph.D.
Assistant Professor
Department of Pediatrics
David Geffen School of Medicine
University of California
Los Angeles
Division of Endocrinology
Mattel Children's Hospital
Los Angeles, California

Peter A. Lee, M.D., Ph.D.
Professor of Pediatrics
Penn State College of Medicine
Hershey, Pennsylvania
Professor of Pediatrics
Indiana University School
   of Medicine
Indianapolis, Indiana
Attending Physician
MS Hershey Medical Center
Hershey, Pennsylvania
Attending Physician
Riley Hospital for Children
Indianapolis, Indiana

Philip D. K. Lee, M.D.
Senior Medical Director
Global Clinical Development
Fertility and Endocrinology
EMD Serono, Inc.
Rockland, Massachusetts

Eric D. Levens, M.D.
Staff Clinician
Program in Reproductive and Adult
   Endocrinology
Eunice Kennedy Shriver National Institute
   of Child Health and Human
   Development
National Institutes of Health
Bethesda, Maryland

Michael A. Levine, M.D.,
   FAAP, FACP
Director
Division of Endocrinology and Diabetes
The Children's Hospital of Philadelphia
Department of Pediatrics
University of Pennsylvania School of
   Medicine
Philadelphia, PA

Karen Lin-Su, M.D.
Assistant Professor of Pediatrics
Mount Sinai School of Medicine
New York, New York

Louis C. K. Low, FRCPCH, FRCP,
   FHKAM
Professor of Pediatrics and Adolescent
   Medicine
The University of Hong Kong
Honorary Consultant
Paediatrics and Adolescent Medicine
Queen Mary Hospital
Hong Kong SAR
People's Republic of China

Anne W. Lucky, M.D.
Volunteer Professor of Dermatology and
   Pediatrics
University of Cincinnati College of
   Medicine
Acting Director
Division of Pediatric Dermatology
Cincinnati Children's Hospital
Cincinnati, Ohio

Vahid Mahabadi, M.D., M.P.H.
Department of Medicine
David Geffen School of Medicine
   at UCLA
Los Angeles, California
Endocrine Fellow
Division of Endocrinology
Harbor-UCLA Medical Center
Torrance, California

Camila Manrique, M.D.
Resident Physician
Department of Internal Medicine
University of Missouri
Columbia, Missouri

Angela D. Mazza, D.O.
Clinical Endocrinologist
The Diabetes Institute
Florida Hospital
Orlando, Florida

Jorge H. Mestman, M.D.
Professor of Obstetrics and Gynecology
Keck School of Medicine
University of Southern California
Los Angeles, California

John E. Morley, M.B., B.Ch.
Dammert Professor of Gerontology
Department of Internal Medicine
Saint Louis University
Director
FRECC
St. Louis VA Medical Center
St. Louis, Missouri

Jon M. Nakamoto, M.D., Ph.D.
Associate Clinical Professor
  (Voluntary)
Pediatrics and Endocrinology
University of California
San Diego, La Jolla, California
Managing Director
Quest Diagnostics Nichols Institute
San Juan Capistrano, California

Maria I. New, M.D.
Professor of Pediatrics/Genetics & Genomic
  Sciences
Director
Adrenal Steroid Disorders Program
Mount Sinai School of Medicine
New York, New York

Saroj NimKarn, M.D.
Assistant Professor of Pediatrics/
  Endocrinology
Mount Sinai School of Medicine
New York, New York

Etty Osher, M.D.
Senior Physician
Institute of Endocrinology
Metabolism and Hypertension
Tel Aviv-Sourasky Medical Center
Tel Aviv, Israel

Anna Pawlikowska-Haddal, M.D.
Assistant Clinical Professor
Department of Pediatrics
Division of Pediatric Endocrinology
University of California, Los Angeles
Mattel Children's Hospital
  at UCLA
Los Angeles, California

Stephanie Smooke Praw, M.D.
Fellow
Department of Medicine
Division of Endocrinology
University of California,
Los Angeles
Los Angeles, California

Rani Radhamma, M.D.
Fellow
Department of Endocrinology
Saint Louis University Hospital
Saint Louis, Missouri

Donna H. Ryan, M.D.
Professor and Associate Executive
  Director of Clinical Research
Pennington Biomedical Research
  Center
Baton Rouge, Louisiana

**Andrew V. Schally, Ph.D., M.D.hc
  (Multi), D.Sc.hc**
Distinguished Leonard Miller Professor
Departments of Pathology and Medicine
University of Miami
Miller School of Medicine
Chief, Endocrine Polypeptide and Research
  Institute
Veterans Affairs Medical Center
Miami, Florida
1983 Nobel Laureate in Medicine

Frederick R. Singer, M.D.
Clinical Professor of Medicine
Geffen School of Medicine at UCLA,
  Los Angeles, California
Director
Endocrine/Bone Disease Program
John Wayne Cancer Institute at Saint John's
  Health Center
Santa Monica, California

Peter A. Singer, M.D.
Professor of Clinical Medicine
Keck School of Medicine
University of Southern California
Los Angeles, California

Jay S. Skyler, M.D., M.A.C.P.
Professor
Division of Endocrinology
Diabetes & Metabolism
Associate Director
Diabetes Research Institute
University of Miami
Miller School of Medicine
Miami, Florida

James R. Sowers, M.D.
Professor of Medicine
Physiology and Pharmacology
Director
MU Diabetes and Cardiovascular Center
Department of Internal Medicine University
  of Missouri-Columbia
Columbia, Missouri

Richard F. Spark, M.D.
Associate Clinical Professor of Medicine
Department of Endocrinology
Harvard Medical School
Director of Steroid Research
Beth Israel Deaconess Medical Center
Boston, Massachusetts

Phyllis W. Speiser, M.D.
Professor of Pediatrics
New York University School of Medicine
New York, New York
Chief of Pediatric Endocrinology
Schneider Children's Hospital
New Hyde Park, New York

Mark A. Sperling, M.D.
Professor of Pediatrics
UPMC University of Pittsburgh
  Medical Center
Children's Hospital of Pittsburgh
  UPMC
Pittsburgh, Pennsylvania

Naftali Stern, M.D.
Professor of Medicine
Sackler Faculty of Medicine
Tel Aviv University
Director
Institute of Endocrinology
Metabolism and Hypertension
Tel Aviv Sourasky Medical
  Center
Tel Aviv, Israel

Emily Swant, M.D.
Medical Student
David Geffen School of Medicine
  at UCLA
Los Angeleca, California

Ronald S. Swerdloff, M.D.
Professor of Medicine
David Geffen School of Medicine
  at UCLA
Los Angeles, California
Chief, Division of Endocrinology
Harbor-UCLA Medical Center
Torrance, California

Shadi Tabba, M.D.
Fellow-PGY-4
Department of Pediatric
  Endocrinology
Diabetes and Metabolism
UPMC University of Pittsburgh
  Medical Center
Children's Hospital of Pittsburgh
  UPMC
Pittsburgh, Pennsylvania

Michael L. Tuck, M.D.
Professor
Department of Medicine
University of California, Los Angeles
Veterans Affairs Medical Center
Sepulveda, California

Srivalli Vegi, M.D.
Geriatric Fellow
Department of Geriatric Medicine
Saint Louis University
Saint Louis, Missouri

Eric Vilain, M.D., Ph.D.
Professor of Human Genetics
University of California
Los Angeles
Attending Physician
Department of Pediatrics
UCLA Medical Center
Los Angeles, California

Christina Wang, M.D.
Professor of Medicine
David Geffen School of Medicine at UCLA
Los Angeles, California
Director
General Clinical Research Center
Harbor-UCLA Medical Center
Torrance, California

**Adam Whaley-Connell, D.O.,
M.S.P.H.**
Assistant Professor of Medicine
Internal Medicine
Division of Nephrology
University of Missouri-Columbia School of
  Medicine
University of Missouri Hospitals and Clinics
Columbia, Missouri

Thomas A. Wilson, M.D.
Professor of Clinical Pediatrics
Chief
Division of Pediatric Endocrinology
State University of New York
Stony Brook, New York

Selma Feldman Witchel, M.D.
Associate Professor of Pediatrics
Department of Pediatric Endocrinology
Children's Hospital of Pittsburgh of
  UPMC/University of Pittsburgh
Pittsburgh, Pennsylvania

Joseph I. Wolfsdorf, M.B., B.Ch.
Professor of Pediatrics
Harvard Medical School
Clinical Director and Associate Chief
Division of Endocrinology
Children's Hospital Boston
Boston, Massachusetts

Sing-yung Wu, M.D., Ph.D.
Professor
Departments of Radiological Sciences and
  Medicine
University of California
Irvine, Irvine, California
Staff Physician
Radiology/Nuclear Medicine
VA-UC Irvine Healthcare System
Long Beach, California

ACKNOWLEDGMENT

J thank Ms. Sirkka Howes, the associate managing editor at Lippincott Williams & Wilkins for her ready availability and tremendous support.

I thank all of my friends and colleagues who have contributed to this fourth edition with their insightful advice and exemplary scholarship. I particularly thank Nancy Herbst, M.A. Ed. for her skillful literary and technical assistance, as well as her unyielding patience and wonderful sense of humor.

I will also never forget the friendship and guidance from Rabbi Bernard Cohen, Ph.D., Dr. Ben Fass, Dr. Al Sils, Neal Schnall, and Rabbi Jay Levy, J.D. Finally, I thank legendary UCLA coach John Wooden for his warm, embracing friendship and transcendent inspiration. Happy 98th birthday, Coach.

N.L.

Basic Science of Clinical Endocrinology

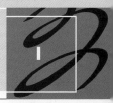

CLINICAL MOLECULAR ENDOCRINOLOGY LABORATORY

Jon Nakamoto and Wayne W. Grody

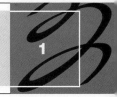

*A*s genetic testing becomes more commonplace in medical decision making, the perceived mystery surrounding "molecular" diagnostics has fallen away, only to be replaced all too often by naïve confidence in the clinical utility of DNA- and RNA-based testing. As with all clinical laboratory testing, the best diagnostic results are achieved after much forethought before any testing is even ordered, and when clinicians understand the limitations and caveats of the testing they use. This is especially true in the area of endocrine disorders, which is still in its infancy as a target of molecular testing, at least compared to such fields as oncology and neuromuscular disorders. Above all, one must ask whether a positive or negative result of the test will actually influence clinical management, and whether the benefits of obtaining this information outweigh the risks. Here, we offer a checklist to help clinicians avoid the most common diagnostic pitfalls and to help ensure rational use of endocrine genetic testing.

I. THE CHECKLIST FOR CLINICIANS
- **A. Purpose:** Is genetic testing appropriate for this patient?
- **B. Probability:** Is the diagnosis likely enough to warrant genetic testing?
- **C. Proper test and procedure:** Which test (and method used to perform that test) is most appropriate?
- **D. Place:** Is there an available laboratory with the proper certifications, quality control, and assistance with diagnostic interpretation?
- **E. Cost/benefit:** Is the benefit worth the potential cost to the patient and society?
- **F. Pitfalls:** Do I know diagnostic pitfalls to watch out for?
- **G. Politics:** Are there legal, regulatory, and ethical currents that might affect my choice of diagnostic approach, or even whether to order the test at all?

II. STARTING WITH THE PURPOSE (STEP 1)
- **A. Proof of diagnosis.** Genetic testing may be useful to provide independent confirmation of a diagnosis made through clinical acumen and biochemical laboratory

testing, although it must be kept in mind that the **positive predictive value** (PPV, probability of disease among patients with a positive test) of most molecular genetic testing is generally better than the **negative predictive value** (NPV, probability of no disease among patients with a negative test). This is not because molecular techniques are inherently inferior at the analytical level, but because they are highly specific and targeted: They will only detect the mutation or gene region examined and will not even assess other potential molecular etiologies of the condition in question. For that reason, in general, negative results on genetic testing should not be used to rule out a clinical diagnosis.

B. **Prognosis.** Knowledge of a specific mutation may be helpful in predicting future outcome. For example, identification of a mutation affecting the glucokinase gene in maturity-onset diabetes of the young, type 2 (MODY2) predicts a much milder progression of pancreatic β-cell dysfunction than other types of MODY.

C. **Pharmacogenetics.** Genetically determined differences in metabolism of and response to different medications may influence dosing decisions. In some cases, specific mutations may influence not only the dose but also the choice of medications: Mutations in the HNF-1α gene (MODY3) are associated with far better response to oral sulfonylurea treatment than are mutations in the HNF-1β gene (MODY5).

D. **Psychosocial benefit.** For conditions in which genetic testing has a strong clinical utility, both the patient and the clinician may benefit from having a firm diagnosis that avoids many of the methodological problems (interferences, population variability, reference interval limitations) inherent in clinical biochemical testing. We have found that even for those disorders with no treatment, there can be a certain psychosocial benefit to finally eliminating the doubts and having a definite diagnosis. In addition, this can save the patient from continuing a futile and sometimes risky search through other specialists and less specific tests.

E. **Presymptomatic diagnosis.** Making a diagnosis of disease prior to the appearance of any symptoms carries potential psychological and even financial risks (e.g., insurability). Thus, presymptomatic diagnosis is often discouraged, especially in pediatrics. However, there are exceptions, such as the testing for RET proto-oncogene mutations in relatives of patients with multiple endocrine neoplasia type 2 (MEN-2A or MEN-2B), where early detection of mutations associated with aggressive disease allows early treatment (e.g., prophylactic thyroidectomy) that can be lifesaving. The decision to pursue such testing is based on the age of onset of the disorder and the overarching question raised at the start: Will a positive result of this test influence clinical management? If there is no preventive intervention that would be done during childhood, then such testing is better deferred until the patient reaches the age of consent.

III. **NEXT STEP: ESTIMATING PRIOR PROBABILITY OF DISEASE.** As noted earlier, genetic testing tends to have a better PPV and worse NPV than more traditional clinical laboratory modalities. Therefore, if the pre-existing risk of disease is very low, genetic testing is most likely to give a noninformative negative result. Conversely, for a diagnosis of very low likelihood, there is a greater chance that any positive result obtained represents a false positive rather than a true positive. Estimates of pretest probability of disease (also called a priori risk) are affected by:

A. **Prevalence** of disease in the population segment (ethnic group, age, sex) to which the patient belongs. Disease prevalence also directly affects the PPV for mutations with **penetrance** (see **Pitfalls**) of <100%.

B. **Presentation.** Certain associated symptoms or signs (biochemical, histologic) may increase the pretest probability of disease, as does presence of early-onset or multifocal disease.

C. **Pedigree.** Family history is helpful in risk assessment and should always be queried prior to ordering a genetic test. A previously affected sibling will greatly raise the probability of a **recessive disorder**, while multigenerational affected cases will raise the likelihood of a **dominant disorder**. Transmission (or lack thereof) through male versus female parents may point suspicion toward **X-linked** or **mitochondrial** disorders. Such patterns are best detected by constructing a detailed pedigree as opposed to a few informal questions about family history. However, recognizing that many clinicians have neither the time nor the background to undertake such an effort, referral to a medical genetics clinic should be considered if familial transmission is suspected. That facility can also facilitate proper ordering of the test, especially if it is an esoteric one, and can provide genetic counseling to the patient and family regarding recurrence risk, testing of other at-risk relatives, and prenatal diagnosis.

IV. STEP 3: PICKING THE PROPER TEST AND PROCEDURE/METHOD

A. Consider right at the beginning whether the available "nonmolecular" diagnostic alternatives should be used first or instead of genetic testing.

1. For example, look for hyperandrogenism first, before using genetic testing for congenital adrenal hyperplasia.

2. On the other hand, favor DNA-based testing if available alternatives do not pick up disease until it actually develops (e.g., C-cell hyperplasia or worse in MEN2/FMTC).

B. Choose a test method of appropriate analytic sensitivity for the intended purpose.

1. For example, **polymerase chain reaction** (PCR) testing for the presence of a cryptic *SRY* gene in Turner syndrome may pick up positive cases that would be missed by standard **cytogenetics** or **fluorescence *in situ* hybridization** (FISH). PCR, by virtue of its exponential amplification of small regions and small amounts of target DNA sequence by repeated cycles of DNA polymerase-mediated replication, is exquisitely sensitive and specific. Whether the increased detection of cryptic Y-chromosomal material by PCR improves the positive predictive value for gonadoblastoma (the primary reason for screening for SRY sequences) remains an open question to be answered by prospective unbiased studies.

2. On the other hand, an *in situ* technique such as FISH may be more informative than PCR for showing the true proportion of cells in a papillary thyroid tumor that contain *RET-PTC* translocations.

C. Choose a test method of appropriate scale for the type of mutation suspected

1. For example, for a single known **point mutation** (single-nucleotide substitution, microdeletion, or microinsertion), as in MEN-2b or 21-hydroxylase deficiency, a targeted approach using PCR amplification of the gene region in question followed by hybridization with an **allele-specific oligonucleotide** (ASO) probe will be most efficient.

2. For disorders in which a small set of point mutations accounts for most or all of the cases as in MEN-2a, **multiplex PCR** amplification of the various gene regions followed by hybridization with a panel of ASO probes covering each of the mutations, often in a **reverse hybridization** format, is an efficient option.

3. For disorders with a greater number of possible mutations that may be found across the gene, as in MEN1, **DNA sequencing** is the "gold standard," casting the widest possible net for detection of whatever unknown mutation may be lurking there.

4. If the gene is very large, it may be more efficient and cost-effective to first perform a **mutation-scanning** technique to survey the gene for potential abnormalities and then sequence only those regions that are suspicious (see Section IV.D).

5. If the suspected mutation is a large deletion of one or several exons or even the entire gene, the most appropriate method will be **Southern blotting**, which is much better at detecting large structural rearrangements than is PCR. In fact, heterozygous deletion of a large gene region will usually be invisible to standard PCR-based sequencing, because only the opposite normal allele will amplify and be sequenced, resulting in a false negative. Because the Southern blot involves gel electrophoresis of total genomic DNA, digested by bacterial restriction enzymes into fragments of several kilobases in size that are then blotted onto a filter membrane for hybridization with a probe, it is especially useful for examining large DNA regions.

6. For disorders characterized by chromosome aneuploides, such as Turner and Klinefelter syndromes, or translocations such as *RET-PTC* in papillary thyroid carcinoma, standard **karyotyping** is the best method for a quick survey of the entire complement of chromosomes. If a specific change is suspected, targeted molecular cytogenetic testing by FISH using the specific probes complementary to the chromosome(s) or breakpoints involved is appropriate. The same approach can be used for targeted detection of specific chromosomal deletions, such as in hypoparathyroidism associated with the 22q11.2 deletion of DiGeorge/velocardiofacial syndrome.

7. For complex clinical situations of unknown etiology, such as nonspecific multiple congenital malformations, the newer technique of **array comparative genomic hybridization** (aCGH) is an efficient method for scanning the entire genome via thousands of probes on a microarray hybridization platform ("DNA chip"), for dosage alterations (copy number variants) between the patient's DNA and a competing normal control DNA sample.

D. Use of Prescreening Methods versus Targeted Mutation Search

1. **Mutation scanning techniques** are designed to detect sequence alterations anywhere along a stretch of DNA by the changes they cause in the topologic structure of the DNA or by their inability to transcribe and translate a full-length protein product. The more common methods used are **single-strand conformation polymorphism** (SSCP), **denaturing gradient gel electrophoresis** (DGGE), **denaturing high-performance liquid chromatography** (dHPLC), and the **protein truncation test** (PTT). The first three typically involve PCR amplification of each exon of the gene, followed by some form of electrophoresis or chromatography to detect aberrant migration of the fragment caused by the sequence alteration. PTT involves in vitro transcription-translation of the patient's gene, followed by analysis of the protein product(s) by polyacrylamide gel electrophoresis. It will pick up nonsense (stop) mutations as well as certain frameshift mutations, large deletions, and RNA splicing mutations because of the truncated protein products produced. It will completely miss all other single-nucleotide substitutions (missense mutations), and therefore it is used primarily for those disorders in which a substantial proportion of the mutations are of the nonsense variety, such as neurofibromatosis. It should be kept in mind that these techniques are quite finicky and are neither highly sensitive nor very specific. Any anomalously migrating exons must be sequenced subsequently for confirmation of a pathologic mutation (as opposed to an electrophoresis artifact or benign polymorphism), and a certain percentage of false negatives, resulting from comigration of a mutant exon with the normal exon, is unavoidable.

2. **PCR and sequencing.** The usual procedure is to amplify all exons of the gene (or those known to contain mutation "hot spots," such as exons 10, 11, and 16, which account for 95% of the RET mutations in MEN2) and sequence the products. In this way, only the coding regions of the gene are analyzed, not promoter regions or introns or upstream enhancers. This may miss mutations of significance (aberrant splicing, promoter mutations). When searching for heterozygous missense mutations, as in MEN2, it is prudent to perform the sequencing in both the "forward" and "reverse" directions (i.e., using both DNA strands as templates), to ensure that any equivocal mutant signals are not missed or overinterpreted.

3. **Comprehensive versus targeted DNA sequencing.** There is an important interpretive difference between those approaches that sequence gene hot spots to detect recurrent, well-documented mutations (as in MEN2) and those that assess every nucleotide in the entire gene (or at least in the coding regions). The latter approach will detect *any* sequence alteration that is present, whether pathologic or not. We now know, through the discoveries of the Human Genome Project, that **single-nucleotide polymorphisms** (SNPs) are remarkably common throughout the genome, in both coding and noncoding regions. Experience with full sequencing of the *BRCA1* and *BRCA2* genes associated with familial breast/ovarian cancer has shown us that for every true disease-causing

mutation, there are many more missense changes of no apparent clinical significance in the genes of all human beings; these are the so-called polymorphisms that make up each individual person's unique DNA "fingerprint" but that do not in themselves disrupt gene function or cause disease. The problem in molecular diagnosis arises when such a missense change is found in a patient at risk, but this particular change has never been seen or reported before. In many cases it can be difficult or even impossible to deduce, in the absence of clinical correlative evidence, whether the change is a true disease-causing mutation as opposed to a benign polymorphism of no clinical significance. One can attempt to do so by considering the nature of the resulting amino acid substitution, the degree of co-segregation of the alteration with the disease state in the family, the evolutionary conservation of the codon in question, and so on, but there are no firm rules that apply in all cases. Needless to say, the ability, or lack thereof, to make this distinction, could have a tremendous impact on the genetic counseling and medical management of the patient and family.

V. STEP 4: FINDING THE RIGHT PLACE TO PERFORM THE TEST

A. Prior knowledge of the genetic aspects of the disease in question allows more rational use of molecular testing. For example, understanding of the relative incidence of different forms of MODY leads to a strategy of screening for HNF-1α (TCF1) mutations prior to genetic analysis of glucokinase or other genes.

B. Preferred nomenclature. Genes may have multiple different names, which may complicate literature searches or attempts to find a testing laboratory. For example, the search for a laboratory offering testing for congenital adrenal hypoplasia should search for both *DAX-1* and *NROB1* gene mutations. A good site to find "official" gene names as well as common synonyms is **GeneCards** (www.genecards.org). As of 2008, more than 24 824 genes were listed. One may search by disease name; for example, the search term "diabetes insipidus" produces a list of 24 genes, with descriptions of each gene, reported benign and pathologic variants, data on the respective protein products, and links to the Human Gene Mutation Database (see later). Another source for synonyms, including both currently preferred and obsolete gene names, is the **Genome Database** at www.gdb.org. Obviously, the use of preferred terms will help when searching for a laboratory offering the desired testing.

C. Performing laboratories. Perhaps the most useful Internet site for clinicians is **GeneTests** (www.genetests.org/servlet/access). This extraordinarily useful resource, funded by the National Library of Medicine and administered by the University of Washington, lists laboratories performing a particular genetic test on either a research and/or clinical basis. The target diseases range from the relatively common, with many testing laboratories listed, to the ultrarare, for which there may be only a single laboratory in the world offering testing. Searches may be performed by disease name, gene symbol, or geographic location of the laboratories. For each laboratory identified, contact information, scope of services offered, laboratory licensure (see next section), and often a link to the laboratory's own Web site are provided. As of early 2008, a total of 607 laboratories testing for 1 527 diseases were featured on the site. Also included on this Web site are two other very useful resources: **GeneClinics**, a directory of genetic disease clinics and the services they offer; and **GeneReviews**, a large set of scholarly, up-to-date summaries of the diseases in question and the modes of testing available. Of course, one may also perform a direct Internet search using any of the powerful search engines (e.g., Google, Yahoo) to reveal candidate laboratories and clinics to contact for further information.

D. Proper certification. Laboratories that provide mutation detection information for clinical diagnostic and management purposes must be certified under **CLIA** (Clinical Laboratory Improvement Amendments). It is a matter of federal law that only CLIA-certified laboratories may provide test results to physicians and patients. So although GeneTests lists many research laboratories that will provide testing for ultrarare disorders as a favor, technically speaking, this is in violation of the law, and both the laboratory and the ordering physician could be held liable if anyone chose to challenge it. Fortunately, regulators have so far chosen to look the other way for such orphan disease tests, realizing that there is no other source of testing for these families to seek out. Moreover, efforts are under way to establish a network of CLIA-certified laboratories dedicated to this sort of testing; further information can be found at www.rarediseasetesting.org/about.php. In addition to CLIA, most high-complexity genetic testing laboratories also submit voluntarily to inspection and accreditation by the **College of American Pathologists** (CAP), which has more stringent and specific criteria for evaluation of molecular genetic laboratories. Further information can be obtained at www.cap.org, and the CAP offices can be contacted directly to inquire whether a certain laboratory has passed inspection and is accredited. Laboratories that perform testing on residents of certain states (e.g., California, New York) must also have that testing certified for those states. The GeneTests Web site provides information about all of the accreditation agencies to which each listed laboratory subscribes, so ordering physicians can make an informed choice about where to send their patient's specimen.

   E. **Professional resources.** An important consideration is availability of expert re-sources (genetic counselors, medical geneticists) who know caveats and limitations of their assays. This information will be listed on the GeneTests Web site entry and on the laboratory's individual homepage. Almost all of the larger academic and commercial genetic testing laboratories recognize the importance of this aspect and have genetic counselors and/or medical geneticists on hand for pre- and posttest consultation with referring physicians. As an alternate source, the Web site of the National Society of Genetic Counselors (www.nsgc.org) features a search function for locating genetic counselors by zip code.

   F. **Other useful Internet resources.** The **Human Gene Mutation Database** (www.hgmd.cf.ac.uk/ac/index.php), is an ongoing catalog of disease-related mutations. As of 2008 there were >57 000 mutations listed in 2 183 genes. **Online Mendelian Inheritance in Man** (OMIM), at www.ncbi.nlm.nih.gov/sites/entrez?db=omim, remains the classic resource for general information about all known genetic dis-eases, the causative genes, the symptoms and signs, and comprehensive literature references.

VI. STEP 5: IDENTIFYING POTENTIAL PITFALLS

   A. **Phenocopy phenomenon.** Overlapping clinical phenotypes may lead to misdi-rected genetic testing. For example, a female with mild hyperandrogenism as a result of polycystic ovary syndrome might be referred inappropriately for testing for a *CYP21A2* mutation because of overlap with nonclassical adrenal hyperplasia.

   B. **Paternity issues.** An eternal problem in genetic analysis is the difficulty of verifying paternity based on history-taking alone, yet it is often essential to have this informa-tion in order to assess risk for genetic disease and appropriate mutation targeting in offspring. Additional testing to determine paternity (using DNA fingerprint-ing techniques) may be helpful but is fraught with legal, social, and psychological risk.

   C. **Promoter and other non–coding-region mutations.** The majority of gene se-quencing tests focus on exons (coding regions) and the boundaries between exons and introns (intervening noncoding regions) where RNA splice-site mutations are most likely to lie. Other regions of DNA may still be clinically relevant: Muta-tions in the promoter (regulatory) region can affect gene expression, and mutations within introns may lead to altered RNA processing during transcription of DNA into RNA. Yet at this time it is still impractical and overly costly to pursue com-prehensive sequencing of these lengthy noncoding regions. Someday, when whole-genome sequencing becomes a reality at the clinical level, this may no longer be an issue, though many other challenges (such as the countless nucleotide variants of uncertain clinical significance that will be found in these regions) will ensue.

   D. **PCR issues**
      1. **Allele dropout** (e.g., nucleotide 656 mutation of the *CYP21A2* gene: When the mutant allele has a G and the wild-type allele is A [heterozygous], the A may

drop out during PCR amplification, with the result that the patient appears to be homozygous for the mutation).

2. **Contamination** is a constant concern when using a technique as powerful as PCR. Laboratories must be extremely vigilant to the possibility of cross-contamination from trace amounts of previously amplified DNA in the laboratory causing false results. These matters are scrutinized by CAP inspectors during laboratory accreditation, and is another reason for choosing a reputable laboratory.

E. Penetrance

1. For example, hemochromatosis: Penetrance may change with age, as in C282Y homozygotes, where females <40 years of age have clinical evidence of iron overload in 39%, rising to 80% in females >40 years old. In contrast, only ~2% of patients with C282Y/H63D compound heterozygous genotype have hemochromatosis. In fact, there has been much controversy over the degree of penetrance of the C282Y/C282Y homozygous state even in males, which is one reason why population screening for this condition has never been launched.

F. Predictive value of the genetic test

1. For example, M918T in the *RET* proto-oncogene essentially proves the diagnosis of MEN2B, making it a clinically valid, targeted mutation test.
2. In contrast, genome association studies often produce candidate single-nucleotide polymorphism (SNP) candidates that have a high rate of false associations with disease, far too many to allow routine clinical use without further clinical validation study.

G. Phase

1. If prenatal DNA analysis reveals two different "severe" mutations in CYP21A2, is the fetus likely to be affected by CAH?
   a. If there is a standard policy of establishing mutations in both parents prior to prenatal testing, the answer is "yes."
   b. If no family studies have been done, the result is ambiguous.
2. If mutations are present on different chromosomes (*"trans"*), yes, the fetus is likely to be affected.
3. If both mutations are present on the same chromosome (*"cis"*), no, the fetus may not be affected.

H. Parental effects

1. For example, PWS (Prader-Willi Syndrome) versus Angelman syndrome depends on loss of paternal versus maternal region of chromosome 15.
2. The concept of uniparental disomy, is a rare event in which both copies of a particular chromosome are inherited from the same parent.

I. Partial prevalence. For example, mosaicism (somatic mutation vs. germline mutation present in certain tissues but absent in others).

J. Sample mix-ups. Sample mix-ups are a potential cause of error in any clinical laboratory test.

VII. POLITICAL AND ETHICAL ISSUES

DNA-based diagnostic testing for genetic diseases is unique from the other areas of molecular diagnostics such as molecular microbiology and molecular oncology. It is primarily in the area of genetic disease testing that issues of privacy and discrimination arise, simply because the test by definition is assessing the patient's fundamental genetic makeup. Although endocrinologists typically order these procedures for purposes of **diagnostic testing** in a symptomatic patient, which raises fewer of these concerns, it is important to remember that the same technology can be used for **presymptomatic testing** of later-onset dominant disorders, **carrier screening** for recessive mutations, and **prenatal diagnosis**. Each of these applications carries its own set of ethical concerns.

A. Genetic discrimination in employment for insurance is always a potential risk, especially for those individuals in small group plans and in the absence of protective legislation. The risk is of most concern in presymptomatic testing of healthy individuals, but problems have been documented with carrier testing in recessive diseases as well. Although the number of such incidents is not great, most genetic counselors feel obligated to warn prospective test subjects of the hypothetical risk.

B. **Abortion** remains a subject of intense religious, political, and constitutional debate in the United States. It is important in the context of prenatal testing in that it must be legal and available in order to justify the expense and potential risk to the fetus of prenatal diagnostic procedures. Prenatal testing for later-onset or treatable diseases, such as MEN, raises its own set of ethical questions, centered around whether the natural history and prognosis (given prophylactic treatment, e.g., thyroidectomy) are of sufficient severity to justify termination of a pregnancy. Some couples in this situation may opt for the procedure of **preimplantation genetic diagnosis** (PGD), in which embryos are produced by in vitro fertilization and then biopsied for single-cell PCR testing. Only embryos not found to carry the mutation(s) in question are implanted in the mother's uterus.

C. **Eugenics** has traditionally referred to "improvement" of the gene pool of the human species through selective or coercive breeding, mandatory sterilization, or genocide. The advent of molecular medicine now raises the possibility of more subtle forms of eugenics based on differential access of certain groups to prenatal diagnosis, in vitro fertilization, gene therapy, and, potentially, human cloning. In routine medical practice, the concern would most likely arise in the context of a family at risk for a testable genetic disease who are not covered for the cost of the testing or subsequent preventive intervention.

D. **Testing of children** who are asymptomatic is generally to be avoided because of potential stigmatization and informed consent issues, unless there is a beneficial medical or surgical intervention that must be started in childhood to be effective. MEN2 is one of the best counterexamples for which predictive DNA testing in early childhood is justified, because of the young age of onset of medullary thyroid carcinoma and the preventive effectiveness of early prophylactic thyroidectomy.

E. **Privacy and confidentiality** must be maintained in all genetic testing situations in order to prevent inadvertent discrimination or stigmatization. In some cases, patients may not want their test results to be placed in the medical record or conveyed to other physicians or family members.

F. **Informed consent** is sometimes appropriate before embarking on certain types of molecular genetic testing, especially predictive tests or those whose clinical utility is not yet fully understood. It should not normally be necessary for routine diagnostic molecular tests in symptomatic patients.

VIII. EXAMPLES

A. **Medullary Thyroid Carcinoma (MTC)/Multiple Endocrine Neoplasia Type 2 (MEN2)**

  1. Father and paternal uncle of a 6-year-old girl had MTC. Should the daughter have genetic testing?
  2. Purpose: Prevent metastatic MTC by early thyroidectomy if test is positive; minimize need for yearly calcitonin or calcium-stimulation challenges if test is negative.
  3. Probability: Autosomal dominant disease with a strong family history suggests at least 50% risk.
  4. Proper test and procedure: Based on information in OMIM, testing should look for mutations in at least exons 10, 11, and 13–16.
  5. Place: GeneCards identifies RET gene as the primary gene of interest, and GeneTests notes 29 labs offering clinical testing of RET.
  6. Penetrance: Very high, and the mutation spectrum is relatively limited.
  7. Phase is not as much of an issue, because this is an autosomal dominant disease.
  8. Conclusion: Molecular genetic testing is clearly indicated.

B. **Maturity-Onset Diabetes of the Young (MODY)**

  1. A father diagnosed with type 2 diabetes mellitus has a daughter diagnosed with diabetes mellitus, assumed to be type 1 despite little or no evidence of autoimmunity. Her glycemic control remains excellent despite relatively small doses of insulin. Is genetic testing indicated?

2. Purpose: Improve knowledge of prognosis and possibly offer alternative (oral hypoglycemic agent) treatment, if certain subtypes of MODY are identified.
3. Probability: Based on the clinical picture (including the family history), the probability of MODY is reasonably high.
4. Proper test and place: GeneTests reveals several CLIA-certified laboratories that perform mutation analysis on some or all of the six different genes associated with different forms of MODY. Testing is expensive but can be approached sequentially rather than looking at all six genes at the same time.
5. Penetrance is high, and inheritance is autosomal dominant for all forms of MODY.
6. Conclusion: Molecular genetic testing is indicated.

C. Multiple Endocrine Neoplasia Type 1 (MEN1)

1. A 45-year-old man is diagnosed with hyperparathyroidism, without other evident endocrinopathies. Family history reveals that his mother had a prolactinoma. Should genetic testing be performed?
2. Purpose: Help estimate risk of additional endocrine tumors in the patient and in his relatives.
3. Probability: Isolated hyperparathyroidism is not uncommon. Family history is suggestive but not sufficient to increase greatly the risk of MEN1 in this patient.
4. Proper test and place: The mutation spectrum of the *MEN1* gene is extremely heterogeneous, requiring complete gene sequencing rather than targeted mutation analysis. This sequencing is available in CLIA-certified laboratories but is expensive. Alternative biochemical tests (serum prolactin, gastrin, insulin, cortisol, urinary 5-HIAA) exist to detect additional endocrine tumors associated with MEN1.
5. Pitfalls: The sensitivity of gene sequencing for detecting MEN1 is well below 100% (estimates range from 60% to 95%), which means that a negative result does not rule out MEN1 or eliminate the need to follow biochemical test results over time. Complete gene sequencing raises the possibility of detecting previously unreported DNA sequence changes whose clinical significance is unknown.
6. Conclusion: Without stronger clinical evidence (e.g., biochemical evidence of an additional endocrine tumor), molecular genetic testing is probably not indicated at this time.

D. Suspected Nonclassical 21-Hydroxylase Deficiency

1. A hyperandrogenic woman has borderline elevation of basal follicular phase 17-hydroxyprogesterone.
2. Purpose: Provide an alternative to cosyntropin-stimulation testing to diagnose nonclassical congenital adrenal hyperplasia (NCCAH). Provide rationale for a trial of corticosteroid treatment.
3. Probability: Would be higher if the 17-hydroxyprogesterone was clearly elevated.
4. Place: GeneTests shows 19 labs offering clinical testing of the CYP21A2 gene.
5. Procedure: Targeted analysis of the top 12 mutations should provide >90% sensitivity.
6. Pitfalls: Phenocopy problem: Could be related to insulin resistance/hyperinsulinism/polycystic ovary syndrome rather than CAH. There are many concerns about rearrangements and deletions in the CYP21A2 gene, an extremely complex locus. Without studying the DNA of the patient's parents, it may not be possible to determine the phase of detected mutations.
7. Conclusion: No clear-cut superiority of molecular genetic testing over biochemical testing in this scenario.

Selected References

Amos J, Grody WW. Development and integration of molecular genetic tests into clinical practice: the U.S. experience. *Exp Rev Molec Diagn* 2004;4:456–477.

Grody WW. Ethical issues raised by genetic testing with oligonucleotide microarrays. *Molec Biotechnol* 2003;23:127–138.

Hoppner W. Clinical impact of molecular diagnostics in endocrinology. *Horm Res* 2002; 58(suppl 3):7–15.

Maddalena A, Bale S, Das S, et al. Technical standards and guidelines: molecular genetic testing for ultra-rare disorders. *Genet Med* 2005;7:571–583.

Nikiforov YE. RET/PTC rearrangement in thyroid tumors. *Endocr Pathol* 2002;13:3–16.

Santoro M, Melillo RM, Carlomagno F, et al. Molecular biology of the MEN2 gene. *J Intern Med* 1998;243:505–508.

Zaykin DV, Zhivotovsky LA. Ranks of genuine associations in whole-genome scans. *Genetics* 2005;171:813–823.

HORMONE-RESISTANT STATES
Mitchell E. Geffner

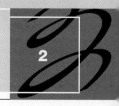

2

I. HISTORY. The concept that hormone resistance could cause endocrinologic dysfunction was first suggested by Fuller Albright and colleagues in 1942 as the mechanism for parathyroid hormone (PTH) unresponsiveness in pseudohypoparathyroidism (PHP). To date, clinical syndromes of resistance have been described for nearly all hormones.

II. GENERAL PRINCIPLES

A. Hormones were originally thought to signal only at sites distant from their glands of origin after transfer via the circulation (**endocrine** action). It is now well known that hormones can act on cells adjacent to their site of origin (**paracrine** action) and even directly on their own cells of origin (**autocrine** action). More recently, it has been shown that certain hormones/growth factors (see later) may act within their cells of origin without ever exiting these cells (**intracrine** action). In theory, resistance to hormone action can involve any or all of these pathways.

B. Growth factors, such as nerve growth factor (NGF), platelet-derived growth factor (PDGF), and epidermal growth factor (EGF), have been traditionally considered distinct from hormones; however, this separation is artificial because many hormones, such as insulin and growth hormone (GH), have both metabolic and growth-promoting/anabolic (mitogenic) activity.

C. Mechanisms of hormone resistance. An older schema divides hormonal resistance into three subtypes: **prereceptor** (resulting from serum factors), **receptor** (resulting from absent or defective hormone binding), and **postreceptor** (resulting from abnormalities beyond the step of hormone binding). This system is overly simplistic and confusing because circulating factors can affect both receptor and postreceptor function. An alternative proposal divides causes of hormonal resistance into two categories.

   1. Intrinsic or primary defects tend to be rare, are genetically mediated within the target cell, and persist in cultured cell models. For example, >50 naturally occurring point mutations in the **insulin receptor** gene have been described, which, depending on the specific abnormality, can affect insulin binding to the receptor, internalization of the insulin–insulin receptor complex, subsequent autophosphorylation of the β subunit of the receptor (see later), or/and phosphorylation of other protein substrates involved in the intracellular signaling cascade.

   2. Extrinsic or secondary defects result from circulating serum factors and are reversible following therapeutic perturbations that remove the resistance-causing factor from the bloodstream. These defects do not persist in cultured cells. Using insulin resistance as the paradigm, extrinsic factors that reduce insulin action include states of counterregulatory hormone excess (e.g., glucocorticoid excess such as occurs in Cushing syndrome), antibodies blocking the insulin receptor (type B syndrome of insulin resistance—see later), and uremia.

D. Molecular characterization of genes coding for hormones and their receptors. Over the past 20 years, numerous genes coding for numerous hormones and growth factors, their corresponding receptors, and portions of their postbinding signaling mechanisms have been localized, cloned, and expressed (Table 2.1). These discoveries and other experimental work have clarified three generic peptide-hormone signaling mechanisms and the general mode of steroid hormone action, and have facilitated the grouping of receptors into superfamilies.

11

| TABLE 2.1 | Gene Products Involved in Genetic Hormone-Resistant States |

Chromosome location	Gene product	Genetic disorder
1p31	Leptin receptor	Morbid obesity
1q21.2	Lamin A	Partial lipodystrophy
2p21	LH/CG receptor	Male pseudohermaphroditism/primary amenorrhea in females
2p21-p16	FSH receptor	"Resistant ovary" syndrome
2q32	Neurogenic differentiation 1	Maturity-onset diabetes of the young
3p22-p21.1	PTH/PTHRP receptor	Blomstrand lethal osteochondrodysplasia
3p24.3	Thyroid hormone receptor β	Dominant-negative thyroid hormone resistance
3p25	Peroxisome proliferator-activated receptor-γ	Partial lipodystrophy
3q21-q24	Calcium-sensing receptor	Benign hypercalcemia (familial hypocalciuric hypercalcemia)
4q21.2	GnRH receptor	Hypogonadotropic hypogonadism
4q31.1	Mineralocorticoid receptor	Autosomal dominant type 1 pseudohypoaldosteronism
5p13-p12	GH receptor	Severe GH insensitivity syndrome (Laron dwarfism)
5q31	Glucocorticoid receptor	Generalized inherited cortisol resistance
6q25.1	Estrogen receptor	Tall stature with osteoporosis in a male
7p14	GHRH receptor	Recessive GH deficiency
7p15-p13	Glucokinase	Maturity-onset diabetes of the young
7p21-p15	CRF receptor	—
7q11.23-q21.11	Peroxisome proliferator-activated receptor-γ	Partial lipodystrophy
8q23	TRH receptor	Central hypothyroidism
9q34.3	1-acylglycerol-3-phosphate O-acyltransferase	Congenital generalized lipodystrophy
11q13	Seipin	Congenital generalized lipodystrophy
12q12-q14	Vitamin D receptor	Familial (vitamin D–resistant) rickets with alopecia
12q12-q13	Aquaporin-2 receptor	Autosomal recessive nephrogenic diabetes insipidus
12q13	ALADIN	ACTH insensitivity
12q13	AMH receptor	Persistent müllerian duct syndrome
12q22-q24.1	Insulinlike growth factor-I	Growth-hormone resistance
12q24.1	Protein-tyrosine phosphatase, nonreceptor-type, 11	Noonan syndrome
12q24.2	Hepatic nuclear factor-1α	Maturity-onset diabetes of the young
13q12.1	Insulin promoter factor 1	Maturity-onset diabetes of the young
14q31	TSH receptor	Familial nongoitrous hypothyroidism
15q25-q26	Type 1 IGF receptor	Intrauterine and postnatal growth failure
16p12.2-p12.1	Amiloride-sensitive epithelial sodium channel	Autosomal recessive type 1 pseudohypoaldosteronism
17cen-q21.3	Hepatic nuclear factor-1β	Maturity-onset diabetes of the young
17q11.2	Signal transducer and activator of transcription 5b	Growth-hormone insensitivity and immunodeficiency
17q11.2	Thyroid hormone receptor a	—
17q12-q22	CRF receptor	—
18p11.2	ACTH (melanocortin-2) receptor	Familial glucocorticoid deficiency

(*continued*)

TABLE 2.1 — Gene Products Involved in Genetic Hormone-Resistant States (*Continued*)

Chromosome location	Gene product	Genetic disorder
19p13.3	G-protein–coupled receptor 54	Hypogonadotropic hypogonadism
19p13.3-p13.2	Insulin receptor	Type A syndrome, Rabson-Mendenhall syndrome, leprechaunism
19q13.2-q13.3	Dystrophia myotonica protein kinase	Myotonic dystrophy type 1
20q12-q13.1	Hepatocyte nuclear factor 4α	Maturity-onset diabetes of the young
20q13.2	Guanine nucleotide-binding protein, α-stimulating activity polypeptide 1	Pseudohypoparathyroidism types 1A and 1B
Xq11.2-q12	Androgen receptor	Partial or complete androgen insensitivity syndrome (testicular feminization)
Xq28	ADH receptor	X-linked nephrogenic diabetes insipidus

ACTH, adrenocorticotropic hormone; ADH, antidiuretic hormone; AMH, anti-Müllerian hormone; CRF, corticotropin-releasing factor; FSH, follicle-stimulating hormone; GH, growth hormone; GHRH, growth hormone–releasing hormone; GnRH, gonadotropin-releasing hormone; IGF, insulinlike growth factor; LH/CG, luteinizing hormone/chorionic gonadotropin; PTHRP, parathyroid hormone–related protein; TRH, thyrotropin-releasing hormone; TSH, thyroid-stimulating hormone.

1. **Generic peptide-hormone signaling mechanisms**
   a. **Receptor autophosphorylation.** As an example, insulin signals by binding to its cell membrane-anchored receptors, leading to the autophosphorylation of its β subunits and the tyrosine phosphorylation of various downstream intermediary proteins (see later). The type 1 IGF receptor, as well as those for EGF and PDGF, are also receptor tyrosine kinases.
   b. **The α subunit of the stimulatory G protein (a-Gs) of adenylyl cyclase,** which serves as an on–off switch that is necessary for the action of various peptide hormones (e.g., PTH) that use cyclic adenosine 3,5-monophosphate (cAMP) as an intracellular second messenger, leads to protein phosphorylation and dephosphorylation of numerous, often cell-specific targets.
   c. **Stimulation of inositol lipid hydrolysis.** G-protein–coupled receptors regulate the activity of every cell in the body by linking to G proteins and activating effectors such as adenylyl cyclase, ion channels, or phospholipase C that lead to increases (or decreases) in intracellular mediator molecules such as cAMP, calcium ions, inositol 1,4,5-trisphosphate, and 1,2-diacylglycerol.
2. **Steroid hormone action.** Steroid hormones enter cells by diffusion, following which they bind to receptor proteins both in the cytoplasm and in the nucleus. Such binding leads to conformational changes of the steroid–steroid receptor complex that result in its activation and heightened affinity to regulatory elements of DNA in the nucleus. This activation of target genes leads to appropriate protein synthesis, which in turn alters cell function, growth, and/or differentiation.
3. **Superfamilies.** Molecular studies have helped us to understand the evolution of receptors and facilitate the grouping of receptors into superfamilies sharing significant amino acid sequence homology. In addition, molecular studies have led to the characterization of specific genetic defects in various receptors responsible for certain hormone-resistant states (Table 2.1).
   a. **Protein tyrosine kinase receptors** include structurally related receptors for insulin and IGF-I. Both insulin and IGF-I receptors (officially known as type 1 IGF receptors) are heterotetramers that possess intrinsic tyrosine kinase activity (see later).

    b. Class 1 cytokine receptors share structurally related extracellular domains and include a diverse group of proteins, including the receptors for GH, prolactin, interleukin-2 (IL-2), IL-3, IL-4, IL-6, IL-7, erythropoietin, and granulocyte-macrophage colony-stimulating factor (GM-CSF).

    c. Seven-transmembrane-helix, G-protein–coupled receptors represent the largest superfamily of receptors known to date and include three subfamilies (rhodopsin/β_2-adrenergic receptors, calcitonin/PTH/PTH-related receptors, and metabotropic glutamate/calcium-sensing receptors). Genes that encode G proteins and G-protein–coupled receptors (GPCRs) are susceptible to loss-of-function mutations that result in reduced or absent signaling by the corresponding agonist and cause resistance to hormone action, thereby mimicking a state of hormone deficiency. The only mutational changes in G proteins that are unequivocally linked to endocrine disorders occur in α-Gs. Heterozygous loss-of-function mutations of α-Gs in the active, maternal allele cause resistance to hormones that act through α-Gs–coupled GPCRs. Loss-of-function mutations involving G-protein–coupled receptors have been described for adrenocorticotropin (ACTH), angiotensin II, antidiuretic hormone (ADH), calcium-sensing receptor, catecholamines, corticotropin-releasing hormone (CRH), follicle-stimulating hormone (FSH), gonadotropin-releasing hormone (GnRH), growth hormone–releasing hormone (GHRH), kisspeptin, luteinizing hormone (LH), PTH, thyrotropin-releasing hormone (TRH), and thyroid-stimulating hormone (TSH). These receptors consist of a single polypeptide chain that is predicted to span the plasma membrane seven times (i.e., it is heptahelical), forming three extracellular and three or four intracellular loops, and a cytoplasmic carboxy-terminal tail.

    d. Ligand-responsive transcription regulators are represented by low-abundance intracellular androgen receptor proteins, which are related to the retinoic acid, thyroid hormone, and vitamin D receptors. Although these receptors have traditionally been thought to reside in the cell nucleus, more recent information suggests that cell-surface receptors may also exist. The hormone-binding domain of these receptors activates the receptor and enables a DNA-binding domain to recognize and bind to specific hormone-regulatory or -response elements in target genes.

    e. Nuclear receptor subfamily 3C consists of glucocorticoid, mineralocorticoid, progesterone, and androgen receptors. Multiple signaling pathways have been established for all four receptors, but the main common pathway involves direct DNA binding and transcriptional regulation of responsive genes.

    f. Transmembrane serine/threonine kinase receptors are of three subtypes. They mediate responses to peptide growth/differentiation factors, including transforming growth factor-β, activins, and anti-müllerian hormone (AMH).

E. Specificity spillover. In states of resistance to traditional hormone action, the serum hormone concentration becomes elevated, on occasion by orders of magnitude, via **negative feedback**. In some cases, it is thought that these high serum hormone concentrations can effect certain unintended actions through a receptor–effector pathway different from, but homologous to, the normal signaling mechanism (i.e., via **specificity spillover** through **"promiscuous receptors"**). For example, in the insulin resistance model, the resultant hyperinsulinemia may induce hyperandrogenism and polycystic ovarian disease, the skin changes of acanthosis nigricans, and hypertrophic cardiomyopathy, all of which may be mediated by a functioning homologous type 1 IGF receptor–effector mechanism in these victimized tissues that responds to the high circulating concentrations of insulin. This phenomenon has also been implicated in certain hormone-*sensitive* states (e.g., insulin stimulates macrosomia in the infant of the diabetic mother through the type 1 IGF receptor, IGF-II secreted from certain nonislet tumors induces hypoglycemia through the insulin receptor, and excess GH in acromegaly produces galactorrhea through the prolactin receptor).

III. SPECIFIC DISORDERS ASSOCIATED WITH HORMONE RESISTANCE: RECEPTORS CONTAINING INTRINSIC TYROSINE KINASE ACTIVITY

A. Insulin

1. General. Insulin exerts its actions mainly in liver, muscle, and adipose tissue, following its binding to cell-surface insulin receptors. The *insulin receptor* gene is located on chromosome 19p13.3-13.2, contains 22 exons, and codes for two slightly different proteins composed of an external α subunit, containing 723 or 735 amino acids, and a transmembrane β subunit of 620 amino acids, containing extracellular and transmembrane domains, and an intracellular domain. Binding of insulin to the extracellular α subunit results in activation of the tyrosine kinase activity of the β subunit, which appears to be the first step of intracellular modifications leading to the actions of insulin. Two major pathways appear to be regulated by insulin, one involving the intracellular phosphorylation of proteins, including, but not limited to, reduced insulin signaling of the insulin receptor substrate (IRS)-1/phosphatidylinositol (PI) 3-kinase pathway, resulting in diminished glucose uptake and utilization in insulin target tissues, and the other involving second messengers such as glycolipids or diacylglycerol. These pathways ultimately lead to activation of the insulin-dependent glucose transporter, GLUT4, and also of multiple enzymes such as glucokinase, glycogen synthase, phosphofructokinase, pyruvate kinase, and pyruvate dehydrogenase.

2. Insulin resistance of uncertain etiology

a. Obesity and type 2 diabetes. Insulin resistance appears to underlie the pathogenesis of type 2 diabetes (with insulin deficiency developing later, presumably secondary to gluco- and/or lipotoxicity). In type 2 diabetes, there is resistance to the ability of insulin to inhibit hepatic glucose output and to stimulate the uptake and use of glucose by fat and muscle; this peripheral insulin resistance is greater in patients with type 2 diabetes than in those with obesity alone. Elevated levels of circulating factors, such as tumor necrosis factor-α (TNF-α) or free fatty acids, have been suggested as possible causes of the insulin resistance of obesity. A reduced number of insulin receptors does not account for the observed insulin resistance but probably reflects physiologic downregulation, which occurs in the setting of concomitant hyperinsulinemia. When the circulating insulin concentration is normal or low in patients with type 2 diabetes, the number of insulin receptors is normal. Both patients with obesity and those with type 2 diabetes have a reversible defect in tyrosine kinase activity of their insulin receptors in skeletal muscle. Impaired insulin-stimulated glucose transport has been demonstrated in muscle and adipocytes of both obese patients and patients with type 2 diabetes. However, the number of insulin-responsive glucose transporters (GLUT-4) in skeletal muscle of patients with type 2 diabetes is normal. In the Mexican American population, single-nucleotide polymorphisms in *calpain 10*, a gene coding for the protein from a large family of cytoplasmic proteases, seems to be responsible for 40% of type 2 diabetes familial clustering. Recent genome-wide association studies have uncovered links between type 2 diabetes (in Finns) and the following loci in an intergenic region on chromosome 11p12, *IGF2BP2*, *CDKAL1*, and *CDKN2A/CDKN2B*, and confirm that variants near *TCF7L2*, *SLC30A8*, *HHEX*, *PPARG*, and *KCNJ111* are also associated with a risk for type 2 diabetes.

b. Insulin resistance, hypertension, hyperlipidemia, and atherosclerosis ("syndrome X"). Originally described in adults in 1988, syndrome X is associated with insulin resistance, along with a series of related metabolic abnormalities consisting of hyperinsulinemia, glucose intolerance, increased very-low-density lipoprotein (VLDL) cholesterol, decreased high-density lipoprotein (HDL) cholesterol, hypertension, and obesity. Of note, this cluster may have its origin in childhood. Recent epidemiologic evidence in several populations suggests that hyperinsulinemia (secondary to insulin resistance) is an independent risk factor for cardiovascular disease. This interrelationship may stem from the ability of insulin to promote smooth muscle proliferation directly within blood vessels, to enhance renal sodium and water retention, to amplify sympathetic tone, to increase VLDL cholesterol, and to reduce HDL cholesterol. The mechanism by which insulin induces these changes in the setting of underlying insulin resistance is unknown.

  c. Polycystic ovarian syndrome (PCOS). This condition is associated with hyperandrogenism and chronic anovulation in conjunction with insulin resistance. The onset of PCOS may be linked to a history of premature adrenarche (early development of pubic and axillary hair) in childhood or to a failure to establish regular menstrual patterns beginning at menarche followed by the development of hirsutism and acne. Insulin resistance is found in both obese and lean women with PCOS, and is associated with *excessive* serine phosphorylation of the insulin receptor in association with decreased tyrosine kinase activity, a defect apparently unique to PCOS. The resultant hyperinsulinemia is thought to play a primary role in the induction of ovarian (and, perhaps, adrenal) hyperandrogenism by an as yet incompletely defined mechanism. In vitro studies show a direct effect of insulin stimulation on ovarian thecal cell production of androgens, whereas in vivo studies aimed at reduction of circulating insulin concentrations (e.g., by administration of diazoxide) are associated with a corresponding decrease in circulating testosterone.

  d. Other associations

  (1) A history of intrauterine growth retardation (which may predispose to future type 2 diabetes)

  (2) Genetic syndromes (e.g., Turner, Klinefelter, and Prader-Willi syndromes, and progeria)

  (3) Degenerative neuromuscular diseases (e.g., myotonic dystrophy [see later] and Friedreich ataxia)

  e. Intrinsic (primary) cellular defects associated with insulin resistance

  (1) Maturity-onset diabetes of the young (MODY)

  (a) Clinical features. MODY is a familial, mild form of type 2 diabetes characterized by early age of onset, autosomal dominant transmission with a high rate of penetrance, and a predominant effect on insulin secretion with at least some degree of insulin resistance.

  (b) Mechanism. MODY is due to one of six monogenic disorders involving: *glucokinase; hepatocyte nuclear factor-4α, 1α, 1β; insulin promoter factor-1α,* and *neurogenic differentiation 1.* With the exception of glucokinase, the others are transcription factors that bind to specific DNA sequences in the promoter region of other genes and regulate expression of their proteins. Glucokinase, on the other hand, is a key regulatory enzyme of pancreatic β cells that catalyzes glucose phosphorylation to glucose 6-phosphate.

  (2) Type A syndrome of insulin resistance and acanthosis nigricans

  (a) Clinical features. Acanthosis nigricans and ovarian hyperandrogenism in women.

  (b) Mechanism. *Insulin receptor* gene mutations in many cases.

  (3) Rabson-Mendenhall syndrome

  (a) Clinical features. Similar to those of the type A syndrome of insulin resistance and acanthosis nigricans, along with dental and nail dysplasia, pineal hyperplasia, precocious pseudopuberty, and accelerated linear growth.

  (b) Mechanism. *Insulin receptor* gene mutations in all cases.

  (4) Leprechaunism (Donohue syndrome)

  (a) Clinical features. Autosomal recessive inheritance, product of consanguineous parents, intrauterine and postnatal growth retardation, dysmorphic facies, lipoatrophy, muscle wasting, acanthosis nigricans, ovarian hyperandrogenism in females, precocious puberty, hypertrophic cardiomyopathy, and early death.

(b) **Mechanism.** *Insulin receptor* gene mutations (homozygous or compound heterozygous in all cases).

(5) **Congenital generalized lipodystrophy (Bernadelli-Seip)**

(a) **Clinical features.** Fat loss beginning at birth, with other features similar to those of the type A syndrome of insulin resistance and acanthosis nigricans, along with fatty liver infiltration leading, in some cases, to cirrhosis; hypertrophic cardiomyopathy; acromegaloidism, and hypertriglyceridemia.

(b) **Mechanism.** This syndrome results from mutations in either *AGPAT2* (encoding 1-acylglycerol-3-phosphate O-acyltransferase) at 9q34, causing increased production of the cytokines, IL-6 and TNF-α; or *BSCL2* (encoding seipin) at 11q13, which functions as a transmembrane protein.

(6) **Partial lipodystrophy (Dunnigan)**

(a) **Clinical features.** Fat tissue affected by lipoatrophy or lipohypertrophy, usually beginning during puberty, with other features similar to those of the type A syndrome of insulin resistance and acanthosis nigricans, along with hepatosplenomegaly, hypertrophic cardiomyopathy, acromegaloidism, and hypertriglyceridemia.

(b) **Mechanism.** Results from mutations of *LMNA* (encoding nuclear lamin) at 1q21-22 or *PPARG* (encoding peroxisome proliferator-activated receptor-γ) at 3p25 or 7q11.23-q21.11.

(7) **Myotonic dystrophy type 1**

(a) **Clinical features.** Unusual form of insulin resistance characterized by weakness and wasting, myotonia, cataract, and often by cardiac conduction abnormalities; adults may become physically disabled and may have a shortened life span, and a congenital form may be fatal.

(b) **Mechanism.** Caused by a CTG trinucleotide expansion in the 3'-untranslated region of the *DM1 protein kinase* gene, resulting in alternative splicing of the *insulin receptor* gene.

f. **Extrinsic (secondary) cellular defects associated with insulin resistance**

(1) **Physiologic states.** Gender (female > male), race (African American, Hispanic, and Native American > Caucasian), puberty (perhaps secondary to increased GH secretion), pregnancy, and old age.

(2) **Abnormal physiologic states.** Infection (including HIV), drugs (e.g., glucocorticoids and GH), stress, starvation, uremia, cirrhosis, and ketoacidosis.

(3) **Endocrinologic causes.** Glucocorticoids (Cushing syndrome), GH (acromegaly), catecholamines (pheochromocytoma), glucagon (glucagonoma), hyperthyroidism, hypothyroidism, and hyperparathyroidism.

(4) **Antibodies blocking the insulin receptor** occur in the setting of a generalized autoimmune diathesis in patients with the **type B syndrome of insulin resistance and acanthosis nigricans** and in patients with **ataxia telangiectasia.**

B. **IGF-I**

1. **General.** Traditional dogma has taught that IGF-I, secreted from the liver, is the major effector of GH action in a classical endocrinologic sense. However, IGF-I, IGF-I–binding proteins, and type 1 IGF receptors are expressed by many different tissues, suggesting that autocrine–paracrine activity may be more physiologically relevant, a finding supported by the observation of normal growth in mice in whom their hepatic *type 1 IGF receptor* gene has been knocked out. IGF-I and IGF-II bind and stimulate the type 1 IGF receptor, the type 2 IGF receptor (IGF-II/mannose 6-phosphate receptor), and, to a lesser extent, the insulin receptor. The type 1 IGF receptor, coded for by a gene located on chromosome 15q25-q26, is homologous to the insulin receptor and is composed of two entirely extracellular α subunits containing cysteine-rich domains and two

transmembrane β subunits containing a tyrosine-kinase domain in their cytoplasmic portion.
2. **Intrinsic defects**
   a. **African Efe Pygmies**
      (1) **Clinical features.** Significant short stature in this population is assumed to be adaptive in nature as a means of survival in the dense low-lying vegetation and high humidity of the jungle; intermittent periods of poor nutrition may also play a role. Depending on nutritional status, random GH levels may be normal or slightly elevated, and IGF-I and GHBP levels normal or low.
      (2) **Mechanism.** Although early studies suggested that GH resistance was responsible for the short stature of African Pygmies, more recent work has demonstrated genetically regulated *combined* GH and IGF-I resistance in African Efe Pygmies. The underlying variation appears to be IGF-I resistance with secondary GH resistance. Neighboring Lese Africans, whose gene pool is intermingled with that of the Efe, show stature intermediate between that of the Efe and non-Pygmy Africans, as well as intermediate in vitro responses (between Efe and controls) to both GH and IGF-I. To date, no mutation has been found in the *type 1 IGF receptor* gene of Efe Pygmies.
   b. Five families have now been described consisting of 12 individuals with heterozygous mutations of the *type 1 IGF receptor* gene who presented with moderate-to-severe postnatal short stature (-1.6 to -5.0 standard deviations [SD] below the mean) in association with intrauterine growth retardation (birth weights between -1.5 and -3.5 SD), variable degrees of facial dysmorphism, small head circumference, and mental development ranging from delayed to normal. In addition, serum IGF-I levels were elevated to varying degrees in affected individuals.
   c. A few children have been described with intrauterine and postnatal growth retardation in association with distal deletions of either **chromosome 15q** or **ring chromosome 15,** thought to perhaps involve the gene for the *type 1 IGF receptor*. IGF-I (combined with both GH and insulin) resistance has also been invoked as a contributory cause to persistent postnatal growth failure in children born SGA (Small for Gestational Age).
3. **Extrinsic defects**
   a. **HIV infection** is associated with in vitro and in vivo evidence of (presumably) acquired, combined IGF-I and GH resistance in both symptomatic adults and children. Such resistance may contribute to the growth disturbances seen in symptomatic HIV-infected children and to the wasting syndrome seen in both children and adults with AIDS.
   b. **Malnutrition** is associated with reversible IGF-I deficiency. In addition, both GH and IGF-I *resistance* have been noted in experimentally-induced protein malnutrition in rats.
   c. The growth delay of **chronic renal failure** stems in part from elevations of IGFBPs leading to IGF-I resistance, which can be overridden with high-dose GH treatment.
   d. **Catabolic states** are associated with IGF-I resistance, perhaps on the basis of elevated circulating and intramuscular concentrations of cytokines, such as TNF-α and various interleukins, which are overproduced in response to cellular injury and appear to cause combined resistance to GH and both IGF-I deficiency and resistance (akin to that observed in malnutrition).

IV. SPECIFIC DISORDERS ASSOCIATED WITH HORMONE RESISTANCE: CLASS 1 CYTOKINE RECEPTORS
A. **Growth hormone**
   1. **General.** The human *GH receptor* gene is located on chromosome 5p13-p12, spans 87-kb pairs (coding for 620 amino acids), and includes 9 exons (numbered 2 through 10), of which exon 2 encodes a secretion signal sequence; exons 3

to 7, a large extracellular GH-binding domain (246 amino acids); exon 8, a single membrane-spanning domain (24 amino acids); and exons 9 and 10, the cytoplasmic domain (350 amino acids). The amino-terminal sequence of the circulating **GH-binding protein (GHBP)** appears to be the proteolytic product of the extracellular binding domain of the GH receptor. GH action is mediated by GH-induced dimerization of the GH receptor, followed by activation of receptor-associated JAK2 tyrosine kinase and cytoplasmic Stat proteins.

2. **Intrinsic defects**
   a. **Severe growth hormone insensitivity syndrome (Laron dwarfism)**
      (1) **Clinical features.** Characterized by moderate-to-severe postnatal short stature, a specific dysmorphic phenotype (including prominent forehead, small face with saddle nose, small hands and feet, sparse hair, high-pitched voice, blue sclerae, and micropenis in boys), high circulating GH concentrations in childhood, very low serum IGF-I levels, and no growth and little IGF-I response to exogenous GH therapy, but with a significant improvement in growth following treatment with recombinant human IGF-I.
      (2) **Mechanisms.** Affected patients have nonsense, frameshift, splice, or missense mutations of the *GH receptor* gene. At least 38 different mutations have been described, most of which are homozygous point mutations or complex gene deletions, and the remainder compound heterozygous mutations. Three different genotype/phenotype relationships have been described.
         (a) Autosomal recessive, product of consanguineous parents, with severe short stature and phenotype, and either typically absent or low, but occasionally normal or even increased, levels of circulating GHBP.
         (b) Dominant-negative form (see later) with moderate short stature and an absent or mild phenotype, and elevated serum level of GHBP.
         (c) GH-GH receptor transduction defects with moderate-to-severe growth failure, variable phenotype, and normal levels of GHBP.
   b. **Partial GH insensitivity.** Some children have been described who manifest mild-to-moderate short stature and the biochemical phenotype of Laron dwarfism (including low levels of serum GHBP), but who lack the usual dysmorphic features. A few of these children have been found to have heterozygous mutations of the *GH receptor* gene, the etiologic relevance of which remains unclear at this time because, within families, the polymorphisms did not align with stature.
   c. **Noonan syndrome.** Approximately 50% of affected children have a demonstrable mutation in the *PTPN11* gene, which regulates production of SHP-2 protein, an essential regulator of several intracellular signaling pathways, including those for GH action and cardiac semilunar valvulogenesis. This mutation may account for the observed low IGF-I and acid-labile subunit (ALS) concentrations found in children with Noonan syndrome, and the lower growth response to GH in children with the syndrome and the mutation compared to those without the mutation.
   d. Several children with idiopathic short stature have been described who, in fibroblast cell lines, exhibit attenuated GH-induced JAK2-dependent phosphorylation and nuclear translocation of Stat3, increases in the cell cycle inhibitor, p21, and decreases in cyclins.
   e. Mutations in the ***Stat5b* gene** have been reported in a few children with **severe short stature** and **immunodeficiency** resulting in loss of GH-induced JAK2-dependent phosphorylation and nuclear localization of Stat5b. Immunodeficiency arises as Stat5b also plays a role in the IL-2 signaling pathway.
   f. Several cases of short stature and X-linked severe combined immunodeficiency (SCID) has been described as a result of loss of the common cytokine receptor γ chain causing decreased GH-induced JAK2-dependent phosphorylation and nuclear localization of Stat5b.
   g. Genetic GH resistance has also been reported in two subjects with severe short stature on the basis of an ***IGF-I* gene deletion**.

3. **Extrinsic defects.** Reversible forms of GH resistance occur in the setting of **malnutrition, liver disease** (especially **Alagille syndrome,** which is characterized by intrahepatic bile duct paucity in association with cholestasis, cardiac disease, skeletal and ocular abnormalities, and a characteristic facies), poorly controlled **diabetes mellitus,** chronic renal failure, and the presence of GH-inhibiting antibodies (which develop in some children with *GH* gene deletions who are then treated with recombinant human GH).

B. **Leptin**

1. **General.** The leptin receptor contains extracellular binding, transmembrane, and variable-length intracellular domains. The human *leptin receptor* gene has been localized to chromosome 1p31. Leptin is produced in adipose tissue, acts on specific receptors in the central nervous system, and is thought to function as an afferent satiety signal in a feedback loop that apparently regulates the appetite and satiety centers in the hypothalamus. Leptin also appears to have a stimulatory role in gonadotropin secretion and fertility.

2. **Intrinsic defects.** At least 11 subjects have been reported with mutations of the *leptin receptor* gene, all of whom presented with early-onset obesity and delayed puberty as a result of hypogonadotropic hypogonadism, in association with consanguinity. Serum leptin levels were generally within the range predicted by the elevated fat mass in these patients. Their clinical features were less severe than those of patients with congenital leptin deficiency.

3. **Extrinsic defects.** Obese humans have higher serum leptin levels than do normal-weight individuals, and these levels correlate with their degree of adiposity. In common obesity, a state of leptin resistance develops in which leptin loses its ability to inhibit energy intake and increase energy expenditure. Following weight loss, serum leptin levels fall.

V. SPECIFIC DISORDERS ASSOCIATED WITH HORMONE RESISTANCE: G-PROTEIN–COUPLED RECEPTORS

A. **Adrenocorticotropic hormone**

1. **General.** The human *ACTH receptor* (preferentially known as *melanocortin-2 receptor* [*MC2R*]) gene, along with that for the related *melanocyte-stimulating hormone receptor,* are located on chromosome 18p11.2. The MC2R receptor is one of the smallest members of this receptor superfamily, being only 297 residues in length and with a predicted molecular weight of 33 kDa in its nonglycosylated form. It is also one of a family of five related receptors (MC1R through MC5R), mutations in four of which are associated with rare human disease. Mutations of MC1R cause various skin and hair abnormalities, along with increased susceptibility to melanoma and other skin cancers, and MC3R and MC4R cause early-onset severe obesity.

2. **Intrinsic defects**

a. **Familial glucocorticoid deficiency (FGD)**

(1) **Clinical.** This rare familial disorder is characterized by autosomal recessive inheritance, skin and mucosal hyperpigmentation, and signs of glucocorticoid insufficiency, but, in general, preserved mineralocorticoid function. Biochemically, this manifests as hypoglycemia and hyponatremia, without hyperkalemia.

(2) **Mechanism.** A genetic classification system has been developed that divides affected individuals into three subtypes. FGD type 1 is caused by mutations of the *MC2R* gene, of which >30 homozygous or compound heterozygous varieties have been described in 25% of affected individuals. FGD type 2 localizes to 21q22.1 and is caused by mutations in melanocyte receptor accessory protein (MRAP), whereas FGD type 3 appears to be linked to a locus on 8q, but the specific gene involved is unknown.

b. **Triple A syndrome**

(1) **Clinical.** This is another rare, familial, autosomal recessive form of primary **adrenocortical insufficiency** with the clinical features of FGD, along with **achalasia** (an inability of the lower esophageal sphincter to

relax, leading to difficulty in swallowing), **alacrima** (absence of tears), neuropathy (mixed upper and lower motor neuropathy, sensory impairment, autonomic neuropathy, and mental retardation), and, in some patients, hyperkeratosis of the palms and soles. Achalasia and alacrima presumably result from an underlying or associated autonomic neuropathy.

    (2) Mechanism. The condition was initially linked to a region on chromosome 12q13, near the *type 2 keratin* gene cluster. Subsequently, the defective gene was found and dubbed *ALADIN* (alacrima, achalasia, adrenal insufficiency neurologic disorder), which codes for a WD protein that localizes to the nuclear pore. To date, >30 mutations have been reported in the gene in 95% of affected individuals.

B. Antidiuretic Hormone
  1. General. The antidiuretic action of ADH or arginine vasopressin is mediated through V_2, cAMP-dependent receptors, whereas its vasoconstrictive action is mediated through V_1, phosphatidylinositol-dependent receptors. The gene for the *human V_2 ADH receptor* has been localized to the X chromosome at band Xq28 and encodes for a receptor protein of 371 amino acids. In response to ADH, intracellular vesicles, containing functional water channels, also known as aquaporin-2 proteins, are inserted into the normally watertight apical membrane of the collecting duct, thereby increasing water permeability. The *aquaporin-2* gene is located on chromosome 12q12-q13.

  2. Intrinsic defects
    a. X-linked nephrogenic diabetes insipidus
      (1) Clinical. This rare disorder is associated with renal tubular resistance to ADH and is characterized by polyuria, polydipsia, and hyposthenuria. In affected families, 50% of males are symptomatic and usually completely unresponsive to ADH. Extrarenal responses to synthetic ADH (DDAVP), including blunted coagulation, fibrinolytic, and vasodilatory effects, are also absent in these patients. Treatment with ADH or its analogs is ineffective. Therapeutic measures are nonspecific; they include hydration and the use of salt restriction and thiazide diuretics, the combination of which is used to reduce urine volume.

      (2) Mechanism. The defect has been found to be caused by mutations involving the *V_2 receptor* gene or the V_2 receptor-transduction process or both. More than 190 mutations have been described.

    b. Autosomal recessive nephrogenic diabetes insipidus. This even rarer form has been reported in the offspring of consanguineous parents and is associated with normal extrarenal responsiveness to DDAVP and a normal *ADH receptor* gene. In contrast, mutations of the **aquaporin-2 gene** have been reported. The recommended therapies are similar to those used to manage the X-linked form of diabetes insipidus.

  3. Extrinsic defects. Secondary or acquired forms of nephrogenic diabetes insipidus may be caused by:
    a. Pharmacologic factors: use of lithium, demeclocycline, and diuretics.
    b. Osmotic diuresis: diabetes mellitus and reduced nephron population (nephritis).
    c. Electrolyte disturbances: hypercalcemia and hypokalemia.
    d. Renal disease: post-obstructive diuresis, renal tubular acidosis, pyelonephritis, papillary necrosis, and sickle cell disease.
    e. Hemodynamic: hyperthyroidism.

C. Calcium-sensing receptor
  1. General. The *calcium-sensing receptor* gene is located on chromosome 3q21-3q24 and encodes a cell-surface protein of 1 078 amino acids that is expressed in the parathyroid glands and in the kidneys. The receptor regulates the secretion of PTH and the reabsorption of calcium by the renal tubules in response to fluctuations in the serum calcium concentration.

  2. Intrinsic defects. Loss-of-function mutations cause autosomal dominantly inherited **benign hypercalcemia,** also known as **familial hypocalciuric**

hypercalcemia. More than 50 different inactivating mutations have been described. Affected individuals are generally asymptomatic, have life-long mild-to-moderate elevations of serum calcium concentrations, and have low urinary excretion of calcium. More rarely, these mutations may cause severe neonatal hyperparathyroidism (presenting before 6 months of age) with marked symptomatic hypercalcemia; without parathyroidectomy, the condition may be lethal. When both are present in the same family, the former appear to represent heterozygous and the latter homozygous forms of the same genetic defect. Functionally, these mutations manifest as a failure to suppress PTH concentrations at expected levels of hypercalcemia as well as inappropriately high renal reabsorption of calcium despite hypercalcemia.

D. **Corticotropin-releasing factor (CRF)**
1. **General.** Genes for the *CRF receptor* are located on chromosomes 7p21-p15 and 17q12-q22. Activation of this receptor in pituitary corticotrophs by CRF regulates ACTH secretion.
2. **Intrinsic defects.** No disease-bearing mutations of the *CRF receptor* gene associated with resistance to CRF have been reported.
3. **Extrinsic defects.** Patients with **depression** manifest a pseudo-Cushing state in which there is reversible dysfunction of the hypothalamic–pituitary–adrenal axis, elevation of basal serum cortisol levels, resistance to the negative-feedback action of dexamethasone on cortisol secretion, and elevated levels of CRF in the cerebrospinal fluid. In addition, depressed individuals manifested a blunted serum cortisol response to administered CRF, consistent with the presence of CRF resistance, the clinical significance of which is unclear. CRF resistance may also occur in females with hypothalamic amenorrhea.

E. **Follicle-stimulating hormone**
1. **General.** The gene for the *FSH receptor* is located on chromosome 2p21-p16 and consists of 10 exons, the last of which, as in the *LH* and *TSH receptor* genes, encodes the entire transmembrane and intracellular domains of the receptor. Activation of this receptor by FSH (follitropin) in the ovary stimulates follicular development and in the testis stimulates spermatogenesis by Sertoli cells.
2. **Intrinsic defects.** *FSH receptor* gene mutations are uncommon. Females harboring an inactivating mutation of the *FSH receptor* gene have a more severe phenotype than those with mutations of the *LH receptor* gene (that is, they have unresponsive ovarian cells and almost completely absent female sex steroid production, resulting in underdeveloped secondary sexual characteristics, amenorrhea, and infertility—often referred to as the **"resistant ovary syndrome"**), in conjunction with elevated serum gonadotropin levels and arrested, but not absent, follicular maturation. Recently, somatic mutations of the *FSH receptor* gene have been described in a series of sex-cord tumors and small-cell carcinomas of the ovary; their role in tumor formation or growth is unknown. Affected males are normally virilized and have small testes, indicating absent or poor spermatogenesis, in conjunction with moderately elevated serum FSH, normal or mildly elevated serum LH, and normal testosterone levels. A total of nine different mutations has been reported. Resistance to FSH also occurs to varying degrees in patients with PHP IA.

F. **Gonadotropin-releasing hormone**
1. **General.** The human *GnRH receptor* gene is located on chromosome 4q21.2 and comprises three exons. Binding of GnRH to its receptor stimulates the activity of phospholipase C and intracellular calcium through G_q/G11 proteins. Activation of this receptor on pituitary gonadotrophs by GnRH stimulates both LH and FSH secretion.
2. **Intrinsic defects.** Nineteen mutations in the *GnRH receptor* gene causing hypogonadotropic hypogonadism have been described. Most are compound heterozygous inactivating missense mutations inherited in an autosomal recessive fashion and are present in ~2% of cases of normosmic hypogonadotropic hypogonadism. Affected individuals present with either no evidence of puberty,

incomplete pubertal development, small testes in males, amenorrhea in females, and/or infertility. As expected, treatment with pulsatile GnRH administration is ineffective, whereas treatment with gonadotropins can induce ovulation in females.

G. Growth hormone–releasing hormone

1. **General.** The human *GHRH receptor* gene is located on chromosome 7p14 and encodes for a 423-amino acid protein. Activation of this receptor on pituitary somatotrophs by GHRH stimulates GH secretion.

2. **Intrinsic defects.** Initially, two perhaps related clusters of individuals from consanguineous kindreds in India and Sindh, Pakistan, and another from Brazil, were described with nondysmorphic, proportionate dwarfism; absence of microphallus and hypoglycemia; and microcephaly, in association with recessively inherited GH deficiency but a normal *GH* gene. These patients have a nonsense mutation of the *GHRH receptor* gene predicted to encode a severely truncated GHRH protein that lacks the spanning domains and the G-protein–binding site. A total of nine different autosomal recessively inherited homozygous or compound heterozygous mutations (missense and deletion) have been reported. Variable degrees of resistance to GHRH have been described in patients with PHP IA. No mutation of the *GHRH receptor* gene has been found in "typical" patients with GH deficiency.

H. Kisspeptin (KiSS-1)

1. **General.** Recent studies have uncovered a role for the GPR54 receptor (located on chromosome 1q32), an orphan receptor of the rhodopsin family, and kisspeptin, its cognate ligand, in pubertal activation, with their respective mRNAs collocalizing in the hypothalamus and GnRH neurons, GnRH-dependent activation of gonadotropins by kisspeptin, and increased hypothalamic KiSS-1 and GPR54 mRNAs at the time of puberty.

2. **Intrinsic defects.** Several large consanguineous families have been reported that harbor inactivating mutations of GPR54 that cause hypogonadotoropic hypogonadism and low sex steroids, with resultant absence of spontaneous pubertal development in affected individuals.

I. Luteinizing hormone

1. **General.** The gene for the LH/chorionogonadotropin (CG) receptor is located on chromosome 2p21 and consists of 11 exons, the last of which, as in the *FSH* and *TSH receptor* genes, encodes the entire transmembrane and intracellular domains of the receptor. Activation of this receptor by LH stimulates gonadal steroid production by ovarian follicles and by Leydig cells of the testis.

2. **Intrinsic defects.** Inactivating mutations of the *LH receptor* gene are rare and may present in males either as 46,XY male pseudohermaphroditism (secondary to an inability of fetal LH/human chorionic gonadotropin [hCG] to induce adequate fetal virilization) in conjunction with Leydig cell hypoplasia or as a milder phenotype characterized by undervirilization and micropenis. Affected females present with primary amenorrhea. Twenty-two distinct loss-of-function mutations have been described. Resistance to LH has been noted in patients with PHP IA.

J. Parathyroid hormone

1. **General.** A common receptor for PTH and the PTH-related peptide (Tharp), also known as the type 1 PTH/PTHrP receptor, has been localized to chromosome 3p22-p21.1. Activation of PTH receptors mobilizes calcium from bone and increases calcium reabsorption by the kidney.

2. **Intrinsic defects**
   a. **Pseudohypoparathyroidism** is defined as resistance to PTH and is most commonly inherited in an autosomal dominant fashion. Affected patients have hypocalcemia, hyperphosphatemia, and elevated PTH levels, and no increase in urinary cAMP or phosphaturia in response to injected PTH. Several forms of PHP have been described, and all are thought to result from intrinsic cellular abnormalities.

(1) Pseudohypoparathyroidism type IA

(a) Clinical. Affected patients have reduced expression or function of α-Gs in the setting of PTH and multihormone resistance (TSH, glucagon, etc.). These patients also have a characteristic phenotype **(Albright hereditary osteodystrophy or AHO)** characterized by short stature, obesity, round facies, short neck, shortened metacarpals and metatarsals, heterotopic subcutaneous calcification or ossification, and mental dullness. It has recently been suggested that the obesity seen in AHO may be the result of resistance to normal epinephrine-mediated lipolysis.

(b) Mechanism. In most patients with PHP IA, heterozygous germline loss-of-function paternally imprinted mutations in the α-Gs gene have been identified. These include base substitutions at a splice junction site, coding frameshift mutations, premature stop codons, large deletions, and even one common 4-bp deletion ("hot spot") in exon 7 in multiple unrelated kindreds. In addition, missense mutations have also been described.

(2) Pseudohypoparathyroidism type IB

(a) Clinical. Affected patients lack features of AHO, have normal expression of α-Gs protein in accessible tissues, and manifest hormonal resistance limited to PTH target tissues. PTH resistance may be limited to the kidney, with PTH responsiveness preserved in the bone, as evidenced by the hyperparathyroid skeletal lesions observed in these patients.

(b) Mechanism. Although the defect is thought to result from an abnormality of the *PTH receptor* gene, none has been described as yet. More recently, linkage has been shown with an unknown paternally imprinted gene that maps to a small region of band 20q13.3, very near the gene encoding for α-Gs. The disease may result from a mutant promoter or enhancer region of this gene that has lost the ability to support expression of α-Gs in the kidney, but not in other tissues and thus leading to the renal resistance to PTH.

(3) Pseudohypoparathyroidism type IC

(a) Clinical. Affected patients have normal α-Gs activity, occasional evidence of the AHO phenotype, and features of multihormone resistance.

(b) Mechanism. This variant is thought to be caused by a postreceptor defect involving PTH action.

b. Blomstrand lethal osteochondrodysplasia. This rare, fatal, short-limbed skeletal dysplasia, characterized by accelerated endochondral and intramembranous ossification, has been found to be caused by an inactivating mutation of the *type 1 PTH/PTHrP receptor* gene.

K. Thyrotropin-releasing hormone

1. General. The *TRH receptor* gene is located on chromosome 8q23. Activation of these receptors on pituitary thyrotrophs by TRH results in TSH secretion.

2. Intrinsic defects. A single patient has been described with central hypothyroidism diagnosed at 9 years of age, in whom there was complete absence of TSH and prolactin responses following administration of synthetic TRH. This prompted molecular analysis of the patient's *TRH receptor* gene, which revealed a compound heterozygous mutation affecting TRH cellular binding and downstream signaling.

L. Thyroid-stimulating hormone

1. General. The *TSH receptor* gene has been mapped to chromosome 14q31 and has two segments: nine exons encoding the amino terminus of the extracellular domain and a large single exon encoding the carboxy-terminal side of the extracellular domain, the serpentine transmembrane portion, and the intracellular domain. The TSH receptor is mainly coupled to α-Gs, leading to stimulation of the cAMP pathway, which mediates the effects of TSH on thyroid gland growth and thyroid hormone secretion.

2. **Intrinsic defects.** More than 30 compound heterozygous or homozygous loss-of-function mutations of the *TSH receptor* gene have been reported. The presenting phenotype ranges from euthyroid hyperthyrotropinemia to, despite development of the thyroid anlage and its normal migration to the mid-neck, congenital hypothyroidism with profound thyroid gland hypoplasia. Intermediate phenotypes have been described as well. The mode of inheritance is autosomal recessive. Resistance to TSH may occur in patients with PHP IA.

VI. SPECIFIC DISORDERS ASSOCIATED WITH HORMONE RESISTANCE: STEROID HORMONES

A. Aldosterone (mineralocorticoid)

1. **General.** The gene for the human *mineralocorticoid receptor* has been mapped to chromosome 4q31.1. It encodes a protein of 984 amino acids. Aldosterone binds to mineralocorticoid receptors located in the distal renal tubule, sweat and salivary glands, and colonic mucosa, stimulating sodium retention and potassium excretion. Secretion of aldosterone is physiologically regulated by the renin-angiotensin system.

2. **Intrinsic defects**
   a. **Type 1 pseudohypoaldosteronism**
      (1) **Clinical.** This form is characterized by salt wasting in infancy, failure to thrive, hyponatremia, and hyperkalemia, and is responsive to supplemental sodium treatment, but not to mineralocorticoid therapy. This disorder is inherited either in an autosomal dominant fashion, affecting only the kidneys, or in an autosomal recessive fashion associated with multifocal target organ unresponsiveness to mineralocorticoids involving kidneys, colon, sweat and salivary glands, and lungs. Markedly elevated serum aldosterone levels are present in all cases, and the plasma renin activity is usually increased. Salt supplementation can often be discontinued after infancy despite persistent absence of aldosterone receptors into adulthood in the autosomal dominant form. Thus, it is presumed that in this form there must be progressive maturation of proximal tubular sodium-conserving mechanisms. Spontaneous remission does not occur in the recessive form.
      (2) **Mechanism.** The autosomal dominant variant of pseudohypoaldosteronism is caused by mutations in the *mineralocorticoid receptor* gene. The autosomal recessive form has been linked to mutations in the gene encoding the amiloride-sensitive epithelial sodium channel (16p12.2-13.1). These channels, normally located in the apical membrane, control sodium reabsorption in the kidneys and colon and regulate fluid secretion in the lungs.
   b. **Type 2 pseudohypoaldosteronism**
      (1) **Clinical.** This form is associated with partial unresponsiveness of the renal tubules to aldosterone, leading to inadequate potassium excretion, metabolic acidosis, hypertension, no renal salt-wasting, low plasma renin activity, and normal or slightly elevated serum aldosterone concentrations. This form of pseudohypoaldosteronism is characterized by chronic mineralocorticoid-resistant hyperkalemia and hypertension.
      (2) **Mechanism.** Unknown.

3. **Extrinsic defects**
   a. Infants with congenital adrenal hyperplasia secondary to 21-hydroxylase deficiency, and *without* associated mineralocorticoid deficiency, often still present with salt-losing crises and hyponatremia, and with mild hyperkalemia. In the untreated state, elevated serum levels of 17α-hydroxyprogesterone and other steroid precursors antagonize mineralocorticoid action and may have a significant role in the salt-wasting state in affected infants.

    b. May occur in infants and children with obstructive uropathy, urinary tract infection, tubulo-interstitial nephritis, sickle cell nephropathy, systemic lupus erythematosus, amyloidosis, neonatal medullary necrosis, and after unilateral renal vein thrombosis presumably secondary to renal tubular injury.

    c. Drugs such as spironolactone block the effects of aldosterone by directly closing the sodium channel in the luminal membrane of the collecting tubular cell.

B. Androgen

  1. General. The human *androgen receptor (AR)* gene spans more than 90 kb and has been mapped to Xq11.2-q12. It comprises eight exons that code for a protein containing 910 amino acids. The AR contains a carboxy terminus that confers specific steroid-binding properties (coded by exons 4 through 8) and a highly conserved (within the family of steroid receptors) cysteine-rich DNA-binding domain (coded by exons 2 and 3). Activation of the AR is required to mediate the biologic actions of testosterone and dihydrotestosterone.

  2. Intrinsic defects

    a. Clinical. In its full form, also known historically as **testicular feminization** and today as **complete androgen insensitivity syndrome**, this disorder causes 46,XY sex reversal and presents in the adolescent age range as primary amenorrhea, little or no pubic and axillary hair, and normal breasts (secondary to peripheral androgen-to-estrogen conversion) in a phenotypically normal female. This condition occasionally presents in the younger child because of the presence of testis-containing inguinal hernias in otherwise normal-appearing girls. Partial resistance to androgen usually presents clinically with ambiguous external genitalia, including perineoscrotal hypospadias, micropenis, and a bifid scrotum, usually in conjunction with undescended testes, in the newborn period and is becoming increasingly referred to as a **disorder of sexual development** or **DSD**. The condition may also present later with pubertal breast development and azoospermia in a male or with a predominant female phenotype with partial labial fusion, clitoromegaly, and normal breast and pubic hair development. Isolated hypospadias may be considered as an expression of androgen resistance, whereas idiopathic micropenis is not. With either presentation, there is a blind-ending vagina and there are no internal genital ducts (because of normal fetal AMH production and action causing regression of müllerian derivatives, and resistance to local androgen action preventing wolffian duct formation). The testes contain normal or increased Leydig cells and seminiferous tubules, but there is no spermatogenesis. Because of the risk of gonadal tumor development (and carcinoma *in situ* in the prepubertal testis), prophylactic orchiectomies are indicated, the optimal timing for which is controversial. Typically, affected postpubertal patients have elevated serum levels of LH, testosterone, and estradiol.

    b. Mechanism. Defects of AR function fall into two categories. The first uniformly causes complete androgen resistance and includes mutations that disrupt the primary sequence of the receptor, resulting in, for example, premature stop codons; frameshift mutations, deletions, or insertions; or alterations of RNA splicing. The second and more common cause is associated with a variable phenotype and is due to single amino acid substitutions within the AR protein, typically occurring in either the hormone-binding domain (the most common cause of androgen resistance) or the DNA-binding domain. More than 300 different mutations have been described.

C. 1,25-Dihydroxyvitamin D$_3$ [1,25(OH)$_2$D$_3$]

  1. General. The human vitamin D receptor is the product of a single gene on chromosome 12q12-q14. It contains 9 exons that encode a C-terminal hormone-binding domain [with high-affinity steroid specificity for 1,25(OH)$_2$D$_3$], a "hinge" region, and a cysteine-rich DNA-binding domain (containing two "zinc fingers"). Activation of this receptor by 1,25(OH)$_2$D$_3$ increases intestinal calcium absorption and increases bone osteoid formation, with other effects on cellular differentiation and immune function.

2. **Intrinsic defects—hereditary vitamin D–resistant rickets (formerly known as vitamin D–dependent rickets, type II)**
   a. **Clinical.** Affected patients with this rare form of rickets present with a constellation of symptoms including early-onset rickets, growth retardation, hypocalcemia, hypophosphatemia, elevated alkaline phosphatase, secondary hyperparathyroidism, and **elevated serum levels of 1,25(OH)$_2$D$_3$.** In addition, severe dental caries, dental hypoplasia, and, in most but not all cases, sparse hair or even total scalp and body **alopecia** frequently occur. The disease can occur in multiple family members of both sexes with a high incidence of parental consanguinity, suggesting autosomal recessive inheritance. Affected patients usually fail to respond to treatment with 1,25(OH)$_2$D$_3$ even at supraphysiologic doses. Therapy with high-dose oral calcium overcomes the receptor defect, normalizes serum calcium, and maintains bone remodeling and mineral apposition. Spontaneous improvement with age also occurs in some affected children.
   b. **Mechanism.** More than 50 mutations of the *1,25(OH)$_2$D$_3$-receptor* gene have been described. These molecular defects typically affect either the hormone-binding or DNA-binding zinc-finger regions, with mutation hot spots identified at conserved sequences among the steroid/nuclear receptor superfamily of ligand-activated transcription factors.

D. **Estrogen**
   1. **General.** Two genes for the human estrogen receptor (ER) have been cloned. ERα is located on chromosome 6q25.1 and encodes a protein containing 595 amino acids, whereas that for ERβ is on 14q and encodes for a species containing 530 amino acids. Activation of the ER effects estrogen actions on the female reproductive system and on bone.
   2. **Intrinsic defects**
      a. **Clinical.** A single case of **estrogen resistance** due to a proven mutation in the *ER* gene has been described in a 28-year-old man (product of a consanguineous marriage) with very tall stature, incomplete epiphysial closure, decreased bone mineral density, and otherwise normal pubertal development. Serum estradiol, estrone, LH, and FSH levels were all increased, whereas serum testosterone concentrations were normal. The patient had no detectable physical or biochemical response to estrogen administration, despite a 10-fold increase in the serum-free estradiol concentration.
      b. **Mechanism.** In the preceding single case, direct sequencing of exon 2 revealed a cystine-to-thymidine transition at codon 157 of both alleles, resulting in a premature stop codon. The patient's parents are heterozygous carriers of this mutation.

E. **Glucocorticoid**
   1. **General.** The cDNAs encoding the human glucocorticoid receptor (GR) predict two protein forms of 777 (GRα) and 742 (GRβ) amino acids, differing at their carboxy termini, with GRα being the classic GR and the role of GRβ not being known. The gene has been mapped to chromosome 5q31. Activation of the GR is required to effect the actions of glucocorticoids.
   2. **Physiologic glucocorticoid resistance.** In the distal nephrons of the kidney, cortisol resistance occurs. More specifically, the human mineralocorticoid receptor can be activated by cortisol, serum concentrations of which exceed those of aldosterone, the natural ligand, by as much as 1 000-fold. To avoid continuous activation of the mineralocorticoid receptor by cortisol, it is converted in the kidney by the enzyme 11β-hydroxylase to cortisone, which does not activate the mineralocorticoid receptor. This localized resistance to cortisol prevents the development of cortisol-mediated hypertension and hypokalemia in normal subjects.
   3. **Intrinsic defects**
      a. **Clinical features. Generalized inherited cortisol resistance** is a rare (usually) autosomal dominant disorder (but occasionally sporadic) that has been reported in several families in which affected members present with

hypercortisolemia but without Cushingoid features. Pituitary and peripheral resistance are balanced so that no features of hyper- or hypocortisolism emerge. Clinical characteristics result from, in females, increased circulating adrenal androgens, which manifest as hirsutism, male pattern baldness, menstrual irregularities, infertility, and masculinization; in boys, sexual precocity; and, in both sexes, increased serum levels of deoxycorticosterone, which cause hypertension and hypokalemia, and, perhaps as a result of relative glucocorticoid receptor deficiency, fatigue. These clinical features respond to dexamethasone therapy. Two sisters have also been reported with combined resistance to glucocorticoids, mineralocorticoids, and androgens, possibly due to a common coactivator defect; they had normal sensitivity to vitamin D and thyroid hormones.

   b. Mechanism. May or may not be associated with abnormalities of the human GR, including decreased receptor number, affinity, stability, and/or translocation into the nucleus.

4. Extrinsic defects

   a. Psychiatric disorders, including depression, anorexia nervosa, and certain types of psychoses, are associated with serum cortisol concentrations as high as those occurring in patients with Cushing syndrome, yet these patients have none of the physical features associated with Cushing syndrome, suggesting a state of glucocorticoid resistance.

   b. HIV. Elevated serum cortisol levels with clinical evidence of glucocorticoid insufficiency have been described in some adults with acquired HIV, in whom wasting, diarrhea, and hyperkalemia are suggestive of adrenal insufficiency. Although decreased glucocorticoid receptors have been found in circulating lymphocytes from these patients, the mechanistic significance of this finding is unclear.

   c. Cushing disease. Pituitary Cushing disease may be caused by glucocorticoid resistance localized to the hypothalamus and/or pituitary. Ectopic Cushing disease frequently is associated with ACTH production that is not suppressed by glucocorticoids.

   d. Inflammatory diseases. Reported autoimmune/inflammatory/allergic diseases associated with glucocorticoid resistance include rheumatoid arthritis, osteoarthritis, systemic lupus erythematosus, Crohn disease, ulcerative colitis, septic shock/respiratory distress syndrome, and bronchial asthma. This effect may be initiated by inflammatory signals such as IL-2, IL-4, IL-13, and TNF-α.

F. Thyroid hormones

   1. General. There are two *thyroid hormone (T$_3$) receptor* genes, designated α and β, which are located on chromosomes 17q11.2 and 3p24.3, respectively. There are developmental and tissue-specific patterns of expression of T$_3$ receptor mRNA. Activation of this receptor affects the various metabolic actions of thyroid hormones.

   2. Intrinsic defects

   a. Clinical. Until recently, patients thought to have thyroid hormone resistance were classified as having either generalized or selective pituitary resistance depending on the absence or presence of symptoms of hyperthyroidism. The term **generalized thyroid hormone resistance** has been applied to a syndrome characterized by elevated serum levels of free thyroid hormones, resistance to thyroid hormone action, and inappropriately normal or elevated and TRH-responsive serum TSH levels. Affected patients may also have attention deficit disorder (60%), stippled epiphyses, short stature, and multiple somatic abnormalities. Whereas patients with generalized thyroid hormone resistance are clinically euthyroid or even hypothyroid, those with the rarer **selective pituitary resistance to thyroid hormones** are clinically hyperthyroid. This variant tends to be inherited in an autosomal dominant fashion and also is associated with inappropriately normal and TRH-responsive serum TSH levels. The somewhat arbitrary classification of patients into generalized and pituitary forms of thyroid hormone resistance implies that clinical examination and routine biochemical measurements together allow clear-cut distinction between the presence and absence of hyperthyroidism. However, it is clear that in both forms there can be variable refractoriness to thyroid hormone action in different tissues, including bone, brain (reflected as degrees of permanent mental deficit), liver, heart, and pituitary gland.

b. Mechanism. These syndromes are usually transmitted in an autosomal dominant fashion. In multiple kindreds with thyroid hormone resistance, an intrinsic heterozygous mutation of the T_3-receptor β gene, involving its ligand-binding domain, has been identified. These mutations fall into the class of **dominant-negative mutations** where the mutant form is coexpressed with a normal receptor but disrupts the activity of the normal receptor. This dominant-negative inhibition by mutant receptors may be corrected in certain tissues by a compensatory increase in the levels of circulating thyroid hormones. More than 100 mutations have been described.

VII. SPECIFIC DISORDERS ASSOCIATED WITH HORMONE RESISTANCE: PEPTIDE GROWTH/DIFFERENTIATION FACTORS THAT ACT VIA TRANSMEMBRANE SERINE/THREONINE KINASE RECEPTORS

A. Anti-müllerian hormone

1. General. The *AMH receptor* gene is located on chromosome 12q13. AMH, also known as müllerian-inhibiting substance (MIS) or factor (MIF), is a hormone produced by immature Sertoli cells, the main action of which prevents development of the fallopian tubes, uterus, and upper vagina in male fetuses prior to 10 weeks' gestation. Postnatal ovarian granulosa cells also produce AMH, although a distinct function has not been recognized in females.

2. Intrinsic defects

a. Clinical. The **persistent müllerian duct syndrome** is a rare form of male pseudohermaphroditism characterized by the presence of a uterus and fallopian tubes in an otherwise normally virilized male. The condition is most often discovered incidentally during repair of an inguinal hernia, at which time the hernia sac is found to contain müllerian remnants.

b. Mechanism. Some boys with this condition have no detectable immunoreactive or bioactive AMH in their serum in conjunction with a mutation in their *AMH* gene. In contrast, other affected boys who express normal amounts of AMH in their serum have been found to have mutations in their *AMH receptor* gene.

Selected References

Beck-Peccoz P, Persani L, Calebiro D, et al. Syndromes of hormone resistance in the hypothalamic-pituitary-thyroid axis. *Best Pract Res Clin Endocrinol Metab* 2006;20: 529–546.

Bichet DG. Nephrogenic diabetes insipidus. *Adv Chronic Kidney Dis* 2006;13:96–104.

Bouillon R, Verstuyf A, Mathieu C, et al. Vitamin D resistance. *Best Pract Res Clin Endocrinol Metab* 2006;20:627–645.

Brown EM. Clinical lessons from the calcium-sensing receptor. *Nat Clin Pract Endocrinol Metab* 2007;3:122–133.

Correia ML, Haynes WG. Lessons from Leptin's molecular biology: Potential therapeutic actions of recombinant leptin and leptin-related compounds. *Mini Rev Med Chem* 2007;7: 31–38.

Hegele RA. Monogenic forms of insulin resistance: apertures that expose the common metabolic syndrome. *Trends Endocrinol Metab* 2003;14:371–377.

Herynk MH, Fuqua SA. Estrogen receptor mutations in human disease. *Endocr Rev* 2004; 25:869–898.

Hughes IA, Deeb A. Androgen resistance. *Best Pract Res Clin Endocrinol Metab.* 2006; 20:577–598.

Huhtaniemi I, Alevizaki M. Gonadotrophin resistance. *Best Pract Res Clin Endocrinol Metab* 2006;20:561–576.

Jain S, Golde DW, Bailey RB, et al. Insulin-like growth factor-I resistance. *Endocr Rev* 1998; 19:625–646.

Jameson JL. Molecular mechanisms of end-organ resistance. *Growth Horm IGF Res* 2004; 14(suppl A):S45–S50.

Khanna A. Acquired nephrogenic diabetes insipidus. *Semin Nephrol* 2006;26:244–248.

Lu NZ, Wardell SE, Burnstein KL, et al. International Union of Pharmacology. LXV. The pharmacology and classification of the nuclear receptor superfamily: glucocorticoid, mineralocorticoid, progesterone, and androgen receptors. *Pharmacol Rev* 2006;58:782–797.

Malchoff CD, Malchoff DM. Glucocorticoid resistance and hypersensitivity. *Endocrinol Metab Clin North Am* 2005;34:315–326.

Malecki MT. Genetics of type 2 diabetes mellitus. *Diabetes Res Clin Pract* 2005;68(suppl 1):S10–S21.

Mantovani G, Spada A. Mutations in the Gs alpha gene causing hormone resistance. *Best Pract Res Clin Endocrinol Metab* 2006;20:501–513.

Metherell LA, Chan LF, Clarke, AJL. The genetics of ACTH resistance syndromes. *Best Prac Res Clin Endocrinol Metab* 2006;20:547–560.

Phillips JA, Prince MA. Applications of new genetic approaches to growth hormone-releasing hormone receptor defects. *Growth Hormone IGF Res* 1999;9:45–49.

Savage MO, Attie KM, David A, et al. Endocrine assessment, molecular characterization and treatment of growth hormone insensitivity disorders. *Nat Clin Pract Endocrinol Metab* 2006;2:395–407.

Schaak S, Mialet-Perez J, Flordellis C, Paris H. Genetic variation of human adrenergic receptors: from molecular and functional properties to clinical and pharmacogenetic implications. *Curr Top Med Chem* 2007;7:217–231.

Seminara SB. Mechanisms of disease: the first kiss-a crucial role for kisspeptin-1 and its receptor, G-protein-coupled receptor 54, in puberty and reproduction. *Nat Clin Pract Endocrinol Metab* 2006;2:328–334.

Tao YX. Inactivating mutations of G protein-coupled receptors and diseases: structure-function insights and therapeutic implications. *Pharmacol Ther* 2006;111:949–973.

van Rossum EF, Lamberts SW. Glucocorticoid resistance syndrome: a diagnostic and therapeutic approach. *Best Pract Res Clin Endocrinol Metab* 2006;20:611–626.

Zennaro MC, Lombes M. Mineralocorticoid resistance. *Trends Endocrinol Metab* 2004;15:264–270.

GENETICS OF ENDOCRINOLOGY
Rena Ellen Falk

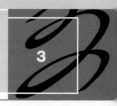

Genetic disease can be divided into four areas: cytogenetic disorders (i.e., autosomal and sex chromosome abnormalities), single-gene disorders, multifactorial disorders, and conditions with nontraditional inheritance.

I. CYTOGENETICS. Approximately 0.7% of live-borns, 5% of stillborns, and 50% of spontaneously aborted fetuses have a chromosomal abnormality. The modal number of chromosomes in humans is 46, including 22 pairs of autosomes and an XX or XY sex chromosome complement. A wide variety of cytogenetic aberrations has been described, many with an associated endocrine dysfunction (Table 3.1). Chromosomal abnormalities can be numeric, structural, or dysfunctional and can involve either the autosomes or the sex chromosomes. An individual with two or more chromosomally distinct cell lines is termed a **mosaic,** a situation often involving the sex chromosomes. The International System for Human Cytogenetic Nomenclature (ISCN, 2005) allows precise descriptions of each heterogeneously stained chromosome according to its number, arm(**p** designating short arm; **q** designating long arm), region, band, and even subband. For example, the notation **2p12** refers to chromosome number 2, short arm, region 1, band 2.

A. Banding techniques. A number of staining procedures are available to produce a specific pattern of bands along the length of each chromosome. The patterns of homologous (paired) chromosomes are identical, with the exception of specific regions in which inherited variants or polymorphisms occur in the normal population, apparently without clinical significance.

1. Q banding. The first heterogeneous staining technique, developed by Cassperson, involved use of a fluorescent dye, quinacrine mustard, to produce regions of varying intensity called **Q bands.** This technique was helpful in rapidly determining genotypic sex, in screening for X–Y or Y–autosome exchanges **(translocation),** and in evaluating a large number of cells when there is a concern that a sex chromosome mosaic may have a Y-bearing cell line. However, fluorescence *in situ* hybridization (FISH) technology (see later) has largely replaced Q banding for these purposes.

2. G banding. After harsh pretreatment, often using the enzyme trypsin, chromosomes stained with Giemsa develop a consistent banding pattern that is similar to the pattern seen with Q banding. G banding is more sensitive and has **replaced Q banding** as the standard staining procedure. G banding is particularly helpful in (a) identifying small structural abnormalities and marker chromosomes (those not obviously matching the banding pattern of a normal chromosome) and (b) defining the breakpoints of structural rearrangements. Dark-staining (G-positive) bands generally contain fewer coding regions (active genes) than light-staining (G-negative) regions. Therefore, small structural abnormalities of G-negative bands may have more profound phenotypic effects than similar abnormalities of dark bands.

3. R banding. R banding, a reverse staining method that generally involves use of Giemsa or the fluorescent stain acridine orange, is most helpful in elucidating nonhomology (nonmatching banding pattern) in the negative- or dull-staining regions of G- or Q-banded chromosomes.

TABLE 3.1	Endocrine Abnormalities in Chromosomal Disorders

Chromosomal disorder[a]	Endocrine abnormality
Down syndrome	Hypogonadism, hyper- or hypothyroidism
Turner syndrome (45,X and variants)	Hypogonadism, hypothyroidism, diabetes mellitus
Klinefelter syndrome (XXY and variants)	Hypogonadism, diabetes mellitus
Trisomy 13	Hypopituitarism, hypogonadism
Trisomy 18	Occasional thyroid or adrenal hypoplasia
Triploidy	Adrenal hypoplasia
del(4p) or Wolf-Hirschhorn syndrome	Hypogonadism
del(18p)	Holoprosencephaly, hypopituitarism
del(7q11.23)—Williams syndrome	Hypercalcemia in infancy
del(11p13)—Aniridia-Wilms tumor association	Ambiguous genitalia, gonadoblastoma
del(15q11q13)—Prader-Willi syndrome[b]	Hypogonadism, diabetes mellitus
del(22q11.2)—VCFS	DiGeorge sequence

[a]A number of rare partial trisomies or monosomies have been associated with hypogonadism with or without a genital anomaly.
[b]Prader-Willi syndrome is also caused by maternal *UPD15* and methylation defects in this region.
del, deletion.

4. **C banding.** This procedure stains centromeric regions composed of constitutive heterochromatin as well as the variable, brightly fluorescent distal portion of the Y chromosome.

5. **T banding.** T banding, which stains telomeric or terminal regions of chromosomes, and **AgNOR** staining, which uses silver nitrate to stain active nucleolus-organizing regions (NORs), may be applied to specific interpretive problems as an adjunct to routine procedures.

B. **Culture techniques.** Variation in the growth media, cell culture time, and use of specific additives to synchronize cell-cycle or to inhibit specific metabolic processes greatly influences the resultant cytogenetic evaluation.

1. **Metaphase analysis.** Most routine cytogenetic analyses require 72- to 96-hour cultures of phytohemagglutinin (PHA)–stimulated peripheral blood lymphocytes. An excellent-quality metaphase preparation should yield at least 500 to 550 bands per haploid set. When more rapid results are needed, a 48-hour culture of lymphocytes or direct preparation of bone marrow is requested. Both of these techniques are adequate for identification of numeric abnormalities, but neither is generally sensitive enough to distinguish small structural abnormalities.

2. **High-resolution analysis.** By using cell synchronization techniques and varying the culture time, one can visualize early metaphase or late prophase chromosomes, which are more elongated and have more bands than standard preparations. Although this technique is quite sensitive, revealing 800 or more bands per haploid set, high-resolution analysis should be reserved for situations in which a structural defect or nonhomology has already been found or for a diagnosis in which a very small structural change has been noted (see Section I.B.3).

3. **Other techniques** helpful to the endocrinologist include the following:
   a. Breakage studies, in which the culture is exposed to a clastogen and a large number of cells are scored for chromosomal breakage and rearrangement.
   b. Cell culture in the presence of folic acid inhibitors or other inducers to elucidate chromosomal fragile sites. These techniques are not used widely in the clinical setting.
   c. Culture of skin or other solid tissues, which may be particularly helpful in the evaluation of sex chromosome anomalies.

C. Molecular cytogenetics. New technology has allowed the implementation of techniques for visualization of specific chromosomes or parts of chromosomes by means of molecular probes.

1. **Fluorescence *in situ* hybridization (FISH).** Oligonucleotide probes, which are complementary to a repetitive or unique DNA sequence, can be hybridized to interphase or metaphase chromosomes. The probes are bound to a fluorescent dye, which allows visualization of a bright fluorescent spot representing each chromosomal region to which the probe has hybridized. This is particularly useful for the detection of aneuploidy in interphase cells, for rapid sex determination or confirmation of trisomy (including prenatal diagnosis), and in cancer cytogenetics.

2. **Chromosome painting.** A set of probes for various markers along the length of a chromosome can be applied to the cells using the FISH technique. The probes "paint" a specific chromosome regardless of its position in the cell or its structural integrity. This technique is especially useful in confirming the origin of small translocations and marker chromosomes.

3. **Single-copy probes.** Molecular probes that hybridize to a specific unique DNA sequence can be used to detect known mutations associated with a defined phenotype. This technique is particularly helpful in detecting **submicroscopic deletions** such as those underlying most cases of Williams syndrome, Prader-Willi syndrome, and velocardiofacial syndrome. The probe signal is visualized by fluorescent microscopy.

4. **M-FISH.** Multiplex FISH (M-FISH) techniques allow visualization of all or parts of all of the chromosomes simultaneously. M-FISH using a subtelomeric probe set is useful in detecting submicroscopic deletions in children with otherwise undiagnosable mental retardation. Recent data suggest that at least 6% of mentally retarded children have subtelomeric deletions that are detectable by M-FISH.

5. **Comparative genomic hybridization (CGH):** CGH is a molecular technique that is rapidly becoming a major clinical diagnostic tool. This technology compares the test (patient) DNA to a standard, and uses a set of molecular probes to identify relative gain or loss of specific chromosomal regions. Visualization is most commonly achieved via a microarray format. Cryptic deletions or duplications identified by CGH can be confirmed by targeted FISH. CGH may replace standard cytogenetic analysis as a diagnostic procedure because it detects numerical abnormalities as well as cryptic duplications, deletions, or more complex abnormalities. CGH is also useful in cancer cytogenetics. However, CGH may identify copy-number variants, which represent inherited polymorphisms and cannot detect balanced structural rearrangements or low-frequency mosaicism.

II. AUTOSOMAL DISORDERS. Complete monosomy for an autosome is generally lethal, most commonly recognized in spontaneously aborted fetuses. In live-borns the effect of trisomy is generally devastating. Mosaicism for an autosomal abnormality generally results in a milder phenotype and can be associated with survival in otherwise lethal conditions. With development of the molecular chromosomal techniques, small deletions and duplications have been recognized with increasing frequency. Parental studies should be performed with appropriate cytogenetic or FISH techniques to exclude balanced rearrangement whenever a structural abnormality is found.

A. Down syndrome occurs with an incidence of 1 in 670 births and is the most common disorder producing malformation and mental retardation. In nearly 97% of cases the cause is trisomy 21 (including nearly 3% with mosaicism for a normal cell line). The remainder result from sporadic or inherited translocations involving chromosome number 21, most commonly occurring as the result of fusion of the centromere of the 21 and another acrocentric chromosome. Many of the phenotypic findings of Down syndrome have been attributed to trisomy of the distal portion of the long arm, segment 21q22. Recurrence risk is ~1% for trisomy 21 and significantly higher for carriers of a balanced translocation. Advanced maternal age is the only risk factor clearly associated with occurrence of trisomy 21. **Endocrine abnormalities**

in Down syndrome include hypogonadism (100% in males), athyrotic and acquired hypothyroidism, and thyroid hyperfunction.

B. Trisomy 18 is variously reported to occur in about 1 in 3 300 to 1 in 10 000 live births. Affected females exceed males by a ratio of at least 3:1; gestational timing is frequently altered (including prematurity and postmaturity). The phenotype in trisomy 18 is more severe than in Down syndrome; only 50% survive to age 2 months, and 10% survive for 1 year. In addition to a characteristic pattern of major and minor malformations, trisomy 18 survivors are profoundly mentally and physically retarded. Aside from deficient growth and hypoplasia of subcutaneous adipose tissue, endocrine abnormalities are relatively uncommon, with thyroid or adrenal hypoplasia occurring in <10% of patients.

C. Trisomy 13 occurs in about 1 in 5 000 live births and is usually associated with a wide spectrum of malformations, many of which are midline defects. Typical facial features include microphthalmia, along with cleft lip and palate or agenesis of the premaxilla, which is the usual concomitant of holoprosencephaly. A number of **endocrine abnormalities** can occur, including hypopituitarism, ectopic pancreas, and gonadal hypoplasia.

D. Other autosomal abnormalities, such as **triploidy** (modal number = 69), **Wolf-Hirschhorn syndrome** (4 short arm deletion), and **18 short arm deletion**, have been associated with increased likelihood of endocrine dysfunction. Of particular note are several well-defined syndromes associated with very small deletions, often requiring high-resolution or molecular studies for demonstration of the defect. These include the **Prader-Willi syndrome** of hypotonia, obesity, small hands and feet, and hypogonadism, in which region 15q11-13 is deleted in ~70% of affected individuals. Etiology of Prader-Willi syndrome is diverse. These 70% have a usually cryptic deletion, 25% have maternal uniparental disomy (UPD), which means that there are two copies of chromosome 15 but they both came from the mother. The remaining 5% have a variety of causes, all related to the same chromosome region, including atypical (usually smaller) deletions and rearrangements, imprinting defects, and, possibly mutation in a gene called SNRPN. **Multiple endocrine neoplasia type 2** (MEN2a; see Chapter 53) which generally segregates as an autosomal dominant in affected families, presents with medullary carcinoma of the thyroid, pheochromocytoma, and variable parathyroid involvement. A small interstitial deletion of 20p has been described in members of several affected kindreds. The **DiGeorge sequence** has also been described in association with the **velocardiofacial syndrome**, which is usually a result of submicroscopic deletion of 22q11.2. Some patients with the **aniridia–Wilms tumor** association (Wilms tumor, aniridia, genitourinary abnormalities, and mental retardation; WAGR) have a deletion of band 11p13. Mental retardation, ambiguous genitalia, streak gonads, other forms of hypogonadism, and gonadoblastoma also occur in this condition. A Wilms tumor locus (WTI) maps to this region and is mutated in patients with **Drash syndrome** (XY gonadal dysgenesis, chronic glomerulopathy, and Wilms tumor). Finally, the **Williams syndrome** of mental retardation, small stature, elfin facies, supravalvular aortic stenosis, and persistent hypercalcemia is caused by a deletion in chromosome 7q11.23. It is important to request cytogenetic analysis in patients suspected of having one of these disorders and to seek molecular studies (FISH) in clinically suggestive cases when chromosome analysis is normal.

III. SEX CHROMOSOME ABNORMALITIES. Monosomy or trisomy of the sex chromosomes is significantly more benign than autosomal abnormalities and may be associated with normal phenotype, as in some trisomy X females. Phenotypic findings are limited, and some sex chromosome abnormalities can be diagnosed only with failure of normal onset of puberty, recognition of aberrant secondary sexual development, or evaluation for infertility or fetal wastage. Screening procedures such as sex-chromatin determination (buccal smear) can be misleading. This is particularly important when there is a Y-bearing cell line in dysgenetic gonads, which implies an increased risk for development of gonadoblastoma. If sex chromosome aneuploidy is suspected, cytogenetic analysis must be performed with evaluation of an adequate number of cells to exclude the possibility of low-frequency mosaicism. In cases where there is a high index of suspicion for a sex chromosome disorder and peripheral blood lymphocyte analysis is normal, evaluation of a second tissue such as skin fibroblasts should be considered. FISH evaluation of a buccal smear may detect mosaicism without need for an invasive biopsy and tissue culture.

A. Turner syndrome, most commonly associated with karyotype 45,X (monosomy X), occurs in 1 in 5 000 live births (1:2 500 females) and produces a variable pattern of craniofacial and visceral malformations. Although the phenotype can be distinguished on the basis of dysmorphic facies, web neck, broad chest, cubitus valgus, and other stigmata, the most consistent and important findings are short stature and gonadal dysgenesis. Despite the relatively mild phenotype in live-born infants, 98% of 45,X concepti are spontaneously aborted.

  1. More than 50% of patients with Turner syndrome have karyotype 45,X. The missing X chromosome is generally paternal in origin; there is no maternal age effect. Various cytogenetic findings are associated with Turner phenotype, including mosaicism for 46,XX, 46,XY, polysomy-X, or a cell line with a structurally abnormal X or Y. The phenotype is modified by the presence of another cell line as well as by the occasional findings of X-autosome translocation. When a Y chromosome is present, sexual ambiguity can occur. Structural abnormalities of the X chromosome include isochromosome of the long arm [i(Xq)], rare isochromosome of the short arm [i(Xp)], deletion of the long arm [del(Xq)], deletion of the short arm [del(Xp)], terminal rearrangement [46,X,ter rea(X;X)], and ring (r)X [46X,r(X)]. In most cases, inactivation of the abnormal X chromosome results in some degree of gene dosage compensation. Mosaicism for a 45,X cell line is a common associate of a structural anomaly. In the case of an X-autosome rearrangement, the karyotype can be balanced or unbalanced. Even when the exchange appears to be balanced, malformation or mental retardation occurs with increased frequency. The normal X is generally inactivated in X-autosome rearrangement. Turner syndrome may occur in association with a structurally abnormal Y chromosome, with or without a 45,X cell line, or with 45,X/46,XY mosaicism. Recurrence risk is generally low, except in the situation of inherited X-autosome translocation and, potentially, in offspring of mothers with a 45,X cell line.

  2. Turner syndrome should be suspected in any newborn with typical stigmata and is often heralded by striking lymphedema or congenital heart disease (~20% have a cardiac defect; 75% of these are ventricular septal defects or aortic coarctation). Any girl with unexplained short stature should be evaluated even in the absence of other stigmata. Finally, girls with failure of normal secondary sexual development, amenorrhea, persistently erratic menses, unexplained infertility, recurrent fetal wastage (three or more episodes), or premature menopause should also be studied. Although gonadotropin levels can be evaluated in early childhood and during the prepubertal age range, the only definitive studies are cytogenetic analysis and CGH. Cytogenetic analysis should include evaluation of at least 30 to 50 cells.

  3. Management of the young Turner syndrome patient includes careful evaluation for associated conditions (especially cardiac, gastrointestinal, or renal malformation, and hearing loss) and appropriate specific therapy as needed. **Autoimmune disorders** are most commonly associated with isochromosome Xq but occur in 45,X individuals as well. Autoimmune thyroiditis, inflammatory bowel disease, diabetes mellitus, and arterial hypertension are common in older children and adults and require long-term treatment. Sudden death from aortic dissection has been reported. Administration of **growth hormone** results in accelerated growth rate and somewhat increased adult height. Such treatment can be initiated as early as 2 years of age and should be considered when growth falls below the 5th percentile. Carbohydrate metabolism should be evaluated periodically, especially during growth-hormone treatment. Low-dose **estrogen replacement** should begin when epiphysial closure is documented, earlier when the psychological state of the patient necessitates institution of pubertal changes. Hormonal replacement should generally begin by age 14 years. Secondary sexual development often remains incomplete. Although infertility is likely, rare Turner syndrome patients achieve spontaneous ovulation and pregnancy. The possibility of fertility is suggested by the spontaneous onset of menses or normal gonadotropin levels before cyclic replacement therapy is started. Limited data suggest an increased likelihood of malformation in the offspring of fertile Turner syndrome patients. Such patients should be counseled carefully about the increased risk of miscarriage and early menopause and should be offered prenatal diagnosis. Finally, as in other situations with a dysgenetic Y-chromosome–bearing gonad, Turner syndrome patients with a mosaic or nonmosaic cell line containing a Y chromosome should undergo removal of the streak ovaries because of the increased risk of gonadoblastoma.

B. Trisomy X (47,XXX) occurs in about 1 in 1 000 female live-borns, is commonly associated with a phenotype in the normal range, and is diagnosed only rarely in early childhood.

1. Although data from prospective, longitudinal studies are limited, the XXX female has a tendency toward tall stature, epilepsy, dull-normal intelligence, delayed language acquisition, menstrual dysfunction, and infertility. Advanced maternal age is well established in association with triple-X populations. Of note, offspring of fertile trisomy X women are unlikely to have chromosomal aneuploidy, suggesting a protective mechanism against development or survival of the aneuploid gamete or zygote.

2. When polysomy X occurs with **more than three X chromosomes** (e.g., 48,XXXX, 49,XXXXX), there is an increasing likelihood of significant mental retardation, dysmorphic features, and visceral or skeletal malformation. These syndromes are rare and generally sporadic.

C. Klinefelter syndrome is usually associated with karyotype 47,XXY and is found in approximately 1 in 700 males. Rarer karyotypes, often associated with polysomy X or Y (with or without mosaicism), also occur. The syndrome of at least two X chromosomes and one Y chromosome constitutes the most common cause of male hypogonadism.

1. **Mosaicism** occurs in ~10% of Klinefelter males and is most commonly associated with karyotype 46,XY/47,XXY. Because the normal cell line can alter the phenotype significantly, 46,XY/47,XXY mosaics can have normal gonadal function and fertility. The additional X chromosome is often maternally derived (60%) and is associated with advanced maternal age. In patients whose additional X chromosome is paternally derived, paternal age distribution is normal.

2. **Phenotypic variability** is typical of Klinefelter syndrome. The most common features are mild increase in stature as a result of disproportionate growth of the lower extremities, and small testes (usually <2 cm) without evidence of abnormal wolffian development. Testicular biopsy might be normal in childhood but becomes progressively more abnormal near or after puberty. Typical findings include tubular hyalinization, Leydig cell hyperplasia, decreased or absent Sertoli cells, and absent or rare spermatogenesis. Even when evidence of spermatogenesis is present, fertility is rare. Secondary sexual characteristics are frequently abnormal, with sparse facial hair, gynecomastia, and a female pattern of fat and hair distribution. As in the 47,XXX patient, intelligence is often normal. Cognitive ability is decreased in comparison with siblings, although the degree of intellectual involvement is mild. Auditory processing and expressive language abilities are especially impaired. Behavior disorders occur more frequently, as do electroencephalographic (EEG) abnormalities or frank seizure disorders. Other conditions associated with Klinefelter syndrome include varicose veins, thromboembolic disease, chronic respiratory disease, osteoporosis, diabetes mellitus, thyroid dysfunction, and, rarely, growth-hormone deficiency or central precocious puberty. There is an increased incidence of extragonadal midline (mediastinal) germ-cell tumors, which usually present in the second to fourth decade. Although the relative frequency of breast cancer is increased compared to normal males, the absolute risk is low, probably about 1 in 5 000.

3. At present there is no viable treatment for infertility in Klinefelter syndrome, though rare patients have fathered children through assisted reproductive techniques (testicular aspiration followed by in-vitro fertilization and intracytoplasmic sperm injection [ICSI]). Testosterone replacement can be implemented between ages 11 and 14 years and is particularly helpful in achieving more complete virilization in the androgen-deficient patient. Adult patients report increased libido after institution of testosterone therapy. Gynecomastia might require surgical attention. Psychological counseling helps to achieve a normal adjustment in Klinefelter patients as well as in other individuals with sex chromosome abnormalities.

D. Of all the sex chromosome abnormalities, the **47,XYY karyotype** has raised the most controversy and public interest.

1. Occurring in 1 in 800 males, this cytogenetic finding is often accompanied by a completely normal phenotype and is rarely ascertained in childhood. The origin of the additional Y chromosome is generally a result of malsegregation at paternal meiosis II. Paternal age is not advanced.

2. Prospective data are limited but support the finding of tall stature with relatively early to mid-childhood growth spurt. Minor malformations can occur with increased frequency, but association of a major malformation is not established. Similarly, electrocardiographic abnormalities, severe cystic acne, and varicose veins have been described, but increased risk for these is unconfirmed. Intelligence is generally within the normal range, with a downward shift in comparison with siblings and the general population. Language acquisition is particularly affected. Aberrant psychosocial development and behavior disorders occur with increased frequency, as does ordinary criminal behavior (i.e., not solely highly aggressive acts). Although gonadal development and function are normal in most XYY males, occurrence of small testes, subfertility, or infertility is known.

3. No specific treatment is indicated in 47,XYY males. Realistic and thorough counseling should be offered when the XYY karyotype is discovered or at the time of prenatal diagnosis. Adults who are newly diagnosed as XYY should be given reassurance and counseling support. Although prenatal diagnosis can be offered to partners of XYY males, their offspring generally have a normal chromosome complement.

IV. SINGLE-GENE DISORDERS

A. Table 3.2 lists a number of multisystem unifactorial (Mendelian) disorders in which endocrine abnormalities are common. Although the terms were initially used to describe the genotype (full complement of genes carried by the 46 chromosomes), the concept of dominant and recessive inheritance is now best applied to the phenotype. In addition to overlap with environmental, multifactorial, and chromosomal disorders, unifactorial disorders often exhibit considerable genetic heterogeneity. For example, both isolated **growth-hormone deficiency** and **panhypopituitarism** can be inherited on an autosomal dominant, autosomal recessive, or X-linked recessive basis. Perhaps the best example of genetic heterogeneity occurs in the numerous disorders associated with **insulin-dependent diabetes mellitus (IDDM, or type 1)** and **non–insulin-dependent diabetes mellitus (NIDDM, or type 2).** Although both **type 1** and **type 2** diabetes occur in association with specific Mendelian disorders, and at least one presentation of type 2 diabetes— **maturity-onset diabetes of the young (MODY)**—occurs as an autosomal dominant disorder, both **isolated type 1 and type 2 diabetes** appear to be highly heterogeneous, with autosomal recessive and multifactorial (including two or more gene loci) modes proposed.

1. A gene is considered dominant if one copy of it is sufficient to result in manifestation of the trait or disorder; the gene is recessive if two copies are required for expression of the phenotype. Examples of codominance are known, particularly in the inheritance of the blood groups. For example, the genes for hemoglobin S and hemoglobin A are codominant, but clinical expression of sickle cell anemia is recessive.

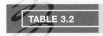

TABLE 3.2	Selected Multisystem Unifactorial Disorders with Endocrine Abnormalities

Acanthosis nigricans (insulin-resistant diabetes mellitus)
Achondroplasia (relative glucose intolerance)
Acrodysostosis (hypogonadism)
Albright hereditary osteodystrophy (hypocalcemia, hypothyroidism, hypogonadism)
Ataxia telangiectasia (hypogonadism)
Beckwith-Wiedemann syndrome (hypoglycemia)
De Sanctis-Cacchione syndrome (hypothalamic dysfunction, hypogonadism)
Johanson-Blizzard syndrome (hypothyroidism)
Kenny syndrome (transient infantile hypocalcemia)
Laurence-Moon-Biedl syndrome (hypogonadism, diabetes insipidus)
Lysosomal storage disorders (short stature, hirsutism may prompt referral)
McCune-Albright syndrome (precocious puberty)
Multiple lentigines syndrome (hypogonadism)
Myotonic muscular dystrophy (diabetes mellitus, thyroid dysfunction)
Neurofibromatosis (precocious puberty, acromegaly)
Noonan syndrome (hypogonadism)
Robinow syndrome (hypogonadism)
Russell-Silver syndrome (fasting hypoglycemia in infancy)
Smith-Lemli-Opitz syndrome (hypogonadism, sex reversal, adrenal hypertrophy, giant islet cells)
Tuberous sclerosis (precocious puberty, hypothyroidism, thyroid adenomas)
Werner syndrome (diabetes mellitus, hypogonadism, hyperthyroidism, adrenal atrophy)

2. A gene can be autosomal or X-linked with resultant differences in the inheritance pattern. Fewer than 30 Y-linked conditions are known, including several related to gender development and fertility.

3. Chromosomes, and their constituent genes, occur in pairs. If an individual has an identical gene at the same locus on each of two paired chromosomes, he or she is **homozygous** for the trait determined by that gene. If the individual has two alternative forms of the gene at the same locus on paired chromosomes, he or she is **heterozygous** for the trait. Such alternative forms, termed **alleles,** can result in normal polymorphism or in a variation of an abnormal phenotype. Because males normally have only one X chromosome, they are **hemizygous** for most X-linked genes.

B. **Autosomal dominant (AD) inheritance** has been implicated in more than 5 000 disorders, most of which result from the action of a rare mutant gene.

1. In general, dominant disorders include abnormalities of structural protein or of gene regulation.

2. **Autosomal dominant disorders** affect both sexes equally, except in sex-influenced or sex-limited conditions (e.g., Opitz syndrome and Opitz-Frias syndrome, both of which are ascertained largely because of the finding of hypospadias).

3. **Dominant disorders** are characterized by variation in expression (clinical phenotype) even within families. Occasional individuals who carry the gene might have no phenotypic findings, in which case the gene is **nonpenetrant.** Although penetrance is generally used as a population genetics concept, both nonpenetrance and minimal expression can result in an apparent "skip generation" or mimic a new mutation in a particular kindred.

4. A **new mutation** for a dominant gene generally results in expression of the trait. Therefore, mutation is important in the genesis of dominant disorders. Paternal age effect has been demonstrated in some dominant disorders, implying that increased paternal age is a predisposing factor for new mutation.

5. Dominant disorders generally follow a vertical pattern within families, except in the case of actual or genetic lethals (those disorders in which fertility is greatly

reduced or absent). The risk of transmission of the gene from an affected individual to his or her offspring is 50%, regardless of the sex of the child or the degree of severity in the parent. Similarly, the parental phenotype does not predict the degree of severity in the offspring. Recurrence risk for apparently unaffected parents of a child with a known dominant disorder is generally low.

6. Disorders of endocrine hyperplasia and neoplasia, as well as other familial cancer syndromes, generally occur as autosomal dominant conditions. Thus, the multiple endocrine neoplasia syndromes (MEN1, 2A, and IIIB; see Chapters 51 and 52), the phakomatoses, and Gorlin syndrome (basal cell nevus syndrome) are inherited as autosomal dominant traits.

C. In >1 800 disorders, **autosomal recessive inheritance** is established or suspected. Expression of a recessive disorder requires absence of the normal allele; the affected individual must be homozygous for the trait or heterozygous for two copies of the mutant genes. Deleterious recessive genes occur rarely in the population.

1. Recessive disorders generally involve genes that determine enzymatic protein and include the classic inborn errors of metabolism.

2. Either sex can be affected, although sex limitation does occur occasionally.

3. Decreased penetrance and extremely variable expression within a family occur much less commonly than in dominant conditions.

4. Although a new mutation can play a role in the occurrence of autosomal recessive disorders, such mutations are demonstrable only when specific heterozygote testing is available. If specific testing is not possible, parents of an affected child are considered **obligate heterozygotes.**

5. Pedigrees of families with autosomal recessive disorders generally show a horizontal relationship among affected members. Affected siblings generally have normal parents and normal offspring. Consanguinity can increase the possibility that the parents share the same rare recessive allele. Recurrence risk to obligate heterozygote parents is 25%. Approximately two thirds of their normal offspring will be carriers of the mutation. Except in the case of a consanguineous union or a relatively common mutant gene (e.g., cystic fibrosis or phenylketonuria), recurrence risk to offspring of an affected parent is quite low; such offspring are obligate heterozygotes (carriers).

6. The majority of endocrine deficiency disorders, inborn errors of protein metabolism and glycogenesis, and lysosomal storage disorders occur as autosomal recessive conditions. The inborn errors of thyroid biosynthesis and the group of disorders that produce congenital adrenal hyperplasia are examples of recessive (largely autosomal) disorders in which glandular hyperplasia occurs as a secondary event as a result of interruption of a normal feedback inhibition loop. Specific therapy, if any, depends on accurate diagnosis. Heterozygote (carrier) testing and prenatal diagnosis are available for most of these disorders.

D. Sex-linked disorders usually are equated with mutation of X-linked genes. Although genes associated with testicular development, sperm production, and height are known to be Y-linked, the range of functions of most Y-chromosome genes has not been characterized definitively. The testis-determining factor (SRY) has been mapped to region 1a on the Y-chromosome short arm (Yp). The gene, which has been highly conserved throughout mammalian evolution, consists of 900 base pairs. It encodes a DNA-binding protein that initiates the developmental cascade involved in testis formation from the undifferentiated gonad. Autosomal genes (e.g., *SOX9*) have a role in male gonadal development as well. Visible or submicroscopic Y-chromosome deletions have been implicated as a major cause of azoospermia and subfertility. At least 495 known or suspected X-linked disorders have been cataloged. In general, X-linked disorders affect males who are related to each other through relatively unaffected (in the case of X-linked recessive [XR]) or more mildly affected (X-linked dominant [XD]) females. Because the male is hemizygous for most X-linked genes, the relationship of gender to severity is expected. **Absence of male-to-male transmission is the hallmark of an X-linked disorder,** because an affected man must pass his Y chromosome to every son.

1. **XR disorders** vary in severity from genetic lethals (e.g., **Lesch-Nyhan syndrome**), in which affected males cannot reproduce, to relatively benign conditions (e.g., male pattern baldness). One third of genetically lethal cases arise as the result of a new mutation, a fact that complicates counseling of women with an apparently negative family history. Lethal XR disorders for which the gene has not been mapped to the X chromosome by cytogenetic, biochemical, or molecular techniques cannot be distinguished from autosomal dominant disorders with male sex limitation (e.g., **testicular feminization**). On average, half the daughters of heterozygous (carrier) females are also carriers, and half the sons are affected. Fertile males affected with an XR disorder have only carrier daughters and normal sons. Examples of **XR endocrine disorders** include adrenal leukodystrophy (a peroxisomal disorder that demonstrates surprising clinical variability), familial panhypopituitarism, rare forms of vasopressin deficiency, nonsyndromic hypoparathyroidism, adrenocortical hypoplasia, and complete or partial androgen insensitivity.

2. **XD disorders** are relatively rare and can be lethal prenatally in hemizygous males. Such an effect has been proposed in several disorders, including incontinentia pigmenti and focal dermal hypoplasia, in which increased spontaneous miscarriages and a paucity of live-born males are well documented. In nonlethal XD disorders there remains an excess of affected females, because a heterozygous female will pass the gene to half of her offspring of either sex, whereas a hemizygous male will pass the gene to all of his daughters and none of his sons. Examples of **XD disorders with endocrine manifestations** include nephrogenic diabetes insipidus and Albright hereditary osteodystrophy (pseudohypoparathyroidism).

3. **Specific treatment modalities,** heterozygote detection, and prenatal diagnosis are available for some X-linked disorders. When specific prenatal testing is unavailable, prenatal diagnosis is limited to sex determination or linkage analysis. In the first case, couples at risk for an XR disorder must opt to continue or terminate pregnancy solely on the basis of the 50% risk that a male fetus will be affected. In the latter situation, molecular markers are used to determine which maternal X carries the defective gene and whether that X or its homolog has been passed to the fetus. Linkage analysis is also useful in diagnosing autosomal dominant conditions.

V. MULTIFACTORIAL INHERITANCE

A. **General principles.** A number of disorders demonstrate familial aggregation without a clear pattern of Mendelian inheritance. Analysis of data from twins studies and population surveys reveals twins concordance or familial recurrence risk higher than expected by chance alone, but lower than predicted for a unifactorial trait, even one with reduced penetrance. The multifactorial model is a mathematical construct that predicts that two or more independent (nonallelic and unlinked) genes will interact in an additive way to create a genetic liability for expression of a specific trait. Interaction of the susceptible genotype with specific environmental effects can then exceed a threshold, resulting in expression of the trait. Although the threshold can be viewed in an all-or-none manner, severity of expression is variable and can be modified by other genetic risk factors, environmental factors, or both.

1. Multifactorial traits often demonstrate an altered sex ratio.

2. Recurrence risk varies with the sex of the affected individual; with the severity of the defect; between families because one family may have a greater genetic liability than another; with the number of affected family members; and with the incidence of the trait in the population.

B. **Multifactorial inheritance** has been implicated in a number of common malformations, including cleft lip (with or without cleft palate), isolated cleft palate, and the myelomeningocele–anencephaly sequence. The relative roles of genotype and environment in the pathogenesis of septo-optic dysplasia, holoprosencephaly, caudal regression, and athyrotic hypothyroidism are less clear, despite progress in identifying genes involved in the pathogenesis of these conditions (especially holoprosencephaly). The latter conditions generally occur as sporadic events in an otherwise normal family, and the recurrence risk appears to be less than that observed for the common multifactorial malformations. However, affected siblings or parents are occasionally described, underscoring the need for careful examination of close relatives of affected individuals. Familial aggregation is well known in the **autoimmune endocrinopathies.** Graves disease and Hashimoto thyroiditis are particularly associated with clustering of symptomatic and asymptomatic family members with positive antibodies.

C. **Environmental disorders with endocrine manifestations** are well known. Rubella embryopathy can be associated with hypopituitarism, isolated growth-hormone deficiency, diabetes mellitus, and hypothyroidism. Fetal hydantoin syndrome can result in hypogenitalism or ambiguity. Hydantoins, retinoids, and alcohol exposure are associated with prenatal and postnatal growth deficiency. Endocrine-acting agents that have a direct adverse effect on fetal outcome include sex hormones and antithyroid agents such as iodides, iodine-131, propylthiouracil (PTU, which may be safer than methimazole), and methimazole. One report compares the relative safety suggests that PTU should be the first-line choice of treatment in pregnancy, with methimazole reserved for cases that do not respond. Methimazole is thought to cause a set of dysmorphic features including scalp defects, and has been associated with increased risk of choanal atresia, esophageal atresia, and at least one case with a limb defect—though the data are not as yet very good.

Finally, maternal metabolic disorders, such as hyperparathyroidism and adrenal or thyroid hyperfunction or hypofunction, can seriously influence fetal viability or neonatal homeostasis. Maternal diabetes mellitus (type 1) is a well-known cause of fetal wastage and increases the risk for specific major malformation. Central nervous system and cardiac malformations, first and second branchial arch defects, caudal regression, and the myelomeningocele–anencephaly sequence are particularly prominent in offspring of diabetic mothers.

VI. NONTRADITIONAL INHERITANCE

A. **Mosaicism.** Both chromosomal and single-gene mutations can be distributed in a subset of cells in all body tissues, in tissues derived from a single embryonic layer, or in germ cells only **(gonadal mosaicism).** Expression of the abnormality depends on the number and distribution of cells in the mosaic cell line.

1. **X inactivation,** which occurs very early in embryonic development, provides gene dosage compensation for most X-linked genes. Females have mosaic expression of all X-linked genes except those that escape X inactivation primarily in the pseudoautosomal region of Xp.

2. **Chromosomal mosaicism** is especially common in the sex chromosome disorders and usually produces a milder phenotype. Asymmetric growth or variable pigmentation is a marker for chromosome mosaicism, particularly when an autosome is involved. Evaluation of cultured skin fibroblasts or interphase cells from a buccal smear is helpful in confirming such diagnoses. Confined placental mosaicism may account for intrauterine growth retardation in chromosomally normal fetuses.

3. **Somatic mutation** with resultant generalized or tissue-specific mosaicism at a single locus can account for patchy distribution of a dysfunctional gene and nonuniform expression of the condition (e.g., segmental neurofibromatosis). An apparent new dominant mutation can recur despite normal parental phenotypes because of **gonadal mosaicism** in one parent.

B. In **uniparental disomy (UPD),** both copies of a particular chromosome pair derive from one parent (i.e., the other parent's contribution is lost). Such cases can occur when a trisomic conceptus loses the extra chromosome (called trisomy rescue) but excludes the single copy of the chromosome derived from the normal gamete.

1. Uniparental disomy has been described in cystic fibrosis, in which both mutations were inherited from the same parent, thus mimicking autosomal recessive inheritance.

2. In 25% to 30% of Prader-Willi syndrome patients with normal cytogenetic and FISH studies, maternal disomy 15 has been demonstrated by molecular

techniques. Molecular analysis demonstrates two maternal chromosomes 15 and no copy of a paternally derived 15.

3. UPD for chromosome 7 has been associated with a clinical phenotype that overlaps the **Russell-Silver syndrome,** although UPD7 accounts for only 6% to 10% of the cases.

4. UPD is also a suggested cause of nonspecific intrauterine growth restriction, mental retardation, and microcephaly, although additional data are needed to confirm this concept and evaluate the extent to which it contributes to these conditions.

C. Genomic imprinting. Some genes or regions of chromosomes can be modified at meiosis such that the expression of a trait is altered and depends on the parental derivation of the gene or chromosomal region.

    1. Chromosomal deletion syndromes can show effects of imprinting. In Prader-Willi syndrome, the 15q11-q13 deletion is always seen in the paternal chromosome 15. Deletion of a similar region of the maternal chromosome 15 produces Angelman syndrome, which can easily be distinguished from Prader-Willi syndrome despite some overlap in phenotype.

    2. Unequal gene expression from the homologous chromosomes may result in genetic "silence" or abnormal expression at a particular locus if the normal allele is not expressed and the homologous allele is defective. For example, in addition to deletion or paternal UPD15, mutation in the maternal copy of the ubiquitin 3A gene (*UBE3A*) on chromosome 15q11-13 results in Angelman syndrome because the normal gene is not expressed from the paternally inherited chromosome 15.

D. Other mechanisms account for some nontraditional inheritance.

    1. Mitochondrial inheritance accounts for some rare conditions that are variable within kindreds, affect males and females, but are always maternally derived. Examples include Leber hereditary optic atrophy and the mitochondrial encephalomyopathies. A number of kindreds demonstrate maternal transmission of some combination of **diabetes**, sensorineural hearing loss, myopathy, central nervous system dysfunction, and retinopathy on the basis of mitochondrial mutation.

    2. Triplet-repeat disorders occur because of expansion of an unstable triplet repeat that interrupts functioning of the gene. Expression of these conditions can depend on which parent transmitted the gene (e.g., juvenile-onset **Huntington disease** occurs only in offspring of affected fathers, whereas **congenital myotonic dystrophy** is limited to the offspring of affected mothers) because some of the triplet repeats are unstable in male meiosis whereas others are unstable during meiosis in the female. Also, these conditions demonstrate anticipation, in which the phenotype becomes more severe and/or the age of onset is earlier in later generations within a kindred.

VII. PRENATAL DIAGNOSIS

A. General principles. Prenatal diagnostic techniques now allow diagnosis of most chromosomal abnormalities and many specific genetic disorders. The use of ultrasound before and during amniocentesis has greatly reduced the risk of the procedure. Chorionic villus sampling (CVS) provides access to fetal tissue during the late first trimester/early midtrimester. This procedure is particularly useful when the fetus is at high risk for a genetic condition that is diagnosable by cytogenetic, biochemical, or molecular techniques. Targeted ultrasound has also been increasingly useful in the evaluation of fetal morphology and growth parameters. Overall risk of major complications following ultrasound-directed amniocentesis is <1 in 200. Risks associated with CVS are not significantly higher in experienced hands. Amniocentesis is no longer recommended before week 13 of gestation, because of an increased risk of spontaneous rupture of membranes, as well as of clubfoot in surviving fetuses.

B. Indications for amniocentesis or CVS vary among prenatal diagnosis programs but generally include the following:

    1. Older maternal age (35 years at term).

    2. Previous child with a chromosomal abnormality.

3. Parent who is a carrier of a balanced chromosomal rearrangement.
4. Parent who is affected with a chromosomal abnormality.
5. Family history of nondisjunction.
6. Parents who are heterozygous for a detectable autosomal recessive disorder, or a parent who is affected by a detectable dominant disorder.
7. Mother who is a carrier of a detectable X-linked disorder or a nondetectable X-linked disorder (fetal sexing).
8. Significant history of fetal wastage (at least three episodes) or a previous child with unexplained multiple congenital anomalies.
9. Previous child or parent affected with a neural tube defect.
10. Abnormal maternal analyte screen (most commonly α-fetoprotein, unconjugated estriol, β-human chorionic gonadotropin, inhibin, or pregnancy-associated plasma protein A).
11. Increased fetal nuchal lucency (neck skinfold thickness) on ultrasound assessment in the late first trimester or early midtrimester.

Selected References

Cassidy SB, Allanson JE, eds. *Management of genetic syndromes.* 2nd ed. New York: Wiley-Liss; 2004.

Chen H. *Atlas of Genetic diagnosis and counseling.* Totowa, NJ: Humana Press; 2006.

Cohen MM, Neri G, Weksberg R. *Overgrowth syndromes.* New York: Oxford University Press; 2002.

Gorlin RJ, Cohen MM, Hennekam RCM. *Syndromes of the head and neck.* 4th ed. New York: Oxford University Press; 2001.

Hall JG, Allanson JE, Gripp K, Slavotinek A. *Handbook of physical measurements.* 2nd ed. New York: Oxford University Press; 2006.

Harper PS. *Practical genetic counseling.* 6th ed. London: Hodder Arnold; 2004.

Jones KL. *Smith's recognizable patterns of human malformation.* 6th ed. Philadelphia: Elsevier Saunders; 2006.

King RA, Rotter JI, Motulsky AG, eds. *The genetic basis of common disease.* 2nd ed. New York: Oxford University Press; 2002.

Lachman RS. *Taybi and Lachman's radiology of syndromes, metabolic disorders, and skeletal dysplasias.* 5th ed. St. Louis: Mosby; 2007.

Nussbaum RL, McInnes RR, Willard, HF. *Thompson and Thompson genetics in medicine.* Rev. reprint 6th ed. Philadelphia: WB Saunders; 2004.

Nyhan WL, Barshop BA, Ozand PT. *Atlas of metabolic diseases.* 2nd ed. London: Hodder Arnold; 2005.

Online Mendelian Inheritance in Man, OMIM™. McKusick-Nathans Institute of Genetic Medicine, Johns Hopkins University (Baltimore, MD) and National Center for Biotechnology Information, National Library of Medicine (Bethesda, MD). www.ncbi.nlm.nih.gov/omim.

Scriver CR, Beaudet AL, Sly WS, Valle D. *The metabolic and molecular bases of inherited disease.* 8th ed. New York: McGraw-Hill; 2001.

Stevenson RE, Hall JG. *Human malformations and related anomalies.* 2nd ed. New York: Oxford University Press; 2006.

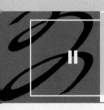

II Hypothalamic-Pituitary Dysfunction

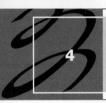

4 ANTERIOR PITUITARY DISEASES
Harold E. Carlson

I. NORMAL ANTERIOR PITUITARY PHYSIOLOGY
A. Anterior pituitary hormones. The normal anterior pituitary gland secretes six well-characterized major hormones.
1. Adrenocorticotropic hormone (ACTH). ACTH has moderate melanocyte-stimulating activity and may account for most of the hyperpigmentation seen in Nelson syndrome and Addison disease.
2. Thyrotropin (thyroid-stimulating hormone [TSH])
3. Luteinizing hormone (LH)
4. Follicle-stimulating hormone (FSH)
5. Growth hormone (GH)
6. Prolactin (Prl).
7. A seventh hormone, **β-lipotropin**, is synthesized along with ACTH in corticotropes as part of a large precursor molecule called **proopiomelanocortin.** The physiology of β-lipotropin is still poorly understood.

B. Feedback system. TSH, ACTH, and the two gonadotropins, LH and FSH, stimulate end-organ target glands to secrete hormones, which in turn exert a restraining negative-feedback effect on their respective pituitary tropic cells. Thus, ACTH secretion is largely controlled by the inhibitory feedback effects of circulating cortisol on the pituitary; similar relationships hold for TSH and thyroid hormones, and for LH-FSH and gonadal steroids. Insulinlike growth factor I (IGF-I; also known as somatomedin C), a GH-dependent growth-promoting peptide, can inhibit GH secretion. In contrast, Prl has no well-defined peripheral product that exerts a feedback effect.

C. Hypothalamic releasing hormones. In addition to the feedback system, the hypothalamus also contributes to pituitary regulation by means of releasing and inhibiting hormones secreted into the hypothalamic-pituitary portal circulation. Several such hormones have been identified.

1. Protirelin, or thyrotropin-releasing hormone (TRH), releases TSH and Prl from the pituitary.
2. Gonadotropin-releasing hormone (GnRH) releases both LH and FSH.
3. Corticotropin-releasing hormone (CRH) stimulates ACTH and lipotropin secretion.
4. Growth hormone–releasing hormone (GHRH) stimulates GH release.
5. Somatostatin inhibits GH and, to some extent, TSH secretion.
6. Dopamine, a potent inhibitor of Prl release, is probably the main factor that physiologically regulates this hormone.

End-organ hormones exert their feedback effects on the hypothalamus as well as directly on the pituitary, although the direct effects on the pituitary are probably more important.

II. HYPOPITUITARISM

  A. **General principles.** Hypofunction of the pituitary can result from disease of the pituitary itself or of the hypothalamus (Table 4.1). In either case there is decreased secretion of the pituitary hormones, with consequent effects on the function of the remainder of the organism. Thus, TSH deficiency produces hypothyroidism without goiter; LH and FSH deficiencies produce hypogonadism; ACTH deficiency leads to hypoadrenalism and poor tanning of the skin; Prl deficiency results in failure of postpartum lactation; and GH deficiency produces short stature and, occasionally, fasting hypoglycemia in children; in adults, GH deficiency may lead to increased abdominal fat, poor energy, reduced muscle mass and strength, dyslipidemia, and impaired psychological well-being. Both GH deficiency and hypogonadism may contribute to fine facial wrinkling.

  B. **Diagnosis.** With some hormones (ACTH, TSH, LH, and FSH), the diagnosis of secondary (i.e., due to hypothalamic-pituitary causes) end-organ hypofunction can easily be established by demonstration of low or inappropriately normal serum levels of the appropriate pituitary hormone concurrent with low levels of the target-organ hormone. Thus, the finding of low or normal serum gonadotropins in the presence of clinical hypogonadism with low serum levels of testosterone or estrogen suggests the diagnosis of secondary rather than primary hypogonadism. To separate hypothalamic from pituitary causes of hypofunction as well as to diagnose GH or Prl deficiency, specific pituitary stimulation tests are needed. However, in many cases it is of no practical importance to distinguish hormonally between pituitary and hypothalamic disorders because the endocrine therapy is the same. Prolactin deficiency is usually of no therapeutic importance in adults; thus, Prl stimulation tests can often be omitted in the evaluation of hypopituitarism. However, documentation of diminished Prl reserve is occasionally useful in supporting the diagnosis of hypopituitarism in adults.

  C. **Pituitary stimulation testing** (Table 4.2)
    1. **GH.** Serum GH levels are normally low throughout most of the day in adults, rising during exercise, sleep, stress, and postprandially. The most useful stimulation tests are insulin-induced hypoglycemia and the combined administration of arginine and GH-RH. Consensus on the criteria for diagnosing GH deficiency in adults is incomplete. Different commercial GH assay kits may produce widely disparate results when the same serum sample is assayed, and GH responses to provocative tests are not entirely reproducible in individual subjects. Nevertheless, most normal adult subjects achieve peak serum GH values of at least 3 to 5 ng/mL in response to stimulation tests; insulin-induced hypoglycemia is probably the most consistent stimulus. In children, the diagnosis of GH deficiency relies on the combination of short stature (more than 2.5 standard deviations below the mean for age), slow growth velocity, delayed bone age, and stimulated serum GH concentrations of <10 ng/mL. Serum IGF-I and IGF-binding protein 3 (IGFBP-3) levels are low in some, but not all, patients with GH deficiency and should not be used as the sole criterion of insufficient GH secretion. Hypothyroid or obese patients often have blunted responses to all GH-provocative agents.

TABLE 4.1	Causes of Hypopituitarism

Infarction
   Postpartum necrosis (Sheehan syndrome)
   Vascular disease (in diabetes mellitus)
   Following pituitary stimulation testing (e.g., TRH, GnRH)
   Head trauma
   Subarachnoid hemorrhage
Infections
   Tuberculosis
   Fungi
   Pyogenic
   Syphilis
   Toxoplasmosis
Granulomas
   Sarcoidosis
   Langerhans cell histiocytosis
Autoimmune lymphocytic hypophysitis
Neoplasms involving pituitary
   Pituitary adenoma
   Craniopharyngioma
   Metastatic or primary carcinoma (rare)
Aneurysm of internal carotid artery
Hemochromatosis
Idiopathic or genetic disorders
   Deficient production of pituitary hormone
   Synthesis of abnormal hormone
Primary hypothalamic disorders
   Tumors (e.g., craniopharyngioma, glioma)
   Granulomas (sarcoidosis, Langerhans cell histiocytosis)
   Midline central nervous system structural anomalies of the hypothalamus
   Genetic or idiopathic releasing hormone deficiency
   Head trauma
Iatrogenic factors
   Stalk section
   Radiation
   Hypophysectomy

GnRH, gonadotropin-releasing hormone; TRH, thyrotropin-releasing hormone.

  2. Prl. Prl secretion is normally low throughout much of the day, rising during sleep or stress and postprandially. Clinically useful provocative tests of Prl release include:

    a. IV TRH (not currently available), which directly stimulates the lactotrope

    b. Dopamine antagonists (e.g., metoclopramide), which block endogenous dopamine, the main Prl-inhibiting factor

  A minimal normal Prl response in any of these tests consists of a doubling of baseline values, with a peak of at least 12 ng/mL. Prl responsiveness is enhanced by estrogen administration and is therefore generally greater in women. Patients with hypopituitarism will have low baseline serum Prl levels that fail to rise appropriately following TRH or other stimuli. In contrast, patients with pure hypothalamic disease will have basal hyperprolactinemia because the intact

| TABLE 4.2 | Pituitary Stimulation Tests |

Hormone	Test agent	Normal response
GH	Insulin, 0.05–0.15 U/kg IV GH-RH, 1 μg/kg IV bolus, plus arginine, 30 g IV	Serum GH >3–5 ng/mL at any time in adults; >10 ng/mL in children
Prl	TRH, 100–500 μg IV, or metoclopramide, 5–10 mg	Doubling of baseline level with peak >12 ng/mL
TSH	TRH, 500 μg IV	Peak value >5 μU/mL
LH and FSH	GnRH, 100 μg IV	Doubling of baseline LH, with peak >10 mIU/mL; 0–30% rise in FSH
	Clomiphene, 100–200 mg/d PO for 5–10 d	50% rise in LH, 30% rise in FSH
ACTH	Insulin, 0.05–0.15 U/kg IV	Peak serum cortisol > 20 μg/dL, with increment >10 μg/dL
	Metyrapone, 2–3 g PO at bedtime	Serum 11-deoxycortisol level >7 μg/dL next morning
	Cosyntropin, 250 μg IV (indirect test)	Peak serum cortisol >20 μg/dL

ACTH, adrenocorticotropic hormone; FSH, follicle stimulating hormone; GH, growth hormone; GH-RH, growth hormone-releasing hormone; GnRH, gonadotropin-releasing hormone; IV, intravenous; LH, luteinizing hormone; Prl, prolactin; TRH, thyrotropin-releasing hormone; TSH, thyroid-stimulating hormone.

lactotropes will have been freed from the tonic inhibitory effect of hypothalamic dopamine; Prl responses can be blunted or normal in such patients.

3. **TSH.** With pure pituitary disease (e.g., posthypophysectomy), serum TSH levels are low and do not rise following intravenous (IV) administration of TRH, which directly stimulates thyrotropes. Patients with pure hypothalamic disease might have low, normal, or even slightly elevated serum TSH in the presence of hypothyroidism, with a normal-sized but delayed TSH peak following TRH administration (see Chapters 28 and 30), presumably reflecting TRH deficiency. The apparent paradoxical occurrence of hypothyroidism despite normal or elevated serum TSH levels by radioimmunoassay is explained by the finding that serum TSH bioactivity is low in such patients; endogenous TRH appears to be needed to confer full bioactivity on the TSH molecule.

4. **Gonadotropins**
   a. **Synthetic GnRH,** a direct stimulator of gonadotropes, is injected intravenously, and LH and FSH responses are assessed. Patients with complete pituitary destruction show low baseline serum LH and FSH levels with no rise after GnRH injection. Subjects with hypothalamic disease generally respond to GnRH, although "priming" doses of GnRH might be needed (400 μg IM daily for 5 days) to fully demonstrate the response.
   b. **Gonadotropin reserve** can also be assessed by testing with oral clomiphene, a competitive estrogen antagonist. In normal adult men and women, clomiphene administration produces a rise in both LH and FSH by blocking the inhibitory feedback effects of gonadal steroids on the hypothalamus. Although it is useful as a research tool, clomiphene testing occasionally has practical applications as well.

5. **ACTH.** The assessment of ACTH secretion has traditionally been indirect because of the difficulty and expense of plasma ACTH measurement.
   a. Recent advances in ACTH radioimmunoassay techniques have made the clinical use of plasma ACTH determinations much more widely available. Indirect assessments have utilized measurements of plasma cortisol, which parallels

plasma ACTH under most circumstances, or urinary free cortisol. In patients with obvious adrenal insufficiency, primary and secondary (hypothalamic-pituitary) adrenal failure can be distinguished by measuring plasma ACTH in the morning (8 to 10 A.M.), when levels are normally highest. In the presence of low serum cortisol concentrations, plasma ACTH will be elevated in patients with primary adrenal failure, whereas low or low-normal levels are seen in patients with secondary adrenal insufficiency.

  b. Provocative testing with insulin-induced hypoglycemia (as described for GH testing; see Section II.C.1) or metyrapone can be used to document lesser defects in ACTH reserve.

   (1) Following insulin-induced hypoglycemia, plasma cortisol should normally rise to levels >20 μg/dL, generally with an increment of at least 10 μg/dL over baseline.

   (2) The short overnight metyrapone test can be performed by giving oral metyrapone (3 g if body weight >60 kg; 2 g if <60 kg) at bedtime with a snack to avoid nausea and measuring serum 11-deoxycortisol at 8 A.M. the next morning. A normal response consists of a serum 11-deoxycortisol level of ≥ 7 μg/dL. If a subnormal rise in 11-deoxycortisol is seen, serum cortisol should be measured in the same sample to assess the adequacy of enzymatic blockade. A serum cortisol level >5 μg/dL suggests poor absorption of the metyrapone, and the test could be repeated with a higher dose of the drug or the response to hypoglycemia assessed.

  c. Cosyntropin testing has been used to assess ACTH secretion indirectly; a **chronic** deficiency of ACTH secretion leads to adrenal atrophy and blunted serum cortisol responses at 30 and 60 minutes following the injection of cosyntropin (synthetic ACTH [amino acids 1–24], 250 μg IV bolus). Results of this test correlate reasonably well with those obtained using insulin-induced hypoglycemia, but the cosyntropin test is performed much more easily. Peak serum cortisol levels are >20 μg/dL in normal subjects. Cosyntropin testing is not useful in evaluating **acute** ACTH deficiency because adrenal atrophy takes several weeks to develop.

 6. Clinical indications for detailed pituitary stimulation testing include:

  a. To assist in the diagnosis of otherwise obscure pituitary or hypothalamic disease

  b. To assess the need for GH replacement therapy

  c. Possibly to determine the feasibility of treating patients with hypothalamic hypopituitarism with GnRH or GHRH

   Note that, with the exception of gonadotropins (for infertility) and GH therapy, the need for hormone replacement therapy is determined solely by clinical status and measurement of end-organ products (cortisol, thyroxine, and testosterone) rather than pituitary hormones.

D. Management of hypopituitarism

 1. In most cases, the hormonal deficiencies of hypopituitarism are treated by supplying the needed end-organ hormones (Table 4.3). Prl replacement therapy is rarely needed and is unavailable in any case. Women with secondary adrenal insufficiency may benefit from dehydroepiandrosterone (DHEA) replacement.

 2. Replacement pituitary hormones are given in only two circumstances.

  a. Human GH is given to GH-deficient pediatric or adult patients with clinical and chemical features of GH deficiency (see Chapters 7 and 9).

  b. Exogenous gonadotropins may be given to stimulate gonadal function in hypopituitary patients who desire fertility. In this situation, human chorionic gonadotropin (hCG) may be used as a substitute for LH; or biosynthetic recombinant human LH can be given; FSH activity can be provided by either urofollitropin or biosynthetic recombinant human FSH preparations.

 3. Patients with hypopituitarism should carry a card or wear a bracelet identifying their hormonal status. Both patients and their families should be capable of administering extra glucocorticoid, either parenterally or orally, in case of severe illness or injury.

TABLE 4.3 Management of Hypopituitarism

Deficient hormone	Therapy
TSH	L-Thyroxine, 0.05–0.2 mg/d PO
ACTH	Oral glucocorticoid, e.g., prednisone, 2.5–5 mg in A.M., 0–2.5 mg in early evening, or hydrocortisone, 10–20 mg in A.M., 5–10 mg in early evening. Mineralocorticoid usually not needed. DHEA, 50 mg in A.M., may benefit adult women
LH and FSH	Men: Testosterone enanthate or cypionate, 200–300 mg IM q2–3 wk, or testosterone transdermal patch, 2.5–5 mg daily, or testosterone transdermal gel, 2.5–10 mg daily Women: Cyclic estrogen and progesterone, e.g., conjugated equine estrogens, 0.625 mg PO daily for days 1–25 of each calendar month with the addition of medroxyprogesterone acetate, 10 mg PO, on days 16–25. Alternatively, an oral contraceptive may be given. For restoration of fertility in either sex, human FSH and either hCG or LH are given by injection, usually for periods of several months.
GH	3–25 μg/kg SC daily in adults (see Chapter 7 for doses in children)

ACTH, adrenocorticotropic hormone; DHEA, dehydroepiandrosterone; FSH, follicle-stimulating hormone; GH, growth hormone; hCG, human chorionic gonadotropin; IM, intramuscular; LH, luteinizing hormone; PO, per os; SC, subcutaneous; TSH, thyroid-stimulating hormone.

III. PITUITARY TUMORS
A. General considerations
1. Types of tumors
a. **Pituitary tumors,** nearly always benign, occur in ~10% of adults; most are small, incidental findings on radiologic studies. The appearance of a pituitary tumor on hematoxylin and eosin staining bears little relationship to its functional status.
b. **Prl-secreting tumors** are the single most common neoplasm, followed by **clinically nonfunctioning tumors** (Table 4.4).
c. **"Chromophobe" tumors** often secrete Prl, GH, or other hormones. Many clinically silent tumors, unassociated with any recognized state of hormone hypersecretion, actually contain or secrete small amounts of gonadotropins or their α and β subunits.

TABLE 4.4 Frequency of Pituitary Tumors

Type of tumor	Relative frequency of occurrence (%)
Prl-secreting	25–30
Clinically nonfunctioning (most secrete gonadotropins or gonadotropin subunits)	25–30
ACTH-secreting	15
GH-secreting	15
Plurihormonal	12
TSH-secreting	2

ACTH, adrenocorticotropic hormone; GH, growth hormone; Prl, prolactin; TSH, thyroid-stimulating hormone.

2. **Signs and symptoms.** Both secreting and nonsecreting tumors can produce signs and symptoms as a result of their space-occupying characteristics and their location. These features, such as headache, visual impairment (typically bitemporal hemianopsia resulting from compression of the optic chiasm), extraocular palsy, hydrocephalus, seizures, and cerebrospinal fluid (CSF) rhinorrhea, are all more common with larger tumors (macroadenomas, >1 cm in diameter) and tumors with extrasellar extension than with intrasellar microadenomas (<1 cm in diameter). Hypopituitarism and diabetes insipidus are also more frequently encountered in patients with large destructive tumors.

Spontaneous hemorrhage into a pituitary tumor occurs in as many as 15% to 20% of patients; about one third of these are clinically recognizable (pituitary apoplexy) and present with headache, decreased vision, extraocular palsies, and other neurologic findings. Evacuation of the hematoma may be needed in severe cases, along with administration of fluids and glucocorticoid supplements.

B. **Radiology of pituitary tumors**
   1. **Magnetic resonance imaging (MRI)** is currently the procedure of choice in documenting the presence and extent of pituitary neoplasms; it is more sensitive than computed tomography (CT) in detecting small tumors. MRI, usually performed both with and without contrast is particularly useful in showing mass effects on the optic chiasm and extrasellar extension. A normal scan does not exclude the presence of a small tumor (e.g., <2 to 3 mm in diameter).

C. **Management of pituitary tumors**
   1. **General principles.** In some patients with small, asymptomatic pituitary tumors, no treatment other than observation and end-organ hormone replacement is indicated. However, many patients require specific therapy to diminish hormone hypersecretion, if present, and to correct or prevent the mass effects of the intracranial lesion. Table 4.5 lists the indications and contraindications for the various methods.
   2. **Surgery.** In general, surgery has historically been preferred when serious anatomic complications exist (e.g., visual field defects) or when immediate correction of hormone hypersecretion is desired. Surgery occasionally damages adjacent structures or results in hypopituitarism.
   3. **Radiation.** Radiotherapy delivered as supervoltage photons from either cobalt-60 or linear accelerator devices, or as heavy particles (protons or α particles) has a slower onset of effect than surgery, generally taking 6 to 24 months for initial benefit to be seen, with progressive improvement over 2 to 10 years. Hypopituitarism is seen in up to 50% of patients 10 to 20 years after radiotherapy. Stereotactic or conformal radiotherapy using cobalt-60 ("gamma knife radiosurgery") or a rotating linear accelerator beam is receiving increasing use; to date, it appears to be no more effective than standard methods, though it results in less radiation damage to adjacent structures.
   4. **Medical therapy.** Dopamine agonists such as **bromocriptine** and **cabergoline** have been shown to lower serum Prl and rapidly shrink many Prl-secreting adenomas; these drugs are often recommended as the sole or adjunctive therapy for such tumors (see Section V). Occasionally, patients with acromegaly or clinically nonfunctioning tumors also demonstrate tumor regression with bromocriptine therapy; in some acromegaly patients, bromocriptine significantly lowers GH as well. Octreotide, a synthetic analog of somatostatin, has been used successfully to reduce GH and TSH secretion from pituitary tumors that produce these hormones, and also frequently partially shrinks such tumors. Synthetic antagonists of GnRH have been used experimentally to inhibit LH-FSH secretion from gonadotropin-producing tumors.
   5. **Preoperative evaluation.** Patients scheduled for hypothalamic-pituitary surgery should not be routinely subjected to an exhaustive preoperative hormonal evaluation because testing needs to be repeated postoperatively. Instead, measurements of serum free thyroxine (T_4) or free T_4 index (because severe untreated hypothyroidism can increase the risks of general anesthesia), IGF-I, and Prl (to detect occult hypersecretion of GH and Prl) should be obtained. Rather

| TABLE 4.5 | Choice of Therapy for Pituitary Tumors |

Radiation therapy

Appropriate for:

Small or medium tumors with minimal or modest suprasellar extension

Patients in whom surgery is contraindicated or refused

Postoperative adjunctive therapy in patients with invasive or incompletely removed tumors

Contraindicated as sole therapy in:

Patients with large suprasellar extensions

Patients with major visual field defects

Acromegaly patients with serum growth hormone levels > 50 ng/mL prior to treatment

Prolactinoma patients who wish to restore fertility

Surgery: transfrontal approach

Appropriate for:

Large suprasellar extensions, especially if dumbbell-shaped with a constriction at the diaphragma sellae, or with lateral suprasellar extension

Patients in whom the transsphenoidal approach to the sella is relatively contraindicated (patients with chronic sinusitis or an incompletely pneumatized sphenoid sinus)

Contraindicated in:

Not generally needed for small intrasellar tumors

Surgery: transsphenoidal approach

Appropriate for:

Microadenomas (<1 cm in diameter)

Tumors associated with extension into the sphenoid sinus or cerebrospinal fluid rhinorrhea

Tumors associated with pituitary apoplexy

Macroadenomas (>1 cm in diameter) with minimal or modest suprasellar extension

Contraindicated in:

Tumors with large dumbbell-shaped or lateral suprasellar extensions

Patients with chronic sinusitis or incompletely pneumatized sphenoid sinus (relative, not absolute contraindications)

Medical therapy with dopaminergic agonists

Appropriate for:

Primary treatment of prolactin-secreting tumors

Rapid correction of neurologic sequelae of large prolactin-secreting tumors

Shrinkage of prolactin-secreting tumors to facilitate ablative therapy

Pregnant patients with prolactin-secreting tumors who experience gestational tumor growth

Adjunctive therapy in patients with acromegaly or TSH-secreting tumors

Contraindicated in:

Nonfunctioning tumors (although a few patients may respond)

Primary treatment of acromegaly, except when ablative therapy is refused

Medical therapy with octreotide

Appropriate for:

Adjunctive therapy in patients with acromegaly or TSH-secreting tumors

Primary therapy in patients with acromegaly when ablative therapy is refused

Contraindicated in:

Other types of tumors

Medical therapy with pegvisomant

Appropriate for:

Patients who have persistent GH hypersecretion following ablative therapy and/or octreotide

Contraindicated as:

Primary therapy in acromegaly except when other therapy is refused

GH, growth hormone; TSH, thyroid-stimulating hormone.

than assess the ACTH reserve preoperatively, most physicians provide supplemental glucocorticoid in the perioperative period and during stressful diagnostic procedures.

6. **Postoperative assessment.** In postoperative patients and in patients receiving radiation or medical therapy alone, the need for hormone replacement should be evaluated by measuring serum testosterone (in men) and the serum free T_4 or free T_4 index, and by assessing the pituitary–adrenal axis with insulin-induced hypoglycemia, metyrapone, or indirectly with cosyntropin. The presence of regular menses in a premenopausal woman usually indicates relatively normal estrogen secretion, and further testing is not needed unless the patient is infertile. Children should have provocative tests of GH secretion (see Chapter 7), as should adults with symptoms of GH deficiency.

7. **Follow-up.** Following initial treatment, patients are seen every 3 or 4 months for 1 year, then every 6 to 12 months. During each visit, signs and symptoms of hormone deficiency or excess should be sought. Serum free T_4 or free T_4 index and serum testosterone (in men) should be tested every 1 to 2 years and ACTH reserve assessed every 2 to 3 years. Patients with pituitary tumors should have follow-up CT or MRI within 6 months of treatment to assess early anatomic changes, and then every 1 to 3 years.

IV. ACROMEGALY AND GIGANTISM

A. **Clinical features.** Hypersecretion of GH produces the typical appearance of acromegaly, with enlargement of the facial features, hands, and feet in most patients. The presence of GH excess prior to the closure of long-bone epiphyses in late puberty leads to increased stature; gigantism can result if the process begins in childhood. Other common symptoms include:

1. Excessive perspiration, perhaps caused by enlarged sweat glands or hypermetabolism.
2. Carpal tunnel syndrome, resulting from compression of the enlarged or edematous median nerve by the fibrocartilaginous tissue of the wrist.
3. Degenerative arthritis, secondary to bony overgrowth and deformity around large weight-bearing joints.
4. Hypertension, perhaps related to salt-retaining effects of GH.
5. Glucose intolerance or diabetes mellitus, reflecting the insulin-antagonistic properties of GH.
6. Hypercalciuria, perhaps secondary to stimulation of 1,25-dihydroxy-vitamin D_3 production by GH.
7. Galactorrhea, resulting either from the intrinsic lactogenic properties of GH or from the presence of a mixed adenoma that produces both GH and Prl.
8. Sleep apnea, both obstructive and central. Increased mortality in acromegaly is attributed to cerebrovascular, cardiovascular, and pulmonary diseases. Additionally, there may be an increased incidence of colon polyps and cancer in these patients.

B. **Diagnosis of acromegaly.** In a patient with a compatible clinical history and appearance, a diagnosis of acromegaly is usually easy to confirm.

1. The best-established test involves the assessment of GH responses to oral glucose. In normal subjects, serum GH is suppressed to low levels (<1 ng/mL; often undetectable) 60 to 120 minutes following the oral ingestion of 50 to 100 g of glucose in solution. Nearly all patients with acromegaly fail to show such suppression and may demonstrate a rise in GH instead.
2. In the absence of serious concurrent illness, serum levels of IGF-I are uniformly elevated in patients with active acromegaly.
3. In addition to dynamic testing, two or three random measurements of serum GH should also be obtained to provide an average pretreatment baseline value.
4. Baseline serum Prl also should be measured in all patients with acromegaly, because up to 40% have a "mixed" pituitary adenoma, secreting both GH and Prl, usually from two separate cell types in the same tumor.

5. After a hormonal diagnosis has been made, patients with acromegaly should also undergo an anatomic evaluation of their sellar contents with MRI and may require a formal visual-field examination if the tumor appears to impinge on the optic chiasm.

C. **Management of acromegaly**

1. Pituitary surgery produces better long-term results than radiotherapy, with ~50% to 60% of patients achieving serum GH values <2 ng/mL and normal serum IGF-I. Surgery also offers the advantage of an immediate lowering of GH, whereas radiation therapy slowly reduces serum GH over many years. In addition, patients with pretreatment serum GH values >50 ng/mL are often left with residual GH hypersecretion after radiotherapy and are probably best treated with surgery as the initial therapy. Factors such as visual-field defects and large suprasellar extensions can also influence the choice of treatment (Table 4.5).

2. Medical therapy is typically given to patients with persistent GH hypersecretion following pituitary surgery. Dopamine agonists, octreotide, and pegvisomant have been successfully used alone or in combination in many patients.

   a. **Dopamine agonists** significantly lower serum GH and IGF-I in a minority of patients (10% to 40%). Unfortunately, there is no means of predicting which patients will achieve significant GH suppression with dopamine agonist therapy. In addition, pituitary tumor shrinkage may occur in ~5% of acromegalic patients who are given dopamine agonists. At present, dopamine agonists are used primarily as adjunctive treatment in acromegaly, following surgery or radiation. Cabergoline appears to be the most useful of the dopamine agonists and is usually begun at doses of 0.25 mg once or twice a week, with doses increased to 1 to 2 mg/week as needed. Rarely, additional benefit is gained by increasing the total daily dose to levels >3 mg/week. In some reports, patients with tumors that cosecreted prolactin were more likely to have significant GH suppression on dopamine agonist therapy.

   b. **Octreotide,** a synthetic analog of somatostatin, has greater efficacy than dopamine agonists in the management of acromegaly, although the requirement for injection makes it much less convenient. A long-acting depot form of octreotide (Sandostatin LAR) is available and is given as a monthly intramuscular injection of 20 or 30 mg. Common side effects include abdominal cramps, loose stools, worsened glucose tolerance, and cholelithiasis. Octreotide normalizes serum GH and IGF-I in 50% to 70% of patients and produces partial shrinkage of GH-secreting adenomas in ~50%. Octreotide therapy is expensive, in the range of $20,000 to $40,000 per year.

   c. **Pegvisomant** is a competitive antagonist of native GH at the cell-membrane GH receptor. It consists of biosynthetic human GH with nine amino acid substitutions that remove its ability to activate the GH receptor without impairing receptor binding; this modified GH molecule is then coupled to polyethylene glycol to prolong its serum half-life. When it is administered to patients with acromegaly, it prevents the binding of native GH to the GH receptor, thereby preventing GH action. IGF-I production falls, and the clinical signs and symptoms of acromegaly are ameliorated. Pegvisomant does not cause shrinkage of the GH-secreting tumor and, theoretically, could result in additional tumor growth by decreasing the effect of native GH to stimulate hypothalamic somatostatin production; for this same reason, it has been observed that secretion of GH (as measured in specific assays) is increased during pegvisomant therapy.

   Pegvisomant is given as a daily subcutaneous injection of 10 to 20 mg; between 75% and 90% of patients will achieve normal serum IGF-I levels. Pegvisomant is relatively free of serious side effects; pain at the injection site, nausea, or diarrhea are each seen in ~10% of patients. Abnormal serum concentrations of liver enzymes have been noted in 1% to 5% of patients; in some individuals, enzyme concentrations have normalized despite continuation of the drug. Frequent monitoring of serum liver enzyme concentrations and bilirubin is recommended during the first year of therapy; pegvisomant may need to be discontinued if severe and persistent elevations are found.

Pegvisomant is detected in routine commercial GH assays, so serum GH measurements cannot be used to monitor disease activity. IGF-1 is measured instead. Tumor size should continue to be monitored by MRI scan every 6 months for at least the first few years of pegvisomant treatment.

Pegvisomant is expensive ($35,000 to $70,000 per year) and is therefore not usually given as initial therapy in acromegaly.

  d. Successful treatment of acromegaly restores serum GH and IGF-I to normal and often results in regression of soft-tissue enlargement, improvement in carpal tunnel syndrome and glucose tolerance, increased energy, and diminution of excessive sweating. Bony changes and osteoarthritis usually do not improve but can stabilize.

 3. Follow-up. Following treatment, patients with acromegaly should have serum GH and IGF-I measured in a random blood specimen every 6 months for 2 or 3 years and then at yearly intervals. Radiologic evaluation of the pituitary tumor and measurement of serum Prl (if previously elevated) should be performed at similar intervals. Serum free T_4 or free T_4 index, testosterone (in men), and ACTH reserve should be tested every 1 to 2 years. Many patients, especially those with residual GH hypersecretion, require ongoing therapy for diabetes mellitus, hypertension, cardiovascular disease, and arthritis, and periodic surveillance for colon polyps and cancer.

V. Prl-SECRETING TUMORS

 A. Clinical features. Adenomas that secrete Prl (prolactinomas) are the most common pituitary tumors. Hyperprolactinemia in women commonly leads to amenorrhea, with or without galactorrhea. Occasionally, women with prolactinomas have spontaneous menses but manifest infertility or a short luteal phase of the menstrual cycle. Men usually manifest decreased libido and potency or symptoms linked to the intracranial-mass lesion. Galactorrhea is uncommon in men, perhaps because the male breast has not been "primed" with endogenous estrogen. The manifestations of hypogonadism in both sexes appear to result principally from the inhibition of GnRH release from the hypothalamus by Prl, with resultant decreased LH and FSH secretion. Some women with Prl-secreting tumors also manifest **hirsutism** and elevated serum androgens; the evidence for Prl stimulation of adrenal androgen production is still controversial. Oral contraceptive use does not appear to cause prolactinomas to develop or enlarge.

 B. Diagnosis

 1. Etiology. In addition to pituitary tumors, hyperprolactinemia occurs in a wide variety of other circumstances (Table 4.6). A careful drug history is of prime importance in the investigation of hyperprolactinemia. Hypothyroidism, pregnancy, and renal failure can be excluded by examination and simple laboratory tests.

 2. Radiologic studies are used to separate patients with pituitary or hypothalamic lesions from those with presumed "functional" hyperprolactinemia. MRI can reveal an intrasellar or suprasellar mass.

 3. Laboratory studies. It is useful to obtain three separate or pooled determinations of serum Prl to account for spontaneous or stress-induced fluctuations in the hormone level. A serum Prl level persistently >200 ng/mL is almost always associated with a pituitary tumor (normal male levels are <15 ng/mL in most laboratories; normal female levels are <25 ng/mL). Because the serum Prl level is roughly proportional to the mass of the tumor, small tumors can cause mild elevations of serum Prl similar to values commonly seen with hyperprolactinemia from other causes (e.g., 30 to 50 ng/mL).

 C. Treatment

 1. Medical therapy with dopamine agonists is the treatment of choice for many patients with prolactin-secreting tumors. Ergot derivatives, such as bromocriptine

TABLE 4.6   **Causes of Hyperprolactinemia**

Altered physiologic states
  Sleep
  Stress
  Postprandial, especially in women
  Coitus
  Pregnancy, including pseudocyesis
  Nursing or nipple stimulation
  Chest wall or thoracic spinal cord lesions
  Hypoglycemia
  Hypothyroidism
  Adrenal insufficiency
  Chronic renal failure
  Cirrhosis
  Secretion of high-molecular-weight prolactin with reduced bioactivity (macroprolactinemia)

Medications
  Phenothiazines
  Butyrophenones (e.g., haloperidol)
  Thioxanthenes (e.g., thiothixene)
  Buspirone
  Olanzapine
  Risperidone and palimperidone
  Ziprasidone
  Quetiapine
  Metoclopramide
  Domperidone
  Sulpiride
  Labetalol
  Monoamine oxidase inhibitors
  Amoxapine
  Reserpine
  α-Methyldopa
  Intravenous cimetidine
  Estrogens
  Opiates
  Verapamil

Decreased delivery of prolactin-inhibiting factor to pituitary
  Pressure on pituitary stalk by sellar or parasellar mass
  Stalk section
  Hypothalamic destruction

Prolactin-secreting pituitary tumors

Ectopic secretion of prolactin by nonpituitary tumors (rare)

Idiopathic

and cabergoline, are potent suppressors of Prl secretion; they promptly lower serum Prl, abolish galactorrhea, and restore normal gonadal function in most patients with hyperprolactinemia from any cause. Bromocriptine and cabergoline also cause anatomic shrinkage of prolactinomas in 60% to 80% of patients, although often this is incomplete. These drugs can thus obviate the need for pituitary surgery or, by partially shrinking large tumors, make surgery easier.

2. **Ablative therapy,** either surgical or radiologic, is no longer the preferred primary mode of treatment for many patients. Because the beneficial effects of radiotherapy are gradual and can require years for full expression, this form of treatment has not been favored for the typical patient with a prolactinoma (i.e., a young woman desiring fertility). Although selective transsphenoidal adenomectomy can be achieved in many patients with microadenomas, a substantial number of such patients (~20%) experience recurrent hyperprolactinemia within 5 years postoperatively; even the initial "cure" rate is low in patients with macroadenoma (~30%).

3. Initial concerns regarding the effects of bromocriptine use during **pregnancy** have been resolved by the finding that to date there has been no evidence of an increase in spontaneous abortions, stillbirths, or fetal anomalies. Although limited experience suggests that cabergoline is also safe during pregnancy, bromocriptine is preferred because more extensive data support its use. Because bromocriptine is usually discontinued once pregnancy is confirmed, there is also the possibility of renewed tumor growth during gestation. Although increased estrogen production during pregnancy does induce pituitary lactotrope hyperplasia, the incidence of clinically significant growth of small prolactinomas during pregnancy appears to be low (~2% to 3%). However, patients with macroadenomas have a somewhat higher risk of complications; those who experience significant tumor growth during pregnancy, with headaches and visual-field problems, can be treated with early delivery or with reinstitution of bromocriptine during gestation, if necessary.

   Thus, women with microprolactinomas who wish to become pregnant can do so, as long as the patient has a clear understanding that there is a small but finite risk of significant tumor growth during pregnancy. The prophylactic use of pituitary radiotherapy prior to conception does not seem warranted in patients with microadenomas but might be useful in patients with large tumors. Radiotherapy does not cause impairment of the subsequent response to bromocriptine.

4. **Bromocriptine** is usually begun at a low dosage (1.25 to 2.5 mg per day, usually at bedtime with a snack, to minimize nausea and orthostatic hypotension), with increments of 1.25 or 2.5 mg every 3 or 4 days until a total dosage of 5 to 10 mg per day is reached (given in two or three divided doses with meals) or serum Prl is normalized. Some patients require larger doses.

   Cabergoline is usually initiated at 0.25 mg once a week and increased as needed to 0.5 mg once or twice a week; higher doses may be given, if necessary.

   Dopamine agonist therapy should be cautiously reduced every 2 to 3 years to assess the need for continued therapy. Recent studies suggest that ~50% of patients appear to be cured of hyperprolactinemia after several years of treatment, particularly patients with a microadenoma who show complete disappearance of the tumor on cabergoline therapy.

5. In men with prolactinomas or in women who do not desire fertility, either radiotherapy or surgery may also be used (Table 4.5). In men, decreased libido and impotence resulting from hyperprolactinemia may not be fully reversed by testosterone administration; these patients may also require lowering Prl to normal by medication or other modalities. Patients with Prl-secreting tumors should receive follow-up as outlined for acromegaly (see Section IV.C).

VI. TSH-SECRETING TUMORS

TSH-secreting pituitary adenomas are uncommon, accounting for <2% of pituitary tumors. Typically, patients with such tumors demonstrate hyperthyroidism with detectable or elevated serum TSH. Serum TSH often shows little response to TRH (see Chapter 31); serum levels of glycoprotein hormone α subunit and the molar ratio of α subunit to TSH are often elevated. About one third of TSH-secreting tumors produce additional hormones, generally GH or Prl. Tumor ablation by surgery or radiation has been the preferred treatment; many patients respond to octreotide with a decrease in serum TSH and some with tumor shrinkage, but only a few respond to dopamine agonists.

VII. GONADOTROPIN-SECRETING TUMORS

In recent years it has been recognized that most clinically nonfunctioning pituitary tumors actually synthesize and secrete LH, FSH, or the subunits (α or β) of these glycoprotein hormones. These tumors are usually large macroadenomas when they are discovered; headaches, visual changes, and, occasionally, hypopituitarism are the typical presenting features. Testicular enlargement has been observed in a few men with FSH-secreting tumors. Serum FSH and, occasionally, LH concentrations are elevated in some cases but more often are normal; serum LH can rise in response to intravenous TRH, a finding that is not observed in normal individuals. The primary treatment is surgical, frequently with adjunctive radiotherapy. Gonadotropin hypersecretion has been suppressed by the administration of a GnRH antagonist (Nal-glu GnRH) in a few cases, but with no effect on tumor size. In a few patients, partial tumor shrinkage has been achieved with octreotide or dopamine agonist administration.

VIII. ACTH-SECRETING TUMORS

The majority of patients with pituitary-dependent <u>Cushing syndrome</u> (<u>Cushing disease;</u> bilateral adrenal hyperplasia) appear to have small (<10-mm) ACTH-secreting pituitary tumors as the cause of their hypercortisolism. Many are cured by selective transsphenoidal adenectomy. In patients with Cushing disease, bilateral adrenalectomy without therapy directed at the pituitary can lead to progressive enlargement of the pituitary tumor, accompanied by intense hyperpigmentation (<u>Nelson syndrome</u>) in 5% to 10% of cases. This presumably occurs because physiologic doses of replacement glucocorticoids exert an inadequate restraining feedback effect on the pre-existing tumor. The ACTH-secreting tumors of Nelson syndrome can behave aggressively and can be difficult to extirpate surgically. For this reason, the best treatment is prevention, consisting of therapy for Cushing disease directed primarily at the pituitary rather than the adrenal. Occasionally, patients with ACTH-secreting tumors respond to bromocriptine or cyproheptadine.

IX. PITUITARY HYPERPLASIA

Patients with untreated primary endocrine end-organ failure (e.g., of the thyroid or gonads) manifest hypersecretion of the appropriate tropic hormone(s) (TSH, LH, and FSH). In some cases, long-standing hormonal hypersecretion is accompanied by sufficient hyperplasia of the pituitary to produce sellar enlargement. It is important to recognize this condition to avoid unwarranted investigation and treatment for a presumed pituitary neoplasm. The elevated pituitary hormone level readily returns to normal following replacement of end-organ hormones (T$_4$ or gonadal steroid), and the pituitary and sella can gradually return to normal size over a period of years.

X. EMPTY SELLA SYNDROME

A. Pathogenesis. When the pituitary gland does not fill the sella turcica, the remaining space is often occupied by CSF, as an extension of the subarachnoid space; such a situation has been called an **empty sella.** The sella can also be enlarged. An empty sella can arise in two ways.

1. A secondary empty sella is found following infarction, shrinkage (e.g., by bromocriptine), or destruction (by surgery or radiation) of a hyperplastic or adenomatous pituitary. In this case, any sellar enlargement was presumably caused by initial expansion of the pituitary tumor. The remaining pituitary can function normally or show residual impairment related to the primary pathologic process or its therapy.

2. More often, an empty sella is found without evidence of pre-existing tumor. In this situation, termed the **primary empty sella,** it is believed that a congenitally incomplete diaphragma sellae (seen in 10% to 40% of normal persons) allows CSF to enter the sella. Normal pulsatile CSF pressures then compress the pituitary and may gradually expand the sella turcica. If intracranial pressure is elevated (e.g., in pseudotumor cerebri), sellar enlargement is more likely to occur. The primary empty sella is most often found in obese, middle-aged women, perhaps because these individuals more commonly have increased CSF pressure.

Pituitary function is usually normal in patients with the primary empty sella; a minority of patients demonstrates diminished gonadotropin or GH secretion, but decreased GH might be a result of obesity rather than pituitary dysfunction. Occasional bona-fide examples of hypopituitarism do occur with the primary empty sella, probably caused by compression of the pituitary stalk with resultant decreased delivery of hypothalamic releasing hormones to the pituitary.

B. Diagnosis. Many cases of empty sella are now detected as an incidental finding during the performance of CT or MRI for other indications; in a few patients, an enlarged sella turcica is found on routine skull radiographs performed for sinusitis, head trauma, or other reasons. Demonstration of CSF within the sella is readily made on MRI or CT; the pituitary gland is usually seen compressed against the posterior or inferior wall of the sella. Endocrine investigation of patients with suspected primary empty sella should be kept to a minimum. In a patient with no endocrine signs or symptoms, measurement of serum Prl, free T_4 or free T_4 index, and testosterone (in men) should be sufficient; patients with endocrine symptoms or with a history suggesting a prior pituitary disorder may require a more detailed evaluation.

C. Treatment. Usually no treatment other than reassurance is required for patients with a primary empty sella. Hormone replacement might occasionally be needed but is more commonly required in patients with a secondary empty sella related to a previous pituitary tumor.

Rarely, visual-field defects may occur in patients with the empty sella syndrome; although the cause is not always clear, it may sometimes be a result of herniation of the optic chiasm into the sella. CSF rhinorrhea facilitated by openings in bony sutures of the sellar floor may also occur. These two rare complications are the only indications for surgery in patients with a primary empty sella. Management of residual pituitary tumor may be necessary in patients with a secondary empty sella.

XI. CRANIOPHARYNGIOMA

Craniopharyngiomas are tumors of developmental origin, arising from the Rathke pouch, but may be clinically unrecognized for many years. The peak incidence is in the second decade. About 55% to 60% of craniopharyngiomas are cystic, 15% are solid, and 25% to 30% are combined. The tumor originates above the sella; as it enlarges, pressure is exerted on the optic chiasm, the hypothalamus, and the pituitary, leading to elevated intracranial pressure, visual defects, endocrine hypofunction (e.g., GH deficiency in children), hyperprolactinemia, and mental changes. Routine skull radiographs can show enlargement or erosion of the sella; 80% of children and 40% of adults have grossly visible supra- or intrasellar calcification. The tumor is usually well defined on CT or MRI. Surgery is helpful in debulking the tumor and in relieving compression of adjacent structures. Radiation therapy permanently controls the tumor in 70% to 90% of patients; surgical and radiation therapies are often combined. Hormone replacement is given as needed (Table 4.3).

Selected References

Agha A, Thompson CJ. Anterior pituitary dysfunction following traumatic brain injury. *Clin Endocrinol* 2006;64:481–488.

Bidlingmaier M, Strasburger CJ. What endocrinologists should know about growth hormone measurements. *Endocrinol Metab Clin N Am* 2007;36:101–108.

Caturegli P, Newschaffer C, Olivi A, et al. Autoimmune hypophysitis. *Endocr Rev* 2005;26: 599–614.

Chakrabarti I, Amar AP, Couldwell W, Weiss MH. Long-term neurological, visual, and endocrine outcomes following transnasal resection of craniopharyngioma. *J Neurosurg* 2005;102:650–657.

Chanson P, Young J. Pituitary incidentalomas. *The Endocrinologist* 2003;13:124–135.

Dekkers OM, Hammer S, deKeizer RJW, et al. The natural course of non-functioning pituitary macroadenomas. *Eur J Endocrinol* 2007;156:217–224.

DeMarinis L, Bonadonna S, Bianchi A, et al. Primary empty sella. *J Clin Endocrinol Metab* 2005;90:5471–5477.

Ezzat S, Asa SL, Couldwell WT, et al. The prevalence of pituitary adenomas. A systematic review. *Cancer* 2004;101:613–619.

Findling JW, Raff H. Screening and diagnosis of Cushing's syndrome. *Endocrinol Metab Clin N Am* 2005;34:385–402.

Gillam MP, Molitch ME, Lombardi G, Colao A. Advances in the treatment of prolactinomas. *Endocr Rev* 2006;27:485–534.

Gittoes NJL. Pituitary radiotherapy: current controversies. *Trends Endocrinol Metab* 2005; 16:407–413.

Greenman Y, Tordjman K, Osher E, et al. Postoperative treatment of clinically nonfunctioning pituitary adenomas with dopamine agonists decreases tumour remnant regrowth. *Clin Endocrinol* 2005;63:39–44.

Levy A. Hazards of dynamic testing of pituitary function. *Clin Endocrinol* 2003;58:543–544.

Lindholm J, Nielsen EH, Bjerre P, et al. Hypopituitarism and mortality in pituitary adenoma. *Clin Endocrinol* 2006;65:51–58.

Lüdecke DK, Abe T. Transsphenoidal microsurgery for newly diagnosed acromegaly: a personal view after more than 1,000 operations. *Neuroendocrinology* 2006;83:230–239.

Melmed S. Acromegaly. *N Engl J Med* 2006;355:2558–2573.

Mingione V, Yen CP, Vance ML, et al. Gamma surgery in the treatment of nonsecreting pituitary macroadenoma. *J Neurosurg* 2006;104:876–883.

Molitch ME, Clemmons DR, Malozowski S, et al. Evaluation and treatment of adult growth hormone deficiency: an Endocrine Society clinical practice guideline. *J Clin Endocrinol Metab* 2006;91:1621–1634.

Prasad D. Clinical results of conformal radiotherapy and radiosurgery for pituitary adenoma. *Neurosurg Clin N Am* 2006;17:129–141.

Saltzman E, Guay A. Dehydroepiandrosterone therapy as female androgen replacement. *Semin Reprod Med* 2006;24:97–105.

Scheithauser BW, Kurtkaya-Yapcer O, Kovacs KT, et al. Pituitary carcinoma: a clinical-pathological review. *Neurosurgery* 2005;56:1066–1074.

Schreiber I, Buchfelder M, Droste M, et al. Treatment of acromegaly with the GH receptor antagonist pegvisomant in clinical practice: safety and efficacy evaluation from the German Pegvisomant Observational Study. *Eur J Endocrinol* 2007;156:75–82.

Sethi DS, Leong J-L. Endoscopic pituitary surgery. *Otolaryngol Clin N Am* 2006;39:563–583.

Shomali ME, Katznelson L. Medical therapy of gonadotropin-producing and nonfunctioning pituitary adenomas. *Pituitary* 2002;5:89–98.

Utz AL, Swearingen B, Biller BMK. Pituitary surgery and postoperative management in Cushing's disease. *Endocrinol Metab Clin N Am* 2005;34:459–478.

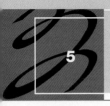

CLINICAL DISORDERS OF VASOPRESSIN

Camila Manrique, Guido Lastra, Adam Whaley-Connell, and James R. Sowers

Normal homeostasis requires a stable internal environment, including a nearly constant tonicity. A great deal of the stability of this internal environment depends on the adequacy and dependability of water metabolism. In spite of the large variation in the intake of water and/or solutes, a remarkable relatively narrow range of osmolality (282 to 298 mOsm/kg) is maintained. This accomplishment is contingent on multiple factors, including functioning of the osmoreceptors, the magnicellular neurons in the paraventricular area that are capable of producing both functional arginine vasopressin (AVP), also known as antidiuretic hormone (ADH), and neurophysins; the presence of functional vasopressin receptors in the kidney; functioning of the tubular cells, which are capable of producing an intact and functional aquaporin; and the maintenance of an adequate medullary osmolarity within the kidney. Vasopressin is involved not only in conservation of water by the kidney when needed, but is also an important component in the thirst mechanism and is a potent pressor. Less important, though essential, is interaction of the thyroid and adrenal glands.

The mechanism of thirst deserves consideration. Thirst can be stimulated as a response to increased extracellular fluid osmolality, through the activation of osmoreceptors located in the hypothalamus, or as a response to depressed plasma volume, through the activation of high- and low-pressure baroreceptors. Despite the existence of these other potential stimulants, the effect of the osmoreceptors stimulation seems to be the principal stimulant of thirst in humans.

I. REGULATION OF VASOPRESSIN SECRETION

A. AVP is a nonapeptide synthesized by specialized magnicellular neurons in the supraoptic and paraventricular nuclei of the hypothalamus. Different stimuli for AVP secretion mainly affect gene transcription and secondarily affect posttranscriptional regulation in these neurons. AVP is transported from the body of the paraventricular and supraoptic nuclei to the posterior pituitary in concert with neurophysins; neurophysins are synthesized as part of the AVP precursor molecule by the transcription of its gene in the short arm of chromosome 20 (20p13). Upon stimulation of the magnocellular neurons, an action potential travels through the neuronal axon toward the posterior pituitary, where it causes calcium influx and endopeptidase activation with release of the content of the neurosecretory granules into the perivascular space and thus into the capillary system of the posterior pituitary.

As neurophysins not only serve a role in hormone transport, disruption of their structure can have two main effects on AVP metabolism. First, there may be a decline in the binding site and hence activity of the endopeptidase responsible for the cleavage of AVP. Second, there may also be a change in the pattern of polymerization of neurophysin and its binding of vasopressin, which in turn may result in a specific enzymatic degradation of the hormone. Both of these effects can theoretically lead to deficiency in the amount of available vasopressin.

B. Stimuli of AVP secretion

1. Plasma osmolality. Plasma osmolality is the main and most important determinant of AVP secretion. Changes in plasma osmolality of as little as 1% are detected by specialized magnocellular neurons in the circumventricular organs and are transmitted to the supraoptic and paraventricular nuclei where AVP is synthesized. Axons from these nerve cells terminate in the distal hypophysial stalk and the posterior pituitary, and release AVP into the circulation. Above a certain osmotic threshold (284.3 mOsm/kg for a young adult), the secretion of AVP is linear with respect to changes in plasma osmolality (a 1-mOsm/kg H_2O increase in plasma osmolality causes an increase in plasma AVP level from 0.4 to 0.8 pg/mL), and a maximal antidiuretic effect (once the maximal urine concentration has been attained) is obtained with increases in plasma osmolality of 5 to 10 mOsm/kg. During regular daily circumstances, spontaneous fluid intake and vasopressin release are the main factors responsible for the maintenance of osmolality.

2. **Arterial underfilling.** Arterial underfilling (bleeding, venous pulling, decreased systemic vascular resistance, third spacing) is another stimulant of AVP secretion. High-pressure mechanoreceptors, located in the aortic arch and carotid sinuses, and low-pressure receptors, located in the atria and in the pulmonary venous system, serve as sensors of volume/pressure status to the magnocellular neurons of the hypothalamus via afferent branches of the vagal and glossopharyngeal nerves. This system is less sensitive than the osmoreceptor system and requires a 5% to 10% reduction in intrathoracic blood volume before it is activated. In spite of this, it may override osmolar regulation and cause hyponatremia when it is elicited. Moreover, these two systems do not function completely independently of each other. A decrease in arterial filling will decrease the osmotic threshold of vasopressin secretion; conversely, an increase in left atrial pressure will raise the osmotic threshold for vasopressin secretion.

3. **Other nonosmotic stimuli.** There are multiple nonosmotic stimuli for the secretion of vasopressin. A very potent one is <u>nausea</u>, which, even without vomiting or a volume-depleted state, can increase vasopressin to 100 to 1 000 times the basal levels. The function of this AVP elevation is unknown, but its presence may account for the vasoconstriction and facial pallor seen during episodes of nausea and vomiting. The elevation in AVP related to nausea may be at least partly responsible for the increase in vasopressin release that has been described with certain medications or in situations in which an emetic response is elicited (e.g., ketoacidosis, motion sickness, acute hypoxia, and vasovagal reactions). Vasopressin physiology is also influenced by multiple drugs (Table 5.1). Of special significance is the ability of central angiotensin-2 and the cytokines, especially interleukin-6 (IL-6), to cause release of vasopressin. This last factor may be

 TABLE 5.1 **Drugs That Influence Arginine Vasopressin Secretion**

Drugs that stimulate AVP secretion	
Acetylcholine	Hypercapnia
Anesthetic agents	Hypoxia
Angiotensin II	Metoclopramide
Barbiturates	Morphine and other narcotics
β-Adrenergic agonists	Nicotine
Carbamazepine or oxcarbazepine	Oxytocin
Clofibrate	Phenothiazines
Clozapine	Prostaglandin E_2
Cyclophosphamide	Serotonin reuptake inhibitors
Ecstasy	Tricyclics
Histamine	Vincristine
Drugs that suppress AVP secretion	
Alcohol	Atrial natriuretic peptide
α-Adrenergic agonists	Phenytoin

AVP; arginine vasopressin secretion.

important in the pathophysiology of the syndrome of inappropriate secretion of antidiuretic hormone (SIADH).

II. EFFECT OF AVP ON THE KIDNEY

A. The kidney is of prime importance in the regulation of water balance and metabolism. This is accomplished through vasopressin-induced increased water permeability and increased urea movement on the collecting ducts, as well as vasopressin-stimulated NaCl absorption in the thick ascending loop of Henle. In the collecting duct, AVP binds to its G-protein–coupled receptor (V2 subtype), with subsequent generation of cyclic adenosine monophosphate (cAMP) and activation of protein kinase A, which in turn phosphorylates aquaporin-2 in serine residue 256, making possible its transport to the apical membrane of the collecting duct cell. The insertion of the aquaporin-2 channel causes H_2O entry to the cell, which is then transported through the basolateral membrane by aquaporin-3 and aquaporin-4, resulting in transcellular water transport. Once the stimulus for H_2O conservation ends, aquaporin-2 is recycled by endocytosis via clathrin-coated pits. Other mechanisms have been reported to limit the vasopressin response, including decreased levels of V2-subtype receptor mRNA and phosphodiesterase-mediated destruction of cAMP (Fig. 5.1).

B. Effect on the permeability to water. The effect of AVP on water permeability is accomplished in both short-acting and long-acting modes, as discussed in the following.

1. Short-term effect. The short-term regulation of water transport is made through the fusion of aquaporin-2–containing intracytoplasmic vesicles with the apical membranes, thereby increasing the permeability of the collecting duct to water. This effect is rapid in onset (within a few minutes) as well as rapidly reversible.

2. Long-term effect. The long-term regulation implies gene transcription and protein expression. This effect is mediated by the phosphorylation of a cAMP response element in the 5′ flanking region of the AQP2 gene with consequent increased gene transcription. This last effect is not rapidly reversible.

C. Effect of AVP on the concentrating mechanism. Vasopressin increases permeability to urea in the inner medullary collecting duct, thereby enhancing the concentration of urea in the medulla of the kidney and maintaining a high medullary interstitial osmotic gradient, and facilitating its own action on the concentration of water. This effect is also mediated by increased intracellular cAMP. Additionally, vasopressin also increases the rate of absorption of NaCl in the medullary thick ascending limb, promoting the <u>countercurrent multiplication mechanism</u> that affects the concentrating ability of the kidney in long-standing deficiency of AVP of any etiology. This, together with the long-term effect on expression of AVP in the collecting duct cells, should be taken into account when interpreting a polyuric patient's "inadequate" response to AVP or its analog.

III. DIABETES INSIPIDUS

A. Definition. Diabetes insipidus (DI) is defined as the passage of a large volume of dilute and hypotonic urine (in general, >30 mL/kg per 24 hours, with urine osmolality <300 mOsm/kg and specific gravity <1.010). This contrasts to the polyuria caused by the osmotic diuresis in diabetes mellitus. DI can result from a relative or absolute deficit of functional AVP (central DI), inability of the kidney to respond appropriately to an adequate amount of circulating AVP (nephrogenic DI), or physiologic suppression of AVP release as a result of water overload (primary polydipsia).

B. Types of DI

1. Central DI (central or neurohypophyseal)

a. Definition. Central DI is a state of hypotonic polyuria resulting from absolute or relatively deficient secretion of AVP in spite of adequate stimuli and with a normal renal responsiveness to AVP.

b. Classification

(1) Complete central DI is characterized by total inability to synthesize or release AVP.

(2) Partial central DI is characterized by an inability to synthesize and/or release an adequate amount of AVP.

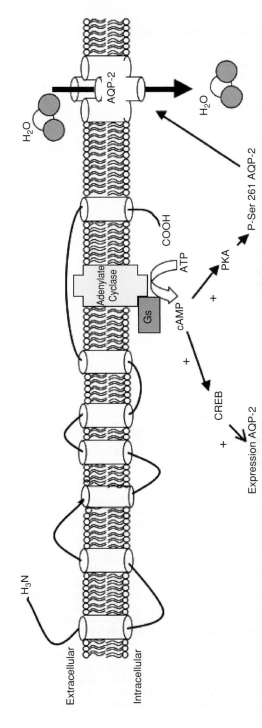

Figure 5.1. Vasopressin binding to its V2 receptor leads to increased cyclic adenosine monophosphate (cAMP) with subsequent activation of protein kinase A (PKA) and stimulation of cAMP response element–binding protein (CREB). PKA activation causes phosphorylation of aquaporin-2 (AQP-2) and translocation to the apical plasma membrane. Phosphorylation of CREB results in increased AQP-2 gene transcription. The final effect is water (H_2O) passage through the AQP-2 channel.

TABLE 5.2	Causes of Central Diabetes Insipidus

Primary causes (not acquired)
Familial (autosomal dominant)
Idiopathic

Secondary causes (acquired)
Traumatic
   Accidental (e.g., head trauma)
   Iatrogenic (e.g., surgery)
Tumors
   Craniopharyngioma
   Primary pituitary tumors
   Metastatic disease (breast cancer, lung cancer)
   Acute leukemia
   Lymphomatoid granulomatosis
   Rathke cleft cyst
   Mixed germ cell tumor (rare)
Granulomatous disease
   Sarcoidosis
   Histiocytosis
   Tuberculosis
Infectious diseases
   Meningitis
   Encephalitis
Vascular
   Aneurysms
   Sheehan syndrome
   Hypoxic encephalopathy
Drugs
   Alcohol
   Diphenylhydantoin
Autoimmune
   Lymphocytic hypophysitis (rare; usually affects anterior adenohypophysis)

   c. Etiology
     (1) Familial central DI is a rare disorder inherited in an autosomal dominant fashion with variable expression and usually presenting during childhood. Most of the genetic defects identified involve the neurophysin molecule, with probable altered packaging of the prohormone in the neurosecretory granules.
     (2) Acquired central DI can result from numerous conditions (Table 5.2). Anterior pituitary tumors rarely cause DI.
   d. Pathophysiology. Polyuria ensues because of the patient's inability to secrete enough AVP to maintain normal water homeostasis. However, polyuria does not occur until 90% of the vasopressinergic neurons are lost. In the presence of an intact thirst mechanism, the resultant hyperosmolality leads to increase in water intake and normalization of plasma osmolality.
   e. Clinical presentation. Patients present with polyuria and polydipsia, often during both day and night. There is often a predilection for cold drinks. Urine output may vary from a few liters to 20 L per day. Serum osmolality and electrolyte balance is determined by the status of the thirst mechanism and the patient's access to water. Indeed, metabolic complications can develop very quickly if the thirst mechanism is impaired (e.g., with altered mental status, under sedation, in nursing home patients). Up to 60% of pituitary surgery

patients present with transitory DI. When DI is the result of surgical or traumatic injury to the hypothalamic-posterior pituitary area, it may be a classical triphasic response. The first phase is transient DI, resulting from axonal shock and inability to propagate action potentials, which presents within 24 hours of the insult and may resolve within days. A possible second phase consists of a SIADH-like phase that may ensue 5 to 7 days after the primary insult and is secondary to unregulated AVP secretion from axonal degeneration. Ultimately, there may be a component of DI that may or may not improve or resolve over time.

f. **Diagnosis.** The diagnosis of central DI involves ruling out other causes of polyuria. Responsiveness to vasopressin does not constitute a diagnosis of central DI, because patients with primary polydipsia and those postoperative patients in positive fluid balance also respond to vasopressin with a decrease in urine output, though with a significant risk of becoming water-intoxicated. Primary polydipsia is a condition characterized by a powerful need to ingest fluid, associated with polyuria, which can result in reduced plasma osmolatity.

The classical picture includes hypotonic polyuria with normal to slightly elevated plasma osmolality and an inappropriately low AVP concentration. This is in contrast to primary polydipsia, in which the serum osmolality is not high and may even be low.

Neuroimaging with magnetic resonance imaging (MRI) of the neurohypophysis may be useful as an adjunctive diagnostic tool. The pituitary stalk can also be evaluated in an MRI. Enlargement is present above 2 to 3 mm and may be caused by infiltrative diseases, infection, or metastasis. The absence of a bright spot in the T1-weighted images of the sella is a characteristic finding in central diabetes insipidus. However, in certain situations, such as early in the course of familial hypothalamic DI, the bright spot may be present.

2. **Nephrogenic DI**

a. **Definition.** Nephrogenic DI is a hypotonic polyuric state resulting from renal insensitivity to the action of AVP. It is characterized by persistent hypotonic polyuria in the presence of adequate levels of AVP and failure of exogenous AVP to significantly decrease the urine volume or increase urine osmolality unless the defect is partial.

b. **Etiology.** Like central DI, this condition also can be familiar or acquired, and can be complete or partial (Table 5.3).

(1) **Congenital nephrogenic DI.** Responsible mutations in two different areas have been identified. Ninety percent of the mutations responsible for the condition involve the vasopressin V2 receptor present in the collecting duct. This usually results in protein misfolding, which in turn prevents the translocation of the receptor to the membrane. The mode of inheritance is X-linked recessive, and heterozygous female carriers may have mild water metabolism impairment with nocturia, noctidipsia, and subnormal urine-concentrating ability. Ten percent of the families with DI have mutations in the aquaporin-2 gene, located in chromosome 12, region q13. Inheritance of this mutation may be autosomal recessive or dominant.

(2) **Acquired nephrogenic DI.** Hypokalemia and hypercalcemia have been classically described as potential causes of DI. In both scenarios there is downregulation of aquaporin-2 expression in the inner medulla and, in addition, hypercalcemia and decreased Na-K-2Cl cotransporter concentration in the outer medulla. Lithium is known to cause DI in 20% of patients taking this medication, secondary to downregulation of aquaporin-2 channels in a cAMP-independent mechanism. Acute renal failure and urinary tract obstruction can also cause nephrogenic diabetes insipidus.

c. **Classification**

(1) **Complete:** Characterized by a complete inability to respond to vasopressin even in pharmacologic doses

(2) **Partial:** Characterized by responsiveness to vasopressin in pharmacologic doses

TABLE 5.3	Causes of Nephrogenic Diabetes Insipidus

Hereditary
Familial X-linked recessive (mutation in V_2 receptor)
Autosomal recessive (mutation in aquaporin gene)
Autosomal dominant (mutation in aquaporin gene)

Acquired
Drugs: Lithium therapy (inhibits production of cAMP? Disruption in short- and long-term regulation of AP), demeclocycline, methoxyflurane
Metabolic: Hypokalemia (decreased sensitivity of adenylcyclase to ADH, affects only long-term regulation of AP-2), hypercalcemia-hypercalciuria (modulate ADH-induced AP-2 regulation via apical calcium sensor receptor)
Postbilateral ureteral obstruction BPH and neurogenic bladder (impaired long-term AP-2 regulation only)
Vascular: sickle cell disease or trait
Infiltrative: amyloidosis
Low-protein diet

ADH, antidiuretic hormone; AP, aquaporin; BPH, benign prostatic hypertrophy; cAMP, cyclic adenosine 3′,5′-monophosphate.

    d. **Pathophysiology.** The basic abnormality in nephrogenic DI is an inability of the collecting ducts to increase their permeability to water in response to vasopressin, and hence impairment in water conservation results with consequent increased plasma osmolality and hypernatremia.

    e. **Clinical presentation.** Familial nephrogenic DI presents very early in infancy, with vomiting, fever, failure to thrive, hypotonic polyuria, and electrolyte imbalances. There may be a family history of other affected males. Obviously, recognition of this disease is imperative to the survival of the patient. The timing of the presentation of the acquired type obviously depends on the underlying disease process or exposure to medication. Acquired nephrogenic DI usually presents with just moderate polyuria (3 to 4 L/min), and if the thirst mechanism is intact, hypernatremia does not ensue.

3. Primary polydipsia

    a. **Dipsogenic DI.** Individuals with dipsogenic DI have a normal osmotic threshold for AVP release but an unusually lower osmotic threshold for thirst than that for AVP release. This abnormality leads to constant hypotonic polyuria because the serum osmolality is maintained at a level below the threshold for vasopressin release. Organic causes such as hypothalamic lesions, especially sarcoidoses, have been described as causative factors.

    b. **Psychogenic polydipsia.** This is a condition of compulsive water drinking seen in individuals with underlying psychological or psychiatric disorders. Unlike patients with dipsogenic polydipsia, these individuals do not have a change in thirst threshold; rather, their polydipsia stems from cognitive impairment resulting from their underlying psychopathology.

4. DI in pregnancy. Transient gestational DI has been reported and is considered to be secondary to increased AVP degradation by placental vasopressinase. Its appearance may be associated with fatty liver of pregnancy and pre-eclampsia.

5. Diagnostic tests for polyuric states. Diagnosis of the etiology of polyuric states may sometimes be straightforward but at other times may be very difficult. Osmotic causes of polyuria, such as hyperglycemia, can be readily identified by clinical history and basic laboratory workup. A history of psychiatric disease in the presence of hypotonic polyuria is highly suggestive of primary polydipsia (i.e., psychogenic polydipsia). Similarly, hypotonic polyuria in the face of increased plasma osmolality and serum sodium excludes the diagnosis of primary polydipsia. In the same way, the sudden development of polyuria after surgical or nonsurgical trauma to the pituitary/hypothalamic area is very suggestive of central DI. In the presence of an intact thirst mechanism, patients are usually ambulatory, not dehydrated, and have normal serum sodium. In this scenario, provocative testing is required to establish a diagnosis. A water deprivation test followed by AVP administration is the most common test used, based on the premise that dehydration stimulates vasopressin release and urine concentration.

6. **Water deprivation test**
   a. **Method.** During the water deprivation test, all fluids are withheld in order to cause dehydration and provide a potent stimulus for maximal AVP secretion (i.e., plasma osmolality >295 mOsm/kg). The duration of fluid deprivation depends on the clinical presentation and may vary from 4 to 18 hours. The test should be done in a room without access to a water source. Patients should be asked to urinate before the test is started and initial body weight recorded immediately after. Thereafter, body weight should be monitored every hour, and urine volume should be recorded. During the time frame of the test, urine osmolality is determined hourly. The test should be discontinued if body weight decreases by 3%, the patient presents with cardiovascular instability, urine osmolality remains stable (three consecutive urine sample osmolalities vary by <30 mOsm/kg), or hypernatremia develops (>145 mmol/L). Once the osmolality has reached a stable value or the patient has lost >2% of body weight, samples are obtained for plasma sodium, osmolality, and vasopressin measurements. Then the patient is given AVP (5 U) or desmopressin (DDAVP) (1 mg) subcutaneously, with subsequent measurement of urine osmolality and urinary volume at 30, 60, and 120 minutes after the injection. The highest value is used to evaluate the patient's response to AVP. For completeness, plasma osmolality should be measured at the beginning of the test, again before the administration of vasopressin or DDAVP, and after the administration of the drug. In individuals with severe polyuria (urine output >10 L per day), water deprivation should be started early in the morning under careful supervision. In patients with less severe polyuria, water deprivation may be started the night before (22:00 hours), because 12 to 18 hours of fluid deprivation may be required.
   b. **Precautions.** Drugs that influence vasopressin secretion or action should be discontinued if at all possible. Caffeine-containing beverages should be avoided on the day of the test, and alcohol and tobacco should be avoided for at least 24 hours before the test. During testing, individuals should be monitored for conditions that may provide nonosmotic stimuli for vasopressin secretion (e.g., nausea, hypotension, or vasovagal reactions).
   c. **Interpretation**
      (1) **Healthy subjects.** In healthy subjects the water deprivation will provide stimulus for maximal vasopressin secretion and maximal urine concentration. Hence administration of additional AVP or its analogs will not lead to >10% increase in the osmolality of the already maximally concentrated urine.
      (2) **Primary polydipsia.** The absence of an increase of urine osmolality above that of plasma osmolality virtually excludes primary polydipsia, provided surreptitious drinking is excluded. In this last circumstance, neither the serum nor the urine osmolality will increase adequately during the water deprivation test. Another clue to surreptitious water drinking during a water deprivation test is an incongruent degree of weight loss in comparison with what would be expected on the basis of urine output during the test.
      (3) **Complete DI.** In both central and nephrogenic complete DI, the urine osmolality does not increase above that of the plasma. The two forms can be further differentiated by the individual's response to the administration of vasopressin or DDAVP. Although there may be some increase in the urine

osmolality in nephrogenic DI, this is usually <10% of the level achieved after dehydration. Patients with central DI usually respond to ADH administration with a >50% increase in urine osmolality.

(4) Partial DI. Individuals with partial DI (both central and nephrogenic) may have urine osmolalities that are higher than their plasma osmolalities after water deprivation. In central DI, however, the measured AVP will be lower than expected for the plasma osmolality, whereas in nephrogenic partial DI it will be appropriate. Adequate plasma AVP can be estimated based on the serum osmolality; that is, $AVP = 0.38 \times$ (plasma osmolality $- 280$) ng/L.

7. **Hypertonic saline infusion.** This method helps to differentiate partial DI from primary polydipsia.
   a. **Method and interpretation.** During this provocative testing, 3% NaCl is infused at 0.1 mL/kg per minute for 1 to 2 hours; subsequently, plasma AVP is measured once the serum osmolality and sodium are >295 mOsm/kg and 145 mEq/L, respectively. Precautions must be taken with individuals who might not be able to handle the increase in volume properly (e.g., patients with congestive heart failure or cirrhosis). When plotted on a nomogram, patients with partial central DI can be distinguished from those with partial nephrogenic DI or primary polydipsia. In patients with nephrogenic DI or primary polydipsia, AVP release in response to hypertonicity is normal, whereas patients with central DI exhibit no or subnormal increases in ADH secretion.

8. **Therapeutic trial of DDAVP.** This procedure is another method by which partial central DI can be separated from partial nephrogenic DI.
   a. **Method and interpretation.** In this approach, a therapeutic trial of DDAVP (10 to 25 μg intranasally or 1 to 2 μg subcutaneously) is given for 2 to 3 days. This will improve central DI while not affecting the patient with nephrogenic DI. Caution must be exercised to avoid water intoxication. Although this is most likely to occur in primary polydipsia, occasionally patients with central DI may also continue to drink large amounts of water out of habit.

9. **Treatment.** Management of DI includes maintaining proper fluid metabolism and balance, educating the patient to adjust the treatment if necessary, and avoiding potentially dangerous situations. Identification and, if possible, correction of underlying acquired pathology when present, should always be considered in the treatment of individuals with DI.
   a. **Maintaining fluid metabolism.** Fortunately, most patients with DI have an intact thirst mechanism and can monitor their own water needs. The problem arises in the few patients who do not belong to this group. Under these circumstances there should be continuous monitoring of fluid intake and careful balancing of water intake and antidiuretic intervention(s).
   b. **Water.** Water intake is the prime target for the management of DI. In any given patient, an adequate amount of water will correct and prevent any of the metabolic derangements that can potentially be caused by DI. Often this is overlooked in hospitalized patients; a simple maneuver, such as having water at the bedside, can prevent consequences of dehydration. The subsequent pharmacologic treatment modalities should be seen as measures that will make the amount of necessary water intake more tolerable and prevent nocturia and sleep deprivation.
   c. **ADH agonists.** ADH agonists should be titrated to minimize sleep disruption caused by nocturia and to minimize breakthrough symptoms throughout the day.
      (1) L-ARGININE VASOPRESSIN. This is the naturally occurring antidiuretic hormone form in humans. Usually administered subcutaneously, it has an onset of action within 1 to 2 hours and a duration of action anywhere between 4 and 8 hours. Because of its potential pressor effect, intravenous administration should be avoided.
      (2) DDAVP [1-(3-Mercaptopropionic acid)-8-D-arginine vasopressin]. This synthetic analog of AVP has modifications of the molecule that result

in a prolonged half-life with reduced pressor activity and relative resistance to degradation by vasopressinase, which makes it the treatment of choice during pregnancy. The agent is about 2 000 times more specific for antidiuresis than the naturally occurring substance. It is available for clinical use in oral, parenteral, and nasal spray forms.

(a) Intranasal application. The onset of action of the nasally applied drug is rapid (45 minutes), with a peak effect evident after 1 to 5 hours and a duration of action of 6 to 24 hours.

 (i) Nasal spray is available in a concentration of 0.1 mg/mL and delivers 0.1 mL (10 μg) fixed dose per spray. One dose has an antidiuretic activity of 40 IU. The usual dose is 1 to 4 sprays per day in a single dose or in two to three divided doses. It is advisable to give the medication at bedtime to prevent sleep disruption due to nocturia and to adjust the dose as needed.

 (ii) Rhinal tube multidose vial comes in a concentration of 0.1 mg/mL and can deliver 5 to 20 μg into a rhinal catheter, from which the drug is blown into the nose.

 (iii) Stimate Nasal Spray is available in a concentration of 0.15 mg/mL and delivers 0.1 mL (150 μg). One dose has an antidiuretic activity of 600 IU.

(b) Parenteral administration. Parenteral administration is 5 to 20 times more potent than intranasal application. Available in a 4-μg/mL solution, the usual dosage is 1 to 2 μg (0.25 to 0.50 mL) given subcutaneously or intravenously twice a day.

(c) Oral administration. Oral forms are available in 0.1- and 0.2-mg tablets. The onset of action is 30 to 60 minutes. This form has the advantage of not requiring refrigeration. Dosage can be started at 0.1 mg at bedtime or divided into two doses per day. The dosage is titrated as needed up to a total of 1.2 mg per day in two or three divided doses.

(d) Other agents

 (i) Chlorpropamide. Chlorpropamide enhances the activity of AVP and possibly also its release, reducing polyuria by 25% to 75% in patients with central DI. It is useful in patients with partial central DI with residual capacity to secrete ADH. The usual dose is 100 to 500 mg PO daily, and the maximal antidiuretic activity will be noticed after 4 days. The risk of hypoglycemia is minimal, and its main advantage is cost.

 (ii) Carbamazepine. Carbamazepine causes the release of ADH. It can be used in partial central DI in doses ranging from 200 to 600 mg per day.

 (iii) Thiazide diuretics. By causing mild volume contraction, Thiazide diuretics reduce the amount of glomerular ultrafiltrate and increase the proximal reabsorption of salt and water. These agents can be used in the management of nephrogenic DI. The usual effective dose is between 50 and 100 mg per day, and the antidiuretic effect can be enhanced by a low-salt diet. Because of the risk of hypokalemia, patients should be evaluated for potassium levels and given potassium supplements if needed.

 (iv) Indomethacin. Indomethacin decreases renal medullary prostaglandin E and thereby enhances cAMP generation secondary to AVP binding to its V2 receptor. Prostaglandin synthase inhibitors may be effective even in patients with nephrogenic diabetes insipidus.

(e) Management of nephrogenic DI. Because of the underlying abnormality, the management of primary nephrogenic DI should not be based on ADH. The most effective treatment is thiazide diuretics and mild salt depletion, but prostaglandin synthase inhibitors can also be considered. Increasing knowledge regarding the role of aquaporin misfolding in the pathogenesis of the congenital nephrogenic DI will probably lead to more effective and specific therapeutic interventions in the coming years.

(f) Management of primary polydipsia. The primary treatment should be behavior modification. Drug treatment with AVP, its analogs, or other agents that increase its secretion or action not only are not indicated but may even be dangerous in view of their tendency to cause water intoxication in individuals who suffer from these disorders.

(g) Treatment during pregnancy. DDAVP is the drug of choice during pregnancy, because the half-life of AVP is reduced as a result of increased vasopressinase activity in the placenta.

(h) Treatment of the patient with altered thirst mechanism. This situation warrants careful and frequent assessment of the patient and design of a plan of fixed fluid intake and antidiuretic drug treatment to maintain a state of balanced water metabolism. In the event of intercurrent febrile illness, one must carefully maintain an adequate fluid balance.

(i) Treatment in the postoperative period. During the postoperative period, special caution should be taken when treating the patient.

> **(a)** First, there should be careful assessment of the patient's water balance, because postoperative polyuria not uncommonly represents diuresis of fluid administered during surgery, which might not be obvious if attention is given only to the current fluid balance.

> **(b)** Osmotic diuresis secondary to glycosuria can be a contributing factor to polyuria, as patients are frequently treated with steroid replacement therapy.

> **(c)** True DI resulting from neurosurgical intervention often has a triphasic pattern as described previously, and caution should be used when administering AVP or DDAVP because water intoxication may ensue. Usually, a dose of 1 to 2 μg of subcutaneous, intramuscular, or intravenous DDAVP is given while closely monitoring plasma sodium, urinary volume, and urine osmolality. The best approach is not to schedule doses of DDAVP, but rather wait to administer the next dose until polyuria reappears.

(j) Treatment of the hypernatremic patient. On occasion, patients with DI may present with hypernatremia because of concomitant illness that impairs their free-water intake. Under these conditions the initial treatment of choice is correction of the fluid deficit with normal saline solution. Once the hypovolemia is corrected, the free-water deficit should be calculated and corrected.

(k) Avoidance of potentially dangerous situations. Another problem arises when a patient with an otherwise intact thirst mechanism is rendered unconscious or is unable to manage his or her own fluid intake because of concomitant illness or other factors. For this reason, patients with DI should carry a medical card or bracelet indicating their potentially life-threatening condition.

IV. SIADH

A. Definition. SIADH is a condition of euvolemic hyponatremia secondary to inadequate AVP secretion, which causes inappropriate urinary concentration and water retention.

B. Pathophysiology

1. Hyponatremia develops in response to AVP (or ADH-like substances) release in spite of low serum osmolality. AVP secretion can occur secondary to ectopic production or pituitary secretion (the latter being responsible for 90% of SIADH cases). Several patterns of AVP secretion in the context of SIADH have been described: (a) random hypersecretion, most commonly seen with ectopic tumors; (b) inappropriate elevated and nonsuppressible basal AVP production;

and (c) reset osmostat, with AVP secretion triggered by a lower-than-normal osmolality.

2. Increased urinary sodium is a contributor to hyponatremia. Water retention–induced pressure natriuresis and increased secretion of atrial natriuretic peptide with secondary natriuresis are possible explanations for this phenomenon.

3. Another common finding of SIADH is hypouricemia secondary to V1 receptor–stimulated uric acid clearance.

4. Interleukin 6 (IL-6) is a proposed causative factor for SIADH during sickness, inflammation, and stress, because it can stimulate AVP secretion. (When it is injected into humans, IL-6 stimulates the secretion of AVP.)

C. Etiology (Table 5.4)

1. **Central Nervous System (CNS) disorders.** Almost any CNS disorder can be associated with SIADH, including vascular events, infections, and metabolic diseases.

2. **Pulmonary conditions.** Many lung pathologies can be associated with SIADH. Whereas in positive-pressure ventilation this is due to the activation of low-pressure cardiopulmonary baroreceptors, the mechanism in other conditions is still not completely understood. As noted earlier, one very plausible candidate is IL-6, because it produces secretion of AVP both in vitro and in vivo.

3. **Neoplasms.** Perhaps the best-understood mechanism of SIADH in neoplastic disease is that seen in small cell lung cancer, in which cancer cells can produce and secrete AVP and ADH/AVP-like substances that possess both immunologic and biological characteristics of AVP.

4. **Pharmacologic agents.** Several drugs are known to augment AVP secretion, enhance its antidiuretic effect, and stimulate renal V2 receptors.

D. Clinical manifestations. Clinical symptoms, when present, are mainly neurologic, but in rare cases rhabdomyolysis can be present. Neurologic symptoms range from vague headache and nausea to seizures, altered mental status, and focal neurologic deficits. These later manifestations are secondary to cerebral edema resulting from water shift into the brain caused by a decreased plasma osmolality. Needless to say, a high index of suspicion is required for proper identification. Although not exclusively so, symptoms occur more commonly when serum sodium drops to <125 mEq/L.

E. Laboratory findings. Hyposmolar hyponatremia with concomitant submaximal dilute urine is the hallmark of SIADH. Often there is a component of urinary uric acid loss with hypouricemia. By definition, diseases that impair free-water clearance are absent (e.g., hypoadrenalism or hypothyroidism). If measured, plasma ADH levels will be inappropriately high for the degree of hyposmolarity but may be within the normal range.

F. Diagnosis. Following are the SIADH diagnostic criteria established by Bartter and Schwartz:

1. Decreased effective osmolality of the extracellular fluid

2. Inappropriate urinary concentration in the presence of hypo-osmolality

3. Clinical signs of euvolemia: absence of signs of hypovolemia (tachycardia, orthostatic changes) and hypervolemia (edema and ascites)

4. Elevated urinary sodium excretion with normal salt and water intake

5. Absence of other causes of euvolemic hypo-osmolality (hypoadrenalism or hypothyroidism)

Additional testing is usually not necessary if the above criteria are met, but occasionally a water load test may confirm the diagnosis. In cases of SIADH, <80% of a water load of 20 mL/kg will be excreted. This challenge should not be done in patients with Na <125 mmol/L or plasma osmolality <275 mOsm/kg because of the risk of worsening the hyponatremia/hypo-osmolality.

Distinguishing the euvolemic from the hypovolemic patient with concomitant renal salt wasting may be a challenge, because urinary sodium concentration and fractional excretion of sodium are identical in these two conditions (Table 5.5). One way to make the distinction is to administer 1 L of 0.9% NaCl intravenously over 24 hours for 2 days. If this improves the hyponatremia by >5 mEq/L, the patient most likely is hypovolemic. In patients with SIADH this

TABLE 5.4   Causes of SIADH

Central nervous system disorders
Head injury
Infections: meningitis, encephalitis, abscess
Cerebrovascular accident
Cavernous sinus thrombosis
CNS neoplasm
Guillain-Barré syndrome
Epilepsy
Porphyria
Hydrocephalus
Shy-Drager syndrome
Multiple sclerosis
Psychosis, delirium tremens

Pulmonary disorders
Infectious: pneumonia, tuberculosis, abscess, empyema
Asthma
Pneumothorax
Cavitation
Positive-pressure ventilation
Cystic fibrosis

Neoplasms
Carcinoma: lung (especially small-cell lung cancer), pancreas, duodenum, bladder, uterine, prostate
Lymphoma, leukemia
Ewing sarcoma, mesothelioma
Thymoma (carcinoid)

Pharmacologic agents
Angiotensin-converting enzyme inhibitors
Carbamazepine
Chlorpropamide
Clofibrate
Cyclophosphamide
Selective serotonin reuptake inhibitors (especially in the elderly)
Haloperidol
Monoamine oxidase inhibitors
Nicotine
Oxytocin
Phenothiazine
Thiazide diuretics
Tricyclic antidepressants

CNS, central nervous system; SIADH, syndrome of inappropriate secretion of antidiuretic hormone.

maneuver does not change the serum sodium concentration or increases it by <5 mEq/L. On the other hand, fluid restriction of 600 to 800 mL per day for 2 to 3 days improves hyponatremia in SIADH but not the hyponatremia in renal salt wasting. Another consideration in the euvolemic hyponatremic patient is cerebral salt-wasting syndrome. It was initially described in subarachnoid hemorrhage patients, and as a cause of hyponatremia, an increase in brain natriuretic peptide has been suggested. Theoretically, the existence of such a syndrome would warrant the supplementation of salt rather than fluid restriction as its primary treatment modality. However, the existence of this syndrome is highly controversial.

TABLE 5.5 Comparison of Various Hyponatremic States

Diagnosis	Volume status	Urinary sodium conc. (mEq/L)	Fractional excretion of sodium (%)
SIADH	Normovolemic	>20	>1
Renal	Hypovolemic	>20	>1
Extrarenal	Hypovolemic	<10	<1
Dilutional hyponatremia	Hypervolemic	<10	<1

SIADH, syndrome of inappropriate secretion of antidiuretic hormone.

G. Treatment. The treatment for SIADH includes correction of the underlying pathology that gave rise to the metabolic aberration if at all possible and management of the hyponatremia. If a medication is identified as a causative factor, it should be discontinued. The therapeutic approach to the hyponatremic patient depends on the following factors: evidence of symptoms, acuteness of onset of hyponatremia, and presence of risk factors for complications resulting from correction of the hyponatremia. Symptomatic disease is most likely to be found with an acute decrease in serum sodium (i.e., a decrease of at least 0.5 mEq/L per hour) and is more commonly seen when serum sodium falls to <125 mEq/L. The duration of hyponatremia should also be taken into account. Whereas chronic hyponatremia (>48 hours) is associated with a higher chance of cerebral demyelinization if it is corrected too rapidly, acute hyponatremia is more likely to lead to the development of cerebral edema if it is not corrected quickly. Other populations at risk for the development of cerebral edema include postoperative premenopausal women, children, elderly women recently started on thiazide diuretics (usually within 2 weeks, although 33% of such cases occur within 5 days), hypoxemic patients, and psychiatric patients with primary polydipsia. Patients at risk for the development of demyelination syndrome include alcoholics, malnourished individuals, elderly women on thiazide diuretics, burn patients, hypokalemia, chronic hyponatremia, and those with serum sodium <120 mEq/L.

1. **Acute symptomatic hyponatremia.** The goal of therapy should be to raise serum sodium at a rate of <0.5 mEq/L per hour up to 125 mEq/L, then fluid restriction is applied. However, in young women with severe symptomatic hyponatremia, a higher rate of correction is often used (1 to 2 mEq/L per hour until sodium reaches 125 mEq/L). The total correction should be <15 mEq per day. Hypertonic saline (3% NaCl) at the rate of 1 to 2 mL/kg per hour is recommended. Addition of a loop diuretic enhances the correction of the hyponatremia by enhancing free-water excretion. Such patients require close neurologic and electrolyte monitoring and should be managed in an intensive care unit.

2. **Chronic asymptomatic hyponatremia.** The simplest available option for the treatment of SIADH, besides correction of the primary cause, is fluid restriction. The nonfood fluid intake is usually restricted to 500 to 1 000 mL per day. The drawback of this method is the high likelihood of the patient's failure to adhere to the regimen. Additional therapeutic strategies involving interference with the AVP renal effect are very appealing, but there are pitfalls identified especially with old nonspecific medications. Demeclocycline (1 200 mg per day initially, followed by 300 to 900 mg per day) or lithium (900 to 1 200 mg per day) has been used. Both of these agents have disadvantages, including a narrow therapeutic window and toxicity for lithium and photosensitivity and toxicity for demeclocycline—this last especially in the presence of hepatic dysfunction. Furthermore, demeclocycline requires 3 to 6 days before its onset of action can be noted. Another way to increase free-water clearance is by administration of a loop diuretic supplemented with 2 to 3 g per day of NaCl and monitoring for hypokalemia. There is the option of inducing osmotic diuresis by administering urea (30 to 60 g per day). However,

this last option has the disadvantage that it may be unpalatable and may cause gastrointestinal symptoms.

Recently, a new therapeutic strategy became available, the aquaretics. These compounds act by blocking binding of AVP to its V2 receptor in the basolateral membrane of the renal collecting duct, promoting free water clearance without Na^+ or K^+ loss. This new class of medications is known as **vaptans** and includes Tolvaptan, a V2-receptor antagonist, Lixivaptan, a V2-receptor antagonist, and Conivaptan, a V1/V2-receptor antagonist. Only Conivaptan is approved by the U.S. Food and Drug Administration (FDA) for panretinal use, but encouraging data recently became available for short-term oral use of Tolvaptan in euvolemic (SIADH) and hypervolemic (cirrhosis, heart failure) hyponatremia. The vaptans have the advantage over diuretics of not causing neurohormonal activation.

Selected References

Addler SM, Verbalis JG. Disorders of body water homeostasis in critical illness. *Endocrinol Metab Clin* 2006;35:873–894.

Chen S, Jalandhara N, Batlle D. Evaluation and management of hyponatremia: an emerging role of vasopressin receptor antagonists. *Nat Clin Pract Nephrol* 2007;3:82–95.

Deen PM. Mouse models for congenital nephrogenic diabetes insipidus: what can we learn from them? *Nephrol Dial Transplant* 2007;22:1023–1026.

Hays RM. Vasopressin antagonists—progress and promise. *N Engl J Med* 2006;355:2146–2148.

Kalelioglu I, Kubat Uzum A, Yildirim A, et al. Transient gestational diabetes insipidus diagnosed in successive pregnancies: review of pathophysiology, diagnosis, treatment, and management of delivery. *Pituitary* 2007;10:87–93.

Knepper MA, Inoue T. Regulation of aquaporin-2 water channels trafficking by vasopressin. *Curr Opin Cell Biol* 1997;9:560–564.

Kovacs L, Robertson GL. Syndrome of inappropriate antidiuresis. *Endocrinol Metab Clin N Am* 1992;21:859–875.

Larsen PR, Kronengberg HM, Melmed S, Polonsky KS, eds. Williams textbook of endocrinology. 10th ed. Philadelphia: Elsevier Science; 2003.

Lauriat SM, Berl T. The hyponatremia patient: practical focus on therapy. *J Am Soc Nephrol* 1997;8:1599–1607.

Legros JJ, Geenen V. Neurophysin in central diabetes insipidus. *Hormone Res* 1996;45:182–186.

Marynger B, Hensen J. Nonpeptide vasopressin antagonists: a new group of hormone blockers entering the scene. *Exp Clin Endocrinol Diabetes* 1999;107:157–165.

Masrorakos G, Weber JS, Magiakou MA, et al. Hypothalamic-pituitary-adrenal axis and stimulation of systemic vasopressin secretion by recombinant interleukin-6 in humans: potential implications for the syndrome of inappropriate vasopressin secretion. *J Clin Endocrinol Metabol* 1994;79:934–939.

McKenna K, Thompson C. Osmoregulation in clinical disorders of thirst appreciation. *Clin Endocrinol* 1998;49:139–152.

Oiso Y. Hyponatremia: how to approach this confusing abnormality. *Intern Med* 1998;37:907–908.

Rai A, Whaley-Connell A, McFarlane S, Sowers JR. Hyponatremia, arginine vasopressin dysregulation, and vasopressin receptor antagonism. *Am J Nephrol* 2006;26:579–589.

Ray JG. DDAVP use during pregnancy: an analysis of its safety for mother and child. *Obstet Gynecol Surv* 1998;53:450–455.

Schrier RW. Body water homeostasis: clinical disorders of urinary dilution and concentration. *J Am Soc Nephrol* 2006;17:1820–1832.

Schrier RW, Fassett RG, Ohara M, et al. Vasopressin release, water channels and vasopressin antagonism in cardiac failure, cirrhosis, and pregnancy. *Proc Assoc Am Phys* 1998;110:407–411.

Schrier RW, Gross P, Gheorghiade M, et al. Tolvaptan, a selective oral vasopressin V2-receptor antagonist, for hyponatremia. *N Engl J Med* 2006;355:2099–2112.

Settle EC. Antidepressant drugs: disturbing and potentially dangerous adverse effects. *J Clin Psychiatry* 1998;59:25–30.

Soupart A, Decaux G. Therapeutic recommendations for the management of severe hyponatremia: current concepts on pathogenesis and prevention of neurologic complications. *Clin Nephrol* 1996;46:149–169.

Swallow CE, Osborn AG. Imaging of sella and parasellar disease. *Semin Ultrasound Comput Tomogr Magn Reson Imag* 1998;19:257–271.

Verbalis JG. Adaptation to acute and chronic hyponatremia: implications for symptomatology, diagnosis, and therapy. *Semin Nephrol* 1998;18:3–19.

Verbalis JG. Disorders of body water homeostasis. *Best Pract Res Clin Endocrinol Metab* 2003;17:4471–1503.

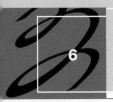

PITUITARY DISORDERS AND TALL STATURE IN CHILDREN

6

Philip D. K. Lee and Norman Lavin

*T*his chapter highlights only those features of pituitary disorders that are unique to or are particularly important in pediatric endocrinology. More detailed reviews of individual disorders can be found in other chapters. Pediatric pituitary hormone disorders involve one or more of all six major anterior pituitary hormones: growth hormone (GH), thyroid-stimulating hormone (TSH), adrenocorticotropic hormone (ACTH), luteinizing hormone (LH), follicle-stimulating hormone (FSH), prolactin (PRL), and antidiuretic hormone (ADH) from the posterior pituitary. Except in the case of PRL, deficient secretion is much more common than excess secretion.

Consideration of pituitary disorders in pediatrics differs from that in adult medicine in several important aspects, including:

1. Types of disorders: an increased frequency of congenital conditions.
2. Etiology: increased proportion of genetic causes and syndrome associations.
3. Clinical presentation: unique emphasis on abnormal growth and sexual development.
4. Diagnosis: different test procedures for children, use of weight-based dosing for pharmaceutical testing agents.
5. Treatment: different treatment regimens for children, including weight-based medication dosing, treatment endpoints (e.g. height and pubertal development), and monitoring procedures.

HYPOPITUITARISM

Overall, GH is the most commonly deficient hormone in pediatric hypopituitarism, occurring either as an isolated deficiency or in combination with other pituitary hormone deficiencies. The prevalence of GH deficiency in the pediatric population has been estimated to be as high as 1 in 3 500. TSH is perhaps the second most commonly deficient pediatric pituitary hormone, occurring in approximately one third of cases of GH deficiency, but rarely occurring as an isolated deficiency. Deficiencies of other anterior pituitary hormones (ACTH, LH, FSH, and PRL) usually occur in association with other pituitary hormone deficiencies. **Panhypopituitarism** generally refers to deficiencies of multiple anterior pituitary hormones. ADH deficiency, or central diabetes insipidus (DI), has an estimated overall population prevalence of 1 in 25 000.

I. ETIOLOGY

    A. Idiopathic. Cases of pediatric hypopituitarism for which no etiology has been definitively identified comprise a large but decreasing plurality of affected individuals. Most of these cases involve idiopathic GH deficiency.

    B. Genetic causes. Following is a partial listing of mutations or deletions of genes that affect pituitary formation during embryogenesis or synthesis of pituitary hormones, resulting in hypopituitarism.

        1. Genes involved in pituitary morphogenesis and predominately genes that code for transcription factors

            a. *HESX1* (chromosome 3p21.2-p21.1). *HESX1* is the earliest embryogenic marker of pituitary development. Mutations have been identified in some patients with septo-optic dysplasia, congenital panhypopituitarism, and isolated GH deficiency (IGHD).

b. *SOX2* (chromosome 3q26.3-q27) and *SOX3* (chromosome Xq27.1). Mutations of *SOX2* present with severe phenotypes including anophthalmia or microphthalmia, pituitary hypoplasia with hypopituitarism (especially GH deficiency and hypogonadotropic hypogonadism), neurodevelopmental delay, and other abnormalities. *SOX3* mutations have been associated with X-linked GH deficiency, often with other pituitary hormone deficiencies, neurodevelopmental delay, and other abnormalities. Mutations in *SOX2* and *SOX3* have been identified in a small number of patients diagnosed with septo-optic dysplasia.

c. *PITX 1* (chromosome 5q31) and *PITX2* (chromosomes 4q25-27). Human mutations of *PITX1* have not been characterized. *PITX2* mutations have been associated with <u>Rieger syndrome</u>, an autosomal dominant condition characterized by short stature, GH deficiency with or without other hormone deficiencies, eye and tooth anomalies, and multiple other anomalies.

d. *LHX3* (chromosome 9q34.3) and *LHX4* (chromosome 1q25.2). *LHX3* mutations have been associated with complete deficiency of all anterior pituitary hormones except ACTH, as well as rigidity of the cervical spine. *LHX4* mutations are associated with GH deficiency, alone or with other anterior hormone deficiencies, cerebellar defects, and abnormalities of the sella.

e. *PROP1* (chromosome 5q35.3). Mutations of *PROP1* are the most commonly identified genetic causes of panhypopituitarism, including deficiencies in PRL, GH, and TSH, with variable gonadotropin deficiency.

f. *PIT1* (aka *POU1F1*; chromosome 3p11). *PITI1* is involved in the regulation of multiple pituitary genes, including those for GH, PRL, TSH, and GH-releasing hormone (GHRH). Phenotype and inheritance patterns depend on the mutation site.

g. *TPIT* (aka *TBX19*; chromosome 1q23-24). *TPIT* is involved in the differentiation of pro-opiomelanocortin (POMC) neurons and, with *PITX1*, in POMC gene expression. Because ACTH is a product of the POMC gene, *TPIT* mutations are associated with the rare autosomal recessive condition of isolated ACTH deficiency.

h. *DAX1* (chromosome Xp21.3-p21.2). *DAX1* is found in the dosage-dependent sex reversal region that is critically involved in phenotypic sex determination. Mutations are associated with X-linked congenital adrenal hypoplasia and male hypogonadotropic hypogonadism. Delayed puberty has been reported in female carriers.

i. *KAL1* (chromosome Xp22.32). *KAL1* codes for anosmin-1, a protein involved in cell migration and adhesion during embryogenesis of gonadotropin-releasing hormone (GnRH) neurons, which have a shared origin with the olfactory neurons. *KAL1* mutations are associated with X-linked Kallmann syndrome, characterized by hypogonadotropic hypogonadism with anosmia or hyposmia.

j. *KAL2* (aka *FGFR1*; chromosome 8p11.2-p.11.1). *KAL2* codes for a fibroblast growth factor (FGF) receptor that may be involved in migration of GnRH neurons during embryogenesis. *KAL2* mutations are associated with the autosomal dominant <u>Kallmann syndrome</u>, manifesting anosmia or hyposmia.

k. *KISS1* (chromosome 1q32) and *GPR54* (aka *KISS1R*; chromosome 19 p13). *KISS1* codes for the protein kisspeptin, whereas *GPR54* codes for the kisspeptin receptor. *KISS1* is expressed in the hypothalamus, whereas *GPR54* has been localized to GnRH neurons; this system may be involved in GnRH secretion. Mutations of these genes have been associated with partial to complete isolated gonadotropin deficiency, without anosmia or hyposmia, in both males and females.

l. *WFS1* (chromosome 4p16). *WFS1* mutations are associated with <u>Wolfram syndrome</u>, a condition associated with diabetes insipidus, diabetes mellitus, optic atrophy, and deafness (aka DIDMOAD).

    m. GNAS1 (chromosome 20q13.3). Chromosome 20q13.3 is part of the imprinted, multigene *GNAS* locus. It codes for the α subunit of $G_s\alpha$, a guanine nucleotide binding protein (G protein). Inactivating mutations of *GNAS1* cause <u>pseudohypoparathyroidism</u> (PHP), a multifaceted condition associated with resistance to hormones that bind to G-protein–coupled receptors, including the pituitary receptors for GHRH (in PHP type Ia) and GnRH (in PHP types Ia and Ic). Activating mutations of *GNAS1* are associated with <u>McCune-Albright syndrome</u> (discussed later).

  2. Genes that code for pituitary hormones and receptors

    a. GH1 (chromosome 17q24.2). *GH1* codes for pituitary GH. Deletions and mutations have been identified in association with IGHD types 1a, 1b, and 2, as well as conditions of "bioinactive" GH.

    b. GHRHR (chromosome 7p14). *GHRHR* codes for pituitary GHRH receptor, a G-protein–coupled receptor. GHRH receptor deficiency leads to pituitary GH deficiency. Mutations have been associated with IGHD type 1b.

    c. FSHB (chromosome 11p14) and **LHB** (chromosome 19q13.32). *FSHB* codes for the FSH β-subunit gene and *LHB* for the LH β-subunit gene. Mutations are extremely rare but have been associated with varying degrees of hypogonadism and infertility. LH levels are reported to be elevated in patients with *FSHB* mutations.

    d. GNRHR (chromosome 4q21.2). *GNRHR* codes for the pituitary GnRH receptor, a G-coupled receptor. Mutations are associated with isolated hypogonadotropic hypogonadism without anosmia or hyposmia, a subgroup of normosmic Kallmann syndrome.

    e. TRHR (chromosome 8q23). *TRHR* codes for the pituitary TSH-receptor. Mutations are extremely rare but have been associated with isolated TSH deficiency.

C. Congenital and syndrome-associated hypopituitarism

  1. Neonatal hypopituitarism. Neonatal hypopituitarism is a broad clinical categorization that includes hypopituitarism with onset in the neonatal period, i.e., from birth to ~1 month of age. In addition to the rare genetic mutations discussed previously and the congenital conditions described later, cases of neonatal hypopituitarism may be associated with perinatal insult and with prematurity, possibly resulting from compromised pituitary blood flow or hypoxia.

  2. Craniospinal malformations. A number of craniospinal disorders have been associated with pituitary hormone deficiencies, particularly GH deficiency. These conditions include spina bifida (myelomeningocele), holoprosencephaly, encephalocele, and Arnold Chiari malformation. Patients with facial clefting (e.g., cleft lip and palate) and other midline craniofacial defects (e.g., choanal atresia, single central incisor, Pallister-Hall syndrome, Robinow syndrome) may also be at high risk for hypopituitarism. Hydrocephalus associated with these or other conditions may also be associated with hypopituitarism.

  3. Empty sella. Empty sella is a condition in which a normal-sized or enlarged pituitary sella is filled with cerebrospinal fluid rather than normal pituitary tissue. This condition is well described in adults but has been recognized in children only relatively recently. The etiology is unclear, although the presence of a normal sella size implies prior occupancy by the pituitary gland. The pituitary gland may be present and flattened or displaced, or it may be partly or completely absent. A high proportion of children with hypopituitarism resulting from a variety of causes may have empty sella on magnetic resonance imaging (MRI). It is unclear whether children with empty sella may also be asymptomatic, as has been reported in adults. Empty sella may be associated with a variety of neurologic symptoms, with or without evidence of hypopituitarism.

  4. Septo-optic dysplasia (de Morsier syndrome). This variably defined condition usually consists of optic nerve hypoplasia, midline craniofacial/brain defects (e.g., absence of the corpus callosum or septum pellucidum), and pituitary hypoplasia. Single (usually GH) or multiple anterior and posterior (ADH) hormone deficiencies may occur. However, the majority of children with optic nerve hypoplasia probably do not have hypopituitarism. A minority of cases of septo-optic dysplasia with hypopituitarism have been associated with mutations of *HESX1*, *SOX2*, and *SOX3*.

5. **Isolated GH deficiency (IGHD).** This is a clinically defined group of conditions involving lack of GH action and severe short stature. IGHD type 1a is typified by autosomal recessive transmission, decreased birth length, neonatal hypoglycemia and cholestatic jaundice, and undetectable serum GH. IGHD type 1b is similar to type 1a but with a milder phenotype and detectable, but low, serum GH. IGDH type 2 typically has autosomal dominant transmission and low serum GH levels. IGHD type 3 is X-linked, with low serum GH levels. The IGHD classification may eventually be replaced by definitive molecular diagnoses. *GH1* mutations have been identified in some patients with IGHD types 1a, 1b, and 2, and *GHRH-R* mutations in IGHD type 1b.

6. **Other syndromes.** GH deficiency with or without other pituitary hormone deficiencies has been reported to occur in a number of congenital syndromes, including Bardet-Biedl, Peters Plus, Prader-Willi, 18p-, and Russell-Silver syndromes, with varying degrees of validation for definitive associations. On the other hand, most congenital syndromes characterized by short stature are not associated with GH or other pituitary hormone deficiencies.

D. **Acquired**

1. **Tumors (benign and malignant)**

   a. **Craniopharyngioma.** Craniopharyngiomas constitute 5% to 15% of pediatric intracranial tumors. They are derived from the embryonic craniopharyngeal ductal epithelium. The onset and pathogenesis are unclear, and neonatal cases have been reported. Peak incidence of childhood diagnosis is between 5 and 14 years of age. Most craniopharyngiomas have both intra- and suprasellar components. They are histologically benign, rarely metastasize, but are often locally invasive and infiltrative. Hypopituitarism and visual disturbances, resulting from mass and pressure effects, are frequent presenting signs in pediatric patients.

   b. **Rathke's cleft cyst.** This is an epithelial, intrasellar cystic lesion that is probably derived from remnants of Rathke's pouch, which is an embryologic progenitor of the pituitary gland. It is often confused or categorized with craniopharyngioma. Most cases are thought to be asymptomatic; however, large cysts may be associated with hypopituitarism. Unlike craniopharyngioma, Rathke's cleft cysts are not invasive, but they may expand, resulting in pressure effects.

   c. **Other central nervous system (CNS) lesions.** CNS lesions may affect pituitary function by causing a mass effect, invading the sella and/or disrupting the pituitary blood supply. They include both benign lesions (arachnoid, dermoid, and epidermoid cysts, nonfunctioning pituitary adenoma, vascular malformation, abscess), lesions related to systemic disease (tuberculosis, sarcoidosis, lymphocytic hypophysitis), or malignant/potentially malignant lesions (germinoma, optic glioma, meningioma).

   d. **Neurofibromatosis type 1 (NF1).** NF1 is a progressive multisystem autosomal dominant disease that affects 1 in 2 000 to 1 in 4 500 people. This disorder results from mutations in the *NF1* gene, located on chromosome 17q11.2, which codes for neurofibromin, a tumor-suppressor protein. Hypophyseal neurofibromas are common and can lead to GH deficiency because of a mass effect.

   Fifty percent of cases are familial and 50% are new mutations. To make the diagnosis, the patient must manifest two of seven listed signs or symptoms as shown in Table 7.1, but young children frequently have only one of the cardinal clinical features. Café-au-lait macules (six or more >5 mm) alone may be enough to diagnose NF1. Other features not listed in the National Institutes of Health (NIH) criteria should be considered in young children, including short stature, macrocephaly, and bright objects on head MRI. Osseous disorders, such as pseudarthrosis, sphenoid wing dysplasia, and dysplastic vertebrae, may also occur.

e. Hyperthyrotropinemia. GH deficiency has been reported in cases of primary hypothyroidism, persisting after normalization of thyroid hormone levels. Pituitary thyrotrope hypertrophy with adverse effects on somatotropes is a postulated mechanism.

f. Infiltrative lesions

(1) Langerhans cell histiocytosis (histiocytosis X) is a disease of unknown etiology involving infiltration of tissues by unusual dendritic monocytes (Langerhans cells or histiocytes). One of three clinical subtypes, Hand-Schüller-Christian disease, occurs primarily in young children and is associated with a seborrheic skin rash (hands, feet, scalp line) with histiocytic invasion of the base of the skull, often involving the pituitary and resulting in diabetes insipidus and exophthalmos. A similar type of clinical picture has been reported in Erdheim-Chester disease, a type of histiocytosis that is thought to be unrelated to Langerhans cell histiocytosis.

(2) Lymphocytic hypophysitis may be observed in association with autoimmune disorders, as discussed later. Severe cases may be associated with pituitary mass effects.

g. Iatrogenic. Treatment of pituitary and other CNS tumors may result in pituitary disorders. In particular, pituitary irradiation is often associated with hypofunction and, rarely, hyperfunction (e.g., precocious puberty). Radiation therapy–associated hypopituitarism is dose-related, can be progressive over several months or years, and, in children, may preferentially affect GH and TSH, although other hormones are also commonly affected.

h. Trauma. Trauma may result from direct trauma (closed or open head injury) to the head as well as motion-related trauma, such as may be observed in cases of child abuse (e.g., shaken-baby syndrome) and motor vehicle accidents. Acute or progressive single (usually GH) or multiple pituitary hormone deficiencies may occur. Trauma may precede GH deficiency/hypopituitarism by many years.

i. Autoimmune. Antipituitary antibodies, lymphocytic hypophysitis, and hypopituitarism have been separately and jointly reported to occur in all of the four types of autoimmune polyglandular syndromes (APS). Perhaps the most frequently reported association in pediatrics is lymphocytic hypophysitis and hypopituitarism (GH deficiency alone or with other deficiencies) or APS1 (also called autoimmune polyendocrinopathy-candidiasis-ectodermal dystrophy [APECED]), a condition caused by mutations in the *AIRE* (autoimmune regulator) gene (chromosome 21q22.3). Antipituitary antibodies and/or autoimmune hypopituitarism have also been reported in association with other autoimmune disorders, including antiphospholipid syndrome and autoimmune connective tissue disorders. However, the specific relationship of pituitary autoimmune markers and clinical pituitary disorders has not been completely defined.

j. Pharmacologic. Suppression of ACTH secretion is associated with supraphysiologic glucocorticoid therapy. GH and TSH secretion may be suppressed by exogenous GH and thyroid hormone treatments, respectively. Suppression of gonadotropin secretion is a desired effect of continuous treatment with GnRH agonists. Pharmacologic hypopituitarism is usually transient and resolves with discontinuation of the causative medication or lowering of the dose to physiologic levels. However, full recovery may be slow, over a period of weeks to months.

II. DIAGNOSTIC EVALUATION FOR HYPOPITUITARY DISORDERS

Testing protocols for diagnostic evaluation of hypopituitarism are discussed in Appendix A and are briefly discussed here only in relation to pediatric considerations. There are few universally accepted guidelines or protocols for evaluation of pituitary function in children. Therefore, clinical acumen and experience are essential elements of pediatric pituitary diagnosis. In some clinical situations, e.g., postpituitectomy or with multiple known hormone deficiencies, minimal, if any, confirmatory diagnostic testing may be required.

A. **General considerations.** A complete history and physical examination are essential. Special attention should be given to accurate measurements of height (with comparison to previous measurements), sexual development, body proportions, dysmorphic features, skin lesions, and neurologic signs and symptoms. An inappropriate decline in height velocity and delayed sexual maturation are common presenting signs of pediatric hypopituitarism.

B. **Imaging.** A bone-age radiograph may provide supportive evidence (usually delayed in hypopituitarism) but is not diagnostic (development may be delayed in other conditions or in healthy children). MRI with and without contrast is the most useful pituitary neuroimaging procedure.

C. **Genetic testing.** A minority of cases of pediatric hypopituitarism are due to identifiable gene mutations. Genetic testing should be considered in apparent familial cases or in cases with specific suggestive features. For instance, a *DAX1* mutation should be considered in an adolescent male with delayed puberty and nonautoimmune primary adrenal insufficiency. Consultation with a pediatric geneticist may be useful prior to consideration of genetic testing. A useful resource is www.genetests. org.

D. **GH.** GH secretion is episodic. Therefore, random levels, which may be very low, are of no utility in assessing GH adequacy. Standard testing involves low response to two pharmacologic stimuli (e.g., insulin-induced hypoglycemia, clonidine, arginine infusion) coupled with low levels of the GH-dependent protein, insulinlike growth factor-I (IGF-I) and its major binding protein, IGFBP-3. Controversies include variable definition of a low versus normal GH response, GH assay variability, and normal GH levels in patients with low IGF-I levels. In addition, GH therapy has been efficacious in promoting growth in short children without GH or IGF-I deficiency, raising questions about the clinical utility of GH or IGF-I levels as a determinant of treatment. Nonetheless, documentation of GH deficiency by standard testing has continued relevance to the evaluation of pediatric pituitary function, and documentation of pituitary GH deficiency may have important implications for management of individual patients.

E. **TSH.** The combination of low serum thyroxine (T4) and very low TSH suggests pituitary TSH deficiency. Low T4 with normal or slightly elevated TSH may be observed in TRH deficiency and in euthyroid sick syndrome. Stimulation of TSH secretion following administration of TRH may have some value in the differential diagnosis of patients with low basal levels of both thyroid hormone and TSH. However, this test has fallen out of favor in pediatrics because of the lack of normative values and the usual co-occurrence of GH deficiency in cases of pediatric TSH deficiency (thereby providing a diagnostic clue). Furthermore, TRH is not readily available commercially in the United States.

F. **ACTH.** Standard testing involves intravenous synthetic ACTH (1-24) and measurement of cortisol levels over 60 minutes; a basal ACTH level can be obtained to distinguish primary adrenal insufficiency. This test relies on the physiologic need for sufficient tonic ACTH secretion to allow rapid synthesis and release of cortisol in response to a pulse dose of ACTH (i.e., simulating a stress response). An adequate test is often defined as any cortisol level (baseline or stimulated) ≥ 20 μg/mL or an increase of ≥ 10 μg/mL above baseline. Controversy has arisen as to the diagnostic sensitivity and specificity of this test for adrenal insufficiency, and particularly for prediction of risk for adrenal crisis, and the relative merits of standard (250 μg) or low ($\sim$1.0 μg) synthetic ACTH (1-24) doses. A more reliable test agent may be metyrapone, which blocks adrenal 11β-hydroxylase and, consequently, cortisol synthesis, resulting in a rise in ACTH secretion. However, the metyrapone test is relatively cumbersome and has been associated with exacerbation of adrenal crisis. ACTH stimulation testing with ovine corticotrophin-releasing factor (oCRF) has also been described but has not been widely accepted.

G. **Gonadotropins.** In the presence of delayed puberty, high basal LH and FSH levels may indicate primary rather than pituitary or hypothalamic hypogonadism. Low basal levels with increases following intravenous administration of synthetic GnRH may provide biochemical evidence of impending puberty. However, if there is a lack of response to GnRH, it may be difficult to distinguish hypogonadotropic hypogonadism from severe constitutional delay of puberty.

H. **PRL.** Diagnostic evaluation of hypoprolactinemia has limited, if any, clinical utility in pediatrics, although a low PRL level may be observed in some of the rare genetic conditions that cause hypopituitarism.

I. **ADH.** The basic principle for diagnosis of **diabetes insipidus** is documentation of inappropriately excessive production of dilute urine in the presence of plasma hyperosmolarity. See Section (p. 83).

J. **Combined testing.** Standard pediatric pituitary testing often involves sequential administration of two GH secretagogs (e.g., a clonidine test followed immediately by an arginine test) after an overnight fast to rule out growth hormone deficiency. Synthetic ACTH infusion at time 0 and measurement of various baseline hormone levels may also be included, to allow assessment of multiple hormone systems. Other types of combined pituitary stimulation testing have been described (e.g., TRH, GnRH, and CRF administrations with GH testing) but are not commonly performed in pediatrics.

K. **Neonatal hypoglycemia.** A special diagnostic situation is the neonate with severe, episodic, unexplained hypoglycemia. A blood sample for GH, cortisol, insulin, and β-hydroxybutyrate levels, obtained during hypoglycemia, can be useful in guiding further evaluation and treatment toward hypopituitarism (low GH and cortisol), hyperinsulinism (high insulin, low β-hydroxybutyrate), or an inborn error of metabolism (elevated β-hydroxybutyrate).

III. TREATMENT OF HYPOPITUITARISM

A. **General principles.** Treatment of pediatric hypopituitarism (and pediatric disease in general) has the goal of optimizing growth, neurodevelopment, and sexual development. All clinically relevant pituitary hormones can be replaced via pharmaceutical agents.

B. **GH.** Biosynthetic human GH, produced via recombinant DNA technology, has been commercially available for treatment of childhood GH deficiency since the mid-1980s. Studies have not shown a relationship of GH therapy to primary, recurrent, or secondary malignancies. Limited data indicate no effect on progression or growth of neurofibromas in neurofibromatosis type 1. Patients with GH deficiency due to *GH1* mutations may develop neutralizing antibodies to exogenous GH.

C. **TSH.** Replacement therapy with once-daily levothyroxine (2–6 μg/kg per day; higher doses per kilogram for infants and young children) is usually adequate in pediatric TSH-deficiency; coadministration of tri-iodothyronine (T3) has not been standard. In pituitary TSH deficiency, monitoring of serum T4 and/or "free" T4 should guide therapy; TSH levels will be low. Normal T4 levels are age-related.

D. **ACTH.** Glucocorticoid, rather than ACTH, replacement therapy is standard. Cortisol (hydrocortisone) doses are usually calculated based on a standard formula, e.g., 6 to 12 mg/m^2 per day with correction for oral bioavailability (e.g., calculated dose × 1.5) and spaced according to the half-life of the medication (e.g., q8–12h). More potent, longer-acting preparations (e.g., prednisone) are typically used for adolescents. Monitoring is based on clinical history (energy levels, etc.) and examination (height, weight, body habitus, etc.); there are no suitable biochemical markers to guide therapy. Mineralocorticoid replacement therapy is usually not required in patients with ACTH deficiency.

Acute adrenal insufficiency is treated with parenteral administration of supraphysiologic doses of glucocorticoid, e.g., >2× replacement dose.

E. **Gonadotropins.** Current treatment for pediatric hypogonadotropic hypogonadism usually involves gonadal replacement therapy (testosterone or estrogen/progestin) beginning in the mid-teens, with consideration of the potential effects of these medications on epiphyseal closure. Gonadal steroid replacement therapy is geared toward enabling completion of sexual development (puberty) and does not facilitate fertility. Monitoring is based on clinical examination, especially height, weight, and Tanner staging.

F. Vasopressin. Vasopressin (or DDAVP) is replacement therapy for diabetes insipidus (see the following section).

 DIABETES INSIPIDUS

DI is a disorder characterized by an inability to maximally concentrate urine. It is caused by a deficiency or defective action of antidiuretic hormone (ADH) or arginine vasopressin (AVP). AVP receptors are now classified as V_1 and V_2 receptors and are present on many organs in the body. There are two major types of DI: (a) central or ADH-deficient DI; and (b) nephrogenic DI. The syndrome of inappropriate ADH secretion (SIADH) is also discussed in this section.

I. CENTRAL DI (DEFICIENCY OF ADH)
  A. Etiology
   1. Primary
     a. Idiopathic.
     b. Defective synthesis or secretion of ADH.
   2. Secondary
     a. Tumors are the most common causes of DI. In children, craniopharyngioma is the most common tumor.
     b. Langerhans cell histiocytosis (LCH), previously called histiocytosis X, refers to a group of diseases that were formerly divided into three categories. The endocrine manifestations occur in the disseminated form (Hand-Schüller-Christian disease). The classic triad of skull defects, DI, and exophthalmos occurs in <10% of patients, but DI occurs alone in 5% to 50%. Other endocrinopathies include hypernatremic hyperosmolar syndrome, growth retardation, hyperprolactinemia, hypogonadism, panhypopituitarism, primary or secondary hypothyroidism, and diabetes mellitus. These result from infiltration of the hypothalamus or posterior pituitary. Magnetic resonance images of patients with LCH and DI show abnormalities of the hypothalamus and absence of the relative hyperintensity of the posterior pituitary.
     c. Infections (such as meningitis) can cause a transient form of DI.
     d. Vascular abnormalities.
     e. Trauma rarely causes central DI in children. An example would be basal skull fracture immediately or after several months following the injury.
     f. Wolfram (DIDMOAD) syndrome is DI associated with diabetes mellitus, optic atrophy, and deafness. It is an autosomal recessive mitochondrial disorder arising on chromosome 4.
   3. Newborn. DI has been reported in patients with asphyxia, intraventricular hemorrhage, intravascular coagulopathy, *Listeria* sepsis, and group B streptococcal meningitis.
  B. Genetics
   1. Familial or sporadic cases can occur.
   2. Both dominant and X-linked recessive inheritance have been described. Mutations have been localized to the vasopressin-neurophysis gene on chromosome 20.
  C. Clinical features
   1. Nocturia and enuresis are common in children. Polyuria and polydipsia as well as dehydration are also found.
   2. Poor weight gain and slow growth rate (secondary to poor caloric intake or decreased level of GH).
   3. Excessive crying.
   4. Vomiting.

5. Constipation.

6. Occasionally, strabismus or double vision.

7. Hypertonic dehydration, leading to stupor or coma in infants or children with impaired thirst mechanism.

D. Diagnosis

1. Inappropriately dilute urine (low specific gravity [e.g., <1.010] or low osmolality [e.g., 50 to 300 mOsm/kg]) in the presence of normal or elevated serum sodium and osmolality. Occasionally, even life-threatening hypernatremia may occur.

2. If fluid is not given overnight, the morning urine specific gravity should be at least 1.018; if it is lower, consider DI.

3. Measure ADH (AVP). Little or no ADH is evident despite dehydration (i.e., a hyperosmolar state voiding hypo-osmotic urine). Patients with partial DI show a subnormal relationship of plasma ADH to plasma osmolality but maintain a normal relationship of plasma ADH to urine osmolality.

4. Skull radiograph and CT or MRI to rule out tumors and vascular abnormalities. The "bright spot" (hyperintense signal) is usually absent in patients with hypothalamic-neurohypophysial tract lesions.

5. Visual-field examination.

6. Laboratory evaluation of all pituitary hormones.

7. Seven-hour water deprivation test. The child must be closely monitored.

   a. No restriction of fluid intake before test.

   b. Regular breakfast, then **NPO** after breakfast.

   c. Weigh patient.

   d. Have patient void to empty bladder at 8 A.M.

   e. Begin test.

      (1) Collect and save hourly urine samples (measure specific gravity of these specimens).

      (2) Send an aliquot of the first-hour urine sample to the lab for osmolality (U_1) immediately.

      (3) Draw blood during the first hour for electrolytes and serum osmolality (S_1) immediately.

   f. As the test progresses: If blood pressure (BP) is low, if pulse increases, or if weight loss exceeds 5% body weight, be prepared to end the test early.

   g. If weight loss exceeds 10%, proceed to **k** (to end the test)—be careful.

   h. If urine volumes decrease markedly and if specific gravity increases to >1.012, consider stopping the test.

   i. During the seventh hour (between 2 and 3 P.M.), send a second aliquot of urine to the lab for osmolality (U_2) immediately.

   j. Draw another blood specimen for electrolytes and serum osmolality (S_2) immediately.

   k. To end the test: To see whether the patient is sensitive to AVP (Pitressin), give a dose of lypressin (Diapid nasal spray) or desmopressin acetate (DDAVP, 1.25 mg or more—nasal spray or oral form) or aqueous Pitressin. Continue to collect urine samples at half-hour intervals; monitor volume and specific gravity. If no changes occur, send an aliquot to the lab for osmolality (U_3), and redraw serum for electrolytes and osmolality (S_3) for a period of 2 hours.

   l. During this last 2-hour period, the patient can be allowed to drink water in quantities of previous half-hour output.

   m. Interpretation of test results

      (1) Normal:

$$\frac{U_1}{U_1} = 0.4 - 4.9$$

$$\frac{U_2}{U_2} = 0.4 - 4.9$$

(2) DI:

$$\frac{U_1}{S_1} = 0.2 - 0.7$$

$$\frac{U_2}{S_2} = 0.2 - 1.0$$

(3) Pitressin-sensitive:

$$\frac{U_3 \text{ will increase}}{S_3 \text{ will remain unchanged or decrease}} => 1.0$$

(4) Pitressin-resistant (nephrogenic):

$$\frac{U_3 \text{ will remain unchanged}}{S_3 \text{ will remain unchanged or increase}} = 0.2 - 1.0$$

(5) Psychogenic polydipsia:

$\frac{U_1}{S_1}$ may look like DI *but*

$\frac{U_2}{S_2}$ will usually normalize or approach normal

- **n.** ADH levels can be measured at the end of the test but may not be helpful in making the diagnosis.
- **o.** If the DI is caused only by an abnormal osmoreceptor mechanism (normal volume receptor), the water deprivation test may be inconclusive.
- **p.** With severe DI, a 3-hour water deprivation test may be diagnostic with an increase in serum osmolality whereas urine osmolality remains below plasma levels. Then administration of DDAVP (as above) will raise urine osmolality.
- **q.** If patient has primary polydipsia, the urine will concentrate during an 8-hour water deprivation test without DDAVP.

E. Differential diagnosis
1. Psychogenic polydipsia (uncommon in children). After large amounts of water are consumed over extended periods, the medullary interstitial gradient becomes more dilute or washes out. Therefore, the concentrating ability of the kidney decreases, resulting in polyuria.
2. Nephrogenic DI.
3. Diabetes mellitus.
4. Renal tubular acidosis.
5. Sickle cell disease.
6. Defect in thirst (dipsogenic DI, adipsia-hypodipsia—absence or blunting of normal thirst).

F. Treatment. The main treatment is replacement of ADH or enhancement of ADH action, in addition to provision of adequate amounts of water.
1. **DDAVP,** which binds to V_2 receptors, is the drug of choice. It is a synthetic analog with a duration of action of 8 to 24 hours, and it is administered by nasal insufflation (1.25 to 10 μg once or twice daily). Smaller doses (0.15 to 0.5 μg per day) are used for children <2 years old. Tablets are now available for oral ingestion. Begin at 0.1 mg and titrate to 0.2 mg as needed.
2. **Lypressin** (aqueous solution) can also be given by nasal spray (one or two sprays in each nostril, three or four doses per day), but it lasts only 2 to 4 hours.
3. **Pitressin in oil,** given intramuscularly, can last for up to 48 to 72 hours. Begin with 0.2 mL (1 U) and increase by 0.2 mL every 1 to 2 days. The range is 0.5 to 1.0 mL. Remember to mix the solution properly.
4. **Chlorpropamide** can be given in a dose of 150 mg/m^2 once daily. Because many patients have some ADH remaining, this drug increases the effectiveness of

the hormone in the distal nephron. The patient should be monitored for hypoglycemia.

5. Infants should be considered separately. The following is recommended:
   a. Low dietary solute load.
   b. Large water intake if thiazides are given.
   c. A single dose of lypressin can be given at bedtime (recommended by some clinicians).
   d. Nasogastric or gastrostomy tube is recommended if adequate hydration is not maintained orally.

6. Mild, partial DI might require only adequate fluid intake and not pharmacologic therapy.

G. Prognosis. Growth and development should ultimately be normal with hormone replacement and adequate fluid intake.

II. NEPHROGENIC DI

In nephrogenic DI, also known as ADH-resistant DI, the patient is unable to form concentrated urine even after vasopressin administration.

A. Pathogenesis. Abnormalities that affect the collective duct may result in DI. Secondary forms of DI are more common than inherited types and include lithium, hypercalcemia, hypokalemia, polycystic kidney, renal dysplasia, sickle cell anemia, chronic pyelonephritis, sarcoidosis, amyloidosis, and urinary tract obstruction. Target organ unresponsiveness is demonstrated by a failure to increase urinary cyclic adenosine monophosphate (cAMP) after vasopressin infusion. The defect is believed to be limited to the V_2 receptors, which mediate the antidiuretic effects on renal tubules. The V_2 receptor gene is on the X chromosome; therefore, males are severely affected whereas females are asymptomatic carriers. (Females can be affected through an X-chromosomal inactivation mechanism.)

B. Genetics. Inheritance is X-linked recessive; therefore males are severely affected.

C. Clinical features. Symptoms and signs begin within the first 3 weeks of life.
   1. Failure to thrive.
   2. Crying constantly; irritable.
   3. Constipation.
   4. Intermittent fever.
   5. Hypertonic dehydration.
   6. Poor growth, poor school performance, and bladder and ureter dilatation in older children. Early recognition and management can prevent hyperosmolality, which in turn can prevent the delayed mental and physical development.
   7. Neurologic impairment if not adequately treated.

D. Diagnosis
   1. Hypernatremia; elevated serum osmolality.
   2. Failure to thrive.
   3. Normal kidney function.
   4. Failure to respond to vasopressin after water deprivation test (i.e., no increase in urine osmolality). (Avoid hypertonic saline infusion test because it may cause or aggravate severe hypernatremia.)
   5. Serum ADH is elevated.
   6. Absent urinary cAMP response after vasopressin administration.
   7. Identify carrier mothers by measuring urine osmolality after a 12-hour period of fluid restriction.

E. Treatment. The general goal is to reduce urine volume and prevent hypertonic dehydration.
   1. Frequent feedings.
   2. Restrict solute such as protein and salt. (Breast milk is preferred to formula because it has a lower osmolar load.) Restrict sodium intake to reduce obligatory water loss by the kidney.
   3. Diuretics such as thiazides, furosemide, ethacrynic acid, and spironolactone all promote sodium excretion but may cause hypokalemia.
      a. Chlorothiazide, 30 mg/kg in three divided doses per day (or 1.0 g/m^2 per day).

b. Hydrochlorothiazide, 3 mg/kg in three divided doses daily (0.1 g/m^2 per day).

c. Recently, the combination of hydrochlorothiazide (2 mg/kg per 24 hours) and amiloride (20 mg/1.73 m^2 per 24 hours; potassium-sparing diuretic) has been shown to be effective therapy for congenital nephrogenic DI, obviating the need for potassium supplements with only minor long-term side effects. The antidiuretic effects of both drugs appear to be additive.

III. SIADH

An inappropriate amount of ADH is produced or released in this syndrome of unknown etiology.

A. Underlying causes

1. Pulmonary (pneumonia, tuberculosis) and cerebral disorders (infection, hemorrhage, trauma) are the most common causes in children.

2. Tumors as a cause are much less common in children than adults.

3. Neonates utilizing mechanical positive-pressure breathing assistance.

4. In some leukemic patients treated with vincristine and cyclophosphamide (Cytoxan).

5. Additional drugs, such as chlorpropamide, some analgesics, and barbiturates.

6. Additional disorders include cardiac disease, severe hypothyroidism, and Addison disease.

B. Symptoms.
Symptoms include weakness, lethargy, and confusion. If water intoxication occurs, vomiting, irritability, and change in personality may follow. If sodium concentration is <110 mEq/L, seizures and coma may occur.

C. Diagnosis

1. Hyponatremia (low serum osmolality).

2. Hypertonic urine compared to plasma (high urine osmolality, 250 to 1 400 mOsm/kg).

3. Normal kidney and adrenal function.

4. Continuous urinary sodium loss even though hyponatremic; urine sodium concentration is usually >30 mEq/L.

5. Elevated serum ADH levels in some cases.

6. Low uric acid levels.

7. Low urine volume.

D. Treatment

1. Fluid restriction.

2. If no improvement, *slowly* administer sodium chloride solution 1.5% to 3% (5 mL/kg) plus furosemide.

3. Treatment of specific causes—e.g., eliminate offending drug or infection.

4. Demeclocycline (blocks the action of AVP on the collecting ducts) and lithium salts are not recommended in children.

IV. HYPEROSMOLAR SYNDROME

A defect in osmoreceptor function results in hypernatremia and serum hyperosmolality.

A. Clinical.
There is a susceptibility to severe dehydration and hyperosmolar coma because the defective thirst mechanism does not stimulate water intake when large urine volume exists with DI.

B. Treatment

1. Adequate fluids

2. Chlorpropamide

PITUITARY HYPERSECRETION

Clinically relevant pituitary hypersecretion is rarely observed in pediatrics. Additional details of these disorders can be found in other chapters.

I. MCCUNE ALBRIGHT SYNDROME (MAS)

MAS is a very rare condition caused by activating mutations of the *GNAS1* gene that codes for the α subunit of $G_s\alpha$, a guanine nucleotide-binding protein (G protein). In relation to activating mutations, *GNAS1* is sometimes referred to as the *gsp* oncogene. The basic features of MAS are polyostotic fibrous dysplasia of bone, café-au-lait hyperpigmented skin spots in a distinct distribution, and hormone hypersecretion. Within the pituitary gland, hyperactivity of the G-protein–coupled receptor for GHRH has been observed in ~20% of MAS patients, resulting in GH hypersecretion and crossover effects, leading to elevated TSH and PRL secretion. The increased growth rate resulting from GH hypersecretion can compensate for the loss of height potential resulting from gonadotropin-independent precocious puberty. Although the pituitary GnRH receptor is also G-protein–coupled, the clinical relevance is unclear because the precocious puberty in MAS is gonadotropin-independent (gonadal steroid production may inhibit FSH and LH hypersecretion).

II. MULTIPLE ENDOCRINE NEOPLASIA TYPE I (MEN I, WERMER SYNDROME)

MEN1 is due to mutation of the *MEN1* gene (chromosome 11q13). MEN I has been associated with pituitary adenomas that hypersecrete GH, TSH, ACTH, PRL, FSH and *a* subunit, as well as extrapituitary secretory adenomas. However, although MEN I is a genetic condition, pituitary adenomas associated with this condition rarely present in the pediatric age group.

III. PITUITARY GIGANTISM

The clinical condition caused by excess GH secretion is termed acromegaly in adults and pituitary gigantism in pediatric populations. Pituitary gigantism is extremely rare, with only a handful of published cases. GH hypersecretion associated with MAS is not usually clinically defined as pituitary gigantism per se. However, *GNAS1* mutations have been identified in GH-secreting adenomas in adults and children. In addition, GH-secreting adenomas may occur in MEN I. However, most cases of pituitary gigantism are caused by GH-secreting adenomas for which genetic defects have not been identified. The diagnosis should be suspected in children with inappropriately rapid height growth for age, especially in the presence of visual or other neurologic signs and symptoms. Cases may also present with diabetes mellitus, with or without ketosis. GH and IGF-I levels are elevated, but these results should be interpreted with caution in adolescents because these levels can be in the acromegalic range during normal puberty. Secretion of other pituitary hormones may be low if there is significant mass effect of the adenoma. Neuroimaging is a key diagnostic tool, although rare cases may be due to ectopic production of GHRH or GH. Neurosurgical debulking and stereotactic radiotherapy are standard first-line therapies. Dopamine agonists (e.g., bromocriptine, cabergoline), octreotide or pegvisomant, and metformin and insulin for the associated diabetes mellitus, may be effective in some cases, although pediatric experience is very limited. This topic is discussed further in Chapter 4.

IV. HYPERPROLACTINEMIA

Pediatric hyperprolactinemia is most often due to a pituitary micro- or macroadenoma, i.e., a prolactinoma. A genetic association has not been identified. In some cases, the prolactinoma itself may cause a mass effect, suppressing secretion of other pituitary hormones and causing visual and neurologic symptoms. In pubertal girls, hyperprolactinemia has been associated with amenorrhea, menstrual irregularity, and galactorrhea; specific symptomatology has not been reported in adolescent boys except, perhaps, galactorrhea. Diagnosis depends on measurement of high PRL levels (e.g., >100 to 200 ng/mL), clinical signs and symptoms, and neuroimaging. Treatment with dopamine agonists, especially cabergoline, may normalize prolactin levels and reduce prolactinoma size. However, neurosurgical intervention may be preferable in cases of macroadenoma, particularly with evidence of optic nerve compression.

Hyperprolactinemia has also been reported with pharmaceutical agents, especially risperidone, an atypical antipsychotic. Treatment with risperidone has been associated with pituitary prolactin hypersecretion and galactorrhea in adolescents of both sexes. Hyperprolactinemia is discussed further in Chapter 10.

V. CUSHING DISEASE

Cushing disease is very rare in pediatrics, with peak occurrence at ~14 years of age; however, it is more common than primary adrenal causes of Cushing syndrome. Nearly all pediatric cases of Cushing disease are caused by ACTH-secreting pituitary microadenomas. The classic presentation of pediatric Cushing syndrome is decreased growth rate and short stature in the presence of inappropriate weight gain. Other typical signs and symptoms are cushingoid facies, hypertension, emotional lability, and unusual fatigue. Diagnosis depends on demonstration of elevated serum and/or urine cortisol in the presence of inappropriately normal or elevated baseline or CRF-stimulated plasma ACTH. MRI and bilateral inferior petrosal sinus sampling are usually performed to confirm the location of the microadenoma. Optimal therapy consists of transsphenoidal pituitary microadenomectomy, followed by pituitary radiotherapy if cortisol levels remain elevated and/or ACTH levels are detectable. Posttherapy hypopituitarism may occur.

VI. TSH HYPERSECRETION

TSH-secreting adenomas are extremely rare in pediatrics. The total published experience in patients <18 years of age is fewer than five cases.

VII. SIADH

See section on SIADH.

VIII. ECTOPIC HORMONES

Ectopic production of hormones that affect pituitary hormone synthesis, e.g., CRF, GHRH, GnRH, is extremely rare in pediatrics.

IX. HORMONE-PRODUCING BRAIN TUMORS IN CHILDREN

- **A. GH-producing tumors** (see Chapter 4)
    1. Gigantism
    2. Acromegaly
- **B. Chromophobe adenomas (rare in children)**
    1. TSH-secreting tumors
    2. FSH-secreting tumors
- **C. Prolactin-secreting adenoma** (see Chapters 4 and 10, and Section IV, Hyperprolactinemia, in this chapter). Patients commonly present with headache, amenorrhea, and galactorrhea. High levels of prolactin can interfere with release of FSH and LH, resulting in hypogonadism.
- **D. Hamartomas.** Hypothalamic hamartomas that secrete GnRH can cause precocious puberty.
- **E. ACTH-secreting pituitary adenomas** (see Chapter 4)
- **F. Pinealomas**

TALL STATURE

In recent years, tall stature has been less of a problem for the endocrinologist because this somatic characteristic has become "culturally advantageous."

- **I. ETIOLOGY.** Tall stature most commonly is constitutional or familial. Other causes include:
- **A. GH-secreting tumors.**
- **B. Marfan syndrome,** which is an inherited disorder characterized by tall stature, thin extremities, malformed eyes and ears, hypotonia, kyphoscoliosis, cardiac valvular deformities, and medionecrosis of the aorta. No specific treatment is available.
- **C. Homocystinuria.**
- **D. Cerebral gigantism (Soto syndrome).** This disorder is characterized by tall stature, prominent forehead, hypertelorism, high-arched palate, large irregular head, antimongoloid slant of the palpebral fissures, mental retardation, and advanced bone age. Endocrine tests are normal.
- **E. Beckwith-Wiedemann syndrome** (omphalocele, macrosomia, macroglossia, hypoglycemia secondary to pancreatic β-cell hyperplasia). This is one of a group of

"overgrowth syndromes" caused by excess of insulinlike growth factor II (IGF-II), encoded by the gene *IGF2*. These children are predisposed to Wilms tumor and carcinoma of the adrenal gland.

F. Untreated prepubertal congenital adrenal hyperplasia (CAH).

G. Klinefelter syndrome (XXY syndrome) includes mental retardation, tall stature, gynecomastia, and small testes.

H. Obesity.

I. Precocious secretion of estrogens or androgens.

II. EVALUATION. Although many causes of tall stature are obvious on clinical inspection, the following tests may be helpful in diagnosis or confirmation.

  A. Screening tests include IGF-I and IGF-binding factor-3 (IGFBP-3), which will be elevated in gigantism.

  B. GH levels are generally elevated in gigantism, but the disorder is verified with a glucose suppression test (i.e., no suppression of GH).

  C. Bone age (all disorders).

  D. Amino acid screen (homocystinuria).

  E. Chromosomes (Klinefelter syndrome).

  F. 17-Hydroxyprogesterone (17-OHP) (CAH).

  G. Glucose (hypoglycemia in Beckwith-Wiedemann syndrome).

  H. Androgens or estrogens (precocious puberty).

III. TREATMENT OF TALL STATURE (see Chapter 21)

Initially these children are taller because of hormone-stimulated advancement of bone age. However, without treatment, early closure of the epiphyses occurs and the ultimate stature is less than it would have been under normal circumstances.

  A. GnRH analogs (treatment of choice for true precocious puberty). The analogs "desensitize" the gonadotropic cells of the pituitary to the stimulatory effect of endogenous GnRH, thus stopping the progression of central sexual precocity. Leuprolide acetate (Lupron Depot) is the only approved Depot preparation in the United States that is given once a month at a dose of 0.25 to 0.3 mg/kg. I usually begin at a dose of 7.5 mg, increasing it every 4 weeks as needed based on clinical, chemical, and radiologic assessment to a maximum of 15 mg. Other long-acting preparations, such as triptorelin (Decapeptyl) and goserelin (Zoladex), are approved for management of precocious puberty in other countries.

  Treatment results in a reduction of both growth rate and bone age advancement. Menses does not begin while the girl is on the medication, and breast size may diminish. Testicular size decreases in boys. Puberty resumes promptly when the analogs are discontinued.

  GnRH analogs are as effective in idiopathic sexual precocity as in children with organic brain lesions. Thus, neurosurgical intervention is not indicated for hypothalamic hamartomas initially, except for associated intractable seizures.

  B. Cyproterone acetate.

  C. Medroxyprogesterone stops menses but does not retard bone age.

  D. Testolactone stops estrogen production from ovarian cysts with cessation of puberty. However, treatment is given four times a day and is not always effective.

  E. Spironolactone

  F. Ketoconazole has been used in boys with gonadotropin-independent precocious puberty by blocking gonadal steroidogenesis. Testotoxicosis, like McCune-Albright syndrome, results from a mutation in testicular Leydig cells. This treatment results in cessation of menses, regression of secondary sexual characteristics, lowering of estrogen levels, and slowing of bone age advancement, but it does not stop the development of ovarian cysts. The dose is 200 mg three times a day. Long-term therapy has not been studied. Side effects include pruritus and, very rarely, liver toxicity.

 SUMMARY

Table 6.1 summarizes the pediatric pituitary disorders described in this chapter.

TABLE 6.1 Pediatric Pituitary Disorders

	Gene locus	GH +/− others	GH	TSH	LH and/or FSH	PRL	ACTH	ADH	Other key features
Hypopituitarism									
Genetic: embryogenesis									
HESX1	3p21.2-p21.1	X							Some cases of septo-optic dysplasia, neonatal hypopituitarism and IGHD
SOX2	3q26.3-q27		X		X				An- or micro-ophthalmia, some cases of septo-optic dysplasia
SOX3	Xq27.1	X							Males; some cases of septo-optic dysplasia
PITX1	5q31	X							Human condition not yet defined
PITX2	4q25-27	X							Rieger syndrome
LHX3	9q34.3	X							Except ACTH; nuchal rigidity
LHX4	1q25.2	X							Cerebellar and sellar defects
PROP1	5q35.3	X							
PIT1 (POU1F1)	3p11	X							Low PRL
TPIT (TBX19)	1q23-24						X		
DAX1	Xp21.3-p21.2				X				Males; congenital adrenal hypoplasia
KAL1	Xp22.32				X				Males; Kallmann syndrome with an/hyposmia
KAL2 (FGFR1)	8p11.2-p11.1				X				Kallmann syndrome with an/hyposmia
KISS1	1q32				X				Hypothalamic gene
GPR54 (KISS1R)	19p13				X				
WFS1	4p16		X						Wolfram syndrome (DIDMOAD)
GNAS1	20q13.3				X			X	Pseudohypoparathyroidism

(*continued*)

TABLE 6.1 Pediatric Pituitary Disorders (*Continued*)

	Gene locus	Typically affected pituitary hormones							Other key features
		GH +/− others	GH	TSH	LH and/or FSH	PRL	ACTH	ADH	
Genetic: hormones and receptors									
GH1	17q24.2	X							Some cases of IGHD types 1a, 1b, 2
GHRHR	7p14	X							Some cases of IGHD 1b
FSHB	11p14				X				
LHB	19q13.32				X				
GNRHR	4q21.2				X				Without an/hyposmia
TRHR	8q23			X					
Congenital conditions and syndromes									
Neonatal hypopituitarism		X							
Craniospinal malformations		X							
Empty sella		X							
Septo-optic dysplasia		X							Optic-nerve hypoplasia, midline craniofacial and brain defects
IGHD types 1a, 1b, 2, 3			X						Genetic defects identified in some cases within various types
Other syndromes		X							See text

Condition	Gene, locus							Comment
Tumors, mass and infiltrative lesions								
Craniopharyngioma		X						
Rathke's cleft cyst		X						
Other CNS lesions		X						See text
Neurofibromatosis type 1	*NF1*, 17q11.2	X						
Hyper-TSH			X					
Langerhans cell histiocytosis				X				Seborrheic rash, exophthalmos
Lymphocytic hypophysitis								See Autoimmune
Other acquired (noncongenital)								
Iatrogenic		X						Radiotherapy, chemotherapy, surgery
Head trauma		X						Open or closed, direct or indirect injury
APS1 (APECED, AIRE)	*AIRE*, 21q22.3	X	X	X				Lymphocytic hypophysitis
APS2, 3, 4		X	X					See text
Other autoimmune		X	X					See text
Pharmacologic			X	X				
Pituitary Hypersecretion								
McCune Albright Syndrome	*GNAS1*, 20q13.3	X	X	X				Activating mutation
MEN Type 1	*MEN1*, 11p13	x	X	?	X	X		Pituitary adenomas usually present in adulthood
Pituitary gigantism		X		X				Usually due to GH-secreting adenoma
Hyperprolactinemia					X	X		Usually due to PRL-secreting adenoma
Precocious puberty				X			X	Usually idiopathic
Cushing disease		X						
SIADH							X	
Ectopic hormones		X	X	X				See text

Selected References

Acerini CL, Tasker RC. Traumatic brain injury induced hypothalamic-pituitary dysfunction—a paediatric perspective. *Pituitary* 2007;10(4):373–380.

Akintoye SO, Chebli C, Booher S, et al. Characterization of *gsp*-mediated growth hormone excess in the context of McCune-Albright syndrome. *J Clin Endocrinol Metab* 2002;87:5104–5112.

Ali O, Banerjee S, Kelly DF, Lee PDK. Management of type 2 diabetes mellitus associated with pituitary gigantism. *Pituitary* 2007;10(4):359–364.

Carillo AA, Bao Y. Hormonal dynamic tests and genetics tests used in pediatric endocrinology. In: Lifshitz F, ed. *Pediatric endocrinology*. Vol 2. 5th ed. New York: Informa Healthcare; 2007:737–767.

Cheetham T, Baylis PH. Diabetes insipidus in children: pathophysiology, diagnosis and management. *Paediatr Drugs* 2002;4:785–796.

Cheung CC, Lustig RH. Pituitary development and physiology. *Pituitary* 2007;10(4):335–350.

Ching J, Lee PDK. Brief review and commentary: diagnosis of pediatric pituitary disorders. *Pituitary* 2007;10(4):327–333.

Eisenbarth GS, Gottlieb PA. Autoimmune polyendocrine syndromes. *N Engl J Med* 2004;351:2068–2079.

Gleeson HK, Shalet SM. The impact of cancer therapy on the endocrine system in survivors of childhood brain tumors. *Endocrine-Related Cancer* 2004;11:589–602.

Hernández LM, Lee PDK, Camacho-Hübner C. Isolated growth hormone deficiency. *Pituitary* 2007;10(4):351–357.

Hoover KB, Rosenthal DI, Mankin H. Langerhans cell histiocytosis. *Skeletal Radiol* 2007;36:95–104.

Jagannathan J, Dumont AS, Jane JA Jr. Diagnosis and management of pediatric sellar lesions. *Front Horm Res* 2007;91:2520–2525.

Kaplan SA. The pituitary gland: a brief history. *Pituitary* 2007;10(4):323–325.

Karavitaki N, Cudlip S, Adams CBT, Wass JAH. Craniopharyngiomas. *Endocrine Rev* 2006;27:371–397.

Kelberman D, Dattani MT. Genetics of septo-optic dysplasia. *Pituitary* 2007;10(4):393–407.

Magiakou MA, Chrousos GP. Cushing's syndrome in children and adolescents: current diagnostic and therapeutic strategies. *J Endocrinol Invest* 2002;25:181–194.

Mantovani G, Spada A. Mutations in the Gs alpha gene causing hormone resistance. *Best Pract Res Clin Endocrinol Metab* 2006;20:501–513.

Mathis D, Benoist C. A decade of AIRE. *Nat Rev Immunol* 2007;7:645–650.

Monzavi R, Kelly DF, Geffner ME: Rathke's cleft cyst in 2 girls with precocious puberty. *J Pediatr Endocrinol Metabol* 2004;17:781–785.

Mullis PE. Genetics of growth hormone deficiency. *Endocrinol Metab Clin North Am* 2007;36:17–36.

Naing S, Frohman LA. The empty sella. *Pediatr Endocrinol Rev* 2007;4:335–342.

Phillips JA III. Genetics of growth retardation. *J Pediatr Endocrinol Metab* 2004;17(suppl 3):385–399.

Ranke MB, ed. *Diagnostics of endocrine function in children and adolescents*. Basel: Karger, 2003.

Savage MO, Storr HL, Chan LF, Grossman AB. Diagnosis and treatment of pediatric Cushing's disease. *Pituitary* 2007;10(4):365–371.

Scully KM, Rosenfeld MG. Pituitary development: regulatory codes in mammalian organogenesis. *Science* 2002;295:22331–2235.

Trarbach EB, Silveira LG, Latronico AC. Genetic insights into human isolated gonadotropin deficiency. *Pituitary* 2007;10(4):381–391.

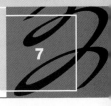

THE PITUITARY GLAND AND GROWTH FAILURE   7
Omar Ali and Pinchas Cohen

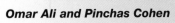

I. **GENERAL PRINCIPLES.** Evaluation and management of growth failure is one of the most common reasons for referral to a pediatric endocrinologist. As in any medical evaluation, thorough history and physical examination will guide the physician in selecting appropriate laboratory tests. We will briefly review the endocrine regulation of growth and the causes of short stature, and then outline the process of evaluating and treating the child who presents with growth failure.

II. **ENDOCRINE REGULATION OF GROWTH**

A. **Growth hormone (GH)** is a 191-amino-acid (22-kDa) protein elaborated by specific somatotropes in the pituitary gland (Fig. 7.1). GH is homologous with some other proteins produced by the pituitary and the placenta, including prolactin, chorionic somatomammotropin (CS; placental lactogen), and a 22-kDa GH variant (hGH-V) secreted only by the placenta. GH is released by the pituitary in a pulsatile fashion that reflects the interplay of multiple regulators including two hypothalamic regulatory peptides: **GH-releasing hormone (GHRH)** and **somatostatin (somatotropin release–inhibiting factor (SRIF).** A third regulatory hormone, **Ghrelin,** is a 28-amino-acid peptide that is secreted in small amounts by the hypothalamus and in much larger amounts by the stomach. The GHRH receptor is a member of the G-protein–coupled receptor family B, also called the secretin family, and has partial sequence identity with receptors for vasoactive intestinal polypeptide, secretin, calcitonin, and parathyroid hormone. Solid tumors that secrete GHRH are a rare cause of GH excess. Ghrelin acts via a separate receptor named the growth hormone secretagogue receptor (GHS-R), and genetic defects in this receptor have been implicated as a cause of some cases of idiopathic short stature.

1. Multiple neurotransmitters and neuropeptides are also involved in the regulation of GH secretion, mostly via hypothalamic pathways. These factors are implicated in the alterations of GH secretion observed in a wide variety of physiologic states, such as stress, sleep, hemorrhage, fasting, hypoglycemia, and exercise, and form the basis for a number of GH-stimulatory tests employed in the evaluation of GH secretory capacity/reserve.

GH secretion is also affected by a variety of nonpeptide hormones, being augmented by androgens, estrogens, and thyroxine, and being suppressed by glucocorticoids.

Once it is secreted into the serum, GH binds to a specific GH-binding protein (GHBP), which is formed by proteolytic cleavage of the extracellular portion of the GH receptor. The Growth hormone receptor is a member of the cytokine receptor family, and activation of the receptor by GH leads to receptor dimerization, followed by intracellular activation of a Janus kinase (JAK2) and other kinases and downstream pathways that then signal to various target genes.

2. Growth hormone has a variety of anabolic and metabolic actions, including stimulation of bone growth, muscle mass, and lipolysis. Some of these effects are due to the direct action of GH on target tissues, but a significant proportion of the anabolic and growth stimulating effects are mediated through another set of hormones called **the insulinlike growth factors (IGFs).**

B. **IGFs** are elaborated under GH control in the liver (which is the primary source of circulating IGFs) as well as other tissues and have growth-promoting actions on

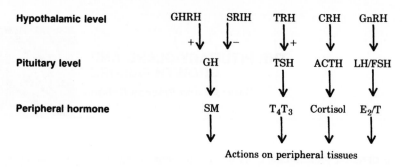

Figure 7.1. Pituitary hormone control and action. ACTH, adrenocorticotropic hormone; CRH, corticotropin-releasing hormone; E2, estradiol; FSH, follicle-stimulating hormone; GH, growth hormone; GHRH, growth-hormone–releasing hormone; GnRH, gonadotropin-releasing hormone; LH, luteinizing hormone; SM, somatomedin; SRIH, somatotropin release–inhibiting hormone (somatostatin); T, testosterone; TRH, thyrotropin-releasing hormone; TSH, thyroid-stimulating hormone; T3, tri-iodothyronine; T4, thyroxine.

a wide variety of target tissues, particularly cartilage and bone. Two major IGFs have been isolated. **IGF-I** is a 70-amino-acid single-chain peptide that is >40% homologous to proinsulin. The other major IGF peptide in human serum is **IGF-II**. This peptide is also homologous to proinsulin and is closely structurally related to IGF-I. Although both IGF hormones have growth-promoting action and coexist in human serum bound to IGF-binding proteins, they have markedly different receptor specificities and presumably fulfill different biologic functions. In addition to stimulating the growth of tissues throughout the body, the IGF peptides, along with GH itself, feed back on the hypothalamus and pituitary gland to control the release of GHRH and somatostatin and the release of GH from the pituitary somatotropes. IGF-1 levels appear to be more closely regulated by GH than IGF-2 levels, and measurements of IGF-1 are a useful indicator of GH activity, though it should be kept in mind that other factors such as nutritional status can affect IGF production. Figure 7.2 shows the mean levels of IGF-1 for boys and girls.

The IGFs bind to a family of **IGF-binding proteins** (IGFBP1 through IGFBP6) that have a wide distribution in various tissues and body fluids. **IGFBP-3** is the most abundant of these binding proteins in postnatal human serum, where it circulates in a ternary complex that consists of IGF, IGFBP-3, and a third protein named **acid-labile subunit (ALS)**. The serum levels of IGFBP-3 are positively regulated by GH, and measurements of this protein are also used as an index of GH activity.

III. NORMAL GROWTH

In humans, linear growth is most rapid in prenatal life, when the embryo grows from a single cell to an average neonatal length of 50 cm in 9 months. This phase of growth is relatively independent of growth-hormone secretion and is minimally affected by hypopituitarism. Instead, size at birth is regulated primarily by maternal and placental factors. After birth, the newborn shifts to a growth rate that is regulated by its own genetic potential and physiologic milieu. Linear growth averages 25 cm in the first year of life, 10 cm in the second, and 7.5 cm in the third. Between the ages of 3 years and the onset of puberty, the minimum annual growth rate is about 5 cm per year, and any child who grows <5 cm in a year deserves an evaluation. Puberty leads to an acceleration of growth in both sexes, with girls entering puberty an average of 2 years before boys and growing an average of 3 cm less during their height spurt. This accounts for the average 13-cm difference in final adult heights between the two sexes.

IV. MEASUREMENT

Accurate measurement is essential in the evaluation of the short child. When feasible, measurement of supine length is employed in children <2 years of age, and erect height

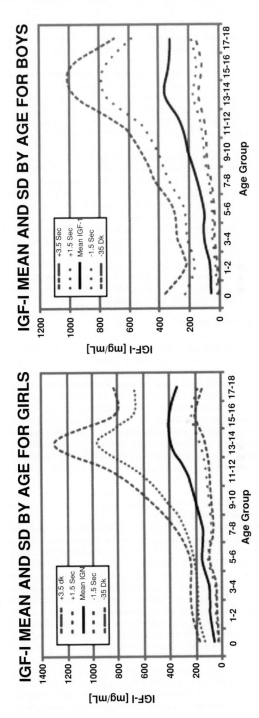

Figure 7.2. IGF-I mean and standard deviation (SD) by age for girls and boys.

is measured in older children. For measurement of supine length, it is best to employ a firm box with an inflexible board against which the head lies and a movable footboard on which the feet are placed perpendicular to the plane of the supine infant. Optimally, the child needs to be relaxed, with the legs fully extended and the head positioned in the Frankfurt plane, with the line connecting the outer canthus of the eyes and the external auditory meatus perpendicular to the long axis of the trunk.

When children are old enough to stand erect (and physically capable of doing so), it is best to employ a wall-mounted Harpenden stadiometer. The patient should be fully erect, with the head in the Frankfurt plane; the back of the head, thoracic spine, buttocks, and heels should be touching the vertical axis of the stadiometer and one another.

Measurement of arm span and sitting height is also important in the evaluation of short stature and should be part of the evaluation of any short child. Height, weight, head circumference (in infants), and height velocity (in children over age 2 years) should then be plotted on standard growth charts. It is also helpful to mark the parents' heights and the <u>mid-parental height</u> (MPH, calculated by adding the height of the parents, subtracting 13 cm in girls and adding 13 cm in boys, and then dividing by 2) on the growth chart so that the child's height can be compared to his or her genetic potential. Two standard deviations (SD) from the mid-parental height are about 9 cm on either side of the MPH, and 95% of children can be expected to fall within this range as adults. Children who are below the 3rd percentile on the growth chart or who are greater than 2 SD below the mid-parental height have short stature and deserve an evaluation. Disease-specific growth charts are available for children with Down syndrome, Turner syndrome, and achondroplasia.

V. CAUSES OF SHORT STATURE
A. Normal variants
1. **Familial short stature.** Children of short parents are likely to be short. Such children typically track along a short growth channel, with normal height velocity, normal body proportions, normal laboratory tests, and normal bone age. Because some pathologic causes of short stature are also familial, an evaluation may still be justified in children who are well below the normal growth charts, even if their growth is consistent with their midparental height.
2. **Constitutional growth delay.** These children are "late bloomers," characterized by short stature, with relatively normal growth rates during childhood, delayed puberty, a delayed pubertal growth spurt, and attainment of normal adult height. Most patients with constitutional delay begin to deviate from the normal growth curve during the early years of life and, typically by age 2 years, are at or slightly below the 5th percentile for height. Such children would be expected to have normal serum IGF-1 and IGFBP-3 concentrations, a normal result of a GH provocative test, and bone age sufficiently delayed to result in normal predicted adult heights.

B. Nutritional Deprivation.
Given the worldwide presence of undernutrition, it is not surprising that inadequate caloric and/or protein intake represents by far the most common cause of growth failure worldwide. **Marasmus** refers to cases with a global deficiency of calories, although often accompanied by protein insufficiency. **Kwashiorkor,** on the other hand, refers to inadequate protein intake, although it may also be characterized by caloric undernutrition. Frequently, the two conditions overlap. The impaired growth characteristic of protein-energy malnutrition is frequently characterized by elevated basal and/or stimulated serum GH concentrations. In generalized malnutrition (marasmus), however, GH concentrations may be normal or even low. In both conditions, nevertheless, serum IGF-1 concentrations are, typically, reduced, indicating some degree of growth-hormone insensitivity.
1. Inadequate caloric or protein intake may also complicate many chronic diseases that are characterized by growth failure, e.g., renal failure, inflammatory bowel disease, cyanotic heart disease, congestive heart failure, central nervous system (CNS) disease, and other illnesses. Some of these conditions may, furthermore,

be characterized by deficiencies of specific dietary components, such as zinc, iron, and various vitamins necessary for normal growth and development.

2. Undernutrition may also be voluntary, as is the case with dieting and food fads. Caloric restriction is especially common in girls during adolescence, as well as in gymnasts and ballet dancers. **Anorexia nervosa** and **bulimia** represent extremes of "voluntary" caloric deprivation and are commonly associated with impaired growth if undernutrition occurs before epiphyseal fusion. Treatment of attention-deficit hyperactivity disorder (ADHD) with stimulant medications is also associated with decreased appetite and possible growth delay (though final adult height is usually normal).

C. **Psychosocial dwarfism.** In psychosocial dwarfism, extreme emotional deprivation is associated with a severe form of failure to thrive. GH secretion is suppressed, but the neuroendocrinologic mechanisms involved have yet to be elucidated. Removal from the harmful environment usually leads to a rapid resolution of growth failure.

D. **Intrauterine growth retardation or small for gestational age (SGA).** About 10% of children born SGA fail to reach normal growth percentiles by 2 years of age. Several studies indicate that GH treatment can lead to improved growth in these children, though these studies are hampered by the inherent heterogeneity of this group of patients, whose poor growth may reflect maternal factors, chromosomal disorders, dysmorphic syndromes, toxins, and so on. These studies have led to the approval of GH treatment for children born SGA who exhibit persistent growth failure. The doses commonly used in SGA children are between 50 and 70 μg/kg per day, and treatment is typically started at age 3 years.

E. **Systemic diseases**

1. **Malabsorption.** Intestinal disorders associated with inadequate absorption of calories or proteins are, typically, associated with growth failure. Accordingly, such conditions, especially gluten-induced enteropathy (celiac disease) and regional enteritis (Crohn disease) must be in the differential diagnosis of unexplained growth failure. Serum concentrations of IGF-1 may be reduced, reflecting the malnutrition.

2. **Cardiovascular disease.** Both cyanotic heart disease and congestive heart failure may be associated with growth failure. Because cardiac defects are usually congenital, many infants have syndromes associated with dysmorphic features and intrauterine growth retardation (IUGR).

3. **Renal disease.** A wide variety of clinical conditions that affect renal function can result in significant growth retardation. Uremia, Fanconi syndrome, and renal tubular acidosis can lead to growth failure before other clinical manifestations become evident. The use of chronic glucocorticoid therapy in the treatment of a variety of nephritic and nephrotic conditions can exacerbate the growth-retardation characteristic of renal disease. Although the growth failure of renal disease is not caused by either GH or IGF deficiency, GH therapy has proven useful in accelerating skeletal growth.

4. **Hematologic disorders.** Chronic anemias, such as sickle cell disease, are characterized by growth failure. Thalassemia, in addition to the consequences of chronic anemia, can also be characterized by endocrine deficiencies resulting from chronic transfusions and accompanying hemosiderosis.

5. **Diabetes mellitus.** Growth failure can be observed in children whose diabetes is under chronically poor control. The so-called **Mauriac syndrome** describes children with diabetes mellitus, severe growth failure, and hepatomegaly resulting from excess hepatic glycogen deposition. This kind of striking growth retardation is unusual in diabetes; and growth failure, in general, is modest.

6. **Inborn errors of metabolism.** Inborn errors of protein, carbohydrate, and lipid metabolism are often accompanied by growth failure, which can be pronounced. Glycogen storage disease, the mucopolysaccharidoses, glycoproteinoses, and mucolipidoses may all be characterized by poor growth. Many inborn metabolic disorders are also associated with significant skeletal dysplasia.

7. **Pulmonary disease.** Cystic fibrosis is the classic example of growth failure associated with pulmonary disease, although poor growth undoubtedly represents

the combined effects of pulmonary and pancreatic dysfunction. Additionally, the appearance of diabetes, the use of steroids, and the presence of frequent infections all contribute to the poor growth in cystic fibrosis. Any condition associated with chronic hypoxemia may result in growth retardation. In children with chronic asthma, the long-term use of glucocorticoids contributes significantly to growth failure.

8. **Chronic infection.** In many developing countries, chronic infestation with intestinal and systemic parasites, such as schistosomiasis, hookworm, and roundworm, contribute to nutritional debilitation and growth failure. Chronic immunodeficiency is also associated with growth failure.

F. **Genetic syndromes.** A large number of genetic syndromes are associated with short stature. Some of the more important ones include the following.

1. **Turner syndrome (TS).** Short stature is the single most common feature of Turner syndrome, occurring more frequently than delayed puberty, cubitus valgus, or webbing of the neck. Mean adult heights in untreated TS range from 142.0 to 146.8 cm The cause of growth failure in Turner syndrome is multifactorial, although the loss of one copy of the homeobox gene, *SHOX* (short stature homeobox-containing gene), is the major contributor. Additionally, **SHOX mutations** appear to be responsible for the mesomelic growth retardation and Madelung deformity characteristic of Leri-Weil dyschondrosteosis, and complete absence of *SHOX* is associated with Langer mesomelic dysplasia. The majority of patients with these disorders have normal GH levels during childhood. Nevertheless, GH therapy is capable of both accelerating short-term growth and increasing adult height in both Turner syndrome and SHOX haploinsufficiency. Early initiation of GH treatment should allow for normalization of growth in childhood, as well as the potential to begin estrogen replacement at a physiologically appropriate age. Treatment of Turner syndrome is discussed in detail in Chapter 21.

2. **Down syndrome.** The encouraging results of GH trials in Turner syndrome have led to studies of GH in other chromosomal disorders, such as Down syndrome. Several preliminary studies have confirmed the ability of GH to accelerate growth in such patients, although ethical issues have been raised concerning the appropriateness of such therapy. No convincing data exist that GH improves neurologic or intellectual function in such patients.

3. **Prader-Willi syndrome.** GH has been shown to improve linear growth in children with Prader-Willi syndrome in several studies. GH treatment also resulted in a reduction of relative fat mass and an increase in fat-free mass. The U.S. Food and Drug Administration (FDA) has recognized Prader-Willi syndrome as an accepted diagnosis for GH therapy, even in the absence of demonstrable GH deficiency.

4. **Russell-Silver syndrome.** Although this syndrome probably represents a heterogeneous group of patients, the "common" findings include IUGR, postnatal growth failure, congenital hemihypertrophy, and small, triangular facies. Other common, nonspecific findings include clinodactyly, precocious puberty, delayed closure of the fontanelles, and delayed bone age. Recently, it has been demonstrated that hypermethylation (termed epimutation) of the IGF2 gene leading to its decreased expression is associated with the majority of cases of this condition.

G. **Osteochondrodysplasias.** These are a heterogeneous group of disorders characterized by intrinsic abnormalities of cartilage and/or bone that share the following features: (1) genetic transmission; (2) abnormalities in the size and/or shape of bones of the limbs, spine, and/or skull; and (3) radiologic abnormalities of the bones (generally). Over 100 osteochondrodysplastic conditions have been identified, based on physical features and radiologic characteristics. Two of the more common forms (achondroplasia and hypochondroplasia) are discussed next.

1. **Achondroplasia.** This is the most common of the osteochondrodysplasias, with a frequency of ~1 in 26 000. Although it is transmitted as an autosomal dominant disorder, 90% of cases apparently represent new mutations. It is caused by a mutation of the gene for fibroblast growth factor receptor 3 (FGFR3),

located on the short arm of chromosome 4. Short stature may not be evident until after 2 years of age, although the deviation from the normal growth curve is progressive. Mean adult height in males and females is 131 and 124 cm, respectively. In addition to short stature, these patients have other abnormalities of the skeleton; including megalocephaly, low nasal bridge, lumbar lordosis, short trident hand, and rhizomelia (shortness of the proximal legs and arms). Radiologic abnormalities include small, cuboid-shaped vertebral bodies with short pedicles and progressive narrowing of the lumbar interpedicular distance. The iliac wings are small, with narrow sciatic notches. The small foramen magnum may lead to hydrocephalus, and spinal cord and/or root compression may result from kyphosis, stenosis of the spinal canal, or disc lesions.

2. **Hypochondroplasia.** Hypochondroplasia has been described as a "milder form" of achondroplasia; however, although the two disorders are both transmitted as autosomal dominant traits, they have not been reported to occur in the same family. Hypochondroplasia has been shown to result from a mutation (Asn540Lys) of the FGFR3 gene, the same gene involved in achondroplasia. The facial features characteristic of achondroplasia are absent, and both the short stature and rhizomelia are less pronounced. Adult heights typically are in the 120- to 150-cm range. As in the case of achondroplasia, short stature may not be evident until after 2 years of age, but stature then deviates progressively from normal. Outward bowing of the legs, accompanied by genu varum, is frequently observed. Lumbar interpedicular distances diminish between L1 and L5 and, as with achondroplasia, there may be flaring of the pelvis and narrow sciatic notches.

Therapy with GH has been studied in several skeletal dysplasias, and modest growth acceleration has been reported. A modest improvement was also seen in the ratio of lower limb length to height. Although GH was well tolerated, it is of note that one patient with atlantoaxial dislocation during GH therapy has been reported. There has also been limited experience with GH treatment of other skeletal disorders, such as dyschondrosteosis, hereditary multiple exostoses, osteogenesis imperfecta, and Ellis–van Creveld syndrome. Because none of these conditions is recognized as an indication for GH therapy by the FDA at this time, GH therapy cannot yet be regarded as standard of care in any of these conditions.

VI. THE GH AXIS AND GROWTH FAILURE

The absolute or relative lack of GH, resulting in a lowering of the IGFs, is an important cause of growth failure in childhood. The incidence of true (absolute) GH deficiency is probably quite low (estimates range from 1 in 4 000 to 1 in 60 000 children), but cases of relative deficiency may be more common. Well-defined forms of GH resistance are all relatively rare, but milder degrees of resistance may underlie an unknown percentage of cases labeled as idiopathic short stature. Defects of the GH–IGF axis include the following.

A. **GH deficiency**

1. **Structural anomalies of the pituitary and hypothalamic region,** for example, holoprosencephaly and septo-optic dysplasia, are associated with multiple pituitary hormone deficiencies, including GH.

2. **Genetic defects in pituitary development or GH secretion.** The pituitary gland develops under the control of a cascade of transcription factors. Genetic defects in these factors usually lead to multiple pituitary hormone deficiencies, but growth-hormone secretion may be the only defect in some cases. The various transcription factors and their associated defects are shown in Table 7.1, which also shows mutations of the GH gene that cause various rare types of GH deficiency.

3. **Acquired lesions of the hypothalamic pituitary region**

    a. **Tumors.** Craniopharyngioma is the most common childhood tumor affecting the pituitary. Other tumors, such as germinomas and gliomas, can also affect the pituitary, though pituitary adenomas are relatively rare in childhood.

TABLE 7.1   GH Stimulation Tests

Stimulus	Dosage	Samples (min)	Comments
L-DOPA (PO)	<15 kg: 125 mg 15–30 kg: 250 mg >30 kg: 500 mg	0, 60, 90	Nausea
Clonidine (PO)	0.15 mg/m²	0, 30, 60, 90	Tiredness, postural hypotension
Arginine HCl (IV)	0.5 g/kg (max 30 g) 10% arginine HCl in 0.9% NaCl over 30 min	0, 15, 30, 45, 60	
Insulin (IV)	0.05–0.1 IU/kg	0, 15, 30, 45, 60, 75, 90, 120	Hypoglycemia; requires supervision[a]
Glucagon (IM)	0.03 mg/kg (max 1 mg)	0, 30, 60, 90, 120, 150, 180	Nausea

Tests should be performed after an overnight fast. It is generally recommended by some authorities that prepubertal children be "primed" with sex steroids [e.g., (1) premarin, 5 mg PO the night before and the morning of the test; or (2) ethinyl estradiol, 50 to 100 μg per day for 3 consecutive days prior to testing; or (3) depot testosterone, 100 mg, 3 days prior to testing]. Patients should be euthyroid at time of testing.
[a]Insulin-induced hypoglycemia is a potential risk of this procedure, which is designed to lower the blood glucose by at least 50%. Documentation of appropriate lowering of blood glucose is recommended. If GHD is suspected, the lower dosage of insulin may be advisable, especially in infants. D50 solutions and glucagon should be available.

    b. Inflammatory infiltrates. Histiocytosis, sarcoidosis, tuberculosis, and other infiltrative disorders can cause pituitary dysfunction in childhood.

    c. Trauma, radiation and chemotherapy can lead to pituitary dysfunction. Exposure to more than 30 Gy of radiation is associated with a very high probability of hypopituitarism.

    d. Idiopathic GH deficiency. Most cases of isolated GH deficiency in childhood still fall into this category. It is worth noting that a majority of the children labeled as GH-deficient in childhood will not be found to be deficient when retested as adults.

    e. GH neurosecretory dysfunction. It has been argued that there exists a group of children with "GH neurosecretory dysfunction," characterized by short stature and poor growth, normal provocative serum GH concentrations, reduced 24-hour serum GH concentrations, and low serum IGF-1 concentrations. These children may be considered GH-deficient, even if they pass provocative GH testing, although the exact diagnostic criteria remain controversial.

B. Growth-hormone insensitivity. Growth-hormone insensitivity is characterized by low IGF levels in the face of normal GH secretion. Causes include the following.

    1. GH receptor abnormalities (Laron syndrome). These patients have mutations involving various portions of the GH receptor so that even though GH secretion might be increased, the action of GH is severely blunted. Mutations in the extracellular portion of the receptor are associated with low GHBP levels, whereas defects in the transmembrane of intracellular portion may be accompanied by increased GHBP levels. These patients respond to treatment with IGF-I, which is now commercially available.

    2. GHR signaling defects. Mutations in STAT5b (a component of the JAK-STAT signaling pathway) have been described in a few cases of growth-hormone insensitivity. These patients have associated immunologic defects and recurrent pulmonary infections.

3. **Primary IGF-1 deficiency.** Severe primary IGF-1 deficiency has been reported in a few rare patients. It is characterized by intrauterine and postnatal growth failure. Additional features include mental retardation and sensorineural deafness. It is possible that milder forms of IGF deficiency are more common and could account for some cases of idiopathic short stature.

4. **ALS deficiency.** Deficiency of the ALS component of the IGF–IGFBP3–ALS ternary complex has been reported as a rare cause of short stature.

C. **Idiopathic short stature (ISS).** Idiopathic short stature can be defined as a condition in which the height of an individual is more than 2 SD below the corresponding mean height for a given age, sex, and population group, without evidence of systemic, endocrine, nutritional, or chromosomal abnormalities. Specifically, children with ISS have normal birth weight and are growth hormone–sufficient. ISS describes a heterogeneous group of children consisting of many presently unidentified causes of short stature. In situations where a specific genetic diagnosis associated with short stature is expected (such as Noonan syndrome or GH insensitivity), the gene(s) of interest should be examined. Online resources such as Genetest (www.genetests.org) identify laboratories capable of performing these tests. Although routine analysis of *SHOX* should not be undertaken in all patients with ISS, *SHOX* gene analysis should be considered for any ISS patient with clinical findings suggestive of *SHOX* haploinsufficiency (e.g., Madelung deformity).

Several countries, including the United States, have recently approved GH therapy of ISS (defined in this case as height greater than **2.25 SD below the mean** for age and sex). It is important to recognize that this is a heterogeneous group of patients and, even though they are grouped under the title "normal short children" or as having "idiopathic short stature," this group will include children who have passed provocative GH testing but are nevertheless IGF-deficient, reflecting the inadequacies of GH testing. The majority of normal short children treated with GH have shown growth acceleration that, generally, is sustained over the first several years of therapy (although attenuation of the response is seen, as in all other instances of GH treatment). Longer-term data are inadequate, however, to address the question of effect of therapy on adult height. Important questions have been raised, additionally, about the financial, ethical, and psychosocial effects of GH therapy on normal short children. No convincing data have been presented that GH treatment of normal short children improves psychological, social, or educational function. On the other hand, it seems unfair to prevent GH therapy of short children who do not meet arbitrary standards on provocative tests that are known to be inadequate. Recent studies on IGF-based dose adjustments in ISS demonstrated increased short-term growth when higher IGF targets were selected, but this strategy has not been validated in long-term studies in terms of safety or final height effects.

VII. OTHER ENDOCRINE CAUSES OF GROWTH FAILURE

A. **Hypothyroidism** is a common cause of short stature, and in children, growth failure may be the first and only sign of thyroid-hormone deficiency. Therefore, evaluation of the thyroid-hormone axis is essential in all children presenting with short stature. Treatment with thyroid hormone restores normal growth velocity, but full catch-up growth does not occur, and long-standing hypothyroidism may be associated with permanent loss of height potential.

B. **Cushing syndrome** is an extremely rare cause of short stature in childhood and is associated with other features of hypercortisolism, including weight gain, hypertension, striae, easy bruising, moon face, and buffalo hump. Determination of midnight salivary cortisol or 24-hour urinary free cortisol can be used as the initial screening test when signs and symptoms suggest the possibility of Cushing syndrome.

VIII. MISCELLANEOUS CAUSES OF GROWTH FAILURE. In addition to the clinical conditions described earlier, GH has been employed in treatment of short stature associated with Noonan syndrome, neurofibromatosis, juvenile rheumatoid arthritis, and a

variety of other conditions associated with postnatal growth failure. In general, such trials have been uncontrolled and have not included sufficient numbers of subjects for adequate evaluation of efficacy, though a review of a large database indicates that many of these conditions might, in fact, be responsive to GH therapy. If, as proposed by Allen and Fost, responsiveness to GH, rather than GHD, should be the most important criterion for GH treatment, then GH therapy for many of these "other" conditions warrants an open-minded, appropriately controlled evaluation.

IX. EVALUATION OF THE SHORT CHILD
A. Step I—Identifying potentially affected children
1. Auxologic abnormalities. **Further evaluation is indicated for children in the following categories:**
   a. Severe short stature (height SDS < -3 SD)
   b. Severe growth deceleration (height velocity SDS < -2 SD over 12 months)
   c. Ht < -2 SD and HV < -1 SD over 12 months
   d. Ht < -1.5 SD and HV < -1.5 SD over 2 years
2. **Risk factors**
   a. History of a brain tumor, cranial irradiation, or other documented organic pituitary abnormality
   b. Incidental finding of pituitary abnormality on MRI
   If any of the above exist, proceed to step 2; if not, follow clinically and return to step 1 in 6 months.

B. Step 2—Screening for GH/IGF deficiency and other diseases
Order a laboratory panel including assessment of bone age, thyroid function, chromosomes (in females), and nonendocrine tests (consider complete blood count, creatinine, erythrocyte sedimentation rate, celiac panel, inflammatory bowel disease screen) and treat any diagnosed conditions as needed. *And*
1. Order an IGF-1 and an IGFBP-3 level.
2. If IGF-1 and/or IGFBP-3 are above the mean, follow clinically and return to step 1 in 6 months.
3. If IGF-1 and/or IGFBP-3 are low, proceed to step 3; but if the MRI is abnormal, GH stimulation is optional.
4. If height < -2.25 SDS, proceed to step 3 regardless of the screening tests.

C. Step 3—Testing GH secretion
This step can be bypassed if a clear GHD risk factor and a severe IGF deficiency are identified. If not, perform two GH stimulation tests. We use clonidine and arginine (Table 7.1), but other options include insulin, glucagon, levodopa and propranolol.
1. If peak GH on both tests is <10 ng/mL, go to step 4.
2. If GH >10 and height is < -2.25 SDS, consider GH treatment for ISS (step 5).

D. Step 4—Evaluating the pituitary
1. **Perform MRI**
   Consider testing the hypothalamic–pituitary–adrenal axis with an ACTH stimulation test or other appropriate test. This is essential in all cases of organic GH deficiency and should be considered on a case-by-case basis in other children.
2. **Testing in the neonate.** The diagnosis of GHD in a newborn is particularly challenging. The presence of a micropenis in a male newborn should always be addressed by an evaluation of the GH axis. A GH level should always be measured in the presence of neonatal hypoglycemia in the absence of a metabolic disorder or other obvious risk factors. All patients with recurrent or persistent hypoglycemia should be evaluated for GH deficiency. A GH level of <20 mg/L during hypoglycemia is suggestive of GHD in the newborn. The use of standard GH stimulation tests is not recommended in newborns, with the exception of the glucagon test, which is safe. An MRI is essential when the diagnosis is suspected, and results may be available sooner than with serum assays. An IGFBP-3 level is of great value for the diagnosis of GHD in infancy, as IGF-1 levels are rarely helpful. In fact, serum IGFBP-3 should be performed as the test of choice in suspected neonatal GHD.

TABLE 7.2	Elements of Monitoring GH Therapy

- Close follow-up with a pediatric endocrinologist every 3 to 6 months
- Determination of growth response (change in height Z-score)
- Monitoring of serum IGF-I and IGFBP-3 levels
- Screening for potential adverse effects
- Evaluation of compliance
- Consideration of dose adjustment based on IGF values, growth response, and comparison to growth prediction models

3. **Therapy.** Daily administration of GH is more effective than giving the same total dose three times weekly. GH injections are best administered in the evening, better mimicking natural physiology and achieving higher GH peaks. The dosage of GH should be expressed in milligrams (or micrograms) per kilogram per day, although consideration should be given to dosing in micrograms per square meter of body surface per day in patients with obesity. GH is routinely used in the range of 25 to 50 μg/kg/day. On this regimen, the typical GH-deficient child accelerates growth from a pretreatment rate of 3 to 4 cm per year to 10 to 12 cm per year in year 1 of therapy and 7 to 9 cm per year in years 2 and 3. This progressive waning of GH efficacy has been observed universally and is still not fully understood.

The emerging consensus is that annual monitoring of serum IGF-1 and IGFBP-3 levels should be part of the routine care of the GHD child receiving rhGH therapy (Table 7.2). Titration of rhGH dose to maintain these growth factors within age-dependent normal limits is physiologically sound and is standard in adult practice. **Periodic monitoring for scoliosis, tonsillar hypertrophy, papilledema, and SCFE** should be performed as part of the regular physical exam during follow-up visits. There are two schools of thought about the duration of treatment. One is that treatment should stop when near-adult height is achieved (Ht velocity <2 cm per year, and/or bone age >16 years in boys and >14 years in girls). Alternatively, therapy can be discontinued when height is in the "normal" adult range (above -2 SD) or has reached another cutoff for the reference adult population (for example, in Australia, the 10th percentile, and elsewhere, the 50th percentile). After attainment of final height, retesting of the GH–IGF axis, using the adult GHD diagnostic criteria, should be undertaken by the pediatric endocrinologist. Standard GH stimulation tests can be performed after an interval of 1 to 3 months off GH therapy.

Selected References

Allen DB, Fost NC. Growth hormone therapy for short stature: panacea or Pandora's box? *J Pediatr* 1990;117:16.

Cohen P, Rogol AD, Howard CP, et al., American Norditropin Study Group. Insulin growth factor-based dosing of growth hormone therapy in children: a randomized, controlled study. *J Clin Endocrinol Metab* 2007;92:2480–2486.

Quigley CA. Growth hormone treatment of non-growth hormone-deficient growth disorders. *Endocrinol Metab Clin North Am* 2007;36:131–186.

Rosenthal S, Cohen P, Clayton P, et al. Ten Streetman perspectives in idiopathic short stature with a focus on IGF-I deficiency. *Pediatr Endocrinol Rev* 2007(suppl 2):252–271.

Walenkamp MJ, Wit JM. Genetic disorders in the growth hormone–insulin-like growth factor-I axis. *Horm Res* 2006;66:221–230.

Wilson TA, Rose SR, Cohen P, et al. The Lawson Wilkins Pediatric Endocrinology Society Drug and Therapeutics Committee. Update of guidelines for the use of growth hormone in children: the Lawson Wilkins Pediatric Endocrinology Society Drug and Therapeutics Committee. *J Pediatr* 2003;143:415–421.

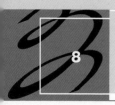

THE ROLE OF IGF-1 IN A SELECTIVE POPULATION OF SHORT CHILDREN
8
Norman Lavin

I. RECOMBINANT IGF-1
Recombinant insulinlike growth factor I (IGF-1) was approved by the U.S. Food and Drug Administration (FDA) in 2005 for use in short children with IGF-1 deficiency, including patients with mutations in the growth hormone receptor, postreceptor signal transduction defects, growth hormone gene deletions with inhibitory growth hormone antibodies, and those with IGF-1 gene deletions or defects. These patients are not growth hormone–deficient and therefore will not generally respond adequately to exogenous growth hormone treatment.

II. ONGOING STUDIES
Ongoing studies are investigating the possible benefits from IGF-1 therapy in idiopathic short stature, Noonan syndrome, leprechaunism, diabetes mellitus, liver disease, neurologic disorders, and critical illnesses.

III. PHYSIOLOGY/BIOCHEMISTRY OF THE IGF-1 SYSTEM
   A. Growth hormone (GH) stimulates production of IGF-1 and insulinlike growth factor binding protein 3 (IGFBP3) in the liver, and growth hormone also promotes proliferation of prechondrocytes and synthesis of IGF-1 at the growth plate. IGFBP3 is produced by the hepatic endothelial and Kupffer cells, whereas the acid-labile subunit (ALS) and IGF-1 are produced by hepatocytes.
   B. Most of the IGF-1 in serum is found in a ternary complex formed by IGF-1, IGFBP3, and the ALS. Less than 1% circulates in the free form. The formation of this ternary complex prolongs the half-life of IGF-1, which thus lasts up to 12 hours, whereas free IGF-1 lasts ~10 minutes. IGFBP3 extends the serum half-life of IGF-1 and also has a role in its distribution.
   C. IGF-1 levels are age-dependent, with low levels at birth, peaking during puberty, and then decreasing with increasing age. Along with low levels in growth hormone deficiency and growth hormone insensitivity, IGF-1 is also decreased in states of malnutrition, catabolism, and some chronic diseases.
   D. Prenatal growth requires IGF-1 and insulinlike growth factor 2 (IGF-2), but not growth hormone. In contrast, postnatal growth needs both growth hormone and IGF-1. Knockout animal models have demonstrated that growth hormone deficiency *and* IGF-1 deficiency affect growth more than that observed in IGF-1 deficiency alone, indicating that growth hormone has growth-promoting activities independent of IGF-1.

IV. DIAGNOSIS OF IGF-1 DEFICIENCY
IGF-1 deficiency is typically associated with elevated growth hormone levels on stimulation, but low or normal levels are also seen. The IGF-1 generation test can be used in differentiating between IGF-1 deficiency that is responsive to growth hormone and IGF-1 deficiency that is not responsive to growth hormone administration. At the current time, this author only occasionally utilizes the IGF generation test because it is not standardized or reproducible.

V. TREATMENT OF IGF-1 DEFICIENCY
In early studies utilizing IGF-1 replacement, growth velocity increased from 4.0 cm per year before therapy to 9.3 cm per year in the first year, 6.2 cm per year in the second

year, and then slowly decreased to 4.8 cm per year after 6 years of therapy. Some studies have reported that the response of children with growth hormone resistance to IGF-1 therapies is of lesser magnitude than is the response of growth hormone–deficient children to growth hormone therapy with respect to growth velocity and adult height. Some possible reasons include: growth hormone is not available to increase IGFBP3 and ALS levels, causing decreased delivery of IGF-1 to target tissues; the lack of growth hormone induced proliferation of prechondrocytes in the growth plate; the absence of growth hormone–induced local IGF-1 production at the growth plate; and the difficulty of using higher doses of IGF-1 because of the risk of hypoglycemia.

VI. SAFETY

A. Hypoglycemia has been reported, but if IGF-1 is administered along with food intake, this adverse effect is very unlikely to occur.
B. Intracranial hypertension can occur in up to 5% of patients.
C. Lymphoid tissue hypertrophy occurs in up to 25% of patients, associated with tonsillar and adenoidal hypertrophy.
D. Anti-IGF-1 antibodies have developed in ~50% of the patients, but they have no effect on growth response.
E. Coarsening of the face has been noted in some patients, particularly during puberty, and both lean and fat mass increase with IGF-1 therapy, in contrast to the response to growth hormone treatment, which manifests an increase in lean body mass and a decrease in body fat.

VII. INDICATIONS FOR IGF-1 THERAPY

IGF-1 deficiency is defined by a height standard deviation score less than − 3.0 and a basal IGF-1 standard deviation score less than − 3.0 and normal or elevated growth hormone response to the growth hormone stimulation test. Some studies are looking at Noonan syndrome because ~50% of Noonan syndrome patients have a mutation in the PTPN11 gene that encodes a non-receptor-type protein tyrosine phosphatase involved in growth hormone receptor signaling. Another group that is being investigated is patients who are growth hormone–deficient but who have a suboptimal response to treatment for at least a year and theoretically may respond to IGF-1 treatment.

VIII. CONCLUSION/AUTHOR'S EXPERIENCE

A. At the time of this writing, I have administered IGF-1 to >30 patients who have primary IGF-1 deficiency manifested by a height standard deviation more than − 3.0 and a basal IGF-1 standard deviation more than − 3.0 with elevated growth hormone response to growth hormone stimulation tests. In every case, there has been improvement of growth velocity to at least a − 1 standard deviation score in height. In another group of six patients, I utilized IGF-1 in those children who had not responded to high doses of growth hormone administration. In five of six of these patients, the standard deviation score improved from − 3 to − 1, and in the one remaining patient the score improved from − 3 to − 2.
B. **Combination therapy.** In a third group of patients, I utilized the combination of growth hormone and IGF-1 in 24 patients who had not responded significantly to either IGF-1 alone or growth hormone alone. The combination has improved their height velocity from − 3 to − 1 standard deviation.
C. Based on the author's initial experience, clinical trials must be undertaken to investigate whether combination therapy should be initiated for these indications.

Selected References

Backeljauw PF, Underwood LE; GHIS Collaborative Group. Growth hormone insensitivity syndrome. Therapy for 6.5–7.5 years with recombinant insulin-like growth factor I in children with growth hormone insensitivity syndrome: a clinical research center study. *J Clin Endocrinol Metab* 2001;86(4):1504–1510.

Chernausek SD, Backeljauw PF, Frane J, Kuntze J, Underwood LE; GH Insensitivity Syndrome Collaborative Group. Long-term treatment with recombinant insulin-like growth factor (IGF)-I in children with severe IGF-I deficiency due to growth hormone insensitivity. *J Clin Endocrinol Metab* 2007;92(3):902–910.

Cohen P, Rogol AD, Howard CP, Bright GM, Kappelgaard AM, Rosenfeld RG; American Norditropin Study Group. Insulin growth factor-based dosing of growth hormone therapy in children: a randomized, controlled study. *J Clin Endocrinol Metab* 2007;92(7):2480–2486.

Savage MO, Attie KM, David A, Metherell LA, Clark AJ, Camacho-Hübner C. Endocrine assessment, molecular characterization and treatment of growth hormone insensitivity disorders. *Nat Clin Pract Endocrinol Metab* 2006;2(7):395–407.

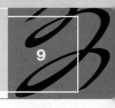

GROWTH HORMONE IN ADULTS
Norman Lavin

9

I. INTRODUCTION
Growth hormone deficiency in adults may lead to cardiovascular risk and increased mortality from cardiac and cerebrovascular disease. Low levels of insulinlike growth factor 1 (IGF-1) may be associated with increased morbidity and mortality from ischemic heart disease and stroke. Treatment with growth hormone and IGF-1 enhances and normalizes vascular and muscle cell proliferation. In animals, it reduces infarct volume and improves neurologic function after ischemia, promotes survival and myelinization of neuronal cells, and stimulates brain angiogenesis in response to hypoxic stimuli.

II. GROWTH HORMONE PHYSIOLOGY
Growth hormone is a protein consisting of 191 amino acids that is synthesized and secreted by cells called somatotrophs, located in the anterior pituitary gland. This hormone controls several complex physiologic processes, including growth metabolism. It is currently used in children as well as in adults. Growth hormone also helps maintain blood glucose within a normal range because it is a counterregulatory hormone to insulin.

Effects are mediated primarily by IGF-1, a hormone that is secreted from the liver, as well as other tissues, in response to stimulation from growth hormone. The growth hormone–promoting effects are primarily the result of IGF-1 acting on its target cells. Growth hormone stimulates the liver to secrete IGF-1, which stimulates proliferation of chondrocytes (or cartilage cells), which results in bone growth in the child. IGF-1 also appears to be a key player in muscle growth. It stimulates both the differentiation and proliferation of myoblasts and stimulates amino acid uptake and protein synthesis in muscle and other tissue.

III. CONTROL OF GROWTH HORMONE SECRETION
Two hypothalamic hormones and one hormone produced in the stomach control growth hormone release and secretion (Table 9.1).
- **A. Growth hormone–releasing hormone (GHRH)** stimulates the synthesis and secretion of growth hormone from the pituitary gland.
- **B. Somatostatin** is a peptide produced by several tissues in the hypothalamus and elsewhere, which inhibits the release of growth hormone.
- **C. Ghrelin** is a peptide hormone secreted from the stomach that binds to receptors on somatotrophs in the pituitary gland and stimulates secretion of growth hormone.
- **D. Growth hormone secretion** is part of a negative feedback system: High levels of IGF-1 lead to suppression of growth hormone by directly suppressing the somatotroph and also stimulating release of somatostatin from the hypothalamus. Growth hormone also inhibits GHRH secretion.

IV. ADULT GROWTH HORMONE DEFICIENCY SYNDROME
Adult growth hormone deficiency syndrome (AGHDS) is a clinical entity characterized by decreased lean body mass and decrease in bone mineral density as well as increased visceral adiposity and an abnormal lipid profile. There is also decreased muscle strength, exercise endurance, and a diminished quality of life. Some data indicate increased morbidity and mortality associated with growth hormone deficiency

TABLE 9.1	Control of Growth Hormone Secretion

Stimulators	Inhibitors
1. GHRH	1. Somatostatin
2. Stage III and stage IV sleep	2. Elevated IGF-1 levels
3. Stressors	3. Hyperglycemia
4. Alpha adrenergic stimuli	4. Elevated free fatty acid levels
5. Fasting	5. Serotonin antagonists
6. Melatonin	6. Corticotropin-releasing factor
7. Estrogens	7. β-Adrenergic stimuli
8. Dopaminergic stimuli	8. Progesterone
9. Exercise	9. ACTH deficiency
10. Serotonin	10. Hyperthyroidism
11. Hypoglycemia	11. Hypothyroidism
12. Interleukin-1, -2, and -6	12. Obesity
13. Levodopa	13. Depression
14. Clonidine	14. Corticosteroids
15. Bromocriptine	15. Amitriptyline
16. Arginine/lysine	16. Substance P
17. Ghrelin	

secondary to cerebral or cardiovascular disease as well as bone fractures. Growth hormone replacement has been shown to reverse many of these abnormalities.

V. EVALUATION

A. IGF-1. Because growth hormone is secreted in an episodic manner, random sampling has little validity in the diagnosis of growth hormone deficiency. A random IGF-1 level, however, can be obtained at any time of the day and is a strong surrogate marker for the level of growth hormone in the absence of catabolic conditions and/or liver disease. Contrariwise, a normal IGF-1 level does not exclude a diagnosis of growth hormone deficiency. Therefore, if it is clinically indicated, growth hormone stimulation tests should be performed. The presence of low levels of three or more pituitary hormones strongly suggests the presence of growth hormone deficiency and, therefore, stimulation testing may not be required in this situation.

B. Stimulation tests

1. Current diagnostic testing involves provocation of growth hormone secretion, including the insulin tolerance test, which is considered to be the "gold standard." This test is fairly risky, particularly in patients with known seizure disorders or cardiovascular disease, and in the elderly. It may result in hypoglycemic seizures and possibly even death. The combination of GHRH and arginine is safe and provides a strong stimulus to growth hormone secretion. Other tests include arginine alone, clonidine, levodopa, and the combination of arginine plus levodopa, but there are not adequate data demonstrating validity, test reliability, and sensitivity or specificity.

2. Because GHRH stimulates the pituitary directly, it can give a false-normal growth hormone response in patients with growth hormone deficiency of hypothalamic origin. In this situation, arginine alone may be used, without concomitant GHRH, using a lower cutoff level. It is still not clear what the lower cutoff level should be, because different centers use different values. Many endocrinologists consider a level of <5.1 μg/L as low on the insulin tolerance test, and <4.1 μg/L as low on the GHRH/arginine stimulation tests.

    3. Obesity or acute overfeeding can markedly blunt the growth hormone response during the insulin tolerance test.

    4. The sequential arginine and GHRH infusion requires 0.5 g/kg of arginine with a maximum dose of 30 g infused in saline over 30 minutes, followed by a single bolus injection of 1 μg/kg of GHRH with a maximum of 100 μg.

  C. Imaging studies. Neurologic imaging (such as magnetic resonance imaging [MRI]) determines the presence of intracranial disease associated with growth hormone deficiency. A dual-energy x-ray absorptiometry (DEXA) scan may be needed to estimate the presence of osteoporosis.

VI. PSEUDO–GROWTH HORMONE DEFICIENCY STATES

  A. Reversible and/or apparent growth hormone deficiency may occur in a cold environment during exercise, postpartum, in obesity, hyperthyroidism, hypercortisolism, Addison disease, congestive heart failure, and protracted critical illness.

  B. A low IGF-1 level in the presence of increased growth hormone secretion, as demonstrated by stimulation tests, may reflect a peripheral resistance to growth hormone.

VII. ETIOLOGY

Adults with growth hormone deficiency can be grouped into three categories:

  A. Previous childhood-onset growth hormone deficiency (transition).

    1. The history of childhood growth hormone deficiency is less predictive of adult growth hormone deficiency because from 26% to 81% of such patients "normalize" growth hormone release in adulthood—that is, even though as children they had abnormal stimulation tests, repeat tests are now normal (the reasons are not clear but may include inadequate growth hormone investigation as a child). Idiopathic causes account for most growth hormone deficiencies in childhood, but there is not total consensus that this entity occurs in adults (see Endocrine Society Consensus Statement). Children with idiopathic growth hormone deficiency are less likely to have permanent growth hormone deficiency as adults and should be retested.

    2. Children who had a congenital anomaly of the pituitary gland or a tumor in the hypothalamic/pituitary region, or previous surgery or radiotherapy in this area, or a proven genetic or molecular defect involving the capacity to secrete growth hormone, probably do not need to be retested.

  B. Acquired deficiency secondary to structural lesions or trauma

    1. Tumors in the pituitary and hypothalamic area may cause hypopituitarism. The most common cause of growth hormone deficiency in adults is a pituitary adenoma, or following specific treatment of the adenoma with surgery or radiation therapy. Irradiation is a common cause of hypopituitarism and may be progressive over time in as many as 50% of patients after a 10-year follow-up.

    2. Other space-occupying lesions, such as craniopharyngiomas, Rathke-cleft cysts, arachnoid cysts, meningiomas, dysgerminomas, metastatic tumors, astrocytomas, or gliomas can result in growth hormone deficiency following surgery and/or radiation.

    3. Growth hormone deficiency is sometimes a result of compression of the portal vessels in the pituitary stalk secondary to an expanding tumor mass, directly or by raised intracellular pressure.

    4. Infiltrative diseases, such as histocytosis, sarcoidosis, and tuberculosis, are additional causes.

    5. The empty-sella syndrome may be associated with endocrine dysfunction, including isolated growth hormone deficiency, as well as multiple pituitary hormone deficiencies.

    6. Traumatic brain injury has been reported to cause growth hormone deficiency in as many as 25% of all patients with sustained brain injury that occurred years earlier (Table 9.2).

TABLE 9.2	Etiology of Growth Hormone Deficiency

1. Pituitary disease: pituitary adenoma, metastatic neoplasm, parasellar surgery, craniofacial irradiation, pituitary apoplexy, head trauma, lymphocytic hypophysitis
2. Hypothalamic etiologies: irradiation, infiltrative processes, primary or metastatic neoplasms, ependymoma, third ventricular cyst, trauma
3. Hypophyseal stalk injury: head trauma, metastatic lesions, infiltrative disease
4. Craniopharyngioma, hypothalamopituitary damage, parasellar lesions: meningioma, central nervous system lymphoma, chordomas, arterial-venous malformation, internal carotid aneurysms
5. Idiopathic isolated growth hormone deficiency of childhood: adult patients with prior childhood diagnosis of growth hormone deficiency
6. Systemic factors: hypothyroidism, Addison disease, high-dose glucocorticoids or Cushing syndrome, obesity, advanced age, hypothermia, acute overfeeding, protracted critical illness.

    C. Adult-onset idiopathic growth hormone deficiency. See Consensus Statement—2007 Endocrine Society.

VIII. CLINICAL
    A. Adult growth hormone deficiency syndrome includes the following signs and symptoms (Table 9.3):
      1. Weakened heart muscle contraction and heart rate
      2. Arterial plaques
      3. Elevated blood pressure
      4. Decreased cardiac ejection fraction and diminished arteriole distensibility
      5. Increased inflammatory markers, such as C-reactive protein (CRP)
      6. Elevated lipids or fats in the blood, such as total cholesterol, low-density lipoproteins (LDLs), and triglycerides
      7. Decreased exercise capacity, probably secondary to decreased cardiac output
      8. Decreased energy
      9. Abnormal body composition
        a. Increased abdominal obesity
        b. Decreased bone density
        c. Increased incidence of fractures and osteoporosis

TABLE 9.3	Symptomatology and Physical Stigmata in Growth Hormone–Deficient Adults

Symptoms	Signs
1. Systemic: fatigue, limited exercise capacity	1. Dyslipidemia: elevated LDL and total cholesterol; variably increased TG and reduced HDL
2. Psychological: impaired mood and social outlook; reduced memory, well-being, and concentration; apathy	2. Osteopenia/osteoporosis
	3. Increased (visceral) body fat; mild insulin resistance
	4. Sarcopenia/muscle weakness; skin thinning
3. Sexual: diminished libido and sexual activity	5. Reduced extracellular fluid space; less sweating
	6. Diminished renal blood flow; low cardiac output; diastolic dysfunction
	7. Mild anemia

HDL, high-density lipoprotein; LDL, low-density lipoprotein; TG, thyroglobulin.

      d. Decreased muscle strength and muscle size
      e. Decreased lean body mass
      f. Increased fat mass
  10. Problems with sleep quality
  11. Decreased social contact
  12. Decreased libido
  13. Weight gain
  14. Psychological symptoms
      a. Shyness
      b. Withdrawal from others
      c. Nervousness or anxiety
      d. Sadness or depression
      e. Feelings of helplessness

IX. PATHOGENESIS

A. Experimental animal infarction models suggest that IGF-1 may promote survival of myocytes exposed to ischemic injury, in part by advancing glucose uptake.

B. IGF-1 has also been identified as a neuroprotective agent. Growth hormone–deficient adults with low IGF-1 levels are at increased risk of cardiovascular disease and have increased carotid artery wall thickness and endothelial dysfunction. Low-normal levels of IGF-1 may predict increased risk of ischemic heart disease and ischemic stroke. Low IGF-1 levels may also increase the risk of developing insulin resistance.

C. In several studies, the **cardiovascular profile** in patients with growth hormone deficiency demonstrated increased incidence of plaque formation, increased intima media thickness, decreased production of nitrous oxide, abnormal lipid profile, inflammatory markers, and development of insulin resistance. Atheromas of the abdominal aorta and of the femoral and carotid arteries were more pronounced in patients with growth hormone deficiency than in the control population. Several studies demonstrated an increased stiffness of arteries in comparison with controls. Böger et al. demonstrated that growth hormone was responsible for endothelial nitric oxide production. Nitric oxide is not only a potent vasodilator but also an inhibitor of LDL oxidation.

D. Atherosclerosis is an inflammatory process, and inflammation markers such as CRP or interleukin-6 (IL-6) are highly sensitive indicators of atherosclerosis. In patients with growth hormone deficiency, CRP is increased.

E. Adults with growth hormone deficiency demonstrate alterations in plasma fibrinolytic balance, including elevated levels of plasminogen activator inhibitor-1 (PAI-1) with decreased tissue plasminogen activator (tPA) activity. These changes may contribute to the increased cardiovascular morbidity in AGHDS.

F. Some articles conclude that the beneficial effects of growth hormone on the cardiovascular system are strongly suggestive but not completely proven.

X. FIBROMYALGIA

A. Growth hormone deficiency may occur in a subset of patients with **fibromyalgia,** which may be of clinical relevance because it is a treatable disorder with demonstrated benefits of treatment. IGF-1 levels are abnormally low in some patients with this disorder. Dinser et al. reported that ~30% of patients with fibromyalgia had an abnormally low response to insulin-induced hypoglycemia and arginine stimulation testing.

B. There are some data showing that a subpopulation of fibromyalgia patients with low serum IGF-1 levels, who also failed the GHRH/arginine test, had improvements in symptomatology when they were treated with growth hormone. Many patients had improvement in functionability, but no patients had complete remission of symptoms or signs. There was a lag of ~6 months before patients started to note improvement. The decision to treat patients with fibromyalgia by growth hormone supplementation must await confirmatory long-term studies of its efficacy and side-effects profile. It is not yet possible to arrive at any definitive conclusion as to the link between the hypothalamic pituitary axis dysfunction in growth hormone deficiency and fibromyalgia.

C. Preliminary studies of growth hormone therapy in a subset of patients with chronic fatigue syndrome and growth hormone deficiency have also shown some encouraging results.

XI. ADIPOSE TISSUE

Adult growth hormone–deficient patients demonstrate increased fat mass, particularly visceral adiposity; and several studies have shown significant decreases in total body fat content in response to growth hormone treatment. These decreases occur in both subcutaneous and visceral fat within 6 months after initiation of therapy. Growth hormone administration increases lipolysis. Untreated adults have decreased lean body mass and, with treatment, an increase in muscle mass ensues.

XII. STRENGTH

Some studies have shown increases in isometric or isokinetic strength. In other studies, exercise capacity and physical performance were improved by treatment, demonstrated by the facts that VO_2 max and maximum work capacity were increased.

XIII. GROWTH HORMONE TREATMENT IN THE ELDERLY

There are many unanswered questions about the use of growth hormone in the elderly, as well as in adults with growth hormone deficiency. Currently, research has brought us to an important beginning in deciphering the actions of growth hormone in this age group. Gotherstrom et al. have described a 10-year prospective study of the metabolic effects of growth hormone replacement in adults. There was a sustained reduction of body fat during the study period, sustained improvement in serum lipid profiles, and lowering of hemoglobin $A1_{1c}$ by the end of the study.

XIV. GROWTH HORMONE AND DIABETES MELLITUS

A. In the study by Gotherstrom study looking at growth hormone–deficient adults, the conclusion was that growth hormone did not affect the risk of diabetes mellitus in patients who had normal body mass index. After 10 years of growth hormone replacement as adults, there was no increased incidence of diabetes or malignancy. Contrawise Growth hormone–deficient patients have increased serum insulin concentration and evidence of insulin resistance. Glucose-clamp studies have confirmed these observations. Patients with an excess of growth hormone may also demonstrate insulin resistance.

B. In a prospective study, a low mean dose of growth hormone normalized serum IGF-1 levels and improved body composition in elderly growth hormone–deficient patients without any significant deterioration in glucose homeostasis.

XV. LIPIDS

Growth hormone replacement reduces visceral fat, and total cholesterol and LDL levels may decrease by 10% to 20%. Sixty-three adults with growth hormone deficiency were assessed after 7 years of treatment. Total cholesterol and LDL decreased and HDL increased, whereas triglyceride concentrations remained unchanged.

XVI. BONE DENSITY

A. Adults

1. Low bone mineral density in adults has been demonstrated in patients with growth hormone deficiency. The age of onset appears to determine the severity of the osteopenia, and the severity of growth hormone deficiency correlates with the severity of osteopenia. There is an increase in the volume of trabecular bone, increased reabsorption, and increased osteolite thickness, suggesting delayed mineralization. Fracture rates up to two to five times greater than normal have been reported in growth hormone–deficient patients. One study looked at 87 patients relative to bone mineral density and showed that growth hormone induced a sustained increase. The mean initial dose of growth hormone was 0.98 mg per day, which was gradually lowered, so that at the end of the study the mean dose was 0.47 mg per day. Growth hormone replacement induced a sustained increase in total lumbar and femur neck bone mineral density (BMD) and bone mineral content as measured by DEXA scan. The authors concluded that 10 years of growth hormone replacement in patients with growth hormone deficiency induced a sustained and, in some cases, a progressive increase in bone mass and bone density.

2. Growth hormone stimulates both bone formation and reabsorption, but with <12 months of treatment the BMD by DEXA scanning may not increase but may actually decrease. After 18 to 24 months of treatment, most studies have shown increases in BMD.

B. Adolescents

1. After discontinuation of growth hormone therapy in children at ages 15 to 17 years, there may be a reduced acquisition of bone mineral content. An important issue, therefore, is whether therapy should be maintained or reinstituted, at least until the subjects reach peak bone mass.

2. There is some evidence that BMD is greater in those who continue growth hormone therapy for an additional 2 years after cessation of growth.

XVII. CARDIOVASCULAR EFFECTS

A. General benefits of growth hormone. Growth hormone has both direct effects on vascular function and also effects mediated through IGF-1 itself. The cardiovascular risk associated with growth hormone deficiency appears to be related to several factors, including hypertension, inflammation, dyslipidemia, and insulin resistance. After administration of growth hormone, there is an increase in flow-mediated dilatation and reduction of arterial stiffness. There is also a slight decrease in blood pressure.

B. Lipids. The administration of growth hormone reduces CRP and improves lipoprotein metabolism. There are increases in high-density lipoprotein (HDL) and decreases in LDL and total cholesterol. Furthermore, growth hormone decreases fat mass and improves insulin sensitivity.

C. Heart and vessel anatomy. Increased intima media thickness and abnormal arterial wall dynamics have been documented in growth hormone deficiency. Growth hormone treatment has reversed these disorders. Some studies show reduced left ventricular, posterior wall, and interventricular septal thickness and left ventricular diameter mass. After growth hormone administration, there were increases in left ventricular mass, left ventricular end diastolic volume, and stroke volume. Changes in these parameters may correlate with reported subjective benefits of increased exercise tolerance and energy.

XVIII. QUALITY OF LIFE

Quality of life is assessed by means of a self-administered survey. Energy and vitality are diminished in growth hormone–deficient patients. Many studies showed definite benefit after patients received growth hormone, whereas in others, improvements were more limited or no improvement was seen.

XIX. ARGUMENTS AGAINST GROWTH HORMONE

A. Safety concerns. Although treatment appears to be safe overall, certain areas require long-term surveillance, such as risks of glucose intolerance and pituitary hypothalamic tumor recurrence and cancer. Although there are benefits in diminishing and decreasing cardiovascular risk factors, reductions in cardiovascular mortality have yet to be demonstrated.

B. Adverse effects. The most common side effects are related to fluid retention as well as paresthesias, joint stiffness, peripheral edema, arthralgia, and myalgia. Carpal tunnel syndrome has been described in as many as 2% of patients. Most of these adverse reactions, however, improve with dose reduction. Benign intracranial hypertension has been linked to growth hormone treatment in children, but only one case has been reported in adults. Gynecomastia has been reported in a very few elderly individuals receiving growth hormone in high doses.

C. **Growth hormone and tumor formation.** There is a concern that growth hormone therapy could lead to tumor recurrence or the development of malignancies. However, an increase in recurrence rates of either intracranial or extracranial tumors has not been demonstrated in AGHDS. There are no published data of long-term observational studies in patients with AGHDS treated with growth hormone that showed any increased incidence of cancer.

D. **Unmasking of thyroid and cortisol deficiency.** Although it is not an adverse effect, growth hormone replacement can cause a lowering of free thyroxine (T4) levels, perhaps because of increased deiodination of T4, enhancing the extrathyroidal conversion of T4 to tri-iodothyronine (T3). Lowering of T4 during treatment with growth hormone, therefore, reflects biochemical unmasking of subclinical central hypothyroidism. Growth hormone treatment has also been found to cause a lowering of serum cortisol levels, revealing central hypoadrenalism that has been masked, likely because of enhanced conversion of cortisone to cortisol during the growth hormone–deficient state. 11β-Hydroxysteroid dehydrogenase type I isoenzyme acts as a reductase that converts cortisone to cortisol and is increased in growth hormone deficiency and reduced by growth hormone replacement. Therefore, free T4 levels and cortisol levels should be monitored during treatment.

E. **Contraindications.** Growth hormone treatment is contraindicated in the presence of an active malignancy. Growth hormone treatment of patients with diabetes mellitus is not a contraindication but may require adjustments in antidiabetic medication.

XX. ARGUMENTS FOR TREATMENT

Growth hormone therapy offers significant clinical benefits in body composition, exercise capacity, skeletal integrity, and quality of life. Growth hormone reduces visceral fat and increases muscle mass and cardiac performance. Total cholesterol and LDL levels decrease, and CRP declines. The effects on cardiac mass are associated with enhanced cardiac performance. An improvement in the lipid profile is often seen after growth hormone treatment. A meta-analysis of several studies documented the effects on total cholesterol, with significant changes more prominent in elderly patients than in the young. Apoprotein B-100 (Apo-B100) is a known independent risk factor for cardiovascular disease that has been shown to decrease after growth hormone therapy. LDL concentrations also decrease.

Arterial distensibility and plaque formation are improved with growth hormone treatment. Growth hormone is also a cytokine, and its receptor belongs to the family of cytokine receptors. Intracellular activation occurs through STAT-4 (the signal-transducing activator of transcription protein 4), a well-known pathway for cytokines. One could speculate that by interfering with the action of proinflammatory cytokines, growth hormone reduces or even reverses intima media thickness and plaque formation. Intima media thickness decreases significantly with growth hormone treatment.

There is improved peripheral vasodilatation and production of nitric oxide. Systolic and diastolic blood pressure measurements decrease slightly but significantly in hypertensive patients.

CRP is a good indicator of cardiovascular risk because it accelerates vascular inflammation by interacting with endothelial receptors. Most patients with growth hormone deficiency have elevated CRP levels. Most, but not all, studies demonstrate a significant decrease of CRP levels with growth hormone replacement.

XXI. TREATMENT

A. Growth hormone dose requirements should be lower in older patients. Higher growth hormone doses are needed to achieve the same IGF-1 levels in women receiving oral estrogen replacement. For ages 30 to 60 years, a starting dose of

300 μg per day is recommended. Daily dosing should be increased from 100 to 200 μg every 1 to 2 months—the goals being an appropriate clinical response, no side effects, and an IGF-1 level in the age-adjusted reference range. Clinical benefits may not become apparent for up to 6 months of treatment. Patients >60 years of age should be started on an even lower dose, such as 100 to 200 μg per day, with slower incremental increases.

B. After maintenance doses have been achieved, monitoring usually occurs at 3- to 6-month intervals. In addition to a normal IGF-1 level for age, monitoring should include a clinical evaluation, assessment of side effects, a lipid profile, a fasting glucose, a free T4 and thyroid-stimulating hormone (TSH), a cortisol level, and, if indicated, a BMD scan. Assessment of quality of life provides another modality for monitoring response to therapy.

C. It is not clear how long one should administer growth hormone therapy. If benefits are being achieved, I would continue the therapy but begin tapering the dose unless clinical goals decline. On the other hand, if there are no apparent or objective benefits after at least 1 year of treatment, discontinuing growth hormone therapy should be considered.

D. Recommendations

   1. Growth hormone dosing regimens should be individualized rather than weight-based.

   2. Growth hormone treatment should start with low doses and be titrated according to clinical response, side effects, and IGF-1 levels.

   3. Growth hormone dosing should take age, sex, and estrogen status into consideration.

   4. During growth hormone treatment, patients should be monitored at regular intervals, such as every 1 to 2 months during dose titration and every 6 months thereafter with a clinical assessment and an evaluation for adverse effects, IGF-1 levels, and other parameters of growth hormone response.

XXII. CONCLUSION

A. The treatment of growth hormone deficiency in adults has been reported to improve quality of life and energy levels, reduce pain, improve depression, enhance self-esteem, improve cholesterol and LDL levels, enhance cognitive psychometric performance, augment stroke volume, improve exercise capacity, and improve muscle strength. Growth hormone therapy offers benefits in body composition, skeletal integrity and quality of life measures. However, reductions in cardiovascular events and mortality have yet to be absolutely demonstrated.

B. Many endocrinologists remain skeptical of using growth hormone as treatment for growth hormone–deficient patients and, therefore, a large fraction of patients who have this deficiency are not treated. It appears that more long-term treatment data will be required to provide reassurance as to whether growth hormone treatment is a safe and necessary form of hormone replacement therapy for adult patients with growth hormone deficiency.

XXIII. FUTURE CONSIDERATIONS

In animal models, IGF-1 promotes survival and myelinization of neuronal cells as well as stimulating brain angiogenesis in response to hypoxic stimuli caused by ischemia or trauma. It is possible that higher serum IGF-1 levels could promote an increased delivery of IGF-1 from the periphery to brain-damaged cells. IGF-1 can cross the blood–brain barrier. Low IGF-1 levels during the acute phase of stroke are associated with a poor outcome or even death. Higher IGF-1 levels, on the other hand, were observed in patients with better outcomes, suggesting a possible neuroprotective role of IGF-1 and its potential use to improve motor and cognitive recovery during rehabilitation after stroke.

The role of growth hormone in normal aging is poorly understood. This is a new area of research, and additional recommendations about risks and benefits will evolve in the near future.

Selected References

Aimeretti G, Ghigo E. Should every patient with traumatic brain injury be referred to an endocrinologist? *Nat Clin Pract Endocrinol Metab* 2007;3(4):318–319.

Bennett RM. Adult growth hormone deficiency in patients with fibromyalgia. *Curr Rheumatol Rep* 2002;4(4):306–312.

Bondanelli M, Ambrosio MR, Onofri A, et al. Predictive value of circulating insulin-like growth factor I levels in ischemic stroke outcome. *J Clin Endocrinol Metab* 2006;91:3928–3934.

Böger RH. Nitric oxide and the mediation of the hemodynamic effects of growth hormone in humans. *J Endocrinol Invest* 1999;22(5 Suppl):75–81.

Burger AG, Monson JP, Colao AM, Klibanski A. Cardiovascular risk in patients with growth hormone deficiency: effects of growth hormone substitution. *Endocr Pract* 2006;12(6):682–689.

Climent VE, Picó A, Sogorb F, et al. Growth hormone therapy and the heart. *Am J Cardiol* 2006;97:1097–1102.

Colao A, Di Somma C, Cuocolo A, Spinelli L, Acampa W, Spiezia S, Rota F, Savanelli MC, Lombardi G. Does a gender-related effect of growth hormone (GH) replacement exist on cardiovascular risk factors, cardiac morphology, and performance and atherosclerosis? Results of a two-year open, prospective study in young adult men and women with severe GH deficiency. *J Clin Endocrinol Metab* 2005;90(9):5146–5155.

Del Monte P, Foppiani L, Cafferata C, et al. Primary "empty sella" in adults: endocrine findings. *Endocr J* 2006;53(6):803–809.

Devin JK, Blevins DK Jr, Verity DK, et al. Markedly impaired fibrinolytic balance contributes to cardiovascular risk in adults with growth hormone deficiency. *J Clin Endocrinol Metab* 2007;92:3633–3639.

Dinser R, Halama T, Hoffmann A. Stringent endocrinological testing reveals subnormal growth hormone secretion in some patients with fibromyalgia syndrome but rarely severe growth hormone deficiency. *J Rheumatol* 2000;27(10):2482–2488.

Endocrine Society Consensus Statement

Follin C, Thilén U, Ahrén B, Erfurth EM. Improvement in cardiac systolic function and reduced prevalence of metabolic syndrome after two years of growth hormone (GH) treatment in GH-deficient adult survivors of childhood-onset acute lymphoblastic leukemia. *J Clin Endocrinol Metab* 2006;91:1872–1875.

Franco C, Johannsson G, Bengtsson BA, Svensson J. Baseline characteristics and effects of growth hormone therapy over two years in younger and elderly adults with adult onset GH deficiency. *J Clin Endocrinol Metab* 2006;91:4408–4414.

Götherström G, Bengtsson BA, Bosaeus I, Johannsson G, Svensson J. A 10-year, prospective study of the metabolic effects of growth hormone replacement in adults. *J Clin Endocrinol Metab* 2007;92(4):1442–1445.

Ho KK; 2007 GH Deficiency Consensus Workshop Participants. Consensus guidelines for the diagnosis and treatment of adults with GH deficiency II: a statement of the GH Research Society in association with the European Society for Pediatric Endocrinology, Lawson Wilkins Society, European Society of Endocrinology, Japan Endocrine Society, and Endocrine Society of Australia. *Eur J Endocrinol* 2007;157(6):695–700.

Kaplan RC, McGinn AP, Pollak MN, et al. Association of total insulin-like growth factor-I, insulin-like growth factor binding protein-1 (IGFBP-1), and IGFBP-3 levels with incident coronary events and ischemic stroke. *J Clin Endocrinol Metab* 2007;92:1319–1325.

Karavitaki N, Warner JT, Marland A, et al. GH replacement does not increase the risk of recurrence in patients with craniopharyngioma. *Clin Endocrinol (Oxf)* 2006;64:556–560.

Le Corvoisier P, Hittinger L, Chanson P, Montagne O, Macquin-Mavier I, Maison P. Cardiac effects of growth hormone treatment in chronic heart failure: A meta-analysis. *J Clin Endocrinol Metab* 2007;92(1):180–185.

McCall-Hosenfeld JS, Goldenberg DL, Hurwitz S, Adler GK. Growth hormone and insulin-like growth factor-1 concentrations in women with fibromyalgia. *J Rheumatol* 2003;30:809–814.

Radovick S, DiVall S. Approach to the growth hormone-deficient child during transition to adulthood. *J Clin Endocrinol Metab* 2007;92(4):1195–1200.

Zucchini S, Pirazzoli P, Baronio F, et al. Effect on adult height of pubertal growth hormone retesting and withdrawal of therapy in patients with previously diagnosed growth hormone deficiency. *J Clin Endocrinol Metab* 2006;91:4271–4276.

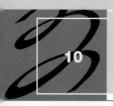

PROLACTIN
Richard F. Spark

10

I. GENERAL PRINCIPLES.

Prolactin (Prl), synthesized in the pituitary lactotrope, is released sparingly into the circulation because its **secretion** is under **tonic inhibition** by a hypothalamic Prl-inhibiting factor, **dopamine.** The tuberoinfundibular neurons of the arcuate nucleus of the hypothalamus produce dopamine, which is transported to the pituitary via the hypothalamic hypophysial portal system. Dopamine binds to specific dopamine receptors on the lactotropes to inhibit pituitary Prl secretion and release. This dopamine-induced inhibition of Prl secretion helps maintain a low circulating serum Prl level of <15 ng/mL. (Normal levels vary in different laboratories.)

A. A **physiologic increase** in serum Prl levels occurs only during pregnancy, when increases in serum estrogen levels exert a direct stimulatory effect on the pituitary lactotrope (overriding dopamine inhibition) to facilitate the secretion of large amounts of Prl into the circulation. This physiologic hyperprolactinemia acts on the breast to stimulate lactation and enables the mother to nurse her child.

B. Elevations in serum Prl levels at times other than pregnancy are indicative of **pathologic hyperprolactinemia,** discussed in Section II. The symptoms and signs of **hyperprolactinemia** are sex-specific.

C. Less common, but of increasing significance, are conditions of inadequate Prl secretion. **Hypoprolactinemia** has proved to be a useful biologic marker for occult hypothalamic or pituitary disorders. Undetectable serum prolactin levels are present when the pituitary gland lactotroph cells are destroyed, as in Sheehan syndrome, whereas low but detectable serum prolactin levels, <4 ng/mL, are found in young men with constitutional delayed puberty (CDP) or idiopathic hypogonadal hypogonadism (IHH). See Section VII.B.

II. HYPERPROLACTINEMIA

A. Clinical presentation. Hyperprolactinemia causes disorders of sexual and reproductive function in men and women. In women, menstrual disorders such as amenorrhea, oligomenorrhea, and infertility resulting from anovulatory cycles or short luteal phase are common, whereas in men, diminished libido, sporadic or complete impotence, and infertility resulting from oligospermia predominate.

B. Galactorrhea. Galactorrhea is defined as discharge of milk from the breast at any time other than the peri- or postpartum period; it occurs in ~70% of hyperprolactinemic women. Elevated serum Prl levels accompanied by adequate circulating estrogen levels are a prerequisite for the development of galactorrhea. Fluid discharge from the nipple similar to galactorrhea can occur in unaffected women who harbor intraductal papillomas or carcinomas and in those who stimulate their breasts.

C. Indications for workup. Indications for determination of serum Prl levels include menstrual disorders and infertility in women, and impotence and infertility in men. Current evidence indicates that hyperprolactinemia interferes with sexual and reproductive function in both sexes by disrupting normal pulsatile secretion of the hypothalamic hormone gonadotropin-releasing hormone (GnRH).

D. Hyperprolactinemia and osteoporosis. In addition to disruption of sexual and reproductive function, untreated hyperprolactinemic men and women suffer from

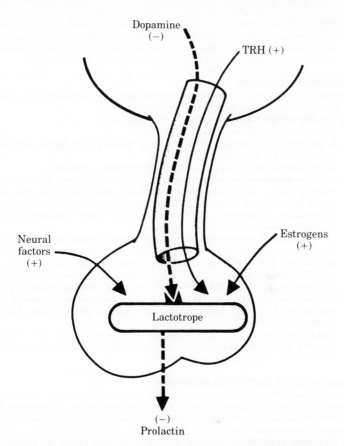

Figure 10.1. Regulation of prolactin secretion. TRH, thyrotropin-releasing hormone.

progressive diminution in bone density and painful osteoporosis, conditions that can be attenuated when serum Prl and gonadal hormone levels are normalized.

Prl is considered to be a "stress" hormone, and modest transient increases in serum Prl levels can be observed after venipuncture, exercise, temporal lobe seizures, and a spectrum of physical and psychological stresses. Repeat serum Prl determinations are required to determine if elevations are evanescent or chronic. Chronic hyperprolactinemia is indicative of an underlying abnormality in the regulation of Prl secretion.

III. REGULATION OF PRL SECRETION (Fig. 10.1)
The dopaminergic inhibition of Prl can be superseded by estrogens, neural stimuli from the nipple, and thyrotropin-releasing hormone (TRH).
- **A. Estrogen** levels increase progressively during pregnancy and in the third trimester reach levels high enough to exert a stimulatory effect on the lactotrope, causing serum Prl levels to increase. The elevated serum Prl levels are critical to prepare the breast for lactation so that the mother can nurse her child.
- **B. Neural influences** initiated by the infant suckling at the nipple stimulate further Prl secretion to maintain breast milk production.

C. TRH, the hypothalamic hormone regulating pituitary thyroid-stimulating hormone (TSH) secretion, also provokes Prl release from the lactotrope and is thought to be responsible for the hyperprolactinemia, galactorrhea, amenorrhea, impotence, and infertility occasionally present in patients with primary hypothyroidism.

IV. HYPERPROLACTINEMIA

Hyperprolactinemia occurring in a nonpregnant euthyroid woman reflects a disruption in the normal physiologic inhibition of Prl secretion.

A. The **physiologic inhibition** of Prl secretion requires:
   1. Normal hypothalamic dopamine secretion
   2. Transport of dopamine to the pituitary lactotrope via the hypothalamichypophysial portal system
   3. An unobstructed dopamine receptor on the pituitary lactotrope

B. Many **medications** commonly used in the treatment of hypertension, nausea and vomiting, gastric atony, and psychiatric disorders cause hyperprolactinemia by depleting hypothalamic dopamine, blocking the dopamine receptor, or antagonizing the dopaminergic inhibition of Prl secretion. Table 10.1 lists medications and clinical conditions known to cause hyperprolactinemia.

On occasion, serum prolactin levels may appear to be elevated in the absence of pituitary pathology or malfunction. This occurs when "macroprolactin," a biologically inactive form of prolactin, is present in serum and interferes with the prolactin assay. To eliminate interference caused by macroprolactin, laboratory directors may add polyethylene glycol (PEG) or rely on some other method to eliminate macroprolactin from the serum sample, allowing for a more accurate estimate of the true prolactin level. Macroprolactinemia my often confound the evaluation of the young woman with polycystic ovary syndrome.

C. Hyperprolactinemia discovered in the course of the evaluation of a woman with infertility or menstrual irregularities and during the evaluation of an impotent or infertile man requires further evaluation.

V. EVALUATION OF HYPERPROLACTINEMIA

Once medical history and appropriate studies rule out medications or miscellaneous causes of hyperprolactinemia (Table 10.1), primary hypothalamic or pituitary disease must be presumed, and anatomic and functional assessments of the hypothalamus and pituitary are in order.

A. Anatomic evaluation. Magnetic resonance imaging (MRI) or computed tomography (CT) provides adequate imaging of the hypothalamus and pituitary gland to determine if pituitary microadenomas, macroadenomas, or craniopharyngiomas are present in the hyperprolactinemic patient. When imaging studies reveal no abnormality, a diagnosis of **idiopathic hyperprolactinemia** must be presumed. Pituitary **microadenomas** appear as small (<10-mm) hypolucent lesions usually in the lateral margins of the pituitary, whereas **macroadenomas** often burgeon to sizes >10 mm and expand superiorly to compress the optic chiasm, laterally into the cavernous sinuses, or inferiorly, eroding the floor of the sella turcica. Craniopharyngiomas that cause hyperprolactinemia by compromising hypothalamic-hypophysial transit of dopamine from the hypothalamus to the pituitary lactotrope appear as cystic calcified masses in the suprasellar area.

B. Functional evaluation. Hyperprolactinemic patients, especially those with pituitary macroadenomas, can have other forms of pituitary dysfunction, including pituitary-adrenal and pituitary-thyroid insufficiency, and should have comprehensive evaluation of pituitary reserve (see Chapters 4 and 5) to determine whether glucocorticoid or thyroid hormone replacement therapy is warranted.

C. Serum gonadotropin levels should be measured because there is a subset of hyperprolactinemic women who have coexistent polycystic ovary syndrome. In this group, normalization of serum Prl levels might re-establish ovulatory menses in some, whereas others might require supplemental clomiphene citrate (Clomid) or metformin to fully normalize reproductive function.

TABLE 10.1	Causes of Hyperprolactinemia

I. Direct stimulation of pituitary lactotrope
   A. Estrogen excess
      1. Pregnancy
      2. Oral contraceptives
      3. Other estrogens
   B. Neural influences
      1. Nipple stimulation
      2. Chest wall trauma or surgery
      3. Thoracic herpes zoster
   C. TRH stimulation
      1. Primary hypothyroidism

II. Dysfunction of dopamine inhibition of prolactin release
   A. Depletion of hypothalamic dopamine
      1. Reserpine
      2. α-Methyldopa (Aldomet)
   B. Blockade of dopamine receptor on lactotrope
      1. Phenothiazines and antipsychotic medications (e.g., Compazine, Thorazine, Stelazine, Mellaril, Haldol, Risperidone)
   C. Dopamine antagonists
      1. Metoclopramide
      2. Sulpiride

III. Primary disorders of hypothalamus and pituitary
   A. Hypothalamus
      1. Craniopharyngioma
      2. Sarcoid and other granulomatous disorders
   B. Pituitary
      1. Idiopathic hyperprolactinemia
      2. Pituitary microadenoma
      3. Pituitary macroadenoma
      4. Pituitary stalk section
      5. Empty sella syndrome

IV. Miscellaneous causes
   A. Chronic renal failure

TRH, thyrotropin-releasing hormone.

   D. For the **hyperprolactinemic man,** serum gonadotropin values can be normal or low. With long-standing hyperprolactinemia, hypothalamic-pituitary testicular function is suppressed and serum testosterone levels fall to hypogonadal levels. Supplemental testosterone therapy will not restore potency in impotent hyperprolactinemic hypogonadal males. Primary treatment to normalize serum Prl levels may restore hypothalamic-pituitary-testicular function, allowing endogenous testosterone secretion to resume and obviating the need for exogenous androgen therapy. However, androgen supplements with either parenteral, transdermal patch, or testosterone gel therapy are warranted and likely to be effective in a man with a pituitary adenoma and normal serum Prl, but persistently subnormal serum testosterone levels.
   E. Evaluation of Prl dynamics in response to provocative stimuli such as TRH, L-dopa, and chlorpromazine or suppression with bromocriptine does not distinguish hyperprolactinemic patients with pituitary tumors from those with idiopathic hyperprolactinemia.
   F. The initial **serum Prl level** should alert the physician to the dimensions of the pituitary lesion.

1. Patients with serum Prl values **>200 ng/mL** usually have substantial pituitary masses.
2. When serum Prl levels are **<200 ng/mL,** idiopathic hyperprolactinemia or pituitary microadenoma is the most likely diagnosis. When hypothalamic lesions, such as craniopharyngiomas, interrupt dopamine transport to the lactotroph, serum Prl levels are usually 40 to 85 ng/mL. A comparable degree of moderate hyperprolactinemia is found in hypothyroidism or drug-induced hyperprolactinemia.

   Marked **elevations** in serum Prl levels comparable to values observed in large pituitary tumors may occur in the **absence of pituitary pathology** when two or more factors coexist, as in the patient with chronic renal failure who is treated with metoclopramide (Reglan).

   The Prl-enhancing properties of metoclopramide have been used to some advantage in mothers who are unable to produce enough breast milk for their nursing babies. With as little as 10 mg of metoclopramide tid, serum Prl levels increase from about 18 to 120 ng/mL, and the volume of breast milk produced each day doubles from 93 to 197 mL.

G. Visual fields. An **expanding prolactinoma** can extend superiorly to encroach on the medial aspect of the optic chiasm, initially causing a superior bitemporal hemianopia, whereas **craniopharyngiomas** compressing the superior margins of the optic chiasm are first evident as an inferior bitemporal hemianopia. Either tumor can progress and cause complete bitemporal hemianopia. Alleviating the pressure on the optic chiasm is critical to preserve vision.

VI. TREATMENT OF HYPERPROLACTINEMIA

A. Bromocriptine has emerged as the initial treatment of choice because this medication can inhibit Prl secretion, normalize circulating Prl levels, and reduce pituitary tumor size.

1. **Action and dosage.** Bromocriptine is a dopaminergic agonist and acts:
   a. In the hypothalamus to slow down dopamine turnover
   b. At the level of the lactotrope, where it binds to the dopamine receptor to decrease Prl secretion and release from the pituitary.

   Initial treatment with 1.25 or 2.5 mg at bedtime with a snack will minimize side effects and might normalize serum Prl levels, but a more common schedule of bromocriptine 2.5 mg twice a day may be necessary to maintain normoprolactinemia.

2. **Indications.** Bromocriptine is effective for Prl-secreting tumors of all sizes. Treatment lowers serum Prl levels and reduces pituitary tumor size, alleviating visual-field defects and other symptoms resulting from prolactinoma expansion. Imaging studies (MRI or CT) can readily demonstrate bromocriptine-induced reductions in pituitary tumor size.

3. **Side effects.** Orthostatic hypotension, nasal stuffiness, nausea, and vomiting are the most common side effects of bromocriptine. They are usually most severe with the first dose, tend to abate thereafter, and can be minimized by taking the medication with a meal.

4. Other dopaminergic agonists, such as cabergoline (Dostinex), are also effective in normalizing serum Prl levels. Cabergoline differs from bromocriptine because it is a long-acting dopaminergic agonist and is effective in normalizing serum Prl levels when administered once or twice weekly. The starting dose is 0.5 mg once weekly. If serum Prl does not normalize with a single dose, a second dose may be added 4 days after the initial dose. Side effects are similar to those of bromocriptine but may be less severe. Indeed, cabergoline has been promoted for use in those patients who are bromocriptine-intolerant.

B. Pituitary surgery is useful for patients with well-circumscribed discrete pituitary microadenomas who desire fertility. It is often necessary in hyperprolactinemic patients when their pituitary macroadenomas compress the optic chiasm, invade the cavernous sinus, or infarct (pituitary apoplexy). Well-circumscribed prolactin-secreting pituitary microadenomas can be extirpated by a transsphenoidal pituitary adenectomy. Postoperatively serum Prl levels fall to normal, galactorrhea ceases, and ovulatory menses resume. Two factors—the size of the pituitary adenoma and the skill of the neurosurgeon—determine the success of pituitary surgery. Smaller (<10-mm) pituitary adenomas are more amenable and larger (>10-mm) pituitary adenomas are less amenable to surgical cure. Initial reports describing "cure rates" of 85% to 90% have been tempered; a still impressive immediate postoperative cure rate of 70% has been cited. Unfortunately, some patients who are believed to be cured after initial pituitary surgery later relapse. More than 50% of the original surgical cures have recurrent hyperprolactinemia within 6 years after surgery. A postoperative serum Prl level <7 ng/mL is a good index of long-term cure, whereas immediate postoperative values of 8 ng/mL or greater appear to herald eventual recurrence of Prl-secreting pituitary adenomas.

C. **Optimal treatment.** Therapy must be individualized. Because both bromocriptine and cabergoline, and pituitary surgery, are effective in lowering serum Prl levels, either may be considered in the treatment of the hyperprolactinemic patient. Bromocriptine has a rapid (within 4 hours) onset of action and has emerged as the initial treatment of choice. Cabergoline, somewhat pricier than bromocriptine, may not always be covered by third-party insurers unless the treating physician can document that bromocriptine was ineffective or was not tolerated by the patient.

Pituitary surgery, when it is effective, has the advantage of being a one-time procedure, but it can be complicated by a disruption of normal anterior and posterior pituitary function, leaving an initially hyperprolactinemic but otherwise normal patient with transient or permanent hypopituitarism and diabetes insipidus. The transsphenoidal operative approach to the pituitary also increases the risk for postoperative meningitis.

Medical and surgical therapy need not be mutually exclusive. In complex cases of patients with large prolactinomas, both bromocriptine and pituitary surgery may be necessary.

A single daily dose of the long-acting nonergot dopamine agonist CV 205-502 has been reported to decrease Prl secretion and pituitary tumor size in patients with Prl-secreting macroadenomas and may prove to be useful in the future. It has a favorable side-effect profile.

VII. HYPOPROLACTINEMIA

Dopamine inhibition of Prl secretion rarely causes serum Prl levels to fall to undetectable levels. Absent or severely inhibited Prl secretion is characteristic of postpartum pituitary necrosis (Sheehan syndrome) and possibly idiopathic hypogonadotropic hypogonadism (IHH). Curiously, bromocriptine-induced suppression of serum Prl levels has a deleterious effect on spermatogenesis as well as baseline and stimulated testosterone production of normal male volunteers, implying that there may be a minimal circulating Prl level required to maintain testicular integrity.

A. **Postpartum pituitary necrosis** occurs when childbirth is complicated by extensive hemorrhage and hypotension. Pituitary size increases during pregnancy, but there is no commensurate increase in vascular supply to the pituitary. When postpartum hemorrhage causes systemic hypotension, blood flow to the pituitary is severely compromised, causing pituitary hypoxia and infarction. Panhypopituitarism can ensue, but characteristically Prl production ceases, leading to agalactia and an inability to nurse.

B. Hormone profiles of young men with **constitutional delayed puberty (CDP)** and IHH are similar, but CDP improves spontaneously whereas IHH requires treatment. Differences in Prl dynamics are believed to help in diagnosis. Low baseline serum Prl levels, unresponsive to TRH or chlorpromazine, are characteristic of the IHH group and differentiate these young men from those with CDP who have normal Prl dynamics. Reassurance is all that is required for CDP patients and their families. Treatment is warranted for IHH patients and should be initiated promptly so that they can avoid the social and physiologic suffering experienced by those who are chronologically adolescent but physically perpetually prepubescent.

Selected References

Besser GM, Parke L, Edwards CR, et al. Galactorrhea: successful treatment with reduction of plasma prolactin levels by bromergocryptine. *Br Med J* 1972;3:669–672.

Boyd AE, Reichlin S, Turksoy RN. Galactorrhea-amenorrhea syndrome: diagnosis and therapy. *Ann Intern Med* 1977;7:165–175.

Bracero N, Zacur HA. Polycytic ovary syndrome and hyperprolactinemia. *Obstet Gynecol Clin North Am* 2001;28:77–84.

Carter JN, Tyson JE, Tolis G, et al. Prolactin-secreting tumors and hypogonadism in 22 men. *N Engl J Med* 1978;299:847–852.

Colao A, Di Sarno A, Sarnacchiaro F, et al. Prolactinomas resistant to standard dopaminergic agonists respond to chronic cabergoline treatment. *J Clin Endocrinol Metab* 1997;2:876–883.

Conley RR. Risperidone side effects. *J Clin Psychiatry* 2000;61:18–20.

Dickinson RA, Seeman MV, Coreblum B. Hormonal side effects in women: Typical versus atypical antipsychotic treatment. *J Clin Psychiatry* 2000;61:10–15.

Ehrenkranz RA, Ackerman BA. Metoclopramide effect on faltering milk production in mothers of premature infants. *Pediatrics* 1986;78:614–620.

Escobar-Morreale HF. Macroprolactinemia in women presenting with hyperandrogenic symptoms. *Fertil Steril* 2004;82:1697–1699.

Greenspan SL, Neer RM, Ridgway EC, Klibanski A. Osteoporosis in men with hyperprolactinemic hypogonadism. *Ann Intern Med* 1986;104:777–782.

Iranamesh A, Mulligan T, Veldhius JD. Mechanisms subserving the physiological nocturnal relative hyporolactinemia of healthy older men: dual decline in prolactin secretory burst mass and basal release with preservation of pulse duration frequency and interpulse interval—a General Clinical Research Center study. *J Clin Endocrinol Metab* 1999;84:1083–1090.

Kavanagh L, McKenna TJ, Fahie-Wilson MN, et al. Specificity and clinical utility of methods for the detection of macroprolactin. *Clin Chem* 2006;52:1366–1372.

Klibanski A, Neer RM, Beitins IZ, et al. Decreased bone density in hyperprolactinemic women. *N Engl J Med* 1980;303:1511–1514.

Koppelman MC, et al. Hyperprolactinemia, amenorrhea, and galactorrhea. *Ann Intern Med* 1984;100(1):115–121.

Legro RS, Bernhart HX, Schlaff WD, et al. Clomiphene, metformin or both for infertility in the polycystic ovary syndrome. *N Engl J Med* 2007;356:551–566.

Oseko F, Nakano A, Morikawa K, et al. Effects of chronic bromocriptine-induced hypoprolactinemia on plasma testosterone responses to human chorionic gonadotropin stimulation in normal men. *Fertil Steril* 1991;55:355–357.

Prolactinomas: bromocriptine rules O.K.? *Lancet* 1982;1:430.

Sartorio A, Pizzocaro A, Liberati D, et al. Abnormal LH pulsatility normalizes after bromocriptine treatment: deconvolution based assessment. *Clin Endocrinol* 2000;52:703–712.

Serri O, Beauregard H, Lesage J, et al. Long term treatment with CV 205–502 in patients with prolactin secreting macroadenomas. *J Clin Endocrinol Metab* 1990;71:682–687.

Serri O, Rasio E, Beauregard H, et al. Recurrence of hyperprolactinemia after selective transsphenoidal adenomectomy in women with prolactinemia. *N Engl J Med* 1983;309:280–283.

Spark RF, Baker R, Bienfang DC, Bergland R. Bromocriptine reduces pituitary tumor size and hypersecretion: requiem for pituitary surgery? *JAMA* 1982;247:311–316.

Spark RF, Pallotta J, Naftolin F. Galactorrhea-amenorrhea syndromes: etiology and treatment. *Ann Intern Med* 1976;84:532–537.

Spark RF, Wills CA, O'Reilly G, et al. Hyperprolactinemia in males with and without pituitary macroadenomas. *Lancet* 1982;2:129–132.

Spitz IM, Hirsch HJ, Trestian S. The prolactin response to thyrotropin-releasing hormone differentiates isolated gonadotropin deficiency from delayed puberty. *N Engl J Med* 1983;308:575–579.

Tindall GT, Barrow LB. Prolactinomas. In: Wilkins RW, Rengachary SS, eds. *Neuro-surgery*. New York: McGraw-Hill, 1985:852.

Tucker H St G, et al. Galactorrhea-amenorrhea syndrome: follow-up of 45 patients after pituitary tumor removal. *Ann Intern Med* 1981;94:302.

Tucker H St G, Lankford HV, Glackard WG. Persistent defect in regulation of prolactin secretion following successful pituitary tumor removal in women with galactorrhea-amenorrhea syndrome. *J Clin Endocrinol Metab* 1980;51:968.

Wass JAH, et al. Reduction of pituitary tumor size in patients with prolactinomas and acromegaly treated with bromocriptine with or without radiotherapy. *Lancet* 1979; 2:66.

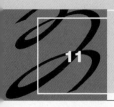

ENDOCRINOLOGY OF PSYCHIATRIC DISORDERS
11

Calvin Ezrin

I. THE ENDOCRINE HYPOTHALAMUS

The hypothalamus is the major interface between the nervous and endocrine systems. Three neurotransmitters—serotonin, dopamine, and norepinephrine—exert important influences on the secretion of hypothalamic regulating factors. They act in the hypophysiotropic area of the endocrine hypothalamus to stimulate or inhibit the activity of the neurons that manufacture peptide hormones that regulate the function of the adenohypophysis. Drug treatment of psychiatric disorders, severe emotional disturbances, and profound malnutrition may significantly impair the function of the endocrine hypothalamus.

II. ANOREXIA NERVOSA

A. Clinical features

1. A profound eating and behavioral disorder producing marked weight loss.

2. The characteristic psychopathology is a morbid fear of becoming fat. Overactivity with deliberate overexercise occurs in order to burn calories and induce weight loss. Typically, activity is solitary, with a strong obsessive character, performed in regular and rigid sequence.

3. A characteristic endocrine disorder is amenorrhea in females and loss of sexual potency and sexual interest in males.

4. In spite of the designation "anorexia," most patients do not complain of actual loss of appetite.

5. Purging behaviors. In addition to food restriction, some anorexia patients use vomiting, laxatives, and diuretics to induce further weight loss. The resultant hypokalemia may cause cardiac arrest, which accounts for some of the considerable mortality associated with this condition.

B. Incidence.
Women constitute ~95% of all cases, with the age ranging from 12 to 30 years. This disorder occurs predominantly in industrialized, developed countries. Sociocultural factors play an important role in the occurrence of this disorder. Fashion models and ballet dancers are at greater risk for the development of this eating disorder than any other professional group.

C. Endocrine disturbances.
Hypogonadotropic hypogonadism manifested by:

1. Secondary amenorrhea.

2. Failure to achieve sexual maturation in prepubertal girls and boys.

3. Osteoporosis and pathologic fractures may result from lack of adequate estrogen at a critical period of bone formation.

4. Thyroid abnormalities. As in other starved states, tri-iodothyronine (T3) is usually reduced because of inhibition of thyroxine (T4) deiodinase, which normally drives conversion of T4 to T3.

D. Diagnosis.
By the time they are brought for help, patients are usually in a state of semistarvation, which they defend as normal. Emaciation increases because of slowly progressive starvation. Hypokalemia suggests laxative and diuretic abuse as well as self-induced vomiting.

E. Differential diagnosis.
A psychological pattern of denial of ill health until wasted to a degree not seen in patients with organic disease who are still able to be active,

distinguishes this condition from patients with other psychiatric and medical diseases. Lesser degrees of hypothalamic hypogonadism, which are sometimes seen with secondary amenorrhea that follows severe emotional upset, can be distinguished by a lack of obsession with thinness. Hypogonadotropic hypogonadism from pituitary or organic hypothalamic lesions is easily distinguished from anorexia nervosa because the morbid pursuit of thinness is lacking.

F. Treatment

1. Hospitalization may be required, depending on the severity of the eating disorder and/or social factors.
2. Careful evaluation and ongoing medical management are essential.
3. Ideally, an eating disorder unit with medical and psychiatric supervision of nursing and nutritional services should be available for seriously affected patients, such as those who have lost >25% of their ideal body weight.
4. Because of the stubborn clinging to the idea that thinness will resolve all of their emotional problems, these patients resist reasonable suggestions to improve their health by regaining weight. Tube feeding or intravenous hyperalimentation may be required for initial treatment in patients who refuse to eat. With improved nutrition, mental attitude toward food often changes, and recovery may then result. A certain number prove incurable, dying of infection that a weakened immune system cannot withstand.
5. Suicide may be a last act of desperation. In those who survive, there is often a long-lasting emotional burden, with lingering depression, social reclusiveness, or schizoid behavior.
6. Psychotherapy and psychotropic drugs are useful adjuncts in most patients, but they are more effective when an improved nutritional state has been achieved.

III. PSYCHIATRIC ASPECTS OF ENDOCRINOLOGY

A review of the psychiatric aspects of endocrine and metabolic practice supports the view that the brain is as likely to be affected by endocrine and metabolic disorders as to cause them.

A. Hypoglycemia

1. Hypoglycemia may manifest as bizarre behavior, aggressive drunkenness, panic attacks, disorientation, and sometimes coma.
2. It is easy to suspect in a patient on insulin, but it may not be recognized early in patients with islet cell tumor or other neoplasm with insulinlike activity (see Chapter 36).

B. Hypothyroidism

1. If it is long-standing and severe, hypothyroidism may present with mental symptoms such as depression, dementia, delusions, and, ultimately, life-threatening coma.
2. If the patient does not respond readily to thyroid replacement, consider some other additional cause for the condition (see Chapter 30).
3. As in other starved states, T3 is reduced because of inhibition of T4 deiodinase, which normally drives conversion of T4 to T3. Because thyroid-stimulating hormone (TSH) remains normal, no treatment is required except improved nutrition, which increases T4 deiodinase.

C. Hyperthyroidism

1. Hyperthyroidism often presents with anxiety, racing thoughts, euphoria, and manic behavior.
2. The diagnosis is usually clinically obvious and is easily confirmed by laboratory testing.
3. Treatment with antithyroid drugs and tranquilizers should be administered before administering radioiodine therapy and surgery (see Chapter 30).

D. Hyperparathyroidism

1. In common with other causes of increased calcium, parathyroid overactivity affects the nervous system via decreased neuromuscular excitability and, ultimately, profound muscle weakness.

2. Mental confusion, drowsiness, and even coma have been observed with very high levels of calcium.
3. Agitation, paranoia, personality disorders, and depression have also been observed.
4. These features disappear promptly on removal of the offending adenoma with restoration of normal serum calcium.

E. Adrenocortical disorders
   1. Cushing syndrome: Profound mental changes may accompany chronic hypercortisolism.
      a. When the disease is caused by **overproduction of cortisol,** there is a high incidence of depression. Suicide is an important cause of death in these patients.
      b. In Cushing syndrome from **exogenous glucocorticoid** therapy, the most common psychological effect is euphoria, although depression is sometimes seen and may be severe.

IV. EFFECT OF PSYCHOTROPIC DRUGS ON ENDOCRINE FUNCTION
   A. Neuroleptic antipsychotic drugs may lead to sufficient depletion of hypothalamic dopamine, which results in excessive secretion of prolactin, producing galactorrhea and amenorrhea.
   B. Lithium
   1. Lithium is widely used to stabilize bipolar affective disorder patients; it may lead to inhibition of thyroid hormone production, resulting in a goiter, often with accompanying hypothyroidism.
   2. Lithium may also cause hyperparathyroidism, affecting calcium homeostasis by several different mechanisms. The most likely is that lithium raises the threshold of the calcium-sensing apparatus within the parathyroid gland, responsible for shutting off parathyroid hormone secretion. Consequently, parathyroid hormone release continues despite elevated calcium levels. Withdrawal of the drug is usually sufficient for control, but PTH, or parathyroid hormone levels, may remain elevated for months and should not prompt inappropriate surgical intervention.
   3. Lithium may produce a type of nephrogenic diabetes insipidus because of its antagonism to the antidiuretic effect of vasopressin.
   C. Atypical antipsychotic drugs. Olanzapine (Zyprexa), risperidone (Risperdal), and quetiapine (Seroquel) have produced significant metabolic side effects, such as weight gain and hypoglycemia, that were not observed to a comparable degree with the original, conventional antipsychotic drugs. These weight-promoting properties appear to be related to stimulation of hypothalamic appetite-enhancing receptors. Because these orexigenic effects cannot be controlled by conventional weight-loss programs, dramatic weight gain, often with type 2 diabetes, may result.

   Appetite-enhancing psychotropic drugs are not indicated for anorexia nervosa when putting on weight could be intolerable and could precipitate an emotional crisis, pushing the patient into further restrictive behavior.

Selected References

Fisher M. Treatment of eating disorders in children, adolescents and young adults. *Pediatr Rev* 2006;27:5–16.

Lambert L. Diabetes risk associated with use of olanzapine, quetiapine, and risperidone in Veterans Health Administration patients with schizophrenia. *Am J Epidemiol* 2006;164:672–681.

Melchior JC. From malnutrition to refeeding during anorexia nervosa. *Curr Opin Clin Nutr Metab Care* 1998;1:481–485.

Slupik RI. Managing adolescents with eating disorders. *Int J Fertil Women's Med* 1999; 44:125–130.

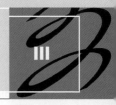

Adrenal Disorders III

THE ADRENAL CORTEX AND MINERALOCORTICOID HYPERTENSION

Naftali Stern, Etty Osher, and Michael L. Tuck

12

CUSHING SYNDROME

I. GENERAL PRINCIPLES

Cushing syndrome refers to a diverse symptom complex resulting from excess steroid hormone production by the adrenal cortex (endogenous) or to sustained administration of glucocorticoids (exogenous). The common clinical features of classical Cushing syndrome include central obesity (90%), hypertension (85%), glucose intolerance (80%), plethoric facies (80%), purple striae (65%), hirsutism (65%), menstrual dysfunction (60%), muscle weakness (60%), bruising (40%), and osteoporosis (40%). Less common features include mental changes, hyperpigmentation, acne, and hypokalemic alkalosis. More subtle presentation of Cushing syndrome may be encountered in early stages or with mild hypercortisolemia, and presenting symptoms may include "common" or moderate weight gain, diabetes, metabolic syndrome, or osteoporosis.

A. Endogenous Cushing syndrome comprises three distinct pathogenic disorders: pituitary (68%), adrenal (17%), and ectopic (15%).

    1. Pituitary Cushing syndrome (Cushing disease) is caused by a small pituitary tumor (microadenoma) that produces excessive amounts of adrenocorticotropic hormone (ACTH). In a small minority of cases, Cushing disease results from a large, usually invasive pituitary macroadenoma.

    2. Adrenal Cushing syndrome results from autonomous cortisol production by an adrenal tumor (adenoma or carcinoma) or by adrenal hyperplasia, which can be macronodular or micronodular. Adrenal Cushing syndrome is associated with suppressed plasma ACTH levels. Adrenal adenomas usually evolve gradually, and by the time of diagnosis, many of the Cushingoid symptoms are present. Dehydroepiandrosterone sulfate (DHEA-S) levels are typically suppressed as a result of suppression of ACTH secretion. Functioning (steroid-secreting) adrenal

131

carcinoma typically evolves rapidly and is often associated with excessive secretion of adrenal androgens, leading to prominent androgenic symptoms in women. ACTH-independent bilateral adrenal nodular hyperplasia is an uncommon group of disorders manifesting as Cushing syndrome. Primary pigmented adrenal nodular dysplasia is a rare disorder in which adrenal pigmented hyperplasia leads to mild and/or cyclic hypercortisolism associated with other endocrine and nonendocrine tumors such as acromegaly, Sertoli cell tumor, and myxoma (Carney complex). Another type of hyperplasia that causes Cushing is massive macronodular adrenal hyperplasia. This condition may be associated with food-dependent hypercortisolism caused by gastric inhibitory polypeptide (GIP) receptors on the adrenal glands. Food intake stimulates GIP, which binds to the ectopic receptors expressed in the adrenal cortex, where it stimulates growth and cortisol secretion. Treatment with long-acting somatostatin has been helpful in some patients. In other cases, anomalous activation of adrenal growth and steroidogenesis is mediated through β-adrenergic receptors, luteinizing hormone (LH) receptors or V1a receptors. Rarely, multiple micronodules in the adrenal produce a similar disorder.

3. **Ectopic Cushing syndrome** results from autonomous ACTH production from extrapituitary malignancies with markedly elevated plasma levels of ACTH. Although numerous malignancies have been associated with this disorder, bronchogenic carcinoma accounts for most cases.

B. **Age and sex** have some diagnostic and predictive value. Adrenal carcinoma is more common in children, pituitary Cushing syndrome is frequently seen in women of child-bearing age, and ectopic Cushing syndrome is more common in adult males.

C. **Obesity,** hypertension, and plethoric facies are common to all forms of Cushing syndrome, but the clinical expression can be highly variable, with no single feature common to all cases. Evidence of virilization (hirsutism, clitoromegaly, temporal balding) is most common in adrenal carcinoma. Hypokalemic alkalosis, myopathy, and sometimes hyperpigmentation occur most often in ectopic Cushing syndrome; and in this form of the disease, the distinguishing clinical features of hypercortisolism are often absent.

D. The **metabolic syndrome** that includes many of the findings characteristic of Cushing (central obesity, hypertension, dyslipidemia, insulin resistance, and atherosclerosis) has been often termed Cushing phenotype. Many patients with the metabolic syndrome have shown mild abnormalities in cortisol metabolism, and subjects with early hypercorticalism can present with features of the metabolic syndrome.

E. The **natural history** of Cushing syndrome can be variable, but if it is unrecognized or untreated, fully manifested disease has a 5-year mortality of 50%. Milder forms of this condition may smolder for years, and gradual transition from pre-Cushing to Cushing syndrome has been encountered. Hypertension and weight gain occur early in this disorder, with variable expression of the other features of hypercortisolism evolving over months to years. Spontaneous remissions have been reported.

F. **Periodic Cushing syndrome,** with predictable cycles of high and normal cortisol levels, can occur in any of the subtypes of Cushing syndrome and should be considered in patients with Cushingoid features when testing fails to demonstrate hypercortisolism.

II. DIAGNOSTIC EVALUATION

Because of a variety of adrenal diagnostic procedures, a stepwise evaluation is carried out in three phases: confirmation of hypercortisolism, differentiation among the three forms of Cushing syndrome, and localization procedures (Table 12.1).

A. **Screening tests for the confirmation of Cushing syndrome**

Unless exceptionally high cortisol values are seen, no single positive test should be taken as sufficient proof for the diagnosis of Cushing syndrome. At least three of the tests listed below should be performed. Sufficient time should be allowed for follow-up and retesting. We consider two positive tests as requiring further workup, i.e., performance of tests intended to differentiate among the various forms of true

TABLE 12.1	Diagnostic Evaluation of Cushing Syndrome

A. Confirmation of hypercortisolism
  1. Overnight dexamethasone suppression test or standard two-day, 2-mg test
  2. Urinary steroid excretion test (urinary free cortisol, 17-hydroxycorticosteroids).
  3. Salivary midnight cortisol or midnight serum cortisol
  4. CRH after low-dose dexamethasone suppression test
B. Differentiation of Cushing syndrome
  1. Plasma ACTH level
  2. High-dose dexamethasone suppression test
  3. Metyrapone test
C. Localization
  1. Adrenal CT
  2. MRI scan (adrenal, pituitary)
  3. Inferior petrosal sinus sampling (IPSS)
  4. Chest CT
  5. Octreotide scintigraphy

Note: In the diagnosis of Cushing syndrome and its etiologies, final interpretation depends on the integration of results from several tests; no single procedure can reliably diagnose this syndrome.
ACTH, adrenocorticotropic hormone; CRH, corticotropin-releasing hormone; CT, computed tomography; MRI, magnetic resonance imaging.

hypercortisolism. A single positive test requires careful clinical consideration and, when appropriate, further follow-up and laboratory reassessment.

1. Overnight dexamethasone suppression test. This test is done in an outpatient setting and is a practical screening test for hypercortisolism.

  a. Procedure

  (1) Dexamethasone, 1 mg PO, given at 11 to 12 P.M.

  (2) Obtain plasma cortisol at 8 A.M. the following morning.

  b. Interpretation. Most laboratories do not presently use the same assays for the measurement of cortisol that served to establish the normal serum cortisol response to dexamethasone suppression as reported in published studies. In general, though, normal subjects should suppress plasma cortisol levels to <1.8 to 2 μg/dL, following 1 mg of dexamethasone administered on the previous night. Cortisol levels in this range may be around the lower detection limit for some assays and should be viewed with caution. Familiarity with the laboratory's performance and methods, repeat testing, or referral to another laboratory, preferably a reference laboratory, are some of the options available to the clinician at this point. Levels between 2 and 7 μg/dL may be difficult to interpret, as they are commonly seen in subjects with mental depression or with alcohol- and stress-induced adrenocortical activation, referred to, collectively, as pseudo-Cushing disorders. Additional forms of testing are therefore recommended under these circumstances. On the other hand, some patients with pituitary Cushing can be quite sensitive to dexamethasone and may sometimes show rather low cortisol levels following administration of dexamethasone. Constitutive variation in the metabolic clearance of dexamethasone and acceleration in dexamethasone metabolism by alcohol and drugs such as nifedipine, rifampin, hydantoin, carbamazepine, phenobarbital, tamoxifen, and topiramate, due to the induction of CYP3A4 enzymes, which also metabolize dexamethasone, can lead to false negative results. Suppression of cortisol can be incomplete in chronic renal failure because of decreased cortisol clearance, or in high-estrogen states because of increased cortisol-binding globulin (CBG) levels. Hence, measurement of plasma dexamethasone, to verify that proper levels of dexamethasone have indeed been attained, can add much to the interpretation of any of the dexamethasone suppression tests.

2. **Urinary steroid excretion.** Absolute elevations of urinary steroid levels can be used to diagnose Cushing syndrome. The measurements are made on baseline 24-hour collections of urine, using creatinine and total volume as estimates of the adequacy of the collection.

   a. **Urinary free-cortisol excretion (UFC)** is the measurement of choice for the initial diagnosis of hypercortisolism. It represents a direct measurement of cortisol that is not bound to plasma protein and is the most reliable and useful test for assessing cortisol secretion rate as long as the assay methods and normal ranges are well defined. Because it is a specific measurement of cortisol rather than of its metabolites, it circumvents problems of variable metabolite excretion. Proper measurement of UFC requires extraction of cortisol from the urinary sample, followed by radioimmunoassay. The upper range is 90 to 100 μg per 24 hours. High-performance liquid chromatography (HPLC)–based methods provide a more specific way to assess UFC, with an upper range of ∼50 μg per 24 hours. Urinary free cortisol is elevated in 95% of Cushing syndrome patients, but only if several samples are assayed. High water intake will elevate the urine free cortisol, as will the drug carbamazepine. Incomplete urine collection, low urine output, and renal failure may cause false negative results. Some authorities advocate reliance on UFC levels exceeding three times the upper limit of the normal range as a proof of true hypercortisolism, but because specificity of detection increases with raised cutoff values, sensitivity is much diminished. We recommend repeat testing over time and consideration of at least two additional screening tests.

   b. **Urinary 17-hydroxycorticosteroids (17-OHCS),** a traditional measure of the metabolites of cortisol, is occasionally of supplementary value. A limitation of the urinary 17-OHCS measurement is the dependence of metabolite excretion on body weight. One advantage of urinary 17-OHCS over UFC is that, unlike UFC, the excretion rate of 17-OHCS is not increased in subjects who drink very large volumes of liquid. Urinary 17-OHCS measurements are elevated in 76% to 89% of cases.

3. **Standard two-day, 2-mg test.** This test provides essentially the same type of information as is derived from the shorter, overnight, 1-mg dexamethasone suppression test, but offers the opportunity to examine more parameters, including urinary excretion of cortisol and its metabolites (17-OHCS) as well as serum cortisol. It may also have higher specificity than the shorter overnight test.

   a. **Procedure**

      (1) **Baseline:** Collect 24-hour urine samples for UFC and 17-OHCS.

      (2) **Day 1:** Administer dexamethasone, 0.5 mg PO q6h, as of 9 A.M. Collect 24-hour urine sample for UFC and 17-OHCS.

      (3) **Day 2:** Administer dexamethasone, 0.5 mg PO q6h, with the last dose administered at 6 A.M. on the morning of day 3. Collect 24-hour urine sample for UFC and 17-OHCS.

      (4) **Day 3:** Collect blood sample for serum cortisol at 8 A.M.

   b. **Interpretation.** Normal subjects show suppression of 24-hour urinary cortisol excretion to <10 μg (27 nmol) per day and in urinary 17-OHCS excretion to <2.5 mg (6.9 μmol) per day. Proper suppression of serum cortisol is considered by most as a better tool in this setting, but it suffers from the same practical limitations outlined for the 1-mg dexamethasone overnight test. The performance of this test is significantly enhanced if dexamethasone is also measured. In normal subjects, serum cortisol should decline to 1.8 to 3.6 μg/dL 6 hours after the last dexamethasone dose (last dose at 3 A.M.; sample collected at 9 A.M.).

4. **Corticotropin-releasing hormone (CRH) after low-dose dexamethasone suppression test.** This test was developed to distinguish between patients with pseudo-Cushing and those with Cushing syndrome. The test is based on the premise that suppression of ACTH by dexamethasone is more profound in normal subjects and depressed patients than in patients with Cushing disease, such that following proper suppression with dexamethasone, serum cortisol cannot

be stimulated by CRH in these patients, but only in subjects with Cushing's disease.

a. **Choice of patients.** This test should be considered only for subjects who show normal suppression following dexamethasone administration but in whom Cushing syndrome continues to be seriously suspected because of clinical considerations or other anomalous (positive) screening test(s) for Cushing states.

b. **Procedure.** Give 0.5 mg dexamethasone at 6-hour intervals for 2 days, as of 12 A.M. on day 1. The CRH stimulation test is initiated at 8 A.M., 2 hours after completion of the last dexamethasone dose (6 A.M.). Both human and ovine CRH are available and can be administered as an intravenous bolus of 1 μg/kg body weight or as a fixed dose of 100 μg intravenously.

c. **Interpretation.** A measurable serum cortisol response to CRH (e.g., cortisol level >1.4 to 2.5 μg/dL measured 15 minutes after CRH administration) identifies patients with Cushing syndrome compared to those with pseudo-Cushing conditions, with a sensitivity of ~90%, but with much lower specificity, ranging overall around 70%, in reports published thus far.

5. **Diurnal variation of circulating cortisol.** Plasma cortisol values are highest from 6 to 8 A.M., declining during the day to <50% to 80% of morning values from 10 P.M. to midnight. This rhythm is typically lost very early in the course of Cushing syndrome.

a. **Salivary cortisol.** The concentration of cortisol in the saliva is correlated with free or biologically active cortisol levels in serum or plasma. A sampling device is available with which saliva can be collected by chewing on a cotton tube for 2 to 3 minutes. This commercially available device is best used at the patient's home, followed by delivery to a reference laboratory the next morning. Cortisol in the saliva is quite stable and can be sent for determination over several days. Testing is done at bedtime up to 11 or 12 P.M., but timing may actually affect the result, as the true nadir of circulating cortisol typically takes place at midnight or even later. A salivary cortisol >5.6 nmol/L is suggestive of true hypercortisolism, but variations in reference values among laboratories and methods (e.g., radioimmunoassay vs. tandem mass spectrometry) requires attention. False positive cases have been noted in older obese hypertensive and/or type 2 diabetic men.

b. **Midnight serum cortisol** seems intuitively to be a direct measure of circulating cortisol, but sample drawing requires hospitalization or some other special setting, with obligatory disruption of normal late-night activities. This in itself may weaken the specificity of the measurement of serum cortisol.

c. **Procedure.** Sampling is best performed with an indwelling needle and with basal conditions maintained for 30 minutes prior to sampling. Because cortisol is secreted in pulsatile bursts, multiple samples are taken: Sampling for cortisol is done at 30-minute intervals between 10 P.M. and midnight. Patients should be in the supine position before and during the study.

d. **Interpretation.** A midnight plasma cortisol of 7.5 μg/dL or greater strongly suggests a diagnosis of Cushing syndrome. Values of 5.0 μg/dL or less are unlikely to be Cushing's syndrome, and values of 2.0 μg/dL nearly exclude Cushing. This test has value in moderate cases of hypercortisolism (where urine free cortisol is normal), especially in distinguishing pseudo-Cushing, in which a normal diurnal pattern can be retained. A timed or spot urinary free-cortisol-to-creatinine ratio at midnight can also be used to establish the presence of hypercortisolism. Also, a midnight "sleeping" plasma cortisol of 1.8 μg/dL or greater is shown to have a 100% diagnostic sensitivity for Cushing syndrome, but specificity at this level is apparently low. In general, it has been difficult to obtain a nonstressed late-night cortisol measurement.

B. **Differential diagnosis of Cushing syndrome:** **is hypercortisolism ACTH-dependent?**

1. **Plasma ACTH**

a. **Basal plasma ACTH.** Improvements in the measurement of plasma ACTH using the immunoradiometric assay (IRMA) offer good sensitivity and specificity in the differential diagnosis of Cushing syndrome. Samples should be taken at 8:00 A.M. under basal condition. Because ACTH is rapidly degraded by circulating peptidases, samples must be chilled and plasma separated, aliquoted, and frozen immediately. The concomitant measurement of ACTH and cortisol offers a rational approach to the differential diagnosis of Cushing syndrome, in that it establishes in a simple preliminary manner whether hyper-cortisolemia, once established and if present at the time of testing, is ACTH-dependent.

(1) **Ectopic or pituitary Cushing.** Whenever basal levels of ACTH are measurable (ACTH values >10 pg/mL) in a patient with high levels of plasma cortisol, ectopic or pituitary Cushing (ACTH-dependent) forms of Cushing syndrome should be suspected. Plasma ACTH is sometimes very elevated in **ectopic Cushing syndrome,** most often because of lung carcinoma, but can be only mildly elevated or normal in patients with bronchial carcinoid tumors. Patients with **pituitary Cushing syndrome** have elevated baseline plasma ACTH values in about half the cases; this elevation is often mild to moderate (50 to 250 pg/mL), with the remainder of patients having levels within the normal range. An important pitfall with ectopic secretion of ACTH relates to the high specificity of the currently used ACTH assays, which may miss even very high levels of slightly modified ACTH molecules formed by the ectopic tissue, which still retains significant bioactivity.

(2) **Adrenal Cushing syndrome.** Undetectable levels of ACTH (ACTH values <5 pg/mL) in the presence of increased plasma cortisol levels suggest the diagnosis of adrenal Cushing syndrome (ACTH-independent).

A common difficult dilemma in the work up of Cushing syndrome is a case of pituitary Cushing with a negative magnetic resonance imaging (MRI) scan of the pituitary (can be up to 50%) and equivocal levels of plasma ACTH versus an ectopic ACTH-secreting tumor, usually a bronchial carcinoid, that might be roentgenographically occult and have equivocal ACTH levels. CRH testing and inferior petrosal sinus sampling is helpful in these cases.

2. **High-dose (8-mg) dexamethasone suppression test.** Administration of large dosages (8 mg/day for 2 days) of the potent synthetic glucocorticoid dexamethasone will suppress urinary or plasma cortisol by >50% of baseline in pituitary but not in adrenal or ectopic Cushing syndrome. The test distinguishes pituitary Cushing syndrome from other causes in ~85% of cases. Some practitioners maintain that the high-dose dexamethasone suppression test has been made obsolete by the availability of reliable methods for the measurement of plasma ACTH, pituitary imaging, and inferior petrosal sinus sampling. The inconvenience of the latter procedure, pitfalls in measuring plasma ACTH, and the high rate of pituitary and adrenal incidentalomas (up to 10% of the general population) comprise sufficient grounds for continued performance of this test.

a. **Procedure**

(1) **Baseline.** Collect 24-hour urine samples for UFC and 17-OHCS.

(2) **Day 1.** Administer dexamethasone, 2 mg PO q6h. Collect 24-hour urine sample for UFC and 17-OHCS.

(3) **Day 2.** Administer dexamethasone, 2 mg PO q6h. Collect 24-hour urine sample for UFC and 17-OHCS.

b. **Interpretation.** Suppression to >50% of baseline of urinary UFC or 17-OHCS on day 2 indicates lack of complete autonomy of ACTH secretion, and is therefore compatible with pituitary Cushing disease or, occasionally, bronchial carcinoid tumor; failure to suppress on 8 mg/day implies adrenal or ectopic Cushing syndrome. **Anomalous responses** to high-dose dexamethasone suppression include the following.

(1) Suppression in ectopic Cushing because of bronchial tumors of low-grade malignancy

(2) Paradoxical increases in 17-OHCS in an occasional case of pituitary Cushing syndrome

(3) Lack of suppression of cortisol and or its metabolites in subjects harboring a large pituitary macroadenoma

This test has a diagnostic sensitivity and specificity of 80% to 85%, so as many as 15% of pituitary Cushing subjects will not be detected by this test. More recent criteria have been established that improve diagnostic accuracy. A decrease from baseline levels in urinary free cortisol of >90% and in 17-OHC excretion of >64% will detect 100% of patients with pituitary Cushing and exclude most ectopic cases.

3. The 8-mg overnight dexamethasone suppression test. This test can be used in place of the 2-day dexamethasone suppression test because it probably has similar accuracy and specificity.

a. Procedure

(1) Obtain a plasma cortisol at 8 A.M. as baseline, then give 8 mg of dexamethasone at 11 P.M. and draw another blood sample for plasma cortisol at 8 A.M. the next morning.

b. Interpretation. More than a 50% reduction in plasma cortisol from the baseline level strongly indicates pituitary Cushing syndrome.

4. CRH stimulation test. CRH, upon its release from the hypothalamus, selectively stimulates the pituitary corticotrope cells to increase ACTH; this is followed by a rise in cortisol. Both human and ovine CRH are available and are administered as an intravenous bolus of 1 μg/kg body weight or as a fixed dose of 100 μg intravenously. This dose increases ACTH and cortisol levels in up to 90% of patients with pituitary Cushing syndrome, because most pituitary ACTH-secreting tumors have CRH receptors. Patients with ectopic or adrenal Cushing syndrome have no ACTH or cortisol response to CRH. This test differentiates ACTH-dependent from ACTH-independent Cushing syndrome but might not always distinguish pituitary (eutopic) from ectopic causes, mostly because some pituitary patients do not respond to CRH. In this situation, a more precise method to localize the source of ACTH, such as inferior petrosal sinus sampling, is required.

5. Limitations of testing procedures for Cushing syndrome. The exact order and number of tests necessary to diagnose and distinguish the presence and type of Cushing syndrome depend on the difficulty of attaining the goal. The perfect approach to the diagnosis of Cushing syndrome is still evolving. In some cases an abnormal overnight dexamethasone suppression test, an elevated plasma ACTH level, and precise localization of the tumor suffice, indicating ectopic, pituitary, or adrenal Cushing syndrome. In other cases, the high-dose dexamethasone test might be needed to establish the etiology of hypercortisolism, or measurement of ACTH during CRH and inferior petrosal sinus sampling. A host of pitfalls (e.g., periodic cortisol production, unreliable laboratory sources, improper handling or transport of ACTH samples, variation in dexamethasone metabolism and cortisol clearance rate, missed doses, inaccurate or incomplete urine collection during dexamethasone suppression) surround these tests. Periodic hormonogenesis in Cushing syndrome with episodic phases of eucorticalism requires repeated testing over time. Depression, alcohol ingestion, and stress produce false positive results (pseudo-Cushing) in basal cortisol and ACTH in the dexamethasone suppression tests. Also, an occasional case of adrenal or ectopic Cushing syndrome displays normal dexamethasone suppression. Increasingly often, cases of Cushing syndrome are detected in the course of the workup of an adrenal incidentaloma on computed tomography (CT) scan, osteoporosis, or unexplained weight gain.

C. Localization procedures

1. Pituitary Cushing syndrome. Magnetic resonance imaging of the pituitary is the initial procedure of choice, as it detects 50% to 85% of pituitary ACTH-secreting microadenomas, with current estimates of resolution reaching as low as 2-mm tumor size. ACTH-secreting pituitary tumors typically (95%) generate a hypointense signal on MRI with no postgadolinium enhancement. Because a minority of ACTH-producing microadenomas (5%) display an isointense signal postgadolinium, care should be taken to obtain pregadolinium images. The sensitivity of CT scanning in the localization of pituitary Cushing disease is much lower and has been estimated at ~40% to 50%, thus rendering CT a suitable choice only if MRI is contraindicated. Because of the significant rate (10%) of pituitary incidentalomas in the general population, caution should be exercised in assuming that the presence of such lesions on MRI establishes the presence of pituitary Cushing disease; biochemical studies must support the diagnosis.

2. **Adrenal Cushing syndrome** is suspected in a subject with suppressed plasma ACTH, blunted ACTH response to CRH, and lack of suppression of urine or plasma steroids by high-dose dexamethasone testing.

   a. **CT scan of the adrenal** is the initial test of choice and reliably identifies most tumors because the surrounding tissue is suppressed and atrophied. One or more lesions can be seen, and they may be uni- or bilateral. Adrenal adenoma or cortisol-producing benign nodules are typically round and of homogeneous density; have a smooth contour, appear well demarcated, and measure <4 cm in diameter. They usually have low unenhanced CT attenuation values of <10 Hounsfield units (HU), which increases only moderately following contrast enhancement, to <37 to 40 HU at 30 minutes. Adrenal carcinoma, on the other hand, is typically unilateral and of nonhomogeneous appearance, larger in size and with higher unenhanced CT attenuation values (>10 HU), rising to >40 HU at 30 minutes after contrast administration.

   b. **MRI** complements the CT scan in some cases but does not offer greater sensitivity for small adrenal lesions. Adenomas are classically isointense with liver on both T1- and T2-weighted MRI sequences and display chemical shift evidence of lipid on MRI. In contrast, adrenal carcinoma is typically hypointensive compared with liver on T1-weighted MRI, but generates high to intermediate signal intensity on T2-weighted MRI.

3. **Ectopic Cushing syndrome**

   a. **Full lung CT and MRI scans** detect a high percentage of ectopic ACTH-secreting tumors in the thorax, such as bronchial carcinoid and small cell carcinoma of the lung, and are therefore the procedures of choice. Detection of these lesions is important because thoracic neuroendocrine tumors (bronchial carcinoid or thymoma) and thyroid medullary carcinoma–producing ACTH can be cured with surgery. Clinical outcome in subjects harboring small-cell lung carcinomas is usually rapidly progressive. Ectopic CRH-secreting tumors have been described, but they usually also contain ACTH, so the tumor behaves in a paracrine rather than endocrine mode. Because some of these ectopic CRH lesions do cause hypercortisolism, it is important to note that they will give a false positive result on inferior petrosal sinus ACTH sampling, because the tumorous CRH utilizes the pituitary ACTH.

   b. **Octreotide scintigraphy.** Some ACTH-secreting neuroendocrine tumors express somatostatin receptors type 2 and/or 5 and may therefore be detected by radiolabeled somatostatin analogs (OctreoScan). However, the likelihood of correct localization of an ectopic ACTH-producing tumor missed by current CT techniques through the performance of an octreotide scan is fairly low. This is also why a positive scan requires confirmation by CT or MRI. While it is not strictly specific for neuroendocrine tumors (false positives may include breast cancer and lymphoma), a positive OctreoScan in the setting of ectopic ACTH secretion likely indicates the presence of a neuroendocrine tumor and may occasionally suggest potential therapeutic response to somatostatin analogs.

D. **Inferior petrosal sinus sampling**

   1. Inferior petrosal sinus sampling is the most reliable means of distinguishing pituitary from nonpituitary ACTH hypersecretion. Sampling for ACTH venous gradients during petrosal sinus catheterization in the areas of pituitary venous drainage may detect a central or eutopic etiology of ACTH. Samples can be drawn before and/or after 100 μg of CRH administered intravenously. Correction for prolactin level in the samples obtained may assist in identifying problems related to localization of the draining catheter and dilution. Administration of CRH may not be necessary if blood samples are obtained closer to the pituitary, from the cavernous sinuses instead of the petrosal sinuses. Such techniques are limited to few

specialized centers and require a skilled invasive radiologist. Samples for ACTH are obtained simultaneously from each inferior petrosal sinus before as well as 2 to 3 and 5 to 6 minutes after CRH.

2. An inferior petrosal sinus (IPS)-to-peripheral (P) ratio >2.0 to 3.0 confirms the presence of a pituitary ACTH-secreting tumor. Subjects who have an IPS:P ratio of 1.8 or less are assumed to have an ectopic source. CRH testing is needed because up to 15% of pituitary tumors will not show an abnormal basal gradient. Correct preoperative lateralization of an ACTH-secreting microadenoma to the right or left hemisphere of the pituitary gland can be accomplished much less frequently than was initially believed, probably because of asymmetric venous drainage in many pituitary glands.

3. The procedure carries some risk, including false positive and false negative results. Direct procedure-related risks are not common but include, besides inguinal and jugular hematomas or transient arrhythmias, rare serious consequences such as perforation of the right atrium, cavernous sinus thrombosis, and cerebrovascular events (0.2%), sometimes with permanent brainstem damage. Hence, IPS should be reserved for clearly equivocal cases such as normal pituitary MRI or the presence of very small pituitary lesions and/or atypical response to dexamethasone and/or CRH.

III. TREATMENT

A. Pituitary Cushing syndrome.

1. **Transsphenoidal adenomectomy** or **hypophysectomy** is the treatment of choice in the majority of patients with pituitary Cushing syndrome. Selective removal of pituitary microadenomas yields an immediate remission rate of 80% to 85%, but remission is <50% for invasive tumors. Surgical damage to anterior pituitary function is rare. Mortality is low and complications occur in ~5% of patients, including diabetes insipidus (usually transient), cerebrospinal fluid (CSF) rhinorrhea, and hemorrhage. Postoperative hypoadrenalism (requiring glucocorticoid replacement therapy) is expected, such that morning (8 A.M.) cortisol levels normally decline to <2 μg/dL within 24 to 72 hours following successful removal of the tumor. Immediate reoperation if postoperative hypocortisolism does not occur is advocated by some, usually resorting to subtotal or total hypophysectomy, but spontaneous delayed decline in serum cortisol in some patients renders this approach questionable. Within the first 5 to 10 postoperative years, significant recurrence is seen, resulting in long-term surgical cure of 60% to 70%.

2. **Pituitary x-irradiation** is an optional form of therapy for patients with pituitary Cushing disease who are either not candidates for surgery or who have failed surgery. The best and fastest results have been reported in children, but despite early reports of low response rate in adults, long-term remission rates in adult subjects who failed surgical attempts may exceed 80%. There is a long lag period before correction of hypercortisolism (6 to 60 months), but symptoms can be controlled in the interim with mitotane, 3 g per day, or enzyme inhibitors. Radiation therapy with protons or α particles yields a higher remission rate and a shorter lag phase. Hypopituitarism and late relapse can occur.

3. **Radiosurgery** is an emerging and apparently effective irradiation technique for Cushing disease after failed transsphenoidal surgery, but relapse is a problem with this therapy as well.

B. Adrenal Cushing syndrome

1. **Unilateral adrenal adenomas** are removed by surgery and have a high remission rate. Because the contralateral adrenal gland is suppressed, glucocorticoid replacement is necessary for several months or years until adrenal function returns (see Adrenal Insufficiency, Section IV).

2. **Adrenal carcinoma.** Surgery is the treatment of choice. The transabdominal approach is preferable because it enables assessment of the extent of the disease and removal of involved organs and because recurrence rate may be higher in subjects undergoing laparoscopic adrenalectomy. For residual disease or inoperable

carcinoma, mitotane can be used as a palliative drug. Further, mitotane may prolong recurrence-free survival in patients with radically resected adrenal cortical carcinoma and is presently recommended even in apparently disease-free subjects following surgery. Starting dose is 250 mg qid and with gradual increase to tolerance levels (24 g/day) should be assisted by monitoring mitotane levels to achieve, whenever possible, therapeutic levels (14 to 25 μg/mL). Severe gastrointestinal effects (nausea, vomiting, diarrhea) occur in 80% of patients. Central nervous system toxicity (somnolence, dizziness, vertigo) is common because mitotane is fat-soluble. Hypercholesterolemia, which usually requires treatment with HMG-CoA reductase inhibitors, often develops as the dose of mitotane is increased toward the effective range. Because hypoadrenalism can occur and because mitotane enhances cortisol clearance and increases CBG, serum cortisol *and* urinary free cortisol should be monitored. In advanced or recurrent disease, chemotherapy consisting of etoposide, doxorubicin, and cisplatin can be added to mitotane, achieving benefit in up to half of subjects treated.

C. Ectopic Cushing syndrome
 1. **Surgery.** Removal of the ACTH-secreting tumor is the treatment of choice but is usually not feasible because of the nature of the underlying process (e.g., carcinoma of the lung). Adrenalectomy can be considered in cases of indolent yet inoperable tumors such as some medullary carcinomas of the thyroid.
 2. **Adrenal enzyme inhibitors** are useful in reducing hypercortisolism in ectopic ACTH syndrome.
    a. **Metyrapone,** an 11-hydroxylase inhibitor, at an average dose of 250 to 500 mg tid, provides an effective means of normalizing cortisol levels. This agent can lead to increases in deoxycorticosterone, which has sufficient mineralocorticoid activity to cause hypertension and hypokalemia.
    b. **Aminoglutethimide,** which blocks the conversion of cholesterol to δ-5-pregnenolone, can also be used starting at 250 mg qid, up to 2 g daily. Because hypoadrenalism can result, monitoring of therapy (plasma cortisol, urinary free cortisol) is mandatory. Aminoglutethimide also enhances the metabolism of dexamethasone and can cause hypoaldosteronism.
    c. **Adrenolytic agents** such as mitotane (medical adrenalectomy) can be used when control cannot be obtained with metyrapone or aminoglutethimide. Mitotane is administered either alone or in addition to the enzyme inhibitors.
    d. **Ketoconazole,** an antifungal agent, is perhaps the **first choice** for antiadrenal therapy, because it is an effective and simple means to control hypercortisolism. This agent blocks steroidogenesis at several levels, the most important being the 20,22-desmolase catalyzing the conversion of cholesterol to pregnenolone. Doses range from 600 to 1 200 mg/day. The major toxicity is hepatocellular, so liver enzyme tests must be followed. It may cause hypogonadism. Patients have been maintained on this agent for years with good responses. Because ketoconazole blocks early (as well as late) in the steroid pathway (cholesterol side-chain cleavage enzyme), there is no accumulation of other potentially toxic steroids. Therapy can be combined with other agents (metyrapone, aminoglutethimide).

ADRENAL INSUFFICIENCY

I. GENERAL PRINCIPLES
  Adrenal (or **adrenal cortical**) **insufficiency** can be caused by:
  A. Primary disease at the adrenal level, involving destruction of >90% of the steroid-secreting cortex (Addison disease).
  B. Destructive process at the hypothalamic-pituitary level, leading to CRH or ACTH deficiency (or both).
  C. Long-term suppression of the **hypothalamic–pituitary–adrenal (HPA) axis** by exogenous or endogenous glucocorticoids followed by inappropriate withdrawal.

TABLE 12.2	Etiology of Chronic Adrenal Insufficiency

Primary
Idiopathic adrenal atrophy (autoimmune adrenalitis, with or without other components of the polyglandular autoimmune syndrome type 1 or 2)
Granulomatous diseases
   Tuberculosis
   Histoplasmosis
   Sarcoidosis
Neoplastic infiltration
Hemochromatosis
Amyloidosis
Following bilateral adrenalectomy
Congenital and genetic hypoadrenalism
ACTH resistance syndromes

Secondary
Tumors
   Pituitary tumor
   Craniopharyngioma
   Tumor of the third ventricle
Pituitary infarction and hemorrhage
Postpartum necrosis (Sheehan syndrome)
Hemorrhage in tumors
Granulomatous diseases
   Sarcoidosis
Following hypophysectomy
Steroid withdrawal

ACTH, adrenocorticotropic hormone.

II. CHRONIC ADRENAL FAILURE (Table 12.2)

A. Primary adrenal failure

1. **Etiology.** Primary adrenal failure evolves only when there is nearly complete destruction or infiltration of the adrenal glands.

   a. **Autoimmune adrenalitis** accounts for ~70% of cases, 50% of whom present with additional forms of autoimmune endocrinopathy, i.e., polyglandular autoimmune syndrome type I or II. Polyglandular autoimmune syndrome type I, also known as **polyendocrinopathy-candidiasis-ectodermal dystrophy (APECD)**, is an autosomal recessive disorder with mutations in the autoimmune regulator gene and is seen in childhood in association with 100% adrenal failure, hypoparathyroidism, and mucocutaneous candidiasis. Hypogonadism and malabsorption may also be present. In the more common type II polyglandular autoimmune syndrome, which is usually comprised of type 1 diabetes mellitus, autoimmune hypothyroidism, primary hypogonadism, and pernicious anemia, autoimmune adrenal insufficiency is a major component (see Table 12.2).

   b. **Infectious disease** is another cause, and disseminated **tuberculosis,** the leading cause of chronic adrenal failure in the first half of this century, now accounts for ~5% of cases. The adrenal glands are usually 100% infiltrated. Rifampin accelerates cortisol metabolism, so higher-dose steroid replacement therapy may be needed. Almost all fungal infections, an exception being candidiasis, can destroy the adrenal gland. **Histoplasmosis** is the most common cause in the United States, and **South American Blastomycosis** is the most common cause in South America. Because ketoconazole but not fluconazole or itraconazole inhibits steroid biosynthesis, it may worsen adrenal insufficiency in someone being treated for a fungal disease. **HIV/AIDS** can be associated with adrenal necrosis, but AIDS by itself does not cause adrenal insufficiency. The usual cause of adrenal insufficiency in AIDS is an associated opportunistic infection, especially cytomegalovirus and tuberculosis. Hyponatremia in AIDS is usually caused by an inappropriate antidiuretic syndrome (SIADH). Hyperkalemia is often related to trimethoprim therapy. Antifungal treatment (ketoconazole), which inhibits steroidogenesis, or concomitant treatment for tuberculosis (rifampin), which accelerates cortisol metabolism, may precipitate hypoadrenalism in these predisposed subjects.

c. **Bilateral adrenal hemorrhage** is being increasingly recognized as a cause of adrenal failure. Initially described in association with severe bacterial infections (e.g., Waterhouse-Friderichsen syndrome in meningococcemia), it is now often seen in very ill patients, particularly in association with anticoagulant therapy. A CT scan shows the classic finding of **bilateral enlargement of the adrenals.** The patient may present with subtle findings of low-grade fever, hypotension, and anemia. The adrenal gland has a rich arterial blood supply drained by only a single adrenal vein. ACTH-induced increase in adrenal blood flow with stress may overwhelm its venous drainage, with subsequent hemorrhage. Patients who have coagulopathies or who are predisposed to thrombosis can also develop adrenal hemorrhage. Heparin-associated thrombosis-thrombocytopenia syndrome is associated with adrenal vein thrombosis. The primary **antiphospholipid antibody syndrome** (lupus anticoagulant) can also be a cause of adrenal insufficiency.

d. **Bilateral metastatic infiltration** of the adrenal glands is common, especially from breast cancer (54%), bronchogenic carcinoma (44%), and renal malignancies (31%). However, most metastatic lesions do not cause adrenal insufficiency.

e. **Adrenoleukodystrophy and adrenomyeloneuropathy** are X-linked causes of adrenal insufficiency in men and are associated with demyelination of the central and peripheral nervous system. In adrenoleukodystrophy (X-ALD), mutations in the ALD gene, which encodes a peroxisomal membrane protein named adrenoleukodystrophy protein (ALDP), and the synthesis of a defective ALDP result in impaired β-oxidation of very-long-chain fatty acids (VLCFAs). Consequently, VLCFAs accumulate preferentially in lipids, primarily in the nervous system and in the adrenal cortex. The very-long-chain fats are thought to infiltrate the adrenals or act as toxins to the adrenal gland, blocking ACTH action. The screening <u>diagnostic test is the measurement of VLCFA</u> concentration in the plasma. Dietary treatment with monosaturated fatty acids is marginally effective. **Adrenoleukodystrophy** is the more severe form, occurring in childhood and advancing to coma and other severe neurologic complications. In **adrenomyeloneuropathy**, which is the milder form seen in adults, $\sim$30% of patients develop adrenal insufficiency. Specific drug therapy aimed to induce the expression of homolog proteins that show some functional redundancy with ALDP, such as ABCD2, may alter these pathways.

f. **ACTH-resistance syndromes** can be induced by mutations that inactivate ACTH receptor action or impair adrenal cortical function or development. Severe forms of the "common" variants of **congenital adrenal hyperplasia,** such as severe to **21-hydroxylase deficiency,** represent one such example. The **triple A syndrome** includes adrenal insufficiency, achalasia, and alacrima and is caused by a mutation in the gene encoding the protein ALADIN, which is part of the nuclear pore complex. The **POEMS** syndrome involves polyneuropathy, organomegaly, endocrinopathy, monoclonal gammopathy, and skin lesions. Mutations in the nuclear receptors **DAX1** and **steroidogenic factor-1** (SF1/Ad4BP, *NR5A1*), which play an important role in adrenal development and function, can lead to <u>adrenal hypoplasia</u>. Mutations in **StAR**, a protein that facilitates the transport of cholesterol into the mitochondria, lead to **congenital adrenal lipoid hyperplasia** with hypoadrenalism and hypogonadism.

    g. Other rare causes. Systemic **amyloidosis** with renal failure can also cause adrenal insufficiency.

B. Secondary Adrenal Insufficiency

1. **High-dose or prolonged glucocorticoid** administration is the most common cause of secondary, or "central" adrenal insufficiency. It is often referred to as tertiary hypogonadism, because of the hypothalamic suppression in this condition.

2. **Common anatomic causes of secondary adrenal insufficiency** include **tumors of the pituitary** gland, compression of the pituitary gland, or pituitary tumor **hemorrhage** (pituitary apoplexy), either spontaneous or during treatment with dopamine agonists. ACTH deficiency is more common in large pituitary tumors and in nonfunctioning macroadenomas than in growth hormone–secreting adenomas. Besides primary pituitary tumors, **metastatic malignancies, craniopharyngiomas, meningiomas,** and other tumors may interfere with the ACTH axis. In these diseases there is usually evidence of other pituitary hormone deficiencies. **Lymphocytic hypophysitis, sarcoidosis, histiocytosis X,** and **hemochromatosis** can destroy the pituitary or hypothalamus. **Postpartum pituitary necrosis** (Sheehan syndrome) and pituitary stalk damage by trauma can cause adrenal insufficiency. Blunt head trauma is a recently recognized cause of hypopituitarism, including secondary hypoadrenalism, and partial to complete ACTH deficiency may persist for months to years.

3. **Genetic diseases leading to developmental abnormalities of the pituitary,** such as mutations of the **Pit-1 and PROP1 genes,** can reduce ACTH and other pituitary hormones. Rare mutations in transcription factors that control early pituitary development, such as HESX1 and LHX4, also can result in variable degrees of hypopituitarism that include ACTH deficiency. Gene mutations of pro-opiomelanocortin (POMC), or prohormone-convertase 1/3, which converts POMC to ACTH, prevent formation of active ACTH.

4. **Congenital defects can lead to ACTH deficiency,** such as **septo-optic-dysplasia,** a midline brain structure developmental abnormality.

5. **Non-glucocorticoid drugs can also induce suppression of the hypothalamic–pituitary–adrenal axis,** e.g., the progestational agent Megace (megestrol acetate) and etomidate, a drug used for sedation and anesthesia.

6. **Successful removal of ACTH-secreting pituitary adenoma or adrenal cortisol-secreting tumor** is usually followed by secondary hypoadrenalism resulting from long standing suppression of the normal corticotrophs . Hypoadrenalism may persist for several months up to many years.

7. Isolated ACTH deficiency may appear in patients who have lymphocytic hypophysitis, presumably an autoimmune disease, which is often linked to recent or current pregnancy.

III. SIGNS AND SYMPTOMS

A. Symptoms of primary and secondary adrenal insufficiency result from glucocorticoid deficiency and include weakness, hypoglycemia, anorexia, weight loss, and gastrointestinal discomfort spanning from mild diffuse tenderness to chronic or acute forms of abdominal pain, vomiting, and diarrhea. Gastrointestinal symptoms are more dominant in primary than in secondary hypoadrenalism, but weight loss is a consistent finding seen in all true cases of adrenal insufficiency. Decreased libido and the loss of pubic and axillary hair are more typical in women, in whom the adrenal is a more dominant source of androgens. With protracted hypoadrenalism, mental changes spanning from memory impairment and unexplained mood changes to depression and psychosis can be seen. Diffuse muscle and joint pain is common. Primary adrenal disease also involves loss of mineralocorticoid-secreting tissue, leading to hypoaldosteronism with sodium wasting, salt craving, hypovolemia, overt or orthostatic hypotension, hyperkalemia, and mild metabolic acidosis. Because the pituitary gland is intact in primary adrenal insufficiency, the lack of cortisol will result in a compensatory increase in ACTH, leading to mucocutaneous **hyperpigmentation** as ACTH binds to the melanocyte receptor 1, which is responsible for pigmentation. The **hyperpigmentation** can be diffuse but is usually spotty, being noted around the lips and buccal membranes and in exposed or pressure areas, e.g., the knuckles, knees, feet, elbows, and belt and brassiere lines. Multiple freckles and generalized tan may be seen along with areas of vitiligo in autoimmune adrenalitis. **Hyperkalemia** occurs in 61% of primary disease, and **hyponatremia** is even more common, because of the combined effect of loss of aldosterone secretion and absence of the physiologic inhibitory effect of cortisol on ADH secretion, leading to water retention. Secondary hypoadrenalism, on the other hand, is accompanied by hyponatremia but not by hyperkalemia.

B. **Secondary adrenal insufficiency.** Clinically, secondary adrenal insufficiency can be quite subtle, presenting only as weakness and fatigue. It does not cause hypoaldosteronism, because the renin–angiotensin system is intact to control aldosterone production from the zona glomerulosa. **Two clinical features** can help distinguish primary from secondary adrenal disease: **(1) hyperkalemia** is not found in secondary disease, but **hyponatremia is common; (2) hyperpigmentation** is also not present in secondary disease, because ACTH and MSH levels are low.

Additional clues of secondary adrenal insufficiency are concomitant symptoms of hypogonadism and hypothyroidism, reflecting deficiencies in luteinizing hormone (LH), follicle-stimulating hormone (FSH), thyroid-stimulating hormone (TSH), and growth hormone (GH).

IV. ACUTE ADRENAL CRISIS
A. **Etiology.** Chronic adrenal insufficiency can evolve into acute adrenal crisis precipitated by severe infection, trauma, or surgery.
B. **Clinical presentation** includes high fever, dehydration, nausea, vomiting, and hypotension that evolves rapidly to circulatory shock. Hyperkalemia and hyponatremia are seen if mineralocorticoid deficiency is present. Elevated blood urea nitrogen (BUN) and sometimes hypercalcemia reflect extracellular fluid loss.

V. SUPPRESSION OF THE HPA AXIS
Chronic glucocorticoid therapy results in suppression of the HPA axis. Individual susceptibility to HPA suppression, with regard to steroid dosage and duration of therapy, is variable. HPA suppression can manifest in several ways, such as weakness, fatigue, depression, and hypotension occurring upon cessation of glucocorticoid therapy. Acute adrenal crisis can ensue during major stressful situations when glucocorticoids have not been appropriately increased. HPA suppression can present as undue prostration during or following relatively minor intercurrent stress or ailments such as mild upper respiratory viral infection. Subjects may present with no overt clinical manifestations and only subclinical or biochemical evidence of HPA suppression (blunted cortisol response to exogenously administered ACTH). The following situations should be considered as producing HPA suppression:
A. Any patient who has taken prednisone at a dosage of 15 to 30 mg daily for 3 to 4 weeks. Suppression of the HPA axis can last for 8 to 12 months after cessation of glucocorticoid therapy.
B. Any patient who received prednisone at a dosage of 12.5 mg daily for 4 weeks. HPA suppression can last for 1 to 4 months after cessation of therapy.
C. Any patient who has been treated with glucocorticoids and exhibits a subnormal response to the ACTH test, regardless of dose and duration of therapy.
D. Any patient with Cushing syndrome who underwent surgery for removal of an adrenal adenoma or carcinoma or transsphenoidal removal of ACTH-secreting pituitary adenoma.

VI. DIAGNOSIS OF ADRENAL INSUFFICIENCY
A. **8 A.M. Serum cortisol, plasma ACTH, and plasma renin activity (PRA).** Unless the patient has low CBG (a fairly uncommon condition), serum cortisol ≤ 3 μg/dL is practically indicative of hypoadrenalism. The ACTH IRMA is a valuable ancillary tool, because ACTH concentration often rises even before significant drops in plasma cortisol occur in primary adrenal failure. When serum cortisol is low,

properly collected and transported plasma ACTH levels should be clearly elevated in primary adrenal insufficiency. A plasma ACTH >50 to 100 pg/mL indicates primary adrenal insufficiency. Low cortisol levels associated with low ACTH concentrations are indicative of secondary hypoadrenalism, and secondary hypoadrenalism is also suggested by the combination of low cortisol levels with inappropriately "normal" plasma ACTH. ACTH level <30 pg/mL is particularly supportive of the diagnosis of secondary adrenal failure. PRA is typically increased in primary but not in secondary hypoadrenalism. *When 8 a.m. serum cortisol is higher than 3 μg/dL, additional testing will be required to confirm the presence of hypoadrenalism.*

B. Rapid ACTH stimulation test (cosyntropin [Cortrosyn] test). Cosyntropin is a potent and rapid stimulator of cortisol and aldosterone secretion. The cosyntropin test can be used on an inpatient or outpatient basis, and time of day and food intake do not alter test results. In a previously undiagnosed patient it can, and indeed should, be performed even in the emergency room, while glucocorticoid replacement with dexamethasone is initiated concomitantly.

1. Procedure

    a. Draw blood for baseline serum cortisol, aldosterone, and ACTH. Aldosterone and ACTH will help differentiate primary from secondary adrenal hypofunction.

    b. Inject 250 μg of cosyntropin either intravenously or intramuscularly. For intravenous injection, dilute cosyntropin in 2 to 5 mL of 0.9% sodium chloride and inject over 2 minutes.

    c. Obtain repeat samples for serum cortisol (and aldosterone) 30 and 60 minutes following ACTH administration.

2. Interpretation. A normal adrenal response to ACTH consists of a rise in serum cortisol to 18 μg/dL or greater. A higher cutoff of 20 μg/dL is also used to increase the sensitivity of the test. A normal response effectively rules out primary adrenal insufficiency. Patients with secondary adrenal insufficiency usually show a blunted response to cosyntropin but occasionally have a normal response. Baseline ACTH levels in primary adrenal insufficiency are high, generally >50 to 100 pg/mL, whereas levels in secondary adrenal insufficiency are low or normal (10 pg/mL or less).

    Evaluation of ACTH-induced aldosterone responses also helps to distinguish primary from secondary adrenal insufficiency. In primary adrenal insufficiency, baseline aldosterone levels are low and there is no response to cosyntropin. In secondary adrenal insufficiency, baseline aldosterone levels may be low or normal, but at 30 minutes there is an increase in plasma aldosterone of at least 4 ng/dL over baseline.

C. The low-dose (1-μg) ACTH test. This test is more sensitive and accurate than the 250-μg dose of ACTH in detecting partial adrenal gland insufficiency, especially in patients with secondary adrenal deficiency. The 250-μg dose of ACTH produces massive pharmacologic concentrations of ACTH, exceeding blood concentrations of 10,000 pg/mL, which is way above the ACTH level seen even under extreme conditions in real life. Therefore, the 250-μg dose tends to test only for maximum adrenocortical capacity and overrides any more partial loss of cortisol function. The 1-μg cosyntropin test should replace the 250-μg dose because it is more likely to detect partial or more subtle forms of adrenal insufficiency, particularly secondary adrenal insufficiency resulting from pituitary tumors or chronic glucocorticoid treatment. Two important limitations of this test should be considered, however: **(1)** standard 1-μg cosyntropin packaging is not commercially available at the present time, and care must be taken to produce the 1-μg dose accurately by serial dilutions; **(2)** the test may be unreliable in the first few weeks after acutely induced secondary hypoadrenalism (e.g., after pituitary surgery), because the evolution of impaired adrenal reserve (cortisol response to ACTH) under these conditions requires some time, yet the HPA axis may already be severely damaged as a result of ACTH deficiency.

D. Single-dose metyrapone test

    1. Purpose. Metyrapone activates the HPA axis by blocking cortisol production at the 11-hydroylase step and lowering cortisol levels. This test is used to establish or confirm the diagnosis of adrenal insufficiency and is particularly useful when secondary adrenal insufficiency is suspected. Often, patients with hypothalamic or pituitary disease have mild symptoms and a normal rapid ACTH stimulation test. Metyrapone is an inhibitor of 11β-hydroxylase, the adrenal enzyme responsible for catalyzing the conversion of 11-deoxycortisol (compound S) to cortisol—the last step in cortisol synthesis. Following metyrapone administration, cortisol synthesis is blocked, levels of cortisol fall, and ACTH release is stimulated, as is the production of adrenal steroids proximal to the enzymatic block as 11-deoxycortisol accumulates. 11-Deoxycortisol can be measured in serum or urine (as tetrahydrol 11-deoxycortisol [THS]).

2. **Procedure**
   a. **Metyrapone,** 2 to 3 g as a single dose, depending on body weight (<70 kg, 2 g; 70 to 90 kg, 2.5 g; >90 kg, 3 g), is given at midnight with a snack to minimize the nausea accompanying metyrapone.
   b. Serum cortisol and 11-deoxycortisol are collected the following morning at 8 A.M.

3. **Interpretation.** A normal response is an increase in serum 11-deoxycortisol of >7 μg/dL; patients with primary or secondary adrenal insufficiency exhibit <5 μg/dL. Cortisol levels should fall below 5 μg/dL to confirm adequate metyrapone blockade. An abnormal metyrapone test in a subject with a near-normal response to the rapid ACTH stimulation test suggests **secondary adrenal insufficiency.** The metyrapone dose needs to be increased in patients who are taking phenytoin (Dilantin), which enhances clearance of metyrapone. Adverse effects of metyrapone include gastric irritation, nausea, and vomiting. The overnight (single-dose) metyrapone test is generally safer than the standard multiple-dose metyrapone test; however, caution must be applied, especially with patients in whom primary adrenal disease is likely, because adrenal crisis can be precipitated. *Hospitalization with proper monitoring of the patient's condition is suggested for this test.* It is advisable to demonstrate some responsiveness of the adrenal cortex to ACTH before initiating a metyrapone test. If the ACTH stimulation test is already markedly blunted, then the metyrapone test may not be necessary.

E. **Diagnosing hypoadrenalism in the critically ill patient.** Partial impairment of the hypothalamic–pituitary–adrenal axis is frequently considered in critically ill patients, especially in association with conditions such as hypotension, hyponatremia, hyperkalemia, or a history of head trauma. Because random serum cortisol levels in the critically ill often reach levels as high as 30 to 60 μg/dL, it is clear that the diagnostic "pass" values of the aforementioned ACTH tests are entirely improper for such patients. Very high cortisol levels should not come as a surprise, as ACTH and cortisol secretion can be turned on, in the critically ill, by acute response circulating factors ("circulating CRH-like factors," e.g., tumor necrosis factor α [TNF-α]) other than ACTH. Based on the serum cortisol response to Cortrosyn, relative hypoadrenalism is reportedly fairly common in the ICU setting. On the other hand, serum free-cortisol response to ACTH test is much less frequently impaired, thus indicating that some critical illnesses modify cortisol binding in the serum because of hypoproteinemia or reduced CBG/CBG-binding capacity. Because no factually substantiated consensus on the diagnostic criteria in this setting exists at the present time, we apply the following principles to the diagnosis and management of hypoadrenalism in the critically ill.

1. Hypoadrenalism cannot be diagnosed using any of the criteria for normalcy used in the noncritically ill.

2. In the interpretation of random serum cortisol, serum protein levels should be considered.

3. When clinical suspicion is reasonably strong, and unless random cortisol level is clearly elevated (e.g., ≥30 to 35 μg/dL), high-dose glucocorticoid replacement therapy should be seriously considered, regardless of the outcome of dynamic testing and if no contraindication to such treatment exists, because it has been shown to benefit some patients under these circumstances.

VII. TREATMENT
A. Chronic adrenal insufficiency
1. **Primary adrenal insufficiency** requires replacement with both glucocorticoids and mineralocorticoids.
   a. **Glucocorticoid replacement** is best given with hydrocortisone. Classically, this agent was given as 20 mg in the morning and 10 mg later in the day. It is now recognized that cortisol production is <30 mg per day, so lower doses should be given, especially because the 30-mg/day dose might decrease bone density and cause other features of chronic hypercortisolism. Because cortisol levels fall markedly at night, some believe that a once-a-day dose is sufficient. Many patients receiving chronic glucocorticoid replacement therapy are candidates for attempted individual dose refinement because of such common confounders as osteoporosis, diabetes, or complaints of easy bruising, subtle puffiness, or increasing waist circumference. The use of hydrocortisone, rather than dexamethasone or prednisone, allows close dose titration based on serial serum cortisol measurements in the course of 8 to 12 hours following oral intake of hydrocortisone. Dose requirements may be higher in extremely obese or very active persons, because cortisol secretion correlates with body surface area and cortisol turnover is increased in obesity. Increased doses are also required if drugs known to enhance the metabolism of glucocorticoids are used concomitantly (e.g., barbiturates, phenytoin, rifampin). Lower doses are indicated in significant liver disease (slow metabolism of glucocorticoids), in geriatric patients, and in those with diabetes mellitus, peptic ulcer, or hypertension. Reliable indices in assessment of glucocorticoid replacement doses include appropriate weight gain and regression of pigmentation.
   b. **Mineralocorticoid replacement** is necessary in primary adrenal insufficiency, and its dose requirements can be variable. The synthetic mineralocorticoid fludrocortisone (Florinef) is given as a single daily dose of 0.1 mg after initial volume and sodium repletion have been achieved. Patients can be started on a liberal sodium intake. Persistent hypotension, orthostatic hypotension, hyperkalemia, or increased PRA indicate that increased doses are needed, whereas hypertension, hypokalemia, or edema indicate dose reduction. Dose changes are in increments of 0.05 mg/day of fludrocortisone.
   c. **Adrenal androgen replacement** may improve overall sense of well-being in both sexes and restore impaired libido in women. DHEA at doses of 25 to 50 mg/day are reportedly well tolerated but is occasionally associated with slight hyperandrogenic phenomena in women. Long-term effects and safety remain untested.
   d. **Patient education** includes instruction to adjust glucocorticoid dosage for mild illnesses and stressful events; in addition, patients should always carry a card or wear a bracelet (Medic-Alert Foundation) indicating their steroid dependency. A traveling kit that provides cortisone acetate-deoxycorticosterone acetate for intramuscular self-injection, and hydrocortisone (100-mg) or dexamethasone (4-mg/mL; Decadron) vials for emergency intravenous administration, is recommended.
   e. **Intercurrent illness** or **stress** requires an adjustment of glucocorticoid therapy but not of mineralocorticoid therapy. For minor illnesses (e.g., respiratory tract infection, dental extraction, unusual physical challenge), glucocorticoid dosage is doubled until the condition has resolved. Vomiting and diarrhea require hospitalization because they preclude oral intake of replacement therapy and result in rapid dehydration. During major stress, the maximum daily glucocorticoid requirement is equivalent to 300 mg of hydrocortisone.
   f. Although the need for any increase in the replacement dose of glucocorticoids during routine surgical procedures has been challenged in a controlled trial, the safety of maintaining the regular dose during elective major surgery has not been sufficiently tested. Traditionally, 100 mg of hydrocortisone is administered intravenously before anesthesia, followed by 100 mg every 8 hours until the patient has stabilized postoperatively. Lower doses (10 mg of

hydrocortisone per hour via continuous intravenous drip) have been also successfully applied in practice, and are perhaps suitable for lesser procedures. Medication is tapered rapidly (3 to 5 days) to the previous dosage. Acute situations do not require higher doses of mineralocorticoids because hydrocortisone at high doses has sufficient mineralocorticoid activity. Major catastrophes or emergencies (e.g., trauma, major emergency surgery, sepsis, myocardial infarction) require treatment as in acute adrenal crisis.

2. Secondary adrenal insufficiency. Secondary adrenal insufficiency does not require mineralocorticoid replacement. Sex hormone replacement may be needed because of the associated gonadotropin deficiency.

B. Acute adrenal (Addisonian) crisis

1. Intravenous hydrocortisone (100 mg) as a bolus.

2. Intravenous saline and glucose.

3. Hydrocortisone, 100 mg every 8 hours as a continuous infusion for the first 24 hours.

4. Hydrocortisone is then tapered during recovery by decreasing one third of the daily dose every day, until a maintenance dosage is reached, preferably within 5 to 6 days. Once the dose of hydrocortisone is <100 mg/day, fludrocortisone (0.1 mg/day) is added.

C. HPA suppression

1. Alternate-day glucocorticoid therapy. During treatment with pharmacologic doses of glucocorticoids, the total daily dose of steroid is best given as a single morning dose to prevent complications, using short-acting glucocorticoids (hydrocortisone, prednisone) but not long-acting agents (dexamethasone, beclomethasone). Short-acting agents given once daily allow time for some HPA recovery between doses, minimizing HPA suppression. When possible, patients are switched from daily to alternate-day regimens. The total daily dose is doubled and given every other morning, such as 50 to 100 mg of prednisone every other day. One method is to shift prednisone from the day off to the day on at daily increments of 5 mg. When the day-off dosage reaches 5 mg, tapering is at 1 mg every other day.

2. Tapering glucocorticoids. Once prednisone is reduced to 5 mg/day, switch to 20–25 mg of hydrocortisone every morning. The short half-life of hydrocortisone allows time for recovery of the suppressed HPA system. The 8 A.M. plasma cortisol is measured monthly; a value of <10 μg/dL indicates continued HPA suppression. Once 8 A.M. plasma cortisol exceeds 10 μg /dL, hydrocortisone can be withdrawn.

3. An ACTH test (1 μg cosyntropin) that shows a normal response demonstrating peak serum cortisol >20 μg/dL indicates recovery of the HPA axis, and all replacement can be stopped. If 8 A.M. serum cortisol is >10 μg/dL but the response to ACTH is still blunted, steroid coverage for major illnesses will be necessary as long as the ACTH test yields a subnormal response.

PRIMARY HYPERALDOSTERONISM

I. General Principles

The human adrenal cortex secretes several steroids with predominantly mineralocorticoid properties, the most important being **aldosterone.** Deoxycorticosterone (DOC) is the most potent mineralocorticoid of the nonaldosterone steroids, demonstrating about one thirtieth the potency of aldosterone. Although the major adrenal glucocorticoid, cortisol, binds effectively to the mineralocorticoid receptor, it has minimum mineralocorticoid potency under normal conditions because of its rapid conversion to cortisone by 11-hydroxysteroid dehydrogenase at the receptor site. However, in excessive amounts cortisol can take on enhanced mineralocorticoid activity.

Under most physiologic conditions, the renin–angiotensin system is the main regulator of aldosterone secretion. Through generation of angiotensin II, this system responds to alterations in sodium and volume status. **Volume depletion** induces the release of renin and the formation of angiotensin II, with subsequent angiotensin II stimulation of aldosterone secretion, leading to retention of sodium and water to restore blood volume. **Volume expansion** leads to reductions in renin, angiotensin II, and aldosterone to facilitate sodium and water excretion. Additionally, potassium and ACTH stimulate aldosterone secretion directly, independent of volume changes. Even small increments in plasma potassium lead to significant stimulation of aldosterone secretion, which, in turn, facilitates renal potassium excretion. Potassium depletion has the opposite effect, lowering aldosterone to minimize potassium excretion.

II. ETIOLOGY.

Primary hyperaldosteronism ("primary aldosteronism"; PA) implies autonomous hypersecretion of aldosterone, whereas in various forms of secondary hyperaldosteronism the stimulus is extra-adrenal. There are at least **five distinct forms**:

A. Adrenal aldosterone-producing adenoma (APA) ($\sim$60% of all cases)

B. Idiopathic hyperaldosteronism (IHA) with bilateral (micronodular) hyperplasia of the adrenals (BAH; 40%).

C. Unilateral micronodular adrenal hyperplasia (1% to 2%)

D. Glucocorticoid-remediable hyperaldosteronism, a rare familial entity characterized by bilateral adrenal hyperplasia (BAH) with reversal of clinical and biochemical abnormalities following glucocorticoid administration.

E. Aldosterone-producing adrenal carcinoma (rare)

III. Prevalence

Until the past decade, the prevalence of primary hyperaldosteronism in the hypertensive population had been estimated at 0.01% to 2.2%, but the prevailing belief now is that the rate may vary between 2% and 15%, depending on the population in question. The rate increases with severity of hypertension, such that it may be $\sim$2% in subjects with mild to moderate hypertension, increasing to as high as 13% or even higher in severe ($>$180/110 mm Hg) or resistant hypertension. Although broadly supported by published data, insufficient consideration has been given in publications favoring such high prevalence of PA to either the dominant effect of aging on systolic pressure or to the fact that hypertension afflicts most of the population after the age of 60 years. None of these estimates represents a true population based study.

IV. CLINICAL FINDINGS

Most of the pathophysiologic findings in primary hyperaldosteronism can be explained by the effects of excessive aldosterone on sodium and potassium transport. Thus one observes increased renal tubular resorption of sodium and water, leading to volume expansion and hypertension, and enhanced renal excretion of potassium and hydrogen ions, leading to hypokalemia and mild metabolic alkalosis.

A. Hypertension is the most prominent and almost universal finding in the disorder and, contrary to previous beliefs, can be mild, moderate, or severe.

B. Hypokalemia is far less common than previously believed, and is present in only half of patients with APA and 17% of those with IHA. If **hypokalemia** is significant ($<$3.5 mEq/L), patients can have symptoms related to potassium depletion, including muscle weakness, fatigue, cramping, and, in severe cases, muscle paralysis. Potassium depletion can produce a renal concentrating defect, leading to **polyuria** and **polydipsia,** which are resistant to vasopressin. Potassium repletion, however, can completely reverse these symptoms.

Chronic hypokalemia also alters the electrical potential of myocardial cells, leading to the electrocardiographic findings of the widened QT interval and U waves in this disease.

C. Hypokalemia impairs insulin secretion from pancreatic β cells and may cause the **diminished glucose tolerance** seen in $\sim$50% of patients with primary aldosteronism. The metabolic syndrome is commonly seen in PA, reportedly afflicting $>$40% of patients.

D. Aldosterone excess results in a **mild metabolic alkalosis,** which is not due to a direct aldosterone effect but seems best correlated with the degree of hypokalemia in these patients.

E. Mild **hypomagnesemia** may be present and appears to result from decreased tubular reabsorption of magnesium. Magnesium deficiency may contribute to insulin resistance in PA.

F. Physical examination of patients with primary hyperaldosteronism reveals few findings. Most typically, edema is almost always absent. When it is present, prolonged hypokalemia may blunt some circulatory reflex responses; consequently, postural hypotension and bradycardia can occur. Nevertheless these are *not* common findings.

V. DIAGNOSIS

A. The classic triad of biochemical criteria for the diagnosis of primary hyperaldosteronism includes **(1)** hypokalemia with inappropriate kaliuresis; **(2)** suppressed plasma renin activity; and **(3)** elevated aldosterone levels that do not fall appropriately in response to volume expansion or sodium load. Although these criteria continue to be important, **active case detection** is now recommended, because of the presumed high prevalence of PA, under the following circumstances:

1. **Spontaneous or diuretic-induced hypokalemia.** Spontaneous or unprovoked hypokalemia of 2.7 mEq/L or less in hypertensive patients is usually due to primary aldosteronism, especially APA. In a patient who does not receive diuretics, urinary potassium excretion >30 mEq in 24 hours in the presence of a serum K^+ concentration <3.5 mEq/L is inappropriately high and is thus indicative of mineralocorticoid excess.

2. **Moderate or severe hypertension,** *particularly in the nonelderly.*

3. **Resistant hypertension.**

4. **Adrenal incidentaloma.**

5. **Family history of hypertension of early onset or cerebrovascular accident at a young age** .

B. Screening tests. Current guidelines of the U.S. Endocrine Society for treatment of patients with PA, cosponsored by the European Society of Endocrinology, the European Society of Hypertension, the International Society of Endocrinology, the International Society of Hypertension, and the Japanese Society of Hypertension, call for use of the **plasma aldosterone/renin ratio (ARR) as the screening test to detect PA in these patient groups.** Although blood pressure–lowering drugs have multiple effects on PRA , in many cases withdrawal of treatment for the purpose of testing is neither feasible, because blood pressure may rise unacceptably, nor necessary, because interpretation can be usually made taking into consideration the known effects of the specific drugs used. Spironolactone and eplerenone as well as high-dose amiloride comprise exceptions to this practice and must be discontinued for at least 6 weeks prior to testing. Additionally, in patients with mild hypertension, drug withdrawal (2 to 4 weeks) prior to testing still appears to be preferable.

1. **Plasma renin activity (PRA).** The chronic hypervolemia of primary hyperaldosteronism accounts for the suppressed renin levels characteristically seen in this disease. However, low renin is actually seen in only **60% to 80%** of patients, perhaps because many hypertensive patients are initially treated with diuretics and vasodilators that stimulate renin activity. Additionally, 25% of the essential hypertension population displays low levels of renin activity of uncertain etiology, and low PRA is observed in the elderly. Among the various assays available, PRA rather than PRC is the preferred method. Because ARR is heavily dependent on PRA and dependence is highest at the low end of the assay range (e.g., lowering measured PRA from 0.2 to 0.1 ng/mL will **double** the calculated ARR), care must be taken not only to collect samples properly, but also to use a reliable laboratory with documented performance and sufficient assay sensitivity at the low range.

2. **Aldosterone measurements.** Aldosterone secretion is suppressed by increased dietary sodium, hypervolemia, and hypokalemia. Plasma and urinary aldosterone

concentrations also decrease with advancing age to 30% to 50% of the values seen in young subjects, making age corrections necessary, especially in evaluating hypertensive patients over the age of 60 years. A significant number of patients with primary hyperaldosteronism (~30%) have basal aldosterone levels that are within the normal range. In patients with serum potassium <3 mEq/L, potassium repletion (200-mEq potassium diet for 5 days or potassium chloride elixir, 60 to 120 mEq daily PO) should be initiated with repeat measurements of aldosterone after repletion. Potassium-ion level itself is a determinant of aldosterone production; therefore, potassium depletion can actually reduce and "normalize" adrenal aldosterone secretion in some patients.

a. For the basal measurement of PRA and aldosterone, patients can be on a regular diet. Sampling should be done in the morning hours, after the patient has been awake for at least 2 hours and in the sitting position for 15 minutes. Blood is collected for PRA in tubes containing EDTA and centrifuged at room temperature to avoid cryoactivation of prorenin to renin.

b. Interpretation of the aldosterone/renin ratio (ARR). Although the ARR is generally recommended as the best screening test, there are no universally accepted trough values that define abnormal ratio levels. Attention should be paid to the following.

(1) Units. Most published cutoff values refer to aldosterone expressed as ng/dL and PRA expressed in ng/mL/h. With this presently most popular unit system, most groups use ratios exceeding 20 to 40 as the cutoff level requiring further diagnostic workup for PA. Less often, PRC (mU/L) rather than PRA is measured and aldosterone levels are provided in SI units (pmol/L), and suggested critical ratios, under these circumstances, range from 70 to 130. Care must be taken to avoid derivatization of ratios based on "mixed units" other than the combinations specified here.

(2) Effect of drugs. Beta-blockers, clonidine, α-methyldopa, and nonsteroidal anti-inflammatory drugs (NSAIDs) suppress PRA and aldosterone and may lead to a false positive ARR; all diuretics, angiotensin-converting enzyme (ACE) inhibitors, angiotensin II receptor blockers (ARBs), and dihydropyridine calcium channel blockers increase PRA and may lead to a false negative ARR. Blood pressure–lowering drugs with minimal effects on ARR include alpha-blockers, hydralazine, and slow-release verapamil. Contraceptives increase PRA but decrease PRC.

(3) Effect of age. PRA declines with age more than aldosterone, leading to higher ARR.

(4) Chronic renal failure is linked to low PRA and high ARR.

(5) Aldosterone levels. In the absence of hypokalemia, low aldosterone levels (<9 ng/dL) are inconsistent with PA. On the other hand, strict requirement for high plasma aldosterone results in a significant rate of false negative cases. Even if aldosterone levels $\geq$15 ng/dL are set as a requirement for the diagnosis in the context of increased ARR, some patients may be unduly excluded.

C. Definitive and confirmatory tests. Given the variability of basal aldosterone levels in this disorder, the nonsuppressibility of aldosterone in response to volume-expansion maneuvers has proved to be a better indicator of primary hyperaldosteronism. Volume expansion via saline infusion, high-salt intake, or mineralocorticoid administration in any condition other than primary hyperaldosteronism suppresses aldosterone levels by >50%. In primary hyperaldosteronism, an additional volume load has only a minimal effect on aldosterone concentration. Spuriously increased ARR may be corrected by the use of one or more of the following tests.

1. Aldosterone suppression tests: salt-volume loading tests. These tests should be deferred until hypokalemia is corrected and are not recommended in individuals with severe hypertension, renal or congestive heart failure, or cardiac arrhythmia.

a. **Saline infusion test**
   (1) Patients should be on a regular diet. Obtain serum K^+ and proceed only if concentration is ≥ 4 mmol/L.
   (2) Obtain baseline aldosterone levels.
   (3) Infuse 0.9% sodium chloride solution for 4 hours (500 mL/hour, a total of 2 L).
   (4) Obtain repeat samples for aldosterone and potassium. Following the infusion, plasma aldosterone will normally drop by at least **50%** or below 5 ng/dL, whereas patients with primary hyperaldosteronism will display postinfusion levels >10 ng/dL.

b. **Oral salt loading test**
   (1) Increase sodium intake to >200 mmol/L and add slow-release potassium chloride tablets to keep serum potassium in the normal range.
   (2) Obtain 24-hour urine collection to verify that the intended intake has been attained.
   (3) Obtain 24-hour urine collection starting on the morning of day 3 for the measurement of urinary aldosterone. Urinary aldosterone excretion >12 to 14 μg in 24 hours is highly suggestive of PA, whereas excretion <10 μg in 24 hours practically excludes this diagnosis.
   (4) HPLC-tandem mass spectrometry is the preferred method for measurements because radioimmunoassays for urinary aldosterone perform poorly in this setting.

2. **Captopril challenge test.** Under normal conditions, inhibition of angiotensin II–converting enzyme leads to acute increase in PRA, because of acute disinhibition of renin release, whereas plasma aldosterone declines because of the reduction in angiotensin II generation. In PA, PRA remains suppressed because of hypervolemia, and plasma aldosterone does not change appreciably because it is secreted autonomously.
   a. After 1 hour in the sitting position, obtain blood for PRA, aldosterone, and cortisol.
   b. Administer 25 to 50 mg of captopril as a single oral dose and keep the patient in the sitting position for 1 to 2 hours.
   c. Draw a second blood sample for PRA, aldosterone, and cortisol.
   d. **Interpretation.** Plasma aldosterone declines by at least 30% in normal subjects, but it is hardly affected in PA. The test is not suitable for patients receiving ACE inhibitors or ARBs. Plasma aldosterone may be decreased in this test in some patients with idiopathic hyperaldosteronism. Equivocal or false negative results are not uncommon.

D. **Tests to differentiate APA and BAH (idiopathic hyperaldosteronism).** Patients with APA respond favorably to surgery, whereas BAH patients do not and require prolonged medical therapy. Thus a preoperative distinction between APA and BAH as the cause of hyperaldosteronism must be made.

1. **Adrenal CT and MR scans.** Once the biochemical diagnosis of primary hyperaldosteronism has been firmly established, CT scans are effective in identifying various adrenal tumors, particularly adenomas with a diameter of 1 cm or more. MRI offers no advantage over CT scan. The results with BAH are variable, ranging from an apparently normal gland to bilateral diffuse enlargement. However, the identification of an adrenal lesion should not be automatically assumed to represent APA, even when the diagnosis of PA has been firmly established. First, adrenal incidentalomas can be seen in as many as 10% of the general population. Second, unilateral adenoma might represent one large nodule in an essentially bilateral disease (BAH). Third, unilateral adrenal hyperplasia may not be identified by these methods. Forth, bilateral nodularity may represent either true bilateral disease or a composite condition with true APA on one side and a nonfunctioning adrenal nodule on the other gland. Finally, small adenomas can be missed by either CT or MRI, leading to erroneous diagnosis of BAH. This is why the concordance rate between CT and the more difficult but accurate adrenal venous sampling for aldosterone does not usually exceed 50% to 60%. CT is still helpful

in identifying the malignant potential of larger lesions (>2.5 cm) through their radiologic features (density in HU units, regularity, etc.) and in identifying the correct adrenal vein to aid in subsequent catheterization during adrenal venous sampling.

2. **Adrenal vein sampling for aldosterone concentration**
   a. In skilled hands and experienced centers, catheterization of the adrenal veins with collection of adrenal vein effluent is the most accurate and definitive means of correct identification of hyperaldosteronism induced by unilateral disease, i.e., APA or unilateral hyperplasia. Sampling can be done through simultaneous catheterization of both adrenals or as a sequential procedure, either unstimulated or stimulated by Cortrosyn injection.
   b. **Interpretation.** Interpretation is highly dependent on the actual protocol used. False lateralization could result from episodic secretion of aldosterone or from dilution effects.
      (1) Episodic secretion of aldosterone can be avoided by simultaneous sampling from both adrenals and is also minimized if samples are collected following injection of ACTH.
      (2) Samples obtained from either side may consist of a variable mixture of adrenal and extraadrenal venous blood (e.g., **"pure"** adrenal blood compared to a "contralateral" **diluted sample**). **Simultaneous measurement of aldosterone and cortisol** in both adrenal veins and in the inferior vena cava (IVC) provides an excellent indicator of sampling-site dilution, using an aldosterone–cortisol ratio to correct for errors induced by the location of the catheter. With continuous Cortrosyn infusion (50 μg of cosyntropin per hour, initiated 30 minutes before catheterization and continued throughout the procedure), a high-side–to–low-side ratio of "cortisol-corrected" aldosterone >4 is indicative of unilateral disease (in most cases, APA). A ratio of <3 suggests bilateral disease. In unstimulated testing, a ratio >2 suggests lateralization. One might also expect that the aldosterone–cortisol ratio should be markedly suppressed on the contralateral side compared with levels from the IVC.

3. **Adrenal radioisotope scanning** with iodocholesterol or NP-59 is often helpful in the differential diagnosis of primary hyperaldosteronism. With 7 days of dexamethasone suppression (0.5 mg, bid), asymmetric uptake is compatible with APA, whereas bilateral uptake favors the diagnosis of BAH. This is not a useful procedure for small APA, but is very useful when the suspected adenoma on CT ≥1.5 cm, especially when access to high-quality adrenal venous sampling is limited, as it is in many parts of the world.

4. **Ancillary tests for equivocal cases**
   a. **Posture test.** APA appears to be quite responsive to ACTH, but not to angiotensin II. The opposite pertains to BAH, in which angiotensin II is the major regulator.
      (1) Procedure for posture test
         (a) Samples for PRA and plasma aldosterone are obtained between 8 and 9 A.M., after the patient has been in the supine position for 30 minutes.
         (b) The patient assumes upright posture and ambulates moderately for 4 hours, at which time samples are collected again.
      (2) Interpretation. Normal subjects assuming upright posture always increase plasma renin activity and, therefore, plasma aldosterone levels, and this is further enhanced with ambulation. Because PRA is suppressed in APA, plasma aldosterone does not respond to posture and declines in association with the diurnal reduction in ACTH (8 A.M. to noon). Patients with BAH show a normal increase (>25% of the baseline value) in aldosterone levels with upright posture, accounted for by a partially intact renin response, and enhanced adrenal gland sensitivity to angiotensin II. However, up to 50% of patients with APA demonstrate posture increases in plasma aldosterone. In fact, the reliability of the test in distinguishing APA and BAH has been questioned in light of recent information that

the magnitude of posture response depends on baseline levels of aldosterone, independent of adrenal pathology. This should therefore be seen as an ancillary procedure and interpreted only in the context of additional functional and imaging procedures.

  b. Plasma 18-hydroxycorticosterone (18-OHB). The immediate precursor to aldosterone biosynthesis is 18-OHB, which, like aldosterone, originates primarily from the adrenal cortical zona glomerulosa. Levels of 18-OHB are particularly high in APA, and plasma 18-OHB concentrations >100 ng/dL indicate that PA is the result of APA; anything less than this value, especially <50 ng/dL, is more likely a result of BAH.

E. Genetic testing. When PA is diagnosed at a young age (e.g., <20 years) and/or in the context of a strong family history of hypertension, stroke at a young age, or familial PA, the diagnosis of **glucocorticoid-remediable hyperaldosteronism (GRA;** also termed **familial hyperaldosteronism type I)** should be considered. This disease results from a chymeric 11β-hydroxylase/aldosterone synthase gene in which the coding sequence of the aldosterone synthase is controlled by the 11β-hydroxylase promoter, thus making aldosterone synthesis sensitive to ACTH rather than to angiotensin II. **Dexamethasone** therapy reverses both high blood pressure and the associated biochemical abnormalities (i.e., hypokalemia, hyperaldosteronism, and hyporeninemia), usually within the first 21 to 28 days of therapy. Genetic testing is now available. For long-term treatment, the lowest dose of dexamethasone effective in controlling blood pressure and correcting the biochemical and hormonal abnormalities should be selected. Negative genetic testing for GRA in a family in whom more than a single member is afflicted with PA, particularly if the inheritance pattern appears to be autosomal recessive, should suggest the diagnosis of **familial hyperaldosteronism type II.** Such patients may have APA or BAH. The underlying mechanism is presently unclear.

VI. TREATMENT

A. APA. Surgical removal of the gland containing the tumor is the treatment of choice. Most adenomas are small, often <1 cm in diameter, and twice as many occur on the left side as on the right. Potassium repletion, either by oral potassium supplementation or by preoperative treatment with the mineralocorticoid antagonist spironolactone (50 to 200 mg/day over 2 to 3 weeks), must be achieved before surgery. Although surgical outcome is imperfect in terms of hypertension control, with cure achieved in <50% of correctly diagnosed subjects, at least partial improvement is the rule in most. Older age, severe preoperative systolic pressure, and the use of multiple blood pressure–lowering drugs are negative predictors of cure. Hypokalemia, on the other hand, resolves within days after surgery. Late recurrence of hypertension, but not hypokalemia, has been reported. Aggressive medical treatment is suggested for patients who do not undergo surgery (see BAH), with attempted treatment to target hypertension as well as all associated risk factors.

B. BAH. Because the surgical cure rate of BAH (normalization of blood pressure) is only **19%,** these patients should be treated medically. Although **spironolactone** (12.5 to 200 mg daily) is the obvious choice, results in BAH have been quite variable, and long-term spironolactone treatment is frequently accompanied by impotence and gynecomastia in males and by menstrual disorders in females. Eplerenone, an alternative mineralocorticoid receptor antagonist that does not interact with the androgen or progesterone receptor, is now available and can be attempted when side effects of spironolactone are intolerable. **Amiloride** (40 mg/day), a potassium-sparing diuretic that acts on renal tubular cells independently of aldosterone activity, has been shown to be a successful therapeutic agent in the treatment of primary hyperaldosteronism. Additionally, dihydropyridine calcium-channel blockers, ACE inhibitors, and ARBs are often effective in PA. Finally, because PA is associated with increased rate of the metabolic syndrome, lifestyle modification and medical treatment of associated risk factors should be rigorously applied when appropriate.

VII. DIFFERENTIAL DIAGNOSIS

Hypertension and hypokalemia as the presenting symptoms are common in other syndromes.

A. Cushing syndrome. Hypertension and hypokalemia may be the presenting symptoms in Cushing syndrome. In Cushing disease, PRA is normal to high and plasma aldosterone is normal (PRA, no increase or decrease; aldosterone, no increase or decrease). In Cushing syndrome secondary to ectopic ACTH secretion, plasma deoxycorticosterone (DOC) reaches high levels in response to excessive circulating ACTH. This weaker mineralocorticoid, originating mainly in zona fasciculata cells, commonly induces a **mineralocorticoid-excess syndrome** that precedes the manifestations of excessive glucocorticoids. The "hypervolemic" state induced by DOC results in suppression of PRA and aldosterone secretion (DOC ↑; PRA ↓; aldosterone ↓).

B. Malignant hypertension. In accelerated or malignant hypertension, excessive hyperreninism secondary to renal damage leads to high levels of aldosterone, frequently **accompanied by hypokalemia** (PRA ↑↑; aldosterone ↑).

C. 11β-Hydroxysteroid dehydrogenase (type 2) deficiency. Because cortisol's affinity for the renal mineralocorticoid receptor is as high as that of aldosterone, and circulating cortisol levels are 1 000-fold higher than those of aldosterone, 11β-hydroxysteroid dehydrogenase type 2, which converts cortisol to cortisone (a molecule incapable of interaction with the mineralocorticoid receptor), is needed to protect the mineralocorticoid receptor from excess activation by cortisol. 11β-Hydroxysteroid deficiency results in an apparent mineralocorticoid excess syndrome secondary to undisturbed access of cortisol to the relatively nonspecific renal mineralocorticoid receptor. This inherited condition, which results in hypertension and hypokalemia, has been described initially in children and more recently in adults. Diagnosis is confirmed by establishing an increased ratio of urinary tetrahydrocortisol (a metabolite of cortisol) to tetrahydrocortisone (a metabolite of cortisone). The glycyrrhizic acid contained in licorice, which induces an acquired form of apparent mineralocorticoid excess syndrome, exerts its effect via inhibition of 11β-hydroxysteroid dehydrogenase.

D. CAH due to either 11α-hydroxylase deficiency or 17α-hydroxylase deficiency. In both conditions, defective cortisol production leads to a compensatory rise in ACTH, which stimulates, in turn, the biosynthesis of the weaker mineralocorticoids produced in the zona fasciculata by cells independent of angiotensin II but sensitive to ACTH (corticosterone ↑; DOC ↑; PRA ↓; aldosterone ↓). The hypertension and hypokalemia are accompanied by virilization in 11α-hydroxylase deficiency and by primary amenorrhea (females) or eunuchoid features or pseudohermaphroditism (males) because of the sex hormone deficiency in 17α-hydroxylase deficiency.

Low doses of dexamethasone appear to be the treatment of choice for both 11α- and 17α-hydroxylase deficiencies. Androgens or estrogens are also added in 17α-hydroxylase deficiency.

E. Liddle syndrome is a rare familial disorder characterized by hypertension and hypokalemic alkalosis in the absence of the excessive secretion of any of the known mineralocorticoids. The primary defect resides in increased reabsorption of sodium chloride and enhanced secretion of potassium in the distal tubule, secondary to various "activating" mutations in the β or γ subunits of the sodium epithelial channel. Hypertension and hypokalemia are relieved by either amiloride (10 to 40 mg daily) or triamterene (100 to 300 mg qd in divided doses), but not by spironolactone. Both PRA and aldosterone are classically low.

F. Low-renin hypertension. Approximately one fourth of patients with essential hypertension demonstrate low levels of PRA. It appears that this traditionally defined subset of patients with "essential hypertension" overlaps, at least to some extent, with BAH patients who do not have clearly increased circulating aldosterone but are detected through increased ARR.

G. Renovascular hypertension. Hyperaldosteronism and hypokalemia secondary to excessive renin stimulation in renovascular hypertension are uncommon, because most of these patients have normal to high-normal peripheral PRA. In severe cases with excessive peripheral PRA, hyperaldosteronism with hypokalemia may be encountered (PRA ↑ or N; aldosterone ↑ or N).

H. Ingestion of exogenous mineralocorticoids. Overdose of fludrocortisone (occasionally prescribed for orthostatic hypotension) or the chronic use of nasal sprays containing α-fluprednisolone (for chronic rhinitis) may result in hypertension and hypokalemia, accompanied by suppressed PRA and aldosterone levels (PRA ↓; aldosterone ↓).

SECONDARY HYPERALDOSTERONISM

I. PATHOPHYSIOLOGY AND ETIOLOGY

Hyperaldosteronism secondary to excessive stimulation of the renin-angiotensin axis is encountered in a variety of clinical instances, all of which are associated with enhanced production and release of renin from the kidney. The most common stimuli for such hyperreninemia are sodium loss or salt deficiency (e.g., sodium restriction, diuretics, diarrhea, salt-losing nephropathy), volume depletion (e.g., hemorrhage, dehydration), or volume redistribution with reduced "central" or "effective" blood volume (i.e., edematous states such as nephrotic syndrome, cirrhosis with ascites, and some stages of congestive heart failure). Very high levels of PRA and aldosterone are normally observed in pregnancy, particularly during the last two trimesters. Excessive intake of potassium can directly increase aldosterone secretion. On rare occasions the hypersecretion of renin is unprovoked, as in Bartter syndrome or renin-secreting tumors.

II. BARTTER SYNDROME

A. Pathogenesis. Bartter syndrome includes a number of genetically transmitted abnormalities in the transport of sodium chloride in the loop of Henle leading to hypokalemia, metabolic alkalosis, hyperreninemia, hyperaldosteronism, and hyperplasia of the juxtaglomerular apparatus. Normally, active sodium chloride transport in the thick ascending loop of Henle occurs via the loop diuretic–sensitive Na-K-2Cl cotransporter at the luminal membrane, which facilitates the entry of sodium chloride to tubular cells; potassium channels which allow back leakage from the cell to the lumen of reabsorbed potassium, so that the Na-K-2Cl cotransport system can be reloaded for continued shuttling of NaCl into the cell; and chloride channels located at the basolateral membrane to allow diffusion of the chloride anions entering the cell via the Na-K-2Cl cotransporter to the interstitial fluid and then further into systemic circulation. Malfunction of any of the components of this system will induce volume contraction secondary to tubular salt loss, which resembles the effect of thiazide diuretics. Hypovolemia comprises a powerful and chronic stimulus for the release of renin, and hence, increased secretion of aldosterone. Further, the resultant enhanced delivery of sodium to the distal tubule elicits, through electroneutral exchange mechanisms, increased excretion of potassium and hydrogen, and hence, hypokalemia and metabolic alkalosis. The latter two are further enhanced by high aldosterone concentrations. Hypertension does not evolve because of the continued "diuretic" effect and because of compensatory formation of vasodilator prostaglandins prostaglandin E2 and prostacyclin, which nevertheless are powerful stimulators of renin secretion. Bartter syndrome, then, can be caused by autosomal recessive mutations in the Na-K-2Cl cotransporter, the luminal potassium channel, and the basolateral chloride channel, which are referred to as Bartter syndrome types I, II, and III, respectively. An acquired form of Bartter syndrome can result from gentamycin treatment.

B. Clinical features. Kaliuresis, hypokalemic alkalosis, hyperreninemia, secondary hyperaldosteronism, and normotension in a nonedematous patient, in whom gastrointestinal potassium and chloride loss and the abuse of laxatives or diuretics have been excluded, establish the diagnosis. Infrequently, hypomagnesemia further complicates these abnormalities.

C. **Gitelman syndrome** results from mutations in the gene encoding the thiazide-sensitive Na-Cl cotransporter in the distal tubule and likewise leads to renal sodium wasting, hyperreninemia, secondary hyperaldosteronism, hypokalemia, metabolic alkalosis, hypomagnesemia, and hypocalcemia.

D. **Treatment principles** are similar in these disorders.

1. **Correction of hypokalemia** is accomplished by the administration of spironolactone, 100 to 300 mg daily, or amiloride (or both). Persistent hypokalemia despite these measures may require a low-sodium diet.

2. **Correction of hyperreninemia and hyperaldosteronism.** Indomethacin (1 to 2 mg/kg/day), ibuprofen (400 to 1 200 mg/day), or aspirin (0.6 to 3.0 g/day) are all effective cyclo-oxygenase inhibitors that will decrease prostaglandins PG12 and PGE2 production, thereby reducing renin and aldosterone secretion.

3. When present, hypomagnesemia should be corrected (10 to 20 mEq magnesium daily). Correction of hypomagnesemia also facilitates the normalization of serum potassium levels.

HYPOALDOSTERONISM

I. HYPORENINEMIC HYPOALDOSTERONISM

Hyporeninemic hypoaldosteronism is most often associated with mild to moderate renal insufficiency, especially in older individuals with varying degrees of hyperkalemia. The most consistent underlying renal disorder has been diabetic nephropathy, although hyporeninemic hypoaldosteronism has also been found in certain interstitial nephropathies. Various disorders of renin synthesis and release have been proposed, including impaired conversion of inactive to active renin, destruction of the juxtaglomerular apparatus, sympathetic nervous system defects, and chronic volume expansion. Hyperkalemia in this entity fails to raise aldosterone secretion because this response apparently requires activation of intra-adrenal renin, which may be impaired as well. ACE inhibitors and NSAIDs, which impair angiotensin II formation or renin secretion, respectively, tend to aggravate this entity or "induce" it in borderline subjects.

A. **Diagnosis.** The diagnosis is made by demonstrating the failure of PRA and plasma aldosterone to increase in response to a combined postural (i.e., 2-hour ambulation) and diuretic test (60 mg furosemide PO, given after baseline levels of PRA and aldosterone have been obtained).

B. **Treatment.** When hyperkalemia is significant and warrants therapy, the treatment choice depends on the patient's blood pressure. If hypertension coexists, furosemide therapy will not only reverse the hyperkalemia but can also restore normal renin and aldosterone secretion after months of therapy. If the patient is hypotensive or presents with orthostatic hypotension, low doses of fludrocortisone should be tried (starting with 0.05 mg daily). It should be noted, however, that the dosage needed is often higher than that used in Addison disease (i.e., 0.2 mg/day).

II. ADDISON DISEASE

Hypoaldosteronism may be the earliest manifestation in Addison disease.

III. HYPOALDOSTERONISM COMPLICATING HEPARIN THERAPY

Heparin treatment, especially when given for a prolonged period, can suppress aldosterone secretion and result in hyperkalemia, presumably by a direct effect on the zona glomerulosa.

IV. TRANSIENT HYPOALDOSTERONISM FOLLOWING UNILATERAL ADRENALECTOMY FOR AN APA

The occurrence of transient hypoaldosteronism following unilateral adrenalectomy for an APA can be minimized by preoperative administration of spironolactone (400 to 600 mg/day), which partially restores the responsiveness of the chronically suppressed renin–angiotensin–aldosterone axis.

V. CONGENITAL HYPOALDOSTERONISM

Congenital hypoaldosteronism results from enzymatic defects in aldosterone synthase, the last enzyme involved in the biosynthetic chain of aldosterone in the zona glomerulosa. This enzyme actually catalyzes three steps, two of which are conversion of corticosterone into 18-hydroxycorticosterone (18-OHB; "18-hydroxylation step"), followed by conversion of the 18-OH group to aldehyde. Mutation in the aldosterone synthase gene impair the ability of the aldosterone synthase protein to catalyze these steps, resulting in type I and type II aldosterone synthase deficiency, respectively. Aldosterone biosynthesis is impaired in both aldosterone synthase deficiency types, while corticosterone of zona glomerulosa origin is excessively produced. The two defects differ, however, in that 18-OHB is deficient in type I but overproduced in type II.

A. Clinical features. The features of this syndrome vary, appearing as volume and sodium depletion, hyperkalemia, and shock in some, and as asymptomatic hyperkalemia in others. It has been described in isolated nomadic tribes with a high rate of consanguinity. Levels of PRA are high in response to volume deficiency.

B. Diagnosis. Specific diagnosis is made by measurements of the ratio of the urinary metabolites of 18-OHB to aldosterone, a procedure limited to special centers.

VI. HYPERRENINEMIC HYPOALDOSTERONISM

The syndrome of hyperreninemic hypoaldosteronism is encountered in critically ill patients. This condition can follow prolonged hypotensive episodes and is manifested by low-grade, unexplained hyperkalemia. The production of cortisol remains intact, whereas both plasma aldosterone and 18-OHB are decreased, suggesting a selective impairment of the zona glomerulosa cells.

PSEUDOHYPOALDOSTERONISM

I. PSEUDOHYPOALDOSTERONISM TYPE I

Pseudohypoaldosteronism type I is a group of rare salt-losing conditions with hyperkalemia, detected in infancy, some of which tend to resolve spontaneously with time. Pseudohypoaldosteronism type 1 is caused by mutations in the α, β, or γ subunit of the sodium epithelial channel (autosomal recessive transmission; severe dehydration, respiratory tract infections; affects all aldosterone epithelial target tissues, i.e., kidney, lung, colon, salivary glands) or by loss of function mutations in the mineralocorticoid receptor (autosomal dominant or sporadic form; generally milder and may improve with time). Acquired forms are encountered in obstructive uropathy and following renal transplantation. Treatment consists of **salt and fluid replacement**.

II. PSEUDOHYPOALDOSTERONISM TYPE II

Pseudohypoaldosteronism type II, also termed **Gordon syndrome** or **familial hyperkalemic hypertension,** is a monogenic form of hypertension with hyperkalemia that results from mutations in WNK kinase 1 and 4, proteins affecting the thiazide-sensitive Na-Cl cotransporter that mediates NaCl reabsorption in the distal nephron. In this syndrome, malfunction of these proteins results in enhanced sodium chloride reabsorption in the distal tubule, volume expansion, hypertension, suppression of renin secretion, and reduced availability of tubular sodium and water for exchange with potassium and hydrogen in the cortical collecting tubular cells. Generally, these patients respond well to treatment with thiazide diuretics.

Selected References

Baid SK, Sinaii N, Wade M, et al. Radioimmunoassay and tandem mass spectrometry measurement of bedtime salivary cortisol levels: a comparison of assays to establish hypercortisolism. *J Clin Endocrinol Metab* 2007;92:3102–3107.

Erickson D, Natt N, Nippoldt T, et al. Dexamethasone-suppressed corticotropin-releasing hormone stimulation test for diagnosis of mild hypercortisolism. *J Clin Endocrinol Metab* 2007;92:2972–2976.

Funder J, Carey RM, Fardella C, et al. Case detection, diagnosis and treatment of primary aldosteronism: an Endocrine Society clinical practice guideline. In preparation.

Pecori Giraldi F, Ambrogio AG, De Martin M, et al. Specificity of first-line tests for the diagnosis of Cushing's syndrome. Assessment in a large series. *J Clin Endocrinol Metab* 2007 Nov; 92(11):4123–4129.

Rossi GP, Bernini G, Caliumi C, et al. PAPY Study Investigators: a prospective study of the prevalence of primary aldosteronism in 1,125 hypertensive patients. *J Am Coll Cardiol* 2006;48:2293–2300.

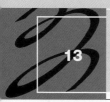

PHEOCHROMOCYTOMAS

Guido Lastra, Adam Whaley-Connell, and James R. Sowers

$\mathcal{P}$heochromocytomas are rare chromaffin-derived, neuroendocrine tumors that manifest most of their symptoms by secretion of excess catecholamines. Most of these tumors arise from the adrenal medulla, but extra-adrenal localization also occurs. These tumors are usually benign; however, malignancy can occur and complicate management. Pheochromocytomas account for ~0.1% of cases of arterial hypertension (HTN), and they are a potentially fatal but correctable cause of HTN.

I. EPIDEMIOLOGY

A. Although it is difficult to ascertain the prevalence and incidence of pheochromocytomas in the United States, reports from the Mayo Clinic between 1950 and 1970 point towards an annual incidence of 0.95 per 100 000 person-years, with almost half of cases identified initially at autopsy. Data from northern Europe yields a lower incidence, ~2.1 per million per year, with 40% of diagnosis made at autopsy. However, newer detection techniques, including mass spectrometric analysis, as well as improved measures of catecholamines secretion, have yielded higher incidences of pheochromocytoma, up to 1.9%, and increased recognition of asymptomatic tumors.

B. Pheochromocytomas display similar frequency in male and female adults. However, in children, ~60% of cases occur in boys, who also have a higher incidence of multiple and extra-adrenal tumors. Ten percent of pheochromocytomas are familial in origin, and in 15 to 20% of patients occur as autosomal dominant inherited disorders, including type 1 neurofibromatosis (NF 1) (Von Recklinghausen disease), Von Hippel-Lindau (VHL) disease, and multiple endocrine neoplasia (MEN) types 2 A and 2 B. Pheochromocytomas can be present in up to 50% of patients affected by MEN 2A, 25% of those with VHL disease, and 5% of individuals with NF 1.

C. Several mutations in the tumor-suppressor VHL gene have been described in patients with VHL disease, and mutations in the RET proto-oncogene in patients provides a powerful screening tool for identification of MEN 2 in patients with pheochromocytomas and/or medullary thyroid carcinomas. NF 1 is associated with inactivating mutations of the NF1 gene, or neurofibromin 1 gene, which is also a tumor-suppressor gene acting through inactivation of *ras* signaling.

II. ANATOMY/BIOCHEMISTRY

A. Pheochromocytomas generally present as benign, vascularized encapsulated lesions, with an average diameter of 5 cm, and a weight of <70 g (Fig. 13.1). It is estimated that ~10% of pheochromocytomas can be malignant, but these numbers oscillate between 5% and 26%. Adrenal pheochromocytomas only rarely are associated with extra-adrenal lesions, and are more frequent in patients >60 years old. On the other hand, extra-adrenal pheochromocytomas present in ~10% of cases (frequency can go up to 23%) tend to affect young adults and present rarely as part of a familial syndrome. The most common extra-adrenal localizations are the superior and inferior para-aortic areas, which occur in ~80% of cases. Tumors have also been described in the thorax, bladder head, neck, and pelvis.

B. Although most pheochromocytomas secrete both epinephrine and norepinephrine, there is usually a predominance of norepinephrine. However, some tumors can produce only norepinephrine, or in rare cases only epinephrine or dopamine. Other substances produced by pheochromocytomas include adrenomedullin (a potent

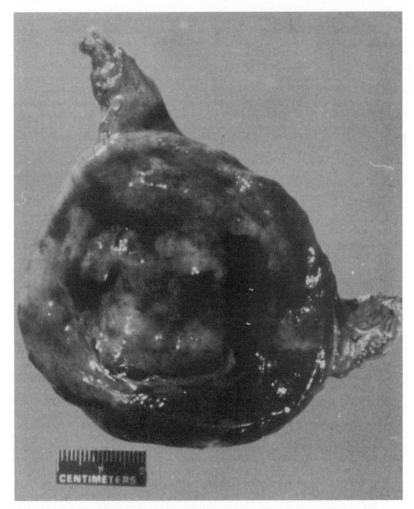

Figure 13.1. Pheochromocytoma of the adrenal gland. Tumor is well encapsulated and exhibits hemorrhagic dark mottling.

vasodilating peptide), as well as chromogranin A and neuropeptide Y, which appear to increase peripheral vascular resistance and enhance the vasoconstricting effect of norepinephrine in the systemic circulation and in the coronary arteries.

III. CLINICAL MANIFESTATIONS

A. There is no correlation among tumor size, circulating levels of catecholamines, and the severity of symptoms and/or hypertension. Most frequently, a pheochromocytoma can present as paroxysmal HTN in up to ~50% of cases. However, patients can also have persistent HTN, or can even be normotensive in ~10% of cases when the amount of catecholamines released into the general circulation is small.

B. Most patients present with paroxysmal or sustained HTN, episodic headaches, palpitations, and diaphoresis. The frequency of these paroxysms is variable, but in up to 74% they occur on at least a weekly basis and their duration is usually

<1 hour, but can last up to 1 week. Adrenergic α-receptor–mediated vasoconstriction results in HTN, facial pallor, and cool moist extremities. Peripheral vasoconstriction and increased catecholamine-induced basal metabolism are responsible for increased temperature, sweating, and flushing. In severe cases, patients can also develop nausea, vomiting, abdominal and/or chest pain, and seizures (Table 13.1). Orthostatic hypotension can also occur, as a result of volume depletion and predominance of epinephrine/dopamine production by the tumor. Pheochromocytomas can also cause left ventricular hypertrophy and cardiac ischemia, which can be identified in characteristic electrocardiographic changes.

IV. SCREENING/DIAGNOSIS

   A. Diagnosis of pheochromocytoma relies on the presence of clinical manifestations as well as laboratory demonstration of excessive production of catecholamines. Patients with pheochromocytoma, and overt symptoms and signs, usually have very high levels of plasma catecholamines, >2 000 pg/mL. On the other hand, because of the heterogeneous nature of the disease, normal levels of catecholamines in asymptomatic patients do not necessarily rule out the diagnosis.
   B. Screening for pheochromocytoma is indicated in patients with severe sustained or paroxysmal HTN, particularly if they are refractory to adequate antihypertensive therapy. Patients with episodic symptoms of headaches, tachycardia, and diaphoresis, even in the absence of HTN, should be screened, as well as patients with hypertensive episodes during parturition, micturition, a family history of pheochromocytoma, MEN syndromes, VHL disease, or NF 1.
   C. Pheochromocytomas secrete varying catecholamines and their metabolites in different concentrations. Numerous assays and techniques are available in the clinical setting to identify patients with pheochromocytoma, including 24-hour urine collection for urinary fractionated metanephrines (normetanephrine and metanephrine), free catecholamines (epinephrine and norepinephrine), and vanilmandelic acid, in addition to plasma levels of catecholamines and metanephrines. None of these tests is 100% accurate because of the imperfect sensitivity and specificity of available tests, but their combination in the appropriate clinical setting will allow the best possible diagnostic yield.
   D. Measurement of 24-hour urine metanephrines and catecholamines is commonly used as a screening test. Urine unfractionated metanephrines measurement has a sensitivity of ~77% and a specificity of 93%, whereas urine VMA has a sensitivity of 64%, and a specificity of 95%. Because of the lower sensitivity of measures of unfractionated metanephrines, determination of urine "fractionated" metanephrines is one of the most commonly used screening tests; it has a sensitivity of 97% and a specificity of 69%. Sensitivity of urine catecholamines is 86% and specificity is 88%.
   E. The emergence of fractionated plasma metanephrines levels by means of high-performance liquid chromatography (HPLC) has significantly contributed to improving accuracy in the diagnosis of pheochromocytoma. Reported sensitivity of this test is up to 99%, with a specificity of 89%, making plasma-fractionated metanephrines a superior test for excluding the presence of pheochromocytoma, because of the very high sensitivity and low rate of false negative values compared to other available options. Furthermore, when combined with other diagnostic procedures, plasma fractionated metanephrines determination has been demonstrated to be an efficient as well as cost-effective diagnostic approach to pheochromocytoma.
   F. False positives can be attributed to stress and ingestion of various substances, including caffeine, acetaminophen, tricyclic antidepressants, phenoxybenzamine, and levodopa, which should be avoided for 2 weeks prior to testing. Renal insufficiency will influence urine catecholamines, leading to elevation in plasma norepinephrine and dopamine, but plasma epinephrine measurements are still reliable for diagnosis.
   G. When the values are equivocal but the clinical suspicion is strong, for example, with plasma catecholamine levels between 1 000 and 2 000 pg/mL, a clonidine suppression test can be performed if the patient is hypertensive. Alternatively, in normotensive patients, a glucagon provocative test can be useful to establish the diagnosis.

TABLE 13.1	Clinical Manifestations of Pheochromocytoma

Symptoms
  Common:
    Headache (72–92%)
    Sweating (60–70%)
    Palpitations with or without tachycardia (51–73%)
    Nervousness (35–40%)
    Weight loss (40–70%)
    Chest or abdominal pain (22–48%)
    Nausea with or without vomiting (26–43%)
    Weakness or fatigue (15–38%)
  Less common:
    Visual disturbances, constipation, warmth, dyspnea, paresthesias, flushing, polyuria,
      polydipsia, dizziness, grand mal seizures, bradycardia (noted by patients), tightness in
      throat, tinnitus, dysarthria, gagging, painless hematuria

Signs
  Blood pressure changes (seen in 98% of patients)
    Sustained hypertension
    Paroxysmal hypertension (which may alternate with hypotension)
    Orthostatic hypotension
    Hypertension induced by a physical maneuver
    Paradoxical blood pressure response to some antihypertensive drugs
    Marked pressor response to anesthesia
  Other signs of catecholamine excess
    Hyperhidrosis
    Tachycardia, arrhythmia, reflex bradycardia, forceful heartbeat
    Pallor of the face and upper part of the body
    Anxious, frightened, troubled appearance
    Hypertensive retinopathy
    Dilated pupils; very rarely, exophthalmos, lacrimation scleral pallor or injection, pupil may not
      react to light
    Leanness or underweight
    Tremor
    Raynaud phenomenon or livedo reticularis; occasionally puffy, red cyanotic hands in
      children; skin of extremities wet, cold, clammy, and pale; gooseflesh, cyanotic nail beds
    Mass lesion in abdomen or neck
    Signs caused by encroachment on adjacent structures or by invasions and
    pressure effects of metastases

Manifestations related to complications of coexisting diseases or syndromes
    Myocardial infarction
    Congestive heart failure ± cardiomyopathy
    Arrhythmias, tachycardia, unexplained hypotension or cardiac arrest following induction of
      general anesthesia
    Shock
    Cerebrovascular accident
    Azotemia
    Hypertensive encephalopathy
    Ischemic enterocolitis ± megacolon
    Dissecting aneurysm
    Severe preeclampsia during pregnancy; fever, shock, or sudden death pre- or postpartum
    Cholelithiasis

(continued)

TABLE 13.1	Clinical Manifestations of Pheochromocytoma (*Continued*)

Mucocutaneous neuromas
Thickened corneal nerves (seen only with slit lamp)
Marfanoid habitus
Alimentary tract ganglioneuromatosis
Neurofibromatosis
Cushing syndrome

H. Finally, measurement of chromogranin A in plasma (elevated in patients with pheochromocytoma) is not affected by medications used to treat hypertension. However, renal function greatly influences the specificity of the test, and a combination with other diagnostic modalities, such as plasma catecholamines measurements, would be required to improve its diagnostic yield.

V. LOCALIZATION/IMAGING

A. Once a biochemical diagnosis of pheochromocytoma is established, its localization can also be challenging. Computed tomography (CT) and magnetic resonance imaging (MRI) are the current methods of choice for localization of these tumors (Fig. 13.2). They have sensitivities of 98% and 100%, respectively, and their specificities are 70% and 67%, respectively. MRI appearance of pheochromocytomas is characterized by distinctive bright signal on T2-weighted images.

B. On the other hand, *meta*-iodobenzylguanidine scintigraphy using radioactive iodine, [123]I (MIBG), has higher specificity (virtually 100%) and positive predictive value, despite poor sensitivity (78%). In patients with biochemically demonstrated pheochromocytoma and equivocal or negative CT scan or MRI, MIBG is indicated to localize the tumor. Rarely, selective arteriography and/or venous sampling to analyze catecholamines concentrations can help in the localization of pheochromocytomas, in cases where noninvasive methods consistently fail.

C. Positron emission tomography (PET) scanning using radioactive isotopes including 6-[18F] fluorodopamine can also be performed as an alternative when other diagnostic studies are equivocal, because of the rapid turnover and metabolism by chromaffin cells compared to MIBG.

VI. TREATMENT

A. Surgery is currently the mainstay of pheochromocytoma treatment. Pharmacologic therapy, however, is necessary to prepare the patient before definitive management. α-Adrenergic blockers, such as phentolamine, or vasodilators such as sodium nitroprusside, are indicated for the management of acute hypertensive crisis or cardiovascular symptoms. After α-adrenergic blockade has been achieved, it is often necessary to incorporate β-adrenergic blockers to help in controlling tachyarrhythmias related to catecholamine excess as well as careful observance of volume status because intravascular volume repletion may be required.

B. Nonspecific α-adrenergic blockers, particularly phenoxybenzamine, have been advocated for long-term blockade, preoperative adjustment of patients, as well as for prevention of hypertensive crisis during surgery because of intraoperative manipulation-induced massive release of catecholamines. Selective α_1-adrenergic receptor antagonists, including doxazosin, terazosin, and prazosin, offer short-term control of symptoms without inducing reflex tachycardia or prolonged postoperative hypotension. Calcium-channel blockers, as monotherapy or combined with the above-mentioned agents, can also be used pre- as well as intraoperatively, because they counteract catecholamines-mediated release of calcium and vasoconstriction.

C. Preoperative adequate medical management aimed at controlling cardiovascular manifestations of pheochromocytoma greatly reduces surgical risk. Patients should

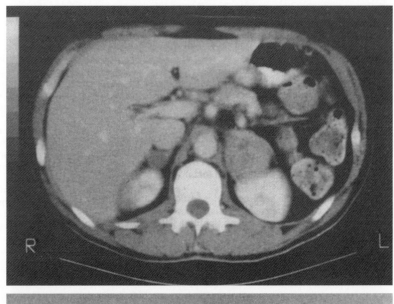

A

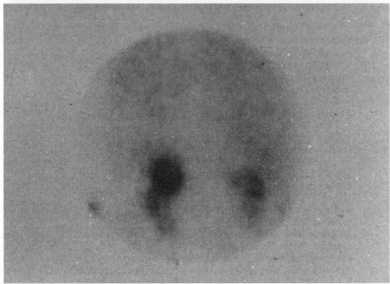

B

Figure 13.2. A: Computed tomographic demonstration of pheochromocytoma in the left adrenal. **B:** MIBG scan, posterior view, localizing the pheochromocytoma to the left adrenal; this location was confirmed by renal scan. MIBG, [131]I-*meta*-iodobenzylguanidine.

be hemodynamically monitored during surgery, and aggressive fluid replacement is indicated, to control intra- and postoperative hypotension. Minimally invasive surgical procedures have largely replaced open adrenalectomy. Laparoscopic adrenalectomy is a safe alternative and has been reported to result in reduced surgical complications, as well as shorter hospital stay and better cosmetic results.

D. Malignant pheochromocytoma

1. Surgical removal of the tumor is the primary therapy for malignant pheochromocytoma. However, metastatic disease can be present at the time of initial diagnosis, and even if there is high variability, the global 5-year survival rate is roughly <50% without treatment. Most available forms of management are palliative and should be directed at controlling cardiovascular complications, as well as tumor bulk-related compressive symptoms. Use of α-adrenergic blockers and later β-blockers is useful in these patients. Severe cases, with extremely high levels of catecholamines can be treated with α-methyl-paratyrosine, but its use is limited because of its toxicity.

2. Metastatic lesions should be resected if possible. Painful skeletal metastatic lesions can be treated with external radiation therapy or cryoablation therapy. Local tumor irradiation with repeated doses of ^{131}I-MIBG has proven to be of therapeutic value. Radiofrequency ablation of hepatic and bone metastases may be effective in selected patients.

3. If the tumor is considered to be aggressive and the quality of life is affected, then combination chemotherapy may be considered. A chemotherapy program consisting of cyclophosphamide (Cytoxan, Neosar), vincristine (Oncovin, Vincasar), and dacarbazine (DTIC-Dome) given cyclically every 21 to 28 days has proven beneficial but not curative in these patients.

Selected References

Beard CM, Sheps SG, Kurland LT, et al. Occurrence of pheochromocytoma in Rochester, Minnesota, 1950 through 1979. *Mayo Clin Proc* 1983;58:802–804.

Bravo EL, Gifford RW Jr. Pheochromocytoma: diagnosis, localization and management. *N Engl J Med* 1984;311:1298–1303.

Bravo EL, Tagle R. Pheochromocytoma: state-of-the-art and future prospects. *Endocrine Rev* 2003;24:539–553.

Canale MP, Bravo EL. Diagnostic specificity of serum chromogranin-A for pheochromocytoma in patients with renal dysfunction. *J Clin Endocrinol Metab* 1994;78:1139–1144.

Eisenhofer G, Bornstein SR, Frerieke MB, et al. Malignant pheochromocytoma: current status and initiatives for future progress. *Endocrine-Related Cancer* 2004;11:423–436.

Eisenhofer G, Walther M, Keiser HR, et al. Plasma metanephrines: a novel and cost-effective test for pheochromocytoma. *Braz J Med Biol Res* 2002;33:1157–1169.

Hakan A. Malignant pheochromocytomas: state of the field with future projections. *Ann N Y Acad Sci* 2006;1073:449–464.

Lam MGE, Lips CJM, Lager PL, et al. Repeated [131I] metaiodobenzylguanidine therapy in two patients with malignant pheochromocytoma. *J Clin Endocrinol Metab* 2005;90:5888–5895.

Lenders JW, Pacak K, Walther MM, et al. Biochemical diagnosis of pheochromocytoma. Which test is best? *JAMA* 2002;287:1427–1434.

Macho P, Perez R, Huidobro-Toro JP, Domenech RJ. Neuropeptide Y (NPY): a coronary vasoconstrictor and potentiator of cathecolamine-induced coronary constriction. *Eur J Pharmacol* 1989;167:67–74.

Pacak K, Eisenhofer G, Carrasquillo JA, et al. 6-[18F]Fluorodopamine positron emission tomographic (PET) scanning for diagnostic localization of pheochromocytoma. *Hypertension* 2001;38:6–8.

Perel Y, Schlumberger M, Marguerite G, et al. Pheochromocytoma and paraganglioma in children: a report of 24 cases of the French Society of Pediatric Oncology. *Pediatr Hematol Oncol* 1997;14:413–422.

Proye C, Thevenin D, Cecat P, et al. Exclusive use of calcium channel blockers in preoperative and intraoperative control of pheochromocytomas: hemodynamics and free catecholamine assays in ten consecutive patients. *Surgery* 1989;106:1149–1154.

Shapiro B, Copp JE, Sisson JC, et al. Iodie-131 metaiodobenzylguanidine for the locating of suspected pheochromocytoma: experience in 400 cases. *J Nuclear Med* 1985;26:576–585.

Sholz T, Eisenhofer G, Pacak K, et al. Current treatment of malignant pheochromocytoma. *J Clin Endocrinol Metab* 2007;92:1217–1225.

Smythe GA, Edwards G, Graham P, Lazarus L. Biochemical diagnosis of pheochromocytoma by simultaneous measurement of urinary excretion of epinephrine and norepinephrine. *Clin Chem* 1992;38:486–492.

Sprung J, O'Hara JF Jr, Gill IS, et al. Anesthetic aspects of laparoscopic and open adrenalectomy for pheochromocytoma. *Urology* 2000;55:339–343.

Strenstrom G, Svardsudd K. Pheochromocytoma in Sweden 1958–1981. An analysis of the National Cancer Registry data. *Acta Med Scand* 1986;220:225–232.

Whahlestedt C, Edvinsson L, Ekblad Hakanson R. Neuropeptide Y potentiates noradrenaline-evoked vasoconstriction: node of action. *J Pharmachol Exp Ther* 1985;234:735–741.

Whalen RK, Althausen AF, Daniels GH. Extra-adrenal pheochromocytoma. *J Urol* 1992;147:1–10.

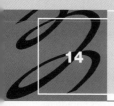

NEUROBLASTOMA

14

Norman Lavin

Neuroblastoma, ganglioneuroblastoma, and ganglioneuroma (known collectively as neuroblastic tumors) are closely related tumors that occur predominantly in children and frequently secrete catecholamines and/or their metabolites.

I. NEUROBLASTOMA

The clinical hallmark of neuroblastoma is heterogeneity; cure rates vary widely according to age, diagnosis, extent of disease, and the biology of the tumor. Some neuroblastomas undergo spontaneous regression, whereas others become highly malignant. Overall survival rates are <40% despite intensive multimodal therapy. The neuroblastoma develops from neural crest tissue and arises from the adrenal gland or along the sympathetic chain. Even though it is a highly malignant neoplasm of early childhood, it has a high spontaneous regression rate when it appears in children <1 year old.

A. Incidence. Neuroblastoma is the second most malignant solid tumor in childhood (brain tumors are first) and occurs most often in children <3 years of age. It accounts for >7% of malignancies in patients <15 years old and for ~15% of all pediatric oncology deaths. The outcome for children with a high-risk clinical phenotype has improved only modestly, with long-term survival still <40%. At least 50% of the tumors arise from the abdomen (35% from the adrenal gland), and 70% of patients have metastases (bone marrow, bone, liver, and skin) at the time of diagnosis. Thirty percent of such tumors arise in the cervical, thoracic, or pelvic ganglia.

B. Clinical presentation

1. The disease is unique because of its broad spectrum of clinical behavior. Although there is extensive overlap, three main clinical profiles are commonly recognized.

a. Localized tumors

(1) Intra-adrenal masses can be discovered incidentally on prenatal ultrasonography. Primary thoracic tumors may be detected incidentally on chest radiographs, whereas cervical masses may be associated with Horner syndrome. Paraspinal tumors can extend into the neural foramina, causing symptoms related to compression of nerve roots in the spinal cord. Up to 5% of patients may have neurologic signs related to cord impingement, including motor weakness, pain, and sensory loss.

(2) Paraneoplastic syndromes are seen more commonly in localized tumors. Secretion of a vasoactive intestinal peptide can result in watery diarrhea and failure to thrive, which resolves with removal of the tumor. Opsoclonus/myoclonus syndrome is evident in 2% to 4% of patients and consists of rapid eye movements, ataxia, and irregular muscle movements. Seventy to eighty percent of these children will have long-term neurologic deficits.

b. Metastatic disease. About half of patients present with evidence of hematogenous metastases. These patients are typically quite ill at presentation. This tumor has a tendency, which has not been explained, to metastasize to the bony orbit, resulting in periorbital ecchymoses (raccoon eyes), proptosis, or both. Bone metastases can result in bone pain, limping, or irritability. Symptoms of catecholamine excess, such as non–renin-mediated hypertension and flushing, often seen in pheochromocytoma, are rare in neuroblastoma.

   c. 4S (4 special) disease. This disease occurs in about 5% of cases. These
   infants have small localized primary tumors with metastases to liver, skin, or
   bone marrow, which almost always regress spontaneously.
2. Clinical presentation includes:
   a. Abdominal mass.
   b. Periorbital swelling.
   c. Weight loss, anorexia.
   d. Bone pain (skeletal metastasis).
   e. Anemia.
   f. Fever.
   g. Signs and symptoms resulting from elevated catecholamines:
      (1) Flushing
      (2) Diaphoresis
      (3) Tachycardia
      (4) Hypertension
      (5) Headaches
      (6) Chronic diarrhea
   h. Opsoclonus/myoclonus. Opsoclonus/myoclonus is a rare syndrome seen in the
   newborn and may be the presenting sign of neuroblastoma. It is also known
   as the "dancing eyes, dancing feet" syndrome because of chaotic eye movements, myoclonus, and ataxia. Autoantibodies against nerve tissue may be
   causative.
C. Laboratory
   1. Urine tests
      a. Vanillylmandelic acid (VMA)
      b. Homovanillic acid (HVA)
         VMA is generally used for screening. However, in 15% to 20% of patients,
         tests are negative for VMA and positive for HVA. Therefore, both tests should
         be ordered. Epinephrine levels are normal.
            The diagnosis of neuroblastoma is based on the presence of specific fea-
         tures of the tumor histology or the presence of the neuroblastoma cells in
         a bone marrow aspirate or biopsy, accompanied by raised concentrations of
         urinary catecholamines. High-risk patients also often have elevated concen-
         trations of serum lactate dehydrogenase, ferritin, or chromogranin, but these
         are relatively nonspecific for the population as a whole. Tumor-specific genetic
         markers and histopathologic assessment are crucial determinants of treatment
         planning.
      c. Cystathionine. Cystathionine is not normally present in urine and, if detected,
      suggests active disease. However, its absence has no significance.
   2. Mass screening. Studies in Japan had previously demonstrated that the pre-
   clinical detection of neuroblastoma at 6 months of age, based on measurement
   of VMA or HVA, is associated with an improved survival of up to 77% cured.
   These infants have higher VMA/HVA ratios than those whose tumors were diagnosed clinically, suggesting more differentiated tumor catecholamine pathways.
   Recently, however, two studies in Germany and North America have shown that
   screening does not reduce mortality. In both studies, almost all tumors detected
   by screening had favorable biologic features. The conclusion is that the cost of
   infant screening and the essentially unchanged mortality rates argue against the
   public health usefulness of mass screening of infants for neuroblastoma.
D. Clinical assessment of disease
   1. Computed tomography (CT) is the preferred method for assessment of tumors in
   the abdomen, pelvis, or mediastinum.
   2. Magnetic resonance imaging (MRI) is better for paraspinal lesions.
   3. *meta*-Iodobenzylguanidine (MIBG) scintiscan. Because MIBG is selectively concentrated in >90% of neuroblastomas, MIBG scintigraphy is a highly specific
   method for assessment of the primary tumor in metastatic disease. Iodine-123 is
   the isotope of choice because of its enhanced image resolution compared with the
   Iodine-131 isotope used previously.

    4. Intravenous pyelography (IVP).
    5. Bone scan or skeletal survey (or both).
    6. Chest radiograph.
    7. Liver scan.
    8. Angiography (?).
 E. Immunocytochemical and polymerase chain reaction (PCR)–based technology. These techniques can detect neuroblastoma cells and neuroblastoma-specific transcripts, such as tyrosine hydroxylase, GD2 synthase, and PgP9.5 in marrow or blood samples at diagnosis and after treatment to assess minimal residual disease.
 F. Treatment (depends on stage). The International Neuroblastoma Staging System (INSS) is used in numerous European and North American countries. Another system is that of the International Neuroblastoma Risk Group (INRG), which can be used for staging presurgically. Both systems define extent of disease by imaging studies and bone marrow morphology. Treatment modalities are
    1. Surgery
    2. Radiotherapy (cobalt-60)
    3. Chemotherapy
    4. Bone marrow transplantation
 G. Prognosis. The younger the child, the better is the prognosis. The survival rate is estimated at 30% to 35%. Patients are followed with serial levels of catecholamines. Tumors are classified as favorable or unfavorable depending on the degree of neuroblast differentiation, Schwannian stroma content, mitosis-karyorrhexis index, and age at diagnosis.
    1. Favorable prognosis is associated with young age and early stage of diagnosis, triploid karyotypes, no 1P abnormalities on N-MyC gene amplification, more mature catecholamine synthesis and excretion, and an excellent clinical outcome despite little or no therapy.
    2. Unfavorable diagnosis is associated with opposite findings to those described above and poor outcome despite multimodality therapy, such as bone marrow transplantation. Favorable neuroblastomas rarely, if ever, evolve into unfavorable types.
        In recent studies, tumors have been classified using the International Neuroblastoma Pathology Classification (INPC) system, a modification of the favorable/unfavorable system.
 H. Comorbidities. Neuroblastoma can be seen with Hirschsprung disease, congenital central hypoventilation syndrome, pheochromocytoma, and neurofibromatosis type I.
 I. New approaches to relapsed disease. Recurrent disease in patients with high-risk neuroblastoma remains a clinical challenge. During the past several years, new agents and techniques have appeared for use in these high risk clinical settings.
    1. Cytoxic agents. Topoisomerase-1 inhibitors, such as topotecan and irinotecan, can be used in the relapse setting. Other drugs in this group include temozolomide and ABT-751 (an oral tubulin-binding agent).
    2. Targeted delivery of radionuclides. Trials of attaching a radionuclide to MIBG, somatostatin analogs, and anti-G antibodies have been shown to be effective for disease palliation.
    3. Immunotherapy. GD2 is a disialoganglioside that is highly expressed in most neuroblastomas, and G_{d2}-targeted therapies using monoclonal antibodies are being studied in clinical trials.
    4. Retinoids. Trials of 13-*cis*-retinoic acid are useful as therapy for high-risk patients.
    5. Angiogenesis inhibitors. Clinical studies have shown varying degrees of success with these new agents.
    6. Tyrosine-kinase inhibitors. These agents have shown a substantial growth-inhibitory effect on neuroblastoma in vivo, and clinical trials are ongoing.
 J. Future Directions. Array-based methods may be used for identifying neuroblastoma-specific molecular targets for novel therapeutics.

II. GANGLIONEUROBLASTOMA

A. Pathology. A ganglioneuroblastoma consists of neuroblasts and mature ganglion cells; it is the product of a transformation from a neuroblastoma.

B. Clinical presentation. In addition to the features described in Section I.B, chronic diarrhea may occur.

C. Laboratory findings. High levels of dopamine, norepinephrine, vasoactive intestinal polypeptides (VIP), and prostaglandins may be present.

D. Radiography/ultrasound/CT/MRI. The presence of paravertebral calcifications and intestinal dilatations in children with intractable diarrhea suggests the presence of a VIP-secreting neural crest tumor.

E. Prognosis. The prognosis is better than that of a neuroblastoma.

III. GANGLIONEUROMA

A. Pathology. Ganglioneuromas are benign and consist of mature ganglion cells.

B. Clinical presentation. In addition to the features described in Section I.B, chronic diarrhea may be evident.

C. Laboratory findings. High levels of dopamine, norepinephrine, VIP, and prostaglandins may be present.

Selected References

Maris JM, Hii G, Gelfand CA. Region-specific detection of neuroblastoma loss of heterozygosity at multiple loci simultaneously using a SNP-based tag-array platform. *Genome Res* 2005;15:1168–1176.

Maris JM, Hogarty MD, Bagatell R, Cohn SL. Neuroblastoma. *Lancet* 2007;369:2106–2120.

Yang ZF, Ho DW, Lam CT. Identification of brain-derived neurotrophic factor as a novel functional protein in hepatocellular carcinoma. *Cancer Res* 2005;65:219–225.

Yu A. Promising results of a pilot trial of a GD2 directed anti-idiotypic antibody as a vaccine for high risk neuroblastoma. *Advances in Neuroblastoma Research* 2004. Conference, Genoa, Italy.

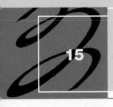

15

CONGENITAL ADRENAL HYPERPLASIA

Naomi Horowitz James, Saroj Nimkarn, Karen Lin-Su, and Maria I. New*

I. PATHOGENESIS

Congenital adrenal hyperplasia (CAH) is a family of autosomal recessive disorders of adrenal steroidogenesis in which there is deficient activity of one of the enzymes necessary for cortisol synthesis. As a result, adrenocorticotropic hormone (ACTH) secretion is stimulated via negative feedback, causing adrenal hyperplasia and overproduction of the adrenal steroids, both those preceding the step that is deficient and those not requiring the disordered enzymatic step. A simplified scheme of adrenal steroidogenesis, showing the series of enzymatic steps required for adrenal steroidogenesis, is depicted in Figure 15.1, and the genes encoding them are shown in Table 15.1.

II. BIOCHEMICAL MARKERS

Heterogeneity in several of these disorders is well recognized, and a range of clinical severity and biochemical abnormality has been documented. The symptoms of each deficiency depend on which steroids are deficient and which are produced in excess. The availability of sensitive and specific radioimmunoassays for the measurement of serum hormone levels has greatly facilitated the diagnosis of these disorders. Serum hormone determinations have largely replaced urinary hormone measurements as the primary method of diagnosis. Urinary hormone measurements can confirm the diagnosis and, with the serum hormone measurements, are useful in monitoring therapeutic response. Determination of which hormones are overproduced and which are deficient and the precursor-product ratio localizes the site of the disordered enzymatic step. Because levels of hormones distal to the enzymatic block (product hormones) may be elevated as a result of peripheral conversion of the markedly elevated hormones prior to the block (precursor hormones), the precursor/product ratios are important in avoiding misdiagnosis because of misleading elevation of product hormones. In the classic (more severe) disorders, basal hormone levels are usually sufficiently elevated to be diagnostic. In the milder, nonclassic disorders, ACTH stimulation is often necessary to pinpoint the deficiency. ACTH 1-24 is administered by intravenous bolus or subcutaneously, usually at a dose of 0.25 mg (25 U), although some investigators have employed a dose of 1 mg (100 U). Following ACTH administration, blood levels are generally measured at 60 minutes, although some investigators use 30-minute levels to aid in diagnosis. Administration of glucocorticoid results in suppression of excessive steroid production. A summary of the clinical and biochemical data in the various forms of CAH is presented in Table 15.2.

III. ENZYME DEFICIENCIES IN CAH

A. Congenital lipoid adrenal hyperplasia (cholesterol desmolase deficiency)

1. **Pathogenesis.** Lipoid adrenal hyperplasia is a rare form of CAH. In this disorder, there is a failure to convert cholesterol to pregnenolone, leading to a marked accumulation of cholesterol esters in the adrenal gland and gonads—hence the name lipoid adrenal hyperplasia. Conversion of pregnenolone to cholesterol requires the 20-hydroxylation and 22-hydroxylation of cholesterol and the scission of the C-20 to C-22 bond to yield pregnenolone. P450scc, formerly called 20, 22-desmolase, is located in the mitochondria. P450scc deficiency affects the

---

*The authors wish to acknowledge Lenore S. Levine, author of this chapter in the previous edition.

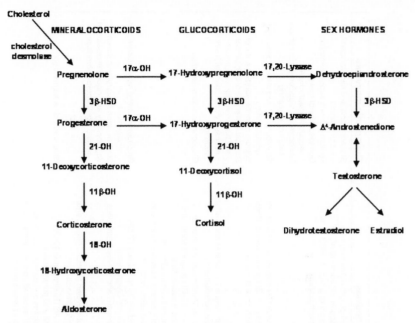

Figure 15.1. Simplified scheme of adrenal steroidogenesis. 17α-OH, 17α-hydroxylase; 3β-HSD, 3β-hydroxysteroid dehydrogenase; 21-OH, 21-hydroxylase; 11β-OH, 11β-hydroxylase.

mitochondria in the adrenal glands and gonads and results in a deficiency of all classes of adrenal and gonadal steroids. There appears to be a single *P450scc* gene, which lies on the long arm of chromosome 15. Mutational analysis of the *P450scc* gene in almost all patients with cholesterol desmolase deficiency has

TABLE 15.1 Enzymes and Genes of Adrenal Steroidogenesis

Enzymatic activity	Enzyme	Cellular location	Gene	Chromosomal location
Cholesterol desmolase (side-chain cleavage)	P450scc (CYP11A1)	Mitochondrion	*CYP11A1*	15q23–24
3β-Hydroxysteroid dehydrogenase	3βHSD (3βHSDII)	Endoplasmic reticulum	*HSD3B2*	1p13.1
17α-Hydroxylase/17, 20-lyase	P450c17 (CYP17)	Endoplasmic reticulum	*CYP17*	10q24.3
21α-Hydroxylase	P450c21 (CYP21A2)	Endoplasmic reticulum	*CYP21A2*	6p21.3
11β-hydroxylase	P450c11 (CYP11B1)	Mitochondrion	*CYP11B1*	8q21–22
Aldosterone synthase (corticosterone 18-methylcorticosterone oxidase/lyase)	P450c18 (CYP11B2)	Mitochondrion	*CYP11B2*	8q21–22

Adapted from Levine LS. Congenital adrenal hyperplasia. *Pediatr Rev* 2000;21:159–170.

TABLE 15.2   Clinical and Hormonal Data

Enzymatic deficiency	Signs and symptoms	Laboratory findings	Therapeutic measures
Lipoid CAH (cholesterol desmolase deficiency)	Salt-wasting crisis, male pseudohermaphroditism	Low levels of all steroid hormones, with decreased/absent response to ACTH Decreased/absent response to HCG in male pseudohermaphroditism ↑ACTH ↑PRA	Glucocorticoid and mineralocorticoid administration Sodium chloride supplementation Gonadectomy of male pseudohermaphrodite Sex hormone replacement consonant with sex of rearing
3β-Hydroxysteroid dehydrogenase deficiency	Classic form: Salt-wasting crisis, male and female pseudohermaphroditism, *precocious pubarche*, disordered puberty	↑↑Baseline and ACTH stimulated *Δ5 steroids* (pregnenolone, 17-OH pregnenolone, DHEA, and their urinary metabolites) ↑ACTH ↑PRA Suppression of elevated adrenal steroids after glucocorticoid administration	Glucocorticoid and mineralocorticoid administration Sodium chloride *supplementation* Surgical correction of genitalia and sex hormone replacement as necessary consonant with sex of rearing
3β-Hydroxysteroid dehydrogenase deficiency	Nonclassic form: Precocious pubarche, disordered puberty, menstrual irregularity, hirsutism, acne, infertility	↑Baseline and ACTH-stimulated 5 steroids (pregnenolone, 17-OH pregnenolone, DHEA, and their urinary metabolites) ↑Δ5/Δ4 serum and urinary steroids Suppression of elevated adrenal steroids after glucocorticoid administration	Glucocorticoid administration
21-Hydroxylase deficiency	Classic form: Salt-wasting crisis, female pseudohermaphroditism, postnatal virilization	↑Baseline and ACTH-stimulated 17-OH progesterone and pregnanetriol ↑↑Serum androgens and urinary metabolites ↑ACTH ↑PRA Suppression of elevated adrenal steroids after glucocorticoid administration	Glucocorticoid and *mineralocorticoid replacement* Sodium chloride *supplementation* Vaginoplasty and clitoral recession in female pseudohermaphroditism
21-Hydroxylase deficiency	Nonclassic form: Precocious pubarche, disordered puberty, menstrual irregularity, hirsutism, acne, infertility	↑Baseline and ACTH-stimulated 17-OH progesterone and pregnanetriol ↑Serum androgens and urinary metabolites Suppression of elevated adrenal steroids after glucocorticoid administration	Glucocorticoid administration

Disorder	Clinical features	Laboratory findings	Treatment
11β-Hydroxylase deficiency	Classic form: Female pseudohermaphroditism, postnatal virilization in males and females, hypertension	↑↑Baseline and ACTH-stimulated compound S and DOC and their urinary metabolites ↑↑Serum androgens and their urinary metabolites ↑ACTH ↓PRA Hypokalemia Suppression of elevated steroids after glucocorticoid administration	Glucocorticoid administration Vaginoplasty and clitoral recession in female pseudohermaphroditism
11β-Hydroxylase deficiency	Nonclassic form: Precocious pubarche, disordered puberty, menstrual irregularity, hirsutism, acne, infertility	↑Baseline and ACTH-stimulated compound and DOC and their urinary metabolites ↑Serum androgens and their urinary metabolites Suppression of elevated steroids after glucocorticoid administration	Glucocorticoid administration
17α-OH/17, 20 lyase deficiency	Male pseudohermaphroditism, sexual infantilism, hypertension	↑↑DOC, 18-OH DOC, corticosterone, 18-hydroxycorticosterone Low 17α-hydroxylated steroids and poor response to ACTH Poor response to HCG in male pseudohermaphroditism ↓PRA ↑ACTH Hypokalemia Suppression of elevated adrenal steroids after glucocorticoid administration	Glucocorticoid administration Surgical correction of genitalia and sex hormone replacement in male pseudohermaphroditism consonant with sex of rearing Sex hormone replacement in female

ACTH, adrenocorticotropic hormone; CAH, congenital adrenal hyperplasia; DOC, 11-deoxycorticosterone; DHEA, dehydroepiandrosterone; HCG, human chorionic gonadotropin; PRA, plasma renin activity.
Adapted from Miller WL, Levine LS. Molecular and clinical advances in congenital adrenal hyperplasia. *J Pediatr* 1987;111:1.

demonstrated normal *P450scc* genes and cDNA sequences. The cause of this disorder is in most cases a mutation in the gene for steroidogenic acute regulatory protein (StAR), a mitochondrial protein that promotes the movement of cholesterol from the outer to the inner mitochondrial membrane. Lipoid adrenal hyperplasia is the only form of CAH that is not caused by a defective steroidogenic enzyme.

2. **Clinical presentation.** The disorder usually presents in the early neonatal period with adrenal insufficiency with cardiovascular collapse, although later presentation has been reported. Because the defect is also present in the gonad, genetic males have a female phenotype, although slight virilization has been reported. A milder, nonclassical form of StAR has been recently reported, in which males had normal genital development. Less severe impairment in ovarian function and spontaneous puberty has been reported in 46 XX patients.

3. **Laboratory findings.** Hormonal evaluation reveals low levels of all adrenal and gonadal steroids and poor response to ACTH and human chorionic gonadotropin (HCG) stimulation (Table 15.2). Imaging studies may demonstrate massive enlargement of the adrenal glands.

B. **3β-Hydroxysteroid dehydrogenase (3β-HSD)/Δ4,5-isomerase deficiency**
   1. **Pathogenesis.** The conversion of pregnenolone to progesterone, 17-hydroxypregnenolone to 17-hydroxyprogesterone, and dehydroepiandrosterone (DHEA) to Δ4-androstenedione requires 3β-HSD/Δ4,5-isomerase, which is located in the endoplasmic reticulum (Δ4,5 represents a double bond between the fourth and fifth positions of a carbon atom). The 3β-HSD gene mediates both 3β-HSD and isomerase activities and is located on chromosome 1. Deficiency of 3β-HSD/Δ4,5-isomerase results in decreased synthesis of cortisol, aldosterone, and the sex steroids synthesized distally to DHEA (Fig. 15.1). Mutations in the type II 3β-hydroxysteroid dehydrogenase gene have been described in patients with this disorder.

   2. **Clinical presentation.** Severe (classic) and mild (nonclassic) forms of this disorder have been reported. The majority of children described with severe 3β-HSD deficiency have manifested salt wasting, although normal aldosterone secretion has been reported.

      The degree of incomplete male differentiation of affected males with the classic form ranges from male phenotype with hypospadias to an almost normal female phenotype, suggesting variable degrees of enzymatic defect in the testes. Normal male secondary sexual development can occur, usually accompanied by gynecomastia.

      Virilization of the external genitalia of an affected female fetus is probably secondary to increased DHEA secretion by the fetal adrenal gland.

      The nonclassic form of this disorder has been diagnosed in individuals presenting in later childhood, at puberty, and in adulthood with signs of androgen excess—early onset of pubic hair, growth and bone age acceleration, menstrual abnormalities, acne, hirsutism, and infertility.

   3. **Diagnosis.** The hormonal diagnosis of 3β-HSD/Δ4,5-isomerase deficiency is based on elevated serum levels of baseline and ACTH-stimulated Δ5 steroids (pregnenolone, 17-hydroxypregnenolone, DHEA, 16-hydroxypregnenolone, 16-hydroxy-DHEA) and elevated Δ5/Δ4 steroid ratios. Elevated Δ5 steroids and elevated Δ5/Δ4 steroid ratios are also found in urine. Diagnosis can be confirmed by molecular genetic analysis.

      a. **Stimulated values.** 3β-HSD activity is most often evaluated by measurement of post-ACTH-stimulated levels of 17-hydroxypregnenolone and DHEA, and the ratios of 17-hydroxypregnenolone to 17-hydroxyprogesterone and DHEA to Δ4-androstenedione. Most laboratories have defined 3β-HSD deficiency as the presence of responses to ACTH stimulation more than 2 standard deviations above the mean of their control population of 17-hydroxypregnenolone and the ratio of 17-hydroxypregnenolone to 17-hydroxyprogesterone.

Although each laboratory must establish its own normal age-appropriate control data, normal adult 60-minute ACTH-stimulated levels of 17-hydroxypregnenolone and DHEA have generally been <1 500 ng/dL and 1 700 ng/dL, respectively, whereas normal values for the ratios of stimulated 17-hydroxypregnenolone to 17-hydroxyprogesterone and DHEA to Δ4-androstenedione have been variously reported as <7 to <11, and <5 to <8, respectively. Patients with classic 3β-HSD deficiency have been reported with ACTH-stimulated 17-hydroxypregnenolone levels of 10 000 to 60 000 ng/dL, DHEA levels of 3 000 to 12 000 ng/dL, and 17-hydroxypregnenolone/17-hydroxyprogesterone and DHEA/androstenedione ratios of 18 to 25 and 18 to 30, respectively. Administration of glucocorticoid results in suppression of the overproduced adrenal steroids (Table 15.2). Mutational analysis of the type II 3β-HSD gene in children with premature pubarche and adult women with hirsutism, diagnosed by previously utilized hormonal criteria, indicated normal 3β-HSD type II genes (gonadal/adrenal specific). Thus, the decreased 3β-HSD activity demonstrated on ACTH stimulation testing was not caused by a mutation in the type II 3β-HSD gene.

    b. Testicular deficiency. The steroidogenic function of the testis can be evaluated by HCG stimulation testing. Protocols for HCG testing vary, with dosages ranging from 1 500 U administered once to 5 000 U given for 5 days. In the presence of testicular 3β-HSD deficiency, testosterone may rise to the normal age-appropriate range, but the markedly increased Δ5/Δ4 ratio is diagnostic of testicular 3β-HSD deficiency.

C. 17α-Hydroxylase/17,20-lyase deficiency

    1. Etiology. It has been demonstrated that the 17α-hydroxylase activity required for converting pregnenolone and progesterone to 17α-hydroxypregnenolone and 17α-hydroxyprogesterone, respectively, and the 17,20-lyase activity, by which 17α-hydroxypregnenolone and 17α-hydroxyprogesterone are converted to DHEA and androstenedione, respectively, are mediated by a single enzyme—P450c17. P450c17 is found in the endoplasmic reticulum. A single *P450c17* gene located on chromosome 10 is expressed in both the adrenals and the gonads. Because it is difficult to distinguish 17α-hydroxylase and 17,20-lyase activities in vivo, cases of P450c17 deficiency have traditionally been reported as 17α-hydroxylase deficiency.

    2. Clinical presentation. 17α-Hydroxylase deficiency (17-OHD) produces a concomitant deficiency of glucocorticoids and sex steroids. As a result of the cortisol deficiency there is increased ACTH secretion, which stimulates excessive 11-deoxycorticosterone (DOC) secretion, resulting in **hypokalemia** and **hypertension.** Females with this disorder present with sexual infantilism, hypertension, and hypokalemia; males present with incomplete male differentiation (male pseudohermaphroditism), hypertension, and hypokalemia. Undiagnosed affected males have usually been raised as females because of their phenotypically normal female external genitalia with a blind-ending vagina and either undescended or inguinal testes. However, ambiguity of the genitalia in genetic males has been observed and male sex assignment reported. Both males and females have decreased or absent axillary and pubic hair. Several patients have demonstrated hypertension in infancy.

    3. Diagnosis. The hormonal diagnosis of 17-OHD is based on the low levels of all 17-hydroxylated steroids with absent or inadequate response to stimulation with ACTH or HCG. There are also elevated baseline and ACTH-stimulated levels of DOC, corticosterone, 18-hydroxycorticosterone (18-OHB), and 18-OH DOC (Table 15.2). Low basal and ACTH-stimulated levels of cortisol (<5 and <10 μg/dL, respectively) and aldosterone (<4 and <10 ng/dL) and markedly elevated levels of corticosterone (30 to 100 times), DOC (10 to 40 times), 18-OHB (10 times), and 18-OH DOC (30 to 60 times) have been reported. Absent or low response of serum androgens to HCG, utilizing varying protocols of administration, confirms the presence of the deficiency in the testis. In the untreated state, plasma renin activity (PRA) and aldosterone are usually suppressed secondary to the excessive DOC secretion and consequent hypervolemia. Glucocorticoid administration results in suppression of the overproduced hormones, reversal of the hypervolemia, and gradual rise in PRA and aldosterone (Table 15.2). Diagnosis can be confirmed with molecular genetic analysis.

4. **Genetics.** The human gene for P450c17 has been cloned and sequenced. Molecular genetic studies of patients with 17-OHD have demonstrated >50 different gene mutations. Base-pair deletions and duplications have been described.

5. **17,20-Lyase deficiency.** A number of cases of deficient 17,20-lyase activity with normal 17α-hydroxylase activity have been reported. These patients demonstrate deficiency of sex steroids but normal glucocorticoid and mineralocorticoid secretion. Females with this disorder present with sexual infantilism and males with male pseudohermaphroditism. Laboratory evaluation reveals elevated levels of 17-hydroxypregnenolone and 17-hydroxyprogesterone, which increase further with ACTH and HCG stimulation. However, sex steroids are decreased and do not increase with ACTH or HCG stimulation. Gonadotropin levels are elevated at puberty. The molecular basis for isolated 17,20-lyase deficiency has been described in a number of patients with mutations in the gene for P450c17.

D. 21-Hydroxylase deficiency

1. **Pathophysiology.** Deficiency of 21-hydroxylase activity (21-OHD) is the most common cause of CAH, accounting for >90% of cases. Failure to adequately 21-hydroxylate 17-hydroxyprogesterone to 11-deoxycortisol (compound S) results in cortisol deficiency, increased ACTH, adrenal hyperplasia, and increased adrenal androgen secretion. The excessive adrenal androgen production, most markedly androstenedione, produces the virilization that is the hallmark of this disorder. Inadequate 21-hydroxylation of progesterone to DOC results in aldosterone deficiency, and salt wasting can occur in ~75% of infants.

2. **Clinical presentation.** CAH resulting from 21-OHD occurs in a severe (classic) form and a mild (nonclassic) form. In the classic form, virilization of the affected female begins in utero and ranges in degree from clitoromegaly, with or without partial fusion of the labioscrotal folds, to complete fusion of the labioscrotal folds with the appearance of a penile urethra. Postnatally there is progression in the signs of androgen excess in males and females: penile and clitoral enlargement, excessive growth, acne, and early onset of pubic hair growth. Bone age advancement exceeding the height/age advancement occurs, and ultimate stature in untreated or poorly treated children is short. In ~75% of patients, there is aldosterone deficiency. Salt-wasting crisis usually occurs in the first weeks of life, although it may occur in later infancy or childhood, usually precipitated by intercurrent illness. Disordered puberty and infertility in patients with CAH are well recognized; however, normal puberty and fertility with successful treatment have been achieved. Children treated when bone ages are >10 years can undergo true precocious puberty when adrenal suppressive treatment is instituted.

   In the *nonclassic form,* symptoms of androgen excess begin in later childhood, in puberty, postpubertally, or in adulthood and may be intermittent. Early onset of pubic hair development, accelerated growth velocity and bone age advancement, acne, hirsutism, menstrual irregularity, and infertility are common presenting findings. Unilateral testicular enlargement as a result of testicular adrenal rest tumors has been reported. It has been suggested that nonclassic 21-OHD is the most common autosomal recessive genetic disorder in humans, with a prevalence in Ashkenazi Jews of 3.7% (1 in 27) and in a diverse white population of 0.1%.

3. **Diagnosis.** The hormonal diagnosis of 21-OHD is based on elevated baseline and ACTH-stimulated levels of serum 17-hydroxyprogesterone and adrenal androgens, particularly androstenedione, and their suppression with glucocorticoid treatment. Measurements of the urinary metabolites pregnanetriol and 17-ketosteroids can provide additional confirmation of the diagnosis. In the classic form, basal 17-hydroxyprogesterone levels are in the range of 10 000 to 100 000 ng/dL; following ACTH stimulation they rise to levels of 25 000 to

>100 000 ng/dL. Androstenedione levels are in the range of 250 ng/dL to as high as 1 000 ng/dL or greater. The aldosterone/PRA ratio (ARR) has been shown to be decreased in cases of even subtle salt wasting and may aid in determining salt-retaining ability.

In the *nonclassic form* of 21-OHD, basal circulating levels of 17-OHP are not as high as in the classic form and may be normal, especially if they are not measured early in the morning. However, following ACTH stimulation there is a diagnostic rise in 17-OHP to levels between ~2 000 and 10 000 ng/dL. Glucocorticoid administration results in a prompt decrease in the elevated steroid concentrations (Table 15.2).

Diagnosis of 21-OHD is confirmed by genetic analysis.

4. **Molecular genetics.** Molecular genetic analysis has demonstrated that there are two human P450c21 genes—*CYP21A1P* and *CYP21A2*. The two genes are highly homologous, but only the *CYP21A2* gene is active. The two 21-hydroxylase genes are located in tandem with two highly homologous genes for the fourth component of complement (C4A, C4B). Several other genes are located in this cluster. Before the identification and sequencing of *CYP21A2*, molecular genetic diagnosis was accomplished through genotypic features of human leukocyte antigen (HLA) markers.

Gene conversions, gene deletions, and point mutations have been reported in patients with 21-OHD. The majority of mutations causing 21-OHD are recombinations between the inactive *CYP21A1P* gene and the active *CYP21A2* gene, resulting in microconversions, accounting for 75% of mutations.

Gene deletions and large gene conversions also occur. Most patients are compound heterozygotes, having a different mutation on each allele. The severity of the disease is determined by the less severely affected allele. The salt-wasting form is found in patients with gene deletions or gene conversions or both; however, point mutations are also found in these patients.

The **nonclassic disorder** is found in patients with a combination of a severe *CYP21A2* mutation (found in the classic form of the disease) and a mild *CYP21A2* mutation (found in the nonclassic form of the disease), or a combination of two mild mutations. Point mutations, gene conversions, and gene duplications have been reported in these patients. A majority of nonclassic alleles are associated with the exon 7 V281L missense mutation.

Several studies have determined the functional effects of mutations in *CYP21A2*. A single amino acid substitution present in patients with nonclassic 21-OHD results in an enzyme with 20% to 50% of normal activity; mutations in patients with the simple virilizing form of 21-OHD result in an enzyme with 1% to 2% of normal activity; and mutations found in salt-wasting 21-OHD result in an enzyme with no detectable activity. The phenotypic expression of the most common 21-OHD genotypes has been well established. However, some instances of genotype-phenotype noncorrelation have occurred; patients with two severe mutations predicted to have the classical form of the disease presented with the nonclassical form, and patients with a severe and a mild mutation, expected to cause nonclassical 21-OHD, had the severe form of the disorder.

E. **11β-Hydroxylase deficiency**
1. **Incidence.** CAH resulting from 11β-hydroxylase deficiency (11β-HSD) accounts for 5% to 8% of reported cases of CAH. It occurs in ~1 in 100 000 births in the general white population. It is more common among Jews of northern African origin and might also be more common in other populations than previously recognized.
2. **Clinical presentation.** A deficiency of 11β-hydroxylase results in a defect in the conversion of 11-deoxycortisol to cortisol and DOC to corticosterone. Similar to 21-OHD, there is virilization secondary to the excessive secretion of the adrenal androgens, resulting in virilization of the female fetus and postnatal virilization of males and females. Hypertension is commonly observed in this disorder, thought to be secondary to increased DOC secretion, sodium and water retention, and volume expansion. Hypokalemia can also be present. Glucocorticoid

administration suppresses the overproduced adrenal steroids (11-deoxycortisol, DOC, androgens), preventing continued virilization and resulting in remission of the hypertension. The external genitalia of the virilized female can be corrected surgically, as in 21-hydroxylase deficiency, and optimal treatment should permit normal growth and pubertal development and fertility.

As with 3β-HSD and 21-OH deficiencies, a **nonclassic form** of 11β-OH deficiency has been described, presenting in later childhood, at puberty, and in adult life with signs of androgen excess: early appearance of pubic and axillary hair, tall stature, advanced bone age, acne, hirsutism, temporal hairline recession, amenorrhea, and infertility.

3. **Diagnosis.** 11β-HSD is diagnosed on the basis of the presence of elevated baseline and ACTH-stimulated serum levels of 11-deoxycortisol, DOC, and androgens (particularly androstenedione) and their suppression with glucocorticoid therapy. Determination of the urinary metabolites tetrahydro-11-deoxycortisol, tetrahydro-11-deoxycorticosterone, and 17-ketosteroids can confirm the diagnosis. As previously stated, each laboratory must establish its own normal control data. However, normal serum levels of 11-deoxycortisol in the range of 11 to 160 ng/dL and of DOC in the range of 3 to 60 ng/dL have been reported. In patients with classic 11β-HSD, 11-deoxycortisol has been reported to be 10 to 40 times elevated (1 400 to 4 300 ng/dL) and DOC 10 to 50 times elevated (183 to 2 050 ng/dL). In the untreated state, plasma renin activity and aldosterone are often suppressed secondary to the sodium and water-retaining effect of the excessive DOC (Table 15.2). An interesting observation is the biochemical and clinical variability in this disorder, with dissociation of hypertension, hypokalemia, and virilization, as well as between 11-deoxycortisol and DOC levels. The pattern of hormonal abnormality in the **nonclassic form** is similar to that in the classic form, with less marked hormonal abnormality (Table 15.2).

4. **Molecular genetics.** Two isoenzymes, P450c11β and P450c18, are encoded by the *CYP11B1* and *CYP11B2* genes, respectively, lying on chromosome 8q21-q22. P450c11β mediates 11β-hydroxylation leading to cortisol synthesis, whereas P450c18 mediates 11β-hydroxylase, 18-hydroxylase, and 18-oxidase activities leading to aldosterone synthesis.

Studies of Moroccan Jewish families with 11β hydroxylase deficiency demonstrated a point mutation in codon 448 in *CYP11B1*, resulting in an arginine → histidine substitution in almost all affected alleles. Other mutations of *CYP11B1* in patients with 11β-HSD have been reported.

IV. MANAGEMENT OF CAH

A. **General principles.** The principles of treatment are outlined in Table 15.2. The standard treatment for CAH is glucocorticoid replacement therapy.

B. **Glucocorticoids.** Hydrocortisone, cortisone acetate, prednisone or prednisolone, dexamethasone, and combinations of these steroids have been used and various schedules recommended. For adults with 21-OHD, 0.25 mg of dexamethasone at the hour of sleep is the preferred treatment. However, in children, hydrocortisone is preferred because dexamethasone may lead to shorter height. The lowest dosage of glucocorticoid that produces adequate androgen (or mineralocorticoid) suppression in those disorders with androgen (or mineralocorticoid) excess should be utilized.

C. **Mineralocorticoids.** Mineralocorticoid therapy, usually in the form of 9α-fludrocortisone (0.1 to 0.3 mg/day), is administered to patients with overt or subtle salt wasting.

D. **Salt.** Sodium chloride, 1 to 3 g/day, is usually administered to an infant with salt wasting to achieve adequate sodium repletion and normalization of plasma renin activity.

E. **Sex hormones.** Sex hormone replacement at puberty is provided to patients with enzyme disorders that result in gonadal steroid deficiency. Such hormone replacement induces development of secondary sex characteristics.

F. **Surgery.** Surgical correction of ambiguous genitalia to conform to the sex of assignment has traditionally been performed within the first year of life when the infant is clinically stable. There is active debate about the timing, the decision-making process, and the need for surgery in disorders of sexual differentiation.

G. Experimental treatments. Analogs of the hypothalamic gonadotropin-releasing hormone (GnRH), in addition to glucocorticoid administration, have been used in the treatment of children with 21-OHD and true precocious puberty. Improvement of final height in children with CAH and true precocious puberty using GnRH and glucocorticoid treatment has been reported. Growth hormone has been used in patients with CAH to improve growth velocity and final height. The combination of growth hormone and a luteinizing-releasing hormone analog was also proven to be highly effective in increasing final height. Positive effects of a combination of an antiandrogen (to block androgen effect), an aromatase inhibitor (to block conversion of androgen to estrogen), and a reduced hydrocortisone dose have also been reported.

V. NEWBORN SCREENING. Screening for CAH resulting from 21-OHD became possible with the development of an assay for 17-hydroxyprogesterone using a heel-stick capillary blood specimen impregnated on filter paper. A number of newborn screening programs have been developed in the United States, Europe, and Japan. Results of screening more than 8 million newborns have been reported. There is a high frequency of CAH resulting from 21-OHD among Yupik Eskimos of southwestern Alaska (1 in 282) and the people of La Reunion, France (1 in 2 141). The worldwide incidence is estimated at ~1 in 14 500 live births and ~1 in 13 500 among whites. Salt wasting is diagnosed in ~77% of newborns. Cost–benefit analysis has indicated that newborn screening for classic 21-OHD is cost-effective.

VI. PRENATAL DIAGNOSIS AND TREATMENT OF CAH RESULTING FROM 21-OHD

A. Prenatal diagnosis. Prenatal diagnosis of CAH resulting from 21-OHD can be performed in the first trimester of pregnancy by molecular genetic analysis of fetal DNA from chorionic villus sampling (CVS) or amniocentesis. CVS is preferred over amniocentesis because the sample can be obtained at the 10th to 11th week of gestation, rather than the 15th or 16th week-of-gestation timeframe for amniocentesis.

B. Prenatal treatment. Prenatal treatment of the female fetus with CAH resulting from 21-OHD has prevented or reduced the degree of virilization of the external genitalia in approximately two thirds of the reported cases. Long-term follow-up into adulthood must be conducted to determine possible long-term complications of this treatment, and studies are currently underway.

1. Maternal side effects. In some mothers, the treatment has resulted in significant side effects, including excessive weight gain and edema, gastrointestinal intolerance, hyperglycemia, hypertension, nervousness or irritability, and striae. These complications resolved after the completion of treatment.

2. Recommended treatment protocol. The current recommended scheme when prenatal diagnosis and treatment are requested is depicted in Figure 15.2. Dexamethasone (20 μg/kg of prepregnancy weight per day in two or three divided doses up to a maximum daily dose of 1.5 mg) should be begun by the ninth week of gestation in order to reduce virilization in the affected female. First-trimester prenatal diagnosis and fetal sex determination by chorionic villus sampling should be performed and dexamethasone continued until term if the fetus is an affected female. This means that to be effective, treatment must be started blind to the sex and diagnosis of 21-OHD of the fetus. If the fetus is proven to be male or unaffected, treatment is discontinued.

VII. PRENATAL DIAGNOSIS/TREATMENT OF OTHER FORMS OF CAH. Prenatal diagnosis of 11β-HSD and lipoid adrenal hyperplasia has been reported. DNA analysis of chorionic villus cells and amniotic cells can be used for the prenatal diagnosis of all forms of CAH. Prenatal treatment of 11β-HSD has been reported in several cases and was effective in reducing virilization in one affected female.

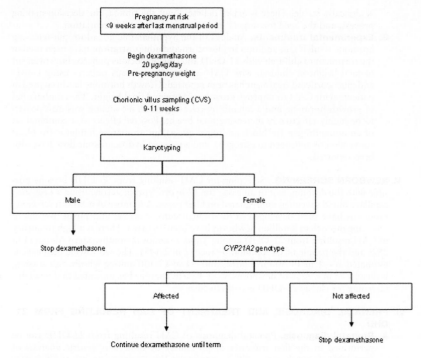

Figure 15.2. Simplified algorithm for prenatal diagnosis and treatment of congenital adrenal hyperplasia resulting from 21-hydroxylase deficiency.

VIII. PRENATAL DIAGNOSIS AND TREATMENT: CONCLUSION. Although the short-term efficacy and safety of prenatal management of CAH has been shown, data are lacking on the long-term effects of prenatal dexamethasone treatment. Studies are currently underway to ascertain the long-term cognitive and medical safety of prenatal treatment.

Selected References

Auchus RJ. The genetics, pathophysiology, and management of human deficiencies of P450c17. *Endocrinol Metab Clin North Am* 2001;30:101.

Baker BY, Lin L, Kim CJ, et al. Nonclassic congenital lipoid adrenal hyperplasia: a new disorder of the steroidogenic acute regulatory protein with very late presentation and normal male genitalia. *J Clin Endocrinol Metab* 2006;91:4781.

Bhangoo A, Wilson R, New MI, et al. Donor splice mutation in the 11beta-hydroxylase (CypllB1) gene resulting in sex reversal: a case report and review of the literature. *J Pediatr Endocrinol Metab* 2006;19:1267.

Crouch NS, Creighton SM. Long-term functional outcomes of female genital reconstruction in childhood. *BJU Int* 2007: doi:10.1111/j.1464.

Forest MG, Dorr HG. Prenatal therapy in congenital adrenal hyperplasia due to 21-hydroxylase deficiency: retrospective follow-up study of 253 treated pregnancies in 215 families. *Endocrinologist* 2003;13:252.

Geley S, Kapelari K, Johrer K, et al. CYP11B1 mutations causing congenital adrenal hyperplasia due to 11 beta-hydroxylase deficiency. *J Clin Endocrinol Metab* 1996;81:2896.

Keen-Kim D, Redman JB, Alanes RU, et al. Validation and clinical application of a locus-specific polymerase chain reaction- and minisequencing-based assay for congenital adrenal hyperplasia (21-hydroxylase deficiency). *J Mol Diagn* 2005;7:236.

Lin-Su K, Vogiatzi MG, Marshall I, et al. Treatment with growth hormone and luteinizing hormone releasing hormone analog improves final adult height in children with congenital adrenal hyperplasia. *J Clin Endocrinol Metab* 2005;90:3318.

Mermejo LM, Elias LL, Marui S, et al. Refining hormonal diagnosis of type II 3beta-hydroxysteroid dehydrogenase deficiency in patients with premature pubarche and hirsutism based on HSD3B2 genotyping. *J Clin Endocrinol Metab* 2005;90:1287.

Motaghedi R, Betensky BP, Slowinska B, et al. Update on the prenatal diagnosis and treatment of congenital adrenal hyperplasia due to 11beta-hydroxylase deficiency. *J Pediatr Endocrinol Metab* 2005;18:133.

New M. Extensive personal experience: nonclassical 21-hydroxylase deficiency. *J Clin Endocrinol Metab* 2006;91:4205.

New M, Carlson A, Obeid J, et al. Extensive personal experience: prenatal diagnosis for congenital adrenal hyperplasia in 532 pregnancies. *J Clin Endocrinol Metab* 2001;86:5651.

New M, Carlson A, Obeid J, et al. Update: prenatal diagnosis for congenital adrenal hyperplasia in 595 pregnancies. *The Endocrinologist* 2003;13:233.

New MI. Inborn errors of adrenal steroidogenesis. *Mol Cell Endocrinol* 2003;211:75.

New MI. An update of congenital adrenal hyperplasia. *Ann N Y Acad Sci* 2004;1038:14.

New MI, Geller DS, Fallo F, et al. Monogenic low renin hypertension. *Trends Endocrinol Metab* 2005;16:92.

New MI, Wilson RC. Steroid disorders in children: congenital adrenal hyperplasia and apparent mineralocorticoid excess. *Proc Natl Acad Sci U S A* 1999;96:12790.

Nimkarn S, Lin-Su K, Berglind N, et al. Aldosterone-to-renin ratio as a marker for disease severity in 21-hydroxylase deficiency congenital adrenal hyperplasia. *J Clin Endocrinol Metab* 2007;92:137.

Nimkarn S, New MI. Prenatal diagnosis and treatment of congenital adrenal hyperplasia owing to 21-hydroxylase deficiency. *Nat Clin Pract Endocrinol Metab* 2007;3:405.

Pang SY, Wallace MA, Hofman L, et al. Worldwide experience in newborn screening for classical congenital adrenal hyperplasia due to 21-hydroxylase deficiency. *Pediatrics* 1988;81:866.

Quintos JB, Vogiatzi MG, Harbison MD, et al. Growth hormone therapy alone or in combination with gonadotropin-releasing hormone analog therapy to improve the height deficit in children with congenital adrenal hyperplasia. *J Clin Endocrinol Metab* 2001;86:1511.

Simard J, Ricketts ML, Gingras S, et al. Molecular biology of the 3beta-hydroxysteroid dehydrogenase/delta5-delta4 isomerase gene family. *Endocr Rev* 2005;26:525.

White P. Steroid 11 beta-hydroxylase deficiency and related disorders. *Endocrinol Metab Clin North Am* 2001;30:61.

Wilson RC, Nimkarn S, Dumic M, et al. Ethnic-specific distribution of mutations in 716 patients with congenital adrenal hyperplasia owing to 21-hydroxylase deficiency. *Mol Genet Metab* 2007;90:414.

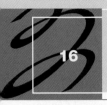

16

HORMONAL HYPERTENSION
Phyllis W. Speiser

I. GENERAL PRINCIPLES
Hypertension is a condition of multifactorial causality that contributes heavily to the risk of coronary artery and cerebrovascular disease, the leading causes of mortality in developed countries. Hypertension is defined as average systolic or diastolic blood pressure above the 95th percentile for age, sex, and height (in children) on at least three occasions. Prehypertension is defined as blood pressures between the 90th and 95th percentiles, whereas normal blood pressure is <95th percentile and/or <120/80. Limited long-term studies have indicated that tracking of blood pressure along centiles occurs when a large cohort of children are followed from early life. About 28% of all North American adults have hypertension defined as blood pressures ≥140/90; the prevalence is higher among Europeans (44%), and American blacks (40%).

II. CHARACTERISTICS OF HORMONAL HYPERTENSION
This chapter deals primarily with hypertension caused by dysfunction of the renin–angiotensin–aldosterone system (for review of adrenal steroid synthesis, see Chapter 15). For heuristic purposes, hypertension has been categorized by Laragh and colleagues as high-, low-, or normal-renin hypertension; only the first category is associated with hypertension caused by disorders of the renin–angiotensin–aldosterone axis (Table 16.1). The exact prevalence of low renin hypertension is subject to dispute, but such patients may comprise a substantial proportion of treatment-resistant hypertensives. At the other end of the spectrum are patients with high plasma renin activity (PRA) and high aldosterone secretion; these patients often have diminished renal blood flow leading to hyperplasia of the renin-secreting juxtaglomerular apparatus.

In this chapter, the following steroid-dependent forms of hypertension will be examined (summarized in Table 16.1):
A. Low-renin hypertension
   1. 11β-Hydroxylase deficiency
   2. 17α-Hydroxylase/17,20-lyase deficiency
   3. Primary aldosteronism
   4. Glucocorticoid-remediable aldosteronism/dexamethasone-suppressible hyperaldosteronism
   5. Apparent mineralocorticoid excess/11β-hydroxysteroid dehydrogenase 2 deficiency
   6. Liddle syndrome
   7. Cushing syndrome
B. High-renin hypertension
   1. Renovascular abnormalities
   2. Juxtaglomerular cell tumors
   3. Bilateral endocrine dysfunction of the kidney

III. LOW-RENIN HYPERTENSION
A. Congenital adrenal hyperplasia (CAH) with steroid 11β-hydroxylase deficiency.
An autosomal recessively inherited homozygous defect in the gene responsible for adrenal cortical 11β-hydroxylation, *CYP11B1*, results in a form of CAH characterized by excessive adrenal androgen and mineralocorticoid production. Interruption of this enzymatic function necessary for the biosynthesis of cortisol by

TABLE 16.1 Forms of Endocrine Hypertension with Suppressed Renin (PRA)

Signs and symptoms	Hormonal findings	Source	Genetics
A. Steroidogenic enzyme defects			
Steroid 11β-hydroxylase deficiency (hypertensive virilizing congenital adrenal hyperplasia): ambiguous external genitalia in newborn females; precocious isosexual development/virilization and rapid growth in both sexes	Aldosterone: elevated serum androgens/urine 17-ketosteroids; elevated serum DOC (mineralocorticoid) and 11-deoxycortisol (S)	Glandular: ZF of adrenal cortex	Mutations in *CYP11B1* gene
Steroid 17α-hydroxylase/17,20-lyase deficiency (congenital adrenal hyperplasia. 46,XY patients have ambiguous or undervirilized external genital appearance, internal blind vagina, no müllerian derivatives. 46,XX patients have lack of secondary sexual development at puberty and primary amenorrhea	Aldosterone: low serum/urinary 17-hydroxysteroids; decreased cortisol, increased corticosterone (B) and DOC in plasma: serum androgens and estrogens low, serum gonadotropins elevated	Glandular: ZF of adrenal cortex and interstitial cells of gonads (Leydig cells in testes—ovarian thecal cells)	Mutations in *CYP17* gene
B. Hyperaldosteronism			
Primary aldosteronism associated with aldosterone-producing adenoma (Conn syndrome): muscular weakness; hypokalemia in sodium-replete state	Elevated plasma aldosterone, 18-OHF and 18-oxocortisol (18-OHF and 18-oxoF): normal 18-OHF/aldo ratio	Adenoma ("clear cell" tumor; suppression of ipsilateral 2G)	Unknown; very rare in children; sex ratio 2.5:1 to 3:1 females/males.
Adrenocortical hyperplasia (as above)	Plasma findings as above; hormonal source established by radiologic scan studies	Focal (micro-/macronodular) or diffuse adrenal cortical hyperplasia (may be uni- or bilateral)	Unknown

(continued)

185

Signs and symptoms	Hormonal findings	Source	Genetics
Idiopathic primary aldosteronism (as above) Deoxycorticosterone-producing tumor (as above)	High plasma aldosterone elevated 18-OHF/aldo ratio; high plasma DOC	Hyperactivity of ZG of adrenal cortex Adenoma/carcinoma	Unknown Unknown
C. Glucocorticoid-remediable aldosteronism: hypokalemia in sodium-replete state	Elevated plasma (and urinary) aldosterone responsive to ACTH and suppressible by dexamethasone within 48 h; steroids 18-hydroxy-11-deoxycortisol (18-OHS), 18-OHF, and 18-oxoF elevated in plasma	Abnormal presence of *CYP11B2* enzymatic activity in adrenal ZF allowing completion of synthesis of aldosterone from 17-deoxysteroids	Hybrid enzyme from chimeric *CYP11B1/B2* gene that (1) is expressed at high level in ZF (regulated like *CYP11B1* gene) and (2) has 18-oxidase activity (functionality of *CYP11B2*)
D. Apparent mineralocorticoid excess; failure to thrive; cardiac conduction changes; + left ventricular hypertrophy and vessel remodeling; some Ca^{2+} ion abnormalities: nephrocalcinosis, rickets	Low plasma ACTH and secretory rates of all corticosteroids; serum F normal because of delayed plasma clearance; extreme hypokalemia and severe early-onset hypertension aggravated by any sodium intake—or by hydrocortisone or ACTH—and responding to spironolactone	High F bioactivity in periphery due to (1) defective oxidase function (F→E) 11β-HSD2 or (2) slow clearance of 5α/β reduction to (allo)dihydro-F	Mutations in *HSD11B2* (placental/kidney isoform)

ACTH, adrenocorticotropic hormone; DOC, deoxycorticosterone; F, cortisol; HSD, hydroxysteroid dehydrogenase; OHF, hydroxycortisol; OHS, hydroxydeoxycortisol; PRA, plasma renin activity; ZF, zone fasciculate.

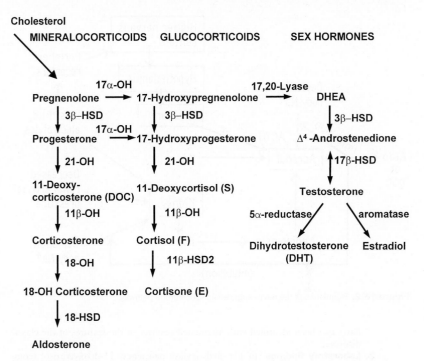

Figure 16.1. Pathways of steroid biosynthesis. OH, hydroxylase; HSD, hydroxysteroid dehydrogenase; DHEA, dehydroepiandrosterone.

the zona fasciculata (ZF) of the adrenal cortex leads to increased production by the ZF of the steroid 11-deoxycorticosterone (DOC) (Fig. 16.1). DOC, a precursor steroid hormone for aldosterone, is a moderately potent mineralocorticoid that causes sodium retention and volume expansion, resulting in hypertension with suppressed PRA (Fig. 16.2). The excess production of adrenal androgens leads to virilization, prenatally in the genetic female and postnatally in both sexes.

The prevalence of steroid 11β-hydroxylase deficiency is ~1 in 100 000 births in the general population. It accounts for 5% to 8% of CAH cases, and may be differentiated from the more prevalent form, steroid 21-hydroxylase deficiency, by the variable presence of hypertension and the absence of salt wasting. The incidence is much higher in Israel (1 in 5 000 to 7 000 births) because of a clustering of cases traced to Jewish families of North African origin, particularly from Morocco and Tunisia, who tend to carry one particular mutation.

1. **Clinical features.** Virilization is the most prominent clinical feature of 11β-hydroxylase deficiency. In this condition, inefficient cortisol synthesis provokes adrenocorticotropic hormone (ACTH) hypersecretion. Accumulation of steroids proximal to the blocked 11β-hydroxylase provides substrate for excessive ACTH-stimulated adrenal androgen secretion. An affected female fetus exposed in utero to excess adrenal androgens will develop ambiguous or frankly masculinized external genitalia. The internal female genital structures, including ovaries and uterus, are intact. Postnatally, continued excessive adrenal androgen production results in premature and inappropriate somatic development in both boys and girls: progressive penile/clitoral enlargement; appearance of axillary, pubic, and facial hair; acne; deepening of voice; and rapid skeletal growth. If adrenal androgens are not suppressed by adequate treatment, early epiphysial fusion results in short stature. Late-onset or nonclassic variants of 11β-hydroxylase deficiency

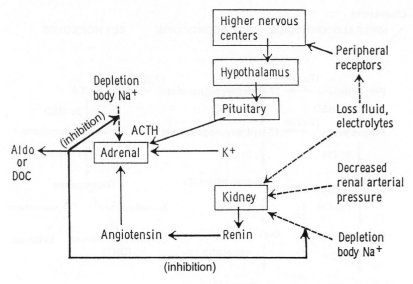

Figure 16.2. Regulation of the renin–angiotensin–aldosterone pathway.

have also been identified with attenuated severity of the features of the classic disorder.

2. **Laboratory findings.** In 11β-hydroxylase deficiency, 11-deoxycortisol (compound S) cannot be hydroxylated to cortisol, and DOC cannot be hydroxylated to corticosterone (Fig. 16.1). Cortisol deficiency leads to endogenous ACTH overstimulation of adrenal androgens that do not require 11-hydroxylation for their synthesis. Dehydroepiandrosterone (DHEA) and androstenedione, themselves weak androgens, are converted mainly in the periphery to testosterone and other sex hormones. Stimulation with exogenous ACTH produces a brisk rise in serum DOC and 11-deoxycortisol to about five times their normal levels, along with elevated levels of DHEA and androstenedione. DOC and its metabolites cause sodium retention, kaliuresis, volume expansion, and hypertension. PRA and, secondarily, aldosterone are suppressed. Twenty-four hour collection of urine will demonstrate elevated levels of tetrahydro-11-deoxycortisol (THS) and tetrahydrodeoxycorticosterone (THDOC), the principal metabolites of compound S and DOC. Urinary 17-ketosteroids are also elevated, reflecting the raised serum levels of adrenal androgens.

3. **Treatment.** Glucocorticoid administration corrects oversecretion of ACTH, DOC (largely a product of the ACTH-responsive ZF), and adrenal-derived androgens. The preferred mode of administration in young children is hydrocortisone in a dosage of 10 to 20 mg/m^2 per day; postpubertal patients can receive more potent and long-acting steroids, such as prednisone or dexamethasone. Reduction of DOC levels produces natriuresis, diuresis, volume contraction, and a rise in renin, which stimulates aldosterone production. Long-standing hypertension that is unresponsive to glucocorticoid administration may require therapy with other antihypertensive drugs, such as calcium-channel blockers. Dietary sodium restriction also helps reduce hypertension in mineralocorticoid-driven hypertension. Mineralocorticoid supplements should not be administered to hypertensive patients. Females with severe forms of virilizing CAH may undergo surgical reconstruction of the external genitalia.

4. **Genetics.** There are two genes (*CYP11B1* and *CYP11B2*) encoding two isozymes, 11β-hydroxylase and aldosterone synthase. The enzyme

11β-hydroxylase, encoded by *CYP11B1*, is responsible for the conversion of DOC to corticosterone and 11-deoxycortisol to cortisol; this gene is defective in 11β-hydroxylase deficiency CAH. Numerous mutations in *CYP11B1* causing 11β-hydroxylase deficiency have been characterized. The type of mutation and the degree of elevation of DOC does not always correlate directly with the presence or degree of hypertension, even when patients carry identical *CYP11B1* mutations. DOC and its metabolites cause sodium retention, kaliuresis, volume expansion, and hypertension. Mutations in *CYP11B1* tend to cluster in exons 6 through 8, but they have been detected throughout the gene in this autosomal recessive condition. Allelic variants consisting of mild mutations account for the nonclassic forms of this disease. In contrast, aldosterone synthase is encoded by *CYP11B2*, which is responsible for converting corticosterone to aldosterone.

A separate set of mutations in *CYP11B2* causes a rare autosomal recessive form of hypoaldosteronism known as **CMO II deficiency** that is characterized by sodium wasting, *hypo*tension, and failure to thrive in infancy. The latter gene and enzyme are intact in CAH resulting from 11β-hydroxylase deficiency.

B. CAH with steroid 17α-hydroxylase deficiency. Homozygous defects in another adrenal cortical gene and enzyme complex required for cortisol and sex hormone biosynthesis, *CYP17*, which encodes steroid 17α-hydroxylase/17,20-lyase, cause a different form of hypertensive CAH. This disorder accounts for perhaps 1% of CAH cases.

1. Clinical features. Combined deficiencies of steroid 17α-hydroxylase/17,20-lyase enzyme result in diminished production of cortisol and of sex steroids; isolated defects in the 17,20-lyase function impair production of androgens and estrogens only. Isolated deficiency of 17,20-lyase activity, therefore, is not a form of hypertensive CAH but is a potential cause of abnormal sexual development.

Because the combined defect is shared by the adrenals and the gonads, the production of all androgens and estrogens is reduced. The phenotype of genetic females is unambiguous; however, no secondary sexual characteristics develop at the age of puberty. The phenotype of genetic males is either ambiguous or female, and a number of these patients have been reared as girls. Males have defective development of internal reproductive organs: blocked androgen production precludes any embryonic wolffian duct development, whereas intact testicular Sertoli cell production of anti-müllerian hormone inhibits formation of female structures.

In both sexes, puberty fails to progress normally because of the lack of sex steroid secretion. This is in direct contrast to 11β-hydroxylase deficiency, which is associated with precocious pubertal development. This diagnosis is often made in young females or apparent females presenting at pubertal age with primary amenorrhea or lack of development of secondary sex characteristics. The disorder can be revealed earlier in 46,XY individuals presenting in infancy or childhood with genital ambiguity, micropenis, hypospadias, and/or cryptorchidism, depending on the severity of the mutation. Patients of both genders can also present with hypokalemia and hypertension as a result of mineralocorticoid excess, i.e., DOC and/or aldosterone in this form of CAH.

Massive overproduction of corticosterone at serum concentrations 30 times normal and higher appears to provide for adequate physiologic response to infection or other stress; as a result, these patients do not experience shock and "adrenal crisis."

2. Laboratory findings. The 17-deoxysteroids, DOC more than corticosterone, are increased in serum and urine. As in 11β-hydroxylase deficiency, aldosterone production, although not enzymatically blocked, is very low, secondary to the suppressed renin attributable to excess DOC. Plasma ACTH levels are less elevated than in other conditions of impaired cortisol production, perhaps as a result of limited feedback response to the presence of this marginal glucocorticoid activity. Exogenous administration of ACTH results in a 5- to 10-fold rise in serum 17-deoxysteroids, including progesterone and DOC, and a blunted cortisol response. Basal levels of C_{19} steroids, precursors of the sex hormones, are generally low in blood and urine. Gonadotropin production is extremely elevated in both sexes because of the absence of any sex steroid feedback.

3. **Treatment.** Glucocorticoid replacement (as in 11β-hydroxylase deficiency) is necessary in prepuberty to suppress DOC production. Sex steroid replacement is initiated at an appropriate pubertal age. In 46,XY patients the testes can be abdominal, inguinal, or labial; if therapy is directed to phenotypic development as a male, the gonads can be preserved and should therefore be placed in the scrotum. Estrogen replacement induces breast development in genetic females, and menstrual cycles can be established with cyclic estrogen and progesterone. As in CAH resulting from 11β-hydroxylase deficiency, refractory hypertension may require additional antihypertensive drug treatment(s) and dietary sodium restriction.

4. **Genetics.** The gene encoding the 17α-hydroxylase and 17,20-lyase activities have been characterized (*CYP17*), and numerous specific defects have been described in association with various disease phenotypes. Mutations selectively reducing lyase activity have also been identified; such mutations produce genital ambiguity in genetic males and sexual infantilism in females, but they do not induce hypertension. Either isolated 17α-hydroxylase or the combined deficiencies of 17α-hydroxylase and 17,20-lyase cause hypertension.

   Polymorphisms that cause excess 17,20-lyase activity may contribute to features of polycystic ovarian syndrome.

C. **Primary aldosteronism.** Primary aldosteronism is the most common specifically treatable and potentially curable form of hormonal hypertension, accounting for ~5% to 15% of all hypertensive patients with a hormonal etiology. This diagnosis should be considered in individuals under age 30 years with mild to moderate hypertension in the absence of obesity.

1. **Clinical features.** Primary aldosteronism is most often the result of a unilateral aldosterone-producing adenoma (APA), a finding in ~5% of all newly diagnosed hypertensive adults, or to bilateral idiopathic adrenal cortical hyperplasia. Adrenal adenomas are mostly solitary, occurring two or three times more frequently in the left gland; multiple adenomas of clinical significance are observed in 10% of cases, and only one fifth of these occur bilaterally. Primary aldosteronism is more likely to be caused by bilateral adrenal hyperplasia in childhood. However, the number of reported cases of primary aldosteronism of either cause in childhood is very small.

2. **Laboratory findings.** The diagnostic markers used in characterizing primary aldosteronism are elevated aldosterone with suppressed PRA; hypokalemia is an inconstant feature. Specifically, a morning ambulatory ratio of plasma aldosterone (nanograms per deciliter) to plasma renin activity (nanograms per milliliter per hour) >20 at baseline, or >30 after challenge with 50 mg of captopril, suggests primary aldosteronism. Plasma or serum aldosterone of >15 ng/dL should also raise suspicions. The diagnosis may be confirmed by failure of aldosterone suppression following saline loading. If the etiologic factor is an adenoma, PRA will not increase in response to postural changes. In contrast, PRA rises after 2 to 4 hours of upright posture in bilateral hyperplasia. Further characterization and localization of the lesion can be accomplished by computed tomography (CT, preferred) and/or magnetic resonance imaging (MRI), followed by bilateral adrenal vein sampling.

3. **Treatment.** Unilateral adrenalectomy is indicated in cases of isolated APA; this may be done laparoscopically. Blood pressure should be well controlled with medications before surgery. Bilateral adrenal hyperplasia is better managed with sodium restriction (<100 mEq/day) and potassium-sparing mineralocorticoid antagonists such as spironolactone (starting at doses of 12.5 to 50 mg twice daily and increasing to 100 to 200 mg twice daily) or, in refractory cases, eplerenone, a more selective mineralocorticoid receptor blocker (starting dose 25 mg twice daily, maximum 50 mg twice daily). Amiloride and hydrochlorothiazide may be used as ancillary therapy.

4. Genetics. Two distinct subtypes of nonadenomatous familial hyperaldosteronism (FH) have been identified. Type I FH (FH-I) is described further below as GRA/DSH and is associated with a hybrid aldosterone synthase gene (*CYP11B2*) responsive to ACTH stimulation. Type II is not linked to *CYP11B2*, and it is not glucocorticoid responsive. FH-II is five times more common than FH-I/GRA, and it has been linked to chromosome 7p22.

D. Glucocorticoid-remediable aldosteronism or dexamethasone-suppressible hyperaldosteronism. Glucocorticoid-remediable aldosteronism (GRA), also known as FH-I, is inherited in autosomal dominant fashion. The diagnosis should be considered in patients with a strong family history of early-onset, severe hypertension, often refractory to first-line antihypertensive drugs such as angiotensin-converting enzyme inhibitors and beta-blockers. Although GRA is usually associated with significant morbidity and mortality at a young age from stroke, some families are more mildly affected.

1. Clinical and laboratory features. Affected patients typically experience the onset of hypertension in childhood or adolescence. Blood pressure control may be refractory to conventional drug therapy. As in several other forms of low-renin hypertension, the electrolyte profile may not be helpful, as most patients do not have hypokalemia. Basal upright plasma aldosterone to PRA ratios are generally >30. The unique feature of this familial disorder (unlike adenomatous hyperaldosteronism or FH-II) is complete and rapid suppression of aldosterone secretion with glucocorticoid administration. Plasma aldosterone <4 ng/dL after suppression with dexamethasone (orally administered, 0.5 mg every 6 hours for at least 48 hours) is diagnostic of GRA. Elevated urinary 18-oxocortisol is an accurate diagnostic tool, but it is not commercially available. There is no abnormality of cortisol secretion.

Aldosterone and PRA responses to sodium manipulations are similar to those in bilateral adrenal hyperplasia or primary hyperaldosteronism resulting from adenoma. There is also unusual regulation of mineralocorticoid secretion by ACTH in GRA patients; in contrast to the response to ACTH administration in normal subjects, in whom the aldosterone response diminishes after 3 days, serum and urinary aldosterone levels continue to rise during 5 days of ACTH administration in these patients. Thus, chronic stress with consequent activation of the hypothalamic–pituitary–adrenal axis increases blood pressure in GRA patients.

2. Genetics. The genetic basis of GRA is a transposition of regulatory elements specific for *CYP11B1* plus exons 1 through 4 (see preceding discussion of CAH-11β-hydroxylase deficiency) onto exons 5 through 9 of *CYP11B2* (Fig. 16.3). The net effect of this mutation is to confer ACTH stimulability on *CYP11B2*, the rate-limiting gene for aldosterone synthesis. Screening of families affected with GRA has identified individuals who carry the mutation with only limited penetrance, confirming that other genetic and environmental factors modify the tendency to develop hypertension, even in the case of a monogenic cause of hypertension.

E. Apparent mineralocorticoid excess

1. Clinical features. Apparent mineralocorticoid excess (AME) is characterized by severe hypertension manifest in early childhood or even infancy, and is associated with low birth weight, failure to thrive, and poor growth. It is a rare autosomal recessive form of low-renin hypertension that is attributable to defects in the 11β-hydroxysteroid dehydrogenase type 2 enzyme (*HSD11B2* gene). The 11β-HSD enzyme consists of two components: 11-reductase (converting inactive cortisone to cortisol, type 1) and 11-oxidase (converting cortisol to inactive cortisone, type 2). The 11-oxidase component is defective in AME. The disorder appears to occur equally in males and females. Although the disease is found in all racial and ethnic groups, there seems to be an excess of Native Americans with AME. There is a high mortality of ~20%, attributed to the unusually malignant hypertension and severe potassium depletion resulting in cardiac arrhythmias.

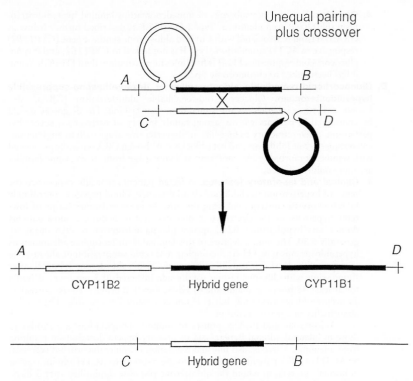

Figure 16.3. Mechanism of misalignment and unequal crossing over in glucocorticoid-remediable aldosteronism (GRA). Note that the gene segment "A–D" contains a third *CYP11* gene with five (regulatory) elements of *CYP11B1* and three (functional) elements of *CYP11B2*. Thus, the hybrid gene is capable of producing aldosterone in response to ACTH stimulation.

Because of the altered enzyme kinetics, the serum half-life of cortisol is prolonged, yet ACTH is suppressed (because of the abnormal cortisol/cortisone ratio at the level of the central glucocorticoid receptors), and patients do not have cushingoid features. Renal damage may occur as a result of nephrocalcinosis in some cases. Other end-organ damage is inevitably observed if hypertension is uncontrolled; this may be reversed by treatment to a limited extent.

2. **Laboratory findings.** The biochemical profile is characterized by low renin (<1 ng/mL per hour) and profound hypokalemia (<3 mEq/L) with metabolic alkalosis. Diagnosis of the disorder is made on the basis of an abnormally low serum cortisone/cortisol ratio; typical patients have abnormal urinary cortisol metabolites (elevation of the THF + 5-THF/THE ratio), representing the major metabolites of cortisol (THF, tetrahydrocortisol) and cortisone (THE, tetrahydrocortisone). These assays are available in specialized noncommercial laboratories. Aldosterone is suppressed. A diagnostic maneuver used only in research studies is the infusion of cortisol labeled with tritium or deuterium at the 11-carbon position with subsequent measurement of labeled water in the urine. Patients affected with AME cannot oxidize cortisol at the 11-position, and thus they have a markedly reduced capacity to produce labeled water in comparison with non-AME hypertensives and controls.

3. **Treatment.** Mineralocorticoid receptor blockade with spironolactone or eplerenone, usually in high doses, results in an initial lowering of blood pressure and an increase in serum potassium. Addition of amiloride or triamterene can

also blunt mineralocorticoid effects by decreasing sodium-channel activity. Potassium supplementation is essential to effective management. Thiazide diuretics are useful in the event of hypercalciuria and nephrocalcinosis. Calcium-channel antagonists may also be effective in the adjunctive treatment of mineralocorticoid hypertension. Kidney transplantation led to a cure in one reported case.

4. **Genetics.** There is a unique interaction among the two isozymes of 11β-HSD, and the mineralocorticoid receptor (MR). The cortisol–cortisone shuttle regulates cortisol availability and binding to the MR. A loss-of-function defect in *HSD11B2* allows cortisol to act as a mineralocorticoid agonist. In brief, the purified MR, or type I receptor, possesses equal affinity for aldosterone and cortisol in vitro. Cortisol is secreted at 1 000 times the rate of aldosterone, yet most people are not hypertensive. The observation that carbenoxolone (11β-glycyrrhetinic acid sodium hemisuccinate) and licorice (glycyrrhetinic acid) produce a hypertensive syndrome similar to AME through inhibition of 11β-HSD2 suggested that this enzyme was critical to the apparent in vivo specificity of the MR for aldosterone. Enzymatic conversion of cortisol by oxidation at the 11-position to the biologically inert cortisone prevents cortisol access to the MR in the renal cortical collecting ducts, the principal site of expression for *HSD11B2* (Fig. 16.4A). Homozygous defects in *HSD11B2* that result in impaired 11β-HSD2 activity cause the hypertensive syndrome of AME by allowing cortisol to interact *ad libitum* with the MR (Fig. 16.4B). Numerous mutations in *HSD11B2* have been detected in AME patients and correlated with biochemical phenotype. Interestingly, polymorphisms in or near *HSD11B2* are associated with salt-sensitive essential hypertension. Mild forms of AME have been reported.

F. **Liddle syndrome.** Liddle syndrome is an autosomal dominant form of low-renin hypertension, distinguished from GRA by an absence of response to glucocorticoid treatment and from AME by a lack of response to mineralocorticoid antagonists. Patients often have early-onset severe hypertension and hypokalemia. Aldosterone is suppressed, even after a low-sodium diet is initiated. The only effective treatments are triamterene, a specific inhibitor of the distal renal epithelial sodium channel (ENaC), amiloride, or renal transplant. Genetic analysis of the *SCNN1 or ENaC* gene reveals mutations in the β or γ subunits, which enhance cell-surface ion-channel expression or increase channel influx, thereby permitting inappropriate sodium retention and consequent hypertension. As in GRA, variable penetrance is observed.

G. **Cushing syndrome and disease.** Cushing syndrome and disease are additional disorders in which hypertension is associated with adrenocortical hyperfunction.

1. **Clinical features.** Cushing syndrome patients have moon facies, pigmented striae, truncal obesity, growth failure in children, impaired glucose tolerance, and low bone mineral density. Virilization is more common in adrenal carcinomas than in adrenal adenomas. Hypertension is a common finding in Cushing syndrome and occurs in up to 80% of adult cases and ~50% of childhood cases. The primary cause of elevated blood pressure is probably sodium retention and expansion of extracellular fluid volume secondary to the mineralocorticoid effect of the excess cortisol. Additional factors associated with the hypertension of Cushing syndrome include obesity and insulin resistance. Peripheral vascular resistance is elevated due to a combination of suppression of vasodilators (e.g., prostaglandins and nitric oxide) and stimulation of pressors (e.g., increased plasma renin substrate, angiotensin II receptors, and enhanced sensitivity to norepinephrine). Aldosterone levels are not usually elevated in Cushing syndrome and are not likely to be implicated in the hypertension, except in the case of an adrenal tumor cosecreting cortisol and aldosterone. Hypertension can lead to congestive heart failure and cerebrovascular accident in Cushing syndrome. As with many cases of secondary hypertension, the hypertension can persist even after a cure of the primary disorder has been achieved. This is attributed to chronic renal changes from the long-standing hypertension. It is of interest that hypertension occurs less frequently in patients treated with glucocorticoids than in spontaneous Cushing disease.

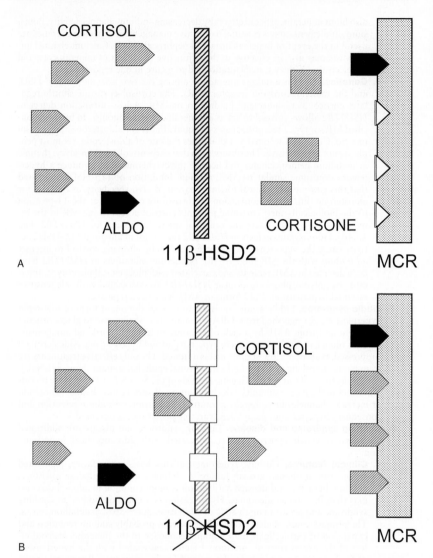

Figure 16.4. Depicted is the epithelial cell of the cortical collecting duct of the renal distal tubule, illustrating the protection mechanism of mineralocorticoid receptors by 11β-hydroxysteroid dehydrogenase type 2 (11β-HSD2). Although aldosterone is a more potent mineralocorticoid than cortisol, the mineralocorticoid receptor binds these hormones with equal affinity. However, cortisol is secreted in milligram amounts daily, whereas aldosterone is secreted in microgram amounts; normal subjects are protected from cortisol overload by the action of 11β-HSD2, as the type 2 isoform of the 11β-HSD enzyme functions unidirectionally to convert cortisol to cortisone **(A)**. Cortisone does not bind to the mineralocorticoid receptor. Aldosterone is not metabolized by the 11β-HSD enzyme because it is a β-lactone and thus has unimpeded access to the mineralocorticoid receptor. However, cortisol saturates the mineralocorticoid receptor in patients with deficient 11β-HSD2 enzyme activity **(B)**. The resulting inappropriate binding of cortisol to the mineralocorticoid receptor causes sodium retention and volume expansion that suppresses plasma renin and aldosterone secretion, and causes potassium excretion and hypokalemia.

Cushing syndrome is rare in children; it is most commonly the result of an adrenal tumor that overproduces glucocorticoid and androgens. In adults, ACTH-dependent Cushing disease is more common.

2. **Laboratory findings.** The diagnosis of Cushing syndrome is suspected based on clinical features. Further diagnostic proof is obtained either by finding high levels of salivary cortisol obtained at midnight, or elevated 24-hour levels of urine-free cortisol on at least two separate occasions. Dexamethasone suppression of cortisol is an important distinguishing feature of adrenocortical hyperplasia. Patients with Cushing disease have elevated peripheral and/or petrosal sinus levels of ACTH associated with pituitary lesions (as detected by MRI). Corticotropin-releasing hormone testing, especially when combined with prior dexamethasone suppression, represents another means of diagnosing this pernicious disease (34). Ectopic ACTH production by tumors should be considered if adrenal hypercortisolism and pituitary sources are excluded.

An adrenal tumor is suspected when hypercortisolemia is not suppressed by dexamethasone and is accompanied by elevated serum and urinary androgens and/or mineralocorticoids. Radiologic studies of the adrenal glands, notably by CT and MRI, are used to document tumors.

3. **Treatment.** Therapy should be directed at identifying and removing the cause for hypercortisolism. Most often, this entails a surgical procedure to remove a tumor. If the patient is not a good surgical candidate, medical treatment with drugs that inhibit cortisol synthesis, such as ketoconazole or mitotane (often necessary in extremely high doses) can be effective. Mifepristone (RU486), which blocks cortisol action, is also effective.

IV. HIGH-RENIN HYPERTENSION

A. **Renovascular abnormalities.** Secondary hyperaldosteronism in children occurs as a result of oversecretion of renin by the juxtaglomerular apparatus. This occurs in the presence of renovascular abnormalities, most commonly fibromuscular dysplasia in the pediatric age group, resulting in renal ischemia. The renovascular abnormality can occur in the main renal artery, in a segmental renal artery, or as a result of coarctation of the aorta. Secondary hyperaldosteronism associated with hypertension can occur after renal transplantation, with genitourinary tract obstruction, or following blunt abdominal trauma. Intra-abdominal or retroperitoneal tumors may cause compression of the renal vasculature with hyperreninemic hypertension. Since the advent of invasive monitoring of premature infants with respiratory distress syndrome, a common complication of umbilical catheter insertion has been thrombosis with consequent hypertension. Other medical conditions associated with renal arterial stenosis include neurofibromatosis and inflammatory arteritides.

B. **Juxtaglomerular cell tumors**
   1. **Clinical features.** A syndrome consisting of hypertension, hyperreninism, and secondary hyperaldosteronism accompanied by failure to suppress renin with high sodium intake suggests the presence of an autonomous tumor of the renin-producing juxtaglomerular cells. Patients with these tumors are often younger than those with essential hypertension and are usually female. The diagnosis is made following visualization of a hypovascular mass on an arteriogram; no arterial stenosis is visible. Other methods of detection include ultrasound, excretory urography, and CT with contrast. In all cases described to date, the blood pressure and plasma renin returned to normal after surgical removal of the tumor.
   2. **Laboratory findings.** In each of the previously described syndromes of high-renin hypertension, PRA is elevated and accompanied by high urinary aldosterone and low urinary sodium excretion. Criteria that suggest renal artery stenosis include diastolic blood pressure >100 mm Hg, elevated peripheral vein renin, and an abnormal renal radionuclide scan during angiotensin-converting enzyme inhibitor administration. Although angiography may be used as both a diagnostic and a therapeutic tool, it is an invasive procedure carrying substantial risk. Magnetic resonance angiography is a noninvasive diagnostic tool, but it cannot

be used therapeutically. Contrast-enhanced Doppler ultrasound is another useful screening test for patients at risk from renovascular hypertension.

3. **Treatment.** Surgical revascularization has resulted in cure or improvement of hypertension in >90% of pediatric cases with renal artery stenoses. Percutaneous transluminal renal angioplasty (PCTRA) and renal arterial stent placement have been relatively less efficacious as alternatives to open surgical correction of reno-vascular lesions. Success rates vary depending on the center and skill of the operator, and potentially carry the risk of vascular perforation. The rate of success with these procedures is also influenced by the extent of disease: Patients with bilateral or multiple stenoses are less likely to be cured, and will probably require surgical revascularization. With a limited stenosis, PCTRA may make the patient amenable to medical management with an angiotensin-converting enzyme (ACE) inhibitor.

C. **Bilateral endocrine dysfunction of the kidney.** In this syndrome, there is severe hypertension, marked hyperreninemia, and hyperaldosteronism. Frequently, there is associated hypertensive encephalopathy and weight loss. The cause of the disorder is unclear. However, hypersecretion of renin occurs equally in both kidneys. The presence of bilateral juxtaglomerular tumors is ruled out by pathologic and arteri-ographic studies. Treatment should be directed at lowering the blood pressure until remission occurs.

D. **Drugs useful in the diagnosis and treatment of high-renin hypertension.** In-hibitors of the angiotensin I–converting enzyme inhibitor are valuable in the diag-nosis and treatment of hypertension. In adults with high-renin hypertension, acute captopril administration produces a dramatic rise in PRA, a fall in plasma aldos-terone, and a fall in blood pressure, reflecting blockage of conversion of angiotensin I to angiotensin II. In general, the long-term blood pressure response parallels the acute blood pressure response. In children, the positive predictive value of acute captopril challenge with peripheral vein PRA measurement has been estimated at <50% for the detection of renovascular disease. Diagnostic accuracy of the ACE inhibitor challenge improves with selective renal vein renin sampling.

Second- and third-generation ACE inhibitors, such as enalapril and ramipril, have now been used extensively in hypertensive children and adolescents. Diag-nosis in such patients has ranged from mild essential hypertension to malignant hypertension of unknown etiology. Although the ACE inhibitors were originally thought to be effective only in high-renin hypertension, they are now favored as first-line agents for various forms of hypertension because of their low incidence of side effects. One important adverse side effect is teratogenicity, and therefore, young women of child-bearing potential should be cautioned to use effective birth control. Recent data suggest that cardiovascular morbidity and mortality can be significantly reduced in high-risk older adult patients treated with ACE inhibitors. Salutary effects include improvement in cardiac function in patients with conges-tive heart failure, reversal of retinopathy, and a decrease in proteinuria in diabetic nephropathy. Adults with diabetic renal disease show improvement in microalbu-minuria and blood pressure when treated with ACE inhibitors. Treatment with an angiotensin II receptor blocker does not confer a similar survival advantage to such patients.

V. SUMMARY

Although hormonal hypertension accounts for a minority of cases of adult and pediatric hypertension (overall perhaps 1%), making a specific diagnosis can aid in designing an effective therapeutic regimen. Furthermore, understanding the cause of the hypertension can help in identifying other affected family members and in providing anticipatory management and genetic counseling in inherited disorders.

Selected References

Auchus RJ. The genetics, pathophysiology, and management of human deficiencies of P450c17. *Endocrinol Metab Clin North Am* 2001;30:101–119, vii.

Auchus RJ, Geller DH, Lee TC, Worthy KM. The function and roles of P450c17 in androgen excess states. *J Pediatr Endocrinol Metab* 2000;13(suppl 5):1271–1275.

Bhangoo A, Wilson R, New MI, Ten S. Donor splice mutation in the 11beta-hydroxylase (CypllB1) gene resulting in sex reversal: a case report and review of the literature. *J Pediatr Endocrinol Metab* 2006;19:1267–1282.

Chu JW, Matthias DF, Belanoff J, et al. Successful long-term treatment of refractory Cushing's disease with high-dose mifepristone (RU 486). *J Clin Endocrinol Metab* 2001; 86:3568–3573.

Clark PA. Nonclassic 11 beta-hydroxylase deficiency: report of two patients and review. *J Pediatr Endocrinol Metab* 2000;13:105–109.

Eide IK, Torjesen PA, Drolsum A, et al. Low-renin status in therapy-resistant hypertension: a clue to efficient treatment. *J Hypertens* 2004;22:2217–2226.

Hajjar I, Kotchen TA. Trends in prevalence, awareness, treatment, and control of hypertension in the United States, 1988–2000. *JAMA* 2003;290:199–206.

Joehrer K, Geley S, Strasser-Wozak EM, et al. CYP11B1 mutations causing nonclassic adrenal hyperplasia due to 11 beta-hydroxylase deficiency. *Hum Mol Genet* 1997;6:1829–1834.

Lavery GG, Ronconi V, Draper N, et al. Late-onset apparent mineralocorticoid excess caused by novel compound heterozygous mutations in the HSD11B2 gene. *Hypertension* 2003;42:123–129.

Lim PO, Young WF, MacDonald TM. A review of the medical treatment of primary aldosteronism. *J Hypertens* 2001;19:353–361.

Magiakou MA, Smyrnaki P, Chrousos GP. Hypertension in Cushing's syndrome. *Best Pract Res Clin Endocrinol Metab* 2006;20:467–482.

Mattsson C, Young WF Jr. Primary aldosteronism: diagnostic and treatment strategies. *Nat Clin Pract Nephrol* 2006;2:198–208.

McMahon GT, Dluhy RG. Glucocorticoid-remediable aldosteronism. *Arq Bras Endocrinol Metabol* 2004;48:682–686.

Mulatero P, di Cella SM, Williams TA, et al. Glucocorticoid remediable aldosteronism: low morbidity and mortality in a four-generation Italian pedigree. *J Clin Endocrinol Metab* 2002;87:3187–3191.

New MI, Levine LS, Biglieri EG, et al. Evidence for an unidentified steroid in a child with apparent mineralocorticoid hypertension. *J Clin Endocrinol Metab* 1977;44:924–933.

Newell-Price J, Bertagna X, Grossman AB, Nieman LK. Cushing's syndrome. *Lancet* 2006;367:1605–1617.

Quinkler M, Stewart PM. Hypertension and the cortisol-cortisone shuttle. *J Clin Endocrinol Metab* 2003;88:2384–2392.

Rich GM, Ulick S, Cook S, et al. Glucocorticoid-remediable aldosteronism in a large kindred: clinical spectrum and diagnosis using a characteristic biochemical phenotype. *Ann Intern Med* 1992;116:813–820.

Rosa S, Duff C, Meyer M, et al. P450c17 deficiency: clinical and molecular characterization of six patients. *J Clin Endocrinol Metab* 2007;92:1000–1007.

Rossi GP, Bernini G, Caliumi C, et al. A prospective study of the prevalence of primary aldosteronism in 1,125 hypertensive patients. *J Am Coll Cardiol* 2006;48:2293–2300.

Stanley JC, Criado E, Upchurch GR Jr, et al. Pediatric renovascular hypertension: 132 primary and 30 secondary operations in 97 children. *J Vasc Surg* 2006;44:1219–1228.

Stowasser M, Gordon RD. Aldosterone excess, hypertension, and chromosome 7p22: evidence continues to mount. *Hypertension* 2007;49:761–762.

Strippoli GF, Craig MC, Schena FP, Craig JC. Role of blood pressure targets and specific antihypertensive agents used to prevent diabetic nephropathy and delay its progression. *J Am Soc Nephrol* 2006;17:S153–S155.

The fourth report on the diagnosis, evaluation, and treatment of high blood pressure in children and adolescents. *Pediatrics* 2004;114:555–576.

White PC, Agarwal AK, Nunez BS, et al. Genotype-phenotype correlations of mutations and polymorphisms in HSD11B2, the gene encoding the kidney isozyme of 11beta-hydroxysteroid dehydrogenase. *Endocr Res* 2000;26:771–780.

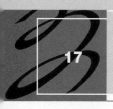

17 PRIMARY HYPERTENSION IN CHILDREN
Norman Lavin

I. INTRODUCTION

It is now apparent that primary hypertension is detectable in the young and occurs commonly. Hypertension may occur at any age in childhood from the newborn period to adolescence. By early detection and appropriate treatment, we may now be able to prevent early- and late-onset arteriosclerotic heart disease.

The purpose of this chapter is to provide recommendations for diagnosis, evaluation, and treatment of hypertension in children based on available evidence and consensus expert opinion. Primary or essential hypertension is much more prevalent than was previously believed. Childhood hypertension predisposes to left ventricular hypertrophy, retinal vascular abnormalities, and cardiovascular disease, including increased risk of coronary heart disease and associated mortality. Because of U.S. federal legislation during the past decade, there has been an increasing number of clinical trials regarding antihypertensive agents in children. In 95% of cases, high blood pressure has no known cause. But this can only be stated if organic disorders, such as kidney disease, are excluded. Children must also be evaluated for additional risk factors, such as sleep apnea, hormonal disorders, abnormal arteries, as well as certain drugs, such as oral contraceptives, steroids, analgesics, nasal decongestants, and cocaine.

More than one fourth of the world's adult population is already hypertensive, and this number is projected to increase to 30% or 1.5 billion people by the year 2025. It is the most common risk factor for cardiovascular morbidity and mortality; however, less than one third of individuals with high blood pressure are adequately treated, and a very high number of people are not even aware that they have hypertension.

Both hypertension and prehypertension have a strong association with obesity, and recently there has been a marked increase in the prevalence of overweight and obese children. The prevalence of hypertension increases progressively with increasing body mass index (BMI). Hypertension is detectable in >30% of overweight children with a BMI above the 95th percentile.

II. DEFINITION OF HYPERTENSION

A. The **definition of hypertension in adults** is based on the level of blood pressure, which is linked to an increase in risk for cardiovascular events. No data are yet available that directly link the threshold level of blood pressure in children with subsequent cardiovascular events, so hypertension in children is defined statistically. It is a systolic or diastolic blood pressure that is equal to or greater than the 95th percentile for age, sex, and height (Tables 17.1A and 1B).

B. The term **prehypertension** designates a level of blood pressure that indicates a heightened risk for development of hypertension. It is defined as systolic or diastolic blood pressure that is between the 90th and 95th percentiles for age, sex, and height. Normal blood pressure is at levels less than the 90th percentile.

C. **Arteriosclerotic cardiovascular disease** begins in early childhood. Fatty streaks and atherosclerotic lesions have been found postmortem in the aorta and coronary vessels of children as young as 6 years of age. The risk factors for this problem include hypertension, dyslipidemia, and obesity. These risk factors may be mild, such as borderline hypertension and mild dyslipidemia.

TABLE 17.1A Blood Pressure Levels for Boys by Age and Height Percentile

Age (y)	Blood pressure percentile	Systolic blood pressure (mm Hg) Percentile of height							Diastolic blood pressure (mm Hg) Percentile of height						
		5th	10th	25th	50th	75th	90th	95th	5th	10th	25th	50th	75th	90th	95th
1	50th	80	81	83	85	87	88	89	34	35	36	37	38	39	39
	90th	94	95	97	99	100	102	103	49	50	51	52	53	53	54
	95th	98	99	101	103	104	106	106	54	54	55	56	57	58	58
	99th	105	106	108	110	112	113	114	61	62	63	64	65	66	66
2	50th	84	85	87	88	90	92	92	39	40	41	42	43	44	44
	90th	97	99	100	102	104	105	106	54	55	56	57	58	58	59
	95th	101	102	104	106	108	109	110	59	59	60	61	62	63	63
	99th	109	110	111	113	115	117	117	66	67	68	69	70	71	71
3	50th	86	87	89	91	93	94	95	44	44	45	46	47	48	48
	90th	100	101	103	105	107	108	109	59	59	60	61	62	63	63
	95th	104	105	107	109	110	112	113	63	63	64	65	66	67	67
	99th	111	112	114	116	118	119	120	71	71	72	73	74	75	75
4	50th	88	89	91	93	95	96	97	47	48	49	50	51	51	52
	90th	102	103	105	107	109	110	111	62	63	64	65	66	66	67
	95th	106	107	109	111	112	114	115	66	67	68	69	70	71	71
	99th	113	114	116	118	120	121	122	74	75	76	77	78	78	79
5	50th	90	91	93	95	96	98	98	50	51	52	53	54	55	55
	90th	104	105	106	108	110	111	112	65	66	67	68	69	69	70
	95th	108	109	110	112	114	115	116	69	70	71	72	73	74	74
	99th	115	116	118	120	121	123	123	77	78	79	80	81	81	82
6	50th	91	92	94	96	98	99	100	53	53	54	55	56	57	57
	90th	105	106	108	110	111	113	113	68	68	69	70	71	72	72
	95th	109	110	112	114	115	117	117	72	72	73	74	75	76	76
	99th	116	117	119	121	123	124	125	80	80	81	82	83	84	84

(continued)

TABLE 17.1A Blood Pressure Levels for Boys by Age and Height Percentile (Continued)

| | | Systolic blood pressure (mm Hg) | | | | | | | Diastolic blood pressure (mm Hg) | | | | | | |
| | | Percentile of height | | | | | | | Percentile of height | | | | | | |
Age (y)	Blood pressure percentile	5th	10th	25th	50th	75th	90th	95th	5th	10th	25th	50th	75th	90th	95th
7	50th	92	94	95	97	99	100	101	55	55	56	57	58	59	59
	90th	106	107	109	111	113	114	115	70	70	71	72	73	74	74
	95th	110	111	113	115	117	118	119	74	74	75	76	77	78	78
	99th	117	118	120	122	124	125	126	82	82	83	84	85	86	86
8	50th	94	95	97	99	100	102	102	56	57	58	59	60	60	61
	90th	107	109	110	112	114	115	116	71	72	72	73	74	75	76
	95th	111	112	114	116	118	119	120	75	76	77	78	79	79	80
	99th	119	120	122	123	125	127	127	83	84	85	86	87	87	88
9	50th	95	96	98	100	102	103	104	57	58	59	60	61	61	62
	90th	109	110	112	114	115	117	118	72	73	74	75	76	76	77
	95th	113	114	116	118	119	121	121	76	77	78	79	80	81	81
	99th	120	121	123	125	127	128	129	84	85	86	87	88	88	89
10	50th	97	98	100	102	103	105	106	58	59	60	61	61	62	63
	90th	111	112	114	115	117	119	119	73	73	74	75	76	77	78
	95th	115	116	117	119	121	122	123	77	78	79	80	81	81	82
	99th	122	123	125	127	128	130	130	85	86	86	88	88	89	90
11	50th	99	100	102	104	105	107	107	59	59	60	61	62	63	63
	90th	113	114	115	117	119	120	121	74	74	75	76	77	78	78
	95th	117	118	119	121	123	124	125	78	78	79	80	81	82	82
	99th	124	125	127	129	130	132	132	86	86	87	88	89	90	90
12	50th	101	102	104	106	108	109	110	59	60	61	62	63	63	64
	90th	115	116	118	120	121	123	123	74	75	75	76	77	78	79
	95th	119	120	122	123	125	127	127	78	79	80	81	82	82	83
	99th	126	127	129	131	133	134	135	86	87	88	89	90	90	91

Age (Year)	BP Percentile	SBP							DBP						
13	50th	104	105	106	108	110	111	112	60	60	61	62	63	64	64
	90th	117	118	120	122	124	125	126	75	75	76	77	78	79	79
	95th	121	122	124	126	128	129	130	79	79	80	81	82	83	83
	99th	128	130	131	133	135	136	137	87	87	88	89	90	91	91
14	50th	106	107	109	111	113	114	115	60	60	61	62	63	65	65
	90th	120	121	123	125	126	128	128	75	76	77	78	79	79	80
	95th	124	125	127	128	130	132	132	80	80	81	82	83	84	84
	99th	131	132	134	136	138	139	140	87	88	89	90	91	92	92
15	50th	109	110	112	113	115	117	117	61	62	63	64	65	66	66
	90th	122	124	125	127	129	130	131	76	77	78	79	80	80	81
	95th	126	127	129	131	133	134	135	81	81	82	83	84	85	85
	99th	134	135	136	138	140	142	142	88	89	90	91	92	93	93
16	50th	111	112	114	116	118	119	120	63	63	64	65	66	67	67
	90th	125	126	128	130	131	133	134	78	78	79	80	81	82	82
	95th	129	130	132	134	135	137	137	82	83	83	84	85	86	87
	99th	136	137	139	141	143	144	145	90	90	91	92	93	94	94
17	50th	114	115	116	118	120	121	122	65	66	67	68	69	70	70
	90th	127	128	130	132	134	135	136	80	80	82	83	84	84	84
	95th	131	132	134	136	138	139	140	84	85	86	87	88	89	89
	99th	139	140	141	143	145	146	147	92	93	94	95	96	97	97

The 90th percentile is 1.28 standard deviations (SD), the 95th percentile is 1.645 SD, and the 99th percentile is 2.326 SD over the mean. For research purposes, the SDs in Table Bl allow one to compute blood pressure Z scores and percentiles for boys with height percentiles given in Table 3 (i.e., the 5th, 10th, 25th, 50th, 75th, 90th, and 95th percentiles). These height percentiles must be converted to height Z scores given by: 5% = −1.645; 10% = −1.28; 25% = −0.68; 50% = 0; 75% = 0.68; 90% = 1.28; and 95% = 1.645, and then computed according to the methodology in steps 2 through 4 described in Appendix B. For children with height percentiles other than these, follow steps 1 through 4 as described in Appendix B.

Adapted from *Pediatrics August 2004, Volume 114 (2), Part 3.*

TABLE 17.1B Blood Pressure Levels for Girls by Age and Height Percentile

Age (y)	Blood pressure percentile	Systolic blood pressure (mm Hg) Percentile of height							Diastolic blood pressure (mm Hg) Percentile of height						
		5th	10th	25th	50th	75th	90th	95th	5th	10th	25th	50th	75th	90th	95th
1	50th	83	84	85	86	88	89	90	38	39	39	40	41	41	42
	90th	97	97	98	100	101	102	103	52	53	53	54	55	55	56
	95th	100	101	102	104	105	106	107	56	57	57	58	59	59	60
	99th	108	108	109	111	112	113	114	64	64	65	65	66	67	67
2	50th	85	85	87	88	89	91	91	43	44	44	45	46	46	47
	90th	98	99	100	101	103	104	105	57	58	58	59	60	61	61
	95th	102	103	104	105	107	108	109	61	62	62	63	64	65	65
	99th	109	110	111	112	114	115	116	69	69	70	70	71	72	72
3	50th	86	87	88	89	91	92	93	47	48	48	49	50	50	51
	90th	100	100	102	103	104	106	106	61	62	62	63	64	64	65
	95th	104	104	105	107	108	109	110	65	66	66	67	68	68	69
	99th	111	111	113	114	115	116	117	73	73	74	74	75	76	76
4	50th	88	88	90	91	92	94	94	50	50	51	52	52	53	54
	90th	101	102	103	104	106	107	108	64	64	65	66	67	67	68
	95th	105	106	107	108	110	111	112	68	68	69	70	71	71	72
	99th	112	113	114	115	117	118	119	76	76	76	77	78	79	79
5	50th	89	90	91	93	94	95	96	52	53	53	54	55	55	56
	90th	103	103	105	106	107	109	109	66	67	67	68	69	69	70
	95th	107	107	108	110	111	112	113	70	71	71	72	73	73	74
	99th	114	114	116	117	118	120	120	78	78	79	79	80	81	81
6	50th	91	92	93	94	96	97	98	54	54	55	56	56	57	58
	90th	104	105	106	108	109	110	111	68	68	69	70	70	71	72
	95th	108	109	110	111	113	114	115	72	72	73	74	74	75	76
	99th	115	116	117	119	120	121	122	80	80	80	81	82	83	83

Age (Year)	BP Percentile	SBP (mmHg) — Percentile of Height							DBP (mmHg) — Percentile of Height						
		5th	10th	25th	50th	75th	90th	95th	5th	10th	25th	50th	75th	90th	95th
7	50th	93	93	95	96	97	99	99	55	56	56	57	58	58	59
	90th	106	107	108	109	111	112	113	69	70	70	71	72	72	73
	95th	110	111	112	113	115	116	116	73	74	74	75	76	76	77
	99th	117	118	119	120	122	123	124	81	81	82	82	83	84	84
8	50th	95	95	96	98	99	100	101	57	57	57	58	59	60	60
	90th	108	109	110	111	113	114	114	71	71	71	72	73	74	74
	95th	112	112	114	115	116	118	118	75	75	75	76	77	78	78
	99th	119	120	121	122	123	125	125	82	82	83	83	84	85	86
9	50th	96	97	98	100	101	102	103	58	58	59	59	60	61	61
	90th	110	110	112	113	114	116	116	72	72	73	73	74	75	75
	95th	114	114	115	117	118	119	120	76	76	77	77	78	79	79
	99th	121	121	123	124	125	127	127	83	83	84	84	85	86	87
10	50th	98	99	100	102	103	104	105	59	59	59	60	61	62	62
	90th	112	112	114	115	116	118	118	73	73	73	74	75	76	76
	95th	116	116	117	119	120	121	122	77	77	77	78	79	80	80
	99th	123	123	125	126	127	129	129	84	84	85	86	86	87	88
11	50th	100	101	102	103	105	106	107	60	60	60	61	62	63	63
	90th	114	114	116	117	118	119	120	74	74	74	75	76	77	77
	95th	118	118	119	121	122	123	124	78	78	78	79	80	81	81
	99th	125	125	126	128	129	130	131	85	85	86	87	87	88	89
12	50th	102	103	104	105	107	108	109	61	61	61	62	63	64	64
	90th	116	116	117	119	120	121	122	75	75	75	76	77	78	78
	95th	119	120	121	123	124	125	126	79	79	79	80	81	82	82
	99th	127	127	128	130	131	132	133	86	86	87	88	88	89	90

(continued)

TABLE 17.1B Blood Pressure Levels for Girls by Age and Height Percentile (Continued)

Age (y)	Blood pressure percentile	Systolic blood pressure (mm Hg) Percentile of height							Diastolic blood pressure (mm Hg) Percentile of height						
		5th	10th	25th	50th	75th	90th	95th	5th	10th	25th	50th	75th	90th	95th
13	50th	104	105	106	107	109	110	110	62	62	62	63	64	65	65
	90th	117	118	119	121	122	123	124	76	76	76	77	78	79	79
	95th	121	122	123	124	126	127	128	SO	80	80	81	82	83	83
	99th	128	129	130	132	133	134	135	87	87	88	89	89	90	91
14	50th	106	106	107	109	110	111	112	63	63	63	64	65	66	66
	90th	119	120	121	122	124	125	125	77	77	77	78	79	80	80
	95th	123	123	125	126	127	129	129	81	81	81	82	83	84	84
	99th	130	131	132	133	135	136	136	88	88	89	90	90	91	92
15	50th	107	108	109	110	111	113	113	64	64	64	65	66	67	67
	90th	120	121	122	123	125	126	127	78	78	78	79	80	81	81
	95th	124	125	126	127	129	130	131	82	82	82	83	84	85	85
	99th	131	132	133	134	136	137	138	89	89	90	91	91	92	93
16	50th	108	108	110	111	112	114	114	64	64	65	66	66	67	68
	90th	121	122	123	124	126	127	128	78	78	79	80	81	81	82
	95th	125	126	127	128	130	131	132	82	82	83	84	85	85	86
	99th	132	133	134	135	137	138	139	90	90	90	91	92	93	93
17	50th	108	109	110	111	113	114	115	64	65	65	66	67	67	68
	90th	122	122	123	125	126	127	128	78	79	79	80	81	81	82
	95th	125	126	127	129	130	131	132	82	83	83	84	85	85	86
	99th	133	133	134	136	137	138	139	90	90	91	91	92	93	93

The 90th percentile is 1.28 standard deviations (SD), the 95th percentile is 1.645 SD, and the 99th percentile is 2.326 SD over the mean.
Adapted from Pediatrics August 2004, Volume 114 (2), Part 3.

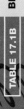

D. Studies show that 85% of children who have essential hypertension have isolated systolic hypertension, whereas diastolic hypertension in children is relatively uncommon and is often secondary to underlying renal disease.

E. Definition of hypertension in children (Tables 17.1A and 17.1B). Blood pressure percentiles are based on gender, age, and height:

1. **Normal:** systolic and/or diastolic blood pressure less than the 90th percentile.
2. **Prehypertension:** systolic and/or diastolic over the 90th percentile but less than the 95th percentile; or the blood pressure exceeds 120/80 even if less than the 90th percentile.
3. **Stage I hypertension:** systolic and/or diastolic blood pressure between the 95th percentile and 5 mm Hg above the 99th percentile.
4. **Stage II hypertension:** systolic and/or diastolic blood pressure over the 99th percentile plus 5 mm Hg.

    Note: The systolic and diastolic blood pressures are of equal importance. If there is some disparity, the higher value determines the severity of the hypertension.

III. PREVENTION

A. Weight/diet. Because obesity is increasing in the population, has more than doubled in the past 20 years, and has a high association with hypertension (detected in children as young as 2 years of age), institution of weight reduction is important to reduce cardiovascular disease. Thirty to 65 percent of cases of hypertension can be attributed directly to obesity. Likewise, obesity is associated with a two- to sixfold increase in risk of occurrence of hypertension. On the average, for each 10 kg increase over ideal body weight, systolic blood pressure rises 2 to 3 mm Hg and diastolic blood pressure rises 1 to 3 mm Hg.

Many obese children have characteristics of the metabolic or insulin resistance syndrome including high blood pressure, abnormal glucose tolerance, and abnormal plasma lipid levels. They are at risk for future cardiovascular disease but improve with an increase in physical activity, diet modification, and control of excess adiposity.

B. Visceral adiposity. Visceral adipose tissue may influence blood pressure by mechanisms in addition to insulin resistance. Some studies have suggested that plasminogen activator inhibitor I may play a role in the relationship between visceral adipose tissue and the risk of hypertension.

C. Salt. Reduction in salt intake also promotes reduction in blood pressure. Even though not every child is sensitive to salt, it is reasonable to restrict sodium intake. This can be done by decreasing consumption of fast foods and refraining from adding salt to cooked foods. The DASH trial (Dietary Approaches to Stop Hypertension) reported results that could be relevant to diet benefits in children. The study demonstrated a decrease in blood pressure with a diet high in fruits, vegetables, and low-fat dairy products.

D. Potassium. Adequate potassium intake has an important role in blood pressure reduction, and low levels of potassium intake may contribute to the development of hypertension.

E. Alcohol. Adolescents who drink alcohol tend to have higher blood pressure levels than those who do not (Table 17.2).

IV. EVALUATION

A. White-coat hypertension is defined as persistent elevation of blood pressure in medical settings but with normal blood pressure at all other times. Ambulatory blood pressure monitoring can be used to make the diagnosis. Recent studies found increased left ventricular mass in ~24% and exaggerated blood pressure response to treadmill in 27% of patients with this type of hypertension. These findings suggest that white-coat hypertension, especially when associated with obesity, is not a simple elevation of blood pressure in response to stress in the medical setting, but may represent a prelude to sustained hypertension with its known long-term consequences.

TABLE 17.2 Clinical Evaluation of Confirmed Hypertension	
Study or procedure	**Purpose**
Evaluation for identifiable causes: sleep history, family history, risk factors, diet, smoking and drinking alcohol; physical examination	Help focus subsequent evaluation
BUN, creatinine, electrolytes, urinalysis, and urine culture	Rule out renal disease and chronic pyelonephritis
CBC	Rule out anemia, consistent with chronic renal disease
Renal ultrasound	Rule out renal scar, congenital anomaly, or disparate renal size
Evaluation for comorbidity; Fasting lipid panel, fasting glucose	Identify hyperlipidemia, identify metabolic abnormalities
Drug screen	Identify substances that might cause hypertension
Polysomnography	Identify sleep disorder in association with hypertension
Evaluation for target-organ damage Echocardiogram	Identify LVH and other indications of cardiac involvement
Retinal exam	Identify retinal vascular changes
Additional evaluation as indicated ABPM	Identify white-coat hypertension, abnormal diurnal BP pattern, BP load
Plasma renin determination	Identify low renin, suggesting mineralocorticoid-related disease
Renovascular imaging Isotopic scintigraphy (renal scan) Duplex Doppler flow studies Three-dimensional CT Arteriography Plasma and urine steroid levels Plasma and urine catecholamines	Identify renovascular disease Identify steroid-mediated hypertension Identify catecholamine-mediated hypertension

ABPM, Ambulatory Blood Pressure Monitoring; BP, blood pressure; BUN, blood urea nitrogen; CBC, complete blood count; CT, computed tomography; LVH, Left ventricular hypertension.
Adapted from Flynn JT. *Differentiation between primary and secondary hypertension in children using ambulatory blood pressure monitoring. Pediatrics* 2004 July;114 (2);Part 3:89–93.

B. Increased serum uric acid has been associated with increased risk for future hypertension in several studies; therefore, it is important to measure uric acid levels in assessing hypertension. The mechanisms that cause hypertension include the direct action of uric acid on smooth muscle and on vascular cells. Uric acid causes hypertension (in a rat model) through activation of the renin-angiotensin system, downregulation of nitric oxide, and induction of endothelial dysfunction in vascular smooth muscle proliferation. There is some evidence suggesting that agents that lower serum uric acid may lower blood pressure and, therefore, with a view to the future, serum uric acid represents a possible new target for the treatment of hypertension.

C. The first step in evaluation, and ultimately treatment, is to distinguish between **essential or primary** and **secondary** hypertension. It is important to rule out secondary causes of elevated blood pressure because these are amenable to specific treatments (Table 17.3). Many laboratory tests should be considered, including

TABLE 17.3 **Examples of Physical Examination Findings Suggestive of Definable Hypertension**

	Finding[a]	Possible etiology
Vital signs	Tachycardia Decreased lower-extremity pulses; drop in BP from upper to lower extremity	Hyperthyroidism, pheochromocytoma, neuroblastoma, primary hypertension Coarctation of the aorta
Eyes	Retinal changes	Severe hypertension, more likely to be associated with secondary hypertension
Ear, nose, and throat	Adenotonsillar hypertrophy	Suggests association with sleep-disordered breathing (sleep apnea), snoring
Height/weight	Growth retardation Obesity (high BMI) Truncal obesity	Chronic renal failure Primary hypertension Cushing syndrome, insulin resistance syndrome
Head and neck	Moon facies Elfin facies Webbed neck Thyromegaly	Cushing syndrome Williams syndrome Turner syndrome Hyperthyroidism
Skin	Pallor, flushing, diaphoresis Acne, hirsutism, striae Café-au-lait spots Adenoma sebaceum Malar rash Acanthosis nigricans	Pheochromocytoma Cushing syndrome, anabolic steroid abuse Neurofibromatosis Tuberous sclerosis Systemic lupus erythematosus Type 2 diabetes
Chest	Widely spaced nipples Heart murmur Friction rub Apical heave	Turner syndrome Coarctation of the aorta System lupus erythematosus (pericarditis), collagen vascular disease, end-stage renal disease with uremia LVH/chronic hypertension
Abdomen	Mass Epigastric/flank bruit Palpable kidneys	Wilms tumor, neuroblastoma, pheochromocytoma Renal artery stenosis Polycystic kidney disease, hydronephrosis, multicystic dysplastic kidney, mass (see above)
Genitalia	Ambiguous/virilization	Adrenal hyperplasia
Extremities	Joint swelling Muscle weakness	Systemic lupus erythematosus, collagen vascular disease Hyperaldosteronism, Liddle syndrome

BMI, body mass index; BP, blood pressure; LVH, left ventricular hypertension.
[a]Findings listed are examples of physical findings and do not represent all possible physical findings.
Adapted from Flynn JT. *Evaluation and management of hypertension in children. Prog Pediatr Cardiol* 2001 Jan;12(2):177–188.

TABLE 17.4	**Underlying Causes of Chronic Hypertension in Children and Adolescents**

Renal	Drugs
Chronic glomerulonephritis	Corticosteroids
Interstitial nephritis	Nicotine
Collagen vascular diseases	Appetite suppressants
Reflux nephropathy	Anabolic steroids
Polycystic kidney disease	Oral contraceptives
Hydronephrosis	
Hypoplastic/dysplastic kidney	
Cardiac and Vascular	**Syndromes**
Coarctation	Airport syndrome
Renal artery Stenosis	Little syndrome
Takayasu arteries	Williams syndrome (renovascular lesions)
	Turner syndrome (coarctation or renovascular)
	Tuberous sclerosis
	Neurofibromatosis (renovascular)
	Adrenogenital syndromes
Endocrine	
Hyperthyroidism	
Pheochromocytoma	
Primary aldosteronism	

Adapted from Falkner B. *Hypertension in Children* 2006 Nov;35(11):795–801.

urinalysis, albumin/creatinine ratio, hematocrit, electrolytes, creatinine with a calculated glomerulofiltration rate, fasting glucose, lipid profile, uric acid, and an electrocardiogram. Underlying causes of hypertension, although uncommon, occur more frequently during childhood than in adults. When a secondary cause is considered, a more extensive evaluation may be necessary. In general, the younger the child and the higher the blood pressure, the more likely it is that the hypertension is a result of an underlying cause (Table 17.4). In the absence of clues directed toward an endocrine or cardiac disorder, the possibility of **renal disease** should be considered in evaluation of all asymptomatic patients with hypertension, because renal disease is the most frequent cause of secondary hypertension in the pediatric population. In addition to the tests listed previously, a renal ultrasound may be considered. Echocardiography is a sensitive means to detect interventricular, septal, and posterior ventricular wall thickening.

D. To rule out **coarctation of the aorta,** every child with hypertension should have upper- and lower-extremity blood pressure measurements. Normally, leg blood pressure levels are slightly higher than arm blood pressure levels, but a child with coarctation will have systolic hypertension in an upper extremity, sometimes absent or decreased femoral pulses, and a blood pressure differential >10 mm Hg between the upper and lower extremities. In other words, if the leg blood pressure is lower than the arm blood pressure, and femoral pulses are weak or absent, consider coarctation of the aorta.

E. Blood pressure should be measured after the patient has been seated quietly for 5 minutes, using a properly calibrated and sized cuff, and the arm should be at heart level. If the cuff is too narrow or too short, the blood pressure may be erroneously high.

F. Smoking or coffee intake can increase systolic blood pressure. Long-term smoking or coffee drinking does not seem to cause persistent elevated blood pressure.

V. GOALS OF THERAPY

A. For children with uncomplicated primary hypertension and no hypertensive target-organ damage, the blood pressure goal should be less than the 95th percentile for age, sex, and height. The blood pressure goal for children with secondary hypertension, diabetes mellitus, or hypertensive target-organ damage should be less than the 90th percentile for age, sex, and height.

B. Furthermore, the goal should be to minimize or limit target-organ damage as a result of hypertension, such as left ventricular hypertrophy. Of the five antihypertensive agents recommended as first-line treatment, calcium antagonists, angiotensin-converting enzyme (ACE) inhibitors, and angiotensin receptor blockers (ARBs) reduce left ventricular mass to a greater extent than do beta-blockers and diuretics. Therefore, not only is treatment duration or achieved blood pressure important to consider, but the choice of drug is also of clinical relevance for treatment of left ventricular hypertrophy that will translate into a reduced rate of cardiovascular complication and improved prognosis. Therefore, reduction of left ventricular hypertrophy becomes a therapeutic goal in primary hypertension that should be addressed.

C. The initial goal should be to introduce nonpharmacological therapy to reduce the blood pressure, which includes exercise and weight reduction.

D. Pharmacotherapy, if needed, usually begins with a single drug. Acceptable drug classes for children include ACE inhibitors, ARBs, beta-blockers, calcium-channel blockers, and diuretics.

VI. NONDRUG THERAPY

A. Exercise. The sedentary, normotensive person typically has a 20% to 50% increased risk of hypertension. Physical activity reduces both systolic and diastolic blood pressure in both normotensive persons and those with hypertension. Regular aerobic exercise in those with hypertension causes an average fall in blood pressure of 4.9/3.8 mm Hg. Moreover, exercise combined with at least a 7% weight loss reduces the onset of new diabetes mellitus in many patients.

B. Salt intake. A reduction in salt intake also promotes reduction in blood pressure. Moderate dietary sodium restriction will reduce blood pressure by ~5/3 mm Hg in individuals with hypertension.

C. Stress management. Although mental stress may immediately increase blood pressure, stress has not been shown to have long-term effects on blood pressure. Current data do not provide convincing evidence for stress management as part of a hypertension prevention or treatment program.

D. Diet and exercise. Dietary modification should be encouraged in patients who have prehypertension as well as in those with hypertension. Treatment should begin with nonpharmacologic interventions, which include weight reduction, exercise, and diet modification. Exercise training lowers blood pressure in both school-age children and adolescents. Power weight lifting should be discouraged in adolescents with hypertension because of its potential to induce marked blood pressure elevation. Participation in other sports should be encouraged as long as blood pressure is under reasonable control and a concurrent examination has been conducted to exclude cardiac conditions.

VII. INDICATIONS FOR USE OF ANTIHYPERTENSIVE DRUGS

A. The indications for initiating antihypertensive drugs include symptomatic hypertension, secondary hypertension, established hypertensive target-organ damage, and failure of nonpharmacologic measures, and/or coexistence in a child or adolescent with dyslipidemia. Pediatric clinical trials of antihypertensive drugs have focused only on their ability to lower blood pressure and have not compared the effects of these drugs on clinical endpoints. The choice of drug for initial antihypertensive therapy, therefore, rests in the preference of the responsible physician.

B. Specific indications for initiating pharmacologic therapy include:
   1. Stage II hypertension
   2. Symptomatic hypertension

3. Secondary hypertension
4. Hypertensive target-organ damage
5. Diabetes mellitus types 1 and 2
6. Persistent hypertension despite nonpharmacologic measures

VIII. PHARMACOLOGIC ANTIHYPERTENSIVE THERAPY (Tables 17.5 and 17.6)
  A. Initiation
   1. Most of the medications used for adults can now be used for children. Efficacy data, however, as well as safety data, are limited for the pediatric population. Medications should be individualized and determined by the degree of hypertension and concomitant medical conditions.
   2. Begin therapy with a single agent and titrate the dose upward until control of blood pressure is obtained. A second medication is added if control is not achieved after using the maximum dose of a single agent. The second drug should be selected from a different class of antihypertensives. Studies in adults, such as the ALLHAT trial, have indicated that a diuretic or a beta-blocker should be the first choice for medication. However, this evidence base is lacking for pediatric patients. Until it is proven otherwise, it is probably advisable to consider ACE inhibitors, ARBs, and calcium-channel blockers as acceptable first-line agents. Table 17.6 provides dosing recommendations for children ages 1 through 17 years. Consider combining drugs with complementary mechanisms of action, such as an ACE inhibitor with a diuretic, or vasodilator with a diuretic or a β-adrenergic blocker. Specific classes of antihypertensive drugs should be used in certain conditions. Examples include the use of ACE inhibitors or ARBs in children with diabetes mellitus and microalbuminuria, or proteinuric renal diseases, and the use of β-adrenergic blockers or calcium-channel blockers in hypertensive children with migraine headaches.
   3. Salt restriction increases the antihypertensive effect of ACE inhibitors. Beta-blockers are contraindicated in children with heart block and asthma and should be used with caution in diabetic patients. ACE inhibitors, calcium-channel blockers, and ARBs appear to be safe and effective. Patient and drug characteristics determine therapy.
   4. It is sometimes difficult to choose a particular drug for a specific indication because few head-to-head comparisons have been performed. There are data, however, showing that certain medications have a benefit relative to the end organ that needs to be most protected.
      a. The ACE inhibitors perindopril and ramipril give protection from future myocardial infarction.
      b. Calcium-channel blockers are marginally better than other treatments to prevent stroke.
      c. ACE inhibitors and ARBs offer improved renal protection and seem to protect from new cases of diabetes.
      d. Beta-blockers/diuretic treatment combinations should be avoided whenever the risk of future diabetes is present.
  B. The renin-angiotensin system
   1. A pathophysiologic approach to the choice of the initial medication might include measuring renin levels. Patients with high renin levels would be considered to have hypertension from renin-mediated vasoconstriction and, therefore, should be prescribed an antirenin agent, such as an ACE inhibitor, whereas patients with low renin levels would be considered to have a volume overload type of hypertension and should be prescribed a diuretic, although this use has not been studied well in children but might be reasonable because of the higher renin levels seen in children with hypertension.
   2. Drugs that affect the renin-angiotensin system are clearly preferred in patients with glomerulonephritis and other forms of renal disease because they may prevent progression to renal failure. Children with type 1 or type 2 diabetes mellitus should be treated with an ACE inhibitor or an ARB because these drugs may prevent the development of diabetic nephropathy. The ACE inhibitors and

| **TABLE 17.5** | Recommended Doses for Selected Antihypertensive Agents for Use in Hypertensive Children and Adolescents |

Class	Drug	Starting dose	Interval	Maximum dose[a]
Angiotensin-converting enzyme inhibitors	Benazepril[b]	0.2 mg/kg/d up to 10 mg/d	QD	0.6 mg/kg/d up to 40 mg/d
	Captopril[b]	0.3–0.5 mg/kg/dose	BID–TID	6 mg/kg/d up to 450 mg/d
	Enalapril[b]	0.08 mg/kg/d	QD	0.6 mg/kg/d up to 40 mg/d
	Fosinopril	0.1 mg/kg/d up to 10 mg/d	QD	0.6 mg/kg/d up to 40 mg/d
	Lisinopril[b]	0.07 mg/kg/d up to 5 mg/d	QD	0.6 mg/kg/d up to 40 mg/d
	Quinapril	5–10 mg/d	QD	80 mg/d
	Ramipril	2.5 mg/d	QD	20 mg/d
Angiotensin receptor blockers	Candesartan	4 mg/d	QD	32 mg/d
	Irbesartan	75–150 mg/d	QD	300 mg/d
	Losartan[b]	0.75 mg/kg/d up to 50 mg/d	QD	104 mg/kg/d up to 100 mg/d
α- and β-Adrenergic antagonists	Labetalol[b]	2–3 mg/kg/d	BID	10–12 mg/kg/d up to 1.2 g/d
	Carvedilol	0.1 mg/kg/dose up to 12.5 mg BID	BID	0.5 mg/kg/dose up to 25 mg BID
β-Adrenergic antagonists	Atenolol[b]	0.5–1 mg/kg/d	QD–BID	2 mg/kg/d up to 100 mg/d
	Bisoprolol/HCTZ	0.04 mg/kg/d up to 2.5/6.25 mg/d	QD	10/6.25 mg/d
	Metoprolol	1–2 mg/kg/d	BID	6 mg/kg/d up to 200 mg/d
	Propranolol	1 mg/kg/d	BID–TID	16 mg/kg/d up to 640 mg/d
Calcium-channel blockers	Amlodipine[b]	0.06 mg/kg/d up to 5 mg/d	QD	0.6 mg/kg/d up to 10 mg/d
	Felodipine	2.5 mg/d	QD	10 mg/d
	Isradipine[b]	0.05–0.15 mg/kg/dose	TID–QID	0.8 mg/kg/d up to 20 mg/d
	Extended-release nifedipine	0.25–0.50 mg/kg/d	QD–BID	3 mg/kg/d up to 120 mg/d
Central α-agonists	Clonidine[b]	5–10 μg/kg/d	BID–TID	25 μg/kg/d up to 0.9 mg/d
	Methyldopa[b]	5 mg/kg/d	BID–QID	40 mg/kg/d up to 3 g/d
Diuretics	Amiloride	5–10 mg/d	QD	20 mg/d
	Chlorothiazide	10 mg/kg/d	BID	20 mg/kg/d up to 1.0 g/d
	Chlorthalidone	0.3 mg/kg/d	QD	2 mg/kg/d up to 50 mg/d
	Furosemide	0.5–2.0 mg/kg/dose	QD-BID	6 mg/kg/d
	HCTZ	0.5–1 mg/kg/d	QD	3 mg/kg/d up to 50 mg/d
	Spironolactone[b]	1 mg/kg/d	QD-BID	3.3 mg/kg/d up to 100 mg/d
	Triamterene	1–2 mg/kg/d	BID	3–4 mg/kg/d up to 300 mg/d

(continued)

| | TABLE 17.5 | Recommended Doses for Selected Antihypertensive Agents for Use in Hypertensive Children and Adolescents (*Continued*) |

Class	Drug	Starting Dose	Interval	Maximum Dose[a]
Peripheral α-antagonists	Doxazosin	1 mg/d	QD	4 mg/d
	Prazosin	0.05–0.1 mg/kg/d	TID	0.5 mg/kg/d
	Terazosin	1 mg/d	QD	20 mg/d
Vasodilators	Hydralazine	0.25 mg/kg/dose	TID-QID	7.5 mg/kg/d up to 200 mg/d
	Minoxidil	0.1–0.2 mg/kg/d	BID-TID	1 mg/kg/d up to 50 mg/d

BID, twice daily; HCTZ, hydrochlorothiazide; QD, once daily; QID, four times daily; TID, three times daily.
[a]The maximum recommended adult dose should never be exceeded.
[b]Information on preparation of a stable extemporaneous suspension is available for these agents.

ARBs have a lower incidence of adverse effects and therefore may be preferable when compliance is a concern.

3. ARBs also reduce the frequency of atrial fibrillation and stroke. This blockade also delays or avoids the onset of type 2 diabetes and prevents cardiovascular or renal events in diabetic patients.

4. Several classes of drugs inhibit the renin-angiotensin system. The renin system can be inhibited at various points, but specific renin inhibitors block the system at its very origin:

    a. Sympatholytic agents or beta-blockers suppress angiotensin II formation by inhibiting renin release from the kidney.

    b. ACE inhibitors reduce the formation of angiotensin II from angiotensin I by inhibiting ACE but not ACE-II or other angiotensin II–forming enzymes.

    c. ARBs antagonize the binding of angiotensin II to the angiotensin receptor, so ACE inhibitors and ARBs are the most important renin-angiotensin system blockers. Renin-angiotensin system blockade reduces insulin resistance, probably because of skeletal muscle profusion, improvement of microvascular changes, and increased profusion of the pancreatic islet cells.

C. Renin blockade

    1. The renin-angiotensin system is an important regulator of cardiovascular and renal function. Inhibitors of the system, such as ACE inhibitors and ARBs, are now first-line treatments for hypertensive target-organ damage and progressive renal disease. ARBs reduce the frequency of atrial fibrillation and stroke.

    2. Renin inhibitors are under investigation and have shown their effectiveness in lowering blood pressure. From the point of view of the biology of the renin-angiotensin system, renin inhibitors offer the potential to inhibit the entire cascade in the system.

    3. Renin inhibitors may be more useful in younger and Caucasian patients because of a more active renin system in this group. Renin inhibitors may also be helpful in patients who are intolerant of ACE inhibitors. Like ACE inhibitors, renin inhibitors behave as vasodilators with the potential to improve the elasticity of the large artery. Conversely, they have the same contraindication as ACE inhibitors and angiotensin receptor blockers, such as pregnancy and bilateral renal artery stenosis.

D. ACE inhibitors

    1. Many of the ACE inhibitors have been studied recently in children, and there are published results available for enalapril, fosinopril, and lisinopril but not for benazepril or quinapril. Blood pressure is reduced in a dose-dependent manner, and there are relatively few adverse effects. Doses range from 0.08 mg/kg per day to 0.6 mg/kg per day.

TABLE 17.6   Antihypertensive Drugs for Management of Severe Hypertension in Children 1–17 Years Old

Drug	Class	Dose[a]	Route	Comments
Most useful[b]				
Esmolol	Beta-blocker	100–500 μg/kg/min	IV infusion	Very short-acting; constant infusion preferred. May cause profound bradycardia. Produced modest reductions in blood pressure in a pediatric clinical trial.
Hydralazine	Vasodilator	0.2–0.6 mg/kg per dose	IV, IM	Should be given every 4 h when given IV bolus. Recommended dose is lower than FDA label.
Labetalol	Alpha- and beta-blocker	Bolus: 0.2–1.0 mg/kg per dose up to 40 mg/dose. Infusion: 0.25–3.0 mg/kg/h	IV bolus or infusion	Asthma and overt heart failure are relative contraindications.
Nicardipine	Calcium-channel blocker	1–3 μg/kg/min	IV infusion	May cause reflex tachycardia.
Sodium nitroprusside	Vasodilator	0.53–10 μg/kg/min	IV infusion	Monitor cyanide levels with prolonged (>72 h) use or in renal failure; or coadminister with sodium thiosulfate.
Occasionally useful[c]				
Clonidine	General α-agonist	0.05–0.1 mg/dose, may be repeated up to 0.8 mg total dose	PO	Side effects include dry mouth and sedation.
Enalaprilat	ACE inhibitor	0.05–0.1 mg/kg per dose up to 1.25 mg/dose	IV bolus	May cause prolonged hypotension and acute renal failure, especially in neonates.
Fenoldopam	Dopamine receptor agonist	0.2–0.8 μg/kg/min	IV infusion	Produced modest reductions in blood pressure in a pediatric clinical trial in patients up to 12 years old.
Isradipine	Calcium-channel blocker	0.05–0.1 mg/kg per dose	PO	Stable suspension can be compounded.
Minoxidil	Vasodilator	0.1–0.2 mg/kg per dose	PO	Most potent oral vasodilator, long-acting.

FDA, U.S. Food and Drug Administration; IM, intramuscular; IV, intravenous; PO, oral.
[a]All dosing recommendations are based on expert opinion or case series data except where otherwise noted.
[b]Useful for hypertensive emergencies and some hypertensive urgencies.
[c]Useful for hypertensive urgencies and some hypertensive emergencies.
Adapted from *Pediatrics* 2004;114(2):Part 3.

2. Because ACE inhibitors and ARBs are associated with favorable effects on renal function and they improve insulin sensitivity, they are ideal first choices in the treatment of patients with both diabetes and hypertension and/or the metabolic syndrome. The combination of an ACE inhibitor with an ARB provides a somewhat greater reduction in proteinuria but little additive effect on blood pressure. Current trials have combined submaximum doses of ACE inhibitors and ARBs, thereby preventing possible adverse effects.

3. In adults, the ACE inhibitors decreased myocardial infarction, cardiovascular disease, and mortality to a greater extent than the results seen with other conventional treatments. Another benefit of ACE inhibitors is that in several studies there was a decrease in the likelihood of the requirement for glucose-lowering therapy in patients receiving the ACE inhibitor versus placebo.

4. In hypertensive patients at risk of developing type 2 diabetes, ACE inhibitors or ARBs should be the first choice for antihypertensive therapy, with calcium antagonists being second-line treatments. Treatment with diuretics and beta-blockers should be avoided in these patients unless comorbidities, such as volume overload or congestive heart failure, require the use of these agents. In patients with diabetic nephropathy, most trials for type 1 diabetics used ACE inhibitors whereas most for type 2 diabetics used ARB-based therapy. By strict evidence-based criteria, ACE inhibitors should be used in type 1 as well as in type 2 diabetes.

E. Beta-blockers

1. β-Adrenergic–blocking agents may precipitate or exacerbate type 2 diabetes. They are effective, however, in the management of ischemic and congestive cardiomyopathies in patients who also have diabetes. The use of the new third-generation beta-blockers, such as nebivolol, that block both α and β receptors, or carvedilol, may prove to be particularly beneficial. These agents cause vasodilatation and an increase in insulin sensitivity.

2. Two cardioselective beta-blockers have undergone pediatric trials: bisoprolol and metoprolol. The starting dose for bisoprolol is 0.04 mg/kg per day. Metoprolol is an extended-release preparation that is given once daily and has been studied in children aged 6 to 16 years. Although asthma and diabetes are contraindicated in β-adrenergic inhibition, this is a β_1-receptor antagonist, which should selectively affect only the cardiogenic receptors.

3. With metoprolol, the greatest reduction of systolic blood pressure occurred with the 1-mg/kg/day dose, whereas the greatest reduction of diastolic blood pressure occurred with the 2-mg/kg/day dose. Overweight children have a somewhat less pronounced antihypertensive response to this medication. Adverse effects included headache, urinary tract infection, cough, nasopharyngitis, and pharyngolaryngeal pain.

F. Angiotensin receptor blockers.

As of this printing, there are two ARBs with completed studies in children: losartan and irbesartan. The losartan study dose was 0.7 mg/kg per day up to 1.55 mg/kg per day. Hyperkalemia was reported in only one individual. These results demonstrated that irbesartan failed to show significant lowering of blood pressure in the age group 6 to 16 years (the FDA review is available). Candesartan and valsartan are being studied at the present time. Valsartan is an ARB that basically inhibits the renin and angiotensin aldosterone system. These blockers improve hypertension and also reduce the incidence of new-onset type 2 diabetes. Valsartan in adults also reduced the incidence of stroke, angina, dissecting aortic aneurysm, and heart failure. The mean dose of valsartan in this study was 75 mg per day.

G. Calcium-channel blockers

1. Calcium-channel blockers (CCBs) or antagonists are a class of drugs that exert their effect by inhibiting the influx of calcium ions across the cell membrane. This results in dilatation of peripheral arterioles. This class of drug can be safely used in children with renal insufficiency or even failure. Side effects include headache, flushing, gastrointestinal upset, and edema of the lower extremities.

2. CCBs are not considered optimal agents for first-line therapy or monotherapy in patients with diabetes, but they have been proven safe and effective in combination with ACE inhibitors, diuretics, and beta-blockers. The first-generation CCBs have not undergone significant pediatric trials, but the newer agents, such as felodipine and amlodipine, have been studied. The felodipine trial had somewhat contradictory results. Amlodipine was found to give significant reductions in systolic blood pressure, with a significant dose/response relationship using a starting dose of 0.6 mg/kg per day. It appears to be safe and effective in the treatment of childhood and adolescent hypertension.

3. Extended-release nifedipine and amlodipine are the two most commonly used oral CCBs in the management of pediatric hypertension. Amlodipine can be made into a solution without compromising its long duration of action. Therefore, it is the CCB of choice for very young children. Oral short-acting nifedipine and intravenous nicardipine are safe and effective CCBs for the management of hypertensive crisis in children. Intravenous nicardipine has been used safely in hospitalized children and newborns.

H. Diuretics, etc. At the time of this writing, there has been no completion of pediatric trials for diuretics, direct vasodilators, centrally acting agents, or α_1-receptor antagonists, despite a long history of their use in the management of childhood hypertension. The exception is sodium nitroprusside.

IX. EMERGENCY TREATMENT FOR HYPERTENSION
Intravenous labetalol, nicardipine, and nitroprusside are effective for treating hypertensive emergencies in children (Table 17.6). There is also an intravenous beta-blocker, esmolol, which has been studied in children (results are found in the FDA review). Intravenous nicardipine has been used safely in hospitalized children and newborns.

X. MIGRAINE
For migraine headaches in a patient with hypertension, consider the use of β-adrenergic blockers or calcium-channel blockers.

XI. INTIMAL MEDIA THICKNESS/MYOCARDIAL INFARCTION/STROKE
ACE inhibitors reduce the rate of progression of carotid intima media thickness. The ACE inhibitors perindopril and ramipril give protection from future myocardial infarction. Calcium-channel blockers are slightly better than other treatments in preventing stroke.

XII. OTHER DRUGS
Orlistat treatment for 4 years accompanied by lifestyle modifications reduced body weight and blood pressure by 4.9/2.6 mm Hg. The cannabinoid-1 receptor blocker, also known as **Rimonaban,** at 20 mg per day, may reduce the blood pressure of some obese individuals.

XIII. DIABETES AND HYPERTENSION
A. Several clinical trials have found that new-onset type 2 diabetes can be reduced by ACE inhibitors and ARBs as opposed to beta-blockers and diuretics. Both ACE inhibitors and ARBs have been shown to reduce cardiovascular events in diabetic patients. In patients who are hypertensive and have a risk for developing type 2 diabetes (family history, high body mass index, or impaired glucose tolerance), ACE inhibitors or ARBs should be the first choice for therapy. Calcium antagonists are the second line of treatment, and treatment with diuretics and beta-blockers should be avoided unless other comorbidities, such as volume overload or congestive heart failure, require the use of these agents.

B. In recent studies, blockade of the renin-angiotensin system reduced the frequency of various diabetic complications including diabetic nephropathy, as well as reducing cardiovascular mortality and morbidity. Blockade of this system prevents the onset of microalbuminuria and reduces proteinuria.

C. Two physiologic systems underlying the adverse effects of hypertension in patients with diabetes are the renin-angiotensin system and the sympathetic nervous system. Therapeutic agents that affect the production of receptor binding of angiotensin-II, such as the ACE inhibitors or ARBs, or block the neurotransmitters that stimulate the sympathetic nervous system, such as beta-blockers, seem to offer particular benefit.

XIV. RENAL DISEASE

Drugs that affect the renin-angiotensin system are clearly preferred in patients with glomerulonephritis and other forms of renal disease because they may prevent progression to renal failure. Children with type 1 or type 2 diabetes should be treated with an ACE inhibitor or ARB because these may prevent the development of diabetic nephropathy. The ACE inhibitors and ARBs have a lower incidence of adverse effects and therefore may be preferable when compliance is a concern. This blockade also delays or avoids the onset of type 2 diabetes and prevents cardiovascular and renal events in diabetic patients.

XV. RESISTANCE TO ANTIHYPERTENSIVE MEDICATIONS
A. Pharmacologic therapy

1. **Definition.** Resistant or refractory hypertension is defined as a blood pressure of at least 140/90 or at least 130/80 in patients with diabetes or renal disease despite adherence to treatments with full doses of at least three antihypertensive medications, including a diuretic. There is literature suggesting that blood pressure goals may be difficult to achieve in as many as 40% of adult patients. Resistant or difficult-to-control systolic hypertension is more common in patients over the age of 60 years than in younger patients. Patients whose hypertension is difficult to control are more likely to have target-organ damage and a higher long-term cardiovascular risk. Heart failure, stroke, myocardial infarction, and renal failure are related to the degree of the elevation in blood pressure.

2. **Management.** Formal studies of the management of resistant hypertension are few, and strategies for control are based largely on observational data from specialty clinics. Suboptimal medical treatment has been shown to be the primary reason for resistant hypertension (Table 17.6).

3. **Treatment**
   a. The general approach is to combine medications from various classes, such as: **(1)** reduce volume overload with diuretics and aldosterone antagonists; **(2)** reduce sympathetic overactivity, such as with beta-blockers; **(3)** decrease vascular resistance through the inhibition of the renin-angiotensin system with the use of ACE inhibitors or ARBs; **(4)** promote smooth muscle relaxation, such as with dihydropyridine, calcium-channel blockers, and alpha-blockers; and **(5)** promote vasodilatation, such as with hydralazine and minoxidil.
   b. Adding additional medications may further lower the blood pressure or overcome compensatory changes in elevated blood pressure caused by the first medication without increasing adverse effects. Some combinations that are effective include: **(1)** a diuretic with an ACE inhibitor, a beta-blocker, or an angiotensin receptor blocker; and **(2)** an ACE inhibitor with a calcium-channel blocker.
   c. Because volume overload is common among patients with resistance, the most important therapeutic maneuver is generally to add or increase diuretic medications. Dyazide diuretics are effective in doses of 12.5 to 25 mg per day if renal function is normal. If the glomerular filtration rate is low, or the creatinine level is >1.5, then loop diuretics should be used, such as furosemide at a dose of 20 to 80 mg per day, or bumetanide at a dose of 0.5 to 2.0 mg daily two to three times per day. Once-daily drug administration may lead to reactive sodium retention mediated by the renin-angiotensin system, with consequent inadequate blood pressure control.

B. Medications that can raise blood pressure. Some medications can elevate blood pressure or antagonize the effects of antihypertensive medication, including sympathomimetic drugs, such as ephedra, phenylephrine, cocaine, and amphetamines. Supplements such as ginseng and yohimbine, anabolic steroids, appetite suppressants, and erythropoietin account for a small percentage of essential hypertension and resistant hypertension. Nonsteroidal anti-inflammatory drugs and cyclo-oxygenase-2 inhibitors may also raise both systolic and diastolic blood pressure.

C. Lifestyle/salt/potassium. Also, determine whether the patient is participating in an exercise and weight-reduction program and is minimizing his or her intake of salt. Low levels of potassium intake may also contribute to insulin resistance. (Table 17.6 summarizes an approach to the optimization of drug therapy in patients with resistant hypertension.)

XVI. LONG-TERM MONITORING
A. Blood pressure measurements

1. Blood pressure should be measured in the physician's office every 2 to 4 weeks until good control is achieved; thereafter, blood pressure measurement can be performed every 3 to 4 months. Home blood pressure measurements should also be incorporated into the treatment plan. Periodic laboratory monitoring may also be required, particularly when a diuretic or agent that affects the renin-angiotensin system is prescribed.

2. Ambulatory blood pressure monitoring can be used in pediatric patients as a method of clinical evaluation and also for long-term monitoring. Its use can facilitate early identification of hypertension, improve 24-hour control for hypertension, and detect more subtle blood pressure abnormalities. One example is that the normal blood pressure pattern during sleep declines by >10% in both systolic and diastolic blood pressure. This decline can be detected by ambulatory blood pressure monitoring. Another use is for "white-coat hypertension."

B. Stroke.
Meta-analysis suggests that ARBs, more than ACE inhibitors, are effective in prevention of stroke beyond blood pressure control. They may exert neuroprotective effects in response to ischemia-induced neuronal injury. The most important factor in stroke prevention is good blood pressure control. The cerebroprotective effects of the angiotensin II receptor stimulation by ARBs have emerged as a further important clinical means to help prevent ischemic stroke.

C. Atrial fibrillation

1. Hypertension is the most important risk factor for atrial fibrillation. Treatment with ARBs reduced the frequency of atrial fibrillation. New atrial fibrillation onset was less frequent in those on ARBs than in those on calcium antagonists. What could be the underlying pathogenic mechanism for renin-angiotensin system blockade prevention of atrial fibrillation? The blockade prevents left atrial dilatation and atrial fibrosis, as well as increasing potassium concentrations, resulting in change in potassium currents and conduction. It also lowers end-diastolic left ventricular pressure, modifies sympathetic tone, and manifests direct antiarrhythmic effects.

2. Statins also help reduce atrial fibrillation, perhaps by reducing the inflammatory state that is also linked to atrial fibrillation.

XVII. CONCLUSIONS

A. Left ventricular hypertrophy is present in up to 30% or 40% of children and adolescents with hypertension. There is also evidence that primary hypertension in childhood is associated with increased carotid intima media thickness, a marker of early arteriosclerosis. Therefore, essential hypertension in children should be considered an early phase of a serious chronic disease that continues into adulthood. Children with elevated blood pressure will continue to have elevated blood pressure as adults.

B. There are many questions that remain unanswered. Certainly, long-term trials are necessary to answer the question of whether antihypertensive medication might affect growth and development in the child. Also, will treatment of children with hypertension using these drugs have any significant health benefits beyond blood pressure reduction?

C. The focus on blood pressure control beginning in a very young age is an important component of health care for children and adolescents.

Selected References

Batisky DL, Sorof JM, Sugg J, et al. Efficacy and safety of extended release metoprolol succinate in hypertensive children 6 to 16 years of age: a clinical trial experience. *J Pediatr* 2007;150:134–139.

Couch SC, Saelens BE, Levin L, et al. The efficacy of a clinic-based behavioral nutrition intervention emphasizing a DASH-type diet for adolescents with elevated blood pressure. *J Pediatr* 2008;152:494–501.

Faulkner, B. et al. *Hypertension in children. Pediatr Ann* 2006 Nov;35(11):795–801.

Flynn JT, Daniels SR. Pharmacologic treatment of hypertension in children and adolescents. *J Pediatr* 2006;149:746–754.

Kaplan NM, Opie LH. Controversies in hypertension. *Lancet* 2006;367:168–176.

Kevey, RE, Kevselis DA, Atallah N, Smith FU. *White coat hypertension in childhood: Evidence for end-organ effect. J Pediatr* 2007 May;150(5):491–497.

Lee S, Bacha F, Arslanian S. Waist circumference, blood pressure, and lipid components of the metabolic syndrome. *J Pediatr* 2006;149:809–816.

Lurbe E, Sorof JM, Daniels SR. Clinical and research aspects of ambulatory blood pressure monitoring in children. *J Pediatr* 2004;144:7–16.

Maggio AB, Aggoun Y, Marchand LM, et al. Associations among obesity, blood pressure, and left ventricular mass. *J Pediatr* 2008;152:489–493.

McNiece KL, Poffenbarger TS, Turner JL, et al. Prevalence of hypertension and pre-hypertension among adolescents. *J Pediatr* 2007;150:640–644.

Moser M, Setaro JF. Resistant or difficult-to-control hypertension. *N Engl J Med* 2006;355:385–392.

The fourth report on the diagnosis, evaluation and treatment of high blood pressure in children & adolescents. *Pediatrics* 2004;114 (2 suppl 4th Report):555–576.

Schmieder RE, Hilgers KF, Schlaich MP, et al. Renin-angiotensin system and cardiovascular risk. *Lancet* 2007;369:1208–1219.

Solomon SD, Janardhanan R, Verma A, et al. Effect of angiotensin receptor blockade and antihypertensive drugs on diastolic function in patients with hypertension and diastolic dysfunction: a randomized trial. *Lancet* 2007;369:2079–2087.

Staessen JA, Li Y, Richart T. Oral renin inhibitors. *Lancet* 2006;368:1449–1456.

AACE Hypertension Task Force. American association of clinical endocrinologist medical guidelines for clinical practice for the diagnosis and treatment of hypertension. *Endo Pract* 2006 Mar–Apr;12(2):193–222.

ADRENAL STEROID EXCESS IN CHILDHOOD
Thomas A. Wilson

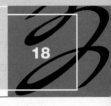

I. GENERAL PRINCIPLES

A. **Divisions of the adrenal cortex.** The mature adrenal cortex is divided into three functional and histologic zones.

1. The **zona glomerulosa** secretes aldosterone and is regulated by the rennin–angiotensin system, serum potassium concentration, adrenocorticotropic hormone (ACTH), and dopamine.

2. The **zona fasciculata** secretes primarily glucocorticoids and is under the control of ACTH alone.

3. The **zona reticularis** secretes glucocorticoids and adrenal androgens. It is under the regulation of ACTH and possibly a putative factor that stimulates the production of adrenal androgens during puberty.

4. In the human fetus, an inner fetal zone exists that dwarfs the adult adrenal cortex. This **fetal adrenal cortex** secretes primarily dehydroepiandrosterone sulfate and pregnenolone sulfate. The fetal adrenal zone involutes within the first 6 months of postnatal existence.

B. **Embryology of the adrenal gland.** Various differentiation factors are involved in the development of the adrenal cortex. Absence of one of these factors, such as SF1 or DAX1, causes **congenital adrenal hypoplasia** (see Chapter 19).

C. **Hormones of the adrenal cortex.** Approximately 95% of the plasma cortisol is bound to transcortin, a carrier protein. Only the unbound portion is metabolically active. Cortisol is secreted in a diurnal fashion with 8 A.M. concentrations in the plasma usually in the range of 11 ± 2.5 μg/dL; values in the evening are generally 3.5 ± 0.15 μg/dL in the nonstressed child. However, this diurnal rhythm might not be well established until after age 1 year. The adrenal glucocorticoids and their metabolites (including pregnanetriol, the major metabolite of 17-hydroxyprogesterone) can be measured in the urine as 17-ketogenic steroids, whereas only the metabolites of cortisol and its immediate precursor, 11-deoxycortisol, are measured as 17-hydroxycorticosteroids, which are therefore more specific. The urinary free cortisol most closely approximates the unbound plasma cortisol concentration and therefore is preferable for assessing cortisol production. Plasma free cortisol concentrations can also be estimated using salivary cortisol concentrations. Metabolites of the adrenal androgens are measured in the urine as 17-ketosteroids. Only about one third of the testosterone secreted is metabolized and excreted as 17-ketosteroids.

D. **Hypersecretion of adrenal steroids** results from:

1. Excess secretion of ACTH by the pituitary.

2. Ectopic secretion of CRF or ACTH from tumors outside the hypothalamic-pituitary axis.

3. Micronodular or macronodular dysplasia of the adrenal.

4. Overproduction of cortisol, aldosterone, adrenal androgens, estrogens, or a combination of these by hyperplastic, adenomatous, or malignant adrenal tissue. The signs, symptoms, and workup depend on which adrenal steroids are secreted excessively. The most common form of adrenal steroid excess in childhood is congenital adrenal hyperplasia, which is discussed in Chapter 19. Adrenocortical tumors occur more frequently in girls and are occasionally associated with hemihypertrophy, urinary tract abnormalities, and tumors in the brain. Carney complex type 1, caused by mutation in the protein kinase A regulatory subunit-1-alpha

219

gene (PRKAR1A) on chromosome 17q (OMIM 160980), is the association of pigmented micronodular adrenocortical disease, pigmented lentigines, atrial myxomas, and schwannomas. Other endocrine tumors may be seen in this syndrome as well. Carney complex type 2 has been mapped to chromosome 2p16 (OMIM 605244).

II. GLUCOCORTICOID EXCESS

A. **Cushing syndrome** is the physical manifestation of excess glucocorticoid action. In children, these manifestations are growth failure, weight gain, muscle weakness, obesity, moon facies, supraclavicular and nuchal fat pads, striae, easy bruising, virilization, hypertension, and glucose intolerance. Rarely, the only manifestation of Cushing syndrome in children is growth failure. **Cushing disease** is Cushing syndrome resulting from excess ACTH secretion from the pituitary. The ectopic production of ACTH is very rare in children but is occasionally seen with tumors of the neural crest, thymomas, Wilms tumors, and pancreatic tumors.

Exogenous obesity is commonly confused with Cushing syndrome. The differential diagnosis is made more difficult by the fact that obese children tend to have mild elevations in 24-hour urinary 17-hydroxycorticosteroid excretion, although urinary free cortisol excretion is normal. A distinguishing clinical feature is the growth velocity, which is suppressed in children with Cushing syndrome but normal or even increased in children with obesity. Biochemical studies, as outlined later, will distinguish Cushing syndrome from other forms of obesity. Patients with AIDS who are taking protease inhibitors may develop the metabolic syndrome and a redistribution of body fat that resembles Cushing syndrome.

Cushing syndrome in the infant and young child is often secondary to an adrenal tumor. In some adrenal tumors and some cases of bilateral adrenal macronodular adrenal hyperplasia, cortisol secretion is dependent on hormones other than ACTH, such as gastric inhibitory peptide (food-induced hypercortisolism), antidiuretic hormone, gonadotropin-releasing hormone, and thyroid-stimulating hormones. Occasionally, hypercortisolism occurs secondary to an activating mutation of the α subunit of the Gs protein, as in the McCune-Albright syndrome (OMIM 174800). Some adrenal cortical tumors are nonfunctional and therefore endocrinologically silent.

B. The **diagnosis of hypercortisolism** is made by demonstrating excess urinary excretion of free cortisol and by demonstrating abnormal regulation of the hypothalamic–pituitary–adrenal axis (Table 18.1). An elevated urinary free cortisol excretion in an unstressed child is highly suggestive of hypercortisolism. Assays and ranges for urinary free cortisol vary among laboratories. Other useful screening tests for hypercortisolism are loss of normal diurnal rhythm in plasma cortisol concentrations and inability of dexamethasone (0.3 to 0.5 mg/m^2, maximum 1 mg) given at 11 P.M. to suppress the 8 A.M. plasma cortisol concentration to <5 μg/dL. More recent data with more sensitive cortisol assays suggest that the morning cortisol should suppress to <1.8 μg/dL. Medications that stimulate the metabolism of dexamethasone, such as many anticonvulsants, rifampin, and aminoglutethimide, may invalidate the dexamethasone suppression test. Because plasma ACTH and cortisol concentrations reach a nadir at 11 P.M. to 1 A.M., a third strategy to screen for Cushing syndrome is measurement of these hormones at that time. This must be done through an indwelling catheter with the patient asleep or relaxed and unstressed. In this setting, a plasma ACTH concentration >7.5 pg/mL and a plasma cortisol >1.8 μg/dL is suggestive of hypercortisolism. As salivary cortisol assays become more readily available, these may supplant serum cortisol measurements.

1. **Etiology.** Once hypercortisolism is established, clarification of the specific cause is made by a variety of tests, as outlined in the following and in Table 18.1, none of which is 100% diagnostic by itself. The first step is to demonstrate whether the hypercortisolism is ACTH-dependent or ACTH-independent. This requires a sensitive and specific assay and placing the sample on ice followed by rapid centrifugation, because ACTH is rapidly degraded by plasma proteases. Elevated or normal plasma ACTH concentrations (>10 pg/mL) in the presence of hypercortisolism suggest that the primary pathology is due to excess ACTH secretion

TABLE 18.1   Diagnostic Approach to the Child with Evidence of Glucocorticoid Excess

Test	Normal range[a]	Adrenal tumor	Hypothalamic/pituitary	Ectopic ACTH	Congenital virilizing adrenal hyperplasia
24-h urinary free cortisol	25–75 μg/m²/d[b]	↑	↑	↔ or ↑	↔ or ↓
24-h urinary 17-OHCS	3 ± 1 mg/m²/d[b]	↑	↑	↑	↔, ↑, ↓
24-h urinary 17-KS	c	↑↑	↔ or ↑	↔ or ↑	↑↑
Diurnal variation	Present	Absent	Absent	Absent	
Cortisol (11 P.M.)	<1.8 μg/mL	>1.8 μg/dL and similar to A.M. cortisol	>1.8 μg/dL and similar to A.M. cortisol	>1.8 μg/dL and similar to A.M. cortisol	
ACTH (11 P.M.)	<7.5 pg/mL	<7.5 pg/mL	>7.5 pg/mL	>7.5 pg/mL	
ACTH (8 A.M.)	<100 pg/mL	<10 pg/ml	↑ or normal	↑ or normal	
Overnight dexamethasone suppression test: 8 A.M. plasma cortisol	<1.8 μg/dL	>1.8 μg/dL	>1.8 μg/dL	>1.8 μg/dL	
Low-dose dexamethasone suppression test	Suppression of serum cortisol to <1.8 μg/dL	No suppression of serum cortisol	No suppression of serum cortisol	No suppression serum cortisol	Suppression of 17-OH progesterone and cortisol
High-dose dexamethasone suppression test	Suppression of serum cortisol to <1.8 μg/dL	No suppression of cortisol	>50% suppression of serum cortisol	No suppression of serum cortisol	Suppression of 17-OH progesterone and cortisol
CRF stimulation test (1 μg/kg (max 100 μg) IV; sample at 0, 15, 30, and 45 min:					
Change in ACTH	↑	↔	↑	↔	
Change in cortisol	↑	↔	↑	↔	
Metyrapone stimulation test	2- to 3-fold ↑ in 17-OHCS[b] and 11-deoxycortisol	No change in 17-OHCS and 11-deoxycortisol	↑↑ in 17-OHCS and 11-desoxycortisol	No change in 17-OHCS and 11-deoxycortisol	

[a] All normal ranges depend on laboratory.
[b] Data from Migeon C. Physiology and pathology of adrenocortical function in infancy and childhood. In: Collu R, Ducharme JR, Guyda H, eds, *Pediatric endocrinology.* New York: Raven Press, 1981:475.
[c] Normal range for 17-ketosteroids [22]:

	24-h 17-KS
Age	
<2 wk	<2.0 mg
1 mo–5 yr	<0.5 mg
6–8 yr	<1–2 mg
Puberty and adulthood	<17 mg (males)
	<13 mg (females)

17-OHCS, 24-h urinary 17-hydroxycorticosteroids; 17-KS, 24-h urinary 17-ketosteroids.

Day	Prescription	Serum cortisol and 24-h urine for free cortisol
1		_____
2		_____
3	Low-dose dexamethasone (30 μg/kg/d [max 2 mg/d] in 4 divided doses)	_____
4	Low-dose dexamethasone (30 μg/kg/d [max 2 mg/d] in 4 divided doses)	_____
5	High-dose dexamethasone (90 μg/kg/d [max 8 mg/d] in 4 divided doses)	_____
6	High-dose dexamethasone (90 μg/kg/d [max 8 mg/d] in 4 divided doses)	_____

TABLE 18.2 Dexamethasone Suppression Test[a]

[a]Test is interpreted as follows:
Normal response: Suppression of urinary free cortisol to <10 pg/mL and 8 A.M. serum cortisol <1.8 μg/dL during low- and high-dose dexamethasone therapy.
Cushing disease: Greater than 50% reduction in urinary free cortisol and 8 A.M. serum cortisol <1.8 μg/dL during high-dose but not low-dose dexamethasone therapy.
Adrenal adenoma, carcinoma, or ectopic ACTH: No suppression of urinary free cortisol or 8 A.M. serum cortisol during either low- or high-dose dexamethasone therapy.
Adapted from Liddle GW. Tests of pituitary-adrenal suppressibility in the diagnosis of Cushing's syndrome. *J Clin Endocrinol Metab* 1960;20:1539–1560.

of pituitary or nonpituitary origin. Consistently suppressed plasma ACTH (<10 pg/mL) concentrations suggest that the primary disorder lies in the adrenal glands. Suppression of plasma cortisol and urinary free cortisol with high-dose dexamethasone (90 μg/kg per day [maximum 8 mg/day] in four divided doses) but not low-dose dexamethasone (30 μg/kg per day [maximum 2 mg/day] in four divided doses) suggests a primary hypothalamic-pituitary disorder. Occasionally, patients with Cushing disease require dosages of dexamethasone >90 μg/kg per day to suppress cortisol production. Lack of suppression to high-dose dexamethasone suggests an adrenal tumor or the ectopic secretion of ACTH (Table 18.2). In the former, ACTH concentrations are suppressed, whereas in the latter situation, ACTH concentrations are elevated. An intact or exaggerated cortisol response to ACTH indicates that the adrenal glands remain under pituitary regulation and suggests a pituitary origin of Cushing syndrome. The ACTH and cortisol responses to corticotropin-releasing hormone (CRH) are generally flat in the ectopic ACTH syndrome and adrenal tumors that secrete cortisol, whereas both responses are intact in Cushing disease. The metyrapone stimulation test is no longer commonly used. A comparison of plasma ACTH concentrations in the inferior petrosal sinus with peripheral and contralateral inferior petrosal sinus concentrations following CRH stimulation may help to lateralize a pituitary microadenoma but may be technically difficult, especially in small children. An inferior petrosal ACTH/ peripheral ACTH ratio >2 without CRH and >3 after CRH is indicative of pituitary Cushing disease. Demonstration of laterality in ACTH concentrations on bilateral inferior petrosal sampling may give an indication of laterality of a pituitary microadenoma, but is not always reliable.

2. **Imaging studies.** Further confirmation of the diagnosis rests on radiographic and scintigraphic studies aimed at anatomically defining the pathology. If Cushing disease is suspected, magnetic resonance imaging (MRI) of the pituitary with gadolinium enhancement is superior to cerebral computed tomography (CT) in

defining a pituitary adenoma but still may not be able to locate a small microadenoma.

If a primary adrenal cause is suspected, abdominal CT, MRI, ultrasound, or scanning of the adrenal glands with I-iodocholesterol may reveal evidence of an adrenal adenoma, carcinoma, or hyperplasia. The latter study produces significant radiation exposure to the adrenal glands. Adrenal CT is generally considered to provide the best radiographic visualization of the adrenal glands.

In-octreotide scan may be useful in identifying the source of ectopic ACTH secretion, such as a bronchial or thymic carcinoid tumor.

C. Treatment. Treatment of hypercortisolism depends on the etiology.

   1. In **Cushing disease**, a radiographically defined pituitary adenoma that does not extend above the sella turcica should be approached transsphenoidally, if possible, and excised leaving the remainder of the pituitary gland intact. If no radiographic abnormalities are found, a microadenoma can still be discovered and removed under direct visualization of the pituitary at surgery; or, if inferior petrosal sinus sampling suggests laterality, a hemihypophysectomy can be performed. If these steps fail to result in cure, the diagnosis should be re-evaluated; if it is still consistent with Cushing disease, pituitary radiation can be used. This should be accompanied by pharmacologic therapy with metyrapone (0.5 to 2.0 g/m^2 per day in four to six divided doses PO) to alleviate the symptoms of hypercortisolism until the response to radiation occurs. Other drugs that reduce cortisol secretion are ketoconazole, aminoglutethimide, mitotane, and etomidate. The former is less toxic and may be used in combination with metyrapone because the two agents work at different enzyme steps to inhibit cortisol secretion. Etomidate may be infused in subhypnotic doses to obtain rapid control of hypercortisolism. Bilateral adrenalectomy, a therapy of last resort, leaves the patient with adrenal insufficiency and results in a significant occurrence of Nelson syndrome (pigmentation of the skin with or without enlargement of the sella turcica secondary to an ACTH-secreting pituitary adenoma).

   2. Adrenal adenomas and carcinomas should be surgically removed if possible. Differentiation based on histology alone is difficult, but large tumors or tumors that have invaded the adrenal capsule are likely to be malignant. Macronodular or micronodular hyperplasia should be treated with bilateral adrenalectomy.

   3. Glucocorticoid coverage: Regardless of etiology, all patients with Cushing syndrome must be covered perioperatively with stress doses of glucocorticoids (hydrocortisone, 40 to 100 mg/m^2 per day in three or four divided doses IV or IM or equivalent), because the remaining pituitary adrenal axis can be suppressed secondary to the primary process, and adrenal insufficiency frequently occurs following removal of the adrenal tumor, pituitary adenoma, or other tumor producing ACTH or CRH. Following the perioperative period, daily glucocorticoid coverage may be gradually withdrawn, but the patient should still receive glucocorticoid coverage for stressful situations such as surgery, trauma, or infection for up to 6 months, as it may take this long for the hypothalamic–pituitary–adrenal axis to recover. A cosyntropin stimulation test is advisable to document recovery of the axis before discontinuation of stress coverage.

   4. Inoperable adrenal tumors can be treated chronically with metyrapone, aminoglutethimide, mitotane, ketoconazole, or mifepristone in an attempt to alleviate the symptoms of hypercortisolism. Mitotane is cytotoxic to adrenal cells and may be useful in the management of adrenal cortical carcinomas.

III. SEX STEROID EXCESS OF ADRENAL ORIGIN

A. Virilizing and feminizing adrenal tumors become apparent in childhood because of the inappropriate development of secondary sexual characteristics and rapid growth. They are found more commonly in females than males and usually produce androgens or both androgens and cortisol. Virilizing adrenal tumors or congenital adrenal hyperplasia should be suspected in boys when secondary sexual characteristics occur in the absence of testicular enlargement. In girls, clitoromegaly, body hair, and amenorrhea develop.

Feminizing adrenal tumors produce gynecomastia in males and gonadotropin-independent breast development or vaginal bleeding in girls. Purely feminizing adrenal tumors are exceedingly rare in childhood.

B. The **diagnosis** of an adrenal tumor producing sex steroids is established by demonstrating elevations in plasma sex steroids, DHEAS and urinary 17-ketosteroids with suppression of gonadotropins. Adrenal adenocarcinomas tend to produce dramatic elevations in plasma concentrations of dehydroepiandrosterone sulfate and in urinary 17-ketosteroids. Dexamethasone administration (30 μg/kg per day in three divided doses for 7 days) does not suppress the elevations in plasma sex steroids and urinary 17-ketosteroids, as it does in normal children and patients with congenital adrenal hyperplasia. Abdominal CT, MRI, or, less commonly, ultrasound may be helpful in localizing the tumor.

C. **Treatment** of choice is surgical removal of the adenoma or adenocarcinoma. The prognosis is best if the tumor is small, well encapsulated, and completely removed. The usefulness of histologic studies in differentiating adrenal cortical carcinomas from adenomas is limited. Mitotane (6 to 10 g/m^2 per day) may be of some use in reducing steroid production in inoperable tumors, but coverage with glucocorticoids must be provided to prevent symptoms of adrenal insufficiency. Often thyroxine therapy is required as well, because mitotane lowers serum thyroxine concentrations. The administration of mitotane is associated with a high incidence of gastrointestinal symptoms, dermatitis, and neurologic side effects such as lethargy, ataxia, and seizures. It also may cause gynecomastia.

IV. ALDOSTERONE EXCESS (Table 18.3)

A. Hyperaldosteronism is rare in childhood. Because aldosterone acts on the distal renal tubule to promote sodium reabsorption and the excretion of potassium and hydrogen ions, hyperaldosteronism results in hypokalemia, metabolic alkalosis, and hypertension. Weakness and polyuria are common manifestations of hypokalemia.

1. **Primary** hyperaldosteronism in children is usually secondary to bilateral hyperplasia of the zona glomerulosa and, rarely, secondary to an adenoma. A rare form of hyperaldosteronism is reversible with glucocorticoid administration. This form of **glucocorticoid-remediable hyperaldosteronism** has been demonstrated to result from a fusion gene resulting in an ACTH-responsive promotor for the aldosterone synthetase gene (OMIM 103900).

2. Hyperaldosteronism also is seen **secondary** to a variety of renal and liver disorders, resulting in hyperreninism (Table 18.3).

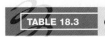

TABLE 18.3	**Causes of Hyperaldosteronism in Childhood**

Primary hyperaldosteronism
Bilateral hyperplasia
Adenoma

Secondary hyperaldosteronism
Glucocorticoid-remediable hyperaldosteronism
Hyperreninism
  Renal parenchymal disease
  Renovascular disease
  Malignant hypertension
  Reninoma
  Bartter syndrome
  Congestive heart failure
  Diuretic administration
  Liver disease with ascites

Pseudohypoaldosteronism

3. **Bartter syndrome** (OMIM 607364) is a disorder of renal tubular chloride reabsorption characterized by failure to thrive, hypokalemia, metabolic alkalosis, and elevations in plasma renin activity, plasma aldosterone concentrations, and urinary prostaglandin excretion.

4. **Pseudohypoaldosteronism** represents a group of disorders involving renal tubular unresponsiveness to aldosterone, resulting in hyponatremia and hyperkalemia despite an elevation in plasma aldosterone concentration. Neither Bartter syndrome nor pseudohypoaldosteronism is accompanied by hypertension.

B. **Liddle syndrome** is a primary renal disorder that can be confused with hyperaldosteronism because patients with Liddle syndrome have hypertension, hypokalemia, and suppressed plasma renin activity. However, the plasma aldosterone concentrations are suppressed in patients with Liddle syndrome, which has been shown to result from an activating mutation of the sodium channel in the renal tubule (OMIM 177200).

C. The **syndrome of apparent mineralocorticoid excess** (OMIM 218030) also causes symptoms and signs of hypermineralocorticoidism without demonstrable elevations in the serum concentrations of aldosterone or deoxycorticosterone. This condition is due to a deficiency of 11β-hydroxysteroid dehydrogenase that results in diminished inactivation of cortisol to cortisone. The resultant accumulation of cortisol activates mineralocorticoid receptors, leading to volume expansion and hypertension. This form of hypertension is also improved by dexamethasone, which suppresses ACTH and cortisol and does not activate the mineralocorticoid receptor as cortisol does.

D. **Diagnosis.** The diagnosis of primary hyperaldosteronism is established by demonstrating hypokalemia and inappropriate hyperkaluria (urinary potassium concentration >20 mEq/L in the presence of hypokalemia) unprovoked by diuretic use, elevated plasma aldosterone concentrations and urinary aldosterone excretion, and suppressed plasma renin activity. Plasma aldosterone concentrations and 24-hour urinary aldosterone concentrations must be interpreted in view of age, posture, and 24-hour urinary sodium intake. If plasma renin activity is not suppressed, one of the disorders listed under hyperreninism in Table 18.3 should be suspected. If CT scans of the adrenal fail to uncover the adenoma, an adrenal scan with I-6β-iodomethylnorcholesterol during the administration of dexamethasone for 7 days before and 5 days after administration of a tracer (to suppress ACTH and the uptake of tracer in the zona reticularis and fasciculata) can help identify an adenoma of the zona glomerulosa.

E. **Treatment.** The treatment for an aldosterone-secreting adenoma is removal. The treatment of choice for bilateral hyperplasia of the zona glomerulosa is spironolactone (1 to 3 mg/kg per day PO in three doses) because adrenalectomy usually does not reverse the hypertension. Glucocorticoid-suppressible hyperaldosteronism should be managed with chronic glucocorticoid therapy in physiologic replacement doses (hydrocortisone, 7 to 20 mg/m^2 per day or equivalent).

Selected References

Arnaldi G, et al. Diagnosis and complications of Cushing's syndrome: a consensus statement. *J Clin Endocrinol Metab* 2003;88:5593–5602.

Batista D, et al. An assessment of petrosal sinus sampling for localization of pituitary microadenomas in children with Cushing disease. *J Clin Endocrinol Metab* 2006;91221–224.

Christopoulos S, Bourdeau I, Lacroix A. Aberrant expression of hormone receptors in adrenal Cushing's syndrome. *Pituitary* 2004;7:225–235.

Godil MA, et al. Metastatic congenital adrenocortical carcinoma: a case report with tumor remission at 3 1/2 years. *J Clin Endocrinol Metab* 2000;85:3964–3967.

Hindmarsh PC, Brook CG. Single dose dexamethasone suppression test in children: dose relationship to body size. *Clin Endocrinol (Oxf)* 1985;23:67–70.

Kobayashi T, Kida Y, Mori Y. Gamma knife radiosurgery in the treatment of Cushing disease: long-term results. *J Neurosurg* 2002;97(5 suppl):422–428.

Krause JC, et al. HIV-associated lipodystrophy in children. *Pediatr Endocrinol Rev* 2005;3:45–51.

Liddle GW. Tests of pituitary-adrenal suppressibility in the diagnosis of Cushing's syndrome. *J Clin Endocrinol Metab* 1960;20:1539–1560.

Lin LY, et al. Assessment of bilateral inferior petrosal sinus sampling (BIPSS) in the diagnosis of Cushing's disease. *J Chin Med Assoc* 2007;70:4–10.

Lucon AM, et al. Adrenocortical tumors: results of treatment and study of Weiss's score as a prognostic factor. *Rev Hosp Clin Fac Med Sao Paulo* 2002;57:251–256.

Magiakou MA, et al. Cushing's syndrome in children and adolescents. Presentation, diagnosis, and therapy. *N Engl J Med* 1994;331:629–636.

Makras P, et al. The diagnosis and differential diagnosis of endogenous Cushing's syndrome. *Hormones (Athens)* 2006;5:31–50.

Martines V, et al. Selective venous sampling in diagnosing ACTH-dependent hypercortisolism. *Radiol Med (Torino)* 2003;105:356–361.

McKusick VA. *Online Mendelian Inheritance in Man (OMIM)*. Baltimore: Johns Hopkins University. www.ncbi.nlm.nih.bov/ornim.

Migeon CJ, ed. Physiology and pathology of adrenocortical function in infancy and childhood. In: Collu DJ, Guyda H, eds. *Pediatric Endocrinology*. New York: Raven Press; 1981:475.

Ribeiro RC, et al. Adrenocortical tumors in children. *Braz J Med Biol Res* 2000;33:1225–1234.

Savage MO, et al. Cushing's disease in childhood: presentation, investigation, treatment and long-term outcome. *Horm Res* 2001;55(suppl 1):24–30.

Simard M. The biochemical investigation of Cushing syndrome. *Neurosurg Focus* 2004; 16:E4.

Storr HL, et al. Clinical and endocrine responses to pituitary radiotherapy in pediatric Cushing's disease: an effective second-line treatment. *J Clin Endocrinol Metab* 2003;88:34–37.

Storr HL, et al. Clinical features, diagnosis, treatment and molecular studies in paediatric Cushing's syndrome due to primary nodular adrenocortical hyperplasia. *Clin Endocrinol (Oxf)* 2004;61:539–553.

Torpy DJ, Stratakis CA, Chrousos GP. Hyper- and hypoaldosteronism. *Vitam Horm* 1999; 57:177–216.

Trilck M, et al. Salivary cortisol measurement—a reliable method for the diagnosis of Cushing's syndrome. *Exp Clin Endocrinol Diabetes* 2005;113:225–230.

Wilson TA, et al. Congenital adrenal hyperplasia. www.emedicine.com, 2006.

ADRENAL INSUFFICIENCY IN CHILDHOOD
Thomas A. Wilson

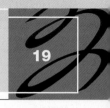

19

I. GENERAL PRINCIPLES

Adrenal insufficiency in children is either congenital or acquired. It can be a result of a primary disorder of the adrenal gland or occur secondary to a deficiency of adrenocorticotropic hormone (ACTH) or corticotropin-releasing hormone (CRH). Secondary adrenal insufficiency is usually associated with deficiencies of other hypothalamic and pituitary hormones.

Presenting complaints of adrenal insufficiency are malaise, weakness, failure to thrive, weight loss, anorexia, hypoglycemia, abdominal pain, vomiting, hypotension, confusion, and coma (Table 19.1). Patients with primary adrenal insufficiency are often pigmented because of the stimulating effect of ACTH on melanocytes, and develop salt craving, hyponatremia, and hyperkalemia secondary to aldosterone deficiency. In contrast, serum aldosterone concentrations are maintained by the renin-angiotensin system, and therefore electrolytes are generally normal in patients with secondary adrenal insufficiency. The exception to this is the dilutional hyponatremia that can develop in any form of severe cortisol deficiency because of impaired excretion of free water resulting from unrestrained ADH secretion.

II. ETIOLOGY (Table 19.2)

Adrenal insufficiency in children has a variety of etiologies, which are summarized in the following.

A. Congenital

1. **Primary congenital adrenal insufficiency**
   a. **Primary congenital adrenal insufficiency** is most commonly caused by deficiency of a protein (usually an enzyme) involved in cortisol synthesis that results in **congenital adrenal hyperplasia.** There are six such proteins described that cause cortisol deficiency. One form, caused by a deficiency of steroidogenic acute regulatory protein (StAR), results in a global inability to produce all adrenal steroids because this protein is required for cholesterol to enter the mitochondria where it can be converted to pregnenolone, thus starting the steroidogenic pathway (OMIM [On Line Mendelian Inheritance in Man] 600617). Congenital adrenal hyperplasia is discussed elsewhere (see Chapter 15).
   b. **Congenital adrenal hypoplasia** results from absence of a differentiation factor that governs development of the adrenal cortex. Well-described forms of adrenal hypoplasia are a consequence of a deletion or mutation of the gene that codes for steroidogenic factor 1 (SF1) ("cytomegalic form"; OMIM 184757) or a mutation or deletion of an X-linked gene, DAX1 ("miniature form"; OMIM 300200). The former condition may also cause XY pseudohermaphroditism. Both forms are associated with hypogonadotropic hypogonadism. Congenital adrenal hypoplasia caused by a defect in DAX1 may be seen as a contiguous gene deletion syndrome with associated glycerol kinase deficiency and Duchenne muscular dystrophy, because the glycerol kinase gene and the muscle dystrophin gene lie in close proximity to DAX1 on the X chromosome. A third form of congenital adrenal hypoplasia is autosomal recessive (OMIM 240200), and a fourth form is associated with intrauterine growth retardation, skeletal dysplasia, and genital abnormalities (IMAGE

227

TABLE 19.1   **Symptoms, Signs, and Laboratory Abnormalities in Adrenal Insufficiency**

Symptoms	Signs	Laboratory abnormalities
Nausea	Tender abdomen	Eosinophilia
Vomiting	Dehydration	Hypercalcemia
Diarrhea	Hypotension	Hyponatremia
Abdominal pain	Shock	Hypoglycemia
Anorexia	Orthostatic	↓ Cortisol
Weight loss	Disorientation	↑ Plasma renin activity
Confusion		
Coma		
Dizziness		
Weakness		
Fatigue		
Symptoms unique to patients with **primary** adrenal insufficiency:		
Salt craving	Hyperpigmentation	↑ ACTH
	Generalized	↓ Aldosterone
	Extensor surfaces	Hyperkalemia
	Palmar creases	
	Gingival margins	

TABLE 19.2   **Causes of Adrenal Insufficiency in Childhood**

Primary adrenal insufficiency (Addison disease)
Acute:
Bilateral adrenal hemorrhage
  With septicemia (Waterhouse-Friderichsen syndrome)
  Without septicemia
    Due to antiphospholipid antibody or hemorrhagic diathesis
Chronic:
  Autoimmune
  Congenital adrenal hyperplasia
  Congenital adrenal hypoplasia
  Infection: tuberculosis, histoplasmosis, cytomegalovirus, HIV
  Medication: ketoconazole, fluconazole, etomidate
  Adrenal leukodystrophy
  Wolman disease
  Congenital unresponsiveness to ACTH

Secondary adrenal insufficiency
Hypopituitarism
Congenital
Acquired
  Tumor
  Trauma
  Radiation
Iatrogenic secondary to chronic steroid therapy or medroxyprogesterone

ACTH, adrenocorticotropic hormone; HIV, human immunodeficiency virus.

syndrome; OMIM 300290). The genetic origins of these later forms remain to be elucidated.

2. **Secondary congenital adrenal insufficiency** results from congenital ACTH or CRH deficiency or can be mimicked by adrenal insensitivity to ACTH caused by a defect in the ACTH receptor mechanism (OMIM 202200, 202355, 300250), which may be associated with alacrima and achalasia (OMIM 231550).

B. **Acquired**

1. **Primary**

   a. **Primary acquired adrenal insufficiency** results from destruction of the adrenal cortex. Historically, the most common cause was tuberculosis. Other infectious diseases, such as histoplasmosis, coccidioidomycosis, cytomegalovirus, and human immunodeficiency virus (HIV) may cause adrenal insufficiency. Currently in the United States, Addison disease more commonly results from autoimmune adrenalitis resulting in destruction of the adrenal cortex. Serum antibodies often directed against the 21-hydroxylase protein may be present.

   b. **Autoimmune Addison disease,** in conjunction with hypoparathyroidism, hypogonadism, keratopathy, vitiligo, alopecia, pernicious anemia, dystrophy of the nails and enamel, and chronic active hepatitis, is inherited as an autosomal recessive trait due to a defect in the autoimmune regulator gene (AIRE) located on chromosome 21q22.3 (autoimmune polyglandular disease type 1, also called APECED; OMIM 240300). Addison disease in conjunction with autoimmune thyroiditis and insulin-dependent diabetes (autoimmune polyglandular disease type 2) is associated with human leukocyte antigens (HLAs) DR3 and DR4. Adrenal insufficiency generally does not appear until adulthood in this disorder.

   c. **Genetic forms of acquired adrenal insufficiency** occur in Wolman disease and adrenoleukodystrophy. Wolman disease (OMIM 27800) is a lipid-storage disease that results in hepatosplenomegaly, malabsorption, and adrenal calcification. Adrenoleukodystrophy (OMIM 300100) is a progressive neurologic disorder with adrenal insufficiency due to a mutation or deletion of ABCD1, an X-linked gene involved in peroxisomal oxidation of long-chain fatty acids.

   d. **Acute adrenal insufficiency from bilateral adrenal hemorrhage** may result from overwhelming septicemia (Waterhouse-Friderichsen syndrome), a hemorrhagic diathesis, anticoagulant therapy, or antiphospholipid antibody.

   e. **Medications** such as ketoconazole and related antifungals and the anesthetic etomidate may cause adrenal insufficiency by interfering with steroidogenesis. Mitotane, an agent used to treat adrenal carcinoma, results in adrenal insufficiency as a result of direct toxic effects on the adrenal cortex.

2. **Secondary adrenal insufficiency** results from any process that interferes with the production or release of CRH from the hypothalamus or ACTH from the pituitary. The most common cause is iatrogenic, secondary to chronic suppression of the hypothalamic–pituitary–adrenal axis from long-term (>2 weeks) glucocorticoid therapy, and may be seen in children on inhalable glucocorticoids for reactive airway disease. Medroxyprogesterone probably causes adrenal insufficiency by suppression of ACTH secretion, similar to glucocorticoids. Full recovery of the axis can take up to 12 months.

   Hypopituitarism with adrenal insufficiency also occurs secondary to a sellar or suprasellar mass, an inflammatory or infiltrative process, surgery, and cranial irradiation. This condition is mimicked by congenital unresponsiveness to ACTH resulting from an absence or alteration of the ACTH receptor (OMIM 202200).

3. **Relative adrenal insufficiency** without adrenal hemorrhage may be seen in the setting of severe sepsis. Studies suggest that some patients with catecholamine-resistant hypotension have a blunted cortisol response to cosyntropin (i.e., a cortisol increment <9 μg /dL) and fare better if treated with glucocorticoids. This issue remains controversial in older patients but is particularly poignant in the setting of low-birth-weight hypotensive infants who may benefit from modest doses of hydrocortisone but who are also at risk of developing gastric perforations

and adverse long-term developmental consequences from exposure to high-dose glucocorticoids.

C. **Hypoaldosteronism** occurs in patients with primary adrenal insufficiency and in some forms of congenital adrenal hyperplasia, but it can also occur as an isolated disorder. Children with enzyme defects in aldosterone synthetase (CYP11B2), which converts corticosterone to aldosterone, present with failure to thrive, salt craving, hyponatremia, hyperkalemia, and hyperreninemia (OMIM 124080). Similar clinical presentations are seen in children with **pseudohypoaldosteronism,** an autosomal recessive or dominant defect in the mineralocorticoid receptor that results in resistance to aldosterone (OMIM 264350) and by mutations of the epithelial sodium channel that render the renal tubule unresponsive to aldosterone (OMIM 177735). Low serum aldosterone concentrations in hypoaldosteronism and high serum aldosterone concentrations in pseudohypoaldosteronism distinguish these conditions.

III. DIAGNOSIS

A high index of suspicion is crucial, because the presenting symptoms of adrenal insufficiency are often subtle and early diagnosis may be life-saving. A history of steroid use, the presence of another autoimmune endocrine disorder (especially hypoparathyroidism), a family history of autoimmune endocrinopathies, or unexplained hypotension or hypoglycemia should heighten the suspicion of adrenal insufficiency. Random serum cortisol concentrations must be interpreted in the context of the clinical condition of the patient. For example, a serum cortisol concentration of 8 to 15 μg/dL in the morning would be normal in an unstressed individual but inappropriately low in a hypotensive, critically ill patient. If the patient's condition permits, an ACTH stimulation test will establish the diagnosis. Otherwise, the patient must first be stabilized with the administration of dextrose, fluids, electrolytes, and glucocorticoids and the diagnosis established subsequently. Infants typically have low baseline serum cortisol concentrations.

A. **Tests of the hypothalamic–pituitary–adrenal axis.** Tests of adrenal function are divided into those that test the entire hypothalamic–pituitary–adrenal axis (Table 19.3) and those that specifically test the function of the adrenal gland itself (Table 19.4). An elevated ACTH concentration (>100 pg/mL) in the presence of an inappropriately low serum cortisol concentration (<5 μg/dL) indicates primary adrenal deficiency or adrenal insensitivity to ACTH. Usually, dynamic stimulation tests of adrenal function are required.

1. **ACTH stimulation tests** (Table 19.4). A 60-minute cosyntropin (Cortrosyn) stimulation test is useful as a screening test for adrenal insufficiency. A normal response is a rise in serum cortisol >9 μg/dL and peak serum cortisol >18 μg/dL. In primary adrenal insufficiency, the baseline serum ACTH is elevated and the cortisol response to cosyntropin is flat. Patients with secondary adrenal insufficiency generally have a blunted cortisol response because of the hypoplasia that occurs in the adrenal in the absence of ACTH stimulation. However, patients with recent acquisition of ACTH or CRH deficiency may still have a normal cortisol response to cosyntropin, because the adrenal gland may not yet be hypoplastic. There is debate as to whether a smaller dose of cosyntropin (1 μg) may be more sensitive in this setting. In the absence of accurate plasma ACTH measurements, a 6-hour IV or 3-day IM ACTH stimulation test (Table 19.4) may be useful to demonstrate a lack of rise in serum cortisol, which is generally preferable to measuring 24-hour urinary 17-hydroxycorticosteroids and free cortisol.

2. **Insulin-induced hypoglycemia** stimulates CRH and ACTH release, which should result in a serum cortisol concentration >18 μg/dL. Patients undergoing this procedure must be monitored closely and the hypoglycemia reversed with intravenous dextrose if unconsciousness or a seizure results from the hypoglycemia. This test is less commonly used instead of the cosyntropin stimulation test (see above) because of the potential for hypoglycemic seizure, but it has the advantage that it directly evaluates the entire hypothalamic–pituitary–adrenal axis.

3. **Metyrapone** inhibits the 11β-hydroxylase enzyme, which converts 11-deoxycortisol to cortisol. In normal individuals, plasma concentrations of ACTH and compound S (11-deoxycortisol) increase following the administration of

TABLE 19.3 Tests of Hypothalamic–Pituitary–Adrenal Function

Insulin tolerance test		
Time	Prescription	Laboratory
0 min	Regular insulin (0.075–0.1 U/kg IV)	Cortisol, blood sugar
15, 30, 45, 60 min		Cortisol, blood sugar
Normal response: 50% decrease in blood glucose and plasma cortisol >18 μg/dL on any sample		
Overnight metyrapone stimulation test		
Time	Prescription	Laboratory
Midnight	Metyrapone (30 mg/kg PO at midnight)	Cortisol, 11-deoxycortisol
8 A.M.		Cortisol, 11-deoxycortisol
Normal response: serum cortisol concentration <8 μg, 11-deoxycortisol concentration >10 μg/dL, and an elevated ACTH		
Glucagon stimulation test		
Time	Prescription	Laboratory
0 min	Glucagon 30 μg/kg (max 1 mg) IV, SC, or IM	Cortisol
60, 80, 120, 150, 180 min		Cortisol
Normal response: serum cortisol >18 μg/dL on any sample		
Corticotropin stimulation test		
Time	Prescription	Laboratory
0 min	Ovine CRH, 1 μg/kg IV	ACTH, cortisol
15, 30, 60 min		ACTH, cortisol
Normal response: peak cortisol >18 μg/dL		

metyrapone. Utilizing this property of metyrapone, several different protocols have been designed to test the integrity of the hypothalamic–pituitary–adrenal axis. **The shorter overnight version of the metyrapone stimulation test** may be useful in screening patients for adrenal insufficiency. The usual dose of metyrapone is 30 mg/kg (maximum of 1 g) PO at midnight. Blood is drawn at 8 A.M. the next morning for cortisol, compound S (11-deoxycortisol), and ACTH. If ACTH is not elevated, the adrenal insufficiency is most likely central. It is often difficult to obtain metyrapone, and this test carries a risk of inducing an adrenal crisis. Therefore, it is rarely used anymore; preference is given to the 1-hour cosyntropin stimulation test.

4. **Glucagon** stimulates the adrenal axis and may be used to assess the adrenal axis.

5. **The corticotropin-releasing hormone (CRH) stimulation test** may be used to assess the pituitary-adrenal axis. This is usually the screening test of preference in evaluating a patient for adrenal insufficiency.

A subnormal rise in serum cortisol concentration in response to hypoglycemia, glucagon, or CRH, or an inadequate increase in serum 11-deoxycortisol concentration following metyrapone establishes a diagnosis of adrenal insufficiency but does not define whether the disorder is primary or secondary. Therefore, either plasma ACTH measurement must be obtained or the adrenal response to ACTH must be tested directly by stimulation with exogenous ACTH.

IV. TREATMENT

A. **Acute adrenal insufficiency** must be managed promptly with IV fluids and glucocorticoids. A solution of 5% dextrose in 0.9% NaCl (450 mL/m^2 in 30 to 60 minutes

| TABLE 19.4 | Tests of Adrenal Function |

Cosyntropin (cortrosyn) stimulation test		
Time	Prescription	Laboratory
0 min	Cosyntropin (0.25 mg/m^2 IV or IM*)	Cortisol
30, 60 min		Cortisol
Normal response: peak plasma cortisol >18 μg/dL		

6-h IV ACTH stimulation test		
Time	Prescription	Laboratory
0 and 6 h	ACTH (25 U IV over 6 h)	Cortisol
Normal response: plasma cortisol >40 $\pm$ 5 μg/dL		

5-Day ACTH stimulation test			
Day	Prescription	Laboratory	
1		24-h urinary free cortisol & 17-hydroxycorticosteroids	Serum cortisol
2		24-h urinary free cortisol & 17-hydroxycorticosteroids	Serum cortisol
3	ACTH gel (25 U/m^2 IM q12h)	24-h urinary free cortisol & 17-hydroxycorticosteroids	Serum cortisol
4	ACTH gel (25 U/m^2 IM q12h)	24-h urinary free cortisol & 17-hydroxycorticosteroids	Serum cortisol
5	ACTH gel (25 U/m^2 IM q12h)	24-h urinary free cortisol & 17-hydroxycorticosteroids	Serum cortisol
Normal response: 5- to 10-fold increase in 24-h urinary free cortisol & 17-hydroxycorticosteroids Peak serum cortisol >40 $\pm$ 5 μg/dL			

*Alternative dose: 1 μg for low-dose cosyntropin stimulation test.

to correct shock, then 3 200 mL/m^2 per day) should be infused. Hydrocortisone (2 mg/kg IV) or an equivalent dose of another glucocorticoid should be given every 6 hours until the patient is stable. Greater amounts of dextrose can be used if necessary to correct hypoglycemia. If hyponatremia or hyperkalemia is present, higher dosages of hydrocortisone (5 mg/kg q6h) can be used for a mineralocorticoid effect, or the patient can start oral fludrocortisone (Florinef) therapy. Deoxycorticosterone acetate (1 to 3 mg per day IM) is very effective as a mineralocorticoid but is no longer available in the United States.

For patients who have not received a diagnosis but who are suspected of having an acute adrenal crisis, the same regimen as outlined previously can be used, but dexamethasone (usually triple maintenance therapy [0.5 to 1 mg/m^2]) may be substituted for hydrocortisone. This allows an opportunity to carry out a cosyntropin stimulation test while the patient is recovering, because dexamethasone will not interfere with the measurement of plasma cortisol concentrations.

B. Chronic treatment

1. Glucocorticoids. Glucocorticoid replacement is designed to replace the normal cortisol production rate, which is estimated to be 6 to 12 mg/m^2 per day. The dosage must be individualized to allow adequate growth but prevent fatigue, malaise, and weakness. Excess glucocorticoid therapy suppresses growth. The oral dosage is approximately twice that of the parenteral. Equivalent dosages of

TABLE 19.5 Glucocorticoid Replacement Therapy: Average Dose

Glucocorticoid	Parenteral (mg/m²/d)	Oral (mg/m²/d)
Cortisone acetate	—	10–20
Hydrocortisone acetate	8–12 (IM only)	—
Hydrocortisone	6–10 (IM or IV)	7–20
Prednisone[a]	—	2–5
Methylprednisolone[a]	1.0–2.0 (IM or IV)	1.5–4
Dexamethasone[a]	0.15–0.25 (IM or IV)	0.2–0.5

[a]Not recommended for infants and small children.

the various steroids are given in Table 19.5. The more potent steroids are best avoided in infants and children because of the difficulty in fine-tuning the dosage to permit adequate growth but prevent symptoms of adrenal insufficiency. The dose of glucocorticoid must be doubled or tripled to cover physically stressful situations (e.g., infections, surgery, and trauma). Patients who have been treated with pharmacologic doses of steroids for more than 2 weeks within the past 6 to 12 months should be given a triple maintenance dose of steroids during times of stress to prevent an adrenal crisis.

2. **Mineralocorticoids.** Only patients with primary adrenal insufficiency require mineralocorticoid replacement therapy. The dosage of mineralocorticoid does not vary with body size because aldosterone secretion varies only twofold from infancy to adulthood. Generally, fludrocortisone acetate, 0.05 to 0.2 mg per day PO is adequate. Unlike glucocorticoids, the dose of fludrocortisone generally does not need to be increased to cover stress. Excessive doses of mineralocorticoid result in hypertension and hypokalemia.

3. **Sodium chloride supplementation** is usually necessary in infants with primary adrenal insufficiency. The usual dosage is 2 to 4 g per day (4 g = 1 teaspoon). Sodium chloride supplements are generally not necessary in older children, who can find access to salt to satisfy their requirement.

4. A **medical alert** bracelet or necklace is advisable for patients with adrenal insufficiency.

5. **Injectable glucocorticoids.** Parents or caretakers should be instructed on how to give injectable glucocorticoids to cover the child's need for cortisol in times of stress or if the child is unable to take medication by mouth. Generally, hydrocortisone, 50 to 100 mg/m² per day, methylprednisolone, 10 to 20 mg/m² per day, or dexamethasone, 1 to 2 mg/m² per day, is sufficient. Hydrocortisone acetate and dexamethasone have the advantage of longer duration of action (12 to 24 hours) than hydrocortisone succinate, which therefore must be repeated every 6 to 8 hours if the child is still unable to take medication orally.

Selected References

Ahonen P, et al. Clinical variation of autoimmune polyendocrinopathy-candidiasis-ectodermal dystrophy (APECED) in a series of 68 patients. *N Engl J Med* 1990;322:1829–1836.

Allen DB. Effects of inhaled steroids on growth, bone metabolism, and adrenal function. *Adv Pediatr* 2006;53:101–110.

Aneja R, Carcillo JA. What is the rationale for hydrocortisone treatment in children with infection-related adrenal insufficiency and septic shock? *Arch Dis Child* 2007;92:165–169.

Berger J, Gartner J. X-linked adrenoleukodystrophy: clinical, biochemical and pathogenetic aspects. *Biochim Biophys Acta* 2006;1763:1721–32.

Bottner A, et al. Comparison of adrenal function tests in children—the glucagon stimulation test allows the simultaneous assessment of adrenal function and growth hormone response in children. [see comment]. *J Pediatr Endocrinol* 2005;18:433–442.

Dahl R. Systemic side effects of inhaled corticosteroids in patients with asthma. *Respir Med* 2006;100:1307–1317.

Dorsey MJ, et al. Assessment of adrenal suppression in children with asthma treated with inhaled corticosteroids: use of dehydroepiandrosterone sulfate as a screening test. *Ann Allergy Asthma Immunol* 2006;97:182–186.

Fujieda K, Tajima T. Molecular basis of adrenal insufficiency. *Pediatr Res* 2005;57(5 pt 2): 62R–69R.

Gezer S. Antiphospholipid syndrome. *Disease-A-Month* 2003;49:696–741.

Linder BL, et al. Cortisol production rate in childhood and adolescence. *J Pediatr* 1990; 117:892–896.

Manglik S, et al. Glucocorticoid insufficiency in patients who present to the hospital with severe sepsis: a prospective clinical trial. [see comment]. *Crit Care Med* 2003;31:1668–1675.

Markovitz BP, et al. A retrospective cohort study of prognostic factors associated with outcome in pediatric severe sepsis: what is the role of steroids? [see comment]. *Pediatr Crit Care Med* 2005;6:270–274.

Mayenknecht J, et al. Comparison of low and high dose corticotropin stimulation tests in patients with pituitary disease. *J Clin Endocrinol Metab* 1998;83:1558–1562.

McKusick VA. *Online Mendelian Inheritance in Man (OMIM)*. Baltimore: Johns Hopkins University. www.ncbi.nlm.nih.bov/ornim.

Ng PC, et al. Reference ranges and factors affecting the human corticotropin-releasing hormone test in preterm, very low birth weight infants. *J Clin Endocrinol Metab* 2002; 87:4621–4628.

Nieman LK. Dynamic evaluation of adrenal hypofunction. *J Endocrinol Invest* 2003;26(7 suppl):74–82.

Oelkers W. Hyponatremia and inappropriate secretion of vasopressin (antidiuretic hormone) in patients with hypopituitarism. *N Engl J Med* 1989;321:492–496.

Powers JM. Adreno-leukodystrophy: a personal historical note. *Acta Neuropathol (Berl)* 2005;109:124–127.

Santhana Krishnan SG, Cobbs RK. Reversible acute adrenal insufficiency caused by fluconazole in a critically ill patient. *Postgrad Med J* 2006;82:e23.

Simm PJ, McDonnell CM, Zacharin MR. Primary adrenal insufficiency in childhood and adolescence: advances in diagnosis and management. *J Paediatr Child Health* 2004;40: 596–599.

Tsigos C. Isolated glucocorticoid deficiency and ACTH receptor mutations. *Arch Med Res* 1999;30:475–480.

Villasenor J, Benoist C, Mathis D. AIRE and APECED: molecular insights into an autoimmune disease. *Immunol Rev* 2005;204:156–64.

Watterberg KL. Adrenocortical function and dysfunction in the fetus and neonate. *Semin Neonatol* 2004;9:13–21.

Wilson TA. Congenital adrenal hyperplasia. www.emedicine.com, 2006.

Zuckerbraun NS, et al. Use of etomidate as an induction agent for rapid sequence intubation in a pediatric emergency department. *Acad Emerg Med* 2006;13:602–609.

Disorders of the Reproductive System

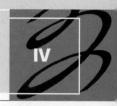

IV

AMBIGUOUS GENITALIA
Selma F. Witchel and Peter A. Lee

20

*A*lthough ambiguous genitalia in a newborn is usually not an impending medical emergency, the inability to ascertain gender and name the infant creates much distress and requires prompt attention. The assessment should be done as part of a team involving the family, providing them with an understanding of the physiology and embryology involved as well as all currently available outcome data of similar patients. Clinicians need a forthright approach that will minimize anxiety while rapidly defining the child's internal and external genital anatomy and elucidating the basis for the ambiguity. Sex assignment can then be made concordant with the child's karyotype, reproductive potential, and molecular basis of the child's disorder of sexual differentiation.

I. MECHANISMS OF DIFFERENTIATION AND DEVELOPMENT
- **A. Fertilization.** In the usual situation, an XX karyotype is associated with a female phenotype, whereas an XY karyotype is associated with the male differentiation. However, infants with genital ambiguity demonstrate that the course of sexual differentiation and development can be influenced by other factors in addition to the genes of the sex chromosome. Defects can occur at the level of the chromosome (e.g., mosaicism such as XX/XY) or within one or more genes mapped to the sex chromosomes or autosomes, or they may reflect environmental factors. Sexual differentiation does not begin until the gonadal ridges differentiate. These tissues begin as undifferentiated paired proliferation of coelomic epithelium and mesenchyme. The structural changes into an early gonad begin in the fourth postfertilization week with the appearance of so-called sex cords. Primordial germ cells (the cells destined to become ova or sperm) then migrate from the yolk sac along the dorsal mesentery into these gonadal ridges (6 weeks).
- **B. Gonadal differentiation**
    1. The embryonic events of gonadal differentiation proceed independently within each gonad. Thus, gonadal histology can differ between sides; and even within a single gonadal ridge, more than one type of gonad can develop. An example

235

is ovotesticular disorder of sexual differentiation, traditionally called <u>true her-maphroditism</u>, in which both ovarian and testicular differentiation occur. Go-nadal histology can range from ovotestis to ovary or testis.

2. In the normal XY male, a specific gene on the short arm of the Y chromosome, <u>SRY</u> (sex-determining region on Y), is the switch that directs differentiation of the indifferent gonad, the sex cords, and surrounding tissues into a testis. Evidence acquired from an XX mouse transgenic for the Sry gene indicated that the *SRY* gene is the only gene on the Y chromosome required for testis determination. Mutations in the *SRY* gene are associated with 46,XY sex reversal.

3. The SRY gene has been identified among those with male differentiation of geni-talia who lack a cytogenetically demonstrable Y chromosome. In such individuals with **46,XX testicular disorder of sexual differentiation,** the presence of the *SRY* gene can often be confirmed by molecular techniques.

4. Multiple genes have roles both upstream and downstream from *SRY*. This com-plex regulatory cascade of sex-linked and autosomal genes includes not only *SRY* but also *DAX1, SOX9, SF1,* and *DHH*. The protein products of these genes function as transcription factors. In humans, duplication of the *DAX1* gene and mutations involving the SRY, SOX9, SF1, and WT1 genes are associated with XY sex reversal. Duplication of SOX9 was identified in a 46,XX infant with pe-nile/scrotal hypospadias and palpable gonads. Duplication of the *WNT4* gene is associated with XY sex reversal.

5. Genes upstream from SRY may be involved in early development of the go-nads and the urinary tract. Steroidogenic factor-1 (SF-1) is essential for gonadal, adrenal, and pituitary development. WT1 is necessary for normal urogenital tract development. <u>Mutations of WT1</u> are associated with <u>Denys-Drash</u> and <u>Fraser syndromes</u>. Deletions of chromosome 9p are associated with XY sex reversal. Although no deleterious mutations have been identified in *DMRT1,* it remains a candidate gene for sex determination because it is expressed in the developing testis and is highly conserved.

6. Mutations of SOX-9 are associated with XY sex reversal females and <u>camp-tomelic dwarfism</u>. Mutations of *DAX-1* are associated with adrenal hypoplasia and hypogonadotropic hypogonadism. *DAX-1* maps to the dosage-sensitive sex reversal locus with duplication resulting in XY females. DAX-1 inhibits expres-sion of *SOX9* resulting in no testis differentiation in XX individuals.

7. WNT-4 is a signaling molecule; it normally upregulates DAX-1 expression. Du-plication of WNT-4 is associated with impaired testicular differentiation and XY sex reversal.

8. As germ cells penetrate the somatic cell matrix of the differentiating gonad, an-other regulatory step can occur. If the karyotype of the germ cell is different from that of the gonad (i.e., an XX germ cell migrating into a developing XY testis), the germ cell will usually not survive and a "sterile" gonad will result. In this model, variants may develop, however, such as a testis containing only XX sperm.

C. **Gonadal development and function.** Testicular organogenesis is rapid, and by the ninth week **testosterone** and **anti-müllerian hormone (AMH)** are being produced. Ovarian organogenesis occurs more slowly; a recognizable structure might not be present until the 17th to 20th week. Following histologic differentiation, the ovary, unlike the testis, may lose its integrity and become a streak if viable, normally meiotic germ cells are not present or are not forming normal follicles. The ovaries of girls with Turner syndrome initially develop follicles that undergo premature degenera-tion/atresia, leaving a streak gonad. Thus, one X chromosome is sufficient for ovarian differentiation, but two X chromosomes are required for maintenance of germ cells and adult ovarian function. Two phases of testicular descent are recognized. INSL3, secreted by Leydig cells, mediates the transabdominal phase, whereas testosterone influences the inguinoscrotal phase of testicular descent. The effects of INSL3 are mediated by its receptor, LGR8.

D. **Internal genital duct development.** The internal genital ducts develop from two different sets of paired mesodermal ductlike structures. Both sets develop alongside each gonadal ridge, and the two ducts are under different control mechanisms. The mesonephric (wolffian) ducts are present in close proximity to the gonadal ridges by 4 weeks, and the paramesonephric (müllerian) ducts develop at 5 weeks in a more lateral position. Testosterone secreted by the ipsilateral testicular Leydig cells stimulates the duct cells to develop into the wolffian-derived structures: epididymis, ductus deferens, seminal vesicle, and common ejaculatory duct. This organization is obvious by 9 weeks and may be complete by 14 weeks. In the absence of locally secreted testosterone, the mesonephric/wolffian duct passively regresses. Thus, wolffian structures further differentiate only on the side with a functional testis; if only one testis is present, this differentiation does not occur on the contralateral side.

The functional testis also secretes AMH, a glycoprotein of Sertoli cell origin that also acts locally and not on the contralateral side to cause degeneration of the paramesonephric duct. When a testis is not present or when there is a lack of production or action of AMH, the paramesonephric duct develops into a fallopian tube and a hemiuterus, which normally fuses later with the contralateral structure, and includes the upper third of the vagina. Failure of testicular AMH secretion or mutations of the AMH gene or the AMH receptor gene are associated with the persistent müllerian duct syndrome (PMDS). Ovarian dysgenesis or exposure to excessive androgens such as in virilizing congenital adrenal hyperplasia does not impair development of the müllerian duct derivatives in an XX fetus.

E. External genital development. The final step in fetal sexual differentiation involves two complex embryonic mechanisms: the development of the excretory system, both urogenital and alimentary, and the development of those elements of the external genitalia directed toward reproductive function and whose appearance ordinarily dictates sex assignment.

1. At about 3 weeks' gestation the cloacal membrane, which closes the hindgut, is already present. An unpaired genital tubercle develops anteriorly, while two genital folds develop laterally. The cloacal membrane then divides into urogenital and anal membranes (6 weeks), and finally into an anterior urogenital groove and a posterior anorectal canal (8 weeks). The genital folds divide into medial urethral folds (surrounding the urogenital groove) and lateral labioscrotal swellings. These steps all occur before the fetus begins true sexual differentiation. Thus, these early embryonic changes are common to both sexes. Congenital anomalies such as imperforate anus, exstrophy of the cloaca, penoscrotal transposition (in which the genital tubercle is below the genital folds), and agenesis of the phallus all occur during this time. When seen, they indicate that an early embryogenic defect occurred, rather than one associated with impaired gonadal development or inappropriate sex hormone milieu.

2. Sexual divergence of the external genitalia occurs after 8 weeks' gestation.

a. In the normal male fetus, circulating testosterone of testicular origin reaches the genital tubercle, where it is converted locally to **dihydrotestosterone (DHT)** by the 5-α-reductase enzyme (type 2). DHT, acting through the androgen receptor, causes rapid elongation of the tubercle. The urogenital groove is also pulled forward, the parallel mucosa folds fuse, and a penile urethra forms by 12 weeks. The genital swellings move caudally, fuse, and form halves of the scrotum. The final glandular urethra (to the tip of the phallus) does not occur until 4 months' gestation, when an invagination of penile ectoderm reaches the formed lumen. This process might not be directly related to testosterone synthesis or action, or it might reflect subtle defects in testosterone secretion, DHT action, or the presence of increased quantities of antiandrogenic steroids such as some synthetic forms of progesterone.

b. In a female fetus, in whom circulating testosterone levels are normally low, the external genitalia, formed during the first 8 weeks of embryologic development, do not manifest significant further differentiation. The genital tubercle remains to form the clitoris (although this organ always has the potential, prenatally or postnatally, to enlarge under the influence of increased androgens). The urethral folds are not pulled anteriorly and form the hood over the clitoris and extend posteriorly, remaining as the unfused labia minora. The genital swellings do not migrate but enlarge to form the labia majora, and the urogenital groove remains open to form the vaginal vestibule. The relative position of the urethral orifice becomes fixed by about 14 weeks, and exposure to androgen thereafter can neither shift the urethral folds anteriorly nor fuse the labia. Therefore, the timing of these events helps to determine when prenatal androgen exposure occurred during gestation. Virilization after 14 weeks may cause clitoromegaly alone, whereas exposure prior to 14 weeks can cause degrees of clitoromegaly, scrotalization of the labia majora, labial fusion, and obliteration of the vaginal vestibule.

II. DIFFERENTIAL DIAGNOSIS OF AMBIGUOUS GENITALIA

The differential diagnosis of genital ambiguity begins with physical examination of the anatomy of the internal and external genitalia. In addition to the physical examination (which may change over time and therefore requires re-examination), radiologic examinations such as contrast retrograde urethrography, ultrasound, fistulography, and, if indicated, cystoscopy with contrast instillation may be helpful. During the physical examination, the symmetry and extent of virilization is assessed. The primordial labioscrotal folds may have developed as labia majora, a fully fused scrotum, or varying degrees of labial–scrotal fusion. The phallus may appear as a clitoris typical of a newborn female, as a penis with the urethral meatus at the tip, as an overdeveloped clitoris or underdeveloped penis with a single or two openings on the perineum. Varying degrees of fusion of the labiourethral folds may be present. The opening may be on the perineum, along the underside of the shaft of the phallus, or with full fusion with the meatus opening at the tip of the glans. The phallus may be markedly enlarged but bound down with an appearance of chordee.

In addition, the evaluation should include the appropriate hormonal determinations and chromosomal studies. When available, identification of genetic mutations is helpful to confirm the diagnosis and for genetic counseling/predictions for future pregnancies. Rarely, stimulation or suppression tests may be indicated during the neonatal period. Exploratory laparoscopy, laparotomy, and gonadal biopsy are necessary in some cases to reach a definitive diagnosis. A trial of androgen therapy may be helpful to ascertain androgen responsiveness. A schematic approach to the infant with ambiguous genitalia is shown in Fig. 20.1, and hormonal abhorrations are summarized in Table 20.1. Some key elements of the physical examination are further discussed below.

The presence or absence of a palpable inguinal or labioscrotal gonad(s) is important, because virilized females will not have a palpable gonad, and incompletely virilized males may have one or both gonads palpable. Some disorders of gonadal differentiation present with a single palpable gonad and asymmetry of the external genitalia, usually with greater scrotalization of the labioscrotal folds on the side of the gonad.

A. No palpable gonads: suspect virilized female. If no gonads are palpable and an ultrasound shows the presence of a uterus, the most likely diagnosis is an XX female infant with virilizing congenital adrenal hyperplasia. Confirmatory tests include steroid hormone determinations and karyotype. Because of the possibility of salt loss as a result of mineralocorticoid deficiency, monitoring of electrolytes for hyponatremia and hyperkalemia is important. The most common of the virilizing forms of congenital adrenal hyperplasia (CAH) is 21-hydroxylase deficiency (with or without adrenal insufficiency and salt loss), which accounts for ~95% of cases. Plasma 17α-hydroxyprogesterone (17-OHP) concentration at 24 hours or thereafter is a most helpful test. Typically, the 17-OHP value is >10 000 ng/dL. Genital development is normal in boys with 21-hydroxylase deficiency. 11β-Hydroxylase deficiency is much less common (<5%) and is associated with elevated 11-deoxycortisol concentrations (compound S). 3β-hydroxysteroid dehydrogenase deficiency is a very rare (<<1%) cause of virilizing CAH among 46,XX infants (it is also associated with inadequate virilization in 46,XY infants). This can be excluded by determining the dehydroepiandrosterone (DHEA) and 17-OH pregnenolone levels. A serum testosterone value should also be obtained to estimate conversion outside the adrenal cortex to this potent androgen. Other rare causes of prenatal virilization of a female fetus include maternal hyperandrogenism, P450 oxidoreductase deficiency, and aromatase deficiency. The genes coding 21-hydroxylase (CYP21), 11β-hydroxylase (CYP11B1),

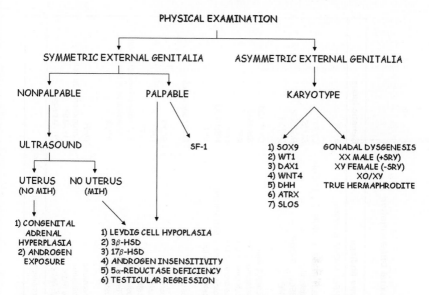

Figure 20.1. Schematic approach to the differential diagnosis of ambiguous genitalia in the infant. CAH, congenital adrenal hyperplasia; IVP, intravenous pyelogram; VCUG, voiding cystourethrogram. (From Lippe BM. Sexual differentiation and development. In: Hershman JM, ed. *Endocrine Pathophysiology: A Patient-Oriented Approach.* 2nd ed. Philadelphia: Lea & Febiger; 1988:118.)

3β-hydroxysteroid dehydrogenase (HSD3B2), P450 oxidoreductase (POR), and aromatase (CYP19) have been mapped and sequenced. Molecular genetic studies can be performed to characterize the molecular defect, which may be helpful for genetic counseling.

Mineralocorticoid deficiency can lead to catastrophic salt loss. In the untreated patient, adrenal insufficiency occurs during the second week of life. Once basal blood samples for steroid and renin measurements have been obtained, hydrocortisone and fludrocortisone acetate therapy can be initiated. If dehydration accompanied by severe hyperkalemia and hyponatremia occurs, intravenous fluid therapy can be instituted. Mineralocorticoid treatment with fludrocortisone acetate (Florinef Acetate), 0.1 to 0.4 mg daily, and glucocorticoid therapy at stress dosages of 25 to 50 mg hydrocortisone IV, IM, or PO for 48 hours (depending on the degree of illness) should be initiated upon confirmation of diagnosis. Subsequently, the dosage should be gradually decreased to physiologic replacement of 25 to 30 mg/m^2 per day in the neonatal period, divided into three doses (at $\sim$8-hour intervals). Over the first year of life, the hydrocortisone dose is decreased to 8 to 18 mg/m^2 per day. Some centers prefer the use of prednisone or dexamethasone. The neonate often requires a greater mineralocorticoid dose, which is typically decreased to 0.1 mg per day. Sodium polystyrene sulfonate (Kayexalate), 1 g/kg per dose, q6h, may be needed to correct life-threatening hyperkalemia. After acute IV therapy, supplemental NaCl may be given orally (3 to 8 mEq per day) as needed to maintain plasma Na levels. Parents of affected children should learn when to administer stress doses and how to administer intramuscular hydrocortisone (Solu-Cortef) for emergency situations. Institution of newborn screening programs has decreased the morbidity and mortality secondary to undiagnosed 21-hydroxylase deficiency. The use of prenatal dexamethasone therapy to decrease virilization of affected female infants remains controversial.

1. If the diagnosis is not congenital adrenal hyperplasia and exposure to exogenous/maternal androgens has been excluded, **genitography** and **abdominal-pelvic**

TABLE 20.1 Genetic and Hormonal Characteristics of Causes of Errors in Sexual Differentiation

Disorder	Phenotype	Hormone findings	Genetic locus
Congenital lipoid CAH	46,XY sex reversal Adrenal insufficiency	↓ 17-PREG, 17-OHP, & cortisol	StAR
17α-hydroxylase/17,20-lyase deficiency	46,XY sex reversal	↑ PREG, ↑ PROG, ↓ 17PREG, ↓ 17-OHP	CYP17
Smith-Lemli-Opitz syndrome	46,XY sex reversal polydactyly/syndactyly	↓ Cholesterol	SLOS
3β-Hydroxysteroid dehydrogenase deficiency	46,XY sex reversal	↑ 17PREG, ↓ 17-OHP	HSD3B2
21-Hydroxylase deficiency	Virilization of 46,XX fetus Adrenal insufficiency	↑ 17-OHP	CYP21
11β-Hydroxylase deficiency	Virilization of 46,XX fetus	↑ 11-Deoxycortisol	CYP11B1
5α-Reductase deficiency	Undervirilization of 46,XY fetus	↑ Testosterone, ↓ DHT	SRD5A2
Androgen insensitivity	Undervirilization of 46,XY fetus	↑ Testosterone, ↑ LH	AR
Leydig Cell hypoplasia	Undervirilization of 46,XY fetus	↑ Testosterone, ↑ LH	LHR
17β-Hydroxysteroid dehydrogenase deficiency	Undervirilization of 46,XY fetus	↑ Androstenedione, ↓ testosterone	HSD17B3
Ambiguous genitalia	46,XY sex reversal Adrenal insufficiency	↓ Testosterone & LH	SF1
Ambiguous genitalia	46,XY sex reversal Hypogonadotropic hypogonadism	↓ Testosterone	DAX1 duplication
Ambiguous genitalia & camptomelic dysplasia	46,XY sex reversal	↓ Testosterone	SOX9
Denys-Drash syndrome	46,XY sex reversal	↓ Testosterone	WT1
Fraser syndrome	46,XY sex reversal	↓ Testosterone	WT1
XY female	46,XX sex reversal	↓ or nl Testosterone	SRY (loss-of-function mutation)
XX male	46,XX sex reversal	↓ Testosterone	Translocation of SRY gene
X-linked α-thalassemia–mental retardation syndrome	46,XY sex reversal	↓ Testosterone	ATRX
Ambiguous genitalia & polyneuropathy	46,XY sex reversal	↓ Testosterone	DHH
Ambiguous genitalia	46,XY sex reversal	↓ Testosterone	Chromosome 9p deletion
Persistent müllerian duct syndrome	46,XY with uterus or uterine remnants	(1) Low AMH (2) High AMH	(1) AMH (2) AMHR2

AMH, anti-müllerian hormone; CAH, congenital adrenal hyperplasia; DHT, dihydrotestosterone; LH, luteinizing hormone; 17-OHP, 17-hydroxyprogesterone.

ultrasound can be helpful to assess for upper vagina, cervix, and uterus, and the interrelationship of the urinary outflow tract and the vagina. Renal anomalies may be present in some undervirilized males and in some neonates with complex congenital anomalies. In the neonate, however, neither intra-abdominal testes nor ovaries are likely to be seen, so nonvisualization does not indicate absence of a gonad. Because the adrenal glands are normally large prior to involution of the fetal zone during infancy, adrenal size estimations may not be helpful in the diagnosis of adrenal hyperplasia.

2. If the imaging studies, hormone determinations, and chromosomes fail to clarify the etiology of the genital ambiguity, **hormonal stimulation tests** with human chorionic gonadotropin (hCG) or adrenocorticotropic hormone (ACTH) may be useful before proceeding to surgical exploration and gonadal biopsy. In the immediate neonatal period, basal gonadotropin and sex steroid hormone concentrations may be sufficient, because of the intrinsic activity of the hypothalamic–pituitary–gonadal axis. Beyond the neonatal period, stimulation testing may be helpful to:

   a. Define a block on gonadal or adrenal hormone production by identifying precursor accumulation or product deficiency. For example, hCG stimulation may elicit increased androstenedione concentrations with low testosterone concentrations in 17β-hydroxysteroid dehydrogenase deficiency resulting from *HSD17B3* mutations.

   b. Suggest the presence of a hormonally competent gonad that was not under maximum stimulation at the time the basal hormones were obtained.

      The difficulty with stimulation tests is that precise protocols and defined normal responses have not been established for the neonatal period and infancy. For example, protocols for hCG are similar to those employed in older children (e.g., 1 000 IU IM for 3 to 5 days, obtaining plasma steroids on day 4 or 6), with unclear criteria to judge a normal response. Similarly, ACTH, administered as cosyntropin (Cortrosyn), can be given (0.25 mg IV) with serum steroids obtained at 30 and/or 60 minutes. Results are then compared to the normal responses established for older children.

3. Mild virilization in the presence of a 46,XY karyotype suggests impaired testosterone secretion. The differential diagnosis includes dysgenetic testis, <u>Denys-Drash syndrome</u>, <u>Fraser syndrome</u>, <u>testicular regression</u>, or <u>DAX-1 or WNT-4 gene duplications</u>.

B. **Asymmetry (gonad on one side only).** Virilized external genitalia in 46,XX infants and undervirilized genitalia in 46,XY infants are generally symmetrical. When the genitalia are asymmetrical, with the labioscrotal folds being fuller on one side, particularly if a gonad is palpable on that side, <u>mixed gonadal dysgenesis or ovotesticular</u> disorder of sexual differentiation (true hermaphroditism) needs to be considered in the differential diagnosis. Normal ovaries do not usually herniate or descend into the lower labioscrotal fold. On the other hand, a testis or ovotestis with its associated gubernaculum can migrate from the pelvis and lodge anywhere along the normal path of testicular descent. The contralateral gonad may be a streak, ovary, or dysgenetic testis.

1. Proceed with genitogram and ultrasonography.

2. The chromosomal karyotype may show mosaicism, such as XX/XY, XX/XO, or XY/X0. However, up to <u>80% of</u> **true gonadal hermaphrodites**, defined as the presence of ovarian follicles and testicular tubules in the same patient (in either one or two gonads) have an <u>XX karyotype</u>.

3. Regardless of the karyotype, sex of rearing depends on clinical judgment, that is, judging the extent of in utero and neonatal central nervous system (CNS) androgen exposure, potential for a functional testis or ovary, and whether the internal anatomy includes a reasonably developed uterus, as well as external genital anatomy. Surgical exploration to determine the full extent of the anatomy may be helpful. For example, patients with ovotesticular disorder of sexual differentiation with one intact ovary and uterus have been fertile, and a female sex of rearing may be considered. Generally, the male ducts for sperm maturation

and delivery are not fully formed, so such individuals cannot be expected to be fertile as males. Nevertheless, a male sex of rearing may be most appropriate for a patient with evidence of considerable androgen exposure before birth, particularly if there is considerable phallic development. The presence or absence of sex chromosomes per se has come to be viewed as less important, the specific genetic deletion perhaps resulting in similar outcome regardless of the presence or absence of a Y chromosome. Thus, some XX true hermaphrodites may be best reared as males, whereas some XY patients with gonadal dysgenesis may best be reared as females.

C. Symmetrically descended scrotal gonads. Because these are almost always testes or ovotestes, suspect incomplete virilized male or gonadal intersex (true hermaphroditism). The differential diagnosis includes defects in testosterone biosynthesis, androgen insensitivity, and Leydig cell hypoplasia. One rare cause of genital ambiguity in 46,XY infants is 3β-hydroxysteroid dehydrogenase deficiency resulting from mutations in the HSD3B2 gene; affected infants are at risk for salt loss secondary to mineralocorticoid deficiency. Leydig cell hypoplasia is an autosomal recessive disorder secondary to mutations in the LHCG receptor gene. Defects in testosterone biosynthesis are also autosomal recessive conditions. Mutations in the androgen receptor mapped to the X chromosome cause androgen insensitivity; inheritance is X-linked.

  1. Ultrasonography is indicated, because varying degrees of müllerian duct–derived development may be present, depending on the amount and timing of AMH secretion.

  2. If microphallus alone is present, suspect either hypopituitarism or a defect in testosterone synthesis or action. Males with hypopituitarism and microphallus often have hypoglycemia and should therefore be monitored closely. In addition, thyroid function should be evaluated to rule out central hypothyroidism. Males with defects in testosterone synthesis can have a similar defect in the adrenal and exhibit salt loss (as discussed previously). The most difficult condition to diagnose and treat is partial androgen insensitivity (PAIS). Inquiry regarding affected maternal relatives can be helpful. Elevated levels of luteinizing hormone (LH), follicle-stimulating hormone (FSH) and testosterone are consistent with PAIS but may not always be demonstrable. Testing may require a genital skin biopsy for androgen receptors and a trial of testosterone to see if the phallus grows. Mutation analysis of the androgen receptor gene can also be done.

  3. When anatomic malformations of the genitalia or rectum are present, the differential diagnoses include CHARGE syndrome, VATER syndrome, IMAGE syndrome, and penoscrotal transposition. These early defects in embryogenesis, involving the formation of the cloaca, anus, and other structures, are usually sporadic. The CHARGE syndrome includes *c*oloboma, *h*eart defect, *a*tresia choanae, *r*etarded growth and development, *g*enetic anomalies, *e*ar anomalies, and possibly hypopituitarism. The VATER syndrome often also includes *v*ertebral *a*nomalies, other bony anomalies, *t*racheoesophageal fistula, and *r*enal problems. IMAGE syndrome is characterized by intrauterine growth retardation, metaphyseal dysplasia, adrenal hypoplasia, cryptorchidism, small penis, and hypercalciuria or hypercalcemia. Penoscrotal transposition can be isolated or associated with imperforate anus.

III. MANAGEMENT OF THE CHILD WITH AMBIGUOUS GENITALIA

Once a diagnosis has been made and a sex assigned, the management of the child and family includes the following approaches.

A. Plans for reconstructive surgery

  1. In the female, it must be decided whether the clitoromegaly is great enough to consider clitoroplasty or clitoral reduction. Importantly, parents need to be informed that some individuals, including those in patient advocacy groups, are suggesting that any such genital surgery be deferred until the child become old enough to make his or her own decisions. Generally, unless the clitoromegaly is minimal enough to anticipate that regression may occur with treatment of the underlying cause of hyperandrogenism, most parents choose surgery. Further, if the position of the urethra is high, surgery may be indicated to provide urinary outflow without risk of recurrent urinary tract infections. The age of surgery varies from the neonatal period to several months of age, when the child is larger and after the results of medical therapy can be seen. When there is agreement between the medical team and parent(s) that surgery is indicated, the goal for the age of surgery has traditionally been prior to a time when the child herself would recognize the ambiguity. Extensive vaginal reconstruction is usually delayed until adolescence, because fixed-form grafts might be necessary, the postoperative period can require the use of dilators, and unless long-term procedures are done on motivated patients, stenosis can occur.

2. In the male, phallic reconstruction is generally a staged procedure, depending on the degree of hypospadias or chordee. Issues of multiple surgeries, the importance of being able to stand to urinate dressed or undressed, and of genital variation should be discussed completely with the parents before surgery is undertaken. If testes are absent, scrotal implants may be considered. However, because the risk of complications is much greater with multiple procedures implanting increasing-sized prostheses, a single implant procedure, with adult-size prostheses placed in adolescence, after early masculinization with androgens, is usually preferable.

3. In the child of either sex who has congenital anomalies, a multidisciplinary approach should be coordinated. Intersex teams involving an endocrinologist, surgeon, and psychologists, together with urology, genetic, gynecologic, and social work representatives, often enhance overall assessment and communication with parents.

B. Mechanisms for interdisciplinary care of the child and family

1. Medical as well as surgical management is often indicated and should be coordinated by the appropriate subspecialist (usually a pediatric endocrinologist). A plan for long-term management should be outlined and educational sessions arranged for the parents. The degree of long-term compliance is often related to the time spent on initial education.

2. Because many of the conditions described are inherited as autosomal recessive or X-linked traits, genetic counseling may be indicated. In addition, the heterogeneity of clinical expression of some disorders (especially those of androgen action) might mandate examination or testing (or both) of family members.

3. The psychological impact of a disorder resulting in ambiguity, as well as a clinical condition requiring long-term medication or multiple surgical procedures, may be devastating for the family (and later for the child). Thus, longitudinal continuity of care and provision for support systems are necessary.

Selected References

Hanley NA, Arlt W. The human fetal adrenal cortex and the window of sexual differentiation. *Trends Endocrinol Metab* 2006;17:391–397. Review.

Lee PA, Houk CP, Ahmed SF, Hughes IA, and the International Consensus Conference on Intersex Working Group. Consensus statement on management of intersex disorders. *Pediatrics* 2006;118:e488–e500.

Lee PA, Stanhope R, guest editors. *Disorders of Sex Development.*Vol. 20, Suppl. 3, 2007.

Wilhelm D, Koopman P. The makings of maleness: towards an integrated view of male sexual development. *Nat Rev Genet* 2006;7:620.

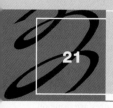

EARLY, PRECOCIOUS, AND DELAYED FEMALE PUBERTAL DEVELOPMENT

Christopher P. Houk and Peter A. Lee

EARLY AND PRECOCIOUS PUBERTY

I. GENERAL PRINCIPLES

Although precocious puberty has traditionally been defined as the early onset of pubertal changes (based on chronologic age), it is critical that pubertal progression and/or a pubertal hypothalamic–pituitary–gonadal (HPG) axis is documented before precocious puberty is diagnosed. Minimal, isolated pubertal changes, such as breast or pubic hair development, do not necessarily indicate the onset of puberty. The diagnosis of precocious puberty in girls requires that early progressive breast development be associated with both an accelerated growth rate (premature growth spurt) and advanced skeletal maturation (determined by a bone-age radiograph). In girls, these early changes may or may not be accompanied by pubic hair.

These caveats make it difficult to make sense of recent studies showing that initial pubertal changes in girls seem to occur at increasingly younger ages. These contemporary studies have also identified distinct racial differences in the timing of puberty, with African Americans showing a tendency to earlier pubertal onset than Hispanics, which in turn begin puberty earlier than Caucasians. Data suggest that the average age of the onset of breast development is around 9.5 years, with as many as 5% of girls showing some breast development before their eighth birthday.

It must be kept in mind that the early onset of nonprogressive breast development is usually a normal variant and does not indicate precocious puberty. When early breast growth is the only physical finding, the diagnosis of **premature thelarche** can be made, and clinical follow-up to monitor for progression is all that is indicated. Although the majority of girls with pubertal onset before their eighth birthday have premature thelarche—particularly those presenting with this sign in the first 2 years of life—isolated premature thelarche may be the first manifestation of progressive precocious puberty. Thelarche may also progress to a poorly described condition referred to as nonprogressive precocious puberty. This nonprogressive precocious puberty is characterized by impressive early breast changes that are not associated with an upturn in growth velocity, advancement in skeletal maturity, or development of a pubertal HPG axis.

When pubic hair develops without breast development, this is not precocious puberty but is referred to as **premature pubarche.** Although premature pubarche may be the first manifestation of adolescent ovarian hyperandrogenism (a sizable portion of these patients later develop the polycystic ovarian syndrome), early development of sexual hair without breast growth or advanced skeletal maturation is usually considered isolated premature pubarche, a consequence of benign **premature adrenarche**—another benign pubertal variant seen in as many as 20% of girls. Other pathologic diagnoses that may initially present with isolated premature pubarche include central precocious puberty, **congenital adrenal hyperplasia,** or sex steroid–secreting tumor—entities that all manifest an undue advancement in skeletal maturity. Accelerated somatic growth that is not accompanied by breast or pubic hair growth is unrelated to sex steroid secretion.

A. **Premature thelarche** (isolated early breast development) is a variant of normal development, presenting most frequently during the first 2 years of life. When it begins after 6 years of age, isolated breast development is most commonly a marker of either nonprogressive or progressive puberty.

1. **Clinical features.** Palpable and visible breast tissue can persist from the neonatal period into the first several years of life, because there is relatively more ovarian sex steroid secreted at this age. Most breast tissue that develops in the first few months of life regresses by the first birthday. Thelarche that appears to progress after the first birthday typically waxes and wanes, usually becoming quiescent around 36 months of age. Although it is unusual, breast growth achieved in infants with isolated premature thelarche may persist until the onset of normal puberty at the usual age. When occurring during mid-childhood (ages 3 to 5 years), thelarche may be the consequence of transient estrogen release by an ovarian cyst. Breast development that occurs as a consequence of ovarian cyst estrogen release typically regresses within a few weeks, as estrogen levels decline, although some patients have shown recurrent ovarian cysts. By definition, isolated premature thelarche is not accompanied by accelerated linear growth or advancement in skeletal maturity.

2. **Treatment.** Treatment is not indicated for isolated thelarche. Counseling and education directed toward understanding the phenomenon and, in the older girl, preventing unhealthy psychological effects of inappropriate-for-age breast development may be needed. The child with isolated thelarche should be followed at 4- to 6-month intervals to ensure that breast development is not the first manifestation of progressive precocious puberty, which subsequently shows progressive breast growth, accelerated growth rate, and advanced skeletal maturation.

B. **Premature pubarche** (early development of sexual hair, pubic or axillary). Isolated early sexual hair occurs as a result of benign **premature adrenarche** (premature pubertal secretion of adrenal androgens). However, early sexual hair may herald significant **hyperandrogenism**. This may involve ovarian hyperandrogenism and may evolve into the polycystic ovarian syndrome or, more rarely, mild forms of congenital adrenal hyperplasia or sex steroid–secreting tumor. In the two latter conditions, growth rate can be significantly accelerated and bone age significantly advanced. In contrast, children with premature adrenarche show a normal growth rate and normal or only mildly advanced skeletal maturities. In females, excessive androgens may cause early progressive sexual hair, acne, oily skin, and, rarely, clitoromegaly, deepening voice, or excessively muscular physique. Without treatment, these characteristics can progress in the pubertal years and result in hirsutism and amenorrhea (see Section I.D).

C. **Precocious puberty** (PP) is present when significant pubertal development occurs, progresses, and is associated with accelerated linear growth (Fig. 21.1). The etiology of gonadotropin-releasing hormone (GnRH)–stimulated or central precocious puberty (CPP) is early onset of pituitary gonadotropin stimulation resulting from early reactivation of the HPG axis. CPP must be differentiated from other causes of early puberty that are not driven by the HPG axis (GnRH-independent or peripheral precocious puberty [PPP]) and from nonprogressive precocious puberty, in which there is early development but no progression. Table 21.1 outlines the etiologic categories of CPP.

1. **GnRH-stimulated, central precocious puberty (pituitary gonadotropin stimulation)** may result from the following:

a. Premature activation of the HPG axis resulting in early onset of pubertal hormonal secretion without central nervous system (CNS) abnormality (also known as idiopathic CPP)

b. Redundant or excessive GnRH-releasing hypothalamic tissue, a **hypothalamic hamartoma**.

c. CNS lesions affecting the balance between stimulatory and inhibitory influences on the HPG axis, with stimulation and upregulation of intermittent GnRH secretory bursts.

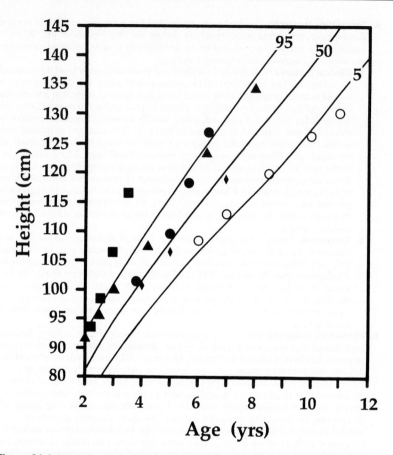

Figure 21.1. Height for age for five girls plotted against 5th, 50th, and 95th percentile standards of height for age from the National Center for Health Statistics. ■, heights of a child with mild 21-hydroxylase deficiency adrenal hyperplasia (note rapid growth acceleration from a young age); ▲, normal tall child growing consistently at the 90th percentile; ●, girl with idiopathic central precocious puberty with the onset of growth acceleration and pubertal changes at 5 years of age; ♦, child with premature adrenarche with no detectable alteration of growth rate; O, child with Turner syndrome and growth deceleration.

   d. Secondary to excessive sustained sex steroid exposure from sex steroid–producing tumors, congenital adrenal hyperplasia, or exogenous sources; such exposure during prepubertal years fosters early maturation of the HPG axis.
   Gonadarche (onset of gonadal pubertal hormone secretion) and adrenarche (onset of pubertal adrenal androgen secretion) are two independent events, which are unrelated physiologically but are usually related temporally. Although the ovaries secrete significant androgen, this may not be significant at the onset of gonadarche. Thus, girls with isolated CPP may present with only gonadarche or estrogen-stimulated findings, such as breast and genital development, without sexual hair. In precocious puberty, as in normal pubertal development, time of menarche cannot be predicted. However, it is generally accepted that menarche is typically reached between 2 and 3 years after first evidence of thelarche. Initial menstrual cycles can be ovulatory, and therefore the potential for fertility exists from menarche onward.

TABLE 21.1 Isosexual Precocious Pubertal Development

I. Pituitary gonadotropin secretion (central or true precocity)
  A. Idiopathic (including sporadic and familial)
  B. CNS abnormalities
    1. Hypothalamic hamartomas (redundant or excessive normal tissue)
    2. Space-occupying lesions (altering stimulatory–inhibitory effects)
      a. Astrocytomas
      b. Arachnoid cysts/suprasellar cysts
      c. Craniopharyngiomas
      d. Ectopic pinealomas
      e. Ependymomas
      f. Optic gliomas (with neurofibromatosis)
      g. Pituitary adenomas
      h. Tumors associated with tuberous sclerosis
    3. Resulting from cerebral damage due to:
      a. Irradiation/chemotherapy
      b. Surgery
      c. Trauma
      d. Encephalitis/meningitis/abscess
      e. Myelomeningocele
    4. Due to cerebral defects associated with CNS anomalies and other neurologic or mental defects
    5. Coincident with hydrocephalus (may be reversible), brain abscess, or granulomas
  C. Secondary to chronic exposure to sex steroids (tumors, untreated congenital adrenal hyperplasia)

II. Sexual steroid–secretion effect independent of pituitary gonadotropin (peripheral precocious puberty and precocious pseudopuberty)[a]
  A. Ovarian tumors (carcinoma, cystadenoma, gonadoblastoma, granulosa cell (may be associated with Peutz-Jeghers syndrome), lipoid, luteoma, sex cord or theca cell)
  B. Adrenal adenomas or carcinomas (rarely secrete estrogens without androgen)
  C. Exogenous sex steroids/gonadotropins[b]
  D. McCune-Albright syndrome (G-protein–activating mutation)
  E. Ectopic gonadotropin-producing tumor (virtually limited to males)
  F. Ovarian cysts[b] (also associated with the normal prepubertal states, premature thelarche, central precocious puberty, and McCune-Albright syndrome)
  G. Gonadotropin-independent puberty, full pubertal maturation, LH-receptor–activating mutation
  H. Gonadotropin-secreting pituitary adenoma
  I. Occasional consequence of chronic primary hypothyroidism likely TSH occupation of FSH receptor[b]

III. Incomplete sexual precocity
  A. Premature thelarche
  B. Premature adrenarche
    1. Premature pubarche may be the first manifestation of hyperandrogen states (CAH, PCOS)

CAH, congenital adrenal hyperplasia; CNS, central nervous system; FSH, follicle-stimulating hormone; LH, luteinizing hormone; PCOS, polycystic ovary syndrome; TSH, thyroid-stimulating hormone.
[a] Vaginal foreign body or tumor (to be ruled out in patients presenting with vaginal discharge or bleeding).
[b] Limited and potentially reversible if of short duration or treated before secondary central precocious puberty occurs.

2. In **GnRH-independent peripheral precocious puberty (precocious pseudopuberty),** clinical presentation is similar to centrally mediated puberty with breast development, sexual hair development, and accelerated linear growth.

    a. **Etiology.** By definition, the etiology is something other than pituitary gonadotropin secretion. The physical development seen results from sex steroid exposure or production that is independent of HPG axis. Causes include autonomous ovarian or adrenal hormone secretion, abnormal gonadotropin stimulation, and exogenous hormonal sources. Endocrine disruptors, particularly chemicals in the environment with estrogenlike effects, have not been shown to significantly affect pubertal onset or tempo.

        (1) Precocious puberty associated with **McCune-Albright syndrome** arises because of ovarian activity resulting from an activating mutation in the G-protein–linked cyclic adenosine monophosphate (cAMP) system. This postconception somatic mutation involves various cell lines and often involves the ovaries. The result is intermittent and autonomous ovarian estrogen secretion that stimulates abrupt pubertal changes that are followed by rapidly falling estrogen levels and withdrawal uterine bleeding. Thus, this syndrome may present with menstrual bleeding despite minimal to no breast development.

        (2) Pubertal development, particularly breast development in girls and testicular growth in boys, may rarely develop with **chronic primary hypothyroidism.** This results from the promiscuous occupation and activation of follicle-stimulating hormone (FSH) receptors on ovarian granulosa cells by the abundant thyroid-stimulating hormone (TSH). The competition of the increased levels of TSH for these FSH receptors appears to stimulate FSH-mediated changes including follicular growth with estrogen secretion as well as ovarian cyst formation and seminiferous tubule growth. In addition, the attendant hyperprolactinemia resulting from increased TRH stimulation as seen in severe hypothyroidism may play a role in breast growth.

        (3) Ovarian and adrenal sex steroid–secreting tumors are rare but may produce dramatic effects as a consequence of estrogen stimulation.

        (4) Exogenous estrogen in foods and cosmetics is regulated and is an unlikely but possible cause. Estrogen-containing medications require more than a single accidental exposure to cause physical pubertal changes.

        (5) Chorionic gonadotropin secretion of tumor origin will cause Leydig cell differentiation and testosterone secretion, resulting in precocious puberty in males. However, the luteinizing hormone (LH) effect of human chorionic gonadotropin (hCG) alone does not result in pubertal changes in females, except at peripubertal ages, because LH and FSH are necessary for estrogen secretion.

    b. **Physical changes.** In peripheral precocious puberty, as in central precocious puberty, pubertal changes can progress rapidly. Withdrawal vaginal bleeding can occur, although ovulation is not expected. Endometrial sloughing can result from excessive estrogen stimulation, fluctuation of estrogen secretion, or a sudden decrease of estrogen effect. Although the bleeding pattern may be regular, it is more often erratic.

3. The sequence of normal pubertal events designated by Tanner staging is summarized in Table 21.2. In central precocious puberty, as in normal puberty, this tempo is variable. In peripheral precocious puberty, the sequence and tempo are related to the magnitude of hormonal stimulation. Central precocious puberty accounts for >90% of all cases of early puberty in girls, and most have no identifiable abnormality and are therefore considered idiopathic. With the availability of more refined imaging, particularly magnetic resonance imaging (MRI), aberrations associated with the central nervous system, including hypothalamic hamartomas, have become more readily demonstrable. Central precocious puberty may be associated with childhood malignancies and their treatment; curiously, these patients may also develop anterior pituitary hormone deficiencies.

TABLE 21.2	Chronologic Sequence of Puberty and Approximate Range for Three Racial Groups		
	Approximate age range (y)		
Tanner stage of development and pubertal event	**Black**	**Hispanic**	**White**
Stage 1			
Prepubertal breasts, papilla elevation only, no pubic hair		Prepubertal	
Stage 2			
Breast budding, elevation of breast and papilla with increased areolar diameter	6.6–11.6	6.8–12.3	8.0–12.5
Pubic hair (long, slightly pigmented hair on labia)	6.7–11.7	7.4–12.7	8.0–12.7
Stage 3			
Further enlargement and elevation of breasts	6.8–12.5	9.5–13.3	10.8–13.3
Pubic hair spread over junction of mons pubis	8.0–12.7	9.7–13.6	8.0–13.6
Menarche	9.7–14.5	10.1–14.5	10.7–14.4
Stage 4			
Breasts: secondary mount projection of areola and papillae (does not always occur)	8.1–14.9	10.7–14.3	10.3–15.5
Adult-type pubic hair; incomplete distribution	7.6–14.3	10.7–15.8	10.6–14.8
Stage 5			
Breast development: mature	9.6–17.5	11.9–13.5	11.3–19.0
Adult quantity and distribution of pubic hair	10.2–18.4	13.5–19.3	12.5–19.7

D. Virilization in females occurs as the result of excessive androgen (hyperandrogenism).

    1. Clinical findings include hirsutism, excessive acne, clitoromegaly, deepening of the voice, an accelerated growth rate or tall stature, excessive muscle development, and a masculine habitus. Although clitoral enlargement is usually the result of a virilizing process, it may rarely occur as a result of regional disease-specific abnormal tissue growth, such as may be seen in neurofibromatosis.

    2. Laboratory findings. Hyperandrogenism is documented by elevated serum levels of testosterone, androstenedione, dehydroepiandrosterone (DHEA), and DHEA sulfate (DHEA-S) for age. Skeletal maturity (bone age) is typically significantly advanced.

    3. Etiology. Causes of virilization in prepubertal and peripubertal girls may result from the milder non–salt-wasting forms of congenital adrenal hyperplasia (CAH), especially 21-hydroxylase deficiency. Mild unexplained virilization during late prepubertal years may herald significant ovarian hyperandrogenism. Other rare causes include androgen-producing tumors (including adrenal adenomas/carcinomas and ovarian arrhenoblastomas), choriocarcinomas, dysgerminomas, and teratomas. Hormone production and malignancy vary for these tumors.

II. Evaluation

Initial assessment of patients with signs of precocious puberty includes a history (searching for factors related to etiology) and a physical examination (documenting growth, extent of sexual development, and identifying abnormal findings). A record of previous heights, such as an accurate growth chart, to identify growth acceleration is most useful.

    A. A child presenting with **only breast development** or **only pubic hair** without growth acceleration (as shown by growth points plotted for the preceding years) usually needs only careful clinical follow-up to monitor for progression and/or an increase in growth velocity.

1. **History** should determine the age at which sexual development was first noticed and explore the possibility of exogenous sex steroid exposure, family pattern of pubertal onset, and the presence of neurologic, dermatologic (café-au-lait patches), or thyroid abnormalities.

2. If previous growth history is not available in a relatively tall child with substantial breast development, a **skeletal age determination (bone-age radiograph)** can be done; if precocious puberty has caused growth acceleration, the bone age will be advanced.

3. In children presenting with breast growth, a **plasma estradiol level** using a sensitive assay (Table 21.3) may help differentiate between the slightly elevated levels seen in isolated benign premature thelarche and the clearly elevated values seen (at times intermittently) in precocious puberty.

4. Patients with pubic hair secondary to adrenarche can be documented by showing an elevated level of plasma **DHEA-S**. Levels of both DHEA-S and DHEA rise significantly at the onset of adrenarche. The half-life of DHEA-S is much more prolonged than that of DHEA, so significant elevation of DHEA-S above prepubertal levels can often be detected before DHEA levels can. On the other hand, DHEA-S has little or no clinical androgenic effect, whereas DHEA is a mild androgen. During early adrenarche, both DHEA and DHEA-S levels are above prepubertal values and are within the normal pubertal ranges. Extreme elevations of DHEA-S/DHEA should prompt consideration of a sex steroid–secreting tumor.

5. **If the bone age is advanced** or if sexual development is not isolated to one physical dimension (such as only breast or only pubic hair), an evaluation should be undertaken. In these cases, precocious puberty is best diagnosed, using GnRH or GnRH analog (GnRHa) testing, hopefully before growth patterns and skeletal age become markedly advanced. A clearly pubertal gonadotropin response, particularly luteinizing hormone, indicates a pubertal hypothalamic–pituitary axis.

   a. **GnRH or GnRHa stimulation testing** involves the intravenous/subcutaneous administration of GnRH or GnRHa with measurement of gonadotropins before and after the injection. GnRH has limited availability and is no longer used routinely for diagnostic purposes; it has been employed in doses of 100 μg or 25 to 50 μg/m^2. More commonly, GnRHa is employed for diagnostic evaluation of precocious puberty. For GnRHa, the subcutaneous aqueous preparation of leuprolide acetate is given at a dose of 20 μg/kg. A child with central precocious puberty will show a rise of gonadotropins—particularly LH—after GnRH stimulation that is of greater magnitude than is seen in prepubertal children. Sampling of gonadotropins at 30 to 60 minutes after GnRHa administration is sufficient for diagnostic testing. The magnitude of the gonadotropin response varies considerably depending on the assays used, although responses among third-generation gonadotropin assays are similar. It is important to know prepubertal and pubertal responses for the gonadotropin assay used. Generally, the rise of LH in the prepubertal female is approximately two- to fourfold above baseline, whereas the pubertal female will show at least an eight- to tenfold elevation above baseline LH. Normal prepubertal females also show a substantial rise of FSH in response to GnRHa (prepubertal males show this to a lesser degree), making the FSH response to the GnRHa stimulation testing less meaningful for evaluating central precocious puberty. Ratios of LH to FSH may be useful in differentiating a prepubertal from a pubertal response using basal or GnRHa stimulated levels. Generally, a ratio of <1 is consistent with a prepubertal state, whereas a ratio >1 suggests puberty.

   b. **A basal level of LH** within the pubertal range may be adequate to make the diagnosis of CPP, but a pubertal response to GnRH/GnRHa stimulation is definitive proof of central sexual precocity. Because gonadotropin response to GnRHa stimulation is the best evidence of a functional pubertal hypothalamic–pituitary-gonadal axis, GnRHa stimulation should be undertaken when basal gonadotropin levels do not clearly indicate puberty.

TABLE 21.3   Approximate Range of Normal Hormone Level for Females at Various Ages and Pubertal Stages

Hormone	Unit	Infancy (1–4 mo)[a]	Infancy (4–12 mo)	Childhood (1–6 y)	Puberty (stages 2–4)	Adult (stage 5)
Serum						
Luteinizing hormone (LH)	mIU/mL	0.05–7.0	0.05–0.8	0.05–03	0.05–11.7[b]	2–12[b]
Follicle-stimulating hormone (FSH)	mIU/mL	0.2–14.0	0.2–14.0	1.0–4.0	1.0–11.0	2.0–11.0
Plasma						
Estradiol (E2)	ng/dL	0.5–5.0	<1.5	<1.07	1.0–8.5	3–10
Dehydroepiandrosterone sulfate (DHEAS)	µg/dL	5–100	5–55	5–55	35–260	75–260
Dehydroepiandrosterone	ng/dL	20–380	20–100	20–140	150–800	150–850
Androstenedione	ng/dL	U–100	U–70	U–50	40–250	80–260
Testosterone (T)	ng/dL	U–12	U–12	U–12	5–60	10–60
Progesterone (P)	ng/dL	U–35	U–35	U–35	U–75[a]	20–75[a]
17-Hydroxyprogesterone (17-OHP)	ng/dL	10–85	10–85	5–85	5–90[a]	15–90[a]
Urinary						
17-Ketosteroids (17-KS)	mg/24 h	U–2	U–1	U–2	2.5–12.0	5–14

U = undetectable, below lower limits of assay.
[a] Preterm levels may vary.
[b] Levels may be greater mid-cycle and in luteal phase.

B. If the findings of a child presenting with sexual hair suggest possible excessive virilization (e.g., clitoromegaly), a pathologic cause must be ruled out. If there is a persistent endogenous source of excessive androgen, plasma **DHEA-S, DHEA, androstenedione,** or **testosterone** levels will be elevated. When plasma levels of any of these hormones are elevated, adrenal hyperplasia, adrenal tumors, ovarian tumors, and other forms of hyperandrogenism must be sought. Mild forms of adrenal hyperplasia can present with minimal but progressive virilization.

C. If a patient presents with the triad of findings indicative of precocious puberty (i.e., **breast and pubic hair development and growth acceleration**), the evaluation should confirm pubertal hormone levels and then determine whether this is gonadotropin-dependent (CPP) or gonadotropin-independent (PPP) sexual development.

   1. History should concentrate on growth patterns and rates (familial forms usually involve males but can affect both sexes), CNS symptoms or abnormalities (present or past), growth history, and possible exposure to exogenous hormones.

   2. Physical examination should document—in addition to anthropometric, neurologic, ophthalmologic, dermatologic, and general findings—sexual maturation (Tanner staging; see Table 21.2), degree of genital maturation, appearance of vaginal mucosa, clitoral and breast size, breast configuration, and, usually only if pelvic ultrasound studies are unavailable, bimanual rectoabdominal examination findings. A pink (vs. red-appearing), vaginal mucosa suggests cellular proliferation resulting from estrogen stimulation. Acne or skin pigmentation should be noted. The examination should also screen for the presence of a goiter or other physical markers of thyroid dysfunction.

   3. Laboratory evaluation

      a. To document precocious puberty and identify the etiologic category causing the early pubertal development, **hormone levels** can be documented (Table 21.3). Serum LH and FSH and plasma estradiol levels (using third-generation assays) should be measured and stratified into prepubertal, pubertal, or supraphysiologic. Plasma DHEA-S and DHEA or androstenedione allow one to classify adrenal androgen production as preadrenarche, postadrenarche (pubertal), or supraphysiologic. Androstenedione levels are less useful for this purpose because this hormone has both ovarian and adrenal sources.

      b. Bone-age radiographs are needed to record skeletal maturation in relation to age and are useful as baseline documentation for comparison with later changes.

      c. A pubertal **basal level of LH** or a pubertal response to **GnRH/GnRHa stimulation testing** (see Chapter 22, Section II.A.5) to verify central precocious puberty (Fig. 21.2), whereas lower levels or a minimal response are indicative of another etiology.

      d. MRI of the cranium is indicated if there is evidence to suggest neurofibromatosis, the McCune-Albright syndrome, or neurologic or ophthalmologic deficits, and when pubertal onset begins at an especially young age.

      e. In documented precocious puberty without known etiology, the MRI of the brain should include coronal views of the sellar and hypothalamic areas to detect otherwise nonapparent CNS abnormalities, such as hamartomas or in the assessment of neurofibromatosis.

      f. Abdominal–pelvic sonography can be used to document ovarian, adrenal, and uterine size and symmetry. It is noteworthy that ovarian cysts may be present in the ovary in association with CPP, forms of peripheral precocious puberty, and the prepubertal child.

      g. Although **electroencephalographic (EEG) abnormalities** occur in the majority of patients with idiopathic precocious puberty, findings are of minimal diagnostic value, so EEG testing is **generally not indicated.**

      h. Other workup may be indicated based on results of the physical and laboratory evaluation. More extensive neurologic assessment, thyroid function tests if **hypothyroidism** is a potential cause, and long-bone radiographs if the **McCune-Albright syndrome** is a possibility, may be indicated.

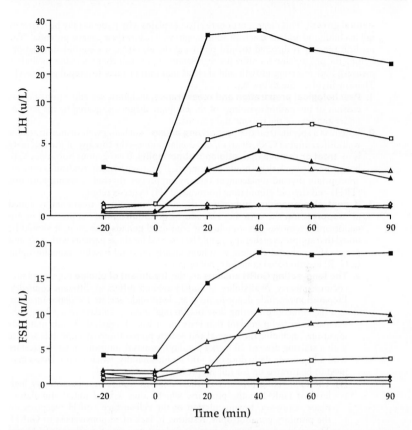

Figure 21.2. Gonadotropin-releasing hormone (GnRH) stimulation of luteinizing hormone (LH) and follicle-stimulating hormone (FSH) in six different clinical situations; 100 μg of GnRH was given as a bolus injection at time 0. ■, responses of LH and FSH in a 5-year-old with idiopathic central precocious puberty; ◊, lack of response in the same patient during suppressive GnRH analog therapy; ▲, response in a 7-year-old girl with premature thelarche; △, response of a normal prepubertal 6 year-old girl; □, minimal response in a 16-year-old hypogonadotropic girl; ◆, lack of response in a 17-year-old girl with hypogonadotropic hypogonadism secondary to a craniopharyngioma. Note scale for LH.

III. MANAGEMENT

A. Premature thelarche and **adrenarche** require only follow-up evaluation at 4 to 12-month intervals for 1 to 2 years to document any progression. Growth rates and, if excessive, bone age can be monitored. If needed, management should include psychosocial counseling of the patient and parents. After adequate assessment, the child and parents need to understand that these conditions can be considered a variant of normal, with the anticipation that current and future development and health will be otherwise normal.

B. Management of precocious puberty is aimed at stopping the untimely pubertal maturation, including menstruation, and reversing the consequences of the accelerated growth rate and skeletal maturation. Suppressive therapy is indicated to avoid the awkward situation in which young children are required to care for menstruation, to prevent the psychological/social consequences resulting from rapid pubertal progression, and to limit the compromise in adult height that may attend precocious puberty. The increased sex steroid levels for age, primarily estradiol, can cause a disproportionately greater advancement in skeletal maturation than overall statural growth. This disproportionate effect explains why patients may be relatively tall in childhood and yet reach an adult height well below their genetic potential. The medical therapy is directed toward removing the excessive sex steroid stimulation, halting the progression (or allowing regression) of pubertal characteristics (including menses), and reverting growth and skeletal maturation rates to prepubertal levels. Therapy involves the following:

1. **Psychological preparation and reassurance,** including sex education and discussion of the pathophysiology of the etiologic diagnosis, geared to the level of understanding of the patient and parents.

2. If there is a specific treatable **underlying cause**—such as a well-demonstrated or well-differentiated CNS, ovarian, or adrenal tumor—the therapy of the precocity is to **treat or remove** that **etiologic abnormality.** If exogenous hormones have been administered, they should be stopped. If primary hypothyroidism is present, appropriate thyroid replacement therapy suppresses thyroid-releasing hormone (TRH) and thyroid-stimulating hormone (TSH) hypersecretion.

3. **If central precocious puberty** is the underlying cause, treatment is aimed at **suppressing** the episodic **release of gonadotropins.** Suppression of gonadotropins removes the stimulus for continued gonadal function. It should be noted that suppressive therapy should be reserved for those patients with early and progressive pubertal changes who have clearly pubertal baseline gonadotropins or GnRHa-stimulated gonadotropin response.

   a. **The long-acting GnRH analogs** are the **treatment of choice** for central precocious puberty. Availability of GnRH analogs differs in different countries. Preparations include depot forms (e.g., leuprolide acetate for depot injection at a recommended starting dose of 300 mg/kg every 28 days or a 50-mg subcutaneous histrelin implant that lasts for at least 1 year), daily subcutaneous injections (including the original and generic preparations of leuprolide acetate with a starting dose of 20 mg/kg per day), or nasal solution (nafarelin acetate with a beginning daily dose of 1 600 μg intranasally, twice a day). Doses may need to be titrated up for full suppression.

      (1) The long-acting property of these analogs results in a persistently high level of GnRH at the pituitary, which, after a brief initial stimulatory phase, causes a downregulation of the cell-surface GnRH receptors on the pituitary gonadotrophs, resulting in lack of responsiveness to GnRH. This induced pituitary nonresponsiveness prevents the release of LH and FSH. Accordingly, episodic gonadotropin secretion ceases, gonadotropins fall, ovarian function is suppressed, and pubertal development and rapid growth rates will slow. Menstruation ceases, although there may be an episode of withdrawal bleeding within the first month of treatment if there has been significant estrogen-mediated endometrial growth.

      (2) Skeletal maturation rate will slow; however, this is often not apparent until after 6 months of suppression. Once a pubertal bone age is attained, there will be minimal progression thereafter until sex steroid exposure resumes. Growth rate will return to a prepubertal velocity (based on skeletal age).

      (3) **Adequacy of suppressive therapy** is **monitored** by random gonadotropin and sex steroid measurements, GnRH or GnRHa stimulation testing, growth rate, bone age, and physical pubertal progression.

         (a) With therapy, sexual characteristics should cease and may regress; growth and skeletal maturation rates should slow to normal for age, and random hormone sampling levels should fall into the prepubertal range.

         (b) If it is unclear whether treatment is adequate, the definite test is GnRH or GnRHa stimulation testing on therapy with measurement of LH and FSH, which should document gonadotropin responses in the prepubertal range. A single sample 1 to 2 hours after the monthly depot injection appears to be sufficient to document suppression. Estradiol levels likewise should also fall into the prepubertal range.

(4) **Side effects** are unusual. None have been clearly shown to be due to the analog itself, although the vehicle may be implicated rarely in a variety of untoward local reactions, including local reactions with induration and sterile abscess formation that may develop into granulomas (with use of the depot injectable preparation and with difficulty inserting or removing the subcutaneous implant).

(5) **After discontinuation of therapy,** pubertal hormone secretion resumes within months, followed by resumption of pubertal development. Growth and skeletal maturation resume, but in most cases no appreciable growth spurt occurs. Following timely and successful GnRHa therapy, adult height will be greater than pretreatment height prediction and will be within range of target (genetically expected) height. Bone mineral density after therapy will be normal for age. Menses begin or resume at an appropriate age, and ovulation and normal rates of fertility have been documented. No long-term sequelae have been identified.

b. **Medroxyprogesterone acetate** (Provera) can still be used in those rare situations in which the goal is merely to stop menstrual periods. It can be administered at doses ranging from 10 to 100 mg (usual dose is 20 to 30 mg) daily PO or 100 to 200 mg IM every 2 weeks. Doses are generally titrated upward as needed. Side effects include those due to glucocorticoid properties with suppression of adrenocorticotropic hormone (ACTH) and cortisol secretion and evidence of a cushingoid state.

C. **Treatment of hyperandrogenic states.** If the hyperandrogenic state is caused by an adrenal or ovarian tumor, treatment is directed toward eradicating the tumor. If it is caused by adrenal hyperplasia, appropriate treatment involves physiologic glucocorticoid and mineralocorticoid replacement therapy. With appropriate treatment, additional virilization will cease and may regress. Optimal treatment for a hyperandrogenic early pubertal girl who is at risk for progression to polycystic ovarian disease is not known.

IV. MISCELLANEOUS CONSIDERATIONS

A. **Ovarian cysts** have been associated with premature sexual development, as part of either central precocious puberty, peripheral precocious puberty, or premature thelarche. Such ovarian cysts are also seen in normal prepubertal children.

1. **Etiology.** Ovarian cysts may be an unusual outcome of the normal prepubertal recruitment and regression of ovarian follicles. Occasional follicles may continue to grow and secrete estradiol rather than following the usual pattern of limited growth and regression. Most cysts are thought to result from sporadic, albeit low-level, gonadotropin stimulation, which occurs in both normal and abnormal development. Therefore, the presence of ovarian cysts is neither indicative nor diagnostic of pathology. However, functional ovarian cysts are able to secrete sufficient estrogen to stimulate early pubertal changes.

2. **Treatment.** In most instances, cysts regress within a matter of months, even in those with central precocious puberty. Functional cysts that cause pubertal changes should be monitored, but their identification should not be followed by immediate surgical resection unless there is an impending surgical emergency. Usually, a repeat pelvic sonogram within 2 to 3 months will verify cyst regression.

B. **The McCune-Albright syndrome** is an entity that classically includes a triad of autonomous endocrinopathies (most commonly precocious puberty), polyostotic fibrous dysplasia, and café au lait skin macules. However, this entity may occur with only one or two of these findings. In this syndrome, ovarian abnormalities may present with vaginal bleeding in the absence of other features of pubertal development as a result of a significant rise of estrogen during cyst rupture that is followed by a sudden fall in estrogen levels.

1. **Associated disorders.** Other endocrinopathies that can coexist include thyrotoxicosis, excess glucocorticoid production, and acromegaly.

2. **Etiology.** The endocrinopathies that occur with this syndrome are the result of autonomous end-organ function without the stimulation of the tropic hormones,

e.g., ovarian function without gonadotropin stimulation. Each of the endocrine glands affected in this condition utilizes cAMP as the second messenger for the signal transduction pathway involving G proteins. The syndrome results from a postzygotic somatic cell mutation in the G protein responsible for coupling tropic hormone receptor–binding intracellular signaling. The result is activation of cAMP without tropic hormone receptor binding.

3. **Treatment.** To date, there is no definitive therapy, but medroxyprogesterone, ketoconazole, aromatase inhibitors, and estrogen receptor antagonists have been tried and have varying efficacy. Because the etiology is independent of pubertal gonadotropin secretion, treatment with GnRH analogs is inappropriate and ineffective unless secondary central precocious puberty ensues. Aromatase inhibitors (including third-generation letrozole and anastrazole, in addition to testolactone) appear to be effective in suppressing estrogen. There are limited data concerning the use of estrogen receptor antagonists (tamoxifen and fulvestrant) regarding effectiveness of blocking estrogen action in this syndrome. Medroxyprogesterone has been used the longest to treat the precocious puberty in this condition. Caution should be used in treating patients with severe bony lesions, as the lesions might be exacerbated as a result of the hypocalcemic effect of the drug.

C. **Precocious puberty with primary hypothyroidism.** The occurrence of sexual precocity in patients with long-term primary hypothyroidism occurs rarely.

1. **Etiology.** The pathophysiology of this disorder appears to involve the promiscuous occupation of the FSH receptor by the TSH molecule when TSH is in abundance. When the hypothyroidism is treated with thyroid hormone and TSH levels are suppressed into the physiologic range, TSH levels return to normal and premature sexual development regresses.

2. **Clinical findings.** The sexual maturation occurring in this syndrome is consistent with a primary FSH effect, the most striking effect being breast development. Full pubertal development does not occur. Multicystic ovaries occur commonly. Skeletal age may be delayed rather than advanced, because of the thyroid hormone deficiency.

3. **Treatment.** Appropriate treatment of the hypothyroidism is followed by regression of changes of puberty.

DELAYED PUBERTY

I. GENERAL PRINCIPLES
The lack of onset of pubertal characteristics (breast or pubic hair development) by age 13 and the lack of menarche by age 15 represents a significant delay. Also, a failure to complete puberty by 4 years after onset is a valid reason for investigation.

A. **Causes** of delayed or inadequate pubertal development are categorized as **hypogonadotropic** or **hypergonadotropic** states (Table 21.4).

B. **Hypogonadotropic states** may be **temporary** (delay in maturation or because of consequences of diseased or malnourished states) or **permanent** (congenital or acquired inability to synchronously secrete GnRH or gonadotropins).

1. **Genetic etiology.** There are several forms of genetic hypogonadotropism, commonly called idiopathic hypogonadotropic hypogonadism (IHH). A genetic syndrome that commonly is associated with permanent hypogonadotropism is the **Kallmann syndrome.** In the classic form, the hypogonadotropism is accompanied by anosmia or hyposmia. This syndrome appears to occur as the result of deficient migration of the GnRH-secreting neurons from their site of origin in the forebrain to the hypothalamus. Defects in the development of the forebrain would be expected to affect both these neurons and the sense of smell. There is, however, considerable variation in expression of this syndrome, and other midline craniofacial and other skeletal abnormalities may be present in patients with hypogonadotropism. It can occur in siblings of either sex. KAL1 gene mutations have been found in about half of males with familial IHH, but not in females with

TABLE 21.4   Delayed or Inadequate Pubertal Development

I. Lack of physical pubertal development
  A. Hypogonadotropic states
    1. Temporary conditions resulting from:
      a. Chronic malnutrition/malabsorption
      b. Chronic systemic disease
        (1) Cardiac
        (2) Gastrointestinal (Crohn disease)
        (3) Hematologic (sickle cell)
        (4) Pulmonary (cystic fibrosis)
        (5) Chronic renal failure
      c. Drug abuse
      d. Emotional stress
      e. Excessive physical stress/overexertion
      f. Exogenous obesity
      g. Malnutrition
      h. Normal variant, constitutional delay of puberty
      i. Psychiatric illness (anorexia nervosa)
      j. Psychosocial dwarfism
      k. Untreated endocrinopathies
        (1) Diabetes mellitus
        (2) Glucocorticoid excess
        (3) Hypopituitarism
        (4) Hypothyroidism
        (5) Isolated growth hormone deficiency
    2. Permanent hypothalamic or pituitary gonadotropin deficiency
      a. Isolated gonadotropin deficiency (nonacquired)
        (1) Pituitary (no LH and FSH response to GnRH)
        (2) Hypothalamic (good LH and FSH response to GnRH)
        (3) Unclear, possibly hypothalamic (partial response to GnRH)
      b. Associated with varying degrees of holoprosencephaly
        (1) Kallmann syndrome with anosmia or hyposmia
        (2) With central maxillary incisor
        (3) With cleft lip or cleft palate
        (4) Septooptic dysplasia (optic nerve hypoplasia)
      c. Associated with multiple pituitary hormone deficiencies
        (1) Panhypopituitarism (hypothalamic defects)
          (a) Genetic mutations
            (i) HESX1 (septo-optic dysplasia)
            (ii) LHX3 (with hypothyroidism and hypoprolactinemia)
            (iii) PROP1 with GH and TSH deficiency and hypoprolactinemia
        (2) Pituitary dysgenesis
        (3) Space-occupying lesions (craniopharyngiomas, Rathke pouch cysts, hypothalamic tumors, pituitary adenomas)
        (4) Absence of corpus callosum
        (5) Following surgery
        (6) Following cranial irradiation
        (7) Following CNS chemotherapy
        (8) Following inflammation
        (9) Infiltrative or destructive processes (autoimmune, hemosiderosis)
      d. Associated with syndromes involving hypothalamic function
        (1) Laurence-Moon-Biedl syndrome with retinitis pigmentosa, dwarfism, mental retardation (polydactyly, obesity)
        (2) Prader-Willi syndrome (neonatal hypotonia, mental retardation, short stature, hypogonadism, obesity)
        (3) Fröhlich syndrome (outdated term referring to hypogonadism and obesity resulting from a variety of causes)
        (4) Also, Alstrom, Börjeson-Forssman-Lehman, Carpenter, CHARGE, Gordon-Holmes spinocerebellar ataxia, multiple lentigines, Noonan and prosencephalon defects (also may include mid-facial cleft, cleft lip or cleft palate, and central incisor)

(continued)

TABLE 21.4	**Delayed or Inadequate Pubertal Development (*Continued*)**

3. Genetic Mutations
   a. KAL1 and FGFR1 or KAL 2 (Kallmann)
   b. Gonadotropin-releasing hormone receptor (GnRHR)
   c. FSHβ isolated FSH deficiency
   d. PROP1 (pituitary deficiency)
   e. HESX1 (septo-opti dysplasia)
   f. DAX1
   g. Prohormone convertase deficiency
   h. Contiguous to Duchenne muscular dystrophy gene
   i. Leptin and LeptinR

B. Hypergonadotropic states: no ovarian function
1. Congenital defects
   a. Gonadal dysgenesis—Turner syndrome (45,X and mosaic forms)
   b. Pure gonadal agenesis (46,XX or 46,XY)—Swyer syndrome
   c. Mixed gonadal dysgenesis (45,X/46,XY)
   d. Steroidogenic enzyme deficiencies
     (1) 17-Hydroxylase/17,20-desmolase
     (2) 17-Ketosteroid reductase
     (3) 3-β-Hydroxysteroid dehydrogenase
     (4) P-450 aromatase
2. Acquired defects: ovarian failure resulting from:
   a. Autoimmune disease
   b. Infection or inflammation
   c. Infiltration (hemochromatosis, sickle cell)
   d. Surgical resection
   e. Irradiation
   f. Chemotherapy
   g. Bilateral ovarian torsion
3. Genetic mutation
   a. FSH Receptor (FSHR)
   b. LH subunit gene mutation

II. Lack of menarche with otherwise apparent normal development
  A. Hypogonadotropic states
    1. Pubertal-aged onset of conditions in I.A.
    2. Lack of maturation of synchrony of hormonal stimulation
  B. Hypergonadotropic states
    1. Acquired defects (see I.B)
    2. Follicular ovarian dysgenesis (resistant ovary syndrome)
    3. Complete androgen insensitivity syndrome (46,XY)
    4. Pregnancy
    5. Polycystic ovarian disease
  C. Physical defects
    1. Absence of vagina or uterus
    2. Obstruction of uterine-vaginal outflow tract

CNS, central nervous system; FSH, follicle-stimulating hormone; GH, growth hormone; GnRH, gonadotropin-releasing hormone; LH, luteinizing hormone; TSH, thyroid-stimulating hormone.

IHH and anosmia. KAL2 (FGFR1) gene mutations have also been described in patients with Kallmann syndrome. Mutations in gonadotropin-releasing receptor have been identified in patients with incomplete IHH. FSH-beta (FSH β) subunit mutations have been found in some patients with pronounced pubertal delay.

  2. Bone age. It may be impossible to tell whether the hypogonadotropism is temporary or permanent until the hypothalamus and pituitary have had ample opportunity to mature. As a general rule, skeletal maturation (bone age) is reflective of hypothalamic–pituitary maturation, so a bone age of 11 years or more in girls should be accompanied by pubertal or adult patterns of gonadotropin secretion. Thus, if levels are prepubertal in a patient who is otherwise healthy and has a bone age of >11 years, and if gonadotropin levels are not elevated, one can assume that permanent gonadotropin deficiency is likely.

3. **Partial pubertal development.** In a patient who presents with some pubertal development and little or no progression, it is also difficult to differentiate delay of development from a partial or acquired hypogonadotropic state. Patients with a prolonged period between the onset of puberty and menarche may be hypogonadal. If the delay is a result of ovarian failure, gonadotropins will be elevated (assuming age and skeletal age at or greater than that when puberty usually occurs). Low gonadotropin levels, however, may be a result of delay in progression of normal maturation or an inability to secrete adequate amounts of gonadotropin. Menarche in females who subsequently have normal fertility can normally be delayed up to 5 years beyond the onset of puberty; however, such a delay is of concern and may herald abnormalities. Although it may be normal for menses to be irregular, infrequent, or anovulatory for 2 years or more after menarche, menses should progressively become more regular during the first 2 years after menarche.

C. **Hypergonadotropism** indicates primary gonadal failure and, once clearly documented, is almost always permanent. This category is the most common cause of pubertal delay in females. Etiologies are listed in Table 21.4. FSH-receptor (FSHR) gene mutations have been identified as a cause of absent breast development and primary amenorrhea.

1. **Turner syndrome** can be defined as the various clinical phenotypes resulting from varying degrees of deletion of one X chromosome. This encompasses a variety of karyotypes, including mosaic patterns with cell lines of 45,X, 46,XX, and 46,XY. Haploinsufficiency of the short-stature homeobox gene (SHOX) in the pseudoautosomal region of the X chromosome is related to many of the features of Turner syndrome.

   a. Patients with Turner syndrome have markedly elevated gonadotropin levels for the first 3 or 4 years of life, with levels dropping toward or within the normal range from approximately ages 5 to 8. Levels subsequently rise to the hypergonadotropic range as age approaches the age of puberty, so elevated levels are present when patients are referred for pubertal delay; FSH levels rise before and to a greater degree than LH levels.

   b. Turner syndrome is the most common cause of primary hypogonadism in girls (physical findings of this entity are listed in Sec II.C).

   c. Generally, the streak gonads that occur in those with the 45,X or 45,X/46,XX karyotypes are not considered to be at risk for developing gonadoblastoma, whereas all patients with a Y chromosome need gonadal resection. If there is genetic evidence of Y chromosomal material, removal of streak gonads should be considered.

2. Turner syndrome should not be confused with **Noonan syndrome,** in which some physical features are similar to those in Turner syndrome, although karyotypes are normal. Noonan syndrome is more commonly diagnosed in males, but it also occurs in females. Females with this condition usually have normal ovarian function.

D. The approach to patients with lack of menarche (see Table 21.4) is initially the same as that to patients with delayed onset or progression of puberty.

1. **Differential diagnosis.** If progression of puberty has been inadequate or incomplete in terms of physical characteristics, both hypogonadism and factors that impede gonadal function are possible (see Table 21.4-I). If physical development appears to be complete, the factors listed in Table 21.4-II should be considered.

2. **Complete androgen insensitivity.** This syndrome results from lack of androgen effect (because of deficiency or defect of androgen receptor or postreceptor mechanisms), so patients are not virilized in utero and do not masculinize at

puberty. These patients, phenotypic females but genetic males, may present with the complaint of primary amenorrhea, although most are diagnosable in infancy or childhood because of inguinal-labial gonads or inguinal hernias. Because of androgen-receptor defects and the resulting lack of feedback, pubertal-aged patients have normal to elevated gonadotropins and significantly elevated androgen levels. Estrogen levels are somewhat elevated for genetic males, and their unopposed effect results in feminization. Patients present as phenotypic postpubertal females with ample breast development and little or no sexual hair. Because of the normal effect of testicular-derived müllerian-inhibiting hormone in utero, the uterus is not present and therefore no menses occur.

II. EVALUATION

A. A blood sample to determine **gonadotropin** status is ordered at the initial visit, even if other laboratory workup is not done. A single serum sample is adequate to document or exclude a hypergonadotropic state.

B. History should review the following:

1. Rates of weight and height gain (see Fig. 21.1).

2. Evidence of current or previous illness, including various systemic diseases, especially subtle gastrointestinal disease (Crohn disease) or undiagnosed or inadequately treated endocrinopathies (hypothyroidism, adrenal insufficiency, and diabetes insipidus).

3. Previous therapy, including surgery, irradiation, and chemotherapy. Gonadotropin levels elevated above the normal range may occur shortly after chemotherapy among oncology patients, with subsequent recovery.

4. Family or pubertal history.

5. Sense of smell.

C. Physical examination should document pubertal development (often different from that reported by patients or parents), height, upper-segment/lower-segment ratios, and general and neurologic findings. The latter should concentrate on fundi, visual fields, and sense of smell. One should search for **stigmata of Turner syndrome.** These include short stature with disproportionately short lower extremities, characteristic facies with micrognathia, epicanthal folds, ptosis, low-set prominent ears, low hairline, high-arched palate, webbed neck, puffy hands and feet, shield chest with widely spaced hypoplastic nipples, cubitus valgus, numerous pigmented nevi, short fourth metacarpals, and abnormal flattened fingernails. A careful genital examination should include inspection and palpation of the inguinal area for masses and visualization of the perineum to determine clitoral size, appearance of vulva, and vaginal opening.

D. Laboratory workup

1. General approach. A single blood sample of **gonadotropin (LH, FSH) determinations** will give values in the low range (consistent with the prepubertal state, hypogonadotropism, or early puberty), in the hypergonadotropic range (clearly elevated above normal adult ranges), or within the pubertal range (this finding suggests that early hormonal puberty has occurred without physical changes). It is most unusual to find borderline elevated levels, but when this occurs, GnRH stimulation is indicated to clarify the result. A hypergonadotropic response is markedly greater than in normal individuals (see Fig. 21.2).

2. Low gonadotropins. If gonadotropin levels are low and there is a history of unusual emotional stress, ongoing excessive physical exertion, inadequate nutrition, or findings suggestive of a systemic condition, the workup should be directed toward diagnosing and correcting the primary abnormality to resolve the hypogonadotropic state.

a. A skeletal age determination (bone-age radiograph) may reflect hypothalamic-pituitary maturation. If **bone age** is less than the normal age of pubertal onset **(10 to 11 years),** it is impossible to determine whether hypogonadotropism is transient or permanent. If the bone age is at or near the age of onset of puberty and there is no concomitant abnormality that could account for hypogonadotropism, a limited workup can be done to try to differentiate the cause. A girl who has had a bone age beyond 11 years for several years and who continues to show low gonadotropin levels likely has permanent hypogonadotropism.

  b. **GnRH or GnRH analog stimulation testing** is seldom helpful in differentiating an etiology of pubertal delay and provides little more information than basal LH and FSH levels. Although complete lack of response of LH and FSH levels suggests a complete pituitary defect, this is rare except in those who have had hypophysectomy or other destruction of the pituitary gland. A clear incremental rise of LH and FSH indicates the ability of the pituitary to respond when stimulated (see Fig. 21.2), but such a response does not discriminate between a hypothalamic problem resulting in an inability to secrete GnRH appropriately and one that is merely immature. Nevertheless, a response clearly well within the pubertal range is more suggestive of potential for normalcy than a minimal rise.

  c. If the bone age is well into the usual pubertal years or if the discrepancy between bone age and chronologic age is great (e.g., bone age 12 years, chronologic age 16 years), low gonadotropin levels are due either to a permanent defect or to one of the situations described in Table 21.4. Assessment of other pituitary hormones (growth hormone, TSH, ACTH, prolactin, vasopressin) should be considered.

3. **Elevated gonadotropins.** If gonadotropins are elevated, a **karyotype** should be done to rule out Turner syndrome. Gonadal dysgenesis can occur with only subtle or no stigmata of Turner syndrome. A 46,XY karyotype may be present in patients with a female phenotype with 46,XY sex reversal, including the syndrome of pure gonadal dysgenesis, the complete androgen insensitivity syndromes, as well as patients with enzyme deficiencies in sex steroid synthesis (see Section **c** following).

  a. If there is a clear explanation of primary hypogonadism (surgical resection, tumor therapy), no further workup is indicated.

  b. To assess autoimmune disease, **antiovarian antibodies** are indicated in addition to an evaluation to determine if workup for associated autoimmune endocrine diseases should be done.

  c. **Enzyme deficiencies** are unlikely to present with pubertal delay. Most will also affect adrenal steroidogenesis and may have previously presented with evidence of adrenal abnormality. Because they represent a form of gonadal failure, hypergonadotropism will be present. If an enzyme deficiency needs to be ruled out, excessive steroid intermediates can be documented. Enzyme deficiencies that block estrogen synthesis include:

    (1) **StAR deficiency** (rare, most unlikely to present with pubertal delay, and likely to present during infancy with adrenal failure; low levels of all intermediate metabolites; both 46,XX and 46,XY individuals have female phenotype).

    (2) **17-Hydroxylase deficiency** (excessive pregnenolone and progesterone; 46,XY patients have a female phenotype, whereas 46,XY patients have genital ambiguity).

    (3) **17,20-Lyase deficiency** (excessive 17-hydroxyprogesterone, 17-hydroxypregnenolone, and progesterone). These two enzymatic conversions are controlled by a single gene and enzyme (P450c17), although in some instances two clinical syndromes may be distinct.

    (4) **17-KS reductase, 3-β-hydroxysteroid dehydrogenase, and P450 aromatase deficiency** will result in lack of or inadequate pubertal development in a 46,XX individual with a female or mildly ambiguous genital phenotype.

E. **Additional assessment for lack of menarche**

  1. **Pelvic examination** and ultrasonography can be done to detect vaginal abnormality, absence of uterus, or abnormal ovarian size.

  2. Karyotype is indicated if the uterus is absent, to rule out androgen insensitivity syndrome.

3. If LH is high and FSH is normal or moderately elevated, rule out pregnancy and androgen insensitivity syndrome and consider the diagnoses of partial ovarian failure and polycystic ovarian disease.
4. Progesterone stimulation can be done if estrogen effect is judged to be adequate by vaginal smear or estradiol levels and if the uterus is documented to be present.
   a. Medroxyprogesterone acetate, 10 mg PO daily for 10 days.
   b. Bleeding 3 to 10 days after administration of the drug indicates an estrogen-primed endometrium; therefore, gonadotropin stimulation has been adequate to stimulate estrogen, and the amenorrhea is a consequence of failure of ovulation and corpus luteum formation.
   c. Lack of bleeding suggests either gonadotropin deficiency or an inadequately developed endometrium. The latter can be ruled out by administration of estrogen plus progesterone with subsequent bleeding.

III. TREATMENT

A. Hypogonadotropic conditions resulting from ongoing physical, emotional, or systemic conditions are generally helped dramatically with replacement therapy. Such therapy is ineffective, or minimally so, however, as long as the underlying abnormality persists. Emphasis should be placed on treating the underlying condition effectively.
B. Sex steroid treatment of apparently normal individuals with delayed puberty (see Sections III.D–III.H) is not indicated for psychosocial or psychosexual reasons. A common reason for starting therapy is to promote more timely physical development.
C. Most patients with **Turner syndrome** are significantly short; although the cause is not understood, it is related to the loss of the SHOX gene.
   1. Although most of these patients are not growth hormone–deficient, treatment with growth hormone increases adult height in most patients.
   2. In pubertal-aged girls, a very-low-dose estrogen plus growth hormone may produce more linear growth and a more timely pubertal development.
D. Current therapy for permanent hypogonadism, whether due to hypogonadotropism or primary gonadal failure, is the same: administration of sex steroids to produce and maintain sexual development. (Obviously, to produce ovulation in patients with potentially functional ovaries, therapy differs.) Because of altered feedback dynamics, it is generally not appropriate to monitor adequacy of therapy of hypergonadotropic individuals by attempting to document suppression of gonadotropins into the normal range.
E. **Therapy** can begin with daily oral estrogen: ethinyl estradiol (0.02 to 0.10 mg daily), Premarin (0.3 to 1.25 mg daily), or estradiol transdermal systems (0.05 to 0.1 mg once or twice a week). Initial therapy can be begun using the lowest oral dose or the low-dose transdermal preparation applied only once a week. This provides a low level of stimulation, allowing gradual changes. Diethylstilbestrol is contraindicated. The original regimen can be continual, although cyclic therapy with the addition of a progestin should be begun within a year or when breakthrough bleeding occurs (see Section III.F). At this point or thereafter, an estrogen–progestin cyclic combination preparation may be used. Therapy should be started when judged to be appropriate based on social and psychological factors and projected adult height, and after other hormonal deficiencies have been addressed. The patient and her parents should be active participants in the decision making on the timing of pubertal induction.
F. Replacement therapy for hypogonadism should eventually involve **cyclic estrogen and progesterone administration,** although an initial period of not more than 1 year of daily estrogen treatment is appropriate. Cyclic therapy should be begun earlier if breakthrough uterine bleeding occurs during daily estrogen therapy. Unopposed estrogen followed by cyclic treatment mimics natural pubertal stimulation and may more rapidly stimulate physical pubertal development.
G. A feasible **cyclic regimen** can involve daily estrogen for the first 21 days of each calendar month. Progesterone (medroxyprogesterone acetate, 5 to 10 mg/day) is added for the last 7 to 10 days of the cycle (days 12 to 21 or days 15 to 21). No

medication is given from day 22 to the end of the month. Menstrual bleeding should begin on calendar day 25. Estrogen should be resumed on the first day of the following month, regardless of the length of the month. An alternative and simpler regimen using low-estrogen birth control pills can be used.

H. Once pubertal development is complete, the patient can choose from a variety of regimens, usually using birth control preparations (BCPs), based primarily on the desired frequency of menses. If monthly periods are desired, preparations including triphasic BCPs can be used. If four periods or fewer per year are chosen, continuous preparations, such as Seasonale, Loestrin, or Prempro can be used, interrupting for a week to allow withdrawal bleeding

I. Patients with potentially normal ovaries might respond to ovulation induction, and those with dysfunctional ovaries but a normal uterus are candidates for **in vitro fertilization.**

Selected References

Dodé C, Hardelin J-P. Kallmann syndrome: fibroblast growth factor signaling insufficiency? *J Mol Med* 2004;82:725–734.

Eugster EA, Clarke W, Kletter GB, et al. Efficacy and safety of histrelin subdermal implant in children with central precocious puberty: a multicenter trial. *J Clin Endocrinol Metab* 2007;92:1697–1704.

Grumbach MM, Styne DM. Puberty: ontogeny, neuroendocrinology, physiology and disorders. In: Larsen PR, Kronenberg HM, Melmed S, Polonsky KS, eds. *Williams Textbook of Endocrinology.* 10th ed. Philadelphia: WB Saunders/Elsevier Science; 2003:1115–1286.

Layman LC. Hypogonadotropic hypogonadism. *Endocrinol Metab Clin North Am* 2007; 36:283–296.

Lee PA, Houk CP. Gonadotropin-releasing analogue (GnRHa) therapy for central precocious puberty and other childhood disorders. *Treatments Endocrinol* 2006;5:1–8.

Lee PA, Houk CP. Puberty and its disorders. In: Lifshitz F, ed. *Pediatric Endocrinology.* 5th ed. New York: Mercel-Dekker; 2006:273–303.

Lee PA, Houk CP. Puberty timing remains unchanged. In: Walvoord E, Pescovitz O, eds. *When Puberty Is Precocious: Scientific and Clinical Aspects.* Totowa NJ: Humana Press; 2007;151–165.

Nathan BM, Palmert MR. Regulation and disorders of pubertal timing. *Endocrinol Metab Clin* 2005;34:617–641.

Reiter EO, Rosenfeld RG. Normal and aberrant growth. In: Larsen PR, Kronenberg HM, Melmed S, Polonsky KS, eds. *Williams Textbook of Endocrinology.* 10th ed. Philadelphia: WB Saunders/Elsevier Science; 2003:1003–1114.

Sedimeyer IL, Palmert MR. Delayed puberty: analysis of a larger case series from an academic center. *J Clin Endocrinol Metab* 2002;87:1613–1620.

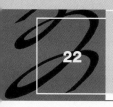

FEMALE REPRODUCTIVE ENDOCRINOLOGY IN ADULTS

22

Eric D. Levens and Alan H. DeCherney

 OVARIAN INSUFFICIENCY

Ovarian insufficiency refers to disorders of deficient ovarian function **within the ovary (primary)** or to disorders **outside the ovaries,** such as disruptions in the hypothalamic–pituitary axis or extragonadal sites resulting in deranged gonadotropin secretion **(secondary).** A follicle-stimulating hormone (FSH) level may be useful when evaluating patients suspected of ovarian insufficiency, because it may assist in localizing the site of the disruption.

I. PRIMARY OVARIAN INSUFFICIENCY (Fig. 22.1)

A. Gonadal dysgenesis. Gonadal dysgenesis represents a spectrum of pathology culminating in bilateral fibrous streak ovaries lacking primary follicles.

1. Pathophysiology

   a. Ovaries of 45,X fetuses are histologically normal until the third month of gestation. The absence or paucity of oocytes in the gonadal streak is a result of accelerated germ-cell atresia.

   b. The oocyte atresia rate is controlled by X-chromosome influences.

   c. The gonadal dysgenesis genotype spans from 45,X (sex chromatin–negative) to apparently normal karyotypes 46,XX and 46,XY (sex chromatin–positive). In between are karyotypes with deletions of chromatin material from sex chromosomes, including X-chromosome deletions of the long (46,XXq⁻) or the short arm (46,XXp⁻). The karyotype may contain more severe deletions, such as a ring X or an X isochromosome.

   d. Genotypic mosaicism consisting of more than one cell population with differing karyotypes may occur as a result of anaphase lag in the first meiotic division or abnormal mitosis after fertilization.

   e. The phenotypic spectrum of gonadal dysgenesis is broad, extending from classic 45,X Turner syndrome stigmata (short stature, primary amenorrhea, and sexual infantilism) to those with a normal karyotype and few or no somatic abnormalities.

   f. Sexual infantilism and short stature are the two most common abnormalities associated with 45,X gonadal dysgenesis and its variants. Short stature may in part be a result of haploinsufficiency of the short-stature homeobox-containing (SHOX) gene. Others features include epicanthic folds, low-set ears, a high-arched or cathedral hard palate, micrognathia, short neck, webbing of the neck, ptosis of the eyelids, shield chest, wide carrying angle of the arms, lymphedema of the dorsum of the hands and feet at birth, shortening of the fourth or fifth metacarpals or metatarsals, hypoplastic nails, osteoporosis, horseshoe kidney, coarctation of the aorta, and red–green color blindness.

   g. The term **pure gonadal dysgenesis** has been used to describe patients with streak gonads, female genitalia, and normal müllerian structures associated with 46,XX or 46,XY (Swyer syndrome) karyotypes. These individuals tend to be sexually infantile but of a normal height and lack the typical Turner stigmata.

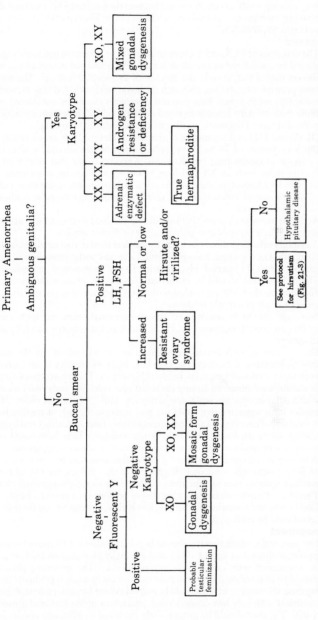

Figure 22.1. Algorithm for the workup of primary amenorrhea. FSH, follicle-stimulating hormone; LH, luteinizing hormone. (Reprinted with permission from Cave WT Jr, Streck W. Amenorrhea. In: Streck W, Lockwood DH, eds. *Endocrine Diagnosis: Clinical and Laboratory Approach.* Boston: Little, Brown; 1983:191–208.)

h. Mixed gonadal dysgenesis represents asymmetric gonadal development with a testis present on one side and a gonadal streak on the other side. These patients may develop wolffian structures and because the fetal testis is functional during fetal life; ambiguous external genitalia may occur. The typical karyotype in this setting is 45,X/46,XY.

2. Diagnosis

a. The diagnosis of 45,X and X-chromatin–positive variants of gonadal dysgenesis should be considered in any adult female with abnormal menstruation who is shorter than 5 feet, even in the absence of dysmorphic features. The majority have primary amenorrhea, although the less severely affected may present with secondary amenorrhea. Pure gonadal dysgenesis should be considered among those with primary amenorrhea and pubertal delay. These patients may be of normal stature. Diagnostic studies should include the following.

(1) Plasma FSH and luteinizing hormone (LH) levels (both are elevated).

(2) A karyotype of 30 to 50 metaphase preparations should be obtained to assist in establishing the diagnosis. Karyotypes are also helpful to identify those with an XY cell line; however, even among nonmosaic 45,X, standard karyotype may not detect a Y-chromosome–containing cell line; strong consideration should be given to performing molecular studies for a Y chromosome.

b. An intravenous pyelogram (IVP) should be obtained to detect renal abnormalities, such as a horseshoe or pelvic kidney or double ureters.

c. A careful evaluation should be made for cardiovascular abnormalities including coarctation of the aorta, bicuspid aortic valve and aortic stenosis, and prolongation of the QT_c interval. Hypertension should be managed aggressively.

d. Thyroid function should be evaluated periodically, because the incidence of autoimmune thyroiditis (Hashimoto disease) is increased in gonadal dysgenesis and can result in hypothyroidism.

e. Bone age should be ascertained before hormonal treatment with estrogen or human growth hormone (hGH) is begun and monitored carefully during treatment.

f. Short stature in 45,X gonadal dysgenesis and its variants is not the result of growth-hormone deficiency. Nevertheless, hGH use results in an increase in both short-term and long-term height achievement. The greatest improvements in stature were observed among those patients receiving early hGH treatment with a delay in estrogen replacement therapy until ≥14 years or older. Of note, studies have suggested that hGH use may increase the risk of conductive and sensorineural hearing loss and may induce higher rates of scolosis and kyphosis.

g. Carbohydrate intolerance and mild insulin resistance have been noted among many Turner syndrome patients; however, recent evidence suggests that insulin deficiency as a result of pancreatic β-cell dysfunction may be a primary feature of Turner metabolic syndrome. Regardless of the etiology, the risk of diabetes mellitus remains two to four times higher than in weight-matched controls. Therefore, glucose tolerance testing should be done on a periodic basis.

h. Conductive and sensorineural hearing loss is also common among these patients and should be evaluated.

3. Management

a. Estrogen replacement therapy should be initiated slowly (0.3 mg of conjugated equine estrogens) at age 14 or 15 and gradually increased to 1.25 or 2.5 mg in conjunction with cyclic medroxyprogesterone. The treatment philosophy should be to simulate the normal pubertal process by using a gradually increasing dose of estrogen, which should be individualized for each patient. Beginning treatment with very low doses permits attainment of the maximal growth potential. The dose should be progressively increased to induce secondary sexual development. In young adulthood, patients frequently switch to oral contraceptives or continuous-combined estrogen/progestin preparations: 100 μg ethinyl estradiol patches daily (young adulthood) and 50 μg (by age 30 to 35 years) with monthly or trimonthly progesterone withdrawal.

b. Assessment of progress should be made with frequent office visits for careful documentation of growth velocity and the attainment of pubertal milestones.

c. Psychological counseling with the goal of improving the individual's sexual self-image is an essential part of the therapeutic program.

d. Surgical correction of the somatic abnormalities may be indicated (e.g., high-arched palate, webbing of the neck, ambiguous genitalia).

e. Those with a Y chromosome or a positive assay for HY antigen should have bilateral gonadectomy because of the high incidence of gonadoblastomas.

f. Careful follow-up is essential because of the projected long-term administration of estrogens. Any abnormal uterine bleeding pattern should be investigated with endometrial sampling.

B. Menopause

1. Pathophysiology

a. **Menopause** refers to the time around menstruation cessation (mean age of 51 years). **Perimenopause** refers to the menopausal transition, which has been divided into early and late based on the variability of the menstrual cycle.

b. Other symptoms and signs of menopause include vasomotor instability, anxiety, depression, irritability, osteoporosis, and conditions associated with epithelial atrophy such as dyspareunia, pruritus, and genitourinary (GU) symptoms.

c. Symptom severity varies among individuals and relates to ovarian estrogen deficiency as well as to personal, familial, and societal attitudes toward aging. Between 25% and 40% of women require medication for menopausal symptom relief.

2. Diagnosis

a. Menopause should be suspected as a cause of amenorrhea in any postpubertal female who has the symptoms listed in Section I.B.1.

b. Hypoestrogenism (estradiol levels average 15 pg/mL) and elevated FSH levels (>20 mIU/mL) is consistent with menopause.

c. Menstruation may cease before age 40 as a result of primary ovarian insufficiency; this condition is termed **premature ovarian failure (POF).** Causes include cytotoxic drugs, irradiation, autoimmune oophoritis, and idiopathic. Expansion of CGG repeats within the FMR1 (*fragile X mental retardation 1*) gene has been associated with fragile X syndrome; whereas premutations in the FMR1 gene have been linked to idiopathic POF.

d. An elevated FSH level does not exclude future ovulation, because patients have been described who show ovulation and even pregnancy after a transient period of elevated FSH levels.

3. Management

a. Indications for therapy

(1) Disabling hot flushes

(2) Severe mucosal atrophy of the GU tract

(3) Osteoporosis

(4) Certain psychiatric symptoms

b. Absolute contraindications to estrogen therapy

(1) Estrogen-dependent tumors, especially of the breast

(2) Acute or chronically impaired liver disease

(3) Thromboembolic disease

c. Relative contraindications

(1) Hypertension

(2) Migraine headaches

(3) Fibrocystic disease of the breast

(4) Chronic thrombophlebitis

(5) Gallbladder disease

(6) Hyperlipidemia

d. General principles of therapy

(1) Not all women require or need estrogen therapy for menopause.

(2) Therapy should be limited to those with severe or disabling symptoms.

(3) No data exist on the safest duration of therapy.

(4) The lowest effective dose should be used, because complications are related to dosage and length of therapy. Progesterone should be used in conjunction with estrogen in those with an intact uterus.

(5) Despite recent evidence suggesting that hormone therapy may convey some cardioprotective benefits in selected populations of women in early menopause, hormone therapy should not be used for the primary or secondary prevention of disease at the present time.

e. Therapy program

(1) Continuous 0.625-mg conjugated equine estrogen and medroxyprogesterone, 2.5 to 5.0 mg, may be used to begin therapy. This dose may be adjusted as symptoms abate or persist.

(2) Cyclic estrogen therapy consisting of 3 weeks on, 1 week off, with a progestational agent (medroxyprogesterone acetate, 5 to 10 mg per day) the last 10 days of estrogen therapy as an option. However, patients should be instructed to expect menstrual flow.

(3) Estrogen alone may be used for women without an intact uterus who are not at risk for developing endometrial hyperplasia.

f. Follow-up of therapy

(1) Any abnormal uterine bleeding should be thoroughly investigated with endovaginal ultrasound and possibly endometrial biopsy.

(2) Regular periodic examination with careful observation for complications should take place every 6 to 12 months.

C. Corpus luteum deficiency

1. Pathophysiology. Deficient corpus luteum function, also termed **luteal phase defect,** remains a controversial diagnosis; nevertheless, it is defined as luteal progesterone production that is inadequate to support the development or to sustain receptive endometrium for implantation. Although they are rarely the cause of primary infertility, luteal phase defects have been implicated as a <u>cause of repeated early miscarriages</u>.

a. Any disturbance of follicular growth and development can produce an inadequate follicle and a deficient corpus luteum.

b. Specific causes include suppressed gonadotropin-releasing hormone (GnRH) production, inadequate FSH level early in the cycle, a deficient ovulatory surge of LH, an inadequate tonic level of LH, deficiency of LH receptors on the cells of the corpus luteum, or the use of drugs to induce ovulation.

c. Secondary causes include severe systemic illnesses, medications (i.e., opioids or nonsteroidal anti-inflammatory agents), endocrinopathies (hyperprolactinemia, hyperandrogenism, or thyroid dysfunction), and endometrial defects.

d. The clinical presentation of the luteal phase defect is recurrent early miscarriages or shortened menstrual cycle length. However, the primary complaints are more likely related directly to the cause, such as galactorrhea or hyperandrogenism.

2. Diagnosis

a. Diagnosis of corpus luteum deficiency depends on documentation of inadequate progesterone production or altered life span of the corpus luteum. Normal basal body temperatures (BBT) should be biphasic, with the luteal phase marked by an increased core body temperature of approximately $1°C$, occurring at the time of corpus luteal function (~12 to 14 days). Chaotic BBT readings in which there are no apparent mid-cycle temperature shifts preceding the onset of menses strongly suggest anovulation.

b. Diagnosis may be made by endometrial histology on the 26th day of the cycle to determine if histologic features are compatible with the menstrual dating. Classically, with inadequate progesterone production, the histologic dating of the endometrium lags behind the menstrual cycle by 2 days or more. There is also disparity in the histologic characteristics of the stroma and glands of the endometrium.

c. A random progesterone level of <3 ng/mL reflects anovulation and is abnormal.

3. Management
   a. Treatment should be directed at correcting the etiologic factor. Hyperprolactinemia can be reversed with bromocriptine (see Chapter 10 for dosage). Inadequate follicle stimulation may be improved with clomiphene or FSH. Certain hyperandrogenic states, particularly those of nontumorous adrenal origin, can be suppressed with a low dose of glucocorticoid, such as dexamethasone, 0.25 mg at bedtime. The initial dose of clomiphene (50 mg per day for 5 days) may be increased to 100 mg and then to 150 mg at intervals of two or three cycles.
   b. Synthetic progestational agents should not be used because they are teratogenic and luteolytic.
   c. The luteal phase defect can also be managed with progesterone suppositories (vaginal or rectal, 50 mg twice a day) to produce a physiologic level of circulating progesterone and lengthen the menstrual cycle by about 3 days.
D. The resistant ovary syndrome
   1. Pathophysiology
   a. An extremely rare cause of primary hypo-ovarianism is resistance to gonadotropins with an unknown etiology. It is characteristically seen in young women with amenorrhea, elevated peripheral gonadotropins, normal secondary sexual characteristics, 46,XX karyotype, and normal immature ovarian follicles who are unresponsive to exogenous gonadotropin administration. The cause for the resistance to gonadotropins is unknown but may be related to abnormalities of the gonadotropin receptors. Resistant ovary syndrome may be <u>distinguished from POF by the presence of ovarian follicles</u>.
   b. Patients with this disorder are not totally estrogen-deficient. The estrogen source is probably from partial stimulation of the follicles and from the peripheral conversion of androgens to estrogens.
   2. Diagnosis. The diagnosis requires documentation of the presence of only unstimulated follicles, which necessitates biopsy of an ovary. The finding of normal peripheral inhibin B levels may also assist in the diagnosis.
   3. Management. Treatment depends on the goal of the patient. If pregnancy is desired and there is evidence of some estrogen production with an occasional LH level higher than the FSH level, the induction of ovulation may be attempted. If pregnancy is not desired, treatment consists of estrogen–progestogen therapy.

II. SECONDARY OVARIAN HYPOFUNCTION (Fig. 22.2)
A. Hypogonadotropism
   1. Pathophysiology
   a. Ovarian hypofunction secondary to low gonadotropin levels is a common cause of menstrual problems and infertility. <u>FSH</u> has been suggested to be the preferred indicator of <u>hypergonadotropic hypogonadism</u>. <u>LH</u> may be the preferred indicator of <u>hypogonadotropic hypogonadism;</u> plasma LH levels <0.5 mIU/mL indicate hypogonadotropism. Altered gonadotropin secretion can result from disturbances in the pituitary or hypothalamus. Hypogonadism in the setting of delayed puberty should warrant consideration of magnetic resonance imaging (MRI) of the brain.
   b. <u>Hypothalamic amenorrhea</u> is the most common variety of hypogonadotropic hypogonadism. The disorder may be functional or may result from an organic lesion such as a tumor from trauma.
   c. Patients with hypogonadotropism can be subdivided into those with deficient estrogen production and those with normal or excessive estrogen production. Conditions that produce hypogonadotropism as a result of primary involvement of the hypothalamic–pituitary axis are usually associated with hypoestrogenism. Examples include **Sheehan disease** (hypopituitarism secondary to a pituitary infarction following obstetric shock because of excessive bleeding), isolated gonadotropin deficiency, space-occupying lesions of the sella turcica, congenital defects, and trauma. Increased estrogen secretion from ovarian tumors and functional cysts of the ovary suppress the secretion of LH and FSH, causing anovulation and hypogonadotropism.

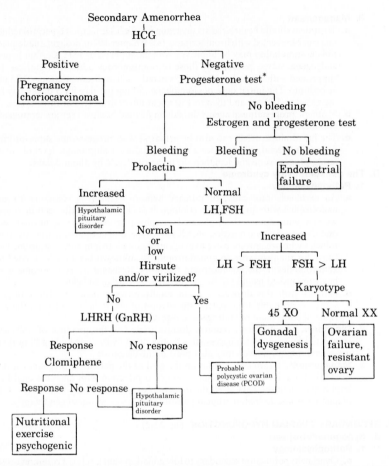

Figure 22.2. Algorithm for workup of secondary amenorrhea. HCG, human chorionic gonadotropin; FSH, follicle-stimulating hormone; GnRH, gonadotropin-releasing hormone; LH, luteinizing hormone; LHRH, luteinizing hormone–releasing hormone. *Obtain LH, FSH. (Reprinted with permission from Cave WT Jr, Streck WF. Amenorrhea. In: Streck WL, Lockwood DH, eds. *Endocrine Diagnosis: Clinical and Laboratory Approach.* Boston: Little, Brown; 1983:191–208.)

2. **Diagnosis.** Secondary hypogonadism causes include stress, sudden weight loss, emotional disturbances, Kallmann syndrome, and "post-pill" amenorrhea.

   a. **Kallmann syndrome** is a congenital hypogonadotropic state resulting from deficient GnRH secretion by the hypothalamus with associated anosmia secondary to olfactory bulb agenesis. Classically, this syndrome affects men as a result of mutations in the *KAL* gene on the short arm of the X chromosome; however, women may present with amenorrhea and anosmia. This may be the result of mutations in numerous genes resulting in X-linked, autosomal dominant or autosomal recessive transmission. Recently, GPR 54 has been implicated in the pathogenesis of GnRH deficiency in the setting of a normal sense of smell.

   b. **Post-pill amenorrhea** represents a heterogeneous group of disorders, including profound suppression from oral contraceptive therapy. Post-pill amenorrhea is also a common presenting complaint of patients who have pituitary microadenomas producing prolactin. The diagnosis of hypothalamic amenor-rhea is one of exclusion; the pituitary must be fully evaluated to exclude it as a source of dysfunction. This may also be the presenting symptom of premature ovarian failure [Section I.B.2(1)].

3. Management

   a. Removal of any organic lesion (e.g., tumor).

   b. Alleviation of the dysfunctional causes, such as weight loss, emotional conflict, and stress.

   c. If fertility is not a consideration and if simple measures are not successful in restoring ovulation, cyclic estrogen–progestogen therapy is indicated but should not be continued indefinitely. Therapy should be suspended for a few months each year to see if function has recovered.

B. Hyperprolactinemia. Hyperprolactinemia may alter ovarian function by a direct effect on the hypothalamus altering the pulsatile secretion of GnRH. Additionally, pituitary GnRH receptors may be decreased as a result of the hyperprolactinemia resulting in reduced gonadotropin release. Moreover, elevated prolactin concentrations may have a lytic effect on the developing corpus luteum, further interfering with ovulation. Correction of hyperprolactinemia usually restores normal function of the hypothalamic–pituitary–ovarian axis.

C. Adrenal disorders

   1. Increased cortisol production reduces the responsiveness to GnRH.

   2. Increased androgen production alters gonadotropin secretion; for example, a patient with virilizing congenital hyperplasia may exhibit a prepubertal GnRH response, resulting in an increased FSH response in comparison with the LH response.

D. Thyroid dysfunction. Disordered thyroid function can cause anovulation with deranged menstruation. Hypothyroidism characteristically causes menometrorrhagia, whereas hyperthyroidism usually causes amenorrhea. Autoimmune thyroiditis may be associated with autoimmune oophoritis.

 OVARIAN HYPERFUNCTION

I. HYPERANDROGENISM (Fig. 22.3)

Hyperandrogenism refers to excessive production of androgens by the ovary or the adrenals or either increased conversion of androgens, particularly testosterone, from steroid precursors by certain peripheral tissues or an increased rate of utilization by androgen-responsive tissues. Hyperandrogenism is a common endocrinopathy and can present clinically as seborrhea, acne, infertility, hirsutism, or virilization. The most common finding associated with hyperandrogenism is the **polycystic ovary syndrome (PCOS).**

A. Polycystic ovary syndrome

   1. Pathophysiology. Polycystic ovary syndrome, also known as Stein-Leventhal syndrome, is a condition in which enlarged ovaries secrete excess androgens as a result of theca and stromal cell hyperplasia. Dehydroepiandrosterone sulfate (DHEAS), the unique adrenal androgen, and the urinary 17-ketosteroids are normal. There is hyperresponsiveness of the androgens to LH (human chorionic gonadotropin). The central abnormality is the increased LH/FSH ratio, which may reflect an abnormality (either primary or secondary) of the central nervous system (CNS) control of LH. Androgen-secreting ovarian tumors, such as luteomas, thecomas, Sertoli-Leydig, and hilar cell tumors must be excluded; despite ovarian androgen hypersecretion, these tumors would not be classified as PCOS. Ovarian hyperandrogenism is associated with the hyperinsulinism of various insulin-resistant states. The elevated insulin enhances the LH-induced ovarian androgen secretion.

   2. Diagnosis

      a. History and physical examination. A thorough history and physical examination are essential, particularly in identifying critical conditions associated

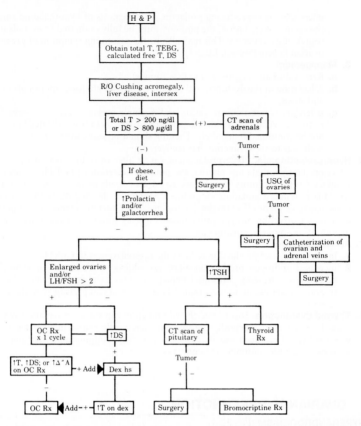

Figure 22.3. Algorithm for the diagnosis and management of hirsutism and hyperandrogenemia. CT, computed tomography; dex, dexamethasone; DS, dehydroepiandrosterone sulfate; FSH, follicle-stimulating hormone; H&P, history and physical examination; LH, luteinizing hormone; OC, oral contraceptive; T, testosterone; TEBG, testosterone-estradiol–binding globulin; TSH, thyroid-stimulating hormone; USG, ultrasonography; Δ^4-A, $\Delta 4$ androstenedione. (Reprinted with permission from Givens JR. Ovaries. In: Wilson J, Foster DW, eds. *Williams Textbook of Endocrinology.* 7th ed. Philadelphia: WB Saunders; 1985.)

with hyperandrogenism, such as Cushing disease, acromegaly, liver disease, intersex states, and androgen-secreting tumors of the ovary or adrenal gland. After excluding other causes of hyperandrogenism, two of the three following must be present to diagnose PCOS: (1) oligo- and/or anovulation; (2) clinical and/or biochemical hyperandrogenism; (3) polycystic ovaries as defined by the presence of 12 or more 2- to 9-mm follicles in each ovary or ovarian volume >10 mm^3. Menstrual history will identify cases of oligo- and/or anovulation.
  b. **Androgen assays.** The diagnosis of hyperandrogenism is dependent on clinical signs or biochemical hyperandrogenism. The biochemical assessment depends on the availability of specific radioimmunoassays including total and/or free testosterone (T). Androstenedione (A) and DHEAS may be measured but are rarely useful in the clinical setting if the total testosterone does not exceed 200 ng/dL.
  c. **Androgen levels.** If total T is >200 ng/dL or if the DHEAS level is >800 μg/dL, an ovarian or adrenal androgen-secreting tumor should be strongly suspected.

Because DHEAS is a marker for adrenal activity, an elevated DHEAS level is presumptive evidence of increased adrenal androgen secretion. Computed tomography (CT) or magnetic resonance imaging of the adrenals and vaginal ultrasonography of the ovaries should be performed. If a suspected tumor is not located, percutaneous differential catheterization of adrenal and ovarian veins with measurement of the appropriate steroids in the effluent blood should be considered.

  d. Clinical hyperandrogenism. Clinical hyperandrogenism may be assessed using the modified Ferriman-Gallwey scoring system.

  e. Transvaginal ultrasound. The ovarian volume typically exceeds 10 mm^3, and each ovary contains 12 or more 2- to 9-mm follicles.

3. Management. Therapy should be determined by the patient's goal.

  a. If fertility is desired, induction of ovulation with <u>clomiphene</u> citrate is the choice of therapy. For dosage, see Section I.C.3.

  b. If fertility is not a goal, low-dose combination <u>oral contraceptive</u> with an estrogen content of <50 μg is the treatment of choice to suppress LH hypersecretion. The usual contraindications for oral contraceptive use should be applied. After one or two cycles of combination oral contraceptive therapy, the T and A plasma levels should be in the normal range if the hyperandrogenism is LH-dependent.

  c. If oral contraceptive therapy is contraindicated, <u>spironolactone</u> may be utilized (give 25 to 200 mg per day until the first day of menses, then stop for 7 days; resume on day 8 and repeat this cycle for 3 to 6 months). If the response is inadequate or absent, increase the dose stepwise to 400 mg per day. Tumors must be surgically removed.

  d. <u>Metformin</u>, 850 to 1 000 mg per day, may be used to correct insulin resistance.

B. Combined adrenal and ovarian hyperandrogenism

1. Pathophysiology. Combined adrenal and ovarian hyperandrogenism may result from deficiency of the steroidogenic enzymes 3β-hydroxysteroid dehydrogenase, which converts the Δ5 to Δ4 compounds, including DHEA to androstenedione, pregnenolone to progesterone, and 17-hydroxypregnenolone to 17-hydroxyprogesterone. This enzyme system is also deficient in the adrenals, but not in the peripheral tissues. Deficiency of the enzyme **17-ketosteroid reductase,** which converts androstenedione to testosterone and estrone to estradiol, is also associated with polycystic ovaries. These patients have high levels of androstenedione and estrone.

2. Diagnosis. The diagnosis of 3β-hydroxysteroid dehydrogenase deficiency remains controversial but nevertheless requires clinical suspicion and documentation of an abnormally high precursor (pregnenolone, 17α-OH pregnenolone, dehydroepiandroandrosterone)/product (progesterone, 17α-OH progesterone, androstenedione) ratio at the three critical steroidogenic steps. A firm diagnosis may not be practical in a clinical setting. Response to therapy can be followed using DHEAS levels.

3. Management. Deficiency of either of these enzyme systems induces androgenic polycystic ovaries as well as androgenic adrenals.

  a. If fertility is desired, the treatment of choice is glucocorticoid suppression using a low dose of dexamethasone (DEX) to suppress the adrenal source of DHEA and DHEAS. The initial dose should be 0.25 mg at bedtime.

  b. The magnitude of the suppression of DHEAS need not be profound. The goal of therapy should be to bring the DHEAS level to within the normal range after 4 weeks of DEX administration. Cortisol level should range from 3 to 5 μg/dL. The overall guiding principle is to use the lowest dose of DEX that will suppress DHEAS levels to between 100 and 200 μg/dL. Some women are exquisitely sensitive to DEX; they may develop some of the symptoms of Cushing syndrome if not carefully followed and the dose of DEX is not adjusted monthly. Some maintain suppression of DHEAS on 0.125 mg taken 3 times a week at bedtime.

  c. Therapy should be discontinued at the end of 1 year to evaluate whether continued therapy is necessary. If the DHEAS is not adequately suppressed with

0.25 mg of DEX, then one can add low-dose contraceptive therapy. This treatment suppresses DHEA from the ovaries and reduces the androgens that were not responsive to DEX.

C. Primary adrenal and secondary ovarian hyperandrogenism

1. **Pathophysiology. Primary adrenal hyperandrogenism,** such as occurs in nonclassic 21-hydroxylase and 11β-hydroxylase enzyme deficiencies, may induce polycystic-appearing ovaries by the increased positive feedback on LH secretion as a result of increased E1 levels derived from the increased secretion of adrenal A.

2. **Diagnosis.** Nonclassic 21-hydroxylase deficiency is diagnosed by comparing the magnitude of an exaggerated response of 17-hydroxyprogesterone following 25 μg of synthetic ACTH to a normogram of the responses of classic and nonclassic enzyme deficiency. Basal T and A are also elevated.

3. **Management.** Treatment consists of adrenal suppression using a low dose of DEX (0.25 mg at bedtime), as previously described.

D. Adrenal hyperandrogenism with decreased ovarian function

1. **Pathophysiology.** The amenorrhea-galactorrhea syndrome is frequently associated with hyperandrogenism. Prolactin induces adrenal androgen hypersecretion but inhibits steroidogenesis in the ovary.

2. **Diagnosis.** Associated with hyperprolactinemia are depressed levels of T and dihydrotestosterone. Circulating DHEAS can be increased.

3. **Management.** Correction of the hyperprolactinemia corrects the androgen excess state from the adrenals and restores normal function of the ovary.

II. HYPERESTROGENISM

A. Pathophysiology

1. The most common cause of estrogen excess is increased conversion from androgens in peripheral tissues, such as liver, skin, and fat.

2. Excess estrogen production in peripheral tissues can result from:
   a. Increased substrate (hyperandrogenism)
   b. Increased percentage conversion of androgens
   c. A combination of the above

3. Ovarian hypersecretion of estrogens results either from primary disease or from secondary hyperstimulation by human chorionic gonadotropin (HCG) secreted by a tumor such as a teratoma or teratocarcinoma. Primary ovarian disorders causing hyperestrogenism include:
   a. Functioning follicular cysts
   b. Granulosa-theca cell tumors of the ovary

B. Diagnosis. Excess estrogen is documented by increased levels in the blood or urine (or both) and by the clinical signs and symptoms resulting from the hormonal derangement, such as isosexual precocious development, advanced bone age, and abnormal uterine bleeding. Gonadotropins may be suppressed and thyroid-binding globulin (TBG) and testosterone-estradiol binding globulin (TEBG) increased. Assay for HCG is positive in those having an ectopic source.

C. Management

1. Therapy is directed to the specific etiologic factor.

2. Tumors of the ovary and tumors associated with ectopic production of HCG should be identified and removed.

3. Hyperandrogenic conditions should be corrected.

4. Efficacy of therapy should be monitored by specific estrogen assays.

Selected References

Arici A, Matalliotakis IM, Koumantakis GE, et al. Diagnostic role of inhibin B in resistant ovary syndrome associated with secondary amenorrhea. *Fertil Steril* 2002;78:1324–1346.

Bondy CA. New issues in the diagnosis and management of Turner syndrome. *Rev Endocr Metab Disord* 2005;6:269–280.

Guzick DS, Carson SA, Coutifaris C, et al. Future trends in infertility treatment: challenges ahead. *Fertil Steril* 1997;68:977–980.

Jaffe RB. Disorders of sexual development. In: Strauss JF, Barbieri RL, eds. *Yen and Jaffe's Reproductive Endocrinology.* 5th ed. Philadelphia: Elsevier Saunders; 2004:463–491.

Legro RS, Barnhart HX, Schlaff WD, et al. Clomiphene, metformin, or both for infertility in the polycystic ovary syndrome. *N Engl J Med* 2007;356:551–566.

Lobo RA. Menopause and aging. In: Strauss JF, Barbieri RL, eds. *Yen and Jaffe's Reproductive Endocrinology.* 5th ed. Philadelphia: Elsevier Saunders; 2004:421–452.

Mastroianni L. Statistically valid infertility research. *Fertil Steril* 1999;72:398–400.

New MI. Extensive clinical experience: nonclassical 21-hydroxylase deficiency. *J Clin Endocrinol Metab* 2006;91:4205–4214.

Rotterdam ESHRE/ASRM-Sponsored PCOS Consensus Workshop Group. Revised 2003 consensus on diagnostic criteria and long-term health risks related to polycystic ovary syndrome. *Fertil Steril* 2004;81:19–25.

Seminara SB, Messager S, Chatzidaki EE, et al. The GPR54 gene as a regulator of puberty. *N Engl J Med* 2003;349:1614–1627.

Soules MR, Sherman S, Parrott E, et al. Executive summary: Stages of Reproductive Aging Workshop (STRAW). *Fertil Steril* 2001;76:874–878.

Wittenberger MD, Hagerman RJ, Sherman SL, et al. The FMR1 premutation and reproduction. *Fertil Steril* 2007;87:456–465.

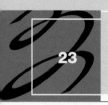

DISORDERS OF SEXUAL DEVELOPMENT IN THE PEDIATRIC AND ADOLESCENT MALE

Louis C.K. Low and Christina Wang

I. NORMAL SEXUAL DEVELOPMENT

A. Fetal

1. **Sex determination.** In humans, the process of sex determination commits the undifferentiated gonads to develop into testes or ovaries, usually by the seventh week of gestation, depending on the presence or absence of the Y chromosome and the sex-determining region on the Y-chromosome gene, SRY. Several transcription-factor genes are required for the early development of the bipotential gonads, including empty spiracles homolog 2 (EMX2), GATA-binding protein 4 (GATA4), LIM homeobox protein 9 (LHX9), steroidogenic factor 1 (SF1), Wilms tumor 1-KTS isoform (WT1-KTS), and chromobox homolog 2 (M33) (Fig. 23-1). SF1 and WT1 act in concert to affect the expression of male specific genes downstream of SRY, and a double dose of the dosage-sensitive sex-reversal adrenal hypoplasia congenita X-linked gene (DAX1) may impair testis development by interfering with the SF1/WT1 synergy. The expression of SRY must reach a threshold level at a critical time in the cascade of early events leading to testis differentiation, before male sex determination occurs; otherwise, the ovary-determining pathway will initiate in the bipotential gonad. However, there are factors downstream of SRY, such as SRY-box 9 gene (SOX9), autosomal genes, and X-linked genes, that are crucial components of the male sex-determining pathway. SRY expression in gonadal somatic cells initiates the differentiation of Sertoli cells, which aggregate around the germ cells to form seminiferous tubular cords and the interstitial space of the testes. Many signaling molecules are required for the differentiation of the peritubular myoid cells, endothelial cells, Leydig cells, and germ cells in the testes. The Leydig cells, fibroblasts, and the typical vasculature of the male gonad make up the interstitial space of the testes. The process of sexual differentiation follows, with the gonads releasing sex-specific signaling molecules or hormones that are responsible for the development of the phenotypic sex of the individual.

  In humans, mutations in WT-1 gene lead to defective development of the external genitalia and the kidneys (Denys-Drash and Frasier syndromes). A double dose of DAX1 gene leads to sex reversal in 46,XY individuals. SOX9 may be required to potentiate the action of SRY, and mutations in SOX9 cause camptomelic dysplasia, an autosomal dominant condition characterized by skeletal, cardiac, and renal abnormalities, and 46,XY sex reversal. 46,XY patients harboring SF1 mutations have sex reversal or ambiguous genitalia together with either normal or impaired adrenal function. A female patient with a heterozygous SF1 mutation was reported to have apparently normal ovarian function and adrenal failure. More information on sex development and its disorders is presented in Chapter 21.

2. **Sex differentiation.** Male phenotypic differentiation is dependent on the action of three hormones: müllerian-inhibiting substance (MIS), testosterone, and dihydrotestosterone. MIS and testosterone are secreted by the fetal testis, and testosterone is converted to dihydrotestosterone by the enzyme $5\text{-}\alpha\text{-reductase}$ within the testis and in peripheral tissues. SF1 regulates adrenal and gonadal expression of many genes and enzymes involved in steroidogenesis. Testosterone biosynthesis by the Leydig cells is controlled by enzymes, and deficiency of these

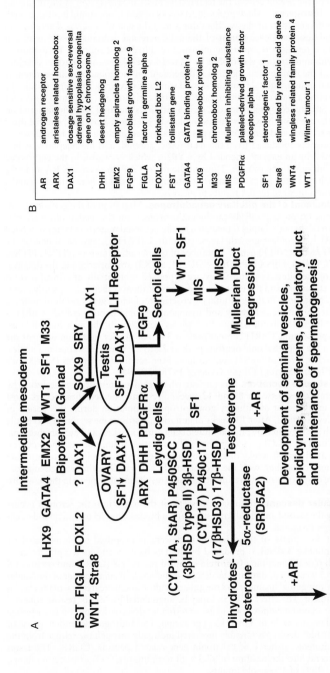

Figure 23.1. A: Pathway of sexual differentiation. **B:** Genes involved in sex development.

enzymes can lead to abnormal genital development in males (Fig. 23.1). MIS produced by the Sertoli cells of the fetal testes causes the regression of the müllerian ducts. Testosterone, which peaks at 20 weeks of gestation, stimulates the growth and differentiation of the wolffian ducts into the epididymis, vas deferens, and seminal vesicles. Development of the male external genitalia from 6 weeks of gestation onwards is under the influence of dihydrotestosterone. Formation of the penis and scrotum is complete by 12 to 14 weeks' gestation. Further development of the male external genital is dependent on the gonadotropin secreted by the fetal pituitary gland from the second trimester onwards. The germ cells in the testes enter a state of mitotic arrest after differentiation and remain so until after birth. Stimulated by retinoic acid, gene 8 (Stra8) is required for meiotic initiation in both sexes. Stra8 expression is stimulated by retinoic acid (RA), and the three major retinoic acid receptor isotypes are expressed in the gonads in both sexes. RA, possibly produced from the fetal testis, adrenal, and mesonephros, is metabolized by an enzyme encoded by CYP26, which is present in the embryonic testis but not in the ovaries. Thus, in the male, CYP 26 decreases RA and Stra 8, resulting in the germ cell entering into mitotic arrest, whereas in the female, activation of Stra8 by RA results in meiosis.

3. **Development of the pituitary gonadotropes.** Migration of the gonadotropin-releasing hormone (GnRH)–producing neurons from the medial olfactory placode to the hypothalamus is mediated by the neuronal migration factors encoded by KAL1, fibroblast growth factor receptor 1 (FGFR1), and nasal embryonic LHRH factor (NELF) genes. A number of transcription factors (PITX1, PITX2, LHX3, LHX4, HESX1, PROP1, POU1F1, SOX3) are important in the development of the pituitary gland. They are expressed sequentially at critical periods of development, and the expression of many of them is then subsequently attenuated. Mutations in these pituitary transcription factors genes result in multiple pituitary hormone deficiency and hypogonadotropic hypogonadism. GnRH is detectable in the hypothalamus by 9 weeks' gestation. In the male human fetus, the hypothalamic GnRH content peak at 34 to 38 weeks' gestation whereas the level in the hypothalamic neurons peak at 22 to 25 weeks' gestation in females, and higher levels of GnRH content have been reported in females (Siler-Khodr TM, Khodr GS. *Am J Obstet Gynecol* 1978:130:795).

4. **Testosterone secretion.** It is unclear what regulates testosterone secretion by the fetal testes between 8 and 12 weeks. Testosterone secretion occurs most likely independent of pituitary gonadotropin stimulation during this period of fetal development. After 13 weeks of gestation, testosterone secretion and penile growth are regulated by pituitary luteinizing hormone (LH) and human chorionic gonadotropin (hCG) present in the fetal circulation. Fetal testosterone secretion peaks at about 20 weeks of gestation and then progressively falls toward late gestation, coinciding with the decline in LH and HCG in the fetal circulation. Failure of testosterone secretion at this time results in micropenis in the newborn infant.

5. **Testicular descent.** In humans, descent of the testes into the scrotum occurs during the second and third trimesters, and a biphasic model of testicular descent has been proposed:
   a. The first phase of transabdominal descent is proposed to be mediated by insulinlike 3 (INSL3) produced by the Leydig cells and its receptor leucine-rich repeat containing G-protein–coupled receptor 8 (LGR8) and occurs at 8 to 15 weeks of gestation. The descent is the result of enlargement of the caudal genitoinguinal ligament and the gubernaculum and by regression of the cranial ligament. The effect of INSL3 may be augmented by MIS or testosterone.
   b. The second inguinoscrotal phase of testicular descent depends on testosterone and occurs at 26 to 35 weeks of gestation. The androgen-dependent phase of testicular descent is possibly mediated indirectly through the release from the genitofemoral nerve of calcitonin gene-related peptide (CGRP). The testes descend into the scrotum in 97.3% of term infants, 79% of preterm infants, and 99% of 1-year-old infants.

B. Infancy and childhood. A transient rise in the circulating LH and FSH concentrations is usually seen in infants of both sexes during the first few months after birth as a result of the rapid withdrawal of placental sex steroids leading to a disturbance of the balance of negative feedback between sex steroids and GnRH release from the hypothalamus. The circulating levels of LH and testosterone, with a smaller elevation of FSH concentrations, increase abruptly after birth and remain elevated for the first 3 months after delivery in male neonates. This minipuberty induces the transformation of gonocytes into Ad (dark) spermatogonia in the process of germ-cell differentiation. This process is impaired in children with cryptorchidism (resulting in an increase in gonocytes) and androgen resistance syndrome. Cryptorchidism is associated with an increased risk of infertility and testicular cancer in adult life. After this period of transient activation of the hypothalamic-pituitary-gonadal axis, it undergoes a long period of relative quiescence until late childhood, when pubertal development occurs. Using highly sensitive immunofluorometric assays, small pulses of GnRH-induced LH and FSH secretion have been detected in prepubertal children as young as 4 years of age with slightly higher values at night than in the daytime. Undetectable or very low apulsatile pattern of LH and FSH concentrations had been described in patients with Kallmann syndrome, but the reliability of spontaneous secretion of gonadotropins in identifying such patients has been called into doubt by the use of highly sensitive gonadotropin assay. Three hypotheses have been proposed to explain the suppression of the hypothalamic-pituitary-gonadal axis during childhood and the mechanism of the onset of puberty. The first is the "gonadostat" hypothesis, based on the concept of changing sensitivity of the regulatory system of gonadotropin secretions to the negative feedback by gonadal sex steroids in childhood and adolescence. The onset of puberty is the result of decreasing sensitivity of the "gonadostat" to the negative feedback of small amounts of gonadal steroids secreted by the gonads during the peripubertal period. The challenge of the "gonadostat" hypothesis comes from the finding that a similar pattern of suppressed circulating gonadotropin levels has been found in agonadal patients. The second hypothesis proposes that the sexual quiescence during childhood before the onset of puberty is a result of central neural inhibition of GnRH release independent of the negative feedback of gonadal steroids. At the onset of puberty, this intrinsic central neural restraint of the hypothalamic pituitary–gonadal axis is inhibited or lessened by stimulating influences. The last hypothesis or "desynchrony theory" proposes that the lack of GnRH stimulation of the pituitary in prepubertal children is a result of the desynchronization of the discharge or "firing" of the GnRH neurons. This hypothesis has some support from in vitro studies in immortalized GnRH neurons.

C. Puberty

1. Gonadarche marks the maturation of the hypothalamic–pituitary-gonadal axis between 9 and 14 years of age in boys. During childhood, there is gradual amplification of GnRH pulse frequency and amplitude that is of great importance in stimulating the secretion of gonadotropins mediating sexual maturation in adolescence. With the onset of puberty, there is increasing pulsatile secretion of LH, initially mainly at night, which is associated with a testosterone rise in boys. In pubertal boys, sleep-entrained pulsatile GnRH secretion every 60 to 90 minutes progresses to become more regular throughout the 24 hours. The pulsatile secretion of LH stimulates the Leydig cells of the testis to produce testosterone, which is then converted either by aromatization to estradiol or by 5α reduction to dihydrotestosterone. Testosterone production from the testes progressively increases, and this hormone is responsible for the development of secondary sexual characteristics and metabolic changes at puberty. The first clinical sign of puberty is testicular enlargement, as shown by a testis length >2 cm or a volume of >4 mL as assessed by the Prader orchidometer. The sexual maturity rating according to Marshall and Tanner is shown in Table 23.1. The adult testes produce about 6 to 10 mg of testosterone per day, with a small amount of testosterone synthesized in extratesticular tissue or via peripheral conversion. LH and FSH are required for the development and maintenance of testicular function. The coordination of testosterone output is under the tight control of both positive

TABLE 23.1 Stages of Puberty in Boys

Stage	Genitals	Public hair	Age Mean	SD	Testicular volume (cm³) Mean	SD
I	Preadolescent: testes, scrotum, and penis are about the same size and proportion as in early childhood.	Preadolescent: vellus over pubes is no further developed than that over abdominal wall (i.e., no pubic hair).			4.98	3.63
II	Scrotum and testes have enlarged, and there is a change in texture of scrotal skin and some reddening of scrotal skin.	Sparse growth of long, slightly pigmented, downy hair, straight or only slightly curled, appearing chiefly at base of penis.	11.7	1.3	6.74	3.54
III	Growth of penis has occurred, at first mainly in length but with some increase in breadth; there has been further growth of testes and scrotum.	Hair is considerably darker, coarser, and more curled and spreads sparsely over junction of pubes	13.2	0.8	14.68	6.32
IV	Penis is further enlarged in length and breadth, with development of glans; testes and scrotum are further enlarged; there is also further darkening of scrotal skin.	Hair is now adult in type, but area covered by it is smaller than in most adults; there is no spread to medial surface of thighs.	14.7	1.1	20.13	6.17
V	Genitalia are adult in size and shape; no further enlargement takes place after stage V.	Hair is adult in quantity and type, distributed as an inverse triangle; there is spread to medial surface of thighs but not up linea alba or elsewhere above base of inverse triangle.	15.5	0.7	29.28	9.10

SD, standard deviation.
Adapted from Marshall WA, Tanner JM. Variations in the pattern of pubertal changes in boys. *Arch Dis Child* 1970;45:13; Daniel WA Jr, et al. Testicular volumes of adolescents. *J Pediatr* 1982;101:1010; Penny R, et al. Overnight follicle stimulating hormone (FSH) and luteinizing hormone (LH) excretion in normal males. *J Clin Endocrinol Metab* 1976;43:1394.

feed-forward and negative feedback mechanisms. FSH and testosterone have little effect in boys until <u>spermarche</u>, when these hormones act on the Sertoli cells to secrete many paracrine factors to support the initiation of spermatogenesis, which involves a process of differentiation from the spermatogonia to the mature spermatozoa. Maintenance of spermatogenesis requires the action of testosterone and the supportive action of FSH. Dihydrotestosterone is not essential in maintaining spermatogenesis, as patients with <u>5α-reductase deficiency have normal spermatogenesis</u> and may be fertile. Sertoli cells are important in supporting germ-cell development and androgen receptor transcription is upregulated by FSH, underscoring a synergistic effect of both FSH and testosterone in spermatogenesis. Mature spermatozoa may be present at Tanner genital stage 3, when the mean testicular volume is 11.5 mL.

The specific mechanisms involved in the timing and onset of puberty are complex and poorly understood. The onset of puberty is triggered by removal or diminution of central inhibition and an increase in stimulation of the GnRH neurons. In addition to changes in transsynaptic stimulatory and inhibitory influences, astroglial inputs via cell-to-cell signaling molecules also play a role in the control of GnRH secretion from the GnRH neurons. Transsynaptic stimulatory modulators of GnRH secretion include glutamatergic innervation, norepinephrine, kisspeptin-1-G-protein–coupled-receptor 54(KiSS1-GPR54) complex, and neuropeptide Y (NPY). Both kisspeptin-1 (KiSS1) and its receptor, G-protein–coupled receptor 54 (GPR54), gene transcripts are upregulated in the hypothalamus with onset of puberty, and kisspeptin-1 is a potent stimulus for GnRH-induced gonadotropin secretion. Mutations in GPR54 cause idiopathic hypogonadotropic hypogonadism, but pituitary responsiveness to exogenous GnRH is preserved, suggesting that GPR54 mutations affect the processing or release of GnRH. There is also some evidence to suggest that KiSS1-GPR54 signaling complex may act as a modulator in the final common path of the cascade of sexual development and maturation events. Transsynaptic inhibitory influences on GnRH secretion include GABAergic and opiatergic innervation, vasoactive intestinal peptide (VIP), corticotrophin-releasing factor (CRF), and melatonin. GnRH neurons and glial cells are intimately related. Transforming growth factor-α (TGFα) and neuregulins (NRG) bind to erbB1 and erbB4 (on astrocytes and tanycytes), respectively, and disruption of TGFα–erbB1 and NRG–erbB4 signaling complexes results in <u>delayed puberty</u>. The TGFα–erbB1 signaling complex has been implicated as the cause of <u>precocious puberty</u> associated with hypothalamic hamartoma. Upstream controlling genes such as Oct2, thyroid transcription factor 1 (TTF1), and enhanced-at-puberty gene (EAP1) can also modulate GnRH neuronal activity. Leptin plays a role in informing the brain of peripheral energy stores and body composition, acting as a permissive signal for the onset of puberty. Body-weight decrease and decrease in body fat following excessive physical training seem only to affect females, not males.

Twins studies have also suggested a genetic influence on the timing of puberty. An effect of nutritional factors and body composition on the time of onset of puberty is supported by the earlier age of puberty in moderately obese children, and by delayed maturation of the reproductive endocrine system in states of malnutrition and chronic illness. Very vigorous physical conditioning and training may independently affect puberty onset and progression in girls but not in boys. Children adopted from developing countries and living in advanced societies have early puberty as a general feature. Exposure to endocrine-disrupting chemicals with estrogen agonistic and androgen antagonistic effects may affect the timing of puberty.

2. **Adrenarche** refers to the increase in the secretion of adrenal androgens, coinciding with the development of the zona reticularis of the adrenal beginning at 7 to 8 years of age in boys. The androgens predominantly secreted are dehydroepiandrosterone <u>(DHEA) and its sulfate</u>. Adrenarche is characterized by maturational increases in 17-hydroxylase and 17,20 lyase and a low 3β-hydroxysteroid dehydrogenase activity of the adrenal gland. The secretion of

adrenal androgens continues to increase until mid-puberty. Adrenocorticotropic hormone (ACTH) rather than pituitary gonadotropins mediates this change. Adrenarche and gonadarche are responsible for pubic and axillary hair development.
3. **Normal values**
   a. **Stages of pubertal development** (Table 23.1)
   b. **Reference levels of sex steroids** (Table 23.2)

II. CLINICAL DISORDERS
A. Undescended testes
1. **Classification**
   a. A **retractile testis** is one that is not located in the scrotum when the child is initially examined but can be easily manipulated into the scrotum. The maneuver should be performed in a warm environment using soap or talcum powder as a lubricant. A retractile testis is the result of a strong cremasteric reflex and is not observed in the neonatal period.
   b. An **ectopic testis** is located in the perineum, medial surface of the thigh, abdominal wall, or, rarely, over the dorsum of the penis. Treatment of this rare condition is always surgical, and patients usually have a poor prognosis for fertility.
   c. A **cryptorchid testis** may be intra-abdominal (10%), in the inguinal canal (20%), or in the superficial inguinal pouch (40%). A testis in the superficial inguinal pouch differs from a retractile testis in that it cannot be manipulated into the scrotum. The remaining cases are obstructed testes (30%) resulting from blockage of the path of descent by a fascial cord between the inguinal pouch and the scrotal inlet.
   d. An **acquired undescended testis** may appear 3 to 4 months after birth, when the gonadotropin levels decline. The condition also occurs in 5- to 10-year-old boys when the elongation of the spermatic cord is inadequate for the change in size of the inguinoscrotal region with growth. Sometimes the fibrous remnant of the process vaginalis impairs the elongation of the spermatic cord.
2. **Clinical features of cryptorchidism**
   a. **Incidence.** Cryptorchid testes are found at birth in 2.7% of term infants and 21% of preterm infants. Spontaneous descent of the testes occurs in the majority of these infants so that only 0.9% of 1-year-old boys have cryptorchid testes. The incidence of cryptorchidism varies in different geographic regions of the world. Recent increases in incidence rate in some European countries have been ascribed to environmental endocrine disruptors including phthalates.
   b. **Pathology.** The histopathology of cryptorchid testes is characterized by a diminution of the number of mature or differentiating germ cells, disturbances of tubular structure, and increases in interstitial tissue by the second and third years of life. Germ-cell abnormality is seen in 2%, 20%, and 45% of testicular biopsies at the time of surgery when orchidopexy is performed at 1, 2, and 4 years of age, respectively. In addition to testicular damage and infertility, there is an increased risk of developing testicular germ-cell tumors (relative risk 5.2). Twelve percent of patients with testicular cancer have a history of cryptorchidism.
   c. **Associated disorders.** Although cryptorchidism can occur in isolation, it may be associated with disorders of sex chromosomes and autosomes, ambiguous genitalia, malformations of the urinary tract, and disorders such as Prader-Willi, Noonan, Bardet-Biedl, Aarskog, and Cornelia de Lange syndromes. Bilateral cryptorchidism can also occur in patients with hypopituitarism or isolated hypogonadotropic hypogonadism.
   d. **Pathophysiology.** An impaired hypothalamic–pituitary-gonadal axis has been proposed as the cause for cryptorchidism but has not been uniformly found by all investigators. An immune cause for cryptorchidism has also been suggested by the demonstration of antigonadotropic cell antibodies in the

TABLE 23.2 Serum Concentrations of Sex Steroids for Normal Related to Tanner Stage of Sexual Development

Stage	T (ng/dL)[a]	DHT (ng/dL)[a]	Delta-4 (ng/dL)[a]	DHEA (ng/dL)[a]	DHEAS (μg/dL)[a]	E_1 (ng/dL)[a]	E_2 (ng/dL)[a]	P (ng/dL)[b]	17-OHP (ng/dL)[b]
I	10 ± 1	3.3 ± 1.3	55.0 ± 7.5	205.4 ± 31.7	41.5 ± 31.7	1.06 ± 0.28	0.75 ± 0.28	36.0 ± 5.0	65.0 ± 5.0
II	85 ± 5	9.2 ± 6.7	60.0 ± 10.0	306.5 ± 91.6	62.7 ± 35.6	1.56 ± 0.31	1.05 ± 0.29	37.0 ± 4.0	67.5 ± 10.0
III	121 ± 17	20.0 ± 10.0	70.0 ± 10.0	402.4 ± 99.7	73.0 ± 48.8	2.14 ± 0.20	1.58 ± 0.53	34.0 ± 4.0	70.0 ± 5.0
IV	493 ± 42	35.0 ± 13.3	95.0 ± 17.5	375.5 ± 98.9	103.0 ± 55.7	3.34 ± 0.62	2.19 ± 0.78	54.0 ± 10.0	95.0 ± 10.0
V	605 (260–1000)	41.7 ± 18.3	117.5 ± 15.0	542.8 ± 112.7	123.4 ± 48.2	3.15 ± 0.70	2.07 ± 0.53	45.0 ± 4.0	140.0 ± 25.0

Delta-4, androstenedione; DHEA, dehydroepiandrosterone; DHEAS, dehydroepiandrosterone sulfate; DHT, dihydrotestosterone; E_1, estrone; E_2, estradiol; 17-OHP, 17-hydroxyprogesterone; P, progesterone; T, testosterone.

[a]Mean value ± standard deviation (range).

[b]Mean value ± standard error of mean (range).

Data from Bidlingmaier F, et al. Plasma estrogens in childhood and puberty under physiologic and pathologic conditions. *Pediatr Res* 1973;7:901; Root AW. Endocrinology of puberty. I. Normal puberty. *J Pediatr* 1973;83:1; Lee PA, Migeon CJ. Puberty in boys: correlation of plasma levels in gonadotropins (LH, FSH), androgens (testosterone, androstenedione, dehydroepiandrosterone and its sulfate), estrogens (estrone and estradiol), and progestins (progesterone and 17-hydroxy progesterone). *J Clin Endocrinol Metab* 1975;41:556; DeParetti E, Forest MG. Pattern of plasma dehydroepiandrosterone sulfate levels in humans from birth to adulthood: Evidence for testicular production. *J Clin Endocrinol Metab* 1978;47:572; Pang S, et al. Dihydrotestosterone and its relationship to testosterone in infancy and childhood. *J Clin Endocrinol Metab* 1979;48:821; Friedman IM, Goldberg E. Reference materials for the practice and adolescent medicine. *Pediatr Clin N Am* 1980;27:193.

serum of cryptorchid boys, infants, and their mothers. In most instances, an inherent testicular dysfunction or dysgenesis may be the cause of cryptorchidism. Cryptorchidism resulting from abnormal production of INSL3, MIS, and testosterone is rare.

3. **Evaluation.** If no testis is palpable in a male infant, the possibilities of 46,XX disorder of sex development (46,XX DSD) and congenital bilateral anorchia should be excluded. Infants with anorchia have normal male external genitalia. Testicular damage resulting from torsion or vascular accident could have occurred after the third month of gestation. These children can be differentiated from children with bilateral intra-abdominal testes by measurement of basal testosterone and the lack of increase in the serum testosterone 72 hours after an intramuscular injection of hCG (5 000 IU/1.73 m^2). About 30% of undescended testes are impalpable. Ultrasonography has a diagnostic sensitivity of 90% to 95% for tests in a canalicular location, but this technique is not adequate for intra-abdominal testes. For the detection of intra-abdominal testes, magnetic resonance imaging (MRI), gadolinium-enhanced magnetic resonance angiography (MRA), or laparoscopy can be used.

4. **Treatment.** No intervention should be considered before 6 months of age because of the possibility of spontaneous descent.

   a. **Medical.** Medical therapy has a limited role in the management of cryptorchidism. This initial enthusiasm for medical therapy has not been confirmed by studies on younger children when cases of retractile testes have been stringently excluded. hCG (1 000 to 6 000 IU per week for 5 weeks) is not particularly effective in children <3 years of age, and intranasal GnRH (1 200 μg per day in divided doses for 4 weeks) is effective in only 20% to 25% of cases, with a significant risk of relapse even after initial descent of the testes.

   b. **Surgery.** Orchidopexy should be performed after 6 months but no later than 18 months of age in patients without spontaneous testicular descent. A biopsy should be obtained at the time of surgery because of the possibility of dysgenetic gonads and malignancy.

5. **Long-term prognosis**

   a. **Retractile testes.** Although retractile testis is generally conceived as a benign condition that does not require treatment, there is increasing evidence that lower average spermatogonia, Sertoli cell number, and increased tubular degeneration are found in retractile testes. There has been a suggestion that hormonal or surgical therapy be offered to patients with retractile testes that do not descend spontaneously.

   b. **Cryptorchidism.** Fertility is significantly decreased after bilateral cryptorchidism and is unrelated to the age of orchidopexy. Fertility is impaired in ~30% of patients with unilateral cryptorchidism, and the risk is increased if the testes were intra-abdominal, there is presence of varicocele, or a partner has a fertility problem. A paternity rate of up to 70% to 90% has been reported in men with unilateral cryptorchidism postorchidopexy. In patients with bilateral cryptorchidism, ~75% have abnormal semen analyses, and the rate of infertility is high. A recent report suggested that low-dose GnRH analog given by nasal spray every other day for 6 months following successful orchidopexy appears to improve spermatograms in adult life as compared to controls. Infertile patients with prior cryptorchidism tend to have higher FSH, lower sperm density, and lower inhibin B levels than fertile patients. There is an increased risk of testicular cancer following bilateral (odds ratio 5.8) or unilateral (odds ratio 2.7) cryptorchidism. Thus, early surgical correction of cryptorchidism is important because (1) any mass in the testis can be detected early, (2) the rate of infertility is decreased, and (3) the risk of cancer of the testis may be decreased.

B. **Micropenis**

1. **Definition.** A micropenis is defined as a penis whose stretched length is >2.5 standard deviations (SD) below the mean stretched penile length of normal

| **TABLE 23.3** | Stretched Penile Length in Normal Males |

	Stretched penile length (cm)	
Normal male	Mean ± SD	Mean − 2.5 SD
Newborn		
30 wk	2.5 ± 0.4	1.5
34 wk	3.0 ± 0.4	2.0
Term	3.5 ± 0.4	2.5
0–5 mo	3.9 ± 0.8	1.9
6–12 mo	4.3 ± 0.8	2.3
1–2 y	4.7 ± 0.8	2.6
2–3 y	5.1 ± 0.9	2.9
3–4 y	5.5 ± 0.9	3.3
4–5 y	5.7 ± 0.9	3.5
5–6 y	6.0 ± 0.9	3.8
6–7 y	6.1 ± 0.9	3.9
7–8 y	6.2 ± 1.0	3.7
8–9 y	6.3 ± 1.0	3.8
9–10 y	6.3 ± 1.0	3.8
10–11 y	6.4 ± 1.1	3.7
Adult	13.3 ± 1.6	9.3

SD, standard deviation.
Data from Lee PA, et al. Micropenis. I. Criteria, etiologies and classification. *Johns Hopkins Med J* 1980; 146:156.

children of the same age (Table 23.3). Undescended testes can be present in children with micropenis.

2. **Etiology** (see Section II.D)
   a. Children with **isolated gonadotropin deficiency** (with or without anosmia) and **congenital idiopathic hypopituitarism** present with micropenis at birth. This is because penile growth in utero is dependent on testosterone secretion, which is regulated by pituitary gonadotropin after 13 weeks of gestation.
   b. It may be seen in children with **congenital central nervous system (CNS) defects,** including midline facial defects, septo-optic dysplasia, and pituitary agenesis.
   c. Many **syndromic disorders** are associated with micropenis. Prader-Willi and Bardet-Biedl syndromes are commonly associated with gonadotropin deficiency. Micropenis resulting from primary hypogonadism is seen in Klinefelter, Noonan, Robinow, Cornelia de Lange, Down, and fetal hydantoin syndromes.
   d. Micropenis resulting from **partial androgen insensitivity** is usually associated with varying degrees of genital ambiguity (see Chapter 20 for diagnosis and management).
   e. **Idiopathic.** In some children, no obvious cause for the micropenis can be found.
3. **Management**
   After evaluation (see Chapter 24, Section II.D), testosterone enanthate, 25 mg IM monthly for 3 doses, can stimulate the growth of the penis into the normal range in infancy and early childhood, thereby reducing problems of psychosexual adjustment for the patient in later childhood. Further assessment and treatment of these patients are required in adolescence.
C. **Gynecomastia** is defined as excessive proliferation of stromal and glandular tissue of the breasts in a male.

TABLE 23.4	Causes of Gynecomastia

1. Physiologic
   - Newborn, puberty, and old age
2. Defects in androgen action or production
   - Androgen resistance syndrome
   - Klinefelter syndrome
   - Congenital anorchia
   - Defects in testosterone biosynthesis
   - Acquired testicular failure
3. Tumors
   - Estrogen-secreting tumors of adrenal gland or testis
   - hCG-secreting tumors
   - Prolactinoma
4. Drugs
   - Spironolactone, cimetidine, digitalis, phenothiazines, tricyclic antidepressants, aromatizable androgens, growth hormone, exposure to hormone-containing cosmetic creams and hair products
5. Endocrine disorders
   - Familial aromatase hyperactivity
   - Obesity
   - Thyrotoxicosis
6. Trauma or refeeding
7. Idiopathic

hCG, human chorionic gonadotropin.

1. **Etiology** (Table 23.4)
   a. **Physiologic gynecomastia** can occur in the neonatal period, at the time of puberty, and with old age. Breast enlargement in newborns results from the effect of maternal or placental estrogen, and most cases resolve in a few weeks. Gynecomastia may be present in 70% of pubertal boys. It is usually bilateral but may be unilateral or asymmetrical. Androgens-to-estrogens imbalance at puberty has been implicated as the cause of pubertal gynecomastia. Enhanced aromatization of androgens to estrogens is important in the pathogenesis of gynecomastia associated with obesity in puberty and aging.
   b. Gynecomastia is present with defects of the androgen receptor in which serum testosterone levels are high while there are defects in androgen action. Gynecomastia can be found in patients with **androgen deficiency,** as in Klinefelter syndrome, congenital anorchia, defects in testosterone biosynthesis, and acquired testicular failure. These conditions are associated with low testosterone concentrations, an elevation of serum LH, and variable increases of serum estrogen as a result of direct testicular secretion or peripheral aromatization of adrenal precursors. The abnormal testosterone–estrogen ratio predisposes the patients to the development of gynecomastia.
   c. Breast enlargement can be caused by estrogen-secreting testicular or adrenal **tumors,** hCG-secreting tumors (germinomas from the liver, CNS, and testis), or prolactinoma.
   d. Gynecomastia can be a result of the effects of **drugs.** Spironolactone inhibits testosterone biosynthesis, and cimetidine blocks the binding of androgen to its receptor. The mechanisms for digitalis-, phenothiazine-, and antidepressant-induced gynecomastia remain unknown. Recently, prepubertal gynecomastia has been reported in children receiving growth hormone (GH) therapy, but the mechanism of this effect of GH remains unknown.

e. Familial aromatase hyperactivity is inherited as an autosomal dominant condition characterized by prepubertal or peripubertal gynecomastia in males and precocious puberty in female members of the family.

f. Idiopathic gynecomastia refers to breast enlargement in prepubertal children in whom no cause can be found despite extensive investigations. In such cases, a careful history is required to exclude the possibility of environmental exposure to estrogens or antiandrogens. The excessive use of tea tree oil and lavender oil has been reported to cause prepubertal gynecomastia.

g. Trauma and recovery from severe **illnesses** associated with weight loss can also cause gynecomastia.

2. Evaluation. A careful history and physical examination will help in evaluating the cause of gynecomastia. Incomplete masculinization indicates androgen resistance or defects of testosterone biosynthesis, and unilateral testicular enlargement is suggestive of testicular neoplasm. Clinical signs and karyotyping will identify Klinefelter syndrome. Prepubertal gynecomastia is rare, and one should look for a pathologic etiology when it occurs. Hormonal assays should include serum testosterone, estradiol, prolactin, LH, FSH, and β-HCG. An elevated serum prolactin in a child or adult usually points to a prolactinoma, but gynecomastia is rare as a primary presentation of prolactinoma.

3. Treatment. The treatment of gynecomastia should be aimed at the underlying disorder. Patients with pubertal gynecomastia should be reassured that the condition persists for only 2 years in 27% of cases and for 3 years in 7.7%. It can be treated with percutaneous dihydrotestosterone (125 mg in a hydroalcoholic gel twice daily for 1 to 4 months) or with an oral aromatase inhibitor such as testolactone (150 mg three times daily for 2 to 6 months) or anastrozole (1 mg daily for 3 to 6 months). Experience with the use of selective estrogen receptor modulators on adolescent gynecomastia is limited. Raloxifene treatment (60 mg daily for 3 to 9 months) has shown promising results, but the long-term side effects are unknown. Medical treatment should be initiated during the rapid proliferative phase within the first year of onset of the gynecomastia, as late treatment is ineffective. An alternative treatment would be surgical or liposuction removal of glandular and adipose tissue if there is no regression after puberty.

D. Delayed puberty

1. Definition. Delayed puberty is a term applied to boys when pubertal changes fail to develop after the age of 14 years (2 SD above the mean age for the onset of puberty).

2. The **etiology** (Tables 23.5 and 23.6) of delayed puberty can be divided into genetic, functional, or organic defects of the hypothalamic–pituitary-gonadal axis. The etiology can be further classified into hypergonadotropic (primary testicular defect) or hypogonadotropic (hypothalamic or pituitary defects) hypogonadism. The discussion of these conditions in this chapter will not be exhaustive.

a. Functional hypogonadism is usually a result of hypothalamic dysfunction of the axis. Acute or chronic systemic disease will suppress the hypothalamic pituitary gonadal axis. Patients with chronic renal failure, connective tissue disorders, cardiac disease, or acquired immunodeficiency syndrome (AIDS) are commonly affected. In such patients, stress, altered nutrition, and inflammatory cytokines play a significant role. Cystic fibrosis, coeliac disease, and chronic inflammatory bowel disease are chronic illnesses that can result in significant undernutrition if the patient is not adequately treated. Chronic elevations of cortisol, catecholamines, or cytokines (such as interleukin-6) resulting from chronic illness and inflammation act in concert to suppress the GnRH–pituitary–gonadal, TRH/TSH/T3, and GHRH/GH/IGF1 axes and to modulate energy metabolism. With chronic illness, progressive hypogonadotropic hypogonadism develops, primarily affecting LH pulse amplitude rather than frequency. These patients have low sex steroid levels. Anorexia nervosa (see Chapter 11), although more common in females, can also occur in males, resulting in delayed puberty because of the effect on the hypothalamic GnRH pulse generator. Severe childhood hypothyroidism can also delay

TABLE 23.5 Genetic Defects in the Three Components of the Hypothalamic–Pituitary–Gonadal Axis

Compartment	Disease	Gene
Hypothalamus	X-linked Kallmann syndrome	KAL1
	Autosomal dominant Kallmann syndrome	FGFR1
	Morbid obesity, hypogonadism	Leptin gene
		Leptin receptor
		Prohormone convertase 1 (PCSK1)
	Adrenal deficiency, hypogonadotropic hypogonadism	DAX1
	Disorder of sexual development, hypogonadotropic hypogonadism	SF1
	Prader-Willi syndrome	del pat chr15q11–13
	Bardet-Biedl syndrome	3 mutant alleles in 2 of 11 genes (BBS genes, MKKS)
Pituitary	Septo-optic dysplasia	HESX1
	Isolated hypogonadotropic hypogonadism	GNRHR
		FSHβ
		LHβ
		G protein-coupled receptor 54 (GPR54)
	Disorder of pituitary organogenesis	PROP1, LHX3, LHX4
		PTX2, SOX3
Gonad	Gonadotropin resistance	FSHR
		LH/HCGR
	Autosomal recessive delay in puberty	Mutations in steroid enzyme pathway genes
	Disorder of sexual development, gonadal dysgenesis	SF1
	Autoimmune polyendocrine syndrome	AIRE
	Galactosemia	GALT
	Cystic fibrosis	CFTR
	Myotonic dystrophy	(CTG)n expansion of DMPK
		(CCTG)n expansion intron 1 of ZNF9
	Noonan syndrome	PTPN11, KRAS, SOS1
	Klinefelter syndrome	47XXY

the onset of puberty. Functional hypogonadism is more common and much better documented in females. Psychotropic drugs such as phenothiazines, risperidone, and tricyclic antidepressants cause a rise in serum prolactin by blocking endogenous dopamine receptors. Abuse of opiates and cocaine leads to anorexia, decreased food intake, and hyperprolactinemia. Constitutional delay in growth and puberty are discussed in Chapters 6, 7 and 8.

b. Hypogonadotropic hypogonadism can present with delayed puberty, failure of progression of puberty, or failure to attain reproductive function, depending on the severity of the gonadotropin deficiency. Despite remarkable advances in our understanding of human hypogonadotropic hypogonadism, the cause in the majority of cases remains unknown.

(1) Nonorganic **isolated gonadotropin deficiency (IHH) patients** have normal growth until adolescence, when their growth starts to fall off because of the absence of sexual development. They have characteristic eunuchoid proportions. Sporadic or autosomal recessive isolated gonadotropin deficiency without anosmia is rare. About half of patients with isolated

TABLE 23.6	Organic and Functional Disorders of the Hypothalamic–Pituitary–Gonadal Axis	

Compartment	Functional	Organic
Hypothalamic	Anorexia nervosa Psychogenic Constitutional delay in growth and puberty Drug use Chronic systemic illness Undernutrition	Hypothalamic and suprasellar tumor Infiltrative disease Head trauma CNS infection Cranial irradiation
Pituitary		Pituitary tumor Pituitary apoplexy Infiltrative disease (lymphocytic or xanthomatous hypophysitis) Hemosiderosis and hemochromatosis Cranial irradiation Congenital hypopituitarism
Gonadal		Chemotherapy and radiation Infection (mumps, sexually transmitted disease) Vanishing testes syndrome/congenital anorchia Trauma (torsion)

CNS, central nervous system.

gonadotropin deficiency do not have a family history of the disorder. Isolated gonadotropin deficiency can be associated with anosmia (<u>Kallmann syndrome</u>), midline facial defects, micropenis (stretched penile length <2.5 cm in neonates and <4 cm in children before puberty), and cryptorchidism.

(a) **Kallmann syndrome (KS)** is an inherited disorder of neuronal migration characterized by hypogonadism and anosmia. Autosomal dominant, autosomal recessive, and X-linked recessive inheritance patterns have been described, indicating heterogeneity. The condition is reported to occur in 1 of 10 00 males and 1 of 50 000 females. The gene underlying the X-linked form of the disease, KAL1, has been localized to chromosome Xp22.3 and encodes a protein named <u>anosmin-I</u>. Anosmin-I is a regionally restricted component of basement membrane and interstitial matrix and acts as a local cue during organogenesis. This extracellular matrix glycoprotein is an adhesion molecule that can modulate neurite growth in a cell-type-specific manner. MRI scans in patients with Kallmann syndrome have demonstrated absence or hypoplasia of the olfactory bulbs, and hypoplastic or rudimentary olfactory sulci. Other symptoms associated with KS include synkinesia, cerebellar ataxia, eye-movement abnormalities, sensorineural deafness, spatial attention abnormalities, spastic paraplegia, and mental retardation. Somatic defects such as cleft lip and palate, renal agenesis, and pes cavus have also been described. The underlying mechanism is a defect in the hypothalamic pulsatile release of GnRH. Serum LH and FSH rise to normal levels with repetitive administration of GnRH in virtually all patients with KS but not in patients with panhypopituitarism. Studies have indicated that the incidence of genetic defects within the coding region of the KAL1 gene in patients with sporadic

GnRH deficiency is low (5% to 8%), suggesting that the X-linked form of inheritance represents the least common form of isolated gonadotropin deficiency.

The autosomal dominant form of Kallmann syndrome is a result of mutations in the fibroblast growth-factor receptor-1 (FGFR1) gene, localized to chromosome 8p11.2-12. There is a wide range of phenotypic spectrum in patients with FGFR1 mutations, and about half of patients have only IHH and hyposmia without other associated features.

(b) **Fertile eunuch syndrome** is characterized by eunuchoidism, normal-size testes, preserved spermatogenesis with absence of mature Leydig cells, and a normal clinical and biochemical androgenic response to HCG. These patients have subnormal testosterone secretion and low-normal basal and GnRH-stimulated serum LH and FSH concentrations. The fertile eunuch syndrome thus represents a less severe form of GnRH deficiency rather than a distinct disorder. It has been reported in a patient with homozygous mutations (Glu106Arg) of the GNRHR gene.

(c) No major abnormality of the GnRH gene has been reported in patients with idiopathic hypogonadotropic hypogonadism. Mutations in the leptin (LEP) gene, leptin receptor (LEPR) gene, and prohormone convertase 1 (PCSK1) gene are rare causes of autosomal recessive hypogonadotropic hypogonadism. Pituitary agenesis or hypoplasia has been reported in a few patients with congenital adrenal hypoplasia, and this has been shown to be due to a loss of function mutations of the DAX1 gene.

(d) Heterozygous GNRH receptor mutations may be found in as high as 20% of familial cases of normosmic IHH patients.

(2) There are now a number of nuclear transcription factors that are known to be important in the embryonic development and definitive function of the anterior pituitary gland. The thyroid transcription factor I gene, PITX 1, PITX 2, and the LIM-class homeodomain transcription factors LHX 3 and LHX 4 are important in the early embryonic development of the pituitary gland. Affected patients have multiple pituitary hormone deficiency and some characteristic somatic features. The homeobox gene HESX I is expressed in prospective forebrain tissue during early embryonic development, which later becomes restricted to the Rathke pouch, the primordium of the anterior pituitary gland. Homozygous and heterozygous missense mutations within the HESXI homeodomain lead to the condition septo-optic dysplasia. Pituitary dysfunction, including hypogonadotropic hypogonadism, is variable and can be progressive, such that long-term endocrine follow-up of these patients is required. Prophet of Pit-I (PROP1) is another pituitary-specific paired–like homeodomain transcription factor that is important in the fetal development of the pituitary gland. Patients with PROP1 gene mutations exhibit secondary hypogonadism in addition to deficiencies of GH, PRL, and TSH. Patients with mutations in the POU1F1 gene do not have gonadotropin deficiency. Both an overdosage of SOX3 (large or submicroscopic tandem duplication of Xq26-27) or underdosage (by expansion of polyalanine tract within SOX3) can result in hypopituitarism. Neuroradiologically, these patients have the features of congenital hypopituitarism, with hypoplastic adenohypophysis, transaction of pituitary stalk, and ectopic position of the posterior pituitary bright signal on MRI. The above gene mutation defects are uncommon.

(3) **Idiopathic hypopituitarism** is a heterogeneous group of disorders that can occur sporadically or can be inherited. Congenital idiopathic hypopituitarism (CH) presents in early infancy with severe fasting hypoglycemia, neonatal hepatitis-like syndrome, hyponatremia, and micropenis in males. Perinatal trauma and hypoxia have been implicated as a cause in 50% to

60% of patients presenting with idiopathic hypopituitarism in later childhood. MRI in patients with congenital hypopituitarism and idiopathic hypopituitarism in childhood may show hypoplasia or absence of the adenohypophysis, transection of the pituitary stalk, and ectopic position of the posterior pituitary. The patients usually have multiple anterior pituitary hormone deficiencies but normal posterior pituitary function. The anterior pituitary secretory responses to hypothalamic releasing factors vary from patient to patient and with time. Rarely, these findings have been reported in patients with mutations in the pituitary transcription factors.

(4) **Prader-Willi** and **Bardet-Biedl** syndromes are commonly associated with gonadotropin deficiency. Prader syndrome is characterized by obesity, hypogonadism, almond-shaped eyes, small hands and feet, and mental retardation. The syndrome can result from deletion of paternal chromosomal 15q11-13, uniparental maternal disomy of chromosome 15, translocation, or a methylation center defect. Bardet-Biedl syndrome is characterized by hypogonadism, obesity, mental retardation, polydactyl, and retinitis pigmentosa. The syndrome occurs when there are three mutant alleles in two of 11 genes (BBS genes and MKKS).

c. **Organic hypogonadotropic hypogonadism**

(1) **Pituitary tumors** are less common in children than in adults. They can be secreting or nonsecreting (functional). The most common pituitary tumors in adults are prolactinomas, followed by nonsecreting tumors, and this is also true in children and adolescents.

(2) **CNS disorders,** including tumors (craniopharyngioma, suprasellar astrocytoma, optic nerve glioma, germinoma, teratoma, and histiocytosis), congenital defects (midline facial defects, septo-optic dysplasia, and hydrocephalus), infection (meningitis and encephalitis), and infiltrative decreases (autoimmune lymphocytic hypophysitis, sarcoidosis xanthomatous hypophysitis), can lead to hypothalamic pituitary dysfunction. A Rathke pouch cyst and empty sella syndrome can also lead occasionally to pituitary dysfunction.

(3) **Radiation treatment** for leukemia or brain tumor can damage the hypothalamic–pituitary axis. The anterior pituitary hormone first affected by radiation is growth hormone, followed by the gonadotropins and ACTH. A radiation dose of <u>2 700 to 3 500 rad is sufficient to produce GH deficiency</u>, and a dose in excess of 4 500 rad can lead to panhypopituitarism. Post–traumatic brain injury hypopituitarism is increasingly being recognized.

(4) Hypogonadotropic hypogonadism can be present in patients with **thalassemia major** and **hemochromatosis** because of iron deposition in the hypothalamus and pituitary as a result of repeated blood transfusions.

d. **Hypergonadotropic hypogonadism** results from primary testicular failure leading to increase in serum LH and FSH. The gonadotropin concentrations may not be markedly elevated in childhood until after adolescence (Tables 23.5 and 23.6).

(1) **Klinefelter syndrome** occurs in 1 in 500 males. The underlying abnormality is the presence of an extra X chromosome (47,XXY), but other karyotypic varieties and mosaicism exist. The classic form of Klinefelter syndrome is a result of meiotic nondisjunction of the chromosomes during gametogenesis. There is evidence that both X chromosomes originate from the mother in 60% of cases. The condition usually presents in adolescence and is characterized by varying degrees of impaired sexual maturation, small genitalia and testes, eunuchoid proportions, gynecomastia, and learning, cognitive, and behavior problems. These children usually have low-normal intelligence. There is an increased risk of thyroid dysfunction, diabetes mellitus, and breast cancer in these patients.

(2) **Noonan syndrome** occurs in 1 in 8 000 births, and the <u>karyotype is normal</u>. Patients exhibit the features of Turner syndrome, such as webbing

of the neck, increased carrying angle of the forearms, short stature, and lymphedema. Other features include ptosis, pectus excavatum, right-sided heart lesion such as pulmonary stenosis, triangular face, and mental retardation. Male patients affected by this condition may have undescended testes or micropenis. Familial cases have shown that the condition is dominantly inherited. The putative gene locus has recently been assigned to chromosome 12q22-qter by linkage analysis. Mutations in PTPN11, encoding the protein tyrosine phosphatase SHP-2, is the cause of 50% of the cases of Noonan syndrome. Noonan syndrome is a disease caused by aberrant signaling through the Ras-GTPase and germline gain-of-function mutations in KRAS (5% of cases) or of the Ras nucleotide exchange factor SOS1 (10% of cases).

(3) Acquired testicular failure can result from viral orchitis caused by mumps, coxsackie virus B, or echovirus. Cytotoxic drugs, especially alkylating agents and methylhydrazines, result in profound disturbance of the morphology of the germinal epithelium. Permanent damage to the germ cells occurs more frequently in postpubertal than in prepubertal boys, because the prepubertal testis is relatively insensitive to the cytotoxic effect of these drugs. Damage can also result from direct testicular irradiation. There is also a high incidence of gonadal dysfunction following the combination regimen of high-dose cyclophosphamide and total-body irradiation used in preparation for bone marrow transplantation. Depending on the dose and type of chemotherapy and the dose of radiation, recovery of the germinal epithelium does occur.

3. Evaluation

a. A **diagnostic evaluation** should be performed when puberty is delayed beyond 14 years of age in boys. Points worthy of note in the history include chronic illness, neurologic symptoms, anosmia, history of hypoglycemia and hepatitis in infancy, and family history of delay of growth and sexual maturation. The physical examination should include a full neurologic evaluation. Impaired vision, nystagmus, microphthalmia, and hypoplastic optic disk on funduscopic examination should suggest a diagnosis of septo-optic dysplasia. Retinitis pigmentosa, polydactyly, and mental retardation in an obese child point to a diagnosis of Bardet-Biedl syndrome. One should also look out for features of other syndromic disorders and midline facial defects. The presence of micropenis indicates gonadotropin deficiency of prenatal onset.

b. **Initial laboratory investigations** should include LH, FSH, testosterone, and other tests such as prolactin, bone age and skull radiographs, and/or MRI, blood count, sedimentation rate, renal and liver function tests, thyroid function, and cortisol levels if indicated. Low FSH and LH levels suggest a problem in the hypothalamus or the pituitary, whereas elevated FSH and LH concentrations suggest a primary testicular defect.

c. **Karyotyping** is performed to confirm the diagnosis of Klinefelter syndrome or Prader-Willi syndrome (deletion of q1.1-q1.3 of chromosome 15% in 50% of cases).

d. **Combined pituitary study** using the arginine/GHRH test, GnRH, and thyrotropin-releasing hormone (TRH) after sex steroid priming should be performed if there is a strong suspicion of hypopituitarism (see Chapter 6). An insulin tolerance test is not recommended for children under the age of 5 years, and more and more investigators prefer the use of an alternative growth-hormone stimulatory test in children, such as the arginine/GHRH test. MRI of the brain should be ordered. Hypopituitarism resulting from an organic cause in the CNS often can be associated with posterior pituitary dysfunction. The possibility of diabetes insipidus, therefore, should be evaluated (see Chapters 5 & 6).

e. The **differentiation of isolated gonadotropin deficiency from constitutional delay** of growth and puberty is a difficult challenge for pediatricians. Clinically, children with isolated gonadotropin deficiency have normal height and growth velocity, whereas children with constitutional delay of growth and puberty are usually short. In both conditions, the basal LH and FSH are low without any disturbance of the secretion of other anterior pituitary hormones. Assessment of the serum LH and FSH response to GnRH is not helpful. An impaired prolactin response to TRH observed in isolated gonadotropin deficiency can be useful in distinguishing this condition from constitutional delay of growth and puberty; but there is a considerable overlap between the two groups. Using a highly sensitive fluoroimmunometric assay, it has been found that nocturnal augmentation of pulsatile LH or FSH secretion (estimated in frequent blood sampling studies) is absent in patients with Kallmann syndrome. Frequent blood sampling is not clinically practical in children.

    f. Genetic studies can be helpful in identifying the genetic defect in familial cases of multiple pituitary hormones deficiencies.

4. Management. Induction of secondary sexual characteristics in patients with hypogonadism can be achieved by replacement with a testosterone preparation at 14 years of age.

    a. Intramuscular testosterone enanthate can be given (50 mg every 4 weeks; then increased by 50 mg every 6 months to a dose of 200 mg every 2 to 3 weeks). Intramuscular testosterone enanthate results in supraphysiologic concentrations of testosterone a few days after injection, followed by a fall to a nadir by 10 to 14 days. In some patients, there may be cyclical skin changes (crops of acne) and mood disturbances (behavior problems).

    b. Newer methods of testosterone administration, which may be suitable for induction of puberty, include transdermal application of **testosterone** via **gels.** The gels have to be specifically tested in children before they can be used.

    c. Oral testosterone undecanoate (not available in the United States) has been reported to be efficacious but may be problematic in adolescents because of lack of absorption without food and problems with compliance.

    d. In older boys or men with hypogonadotropic hypogonadism, **hCG** or recombinant human LH **(r-hLH)** and pulsatile GnRH infusion are alternatives to testosterone enanthate replacement when fertility is desired (see Chapter 24). HCG or hLH should be given in an initial dose of 1 000 IU twice weekly by intramuscular injection; the dose is increased to 2 000 to 3 000 IU twice weekly over a period of 2 to 3 years. HCG alone induces only moderate increase in the size of the testes, to about 8 mL. Human menopausal gonadotropin (HMG) or **recombinant human FSH,** 75 IU by intramuscular route, two to three times per week, might be required to induce spermatogenesis and further growth of the testes during the second and third years or when fertility is desired. Recombinant hCG, hLH, and hFSH can also be given by the subcutaneous route.

    e. GnRH given in a **pulsatile** manner every 90 minutes subcutaneously or intravenously using a portable programmable infusion pump would be the most physiologic way to induce puberty in hypogonadotropic hypogonadal boys. However, this form of treatment is expensive and technically difficult to administer. Pulsatile GnRH (2 to 20 μg) subcutaneously every 90 minutes can be used to induce spermatogenesis in males with hypothalamic hypogonadotropic hypogonadism, but this is no more effective than the combination of gonadotropins.

    f. In patients with combined growth hormone and gonadotropin deficiency, puberty should be induced only after growth-hormone replacement therapy, when the bone age is >12 years, or when the growth velocity falls below 3 cm a year while on growth-hormone treatment. Some have advocated an increase in the dose of growth hormone at the time of pubertal induction, but this may only accelerate the rate of pubertal development without increasing final height.

    g. Patients with constitutional delay of growth and puberty (CDGP) can be reassured; however, treatment is frequently offered because the patient experiences significant social and psychological distress. Patients in whom short stature is the dominant problem can be offered oxandrolone (1.25 to 2.5 mg) at night for 3 to 4 months or a more prolonged course using a lower dose (0.05 mg/kg per day). Such a regimen allows earlier growth acceleration without compromising final adult height. In cases where absence of sexual development is causing social/psychological difficulties, testosterone enanthate (100 mg IM monthly for three doses) will bring about some penile enlargement and pubic hair growth. A further short course of testosterone can be given after 3 to 4 months. Frequently, spontaneous pubertal development occurs within a year of starting testosterone treatment. In a randomized controlled trial, letrozole (a specific aromatase inhibitor) in a dose of 2.5 mg orally daily together with testosterone therapy has been shown to improve the final height of adolescents with CDGP compared to those treated with testosterone alone. However, the potential deleterious side effects on bone density have to be taken into account when manipulating growth by inhibiting estrogen action.

E. Precocious sexual development (see Chapter 23)

   1. Definition. Puberty is considered precocious if secondary sexual characteristics occur before the age of 9 years in boys. The rapid increase in growth and sexual maturation may provoke serious behavioral and emotional problems. The most important long-term consequence in these children is short stature, because rapid skeletal maturation leads to early epiphyseal fusion. In true or **central precocious puberty,** there is premature activation of the hypothalamic–pituitary–gonadal axis. **Incomplete (pseudo-, peripheral) precocious puberty** refers to development of secondary sexual characteristics in boys before age 9 as a result of autonomous secretion of androgens or hCG.

   2. Etiology

   a. Central precocious puberty (Table 23.7)

   (1) Idiopathic central precocious puberty (CPP) is diagnosed when no organic cause can be found for the disorder. It accounts for 10% to 75% of all cases in boys, which is in contrast to girls, in whom >90% of cases are idiopathic. The slowly progressive variant of central precocious puberty, which is well documented in girls, may also occur in male adolescents. In a study from Israel, about half the boys with CPP ($n = 21$) and early puberty ($n = 44$) have the slowly progressive variant. They have a prolonged course of puberty, and their final height is not impaired.

   (2) CNS lesions are a common cause of central precocious puberty. CNS lesions or tumors (glioma, ependymoma, astrocytoma, hypothalamic hamartoma, germinoma, teratoma) in the posterior hypothalamus, tuber cinereum, third ventricle, and pineal region can disturb the regulatory mechanism by infiltration, compression, or interruption of neuronal connections within the hypothalamic–pituitary–gonadal axis to cause precocious puberty. In some patients, hypothalamic hamartoma may be a source of GnRH. Activation of the TFGα-erbB1 signaling complex has been implicated in precocious puberty caused by hypothalamic hamartoma. Patients with hypothalamic hamartoma typically develop "gelastic" seizures that are quite resistant to anticonvulsant treatment. **CNS infection** can cause early sexual development and can be associated with the presence of hydrocephalus. Sexual precocity following **head injury** may also occur, although hypopituitarism is more common.

   (3) Juvenile hypothyroidism is a well-known but very rare cause of precocious puberty. The pathogenesis is unknown. It can be associated with hyperprolactinemia and galactorrhea. This syndrome has been postulated to be the result of a hormonal overlap phenomenon, with overproduction of gonadotropins as well as TSH. As alternative hypothesis is that the condition arises from weak intrinsic FSH activity associated with extreme TSH elevation. Early sexual development as a result of overtreatment of thyrotoxicosis with propylthiouracil has also been reported.

   (4) Any **virilizing condition** can cause early activation of the hypothalamic–pituitary–gonadal axis because of exposure to androgens leading to rapid

TABLE 23.7 Etiology of Central Precocious Puberty

Idiopathic	Sporadic
	Familial autosomal dominant (rare)
CNS tumors	Optic and hypothalamic gliomas
	Hypothalamic hamartoma
	Ependymoma
	Pineal-region tumor
CNS lesions	Hydrocephalus
	Septo-optic dysplasia
	Arachnoid cyst
	Cerebral atrophy
	Head trauma
	Epilepsy
CNS infection	meningitis, encephalitis, abscess
Cranial irradiation and cancer chemotherapy	
Fetal alcohol syndrome	
Maternal uniparental disomy of chromosome 14	
Hypothyroidism	
Williams syndrome	
Secondary to virilizing disorders such as congenital adrenal hyperplasia, hormone-secreting neoplasms	

CNS, central nervous system.

advancement of bone age. Patients with congenital adrenal hyperplasia (CAH) are exposed to excessive amounts of adrenal androgens. If glucocorticoid suppression is inadequate, this may lead to accelerated skeletal maturation, which may <u>trigger the onset of central precocious puberty</u>. This form of precocious puberty frequently complicates the treatment of patients with CAH.

- **b. Incomplete (pseudo-, peripheral) precocious puberty** (Table 23.8)
  - **(1)** Virilizing **congenital adrenal hyperplasia** causes precocious pseudopuberty because of increased adrenal androgen production resulting in sexual maturation (e.g., 21-hydroxylase, 11-hydroxylase deficiency).
  - **(2)** Virilizing **adrenal tumors,** usually adrenocortical carcinoma, are rare in childhood (see Chapter 18).
  - **(3) Cushing syndrome** as a cause of virilization is also rare.
  - **(4) Interstitial cell (Leydig cell) tumors** of the testes secrete testosterone and typically present with unilateral testicular enlargement. They are usually benign. Tumors can arise from adrenal rest tissue in the testes, or the adrenal rest tissue can increase in size during adrenarche or secondary to congenital adrenal hyperplasia, leading to testicular enlargement. Although most Leydig cell tumors presenting with incomplete precocious puberty are sporadic in nature, somatic activating mutations of the stimulatory G protein (Gsp oncogenes) resulting in constitutively activation of the LH receptor may result in Leydig cell hyperplasia and tumor.
  - **(5) HCG** can be produced by hepatoblastomas, retroperitoneal tumors, and germ-cell tumors. HCG-secreting tumors account for 4% of cases of sexual precocity in males and are reported <u>more commonly in Oriental people</u>. Frequently, germ-cell tumors are intracranial and show marked contrast enhancement on CT brain scan because of their high vascularity. Elevated levels of α-HCG and β-fetoprotein can be found in the blood and cerebrospinal fluid. These patients have pubertal testosterone concentrations,

TABLE 23.8	Causes of Incomplete Precocious Puberty in Boys

1. Gonadotropin-independent sexual precocity
   - Familial male-limited precocious puberty (FMPP)
   - McCune-Albright syndrome and other activating GNAS gene mutations
   - DAX1 gene mutation
2. Premature adrenarche
3. hCG-secreting tumors located within and outside (hepatic, testicular, and retroperitoneal) the central nervous system
4. Increased androgen secretion from the adrenal gland or testes
   - Congenital adrenal hyperplasia
   - Virilizing adrenal tumors
   - Leydig cell adenoma (may contain somatic activating mutations of LHR or Gsp oncogenes)
   - Corticosteroid resistance syndromes
5. Heterosexual development
   - Feminizing adrenal tumors
   - Environmental exposure to estrogen and drugs
   - Familial aromatase hyperactivity
   - 3β-hydroxysteroid dehydrogenase and 17-ketoreductase deficiency

mildly elevated serum LH (because of cross-reaction with hCG in some radioimmunoassays), which does not increase in response to GnRH stimulation; and suppressed serum FSH levels.

(6) Premature adrenarche has conventionally been defined as the development of pubic hair with or without axillary hair before the age of 9 years in boys. In the United States today, boys have testicular and pubic hair development at a younger age than in the past. Girls are affected 10 times as frequently as boys, but no explanation for the unequal sex ratio has been forthcoming. An increase in frequency of premature adrenarche has been reported in children with cerebral dysfunction, and both sexes are equally affected in such cases. Premature adrenarche is also more frequently observed among children with obesity and Prader Willi syndrome. In some patients, the early development of sex hair is associated with normal adrenal androgen concentrations for their chronologic age, suggesting that premature adrenarche may be the result of increased sensitivity to androgens in peripheral tissues. Premature sex hair development is associated with increased body odor as well as oily skin and hair, but there is no penile enlargement. Premature adrenarche has no adverse effects on the onset and progression of gonadarche or on final adult height. These children tend to have advanced bone age at the time of diagnosis or during the initial follow-up period.

The serum DHEA and DHEAS levels in children with premature adrenarche are higher than normal for their chronologic age, but the levels are still in the normal pubertal range. These children may have impaired insulin sensitivity, increased serum total and free IGF-1 concentrations, and unfavorable lipid profiles. Investigation should be carried out to exclude other causes of androgen excess, such as adrenal, testicular, or hCG-secreting tumors, or mild/occult defects of adrenal steroidogenesis, because premature adrenarche is a diagnosis of exclusion. Patients with borderline elevation of adrenal steroid precursor concentrations (17α hydroxyprogesterone, 17-OHP, >6 nmol/L) should undergo an ACTH stimulation test (250 μg Synacthen IV and measuring the 17-OHP levels at 30 and 60 minutes). An ACTH-stimulated 17-OHP level >30 nmol/L is diagnostic of late-onset 21-hydroxylase deficiency. The prevalence of late-onset CAH among patients with premature adrenarche is not well defined and ranges from 7% to >40%.

(7) <u>Familial male-limited precocious puberty (FMPP)</u>, formerly known as <u>testotoxicosis</u>, is a form of gonadotropin-independent sexual precocity characterized by sexual development with pubertal sex hormone concentrations and spermatogenesis in the absence of a pubertal pattern of pituitary gonadotropic secretion. In contrast to patients with central precocious puberty, patients with FMPP have elevated serum testosterone levels in the absence of pulsatile, nocturnal LH (immunoreactive and bioactive), and FSH secretion or pubertal gonadotropin response to GnRH. Testicular biopsies have revealed an abundance of mature Leydig cells with variable degree of spermatogenesis and seminiferous tubule maturation as well as germ-cell degeneration in some tubules. Testicular Leydig cell nodules have been reported in some patients. The pattern of inheritance supports a sex-limited autosomal dominant transmission with >90% penetrance, and female carriers do not have any endocrine abnormalities. The condition is a result of activating mutations in the third cytoplasmic loop, transmembrane helix II, V, and VI of the LH receptor. The Gsα-protein subunit couples >20 different receptors to stimulation of adenylate cyclase, and mutation in this gene can result in loss of function (pseudohypoparathyroidism type 1a) or gain in function as in McCune-Albright syndrome. Recently, two boys with McCune-Albright syndrome and gonadotropin-independent sexual precocity have been described. Concurrent occurrence of pseudohypoparathyroidism type 1a and gonadotropin-independent precocity has been reported in two boys who were found to have a unique point mutation in the guanine nucleotide-binding protein subunit Gsα gene. This mutant protein has been shown to be constitutively active at a "low" temperature of 32°C, but the protein rapidly denatures with loss of function at the usual "core" temperature of 37°C. These patients present with early development of secondary sexual characteristics between 3 and 5 years of age and are indistinguishable clinically from patients with true precocious puberty.

(8) Primary adrenal insufficiency and gonadotropin-independent precocious puberty were reported in a 2-year-old Brazilian boy with a G-nucleotide insertion between nucleotides 430 and 431 in exon1 in the DAX1 gene, resulting in a frameshift mutation and a premature stop codon at position 71 of the DAX1 gene. Steroid replacement led to a decrease in testicular size and return of testosterone levels to prepubertal level.

(9) **Androgens** prescribed in the past for aplastic anemia may cause accelerated growth and penile enlargement.

3. Diagnosis

a. A detailed history should uncover the timing of the onset of excessive growth, body odor, oiliness of skin and hair, pubic hair, and genital development. History of CNS infection and the pattern of sexual development in other family members may be helpful. Children with a CNS cause for the sexual precocity frequently have neurologic symptoms.

b. In the **physical examination**, the height, weight, and pubertal staging must be accurately documented. Penile enlargement without significant testicular enlargement is helpful in identifying patients with incomplete precocious puberty. Hypertension, abdominal mass, and cushingoid features are suggestive of an adrenal tumor. A full neurologic evaluation and funduscopic examination are essential. Unilateral testicular enlargement is suggestive of a testicular malignancy.

c. **Hormonal assays** should include serum testosterone and basal and peak serum LH and FSH response to GnRH. Patients with central precocious puberty have a peak serum LH and FSH in the pubertal range, with the LH response greater than the FSH response. The interpretation of the serum LH and FSH concentrations as indices of pubertal gonadotropin levels depends on the type of assays that are used for their measurements. Using a conventional radioimmunoassay, it was found that even an LH/FSH ratio of 3 was not sensitive enough to establish a diagnosis of precocious or normal puberty in boys. With the use of two-site fluoroimmunometric assay or other sensitive immunochemiluminometric (ICMA) assays, a basal LH cutoff of 0.6 IU/L and a GnRH-stimulated LH >9.6 IU/L have been found to be sensitive indices to establish a male pubertal gonadotropin profile. Although the GnRH test is helpful in distinguishing incomplete from central precocious puberty, it is not helpful in identifying the underlying CNS pathology. Additional hormone tests, including thyroid function as well as adrenal steroids, should be ordered if adrenal tumor or hyperplasia is suspected.

d. Bone-age radiography and CT or MRI brain scan should be performed on all patients with suspected central precocious puberty. CT scan or MRI of the adrenal area is indicated if the presence of an adrenal tumor is suspected.

e. All patients with midline CNS tumors and sexual precocity should have a measurement of β-HCG and of α-fetoprotein in the serum and also in the cerebrospinal fluid, if possible, to exclude the existence of germ-cell tumors.

f. Molecular genetic studies will be helpful in patients with gonadotropin-independent sexual precocity.

4. Treatment

a. Central precocious puberty. One possible sequela of CPP is a variable attenuation of adult stature depending on the age of onset. Although treatment with medroxyprogesterone acetate and cyproterone acetate can suppress pubertal development effectively in children with precocious puberty, neither has any effect on skeletal maturation and hence eventual adult height. They are no longer recommended for treatment of CPP. Indications for GnRH-analog treatment for CPP include **(1)** CPP with one or two signs of puberty before the age of 9 years; **(2)** pubertal GnRH-stimulated gonadotropin levels; **(3)** rapidly progressive puberty; **(4)** compromised predicted adult height; and **(5)** psychological or behavioral reasons.

(1) Recent experience with depot GnRH agonists (depot leuprolide acetate, 100 to 150 μg/kg, and depot triptorelin, 80 to 100 μg/kg) given IM every 4 weeks has shown that these preparations are equally effective and they are currently the preferred treatment. Treatment can be discontinued at 11 to 12 years of age, and there is prompt reactivation of the hypothalamic–pituitary–gonadal axis, allowing puberty to progress. The height gain from cessation of therapy to final height is negatively correlated with the bone age at the end of treatment, and boys will grow about 9.9 ± 3.3 cm after interruption of treatment. Though GnRH antagonist has not been used in central precocious puberty, the development of orally bioavailable nonpeptide GnRH antagonist (and agonists) may lead to simpler and more acceptable delivery methods.

(2) Successful suppression of puberty has been achieved with 3-month depot leuprorelin (11.25 mg), 2-month long-acting goserelin (20 ladex LA, 10.8 mg) or 3-month depot triptorelin (11.25 mg), but the efficacy of these long-acting depot preparations in improving final adult height has not been adequately documented.

(3) Subnormal growth velocity, which is occasionally observed in some children with precocious puberty treated with a GnRH agonist, is likely to be due to "catch-down" growth; or these patients have already passed the pubertal growth spurt because of the advanced skeletal maturation. The subnormal stimulated and spontaneous growth hormone concentrations observed can be secondary to the elevated body mass index in these patients. Serum IGF1 levels are usually normal in such children.

(4) Final heights in treated children are greater than the historical controls. In a recent review, 78% of patients treated with depot GnRH analog reached a final height in their target height range, and they had normal body proportions. Therapy offers the greatest advantage for those children in whom the onset of puberty occurs before the age of 6 years, those who demonstrate rapidly accelerating bone age, those with the lower genetic height potential, or those with the largest difference between the target and predicted height. Obesity occurs with a high rate in boys with CPP and does not appear to be related to long-term gonadal suppression by GnRH analog. No negative effects on bone mineral density or fertility have been reported. Semen analysis in a limited number of CPP patients treated with GnRH analogs had revealed normal sperm count, motility, and morphology. However, in boys with CPP resulting from hypothalamic hamartoma and treated with GnRH-analog, the testicular volume remained smaller than normal posttreatment and took up to 5 years after stopping treatment before the testicular size became normalized. Treated patients should be followed up into adulthood.

(5) Patients with CPP with poor predicted adult height despite GnRH analog treatment can be <u>treated with growth hormone</u>. Preliminary results are encouraging.

(6) Children with an organic cause for their central precocious puberty should have treatment of their underlying pathology in addition to GnRH agonist therapy. Both boys and girls with CPP have been found to have hypothalamic hamartomas, which are slow-growing and seldom associated with neurodevelopmental or gross neurologic deficit. Young patients with hamartoma of the tuber cinereum typically present with gelastic seizures that respond poorly to anticonvulsants. Conventionally, surgery is not recommended, and conservative symptomatic management with anticonvulsants for epilepsy and GnRH-analog for precocious puberty has been the treatment of choice. Occasionally, such children progress to having intractable seizures despite anticonvulsant treatment in later childhood and adolescence. An innovative surgical approach (trans-callosal, trans-septal, trans-ventricular) through the third ventricle under stereotactic and magnetic resonance guidance has allowed safe and complete removal of these hamartomas and control of the intractable seizures.

b. Incomplete precocious puberty. Among patients with incomplete precocious puberty are those with <u>premature adrenarche</u> who do not require any treatment. Treatment of patients with an <u>androgen-secreting</u> tumor should be directed at the tumor. Patients with <u>congenital adrenal hyperplasia</u> should be given glucocorticoid and mineralocorticoid replacement. GnRH analog treatment can be started if central precocious puberty develops during the treatment of CAH. <u>Leydig cell tumors</u> of children are always benign, but radical orchiectomy remains the treatment of choice. <u>Intracranial germ-cell tumors</u> are very radiosensitive, and combination chemotherapy is advised if ventriculoperitoneal shunting is done for hydrocephalus. Even after definitive treatment for incomplete precocious puberty, spontaneous onset of central precocious puberty can occur because of the advanced skeletal maturation. GnRH agonist therapy is indicated if that occurs.

c. Children with <u>familial male-limited precocious puberty (testotoxicosis)</u> can be treated with medroxyprogesterone acetate (100 to 150 mg IM every 2 weeks) or ketoconazole, an antifungal agent that blocks androgen synthesis (200 mg q8h). Adult height exceeded pretreatment predicted height by 5 to 13 cm in 5 patients with FMPP treated with ketoconazole for a mean duration of 6.2 years. A combination of spironolactone, which blocks androgen action (1 to 3 mg/kg q12h), and testolactone, an aromatase inhibitor (5 mg/kg q6h, increasing to 10 mg/kg q6h), can also achieve short-term and medium-term control of testosterone secretion. Measurement of testosterone and estradiol levels is not helpful in monitoring treatment with this combination of drugs. Elevation of circulating gonadotropins when a patient is treated with ketoconazole or spironolactone/testolactone combination can be managed by the addition of GnRH agonist therapy. The results of 6 years of treatment with spironolactone, testolactone, and deslorelin in FMPP have been encouraging.

Selected References

Acherman JC, Ozisik G, Meeks JJ, Jameson JL. Genetic causes of human reproductive diseases. *J Clin Endocrinol Metab* 2002;87:2447–2454.

Bin-Abbas B, Conte FA, Grumbach MM, Kaplan SL. Congenital hypogonadotropic hypogonadism and micropenis: effect of testosterone treatment on adult penile size. Why sex reversal is not indicated. *J Pediatr* 1999;134:579–583.

Brennan J, Capel B. One tissue, two fates: molecular genetic events that underlie testis versus ovary development. *Nat Rev Genet* 2004;5:509–521.

Britto VN, Batista MC, Borges MF, et al. Diagnostic value of fluorometric assays in the evaluation of precocious puberty. *J Clin Endocrinol Metab* 1999;84:3539–3544.

Butler GE, Sellar RE, Walker RF, et al. Oral testosterone undecanoate in the management of delayed puberty in boys: pharmacokinetics and effects on sexual maturation and growth. *J Clin Endocrinol Metab* 1992;75:37–44.

Delemarre Van de Waal HA, Odink RJ. Pulsatile GnRH treatment in boys and girls with idiopathic hypogonadotropic hypogonadism. *Hum Reprod* 1993;8(suppl 2):180–183.

Denburg MR, Silfen ME, Manibo AM, et al. Insulin sensitivity and insulin-like growth factor system in prepubertal boys with premature adrenarche. *J Clin Endocrinol Metab* 2002;87:5604–5609.

Hadziselimovic F, Herzog B. Treatment with a luteinizing hormone-releasing hormone analogue after successful orchidopexy markedly improves the chance of fertility in late life. *J Urol* 1997;158(suppl 342):1193–1195.

Hutson JM, Hasthorpe S. Abnormalities of testicular descent. *Cell Tissue Res* 2005;322: 155–158.

Lawrence SE, Faught KA, Vethamuthu J, Lawson ML. Beneficial effects of raloxifene and tamoxifen in the treatment of pubertal gynecomastia. *J Pediatr* 2004;145:71–76.

Layman LC. Human gene mutations causing infertility. *J Med Genet* 2002;39:153–161.

Lee PA, Coughlin MT, Bellinger MF. Paternity and hormone levels after unilateral cryptorchidism: association with pretreatment testicular location. *J Urol* 2000;164:1697– 1701.

Leschek EW, Jones J, Barnes KM, et al. Six year results of spironolactone and testolactone treatment of familial male limited precocious puberty with addition of desorelin after central puberty onset. *J Clin Endocrinol Metab* 1999;84:175–178.

Low LCK, Wang Q. Gonadotropin independent precocious puberty. *J Pediatr Endocrinol Metab* 1998;11:497–507.

Ojeda SR, Lomniczi A, Mastronadi C, et al. Minireview: the neuroendocrine regulation of puberty: is the time ripe for a system biology approach? *Endocrinology* 2006;147:1166– 1174.

Parks JS, Brown MR, Hurley DL, et al. Heritable disorders of pituitary development. *J Clin Endocrinol Metab* 1999;84:4362–4370.

Partsch CJ, Heger S, Sippell WG. Management and outcome of central precocious puberty. *Clin Endocrinol* 2002;56:129–148.

Rohrich RJ, Ha RY, Kenkel JM, et al. Classification and management of gynecomastia: defining the role of ultrasound-associated liposuction. *Plast Reconstr Surg* 2003;111:909– 923.

Root AW. Magnetic resonance imaging in hypopituitarism. *J Clin Endocrinol Metab* 1991;72:10–11.

Seminara SB. Mechanisms of disease: the first kiss-a crucial role for kisspeptin-1 and its receptor, G-protein-coupled-receptor 54, in puberty and reproduction. *Nat Clin Pract Endocrinol Metab* 2006;2:328–334.

Seminara SB, Hayes FJ, Crowley WF Jr. Gonadotropin-releasing hormone deficiency in the human (idiopathic hypogonadotropic hypogonadism and Kallmann's syndrome): pathophysiological and genetic considerations. *Endocr Rev* 1998;19:521–539.

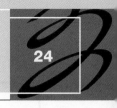

I. GENERAL PRINCIPLES

The human testis is an organ with dual function, endocrine (hormone production) and exocrine (sperm production). The testis is composed of parenchyma, which is surrounded by a solid capsule (tunica albuginea). Extension of tunica albuginea into the testicle as fibrous septa creates 200 to 300 pyramidal lobules, which contain coiled seminiferous tubules. Each testis contains 600 to 900 seminiferous tubules with an approximate length of 200 to 300 m and occupies 80% to 90% of the testicular mass. It has a huge reproductive capacity, with production of 10 to 20 million spermatozoa daily during male reproductive life. The seminiferous tubules are composed of Sertoli cells and germinal cells. The seminiferous tubules are interspersed within an interstitial space containing androgen-producing Leydig cells, blood vessels, lymphatics, nerves, macrophages, and fibroblasts. Testicular function is regulated by a series of closed-loop feedback systems consisting of six main components: (a) extrahypothalamic central nervous system (CNS), (b) hypothalamus, (c) pituitary gland, (d) testes, (e) sex steroid-sensitive end organs, and (f) sites of androgen transport and metabolism.

A. Hypothalamic pituitary function (Fig. 24.1)

1. **Extrahypothalamic central nervous system.** Extrahypothalamic brain tissues have both stimulatory and inhibitory effects on reproductive function. In the midbrain, cell bodies containing the biogenic amines, norepinephrine (NE) and serotonin (5-hydroxytryptamine; 5-HT), as well as other neurotransmitters, are connected to many areas of the hypothalamus, including the preoptic, anterior, and medial basal areas where gonadotropin-releasing hormone (GnRH)–containing neurons are located.

2. **Hypothalamus**
   a. **Pulsatile secretion of GnRH.** The hypothalamus is the integrating center for the regulation of GnRH. GnRH is a decapeptide released in predetermined regular pulses, which peak every 90 to 120 minutes into the portal circulation to stimulate pituitary gonadotropin synthesis and release. GnRH has a half-life of 5 to 10 minutes and, because of its low systemic concentration, is not easily measured in the systemic circulation. The pulse frequency of hypophysial GnRH release is important in determining the relative ratio of luteinizing hormone (LH) and follicle-stimulating hormone (FSH) released into the circulation. <u>Continuous administration</u> of GnRH causes cessation of gonadotropins (LH, FSH) production, through inhibitory downregulation of GnRH receptors. Inhibition of gonadotropic secretion results in decreased serum testosterone and estradiol levels and thus has therapeutic applications in sex steroid–dependent conditions such as prostate carcinoma, endometriosis, and precocious puberty. On the other hand, physiologic <u>pulsatile administration</u> of GnRH can establish normal production of LH and FSH in patients with hypothalamic-induced hypogonadism, such as those with Kallmann syndrome.
   b. **GnRH regulation.** The extrahypothalamic CNS, circulating androgens, and circulating peptide hormones such as prolactin, activin, inhibin, and leptin regulate GnRH synthesis and release. Local modulators of GnRH secretion include a number of neuropeptides, catecholamines, indolamines, nitric oxide, excitatory amino acids, dopamine, neuropeptide Y, vasoactive intestinal

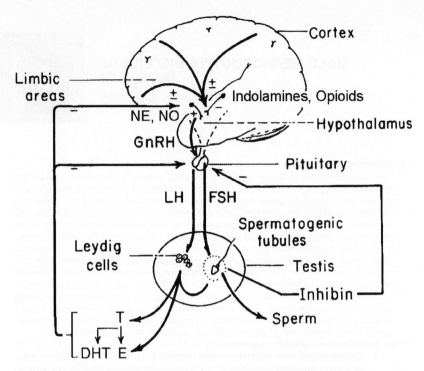

Figure 24.1. Hypothalamic–pituitary–testicular axis in the male. The hypothalamus is the integrating center for central nervous system (CNS) regulation of gonadotropin-releasing hormone (GnRH). Extrahypothalamic CNS input has both inhibitory and stimulatory influences on GnRH secretion. Neurotransmitters such as norepinephrine (NE), dopamine (DA), opioid peptides, γ-aminobutyric acid (GABA), serotonin, and melatonin serve as regulators of GnRH synthesis and release from hypothalamus. The human testis is a dual organ with endocrine and reproductive functions. Testicular function is regulated by a series of closed-loop feedback systems involving higher centers in the CNS, hypothalamus, pituitary, and testicular endocrine and germinal compartments. DHT, 5α-dihydrotestosterone; E, estradiol; FSH, follicle-stimulating hormone; LH, luteinizing hormone; NO, nitric oxide; T, testosterone. (Reprinted from Swerdloff RS, Wang C. The testes and male sexual function. In: Goldman L, Ausiello D, eds. *Cecil Textbook of Medicine.* 22nd ed. Philadelphia: WB Saunders; 2004:1472–1483.)

polypeptide (VIP), and corticotropin-releasing hormone. Testosterone (T), directly or by its metabolic products, estradiol (E_2) and dihydrotestosterone (DHT), has an inhibitory effect on GnRH, LH, and FSH secretion.

3. **Pituitary gland.** LH and FSH are large glycopeptides that, like thyroid-stimulating hormone (TSH) and human chorionic gonadotropin (hCG), are created from α and β chains. The α chain is identical in all four hormones, but the biologic effects are exerted by the β chain. The α and β chains are encoded by genes on different chromosomes. The α chain is encoded by a gene on chromosome 6 (6q12.21), FSH-β on chromosome 11 (11p13), and LH-β and hCG-β on chromosome 19 (19q13.32). LH and FSH are produced by gonadotropin cells in the pituitary gland and are secreted in a pulsatile pattern.

   a. LH binds to specific, high-affinity surface membrane receptors on Leydig cells. Binding is followed by G-protein–mediated events that stimulate testosterone production within the testes. LH has a half-life of ~20 minutes, versus that of FSH of 3 hours and hCG of 5 hours.

   b. FSH binds to receptors on Sertoli cells, stimulating production of a large number of specific proteins including androgen-binding protein, inhibin, activin, plasminogen activator, γ-glutamyl transpeptidase, and protein kinase inhibitor. FSH, in conjunction with testosterone produced by Leydig cells, works synergistically to promote spermatogenesis and to inhibit germ-cell apoptosis.

  c. **Gonadotropin regulation.** As stated previously, gonadotropin release is regulated by the pulsatile release of GnRH. The feedback regulation of LH production in man occurs by testosterone and its metabolites estradiol and dihydrotestosterone. Testosterone mainly inhibits GnRH at the hypothalamus with mild suppressive action on LH, whereas estradiol has inhibitory effect at both the hypothalamus and pituitary levels. Inhibin and activin are glycoproteins involved in regulation of FSH secretion. Inhibin B, produced by Sertoli cells, enters the peripheral circulation and inhibits pituitary secretion of FSH. Activin stimulates FSH secretion and spermatogenesis. Both inhibin and activin are also thought to act locally as paracrine regulators of spermatogenesis.

B. Testes function

  1. Steroid hormone production and action

  a. **Testosterone production and secretion** (Fig. 24.2). The testes are composed of interstitial steroid-secreting cells (Leydig cells) and seminiferous tubules containing Sertoli cells and germ cells. Under the regulation of LH, Leydig cells are the main source of $\sim$7 mg of testosterone produced each day. The parent substance of testosterone biosynthesis is cholesterol, which is mainly produced and stored in vacuoles of Leydig cells. Testosterone synthesis occurs through the $\Delta 4$ or $\Delta 5$ pathway, with the rate-limiting step being the LH-inducible conversion of cholesterol to pregnenolone by the enzyme P450scc, cholesterol 20, 22-hydroxylase:20, 22 desmolase activity (side-chain cleavage enzyme). The majority of produced testosterone is immediately released to the blood, mainly via the spermatic vein, and smaller amounts are transported in the lymphatic system. In eugonadal men, $\sim$95% of circulating testosterone is produced by the testes. The testes also produce equimolar amounts of epitestosterone, which is an inactive epimer of testosterone. The ratio of testosterone to epitestosterone in urine is used as a marker for exogenous testosterone in athletes who are doping.

  b. **Testosterone transport and binding proteins.** The majority of circulating T is bound either strongly to sex hormone–binding globulin (60%) (SHBG) or loosely to albumin (37%), whereas 2% to 3% remains unbound (free testosterone). Unbound and albumin-bound T are available for cellular entry and are referred to as **bioavailable testosterone.** Despite binding to SHBG, the half-life of T in blood is only 10 minutes, and it is catabolized efficiently by the liver and eliminated via the urine as 17-ketosteroids and sulfates.

  Circulating SHBG is a large glycoprotein, which is encoded by a gene on chromosome 17 and produced by the liver. SHBG may also be produced in other tissues such as prostate and mammary glands, where it may have local functions. Hepatic production of SHBG is influenced by a number of physiologic and metabolic factors.

  (1) Sex steroids are important modulators of SHBG synthesis; **estrogens stimulate whereas androgens inhibit SHBG production, which explains the higher level of SHBG in women.** The estrogen/androgen ratio is a major determinant of the hepatic production of SHBG.

  (2) In patients with hepatic cirrhosis, estrogen levels are maintained despite a fall in androgen levels, leading to an increase in circulating SHBG. Because elevated SHBG levels tend to increase the total T levels without affecting the free or bioavailable T concentrations, total T levels may be normal in the presence of a moderate decrease in T secretion.

  (3) Thyroid hormones influence SHBG levels. Decreased concentrations of thyroxine (T_4) or tri-iodothyronine (T_3) diminish SHBG, whereas hyperthyroid states are associated with high binding protein concentrations.

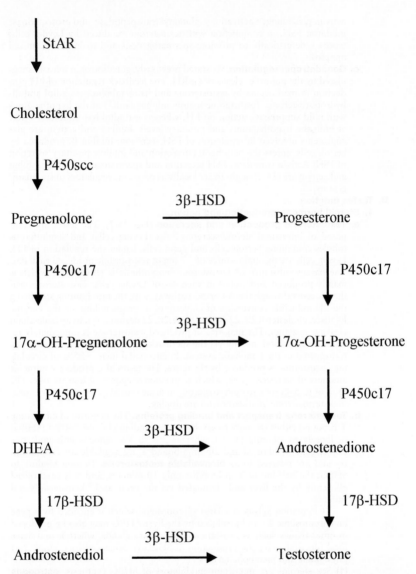

Figure 24.2. Testosterone synthesis in the testis. Steroidogenic acute regulatory protein metabolizes cholesterol from cellular stores to the mitochondria. Intratesticular pathways for synthesis of testosterone. Whereas both the ∆5 **(left)** and ∆4 **(right)** pathways exists the ∆5 pathway predominates in the testes. (Reprinted from Swerdloff RS, Wang C. The testes and male sexual function. In: Goldman L, Ausiello D, eds. *Cecil Textbook of Medicine.* 22nd ed. Philadelphia: WB Saunders; 2004:1472–1483.)

    (4) Body mass and degree of adiposity influence SHBG concentrations. SHBG levels are **low** in obese and acromegalic patients. Much of this effect is **mediated by insulin, which is increased in such patients.**
   c. T conversion to E$_2$ and DHT (Fig. 24.3). Daily testosterone production is 5 to 7 mg (5 000 to 7 000 μg) per day. About 40 μg of estradiol (E$_2$) is

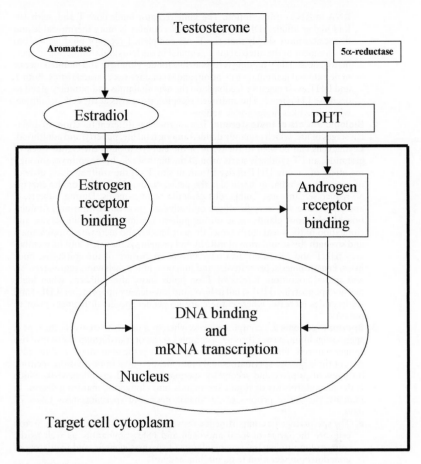

Figure 24.3. Conversion of testosterone to estradiol and dihydrotestosterone, and genomic effect on target tissue.

produced daily in a eugonadal adult male. Three fourths of this is derived from peripheral aromatization of T by the enzyme **aromatase**, and the rest (~10 μg) is secreted directly by the testes (Leydig cells). Dihydrotestosterone (DHT) (350 μg) is mainly derived from peripheral conversion of T by **5α-reductase**. Two isozymes of 5-reductase have been identified in humans. Type I is predominantly found in the skin, liver, and testes, whereas type II 5α-reductase predominates in the reproductive tissues, genital skin, and epididymis. T thus serves as a prohormone for both E_2 and DHT.

d. **Androgen receptor (AR) binding.** The androgen receptor gene is encoded by eight exons (A to H) on the long arm of the X chromosome near the centromere (Xq11-12), and is expressed on androgen-sensitive organs. The androgen receptor is a polypeptide consisting of 910 amino acids, and, like other steroid and thyroid hormone receptors, is a DNA-binding protein. The AR protein is distributed in both the cytoplasm and the nucleus. Its activity is ligand-dependent and transcription-regulating. The androgen receptor is a typical steroid receptor consisting of three main regions: a steroid-binding site, a DNA-binding site, and a regulatory region that influences messenger

RNA (mRNA) transcription. The same receptor binds both T and, with 10-fold higher affinity, DHT. The DHT–AR complex is more thermostable and dissociates more slowly than the T–AR complex. T-receptor binding leads to development of the internal male genitalia in the fetus and stimulation of spermatogenesis. DHT binding is responsible for development and maintenance of male external genitalia, virilization, and secondary sex characteristics. Both T and DHT exert negative feedback on the hypothalamus and pituitary gland to decrease LH release. The androgen receptor also exists at the cell membrane, where it evokes nongenomic actions.

2. **Biologic effects of testosterone:** Testosterone has different functions in different stages of life, which is mainly divided among fetal life, puberty, and adulthood. Leydig cells can be seen in the testis of the embryo around the eighth week of gestation, and T synthesis starts around the ninth week. In the embryo, through the effect of mainly DHT derived from in situ T on the wülffian duct, growth of external genitalia, in particular the penis, occurs. Lack of T or the enzyme 5a-reductase can cause ambiguous genitalia or micropenis. During puberty, T and DHT have very specific effects on body-hair growth (virilization), stimulation of sebaceous glands (acne during puberty), stimulation of the larynx and elongation of the vocal cords (voice drop or break), and increase of muscle mass and strength (by stimulation of mRNA and protein synthesis). T and its metabolites (DHT and estradiol) also have effects on closure of the epiphysis, bone mass, hematopoiesis, prostate size and function, libido, behavior, aggressiveness, and spatial cognition. Effects of T on lipids show after puberty, when high-density lipoproteins (HDLs) fall in boys, and low-density lipoproteins (LDLs) and triglycerides increase, whereas there are no gender-specific differences prior to puberty.

3. **Spermatogenesis** is a complex process whereby a primitive stem cell, the type A spermatogonium, passes through a complex series of transformations to give rise to spermatozoa. The maturation of the germ cells in the seminiferous tubule consists of three phases: spermatogonial multiplication by mitotic division; meiotic divisions of primary and secondary spermatocytes; and spermiogenesis, which is the metamorphosis of round spermatids into elongating maturing sperm. In humans, the entire process of spermatogenesis and spermiogenesis takes 72 days.

   a. The spermatogenic compartment consists of the Sertoli and germ cells. Sertoli cells are the target of local androgen and FSH stimulation, as well as the source of multiple paracrine regulators of spermatogenesis, and regulators of gonadotropin secretion (e.g., inhibin, activin).

   b. LH or hCG administration stimulates an increase in intratesticular T and promptly initiates spermatogenesis. In the congenital and complete form of hypogonadotropic hypogonadism, treatment with hCG alone does not result in maturation of the seminiferous epithelium beyond the spermatid stage. In these patients, FSH alone will not initiate spermatogenesis, but FSH administration to hCG-primed hypogonadal men results in completion of spermatogenesis. Thus, FSH appears to be essential for spermiogenesis (development of spermatids into mature spermatozoa). Once LH or hCG has induced spermatogenesis, additional FSH is not required for maintenance of spermatogenesis. Thus, in hypogonadotropic subjects primed with hCG and FSH, spermatogenesis can be maintained by hCG alone. Furthermore, in patients with incomplete or acquired hypogonadotropism (previously exposed to FSH), hCG alone may reinstate close to normal sperm counts.

4. **Paracrine control of testicular function and Leydig cell–Sertoli cell interaction.** The results of numerous studies suggest the existence of an **intratesticular Leydig cell–Sertoli cell axis**. The precise nature of this interaction remains unclear, but recent studies suggest that Sertoli cells exert both inhibitory and stimulatory influences on Leydig cells. It has been proposed that Sertoli cells may be the source of a large number of peptides that have paracrine-regulatory activity on both the Leydig cells and the germinal elements. The interaction between

the Sertoli cells and the maturing germ cells might be responsible for the orderly events of spermatogenesis.

II. MALE REPRODUCTIVE DISORDERS
Male reproductive disorders are discussed under the following broad categories:
- Hypogonadism
- Infertility
- Varicocele
- Male sexual dysfunction
- Gynecomastia

A. Hypogonadism. Hypogonadism refers to a state of absolute or relative androgen deficiency. Major diagnostic categories are listed on Table 24.1; these include primary hypogonadism (testicular insufficiency), secondary or hypogonadotropic hypogonadism (resulting from decreased GnRH or LH production), and androgen insensitivity (decreased action of androgens on target tissues).

    1. Clinical manifestations of androgen deficiency. The time of onset of androgen deficiency influences clinical features.

        a. Fetal onset. Differentiation of the genitalia along male lines is an androgen-dependent process that occurs during the first trimester of gestation. During this time, placental hCG binds to LH receptors on Leydig cells and promotes T secretion. By the 13th week, pituitary secretion of LH in conjunction with hCG continues to stimulate T secretion. T deficiency or end-organ unresponsiveness during this critical developmental period results in pseudohermaphroditism. The degree of sexual ambiguity is determined by the extent of the androgen deficiency and can range from hypospadia to phenotypically female external genitalia (with a short vagina). If androgen secretion or action is diminished before birth but after the genitalia have differentiated along male lines,

TABLE 24.1   Classification of Male Hypogonadism

Hypothalamic-pituitary dysfunction
Idiopathic GnRH deficiency, Kallmann syndrome, Prader-Willi syndrome, Laurence-Moon-Biedl syndromes (multiple)
Hypothalamic deficiency, pituitary hypoplasia
Trauma, postsurgical, postirradiation
Tumor (adenoma, craniopharyngioma, others)
Vascular (pituitary infarction, carotid aneurysm)
Infiltrative (sarcoidosis, histiocytosis, tuberculosis, fungal infection, hemochromatosis)
Systemic illness, malnutrition, anorexia nervosa
Autoimmune hypophysitis
Drugs (drug-induced hyperprolactinemia, sex steroids)

Testicular disorders (primary Leydig cell dysfunction)
Chromosomal (Klinefelter syndrome and variants, XX male gonadal dysgenesis)
Defects in androgen biosynthesis
Orchitis (mumps, HIV, other viral, leprosy)
Cryptorchidism
Myotonia dystrophica
Toxins (alcohol, opiates, fungicides, insecticides, heavy metals, cotton seed oil)
Drugs (cytotoxic drugs, ketoconazole, cimetidine, spironolactone)
Systemic illness (uremia, liver failure)

End-organ resistance (impaired androgen action)
Androgen receptor defects
Postreceptor transduction abnormalities
5α-Reductase deficiency

a small but anatomically intact phallus (microphallus) may be seen. The latter situation can be seen in congenital GnRH deficiency.

b. Prepubertal onset. During the prepubertal period, GnRH, LH, and FSH are secreted at low levels. Puberty is heralded by increased nocturnal pulsation of GnRH and pituitary gonadotropins. The increase of LH and FSH leads to androgen production and spermatogenesis. The testes increase in size from 1 to 2 mL to 15 to 35 mL by adulthood, and secondary sexual characteristics develop. If androgen deficiency begins after fetal development but prior to the completion of puberty, the clinical presentation is that of delayed puberty, and secondary sex characteristics will fail to develop. The lack of T and its metabolite (E_2) results in delayed epiphysial closure. Thus, growth of the long bones continues, and the patient develops eunuchoid proportions (arm span at least 2 cm more than height and heel-to-pubis measurement more than 2 cm greater than pubis-to-crown measurement). If there is concomitant growth-hormone deficiency, a eunuchoid habitus may not be present.

c. Postpubertal onset. Because these patients have proceeded through normal pubertal maturation, they have normal body measurements and normal voice but present with sexual dysfunction (i.e., decreased libido, impotence, and infertility), osteoporosis, anemia, muscle weakness, depression, and lassitude. These symptoms may be associated with loss of secondary sex characteristics (i.e., decreased facial, pubic, and body hair; decreased muscle mass and strength; increased adiposity; and small, soft testes). Gynecomastia can result from imbalance of serum T and E_2 (decreased T/E_2 ratio). The absence of chest hair, a sparseness of pubic hair, female escutcheon, and fine wrinkling of skin, suggest severe long-standing hypogonadism. Less severe defects produce more subtle changes.

2. Diagnosis of underandrogenization

a. History. A detailed developmental history pertaining to testicular descent, timing of puberty, frequency of shaving and body-hair development, sinopulmonary complaints, and medical history focused on past and present systemic illnesses, sexually transmitted diseases, orchitis (in adulthood), prior irradiation treatment, prostate surgery, and drug use is important. A detailed sexual history regarding libido, erectile and ejaculatory function, masturbation, coitus, and fertility should be obtained.

b. Physical examination includes assessment of height, span, hair pattern, fat distribution, and skin exam for wrinkling and acne. The genitourinary exam should include penis length, urethral integrity for hypospadia, digital rectal exam of the prostate (small, underdeveloped in prepuberty and atrophy of prostate in postpuberty hypogonadism), and scrotal exam for pigmentation, wrinkling, contents, proper fusion, and testicular descent. The normal size of testes ranges from 3.6 to 5.5 cm in length, 2.1 to 3.2 cm in width, and 15 to 35 mL in volume in Caucasian and African American men. In assessing T-responsive body hair, the clinician must take into account the patient's genetic and racial background. Whereas Caucasians may need to shave daily, African Americans, Asians, and Native Americans may shave less frequently. Last, but not least, the clinician needs to assess musculoskeletal system for underdevelopment, lack of or decreasing strength, muscle atrophy, excessive eunuchoid growth, and bones for osteopenia or osteoporosis.

c. Testosterone level. The clinical suspicion of low T secretion can be confirmed by measuring the serum total T level (normal range ~280 to 1 000 ng/dL). Because T is secreted in a pulsatile manner, a more accurate measurement of serum T may be obtained by separate or optimally by pooling three blood samples taken ~20 minutes apart. Low serum T concentrations in the absence of clinical manifestations suggest a low SHBG level, which can be either a congenital or an acquired defect. A normal free T or bioavailable T measurement (albumin-bound and free T) is helpful in such cases.

d. Anatomic localization of underandrogenization defect. If serum T concentration is low (in the absence of low SHBG), the diagnosis of hypogonadism

TABLE 24.2 Summary of Hormone Levels and Treatment in Major Diagnostic Categories of Hypogonadism

Category of hypogonadism	FSH	LH	T	Treatment
Hypogonadotropic hypogonadism	↓	↓	↓	HCG or T to virilize, HCG and HMG for fertility
Primary testicular insufficiency	↑	↑	↓	T to virilize only
Isolated germinal cell damage	↑/N	N	N	None
T resistance	↑/N	↑/N	↑/N	None

FSH, follicle-stimulating hormone; HCG, human chorionic gonadotropin; HMG, human menopausal gonadotropin; LH, luteinizing hormone; N, normal; T, testosterone; ↑, increased; ↓, decreased.

is confirmed, and the evaluation proceeds to identification of the anatomic level of defect. If underandrogenization exists in the absence of lower serum T levels, androgen resistance is suspected. A classification of underandrogenization according to the major sites of organ impairment is provided in Table 24.1. A summary of the laboratory changes in hypogonadism according to anatomic site is provided in Table 24.2.

(1) Primary hypogonadism. Primary testicular insufficiency is characterized by low serum T levels accompanied by elevated serum concentrations of LH and FSH. The disorder can result from a long list of conditions, including chromosomal abnormalities such as Klinefelter syndrome; enzymatic defects of androgen synthesis; acquired defects as a result of trauma, infection, infiltrative diseases, autoimmune destruction, certain drugs, and malformations such as cryptorchidism and anorchia. The androgen deficiency is usually accompanied by damage to the seminiferous tubules, resulting in azoospermia and infertility.

(2) Secondary hypogonadism. Hypogonadotropic hypogonadism is characterized by low serum T levels and low serum concentrations of LH and FSH. Low gonadotropin secretion can result from impaired hypothalamic secretion of GnRH or as a result of direct pituitary dysfunction. Functional defects may occur as a response to severe stress or illness, malnutrition, or drugs. Acquired destructive processes of the hypothalamus and pituitary gland include neoplasia, infiltrative processes, trauma, and irradiation. Hyperprolactinemia of any cause can produce hypogonadotropic hypogonadism, primarily by suppressing GnRH and LH secretion. Isolated GnRH deficiency, such as that associated with Kallmann syndrome and idiopathic hypogonadotropic hypogonadism, has been described. An algorithm for evaluation of such patients is suggested in Figure 24.4.

(a) The distinction of hypothalamic from pituitary causes can be difficult. GnRH measurements are not practical because of the location in the portal system, low systemic concentration, and short serum half-life (5 to 10 minutes). GnRH deficiency may be suggested if androgen deficiency is accompanied by anosmia (Kallmann syndrome) or diabetes insipidus. Findings such as visual-field defects and panhypopituitarism are more suggestive of pituitary disease. Further resolution requires magnetic resonance imaging (MRI) of the sella (hypothalamic-pituitary region) with and without contrast material.

(b) Because both hypothalamic and pituitary disease can result in a blunted or absent response of LH and FSH to an acute bolus of GnRH, this should not be used to distinguish hypothalamic and pituitary disorders. However, priming the pituitary with multiple properly spaced injections of GnRH will result in stimulation of LH secretion in patients with hypothalamic GnRH deficiency and could be

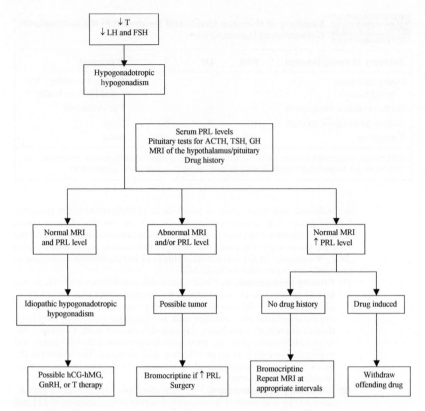

Figure 24.4. Evaluation and treatment of a patient with hypogonadotropic hypogonadism. ACTH, adrenocorticotropic hormone; FSH, follicle-stimulating hormone; GH, growth hormone; HCG, human chorionic gonadotropin; HMG, human menopausal gonadotropin; LH, luteinizing hormone; LHRH, luteinizing hormone–releasing hormone; T, testosterone; TSH, thyroid-stimulating hormone. (Modified from Swerdloff RS, Boyers SP. Evaluation of the male partner of an infertile couple: an algorithmic approach. *JAMA* 1982;247:2418. Copyright 1982 American Medical Association.)

of value in separating such patients from those with pituitary disease if localization of the primary defect is unclear. Because most patients with a pituitary basis for secondary hypogonadism have either hyperprolactinemia or a mass lesion on MRI, distinguishing between hypothalamic and pituitary causes by GnRH pulsing is rarely indicated.

(3) End-organ resistance: Androgen resistance is caused by sporadic or familial mutations of the androgen receptor gene, which is located on chromosome X (Xp11-12), and ~250 different gene mutations have been recognized. It is estimated that 1 in 20 000 to 64 000 newborns has the AR defect. End-organ resistance to T can occur as a result of the absence or instability of T receptors (receptor defect), or failure of receptor-bound T to influence DNA-dependent RNA synthesis (postreceptor defect). Androgen receptor defects appear to be the most common cause of T resistance and have a characteristic hormonal pattern with elevated serum T and LH levels. Such patients often present with clinical manifestations ranging from complete <u>testicular feminization</u> (external genitalia are female, with the presence of testes in the inguinal canal) to <u>Reifenstein syndrome</u>

(identifiable as male at birth, with moderately ambiguous genitalia, gynecomastia, and azoospermia) and infertile-man syndrome (mild form with male external genitalia and descended testis with defective spermatogenesis and oligospermia). DHT should be measured when there is abnormal differentiation of external genitalia. Gynecomastia is common and is a result of excessive production of E_2 from both aromatization of circulating T and direct hypersecretion by the testis.

(4) **5α-reductase deficiency** is a disorder of sexual differentiation due to a mutation of the gene for the enzyme 5α-reductase type II located on chromosome 2, which converts T to DHT. Despite a 46,XY karyotype, because of the lack of enzyme activity, these patients do not have a normal male phenotype, and the external genitalia may appear female. The testes are usually located in the labia majora, inguinal canal, or abdomen. The level of T is high, with low to undetectable DHT levels. DHT replacement is the potential treatment, although it is not approved by the U.S. Food and Drug Administration (FDA) for this purpose.

(5) **Delayed puberty** is defined as when puberty has not started by age 14 in boys (2.5 years standard deviation from the norm). It is often challenging and difficult to distinguish delayed puberty from hypogonadotropic hypogonadism in the prepubertal age, thus it is a diagnosis of exclusion. Among hypogonadotropic males, basal serum LH, FSH, and T concentrations and the gonadotropin response to GnRH are indistinguishable from those of prepubertal boys. The following may be helpful.

(a) Measure serum LH levels using the newest generation of highly sensitive immunofluorescent assays, which are often capable of separating normal prepubertal from hypogonadotropic concentration.

(b) Progressive testicular growth and onset of virilizing signs indicate that puberty is progressing normally.

(c) The presence of nocturnal LH release in early pubertal boys may help to establish that puberty has been initiated.

(d) In isolated hypogonadotropism, levels of adrenal steroids (dehydroepiandrosterone sulfate; DHEAS) are normal relative to chronologic age. In constitutional delay, bone age is delayed and serum DHEAS concentration is low.

(e) Careful analysis of a growth chart can be useful. Patients with constitutional delay in puberty have a history of slow growth velocity throughout childhood. In hypogonadotropism, growth velocity is normal in childhood and is normal or slightly slower during the prepubertal growth spurt, even though these individuals may eventually be taller with eunuchoid proportions.

3. **Treatment of androgen insufficiency.** The requirement for androgens varies at different stages of life, and it must be adjusted accordingly based on disease state, age, and current reproductive needs of the patient. Indications for androgen therapy are given in Table 24.3. Androgen replacement has risks and benefits, which again differ in different situations and stages of life. The benefits and risks of androgen replacement are summarized in Table 24.4. In general, if the hypogonadism is caused by extratesticular factors, attempts should be made to correct these. Otherwise, libido, potency, and secondary sex characteristics can be restored by androgen replacement therapy. Patients with hypothalamic or pituitary processes causing secondary hypogonadism should be treated with testosterone to restore virilization or with either gonadotropins (human menopausal gonadotropin, hCG) or pulsatile GnRH replacement therapy if restored fertility is required. It is important to emphasize that the gradual decline of T secretion can lead to the insidious onset of symptoms such as loss of libido and potency, tiredness, lack of ambition and drive, hot flushes, and depression. Many of these symptoms can be attributed to other causes; therefore, it is important to establish the diagnosis by the measurement of T and LH levels. It is equally important to realize that a patient who has never had adequate T secretion may claim that the

TABLE 24.3 Indications for Androgen Therapy

Androgen deficiency (primary and secondary hypogonadism)
Delayed puberty in boys
Transsexuality (female → male)
Elderly men with low testosterone levels
Angioneurotic edema
Microphallus (neonatal)
Other possible uses or under investigation:
  Hormonal male contraception
  Wasting disease associated with cancer/HIV/chronic infection
  Postmenopausal female (in combination with estrogens)

levels of libido and potency he experiences are normal, because he does not have a basis for comparison.

a. Methods of androgen replacement. There has been a recent surge of scientific and pharmaceutical interest in androgen replacement therapy, leading to the development of a number of novel preparations (Table 24.5). Testosterone is available in different forms and serves as a hormone and prohormone, which is converted to DHT by 5α-reductase and estradiol by aromatase. Patients need to be evaluated 3 months after treatment initiation and then annually for response to treatment as well as adverse effects.

(1) Testosterone esters (injectable forms): Adequate replacement therapy can be achieved with parenteral depot testosterone esters, such as testosterone enanthate and cypionate, but these result in nonphysiologic peaks and troughs. Treatment usually commences with intramuscular injections of T enanthate or cypionate in a dosage of 75 to 100 mg weekly, or 150 to 200 mg every 2 weeks. Serum T levels should be within the mid-normal range when measured 5 to 7 days after an injection, and the patient should be free of symptoms of androgen deficiency throughout the interval between injections. For monitoring, measure serum testosterone levels midway between injections. If the serum T level is >700 ng/dL or <350 ng/dL, the physician will need to adjust the testosterone dose or frequency. The patient is then encouraged to give his own injections. The optimum

TABLE 24.4 Benefits versus Risks of Androgen Replacement Therapy

Benefits	Risks (potential)
↑ Sexual motivation and performance	Acne, oiliness of skin
↑ or maintains secondary sexual characteristics	Gynecomastia (aromatizable androgens)
↑ Muscle mass and strength	↑ Hematocrit
↓ Body fat including visceral fat	Sleep-related breathing disorders, apnea
↓ Bone resorption, ↑ bone formation, and maintains bone mass	↓ HDL cholesterol, ↓ HDL-to-total cholesterol ratio (cardiovascular risk?)
Improves mood parameters	Aggravates benign prostatic hypertrophy (?)
Improves quality of life (?)	Stimulation of existing cancer of the prostate
Improves or prevents deterioration of cognition (?)	

HDL, high-density lipoprotein.

| **TABLE 24.5** | **Androgen Preparations** |

Type	Currently available in the United States	Under development
Injectables	Testosterone enanthate, cypionate, cyclohexane carboxylate (200–250 mg every 10–21 days, 100 mg every wk) Mixture of esters (e.g., testosterone propionate, testosterone phenylpropionate, testosterone isocaproate, testosterone decanoate)	Testosterone undecanoate injections (1 000 mg once every 6–12 wk) Testosterone buciclate (12–24 wk) Testosterone microspheres (6–11 wk)
Oral	Methyltestosterone[a]	Testosterone undecanoate (120–240 mg/d in divided doses)
Buccal	Transbuccal testosterone tablets (60 mg/d in divided doses)	
Implants	Testosterone pellets (100–200 mg, 3–6 inserted once every 4–6 mo)	7α-Methyl-19 nortestosterone (minimally 5α-reduced)
Transdermal	Testosterone gel (1% T hydroxyalcohol-based gel, 5–10 g/d) Nonscrotal patches (two 2.5-mg patches or one 5-mg patch testosterone per day	Dihydrotestosterone gel (2% hydroxyalcohol-based gel, 10 g/d) MATRIX testosterone patches (60 cm^3) every 2 d

[a]Associated with severe hepatotoxicity.

interval for injections varies considerably, but 10 to 17 days is usual. T:DHT and T:E$_2$ ratios are in the normal range in this mode of replacement if replacement is physiologic. **Testosterone undecanoate (TU)** in oil is an injectable long-acting formulation; TU in oil is available in Europe under the brand name of Nebido but is not currently approved by the FDA, as it is still in clinical trials in the United States. The dosage in Europe is 1 000 mg IM followed by another 1 000 mg in 6 weeks and then 1 000 mg every 12 weeks. The advantage is less frequent injections, but the volume of the injection is large (4 mL).

(2) Transdermal delivery. The transdermal scrotal patch delivers 6 mg of T per day and has been shown to produce steady serum concentrations in many but not all androgen-deficient men. Application requires shaving of scrotal hair. T:E2 ratio is normal but T:DHT ratio is significantly lower, because of the high level of 5α-reductase in scrotal skin, which results in an increased level of DHT. Two types of nonscrotal patches are available. They deliver 2.5 to 5 mg of T per day. One of the patches has been reported to cause irritation at the application site in 30% of patients. T:DHT and T:E$_2$ levels are in the physiologic male range. Two testosterone gels (AndroGel and Testim) are currently available in the United States. The usual dose is between 5 and 10 g of 1% hydroalcoholic gel, which deliver 50 and 100 mg of testosterone. Consistent blood levels are attained within a few days and the treatment is well tolerated, with <10% of patients complaining of skin irritation. Serum DHT levels are higher, thus the T:DHT ratio is lower in treated groups.

(3) Oral preparations. Most oral testosterone preparations are absorbed into the portal circulation and rapidly degraded by the liver. Synthetic oral 17-alkylated androgens, such as methyltestosterone, fluoxymesterone, and oxymetholone, are not recommended because they produce only partial androgenization. Methyltestosterone and fluoxymesterone have been associated with several hepatic disorders, including cholestatic jaundice, liver cell carcinoma, and the rare vascular disorder peliosis hepatis. **Testosterone undecanoate** (non-17-alkylated) is an oral testosterone preparation; it has the advantage of lymphatic absorption, thus bypassing first-pass metabolism in the liver. The dose ranges between 40 and 80 mg orally 2 or 3 times daily with meals. It is widely used in Europe and Asia with favorable results as well as a favorable side-effect profile. It had variable clinical response in the same individual on different days, as it is very dependent on the fat in the diet for optimal absorption. The formulation has been modified for longer action and is undergoing additional clinical trials in the United States.

(4) T implants Four to six 200-mg pellets are implanted subcutaneously. They are capable of maintaining physiologic levels of T for 5 to 6 months but are not widely used in the United States, although they are popular in the United Kingdom and Australia.

(5) Dihydrotestosterone is used in Europe in the form of a topical gel. It is particularly useful in men with 5α-reductase deficiency, prepubertal gynecomastia, microphallus, and delayed puberty because it **cannot be aromatized to estrogen.** It has not been associated with gynecomastia, and reports have suggested an actual decrease in prostate size. This may be advantageous in older men at risk for obstructive uropathy; however, because DHT is not aromatized to E_2, long-term effects on bone density, cardiovascular disease, and cognition are not known.

b. Potential adverse effects. Androgen replacement is contraindicated in patients with androgen-sensitive neoplasia (breast and prostate carcinoma). Prostate enlargement is a potential complication, and patients with symptomatic prostatic hypertrophy should have surgical correction or medical control prior to starting replacement. It is important to measure prostate-specific antigen and prostate size by digital rectal examination annually while on replacement. Development of or pre-existing polycythemia (hematocrit >52%) is an indication to withhold androgen replacement, because androgens increase red cell production either by stimulating erythroid precursors or by stimulating erythropoietin secretion. Because of neuromuscular effects of testosterone on the upper airway, apneic sleep disorders may be exacerbated by androgens. Other side effects include gynecomastia secondary to aromatization to E_2, fluid retention, and acne. High-density lipoprotein (HDL) cholesterol levels may be lowered; however, the long-term cardiovascular consequences are not known.

c. Management of primary testicular failure. Unfortunately, the majority of testicular disorders causing androgen deficiency are irreversible. Consequently, treatment consists of androgen replacement therapy alone.

d. Management of secondary hypogonadotropic hypogonadism. The initial aim in management is always to exclude tumors of the pituitary or hypothalamus, along with other treatable causes, such as thyroid disease, hyperprolactinemia, and offending drugs, by the appropriate investigations. Treatment of men with congenital hypogonadotropic hypogonadism usually begins at puberty. If fertility is not desired, T replacement can be given (as described above) to achieve masculinization without concern for any irreversible compromise of testicular function. If fertility is desired, subsequent management involves replacement therapy with gonadotropins or GnRH infusion.

(1) Treatment with gonadotropins. When fertility is desired, T is withdrawn, and injections of hCG (purified from the urine of pregnant women) (1 500 IU) are given 2 to 3 times a week for ~6 months. **hCG acts as LH** in binding to LH receptors and increasing testicular T production. If semen analyses show that sperm production has not commenced or is <7 to 10 million per milliliter, FSH, in the form of human menopausal gonadotropins (hMG, which is purified from the urine of postmenopausal women) or recombinant FSH, 75 IU 3 times a week, is added to the hCG regimen. Because FSH or hMG is more expensive than hCG, treatment usually begins with hCG alone, but combined therapy is often needed for 12 to 15 months. Once spermatogenesis is initiated, hCG alone may maintain normal sperm count. Recombinant human hCG and recombinant human FSH is now available (hFSH) with identical biologic and pharmacokinetic activities. Predictors of success are the testicular volume (>8 mL with better response vs. <4 mL with poorer outcome) and time of onset (onset of hypogonadism prior to puberty with less favorable outcome than after puberty).

(2) Pulsatile administration of GnRH for treatment of hypothalamic hypogonadotropism. Pioneering studies in a hypogonadotropic model demonstrated that GnRH could stimulate appropriate gonadotropin secretion only when the hormone was administered in an episodic mode and at a physiologic frequency. Continuous administration was completely ineffective in evoking the desired pattern of gonadotropin discharge. Using such a regimen of long-term episodic GnRH administration by means of a portable pump with an initial dose of 25 ng/kg per pulse every 2 hours subcutaneously, it has been possible to restore spermatogenesis in men with Kallmann syndrome and to induce clinical and biochemical changes of puberty in patients with delayed puberty because of hypothalamic GnRH deficiency. A similar approach has been used with success in inducing ovulation in women with hypothalamic amenorrhea associated with idiopathic GnRH deficiency, anorexia nervosa, or competitive exercise. Although subcutaneous administration of GnRH has been reported to be effective, it is less practical and less effective than gonadotropin therapy.

e. End-organ resistance. There is no known effective therapy for the eunuchoidism resulting from androgen resistance. Patients with male phenotypes and gynecomastia usually require cosmetic surgery to remove breast tissue and to correct the more severe degrees of hypospadia.

4. Specific disease states associated with primary hypogonadism:

a. Klinefelter syndrome. Klinefelter syndrome is the most common disorder of sexual differentiation, occurring in about 1 of 500 to 1 000 men. It has been reported that ~10% of individuals with Klinefelter syndrome are diagnosed by karyotype screening at birth and childhood, and overall only 25% are diagnosed during life. The primary abnormality is the presence of two or more X chromosomes, usually in the form of a 47,XXY chromosomal complement (the classic form) or, less commonly, 46,XY/47,XXY (the mosaic form). The additional X chromosome(s) may be a result of nondisjunction during gametogenesis or nondisjunction in the zygote during mitosis.

(1) Classic form. Before the onset of puberty, the hypothalamic-pituitary-testicular axis functions normally. By age 12 to 14 years, impaired Leydig cell function results in decreased T, increased gonadotropins, and hypogonadism. Testicular biopsy reveals pathologic hyalinization and fibrosis of the seminiferous tubules. Decreased testicular size and defective spermatogenesis are present in almost all patients with the classic form. Clinically, it is characterized by an unequivocally male phenotype, small penis size, small firm testes (with median volume of 4 mL, and always <12 mL), azoospermia, and decreased male-pattern body and facial hair. If Leydig cell failure occurs prior to puberty, then patients manifest eunuchoid features. Gynecomastia is common and may be due to increased peripheral conversion of T to E_2 as well as decreased clearance of estrogens. Most patients come to medical attention after puberty with complaints of dyslexia, infertility, or gynecomastia. Obesity and varicose veins occur in one third to one half of patients with Klinefelter syndrome. There is an increased incidence of learning disability and social maladjustment, subtle abnormalities of thyroid function, diabetes mellitus, and abnormalities of pulmonary function. Taurodontism is common and may be associated with early tooth decay. Incidence of breast cancer is 1 in 5 000, about 20 times that of normal men but only one fifth that of women. Screening mammography is not recommended because of the low incidence. There are also higher incidences of germ-cell tumors and autoimmune disorders. These patients generally have a male psychosexual orientation and are capable of functioning sexually as normal men.

(2) **Mosaic form.** About 10% of patients with Klinefelter syndrome have the mosaic form, a less severe form of the disorder. As many as one fourth of these patients have normal testicular size, and only half have complete absence of spermatogenesis accounting for rare instances of fertility. Mosaicism may be limited to the testes and thus can only be diagnosed by testicular biopsy.

(3) The diagnosis of Klinefelter syndrome in patients with the classic 47,XXY is suggested by elevations of LH and FSH, and a low to normal T. A careful history will almost always demonstrate learning disabilities and varying degrees of dyslexia. From a standard laboratory perspective, a **high FSH level** (because of germinal compartment failure) is the best demarcator between patients with Klinefelter syndrome and normal men. If FSH is elevated, the condition can be rapidly confirmed by buccal smear and detection of Barr bodies (extra X chromosome), a chromosomal analysis performed on peripheral blood leukocytes, or by FISH. Mosaicism can be missed in some patients in whom the mosaic pattern is limited to the testes. Under these circumstances, only a chromosomal analysis of testicular cells provides a definitive diagnosis.

(4) Treatment with testosterone will lead to masculinization and improvement of symptoms of hypogonadism; however, **infertility is irreversible,** despite hormone therapy.

b. **Gonadal dysfunction in patients treated with cancer chemotherapeutic agents.** With the advent of multiagent chemotherapy for malignant disorders and the ensuing increased survival, it has become apparent that germinal aplasia and resulting infertility may be a common side effect. Chemotherapeutic agents are not equivalent in their potential gonadal toxicity. The side effects depend not only on the specific class of drug used but also on the total dose used. Alkylating agents (cyclophosphamide, thiotepa, chlorambucil, nitrogen mustard, and melphalan) as a class produce dose-dependent germinal depletion. Procarbazine, most commonly used in the management of lymphoma, produces permanent germinal aplasia. Doxorubicin hydrochloride (Adriamycin) (500 mg/m^2), vincristine, and high-dose methotrexate do not have these side effects in humans.

c. Radiation produces reversible germinal depletion between 50 and 400 rad; above 500 rad, germinal aplasia is usually permanent.

d. **Endocrine disruptors (ED).** These are man-made drugs, toxins, and synthetic chemicals as well as natural phytoestrogens, which act on the endocrine system by mimicking, blocking, and/or interfering in some manner. They can cause gonadal toxicity by effect on the germinal epithelium, which is a rapidly dividing tissue like bone marrow and gastrointestinal tract, and susceptible to damage.

(1) **Marijuana.** There is evidence that marijuana not only **lowers the plasma T level** by decreasing GnRH production but may also produce **gynecomastia** and **altered germinal maturation** in the testes. Crude marijuana contains plant estrogens that interfere with gonadal function, but there is little evidence that purified tetrahydrocannabinol has any direct effect.

(2) **Fetal exposure to diethylstilbestrol (DES) and medroxyprogesterone acetate (MPA; Provera).** Fetal exposure to DES and MPA can produce significant abnormalities of the male genital tract. In both rodents and humans, DES produces an increased incidence of epididymal cysts and testicular atrophy. MPA likewise can be associated with abnormalities of

the external genital apparatus. Accordingly, a maternal history of drug exposure can be helpful in evaluation of the infertile male.

(3) Miscellaneous. Each year the list of environmental toxins shown to produce adverse effects on the testes grows. Dibromochloroperine, boron, dioxin (Agent Orange), and kepone are some of the better-known toxins.

5. **Specific hypothalamic syndromes characterized by hypogonadotropic hypogonadism**

a. **Kallmann syndrome.** Hypogonadotropic hypogonadism was first recognized by Kallmann, Schoenfeld, and Barrera in 1944. Kallmann syndrome has different genetic modes of transmission (X-linked, autosomal dominant with variable penetration, and autosomal recessive) and is characterized by isolated GnRH deficiency. During normal fetal development, GnRH neurons begin migration from the olfactory placode to the arcuate nucleus of the hypothalamus. Migration is interrupted or absent in Kallmann syndrome because of mutations in the KAL1 gene, which encodes **anosmin,** a cell-adhesion protein that mediates migration. Approximately 50% of these subjects have midline craniofacial defects (anosmia or hyposmia, cleft lip and palate), and may manifest increased frequencies of sensorineural deafness and ataxia, and renal defects. MRI of the brain may show anomalous or absent olfactory bulbs in up to 75% of cases. Women are affected much less frequently than men (4:1 male-to-female ratio). This makes the X-chromosomal inherited variant the most common form. A positive family history is present in ~50% of cases; relatives may have hypogonadism, and many manifest only one of the associated midline defects. In teenagers who fail to enter puberty, these clinical markers can be useful in differentiate Kallmann syndrome from constitutional delay of puberty.

b. **Fertile eunuch syndrome (Pasqualini syndrome).** This term has been used to describe patients with partial GnRH deficiency that is enough to stimulate normal levels of FSH, but the LH levels are not completely normal, leading to eunuchoidism and delayed sexual development but normal-sized testes. These individuals appear to have sufficient gonadotropin to stimulate enough intratesticular T production for spermatogenesis but not enough circulating T to adequately virilize the peripheral tissues. **Despite the name, these patients are frequently infertile.**

c. **Functional hypogonadotropism**

(1) Marked weight loss in patients with chronic diseases such as malabsorption syndrome in gastrointestinal diseases (i.e., celiac disease), chronic renal insufficiency, tumor cachexia, severe systemic illnesses, and **anorexia nervosa** are associated with hypogonadotropic hypogonadism. The underlying mechanisms remain to be elucidated but likely involve a combination of cytokine and/or glucocorticoid effects. One mechanism is decreased secretion of GnRH and consequent reduction in LH and FSH, which in turn causes T production and spermatogenesis to cease. This may be a result of leptin deficiency secondary to lack of enough adipocytes, which provides feedback to the hypothalamus indicating that the body fat is inadequate for reproduction. With correction of the underlying disorder and restoration of normal weight, usually long-term therapy is not required.

(2) Exercise and stress also affect the hypothalamic–pituitary axis. Basal T levels were lower than normal in a study of joggers and fell markedly after completion of a marathon. T levels also fell in military personnel studied during stressful periods at officer candidate school. Women involved in strenuous exercise (e.g., joggers, athletes, and ballet dancers) can develop hypothalamic amenorrhea in a manner similar to that seen with anorexia nervosa. Pulsatile administration of GnRH restores normal gonadotropin secretion and menstrual cycles in these patients, suggesting a defect in hypothalamic GnRH secretion.

d. **Miscellaneous hypothalamic syndromes.** Acquired hypogonadotropic hypogonadism can result from structural lesions affecting the hypothalamus (e.g., craniopharyngiomas and germinomas) and head trauma. In the majority of cases, hypogonadotropism as a result of infiltrative processes of the hypothalamus (e.g., sarcoidosis and hemochromatosis) has been shown to be that of GnRH deficiency. A few individuals have a pituitary cause, with impaired pituitary response to GnRH administration. The etiologic progression of hypogonadotropism seen in association with Prader-Willi and Laurence-Moon-Biedl syndromes appears to be caused by hypothalamic dysfunction in most cases. **Prader-Willi syndrome** and **Angelman syndrome** are rare syndromes (1:20 000) characterized by combination of marked hypotonia, secondary hypogonadism, hyposomia, oligophrenia, facial dysmorphism, obesity, and type 2 diabetes mellitus. Prader-Willi syndrome is caused by a deletion on the long arm of the paternal chromosome 15, whereas in Angelman syndrome the maternal chromosome 15 is deleted (15q11-13). There is no definitive treatment, and because of reduced cognitive abilities and abnormal behavior, testosterone should be administered with caution. Life expectancy is decreased because of extreme obesity, which increases the risk of cardiovascular disease. **Laurence-Moon-Biedl syndrome** is an autosomal recessive disorder characterized by obesity, hypogonadism, oligophrenia, retinitis pigmentosa, and polydactylism. At birth, undescended testes, micropenis, and hypospadia are frequently observed.

6. **Male senescence.** Unlike the abrupt gonadal failure of female menopause, men have a gradual decline in circulating androgens, adrenal androgen precursors, and growth hormones, which has been shown in a number of cross-sectional and longitudinal studies such as The Baltimore Longitudinal Study of Aging and The Massachusetts Male Aging Study (Table 24.6).

   a. Both total and free T gradually decline and are associated with elevated serum LH and FSH levels, indicating a primary defect within the testes. A second, partial defect in hypothalamic GnRH secretion may also exist, resulting in a blunted rise in LH and FSH relative to the lowered serum T concentration. The effects of low testosterone are similar to those observed in younger men. These include decreased muscle mass, muscle strength, bone density, libido, and erectile function, and depressed mood. Body fat, especially visceral fat, is increased. E_2 is increased as a result of T aromatization in adipose tissue. Screening of older male population for low T level is not recommended, but testing should be utilized for men who have signs and symptoms of androgen deficiency. Replacement therapy with testosterone has been shown to increase lean body mass, grip strength, bone density, quality of life, sense of well-being, and libido. However, erectile dysfunction is multifactorial in origin, with impaired vasodilatory function in the penis being a predominant factor

 TABLE 24.6 Hormonal Changes with Aging

GnRH-LH/FSH-T	CRH-ACTH-DHEA/S	GHRH-GH/IGF-1
↑ LH,[a] FSH	No change in ACTH	↓ GHRH message and receptor
↓ T (↓ Leydig cells)	↓ DHEA and DHEAS	↓ GH secretory pulses
↓ Free T	↓ DHEA and DHEAS response to ACTH ↓	↓ Circulating GH
↑ SHBG		↓ Serum IGF-1

[a] ↓ LH pulse amplitude and ↓ responsiveness to GnRH.
ACTH, adrenocorticotropic hormone; CRH, corticotropin-releasing hormone; DHEA, dihydroepiandrosterone; DHEAS, DHEA sulfate; FSH, follicle-stimulating hormone; GH, growth hormone; GHRH, growth hormone–releasing hormone; GnRH, gonadotropin-releasing hormone; IGF-I, insulin-like growth factor type I; LH, luteinizing hormone; SHBG, sex hormone–binding globulin.

in many older men. Thus, erectile dysfunction is often not improved despite androgen therapy.

b. Androgen precursors DHEA and DHEAS also decrease with age. Small studies have reported that **DHEA** administered to aging animals and humans may improve sense of well-being, enhance memory, decrease body fat, reduce risk of cardiovascular disease, prevent cancer, and provide beneficial effects on immune function. DHEA is sold as a dietary supplement in the United States and is available without prescription.

c. Hormonal changes may contribute to male frailty; however, it is not known whether the changes represent a physiologic or a pathologic process. There is ongoing debate as to whether androgen replacement is beneficial in male senescence, but new guidelines recommend it for symptomatic men with classical androgen deficiency (see above). On the other hand, experts recommend against T therapy in patients with breast or prostate cancer, palpable prostate nodule or induration, prostate-specific antigen (PSA) >3 ng/dL, symptomatic severe benign prostate hyperplasia, erythrocytosis (hematocrit >52%), hyperviscosity, untreated obstructive sleep apnea, and uncontrolled severe heart failure.

B. Male infertility. Infertility is defined as a lack of conception following 1 year of frequent unprotected intercourse. The causes of male infertility can be divided into six main areas (Table 24.7): (1) hypothalamic disease (secondary hypogonadism) accounting for 1% to 2% of causes; (2) testicular disease (primary hypogonadism), 30% to 40%; (3) posttesticular defects (disorders of sperm transport), 10% to 20%; (4) sexual dysfunction, 1% to 2%; (5) systemic illnesses (uncommon); and (6) nonclassifiable, 40% to 50%. All evaluations for infertility must include a thorough assessment of both the man and the woman, because in many cases abnormalities of reproductive function exist in both partners. A population-based study by the World Health Organization (WHO) found the following distribution of causes when evaluating infertile couples: male factors 23%, ovulatory dysfunction 18%, tubal damage 14%, endometriosis 9%, coital problems 5%, cervical factors 3%, and unexplained 28%.

1. Evaluation. An algorithmic approach to the evaluation of a man for infertility is presented in Figure 24.5.

a. History. History should focus on sexual development, puberty, school performance, symptoms of hypogonadism (loss of body hair, loss of libido), chronic illnesses, infections, sexually transmitted diseases, previous surgery, drug and environmental exposures, and a detailed sexual history. Many drugs are associated with impaired spermatogenesis and/or Leydig cell dysfunction. Among them, the most important are the alkylating drugs (cyclophosphamide and chlorambucil). Antiandrogens (flutamide, cyproterone, spironolactone), ketoconazole, and cimetidine cause testicular dysfunction by inhibiting testicular androgen production or action (Carlson et al., 1981). Environmental toxins may be an underappreciated cause of infertility. The pesticide dibromochloropropane is a well-known cause, as are lead, cadmium, and mercury (Schrag and Dixon, 1985). The possibility that chemicals with estrogenic activity, including phytoestrogens, may lower sperm counts has attracted much attention recently, although direct proof of an effect is lacking. The suspicion of such an effect originated with observations that sperm counts had decreased over the last several decades. However, a recent meta-analysis suggested that while decreases in sperm counts have occurred on a local basis, there has been no worldwide decline (Becker and Berhane, 1997).

b. Physical exam should include assessment of secondary sex characteristics, developmental defects, gynecomastia, and detailed genitourinary exam.

c. Semen analysis. Semen analysis is the cornerstone in the assessment of a male partner of an infertile couple. A normal semen analysis should prompt a thorough evaluation of the female partner. The semen sample should be collected in a standardized manner and assessed as described by the WHO *Laboratory Manual for the Examination of Semen and Sperm–Cervical Mucus*

| TABLE 24.7 | Common Causes of Male Infertility |

Cause	Percent of patients
Hypothalamic pituitary disease	1–2
Isolated hypogonadotropic hypogonadism	
Hypopituitarism (tumors, hyperprolactinemia)	
Hemochromatosis, others	
Testicular dysfunction	30–40
Chromosomal (XXY or variants)	
Cryptorchidism	
Varicocele	
Orchitis (mumps, tuberculosis, cytomegalovirus)	
Drugs (alkylating agents and other cytotoxic drugs)	
Irradiation	
Toxins	
Hyperthermia	
Autoimmune testicular disease	
Y-chromosome deletions or substitutions	
Sexual dysfunction	1–2
Retrograde ejaculation	
Erectile dysfunction	
Problems with sperm transport	10–20
Epididymal obstruction/dysfunction	
Congenital absence of the vas	
Young syndrome	
Vasectomy	
Systemic illness	Less common
Debilitating disease (e.g., renal failure, liver failure, HIV)	
Not known	40–50

Data from Baker HWG. Male infertility. In: De Grout LJ, ed. *Endocrinology*. Philadelphia: WB Saunders; 1994:2404. De Kretser DM. Male infertility. *Lancet* 1997;349;787.

Interaction (1999). At least 2 days of sexual abstinence is recommended prior to collection of the specimen in a clean container. The semen specimen should be kept warm (as close to body temperature as possible) and transported to the laboratory within 2 hours of collection. Because there is considerable variation in the characteristics of semen specimens obtained from a given patient, any abnormal semen analysis should be repeated after an appropriate period of abstinence. Table 24.8 lists the parameters assessed in a basic semen analysis, and normal reference ranges are listed in Table 24.9. Evaluation of the semen specimen includes assessment of the following.

(1) **Volume.** The normal volume varies between 2 and 5 mL. A low volume with azoospermia or oligospermia may be caused by genital tract obstruction. Congenital absence of vas deferens may be diagnosed by physical examination and a low semen pH, whereas ejaculatory duct obstruction is diagnosed by finding dilated seminal vesicles on transrectal ultrasound.

(2) **pH.** The normal range of pH is 7 to 8. A low pH suggests occlusion of the ejaculatory ducts or contamination of the specimen with urine. An alkaline pH raises the question of acute diseases (i.e., infection) of the secondary sex glands.

(3) **Microscopy for debris and agglutination.** The presence of agglutination suggests autoantibodies to sperm. This should be confirmed by the mixed

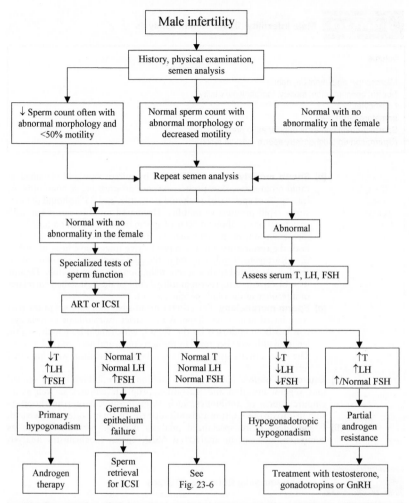

Figure 24.5. Algorithmic approach to the diagnosis and management of male infertility. ART, assisted reproductive technology; FSH, follicle-stimulating hormone; ICSI, intracytoplasmic sperm injection; LH, luteinizing hormone; T, testosterone. (Reprinted from Swerdloff RS, Wang C. The testes and male sexual function. In: Goldman L, Ausiello D, eds. *Cecil Textbook of Medicine.* 22nd ed. Philadelphia: WB Saunders; 2004:1472–1483.)

antiglobulin reaction or the immunobead test. A clinically significant immune disorder is suggested when >50% of spermatozoa are coated with autoantibodies.

(4) Sperm count, motility, and morphology

   (a) A normal sperm count is defined as >20 million per milliliter of semen or a total sperm count of >40 million, although a moderate decrease (moderate oligospermia) in sperm concentration (10 to 20 million per milliliter) is compatible with fertility provided sperm motility and morphology are normal. A sperm count of <5 million per milliliter is defined as severe oligospermia. Azoospermia is the complete absence of sperm.

TABLE 24.8	Male Infertility: Basic Semen Analysis

Volume
pH
Microscopy: agglutination, debris
Sperm: concentration, motility, morphology, vitality
Leukocytes
Immature germ cells
Sperm autoantibodies (if agglutination present)
(Sperm/semen biochemistry sperm function tests)

(b) **Sperm motility.** Sperm is assessed by microscopy and classified as rapid progressive, slow progressive, nonprogressive, or nonmotile. At least 50% of spermatozoa should be motile, and 25% should demonstrate rapid progressive motility. Decreased motility can occur with structural or metabolic defects of sperm or can represent a hostile semen environment. Specific defects of ciliary structure or function in both the respiratory and the reproductive tracts have been identified (i.e., <u>Kartagener syndrome</u>, <u>immotile cilia syndrome</u>), resulting in infertility associated with a severe reduction in sperm motility. Despite its subjective nature, sperm motility is one of the best semen correlates of infertility in the oligospermic patient.

(c) **Sperm morphology.** The criteria for normal morphology in the past were based mainly on shape. A new strict morphologic criteria system has been endorsed by the WHO, which includes length, width, length/width, area occupied by the acrosome, and neck and tail defects. The strict criteria appear to have a better correlation with impaired fertility.

(5) **Leukocyte count.** Elevation (>1 million per milliliter in the semen) may suggest infection and warrant appropriate cultures as well as an empiric course of antibiotics, such as erythromycin or trimethoprim–sulfamethoxazole. Culture and antibiotic treatment are often of low yield.

(6) If indicated, more specialized analysis may be performed, such as computer-aided sperm analysis (CASA), sperm biochemistry analysis

TABLE 24.9	Semen Analysis: Reference Ranges

Parameter	Reference range
Semen volume	>2 mL
Sperm	
Concentration	>20 million/mL
Total count	>40 million/ejaculate
Motility	>50% motile
	>25% rapid progressively motile
Morphology	>15% normal[a]
Vitality (live)	>75%
Leukocytes	<1 million/mL

[a]This value is based on using the strict criteria for assessment of sperm morphology in studies using in vitro fertilization as an endpoint.
Modified from WHO: *Laboratory Manual for Examination of Human Semen and Sperm Cervical Mucus Interaction.* 4th ed. Cambridge, UK: Cambridge University Press; 1999.

(including fructose), sperm function tests such as the acrosome reaction, and penetration assays such as the zona-free hamster penetration test.

d. Hormonal assessment. All abnormal semen analyses should be repeated. If the repeat analysis shows severe oligospermia or azoospermia, basal serum T, LH, and FSH should be measured on a morning serum sample to rule out hypogonadism. The evaluation and management of patients with primary (high LH, FSH, low T) and secondary (low LH, FSH, T) Leydig cell dysfunction and end-organ resistance to androgen have been discussed in Section II.3. If LH is low, the serum prolactin level should be measured to rule out prolactin-induced hypogonadotropism. Patients with isolated FSH elevations have isolated germinal compartment failure and respond poorly to therapy. An algorithm for the workup and treatment of males with normal hormonal values is given in Figure 24.6.

e. Azoospermia with normal-sized testes, serum T, LH, and FSH. These patients usually have retrograde ejaculation or an obstruction of the ejaculatory system. A postejaculation urine sample should be checked for spermatozoa.

(1) Retrograde ejaculation is suspected by the presence of autonomic neuropathy and is most commonly seen in patients with <u>diabetes mellitus</u>. The presence of large numbers of sperm in postejaculation urine specimens confirms the diagnosis.

(2) Obstructive azoospermia. The absence of sperm in the postejaculation urine suggests obstructive azoospermia or impaired spermatogenesis. Recognition of obstructive disorders is important because therapy must be directed to surgical correction of the disorder.

(a) The combination of absence of vas deferens (normally palpable in the scrotum as an elongated tube) on physical exam, low seminal fluid volume, and acidic pH is suggestive of congenital absence of vas deferens and seminal vesicles. Congenital <u>absence of the vas deferens</u> is associated with the <u>cystic fibrosis regulator gene (CFRG)</u> in Caucasian men. Seminal fructose, normally produced by the seminal vesicles and transported into the vas deferens by the ejaculatory ducts, is absent on biochemical analysis.

(b) If semen fructose is normal, a high percentage of these cases will prove to have an obstruction of the epididymis proximal to the entry of the ejaculatory ducts. The finding of normal-size testes with or without palpable enlargement of the caput epididymis almost certainly indicates obstructive disease. If surgery is contemplated, exploration of the scrotum with visualization of the epididymis may demonstrate epididymal obstruction, and microsurgical correction of the obstruction or collection of spermatozoa for intracytoplasmic sperm injection (ICSI) may be attempted.

(c) If exploration fails to demonstrate an obstruction, then testicular biopsy may be required to determine intratesticular defect.

f. Oligospermia with normal-sized testes, serum T, LH, and FSH. A normal hormonal pattern is seen in the majority of oligospermic patients. Varicocele, reproductive tract infection, and sperm antibodies should be ruled out by physical exam and laboratory tests before the diagnosis of idiopathic infertility is made. Varicocele will be discussed separately in Section C. The remainder of these patients with oligospermia and normal hormonal profile are categorized as having idiopathic oligospermia and account for most male infertility.

g. Normal sperm count but impaired sperm morphology or motility.

(1) Dead sperm (necrospermia) can be identified with supravital stains or assessed indirectly by the hypo-osmotic swelling test, which assesses the fluidity of the plasma membrane.

(2) Abnormal sperm motility or morphology is usually seen in oligospermic specimens but can occur in men with normal counts. Abnormal forms indicate impaired spermatogenesis.

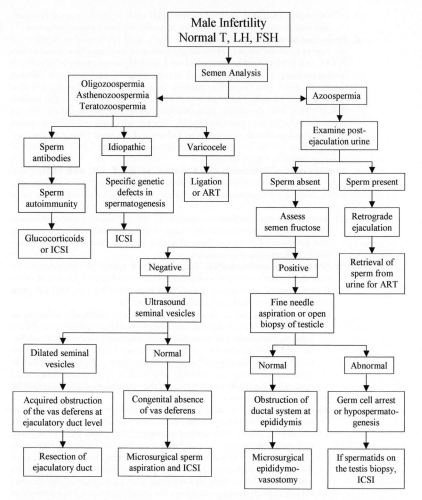

Figure 24.6. Algorithmic approach to the diagnosis and treatment of male infertility in patients with normal serum hormone concentrations. (Reprinted from Swerdloff RS, Wang C. The testes and male sexual function. In: Goldman L, Ausiello D, eds. *Cecil Textbook of Medicine.* 22nd ed. Philadelphia: WB Saunders; 2004:1472–1483.)

2. **Treatment.** It is essential that the female partner be thoroughly evaluated along with the male partner. Treatment of a female partner can often compensate for male-factor subfertility of mild to moderate decreases in semen parameters.

   a. There are a number of causes of irreversible infertility with no available therapy. This is true for most instances of primary hypogonadism or those involving damaged seminiferous tubules, including Klinefelter syndrome, microdeletions of the Y chromosome, Sertoli-cell only syndrome, and idiopathic infertility associated with azoospermia.

   b. Secondary hypogonadism may be managed with gonadotropins, GnRH infusions, and correction of underlying causes as outlined in Section II.3.d.

c. Assisted reproductive techniques (ART)

(1) Intracytoplasmic sperm injection (ICSI). This technique involves the direct injection of a single spermatozoon into the cytoplasm of a human oocyte. The overall fertilization rate is ~60%, and the clinical pregnancy rate per cycle is between 20% and 40%. ICSI can be performed with sperm obtained from ejaculate, epididymal aspiration, testicular biopsy, or fine-needle aspiration.

(2) Intrauterine insemination and in vitro fertilization have low efficacy rates.

(3) The introduction of ICSI has made it possible for men with severe oligospermia and azoospermia to father children, but the genetic risks must be considered. Examples include transfer of the *CFRG* gene and microdeletions of Y chromosome. Genetic counseling and molecular genetic tests should be undertaken prior to ICSI therapy. Fortunately, to date, there has been no reported increase in the incidence of birth defects with ICSI in comparison with natural conception.

C. Varicocele. A varicocele is an abnormal tortuosity and dilatation of the veins of the pampiniform plexus within the spermatic cord. Incompetence of the venous valvular structure produces increased hydrostatic pressure and dilatation of the veins. Because the left spermatic vein inserts directly at a right angle into the left renal vein, the left side is more prone to varicosity; therefore, **90% of varicoceles occur on the left side**. Right-sided varicoceles have been described, but they are usually associated with bilateral varicosity because collateral veins permit venous reflux from the left.

1. Detection. Moderate-sized to large varicoceles are easily detected by physical examination of the spermatic cord. Small varicoceles usually enlarge when the patient is asked to perform a Valsalva maneuver. Occasionally, mild exercise or standing for 30 minutes can be used to bring out a latent varicocele. In the past, equivocal physical findings have been confirmed by retrograde venography. However, ultrasonography, thermography, and radionucleotide methodology are now commonly used as noninvasive alternatives to corroborate the diagnosis.

2. Infertility and indications for varicocelectomy. The role of varicocele in the etiology of infertility remains controversial.

a. Incidence. A varicocele is present in ~10% to 15% of the male population, and the majority of these men have no testicular dysfunction or infertility. Therefore, physicians must be relatively conservative in their diagnostic and therapeutic approaches to men with varicocele. The presence of a varicocele alone is not evidence of testicular dysfunction and therefore does not constitute an indication for varicocelectomy. However, among infertile men, the incidence of varicocele has been reported to be 20% to 40%, suggesting an etiologic link.

b. Selection for treatment. Although the presence of varicocele can be associated with normal semen parameters and normal fertility, most men with varicocele and presumptive infertility have abnormal semen parameters, including low sperm concentration and abnormal sperm morphology. The causal relationship between varicocele and male infertility has been ascribed to increased testicular temperature, delayed removal of endogenously produced toxic metabolites, hypoxia, and stasis. A 1992 WHO study of 9 034 men found varicocele to be associated with increase in abnormal semen, decreased testicular volume, impaired sperm quality, and a decline of Leydig-cell hormone secretion. Interestingly, spontaneous pregnancies were equal in couples with and without a varicocele. Treatment of a varicocele by surgery or vein embolism/occlusion has been reported to improve semen quality; however, whether varicocele ligation will improve pregnancy rates in the female partner remains controversial. A large prospective study by the WHO compared pregnancy rates among infertile couples in which the male partner with a varicocele underwent immediate varicocele ligation, as opposed to ligation delayed for 1 year. The study suggested that varicocele ligation was beneficial, with a 34.8% first-year cumulative pregnancy rate in the immediate-treatment group, compared with 16.7% in the delayed-treatment group. However, there were flaws in the design and follow-up of patients in this trial. Furthermore, the first-year cumulative pregnancy rate of the delayed-treatment group was only 20%. Other studies have suggested that there are no significant differences in spontaneous pregnancy rate between couples treated for varicocele and untreated couples. Therefore, the use of varicocele ligation should be presented to the infertile couple with knowledge of yet uncertain efficacy. If there is a response to ligation, the response rate may be better in younger couples and in couples whose infertility is of shorter duration. The presence of atrophic testes, elevated FSH, and severe oligospermia/azoospermia suggests severe germinal damage, and consequently treatment for the varicocele is unlikely to aid fertility.

D. Male sexual dysfunction. Normal sexual function is a complex process that is dependent on higher cortical centers of the brain, which control fantasy and sexual thought; the autonomic nervous system, which controls erection and ejaculation; the pelvic vascular flow; and hormonal balance. Sexual dysfunction may be a manifestation of a decreased libido, erectile dysfunction, ejaculatory difficulties, or a combination of these factors.

1. Reduced libido may result from psychological factors such as depression, anxiety, and relational problems, or it may be caused by medical conditions such as hypogonadism or the effects of medications.

2. Ejaculatory difficulties

a. Premature ejaculation (ejaculation within 2 minutes of vaginal penetration) is more common in younger men. Psychological factors including anxiety or medications (especially adrenergic agents) are common causes.

b. Retrograde ejaculation is associated with neurologic impairment, especially diabetes mellitus or following prostatic surgery.

c. Anorgasmia may be attributable to psychological, neurologic, or medical causes. Selective serotonin reuptake inhibitors used for the treatment of depression are a class of medication associated with anorgasmia.

3. Erectile dysfunction. Erectile dysfunction is defined as the inability to maintain an erection of sufficient duration and firmness to complete satisfactory intercourse.

a. Normal erectile physiology. Nerve impulses prompted by excitatory stimuli travel from higher areas of the brain, down the spinal cord, to the thoracolumbar cortex. This leads to parasympathetic relaxation of the penile arterioles and cavernosal smooth muscles as a result of increase in endothelium-derived relaxing factor (nitric oxide). Expansion of the cavernosal muscles leads to compression of the penile venous outflow against the tunica albuginea, causing further expansion of the penis. Tactile sensation from the shaft results in additional parasympathetic stimulation.

b. Etiology. Causes of erectile dysfunction include psychological factors (more common in younger men), vascular insufficiency (more common among older men), neuropathy, hormonal impairment (hypogonadism, hyperprolactinemia), generalized fatigue from systemic illnesses, or use of drugs (antihypertensives, antihistamines, psychotropics). Erectile dysfunction may be multifactorial in origin and may be difficult to treat. For instance, although testosterone levels decrease with aging, the increased incidence of atherosclerosis leads to vascular disease and may play a more prominent role in erectile dysfunction in the elderly.

c. Evaluation. Couples should be evaluated together, at least in the initial visit(s), to ascertain chemistry and interrelational dynamics. A complete social, medical, and sexual history, including drug and medication history, should be obtained and a detailed physical examination performed. The presence of morning erections, by history or documented with the use of a RigiScan portable home monitor, may aid differentiation between organic and psychological causes. Obvious associated conditions, such as paresis, developmental defects, or atrophic testes, may infrequently be found on examination. Blood work entails a chemistry panel and glucose, serum testosterone level, and thyroid function tests if indicated. More specialized tests, such as the penile brachial index, penile injection of 10 mg prostaglandin E_1 (PGE_1) or 10 mg papaverine, may be used to assess vascular sufficiency. Bioesthesiometry or electromyography can be used to assess sensory innervation and the presence of neuropathy.

d. **Medical management.** Cells in the corpus cavernosum produce nitric oxide (NO) during sexual arousal in response to nonadrenergic, noncholinergic neurotransmission. NO stimulates the formation of cyclic guanosine monophosphate (cGMP), which leads to relaxation of smooth muscle of the corpus cavernosum and penile arteries, engorgement of the corpus cavernosum, and erection. Oral phosphodiesterase-5 inhibitors (sildenafil, vardenafil, and tadalafil) lead to persistent cGMP-stimulated relaxation of the corpora cavernosa. If taken 1 to 2 hours before intercourse, they are effective in 60% to 80% of patients. Response rate in men with diabetes mellitus is somewhat lower ($\sim$50%). The most serious side effect is cardiovascular collapse, especially in those with underlying coronary artery disease or on nitrates. Trazodone, which has serotonergic and α-adrenergic properties, may be effective in a third of patients but causes sedation. Intracavernosal injections of PGE_1 (papaverine) and PGE_1 intraurethral suppositories are available. Surgical treatments include penile implants or revascularization procedures. Revascularization of the penis and venous ligation for venous leakage has a high rate of failure and is recommended only under special circumstances.

E. **Gynecomastia.** Gynecomastia refers to male breast enlargement because of proliferation of glandular and stromal tissue. It is a common disorder affecting $\sim$70% of pubertal males. More than 30% of men >40 years old have some palpable breast tissue.

1. **Normal breast development.** In both male and female fetuses, epithelial cells proliferate into ducts that will eventually form the areola of the nipple at the surface of the skin. The milk line appears at about 10 weeks of gestation and the nipple at about 20 weeks. At $\sim$25 weeks of gestation, branching of the primordial ducts begins. The major period of proliferation of the ductal apparatus is between 32 and 40 weeks of gestation. Male and female breasts are equivalent at birth, and the male breast, when stimulated by estrogen, will progress through the same stages of development as the female breast. Up to 90% of male newborns have transient gynecomastia as a result of exposure to high maternal levels of hCG, estrogen, and progesterone, which stimulate breast tissue.

2. **Detection of gynecomastia.** All patients require a thorough history and physical exam. Special attention should be given to medications, drug and alcohol abuse, and other chemical exposure. Presence of systemic illnesses, such as hyperthyroidism, liver disease, and renal failure should be sought. Rapid, recent breast growth should be more concerning. Finally, the clinician should inquire about fertility, erectile dysfunction, and libido in order to evaluate hypogonadism as a potential cause. Physical examination should be done in supine position with palpation from the periphery to the areola and can usually distinguish glandular tissue from pseudogynecomastia (adipose or other nonglandular tissue) on the basis of texture and shape of the breast. Glandular tissue is rubbery, with mild nodularity, and spreads radially from underneath the areola. Comparison of the breast with nearby subcutaneous tissue provides a definitive diagnosis. The glandular mass should be measured in diameter, which is diagnosed by the finding of subareolar breast tissue of 4 cm or greater. Gynecomastia is usually bilateral but may be asymmetric. It is important to differentiate unilateral gynecomastia from carcinoma of the breast. Concerning findings include unusual firmness, a fixed mass, skin dimpling, nipple retraction and bloody nipple discharge, ulceration, and local adenopathy. Testicular exam is essential. Bilateral small testes are indicative of testicular failure, whereas testicular asymmetry or mass suggests the possibility of neoplasm. Visual-field impairment may suggest pituitary disease.

3. **Classification**
   a. Pseudogynecomastia
      (1) Adipose tissue
      (2) Neoplasm
      (3) Neurofibromatosis
   b. Gynecomastia
      (1) Newborn: physiologic exposure of fetus to estrogens
      (2) Prepubertal onset
         (a) Drugs
         (b) Idiopathic
         (c) Neoplasms (feminizing adrenal carcinoma)
      (3) Pubertal onset
         (a) Normal external genitalia
            (i) Pubertal gynecomastia
            (ii) Klinefelter syndrome
            (iii) Pubertal macromastia
         (b) Ambiguous external genitalia
            (i) Mixed gonadal dysgenesis
            (ii) Androgen-resistant syndromes
            (iii) Testosterone biosynthetic defect
            (iv) True hermaphroditism
      (4) Postpubertal onset
         (a) Idiopathic
         (b) Testicular failure
         (c) Drugs: alcohol, spironolactone, estrogens, digitalis preparations, androgens, chorionic gonadotropin, cimetidine, flutamide, mitotane, methyldopa, isoniazid, phenothiazine, amphetamines, diethylpropion, reserpine, marijuana, diazepam, and cytotoxic agents
         (d) Cirrhosis
         (e) Thyrotoxicosis
         (f) Chronic renal failure
         (g) Refeeding after starvation
         (h) hCG-secreting neoplasms
         (i) Leydig cell tumors
         (j) Feminizing adrenal carcinoma
4. **Pathophysiology.** The common denominator in disorders characterized by gynecomastia is an imbalance between circulating estrogens and androgens. Estrogens have a stimulatory effect on breast tissue, whereas androgens have an inhibitory role. Relative or absolute excess of circulating estrogens or a deficiency of circulating androgens leads to breast enlargement. Mechanisms for this imbalance include increased production of estrogens, increased aromatization of estrogen precursors, displacement of estrogens off SHBG, drugs with estrogenlike effect, and exogenous estrogen exposure. Decreased circulating androgens may result from decreased synthesis, increased metabolism, or a relative deficiency associated with androgen-resistant syndromes.
5. **Specific clinical syndromes**
   a. **Puberty.** Gynecomastia develops in ~70% of normal boys during puberty, although most patients are asymptomatic. The condition usually begins between 12 and 15 years of age and spontaneously abates in 90% of those afflicted within 3 years of onset. Serum E_2 concentrations are often high in relation to T in boys with pubertal gynecomastia, resulting in a high E_2/T ratio. This ratio returns to normal adult values as puberty progresses. The diagnosis of pubertal gynecomastia is made by recognition of the clinical setting, that is, onset of breast enlargement in an otherwise healthy pubertal male.
   b. **Adulthood.** About 30% to 40% of patients over the age of 40 have some palpable breast tissue. With advancing age, circulating concentrations of total and free T decrease along with a rise in serum LH. However, serum E_2 concentrations are maintained, resulting in an altered E_2/T ratio. Increasing

adiposity may also contribute by increasing peripheral aromatization of androgens to E_2. Finally, SHBG increases with age in men. Because SHBG binds estrogen with less affinity than testosterone, the bioavailable estradiol-to-T ratio may increase in the obese older male. Diagnosis requires exclusion of other causes of gynecomastia.

c. **Hypogonadism.** Gynecomastia occurs more commonly in men with primary testicular failure but can also be seen in patients with secondary hypogonadism. Serum T concentrations are low, whereas serum estrogens are usually normal or slightly elevated, resulting in an increased E_2/T ratio.

   (1) In primary testicular failure such as <u>Klinefelter syndrome</u>, serum T level is reduced and serum LH is increased. A high LH level stimulates aromatase activity in the testes, resulting in increased testicular E_2 production and an increased E_2/T ratio. In secondary hypogonadism, e.g., <u>Kallmann syndrome</u>, low levels of T and unopposed estrogen effects from the normal conversion of adrenal precursors to E_2 result in increased E_2/T ratio.

   (2) Serum prolactin is normal in most patients with gynecomastia, and enlarged breasts do not develop in most patients with hyperprolactinemia. Prolactin may occasionally contribute to gynecomastia by causing secondary hypogonadism and alterations in the ratio of circulating estrogens to androgens.

d. **Cirrhosis.** Approximately 50% of patients with cirrhosis have gynecomastia; 65% have testicular atrophy; and 75% experience decreased libido. The T production rate is decreased, although total serum T concentrations may not reflect this decrease because of increased SHBG. Adrenal androstenedione production rate is increased, which may result in higher estradiol levels. Serum E_2 levels are high-normal, but serum estrone (E_1) levels are quite elevated because of increased peripheral conversion of androstenedione to E_1. Thus, increased aromatization of an abundant adrenal substrate along with impaired T secretion leads to a high estrogen/androgen ratio.

e. **Thyrotoxicosis.** Approximately 30% of men with Graves disease have clinically detectable gynecomastia, and 80% have histologic evidence of gynecomastia on biopsy. Gynecomastia regresses when euthyroidism is restored. Patients often have elevated estrogen, which might be the stimulatory effect of thyroid hormone on peripheral aromatase activity. Thyroid hormones also increase SHBG. This results in elevation of both total serum T and E_2. Because serum T binds more avidly than E_2 to SHBG, free E_2 may be relatively increased compare to free T, resulting in an increased E_2/T ratio.

f. **Hormone-secreting tumors**

   (1) Feminizing adrenal carcinoma. This is a rare tumor that directly secretes E_2. The incidence of gynecomastia is close to 100%. Other adrenal neoplasms can secrete excess dehydroepiandrosterone, dehydroepiandrosterone sulfate, and androstenedione that can then be aromatized peripherally to estradiol.

   (2) Leydig cell tumor. Leydig cell tumors constitute only 1% to 3% of all testicular tumors. Approximately 25% of the reported cases have had associated gynecomastia. These tumors are associated with isosexual precocity (if they occur prior to puberty) and may secrete E_2 directly. Less than 10% of Leydig cell tumors are malignant, but when present, metastatic sites include the lung, liver, and retroperitoneal lymph nodes.

   (3) Germ-cell tumors. These are the most common cancers in males between the ages of 15 and 35, and they are divided into <u>seminomatous and nonseminomatous subtypes</u>. A variety of malignant tumors originating in the germinal elements of the testis as well as extragonadal germ-cell tumors have been shown to secrete hCG, which stimulates aromatase activity in Leydig cells to produce an excess of E_2. Nontesticular tumors can also produce hCG and stimulate E_2 by the same mechanism.

   (4) Certain chorionic tumors and hepatocellular carcinoma may transform circulating precursors into estrogens.

g. Refeeding gynecomastia. Prisoners of war during World War II, when refed, acquired tender gynecomastia that regressed spontaneously within 1 to 2 years. Similarly, gynecomastia can develop during recovery from anorexia nervosa, starvation, or any prolonged illness accompanied by substantial weight loss. The mechanism of refeeding gynecomastia is unclear. In men with hypogonadism as a result of malnutrition, both the gonadotropin secretion and Leydig cell function appear to be impaired. During refeeding, pituitary and gonadal function return to normal.

h. Drugs. A significant percentage of gynecomastia is caused by medications or exogenous chemicals, which occur mainly by several mechanisms:

(1) synergistic action with estrogen because of intrinsic estrogenlike properties of the drug,

(2) the production of increased endogenous estrogen, or

(3) excess supply of an estrogen precursor (e.g., T or androstenedione) that can be aromatized to estrogen.

(a) Spironolactone, cimetidine, and flutamide can produce gynecomastia by competitive displacement of DHT from its intracellular receptor (androgen receptor blocker). Spironolactone has the ability to block androgen production by inhibiting enzymes in the T synthetic pathway (i.e., 17α-hydroxylase and 17,20-desmolase), like ketoconazole. Spironolactone also can displace estradiol from SHBG, increasing free estrogen level.

(b) Digitoxin has inherent estrogenlike properties. In contrast, digoxin does not act as an estrogen agonist. It may occasionally produce gynecomastia through a "refeeding" mechanism in debilitated men with congestive heart failure.

(c) T administration, probably by its conversion to estrogens, may cause gynecomastia. However, nonaromatizable androgens, such as methyltestosterone, have been reported to produce gynecomastia, suggesting that additional mechanisms may be operative.

(d) A wide variety of agents that act on the central nervous system can raise serum prolactin, induce a secondary hypogonadal state (GnRH deficiency), and cause gynecomastia.

(e) Many chemotherapeutic agents, such as busulfan, nitrosourea, and vincristine, may cause Leydig cell and germ cell damage, resulting in primary hypogonadism.

(f) Alcohol causes gynecomastia by several mechanisms; it is associated with increased SHBG and decreases free T, thus increasing the E_2/T ratio. Alcohol also increases hepatic clearance of T and has a direct toxic effect on testes.

(g) Protease inhibitors used in the treatment of HIV infection are associated with gynecomastia.

6. Evaluation of the patient with gynecomastia

a. Exclude breast carcinoma. Localized areas of irregularity, firmness, or asymmetry in the mass suggest the possibility of early breast carcinoma and should be an indication for biopsy. In advanced stages, signs such as ulceration and adenopathy may be evident.

b. Recent or symptomatic gynecomastia is more likely to be clinically important and requires further evaluation. If the gynecomastia is of long duration and is asymptomatic in an otherwise healthy male, the patient can initially be followed without treatment.

c. A thorough drug history is important. In a Veterans Administration hospital study, more than 60% of patients were found to be receiving one or more medications associated with breast enlargement.

d. Gynecomastia may be the first sign of a hormone-secreting tumor of the testis or adrenal gland. The testes should be examined carefully for neoplasms. A variety of tumor markers are useful as screening tests, for example, measurement of β-hCG for hCG-secreting tumors of the testis or serum DHEAS for adrenal carcinoma.

e. **Laboratory evaluation.** In general, all patients with gynecomastia should have **serum T, estradiol, LH, FSH, and β-hCG** measured, and then, in light of the history and physical exam, further testing should be tailored. If i-hCG and E_2 are markedly elevated, this suggests a neoplasm. In this case, testicular ultrasound is warranted. If no testicular source is detected, additional imaging studies are required to detect nontesticular tumors that produce β-hCG. If T is low but LH is high and E_2 is normal-to-high, this indicates primary hypogonadism, and if the history suggests Klinefelter syndrome, a karyotype is needed for a definitive diagnosis. On the other hand, low T, low LH, and normal E_2 levels imply secondary hypogonadism, and hypothalamic and pituitary causes should be investigated. If T, LH, and E_2 are all elevated, then diagnosis of androgen resistance should be considered.

7. **Treatment.** Gynecomastia of long-standing duration might not regress with medical treatment, and reduction mammoplasty or liposuction is required if the gynecomastia is cosmetically or psychologically disabling. Gynecomastia associated with some conditions, such as puberty and refeeding, is usually transient, and these patients need only be observed. In many other conditions, correction of the underlying cause can lead to regression of gynecomastia.

   a. There are three classes of medical treatment for gynecomastia: **androgens** (testosterone, dihydrotestosterone, and danazol), **antiestrogens** (clomiphene citrate and tamoxifen), and **aromatase inhibitors** (testolactone).

   b. In patients with hypogonadism because of primary testicular dysfunction, T can be administered to decrease progression of gynecomastia, presumably by suppressing LH-mediated secretion of E_2 from the testes and restoring the T/E_2 ratio. Exogenous testosterone may itself produce gynecomastia by aromatization to E_2.

   c. Danazol appears to be less effective than tamoxifen in clinical trials. In Europe, DHT preparations are available and are associated with some success.

   d. The role of **antiestrogens (tamoxifen** and **clomiphene)** in the management of gynecomastia remains unclear despite encouraging reports. A short-term trial may be attempted to reduce breast size. The relapse rate is high, and the cost of long-term use of tamoxifen for this cosmetic disorder limits its widespread use.

   e. Aromatase inhibitors such as **testolactone** can be effective in the early proliferative phase of the disorder, but further studies are needed with more potent aromatase inhibitors such as letrozole, fadrozole, anastrozole, or formestane.

Selected References

AACE clinical practice guidelines for the evaluation and treatment of hypogonadism in adult male patients. *Endocr Pract* 2002;8:439.

AACE clinical practice guidelines for the evaluation and treatment of male sexual dysfunction. *Endocr Pract* 2003;9:77.

Bhasin S, Cunningham GR, Hayes FJ, et al. Testosterone therapy in adult men with androgen deficiency syndromes: an Endocrine Society clinical practice guideline. *J Clin Endocrinol Metab* 2006;91:1995–2010.

Burnett AL, Lowenstein CJ, Bredt DS, et al. Nitric oxide: a physiologic mediator of penile erection. *Science* 1992;257:401–403.

Carlson HE, Ippoliti AF, Swerdloff RS. Endocrine effects of an acute and chronic cimetidine administrations. *Dig Dis Sci* 1981;26:428.

Flynn MA, Weaver-Osterholtz D, Sharpe-Timms KL, et al. Dehydroepiandrosterone replacement in aging humans. *J Clin Endocrinol Metab* 1999;84:1527–1533.

Griffin JE, Wilson JD. The syndromes of androgen resistance. *N Engl J Med* 1980;302:198.

Gruntmanis U, Braunstein GD. Treatment of gynecomastia. *Curr Opin Invest Drugs* 2001; 2:643.

Hajjar RR, Kaiser FE, Morley JE. Outcomes of long-term testosterone replacement in older hypogonadal males: a retrospective analysis. *J Clin Endocrinol Metab* 1997;82:3793–3796.

Handelsman DJ, Liu PY. Klinefelter's syndrome—a microcosm of male reproductive health. *J Clin Endocrinol Metab* 2006;91:1220.

Hayes FJ, Seminara SB, Crowley WF. Hypogonadotropic hypogonadism. *Endocrinol Metab Clin N Am* 1998;27:739–763.

Kaufman JM, Vermeulen A. Declining gonadal function in elderly men. *Bailliere's Clin Endocrinol Metab* 1997;11:289–309.

Khorram O, et al. Reproductive technologies for male infertility. *J Clin Endocrinol Metab* 2001;86:2373.

Lanfranco F, Kamischke A, Zitzmann M, Nieschlag E. Klinefelter's syndrome. *Lancet* 2004; 364:273.

Morales AJ, Haubrich RH, Hwang JY, et al. The effect of six months treatment with a 100 mg daily dose of dehydroepiandrosterone (DHEA) on circulating sex steroids, body composition, and muscle strength in age-advanced men and women. *Clin Endocrinol* 1998;49:421–432.

Nieschlag E, Hertle L, Fischedick A, et al. Update on treatment of varicocele: counseling as effective as occlusion of the vena spermatica. *Hum Reprod* 1998;13:2147–2150.

Rommerts FFG, Focko FG. Testosterone: an overview of biosynthesis, transport, metabolism and action. In: Nieschlag E, HM Behre HM, eds. *Testosterone Action Deficiency Substitution*. Berlin: Springer-Verlag; 1990:1–22.

Salameh WA, Swerdloff RS. *Encyclopedia of Neuroscience, Neuroendocrine Control of Reproduction*. 3rd edition. New York: Elsevier; 2004.

Seftel AD, Mohammed MA, Althof SE. Erectile dysfunction: etiology, evaluation, and treatment options. *Med Clin North Am* 2004;88:387.

Sih R, Morley JE, Kaiser FE, et al. Testosterone replacement in older hypogonadal men: a 12-month randomized controlled trial. *J Clin Endocrinol Metab* 1997;82:1661–1667.

Swerdloff RS, Ng J, Kandeel FR. Gynecomastia. In: Kandeel F, ed. *Male Reproductive Dysfunction: Pathophysiology and Treatment*. New York: Informa Healthcare USA; 2007:519–528.

Swerdloff RS, Wang C. Evaluation of male infertility. *UpToDate* 8(1).

Swerdloff RS, Wang C. The testes and male sexual function. In: Goldman L, Bennett JC, eds. *Cecil Textbook of Medicine*. 21st ed. Philadelphia: WB Saunders; 2004:1472–1483.

Swerdloff RS, Wang C, Kandeel FC. Evaluation of the infertile couple. *Endocrinol Metab Clin N Am* 1988;17:301–331.

Swerdloff RS, Wang C, Sokol RZ. Endocrine evaluation of the infertile male. In: Lipschultz L, Howards S, eds. *Infertility in the Male*. 2nd ed. St. Louis: Mosby; 1991:211–222.

Vermeulen A. Andropause. *Maturitas* 2000;34:5–15.

Vermeulen A, Goemaere S, Kaufman JM. Testosterone, body composition, and aging. *J Endocrinol Invest* 1999;22:110–116.

Wang C, Swerdloff RS. Androgen replacement therapy. *Ann Med* 1997;29:365–370.

Wang C, Swerdloff RS. Androgens. In: Smith CM, Raynard AM, eds. *Textbook of Pharmacology*. Philadelphia: WB Saunders; 1991:683–694.

Wang C, Swerdloff RS. Evaluation of testicular function. *Bailliere's Clin Endocrinol Metab* 1992;6.

Wang C, Swerdloff RS, Iranmanesh A. Transdermal testosterone gel improves sexual function, mood, muscle strength, and body composition parameters in hypogonadal men. Testosterone Gel Study Group. *J Clin Endocrinol Metab* 2000;85:2839–2853.

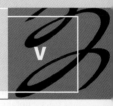

Mineral Disorders

V

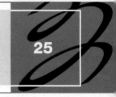

DISORDERS OF CALCIOTROPIC HORMONES IN ADULTS

25

Frederick R. Singer and Arnold S. Brickman

I. CALCIOTROPIC REGULATORY HORMONES AND FACTORS

Calcium and phosphorus homeostasis may be modulated in large part through three hormones that exert actions at the intestine, kidney, and bone: parathyroid hormone (parathyrin, PTH), vitamin D, and calcitonin, although the role of calcitonin in man remains less certain. Other calciotropic factors have been identified through their presence in several pathologic states and may have a role in modulating divalent ion metabolism under physiologic conditions. A partial list of these includes magnesium; parathyroid hormone–related peptide (PTHrP); various cytokines and growth factors such as interleukin-(IL) 1, 2, and 6; transforming growth factors α and β; the superfamily of tumor necrosis factors, including RANK, RANK ligand (RANKL), and osteoprotegerin; platelet-derived growth factor; and the family of insulinlike growth factors and related binding proteins.

A. Parathyroid hormone

1. Modulating factors. Human PTH is an 84-amino-acid polypeptide **(intact PTH 1-84)** secreted by the parathyroid glands under acute modulation by the level of ionized calcium perfusing the glands. PTH secretion is inversely related to the extracellular concentration of calcium. The level of calcium is "sensed" by a G-protein–coupled receptor in the cell surface **(calcium-sensing receptor [CSR]).** Calcium ion acts as an agonist to the CSR. A rise in extracellular calcium concentration activates the CSR, which, through a series of intracellular events, suppresses the secretion of PTH. Long-term stimulation can suppress parathyroid cell proliferation. Serum calcium levels also modulate transcription of the *PTH* gene. Extracellular and tissue levels of magnesium also can modulate PTH secretion, with both high levels and low levels or tissue depletion suppressing secretion. Calcitriol **(1,25-dihydroxycholecalciferol [1,25(OH)$_2$D$_3$]),** but not its precursor, 25-OHD$_3$, has been shown to modulate transcription activity of the *PTH* gene and production of the prohormone form of PTH. Finally, although serum phosphorus has been thought to have no direct effect on PTH secretion, studies have suggested that high levels of phosphate ion stimulate PTH synthesis independent of effects of the ion on $1,25(OH)_2D_3$ production. Although the classic target organs for PTH are bone and kidneys, receptors for the hormone have been identified in a variety of other tissues, a fact that should be kept in mind when considering other possible actions of PTH.

2. **Structure.** The *PTH* gene resides on chromosome 11 and codes for a precursor polypeptide, <u>preproPTH</u>, which undergoes sequential cleavages to form the mature secreted form of the hormone (PTH 1-84). PTH 1-84 is also metabolized in the parathyroid glands and at extracellular sites (e.g., liver, kidney, bone) forming **carboxy-terminal (C-terminal)** and **amino-terminal (N-terminal) fragments.** Both PTH 1-84 and the N-terminal fragment (containing at least the first 32 amino acids) are biologically active. Some studies in vitro have also demonstrated selective biologic activity for C-terminal peptides, although the physiologic significance of these observations remains to be established. C-terminal fragments are disposed of by glomerular filtration and subsequent degradation by the kidney. Under conditions of reduced renal function, disappearance of the C-terminal fragment is prolonged. Reduction of renal function has less effect on plasma clearance of the N-terminal fragment, which is filtered by the kidney and removed by peritubular uptake and metabolism at sites of action. Radioimmunoassays have been developed to measure PTH 1-84 and both C-terminal and N-terminal fragments. In addition, a midhormone peptide sequence–specific assay has been developed. Assays for PTH 1-84 are quite useful because levels are not affected by underlying renal insufficiency. It has been previously demonstrated that the most used commercial <u>intact PTH assay</u> (Nichols Institute intact PTH) also measures nonintact hormone fragments. Improved PTH 1-84–specific assays were subsequently developed.

3. **Action.** PTH acts at bone to modulate osteoblastic activity directly and osteoclastic activity indirectly through coupled bone remodeling activity. Only the osteoblast has receptors for PTH. At the kidney, PTH modulates transtubular transport of phosphorus, calcium, bicarbonate, and magnesium ions. The major effect of PTH on the intestinal transport of calcium is indirect, e.g., through its regulatory function on formation of calcitriol from its precursor, 25-hydroxycholecalciferol [25(OH)D].

B. **Vitamin D**

1. **Vitamins D_2 and D_3**

   a. Vitamin D is a general term that has been used to refer to the concerted activity of several different metabolites of cholecalciferol (vitamin D_3) and ergocalciferol (vitamin D_3). The metabolites are sterols whose production occurs in several different organs. Vitamin D_3 is synthesized in the epidermis, whereas vitamin D_2 comes from plants and yeasts and has been synthesized to fortify various foods and vitamin products. In general, the biologic activity of vitamin D_2 and its metabolites is equal to that of vitamin D_3. For purposes of diagnostic testing, separate measurements of vitamins D_3 and D_2 are preferred.

   b. Vitamin D_3 is a **prohormone** produced in the epidermis from conversion of **7-dehydrocholesterol (7-DHC; provitamin D_3)** to **pre–vitamin D_3,** reactions requiring absorption of ultraviolet radiation and thermally induced isomerization. It (vitamin D_3 + vitamin D_2) circulates in small amounts (1 to 2 ng/mL) bound to a single **vitamin D–binding protein (DBP),** which binds and transports all vitamin D sterols. A number of factors can influence the production of vitamin D_3 in the skin, including melanin pigmentation, age, season, and geographic latitude. Because aging reduces epidermal levels of 7-DHC, inadequate production of vitamin D_3 contributes to depletion, particularly in elderly persons during the winter months. Prolonged use of sunscreens can contribute to development of vitamin D_3 deficiency. In contrast, vitamin D intoxication is *not* known to occur with excessive sun exposure in otherwise healthy individuals.

2. **Calcidiol.** Vitamin D is metabolized in the liver by a **cytochrome P450 hydroxylase** to form 25(OH)D **(calcidiol).** Quantitatively, it is the major circulating vitamin D metabolite. Because its formation in the liver is not tightly regulated,

there may be wide physiologic and nonphysiologic fluctuations in circulating levels. Clinically and diagnostically, measurement of plasma levels of 25(OH)D are used to indicate the "vitamin D status" of an individual (delineation of vitamin sufficiency, depletion, or intoxication, with the latter being attributable to excessive administration of vitamin D_2/D_3. Depending on geographic location, levels of 25(OH)D undergo seasonal variation, with the highest levels occurring during the summer and the lowest levels during the winter and early spring. Normal levels are now thought to range from 30 to 60 ng/mL. There has been some experimental evidence that 25(OH)D is hormonally active, but there is no general agreement on the issue. The metabolite is approximately 1/10 to 1/100 as active as $1,25(OH)_2D$ (**calcitriol**), depending on the in vitro or in vivo assay utilized. Synthetic $25(OH)D_3$ is available for clinical use in a 20-μg dose. Recent evidence indicates that the blood half-life of $25(OH)D_3$ is three to four times as long as that of $25(OH)D_2$.

3. **Calcitriol.** Under physiologic conditions, 25(OH)D undergoes a second hydroxylation in the kidney to either $1,25(OH)_2D$ or $24,25(OH)_2D$, the former considered to be the hormonally active form of vitamin D.

   a. A possible physiologic function for **24,25(OH)₂D** in humans is controversial, with some evidence suggesting that this metabolite has a function in formation of cartilage and skeletal remodeling. Its formation has also been regarded as a disposal pathway, utilized when the need for calcitriol synthesis is decreased. It circulates at levels 100 times greater than that of calcitriol.

   b. Enzymatic formation of calcitriol **25(OH)-1α-hydroxylase** is very tightly regulated, involving factors such as levels of PTH, dietary intake, extracellular concentrations of calcium and phosphorus, the level of calcitriol itself, and possibly (directly or indirectly) other hormones, including calcitonin, estrogen, insulin, and growth hormone. Calcitriol secretion is modulated by PTH and extracellular and intracellular levels of phosphorus, calcium, and magnesium. Hypophosphatemia, hypocalcemia, and elevated levels of PTH stimulate secretion. In addition to the kidney, other tissues, such as monocytes, macrophages, lymphocytes, and skin cells, may express 25(OH)-1α-hydroxylase activity and produce calcitriol under pathologic conditions. In the latter setting, secretion of calcitriol is not under physiologic regulation. During pregnancy, the placenta can also produce the hormone.

   c. Calcitriol is recognized as the most active natural metabolite stimulating active intestinal transport of calcium and phosphorus. In bone, calcitriol promotes formation of osteoclasts from stem cells, although mature osteoclasts lack vitamin D receptors. In contrast, mature osteoblasts possess vitamin D receptors and respond to calcitriol by producing a number of cytokines and other humoral factors. The latter then can modulate osteoclastic activity. Calcitriol promotes bone mineralization by maintaining extracellular divalent ion concentrations in a physiologic range that allows deposition of calcium hydroxyapatite in osteoid.

4. **Vitamin D receptors.** High-affinity nuclear receptors for calcitriol have been identified in a large number of target tissues for vitamin D. These include tissues other than intestine, bone, and kidney. Receptors have been identified in the pancreas, skeletal muscle, vascular smooth muscle, epidermal keratinocytes, hematopoietic cellular elements, and lymphocytes, as well as in other cells of the immune system. This indicates that vitamin D sterols have cellular functions other than regulation of extracellular divalent ion concentrations.

C. **Calcitonin**

1. **Action.** Calcitonin is a 32-amino-acid peptide produced primarily by **parafollicular C cells** of the thyroid gland. Other neuroendocrine cells also have the capacity to produce calcitonin. Like PTH, cellular secretion of calcitonin is modulated by a CSR. However, secretion by the thyroid C cells is stimulated by a rise in extracellular calcium and inhibited by a fall in calcium. In addition, calcitonin secretion also may be modulated by several gastrointestinal hormones, including gastrin.

a. Calcitonin reduces bone resorption by <u>inhibiting osteoclastic activity</u>. It also has been found to have a positive effect on bone formation in some animal studies, but evidence for this in humans is lacking.

b. At the kidney, calcitonin <u>reduces tubular reabsorption of both calcium</u> and <u>phosphorus</u>, producing a modest increase in excretion of both ions. The former may contribute to the hypocalcemic effect of pharmacologic doses of calcitonin.

c. A homeostatic function of calcitonin may be to buffer calcium absorbed through the intestine. The net effect of the stimulation of calcitonin secretion (or exogenous administration) is a lowering of serum levels of both calcium and phosphorus.

d. In women, **estrogen** may also play a role in maintaining calcitonin's secretory capacity. There is some evidence that in estrogen-deficient states (natural or artificial menopause), the calcitonin level is decreased, thereby affecting the accelerated menopausal bone loss.

2. Clinical application. Measurement of circulating levels of calcitonin has limited clinical application. However, calcitonin is the major tumor marker for **medullary carcinoma of the thyroid gland.** Basal as well as pentagastrin- and calcium-stimulated calcitonin secretion is utilized to assess tumor activity.

3. Calcitonin gene–related peptide (CGRP) is a 37-amino-acid peptide that is produced by alternative expression of the calcitonin gene. Secreted by neuroendocrine cells, it acts as a neurotransmitter and has vasodilatory action. It probably contributes little of skeletal and extracellular divalent ion homeostasis but binds weakly to the calcitonin receptor.

D. PTHrP

1. PTHrP was originally discovered as a circulating factor responsible for the development of hypercalcemia in patients with various malignant disorders (humoral hypercalcemia of malignancy). Elevated circulating levels of PTHrP have been demonstrated in 50% to 80% of patients with <u>malignancy-associated hypercalcemia</u>.

The gene coding for PTHrP is situated on chromosome 12 and is thought to share its ancestral origin with the *PTH* gene situated on chromosome 11. PTHrP is a much larger molecule than PTH and is synthesized in three different polypeptide isoforms. These are produced by alternative messenger RNA (mRNA) splicing **(PTHrP 1-139, PTHrP 1-141,** and **PTHrP 1-173).** In addition, subsequent processing of the PTHrP molecule results in production of various peptide fragments with distinctly different biologic actions.

2. Action. PTH and PTHrP have structural homology at only 8 of the first 13 amino acids of the amino terminus, which explains the similarity in some of their biological activities. Both PTH and amino-terminal fragments of PTH bind with high affinity to a common receptor **(PTH/PTHrP receptor)** and produce common physiologic actions. A second PTH receptor has now been identified with high binding affinity only for PTH, and a receptor for carboxyl-terminal PTH has also been described. A unique cell receptor for PTHrP has not been identified, although specific receptors for some of its fragments apparently exist.

Under normal physiologic circumstances, PTHrP probably circulates in much lower levels than PTH, although with present assays it is not measurable in normal individuals. A major role in the maintenance of normal divalent ion homeostasis has not been demonstrated. However, a large body of evidence indicates that PTHrP has important physiologic functions in <u>growth regulation</u> in developing fetal and adult tissues. These are local (autocrine and paracrine actions) rather than systemic actions of the hormone or its peptide fragments. PTHrP has been demonstrated in numerous tissues, including cartilage, skeletal and cardiovascular musculature, central nervous system (CNS) tissues, distal renal tubules, placenta, prostate, breast, epidermis, and hair follicles. With respect to the breast, PTHrP appears to have roles both in <u>morphogenesis and in lactation</u>. High concentrations of PTHrP have been shown in human milk. Other observations suggest that PTHrP functions in utero to modulate mineral homeostasis across the placenta and in the developing fetus. **Elevated levels of PTHrP** may be one cause of **hypercalcemia of infancy.**

E. **Fibroblast growth factor 23.** Fibroblast growth factor 23 (FGF23) is a systemic factor which in recent years has been found to be an important regulator of the serum phosphorus concentration and a factor in the pathogenesis of both hypophosphatemic and hyperphosphatemic disorders. The FGF23 gene produces a 251-amino-acid peptide with a 24-amino-acid signal peptide. The protein appears to be produced primarily in bone and, unlike other members of the FGF family, it functions as a hormone rather than a local factor. FGF23 binds to several FGF receptors and the protein Klotho, but knowledge of its mechanism of action is incomplete. Elevations of serum FGF23 lower the serum phosphorus concentration and serum $1,25(OH)D_2$. FGF23 appears to be the causative factor in a number of hypophosphatemic disorders, including **autosomal dominant hypophosphatemic rickets/osteomalacia, tumor-induced rickets/osteomalacia, X-linked hypophosphatemic rickets/osteomalacia, and autosomal recessive hypophosphatemic rickets/osteomalacia. Familial hyperphosphatemic tumoral calcinosis** is associated with low levels of full-length FGF23 in the circulation, further evidence for the importance of the protein in phosphorus homeostasis.

II. DISORDERS ASSOCIATED WITH HYPERCALCEMIA

A. **Clinical features of hypercalcemia.** The clinical presentation of hypercalcemia can range from that of a mild asymptomatic disorder detected during routine examination to a severe, potentially life-threatening condition requiring emergency medical management. However, to a large extent, symptoms and signs associated with hypercalcemia are a reflection of the patient's age, the underlying primary disease process, concurrent medical disorders, and the degree, duration, and rate of development of elevated calcium. Gradually developing severe hypercalcemia in a younger individual may be surprisingly well tolerated with minimal symptoms, whereas mild to moderate hypercalcemia developing acutely may be associated with severe symptoms. Elderly patients are frequently sensitive to mild elevations in serum calcium. Most symptoms reflect disturbances in the renal, gastrointestinal, cardiovascular, neuromuscular, and central nervous systems.

1. **CNS.** Symptoms referable to hypercalcemia-induced disturbances in the neuromuscular system and CNS include weakness, fatigue, lassitude, anorexia, depression, and confusion, and, in severe cases, stupor and coma. Impairment in cognitive function is common, particularly in the elderly, even in cases of mild elevation in serum calcium. Agitated behavior, including frank psychosis, can occur with serum calcium levels >14 to 15 mg/dL.

2. **Cardiovascular system.** Possible disturbances in the cardiovascular system include hypertension, bradycardia, nonspecific cardiac arrhythmias (shortened QT interval on the electrocardiogram), and increased sensitivity to digitalis glycosides. If intravascular volume is not maintained, hypotension may occur.

3. **Renal.** Alterations in renal function include impaired urine-concentrating capacity, polyuria (with consequent polydipsia), reduced glomerular filtration rate, nephrocalcinosis, and nephrolithiasis. Depending on the primary disorder, urinary calcium excretion can vary from low to markedly elevated. Nephrocalcinosis and/or nephrolithiasis can occur particularly in conditions associated with chronic hypercalcemia.

4. **Gastrointestinal.** Gastrointestinal disturbances range from nausea, vomiting, and anorexia to symptoms of gastroesophageal reflux with or without the presence of peptic ulcer disease to constipation. Acute pancreatitis is an uncommon but serious presenting condition of hypercalcemia.

B. **Causes of hypercalcemia.** A differential diagnosis for hypercalcemia includes an extensive group of disorders (Table 25.1). A thorough medical history and a few readily available diagnostic tests usually can reduce the list of possible causes. The most common disorders include primary hyperparathyroidism, malignancy, granulomatous diseases, and medications. A useful approach is to classify disorders according to the altered physiologic condition responsible for the development of

TABLE 25.1	Classification of Causes of Hypercalcemia according to Pathogenesis

Increased release of calcium from bone
Primary hyperparathyroidism
Exogenous PTH therapy
Malignancy
    Humoral hypercalcemia of malignancy (tumor production of PTHrP)
    Osteolytic bone metastases
    Tumor-associated ectopic cytokine production
    Ectopic tumor-produced PTH
Immobilization
Thyrotoxicosis
Vitamin A intoxication

Reset parathyroid calcium sensor-receptor
Familial hypocalciuric hypercalcemia
Lithium

Increased intestinal absorption of calcium
Autonomous hyperparathyroidism of diverse etiologies
Vitamin D intoxication
    Chronic granulomatous disease [extrarenal $1,25(OH)_2D_3$ formation]
Malignancy [extrarenal $1,25(OH)_2D_3$ formation]

Decreased renal calcium excretion
Familial hypocalciuric hypercalcemia
Acute renal failure
Milk–alkali syndrome

Decreased uptake of calcium by bone
Aluminum toxicity

Pseudohypercalcemia
Hyperalbuminemia
Macroglobulinemia of Waldenström
Myeloma
Hyperlipidemia

Miscellaneous causes or uncertain pathogenesis

Adrenal Insufficiency	Thiazide diuretics
Pheochromocytoma	Theophylline, aminophylline
VIP-producing pancreatic tumors (VIPoma)	Estrogens and antiestrogens
Parenteral hyperalimentation	Tamoxifen
Hemodialysis (high-Ca dialycate)	Androgens
	Growth hormone

PTH, parathyroid hormone; PTHrP, parathyroid hormone–related peptide; VIP, vasoactive intestinal polypeptide.

hypercalcemia: **(1)** increased release of calcium from bone (increased resorption); **(2)** increased intestinal absorption of calcium; **(3)** a combination of increased intestinal calcium absorption and bone resorption; and **(4)** decreased urinary excretion of calcium.

In a few conditions, the mechanism of hypercalcemia remains poorly characterized.

1. **Primary hyperparathyroidism (PHP).** PHP is the most common cause of hypercalcemia in an unselected clinical setting. Both sporadic and familial forms of disorder occur, the latter being very uncommon to rare, with autosomal dominant inheritance demonstrated in most cases. Solitary **parathyroid adenomas,**

single or multiple, are found in 80% to 85% of cases, and two parathyroid adenomas are found in 1% to 2% of patients. **Parathyroid hyperplasia** involving all glands occurs in 15% to 20% of patients. **Parathyroid carcinoma** is rare, occurring in <1% of cases. Benign **parathyroid cysts** are rarely associated with hypercalcemia, although the high levels of PTH can be demonstrated in aspirated cyst fluid.

Hereditary forms of PHP occur as both isolated parathyroid disorders or in association with other genetically determined conditions. **Multiple endocrine neoplasia type 1 (MEN1/Wermer syndrome)** is a distinct disorder in which PHP is the most common feature (occurring in >95% of cases), but in which concomitant enteropancreatic and pituitary neoplasms may also occur with high frequency (frequency varying among different kindreds). The most common pancreatic lesions are **gastrin-(Zollinger-Ellison syndrome)** and **insulin-producing tumors.** The most commonly encountered pituitary tumor is **prolactinoma.** A variety of other substances may be produced by these respective tumors (pancreas—**glucagon, vasoactive intestinal polypeptide, pancreatic polypeptide;** pituitary—**growth hormone, ACTH),** but these associated syndromes occur less commonly. **Adrenal hyperplasia** and **thyroid adenomas** have also been described in some kindreds. The development of MEN1 has been linked to the expression of an inactivating mutation of a tumor suppressor gene **(Menin/MEN1 gene)** that is localized to **chromosome 11q13.** The clinical expression of PHP in MEN1 is similar to that of sporadic PHP, but it tends to occur at younger ages and with equal frequency in both sexes. Although solitary parathyroid adenomas have been described in MEN1, it is usually characterized by the presence of multiglandular parathyroid hyperplasia. Parathyroid carcinoma has been reported but is rare in MEN1.

Multiple endocrine neoplasia type 2a (MEN2a/Sipple syndrome) is a distinct disorder characterized by the expression of medullary carcinoma of the thyroid (~100% of cases), bilateral pheochromocytomas (up to 50% of cases), and parathyroid hyperplasia (50% to 70% of cases). Clinical PHP tends to be mild in MEN2. The syndrome is caused by an **activating mutation of the RET proto-oncogene on chromosome 10.** Commercial genetic tests are available for identification of individuals at risk for both MEN1 and MEN2a.

Other familial syndromes associated with PHP include **hyperparathyroidism–jaw tumor syndrome (HJTS)** and **familial isolated PHP.** HJTS is an autosomal dominant disorder characterized by early-onset (childhood to adolescence), often severe, PHP. Recurrent adenoma and parathyroid carcinoma have been described. The bone lesions associated with HJTS occur as punched-out cystic lesions in the mandible and maxilla ranging from small asymptomatic cysts to large disfiguring masses. They differ from the classical "brown tumors" of PHP in that they lack osteoclasts. Various types of renal tumors, including Wilms tumor and hamartomas, have been described in different kindreds. Mutations in the tumor-suppressor protein parafibromin are responsible for HJTS as well as some kindreds with familial isolated PHP and parathyroid cancer.

a. **Pathophysiology of PHP.** In individuals with parathyroid adenomas, the set point for calcium-induced suppression of PTH secretion is altered or "shifted" so that the level of hormone secreted is inappropriately increased for the level of calcium (e.g., a loss of feedback control). The calcium set point for PTH secretion (effected by the CSR) is an ionized calcium level of 4 mg/dL (1 mmol/L). In PHP resulting from hyperplasia of the parathyroids, the calcium set point is normal but the number of PTH secreting cells is increased. The genetic alterations that contribute to development of parathyroid adenomas remain elusive for the majority of cases. In a small number of tumors a mutation resulting in rearrangement of the cell growth promoter, **the proto-oncogene PRAD1 (cyclin D1),** has been identified. This genetic rearrangement results in a location of a cell growth–regulating element proximal to the gene controlling PTH synthesis. Activation of *PTH* gene expression thus also promotes cell growth. Separate studies have shown increased levels of *PRAD1* in up to 20% of tumors. The MEN1 tumor-suppressor gene has also been identified in some sporadic adenomas.

With excess PTH, bone remodeling is increased and there is increased release of calcium, contributing to the generation of hypercalcemia. At the kidney, the tubular threshold for phosphate reabsorption is lowered, augmenting phosphaturia and contributing to the development of hypophosphatemia. Tubular reabsorption of calcium is increased, but the net effect on urinary excretion of calcium is balanced by the increased filtered load of calcium as a function of the degree of hypercalcemia. Both excess PTH and hypophosphatemia stimulate calcitriol production and augmentation of intestinal absorption of calcium. Hypercalciuria and augmented intestinal absorption of calcium are present in 40% and 60% of patients, respectively.

b. **Clinical features of PHP** (Table 25.2)

(1) In Rochester, Minnesota, between 1993 and 2001, the overall age- and sex-adjusted rate of primary hyperparathyroidism was 21.6 per 100 000 patient years, a nearly fourfold lower rate than from 1974 to 1982. The disorder occurs at all ages, with a peak incidence between the ages of 60 and 70 years.

(2) Currently, >50% of diagnosed patients are asymptomatic, with hypercalcemia discovered fortuitously. On close examination, many of these patients may be found to have subtle clinical features attributable to hypercalcemia and/or elevated PTH levels. In younger patients there is frequently a poor relationship between the degree of hypercalcemia and the presence or absence of symptoms.

(3) Severe metabolic bone disease **(osteitis fibrosa cystica),** with development of bone cysts, brown tumors, and marrow space fibrosis, is now uncommon in PHP. Severe skeletal disease is more likely to be found in patients with underlying renal insufficiency or familial disorders such as HJTS. Regardless of the severity of the bone disorder, bone biopsy shows qualitative histologic features characteristic of PHP in most cases. **Osteopenia** is now the most commonly observed skeletal abnormality in PHP, present in ~30% of cases, depending on the method of assessment. There is evidence that fracture rates at the forearm, hip, and spine are increased.

(4) **Calcium nephrolithiasis** or **nephrocalcinosis** is present in 40% to 50% of patients with symptomatic PHP. In contrast, <5% of calcium stone formers have PHP. Renal stone disease tends to occur in younger patients with PHP, with a reported peak incidence in the third and fourth decades. Correlations can be demonstrated between the presence of stone disease and both the degree of hypercalciuria and the elevation of calcitriol level.

(5) **Hypertension** has been reported in **30% to 50% of patients with PHP.** It remains unclear whether this differs from the prevalence in the general population when corrected for age, sex, and race. It is also not known whether the incidence of hypertension in PHP is greater than in other causes of hypercalcemia. Acute elevation in serum calcium levels is associated with a rise in blood pressure in normal individuals.

c. **Diagnosis.** Clinical suspicion is a major consideration in the diagnosis of PHP.

(1) **Hypercalcemia** is present in the majority of patients. In cases in which serum calcium is intermittently normal or only marginally elevated, determination of ionized calcium is a useful adjunct to confirming the presence of hypercalcemia. Some patients may have persistent normocalcemia **(normocalcemic PHP),** which can represent a transient phase in the natural history of the disorder. Rarely, the presence of vitamin D deficiency with osteomalacia masks hypercalcemia. Treatment with replacement doses of vitamin D will unmask PHP in this setting **(vitamin D challenge test)**.

(2) **PTH levels** can be measured using a number of highly sensitive assays, the most useful being those that measure the **intact hormone** (PTH 1-84).

| TABLE 25.2 | Spectrum of Clinical Features of Hyperparathyroidism according to Organ Systems |

Central nervous system
Fatigue, lassitude
Depression
Memory impairment
Dementia
Psychosis
Coma

Ocular
Cataracts
Band keratopathy

Gastrointestinal
Peptic ulcer disease
GERD, cholelithiasis
Pancreatitis
Constipation

Skeletal
Osteopenia
Osteoporosis
Fractures
Bone cysts
Brown tumors
Marrow fibrosis
Osteosclerosis

Neuromuscular and articular
Myopathy
Gout
Pseudogout
Chondrocalcinosis
Erosive arthritis

Cardiovascular
Hypertension
Left ventricular hypertrophy
Shortened QT interval
Arterial stiffness
Arrhythmias
Vascular and cardiac calcifications

Renal
Polyuria
Urine-concentrating defect
Nephrolithiasis
Renal tubular acidosis

Miscellaneous
Anemia
Fever of unknown origin

GERD, gastroesophageal reflux disease.

They employ one-or two-site radioimmunoassay techniques, respectively. It is essential that serum or ionized calcium be measured simultaneously with PTH. In most cases this is sufficient for diagnosis.

(3) Measurement of the urinary excretion of total or **nephrogenous cyclic adenosine monophosphate (cAMP)** provides an assessment of PTH action on the kidney. With the development of sensitive and clinically useful assays for PTH, measurement of cAMP excretion is seldom used as a diagnostic aid in PHP.

(4) **Urinary calcium excretion** varies from normal to elevated in PHP, depending on the level of serum calcium, filtered load of calcium by the kidney, intestinal absorption of calcium, dietary intake, and effect of PTH on tubular reabsorption of calcium. Because most non-PHP causes for hypercalcemia are associated with the presence of hypercalciuria, normal urinary calcium excretion in the presence of hypercalcemia is frequently of greater diagnostic value than the presence of increased urinary calcium. In PHP, the degree of hypercalciuria correlates with elevated levels of $1,25(OH)_2D$.

(5) **Hypophosphatemia** is present in ~50% of cases and is associated with a lowered **renal threshold for phosphorus reabsorption,** that is, the **tubular maximum for phosphorus reabsorption (TmP)** expressed as a function of glomerular filtration rate (GFR) **(TmP/100 mL GFR).**

(6) An elevated serum **chloride/phosphorus ratio** (normal >32) occurs in 60% to 70% of patients with PHP, indirectly reflecting the effect of PTH as lowering the tubular maximum for bicarbonate excretion (mild elevation in serum chloride and depression of serum bicarbonate).

(7) **Biochemical markers of bone remodeling** are typically increased in PHP (e.g., **formation markers—osteocalcin** and **alkaline phosphatase;** and resorption markers—**hydroxyproline, deoxypyridinoline, collagen _N_-telopeptide** and **collagen C-telopeptide**). These alterations may on occasion be helpful in distinguishing PHP from other disorders associated with hypercalcemia.

d. Preoperative and intraoperative parathyroid localization procedures. Routine utilization of techniques for attempting localization of parathyroid tumors prior to the initial surgical exploration have gained popularity in recent years, although success rates associated with first-time parathyroid surgery, when performed by highly experienced endocrine surgeons are ~90% to 95%.

(1) Depending on the experience of the technologist, **ultrasonography** localizes parathyroid enlargement in up to 80% of cases. Recently, intraoperative ultrasonography performed by surgeons has also proved successful in localizing abnormal parathyroid glands. Magnetic resonance imaging (MRI) is similar to ultrasound in detecting parathyroid abnormalities, but its high cost is a drawback. Computed tomography (CT) imaging is also an effective but expensive technology.

(2) **^{99m}Tc-sestamibi scintigraphy** has become widely used as a sensitive localization procedure (sensitivity ~80%) for parathyroids. Because all noninvasive localization procedures are associated with false-positive and false-negative results, confirmation of findings with two procedures can offer greater confidence in test results.

(3) **Parathyroid angiography,** particularly when combined with selective venous sampling to identify a gradient in PTH levels, can localize hyperplastic glands or an adenoma in most cases (80% to 95%). Cost and available expertise are limitations in routine utilization of these techniques.

(4) **Intraoperative parathyroid localization** is now common in many centers using ^{99m}Tc-sestamibi imaging. A hand-held gamma-radiation detector **(gamma probe)** can often rapidly locate an abnormal gland. When combined with intraoperative ultrasound, the detection of adenomas is ~90%. Intraoperative PTH levels can be measured following removal of suspicious lesions. A decrease of >50% 10 minutes after removal of an abnormal gland nearly always indicates correction of hyperparathyroidism. Patients with hyperplasia require multiple gland removal before PTH levels are appropriate.

e. Medical management

(1) Surgical removal and angiographic ablation (selective infarction) of the parathyroid glands are the only definitive treatments for PHP.

(2) **Transcutaneous injection of adenomas with alcohol** has been carried out in several centers using ultrasound. The procedure has been associated with a high incidence of complications, such as injury to the recurrent laryngeal nerve.

(3) Patients who are poor surgical risks, who have had previous unsuccessful surgery, or who decline surgical intervention can benefit from medical treatment.

(a) Administration of **orthophosphate salts** in doses providing 1 to 3 g per day of phosphorus can control hypercalcemia as well as certain forms of nephrolithiasis (e.g., calcium oxalate, calcium hydroxyapatite) in some patients. This form of treatment should not be undertaken in patients with renal insufficiency, with serum calcium >12 mg/dL, or under conditions of habitual poor hydration. Treatment with phosphate salts can enhance calcium phosphate renal stone formation. In addition, treatment with orthophosphate salts might increase levels of PTH. In practice, this form of therapy is seldom used.

(b) <u>Estrogen</u> has been shown to antagonize PTH-mediated bone resorption. Several studies in postmenopausal women treated with estrogens with or without progesterone have demonstrated reduction in serum calcium levels without significant effects on levels of PTH.

(c) The bisphosphonate **alendronate** has been convincingly shown to preserve bone density in patients with primary hyperparathyroidism. Maintenance of normal serum calcium levels with chronic bisphosphonate therapy has not been convincing, although acute decreases in high serum calcium levels are readily achieved with intravenous **pamidronate.** The safety of management of PHP with bisphosphonates has not been established.

(4) **A new class of drugs (calcimimetics)** that act as calcium sensor-receptor agonists has been developed. Administration of calcimet to patients with PHP has been shown to reduce both serum calcium and PTH levels for up to 5 years. Despite this, it cannot be first-line treatment because there is no evidence that it produces the same benefits as surgical cure, such as improvement in bone density. It is appropriate to consider its use if patients refuse surgery or have medical contraindications for surgery. As yet, this agent has only been approved by the U.S. Food and Drug Administration (FDA) for dialysis patients and for patients with primary hyperparathyroidism resulting from parathyroid carcinoma.

2. Familial hypocalciuric hypercalcemia (FHH). Also known as **familial benign hypercalcemia,** FHH is an uncommon disorder that can be confused with PHP. It may represent 1% to 2% of cases of asymptomatic hypercalcemia. The major clue to the diagnosis is a family history of hypercalcemia, sometimes in individuals who have undergone unsuccessful exploratory parathyroid surgery.

a. Inheritance is autosomal dominant and is **expressed very early in life,** with hypercalcemia sometimes detected within the first few days. Sporadic cases have also been described. In the majority of cases of FHH studied, the presence of an **inactivating (loss-of-function) mutation of the CSR** has been demonstrated. A number of different mutations have been identified in different kindreds and have been mapped to genes on the **long arm of chromosome 3,** as well as on both the **long and short arms of chromosome 19.** These CSR mutations cause a shift in the set point for suppression of PTH secretion, resulting in a higher threshold of serum calcium to suppress hormone secretion and the presence of mild to moderate hypercalcemia. The presence of the mutated CSR in the kidney produces a variable reduction in urinary calcium excretion, often to the level of hypocalciuria.

b. Biochemical features include variable degrees of reduced urinary calcium excretion ("hypocalciuria"), hypercalcemia, hypomagnesuria, and hypermagnesemia. Urinary calcium excretion is usually expressed as the **ratio of calcium clearance to creatinine (CCa/CCr)**, which is a more sensitive index of renal calcium excretion than total urinary calcium. The CCa/CCr in FHH is usually <0.1, allowing discrimination from PHP. Serum phosphorus levels are variable. PTH levels are normal to slightly elevated, as is urinary cAMP excretion. Levels of vitamin D metabolites are normal.

c. Patients with FHH lack the clinical features of PHP or MEN syndrome. Serum calcium levels are generally mild to moderately elevated, with clustering of similar levels of calcium in affected individuals in families. Acute and recurrent pancreatitis has been described in individuals and within kindreds that have higher degrees of hypercalcemia. Response to parathyroid surgery in FHH is invariably poor, thus underscoring the need to distinguish the disorder from PHP prior to undertaking surgical exploration. The development of recurrent pancreatitis in FHH may necessitate total parathyroidectomy. At surgery, the parathyroids can have the appearance of chief-cell hyperplasia **(pseudoadenomatous chief-cell hyperplasia)**.

d. Neonatal severe primary hyperparathyroidism (NSPHP). See Chapter 27.

3. Hypercalcemia of malignancy (HCM). HCM is the most common cause of hypercalcemia in hospitalized patients. The pathogenesis of HCM is multifactorial, varying among the different types of malignancy. Hypercalcemia occurs most commonly in patients with various squamous cell carcinomas, breast cancer, renal cell carcinoma, bladder carcinoma, multiple myeloma, and various lymphomas. It is uncommon in certain malignancies, such as colon and prostate cancers. Development of hypercalcemia was considered a poor prognostic sign because it occurred late in the course of malignancy; however, advances in treatment for various types of cancers are changing this perspective. As with other hypercalcemic disorders, dehydration, immobilization, and treatment with certain drugs (e.g., thiazide diuretics, lithium, vitamin D) can contribute to or potentiate development of HCM. Other **specific** causes include:

- Direct invasion of bone (local osteolysis)
- Tumor production of one or more circulating factors that augment osteoclastic resorption of bone (humoral hypercalcemia of malignancy)
- Ectopic production of $1,25(OH)_2D_3$
- Concomitant malignancy
- PHP or granulomatous disorders
- Treatment with estrogen or antiestrogens (tamoxifen)

a. Tumor-associated local osteolysis accounts for hypercalcemia in about 20% to 40% of cases.

(1) Although direct resorption of bone by malignant cells has been hypothesized, most investigators do not believe this is the case.

(2) A number of locally produced **osteoclast-activating factors (OCFs)** that activate osteoclastic resorption of bone (e.g., by a paracrine pathway) have been identified. Such factors may be produced by or under the influence of malignant cells acting on *in situ* bone cell elements. They comprise, **parathyroid hormone–related protein (PTHrP)**, prostaglandins of the E series, and several cytokines, including **tumor necrosis factor-α (cachectin) and -β (lymphotoxin), transforming growth factors-α and -β**, and several **interleukins (IL-1α, IL-1β, and IL-6)**. The pathogenesis of bone lesions in multiple myeloma is particularly complex, as recent studies have identified **RANK ligand, macrophage inflammatory peptide 1α** and **IL-3** as likely mediators of bone resorption and a suppression of **OPG** secretion as a contributory mechanism.

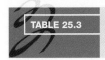

TABLE 25.3	Comparison of Biochemical Features of Primary Hyperparathyroidism, Humoral Hypercalcemia of Malignancy (Ectopic PTHrP Syndrome), and Familial Hypocalciuric Hypercalcemia

Feature	PHP	HHM	FHH
Serum Ca	I	I	I
PTH	I	D	N/sl.I
PTHrP	N	I	N
CSR set point	I/N^a	N	I
Serum phosphorus	D/N	D	N/sl.D
TmP/GFR	D	D	N
Serum chloride	N/I	N/D	N
Urinary calcium	I/N	I	D
Urine NcAMP	I	I	N/sl.I
1,25(OH)$_2$D$_3$	I/N	D	N
Osteocalcin	I/N	D	N
Urine N-telopeptide collagen cross-links	I/N	I	N

CSR, calcium sensor receptor; D, decreased; I, increased; FHH, familial hypocalciuric hypercalcemia; HHM, humoral hypercalcemia of malignancy; NcAMP, nephrogenous cyclic adenosine phosphate; PHP, primary hyperparathyroidism; PTH, parathyroid hormone; PTHrP, parathyroid hormone–related peptide; sl.D, slightly decreased; sl.I, slightly increased.
^{a}The CSR set point is normal in idiopathic parathyroid hyperplasia.

- **b. Humoral hypercalcemia of malignancy (HHCM)** refers to a condition in which a malignant tumor produces one or more circulating factors that cause hypercalcemia in the absence of evidence for skeletal metastasis. HHCM accounts for malignancy-associated hypercalcemia in 40% to 50% of cases. The term **pseudohyperparathyroidism** was originally used to describe this condition.
  - **(1)** It is now recognized that tumor production of a PTHrP is the major cause of HHCM. Elevated circulating levels of PTHrP have been reported for a number of malignancies, utilizing several different commercial assays.
  - **(2)** PTHrP-mediated hypercalcemia is associated with low to undetectable PTH, hypophosphatemia due to a lowered TmP/GFR, increased urinary nephrogenous cAMP excretion, and relative hyper-calciuria. However, in contrast to PHP, levels of 1,25(OH)$_2$D are low or reduced (Table 25.3).
- **c.** Tumors capable of producing a peptide that is immunologically and physiologically identical to native PTH (e.g., **ectopic primary hyperparathyroidism**) are rare. Proof of occurrence includes extraction of PTH from the tumor, demonstration of an arteriovenous gradient for PTH across the tumor, detection of mRNA for PTH in tumor cells, production of PTH by cultured tumor cells, and, optimally, cure of hyperparathyroidism with obliteration of the malignancy. Patients whose ectopic PHP meet such criteria include those with **squamous carcinoma of the lung, ovarian adenocarcinoma, thymoma, papillary carcinoma of the thyroid,** and **small-cell carcinomas of lung and ovary**.
- **d.** Hypercalcemia caused by **extrarenal production of 1,25(OH)$_2$D** affects patients with lymphoproliferative malignancies, including **Hodgkin disease, B-cell lymphomas, and Burkitt lymphoma.** The malignant lymphoid cell is the site of 1α-hydroxylase activity. In some cases of **T-cell lymphoma,** hypercalcemia may be attributed at least in part to tumor production of calcitriol; however, in other cases, the **predominant factor appears to be ectopic production of PTHrP**.
- **e.** Some squamous cell or poorly differentiated carcinomas have been reported to produce high levels of an E prostaglandin (PGE-M). Tumor production

TABLE 25.4 Tumors Associated with Ectopic Production of 1,25(OH)$_2$D$_3$

Malignant disorders
B-cell lymphoma
Hodgkin disease
Myeloma (uncommon)
Lymphomatoid granulomatosis

Chronic granulomatous disorders
Infectious diseases
  Tuberculosis
  Histoplasmosis
  Coccidioidomycosis
  Candidiasis
  Cat-scratch fever
  Leprosy
Noninfectious conditions
  Sarcoidosis
  Foreign-body granulomata (silicon, paraffin, lipoid pneumonia)
  Berylliosis
  Eosinophilic granuloma
  Wegener granulomatosis

of **prostaglandin** E2 has been described in some patients with renal carcinoma. Treatment with **aspirin** or **indomethacin (prostaglandin synthetase inhibitors)** has resulted in a concomitant reduction of high urinary levels of PGE-M and control of hypercalcemia. This does not appear to be a common mechanism for HCM and contrasts with prostaglandin-mediated local osteolysis.

  f. Treatment of some women with breast cancer with estrogen or tamoxifen can produce a **hypercalcemic flare.** The mechanism is not well understood.

4. Granulomatous diseases (Table 25.4)

  a. Hypercalcemia occurs in ~10% of patients with active pulmonary sarcoidosis; hypercalciuria is detected even more frequently, in up to 50% of cases. A correlation can be shown between the degree of severity of sarcoidosis or elevation in levels of angiotensin-converting enzyme and degree of hypercalcemia.

    (1) Patients with sarcoidosis have been shown to have elevated circulating levels of 1,25(OH)$_2$D. The cause has been shown to be ectopic production of 1,25(OH)$_2$D by granuloma macrophages containing a 25(OH)-vitamin D-1α-hydroxylase, similar to that in the kidney. Normal physiologic regulation of calcitriol formation is absent in granulomatous tissue. The increased sensitivity to vitamin D derived from dietary intake or solar exposure and classically described in sarcoidosis can be explained as rapid and unregulated conversion of precursors to the active metabolite. Circulating levels of calcitriol also correlate with disease severity.

    (2) Treatment with steroids is both rapid and highly effective in controlling the hypercalcemia and hypercalciuria of sarcoidosis. A **steroid suppression test** for hypercalcemia has been used to distinguish sarcoidosis from PHP. This test is performed by administration of 150 mg of hydrocortisone (or 40 to 60 mg of prednisone) daily for 7 to 10 days. Serum calcium levels in patients with sarcoidosis invariably drop during treatment, usually within 3 days, whereas individuals with PHP usually show no change. This test cannot identify the rare patient who has both disorders. Because patients with uncomplicated sarcoidosis have low levels of PTH, this measurement usually allows differentiation from PHP.

(3) **Chloroquine, hydroxychloroquine,** and **ketoconazole** have also been shown to reduce $1,25(OH)_2D$ production and control both hypercalcemia and hypercalciuria in patients with sarcoidosis.

(4) In addition to the above-described measures, reduction in sun exposure, avoidance of excessive exogenous vitamin D intake, and control of dietary calcium intake to not more than 1 000 mg per day are efficacious in the control of hypercalciuria and hypercalcemia.

b. Hypercalcemia has also been reported in a number of other granulomatous diseases (Table 25.4). Elevated serum levels of $1,25(OH)_2D$ have been documented in most of these conditions. The mechanism of ectopic production of calcitriol may be similar to that of sarcoidosis. However, other mechanisms for altered calcium homeostasis may be operative, because low levels of calcitriol in the presence of hypercalcemia have been described in isolated cases.

Treatment with steroids, hydration, and reduction of dietary calcium intake may be useful and effective in controlling hypercalciuria and hypercalcemia in the various granulomatous disorders.

5. Vitamin D intoxication

a. Development of hypercalcemia during prolonged treatment with pharmacologic doses of vitamin D generally results from accumulation of high levels of $25(OH)D$, but can also result from excessive dietary intake of calcium supplements or dairy products. Vitamin D intoxication has also been described in individuals ingesting dairy products erroneously fortified with excessive amounts of vitamin D. Despite plasma levels of $25(OH)D$ that can be 5 to 10 times normal in vitamin D–intoxicated patients, the levels of $1,25(OH)_2D$ are usually, but not invariably, normal or only slightly elevated. In this setting, hypercalcemia and hypercalciuria develop as an apparent consequence of the mass action effect of high levels of $25(OH)D$ acting at vitamin D receptors in the intestine and possibly skeletal sites. Because of the storage and slow release of $25(OH)D$ in muscle and adipose tissue, high circulating levels and the potential for symptomatic vitamin D intoxication can persist for weeks to months after discontinuation of the medication.

b. In comparison with the risks associated with vitamins D_3 and D_2, the potential for development of hypercalcemia during treatment is greater with more potent compounds, such as $25(OH)D_3$, $1,25(OH)_2D_3$, and the synthetic compounds **dihydrotachysterol** and **1α-hydroxyvitamin D_3** (both metabolized in the liver to their biologically active forms, respectively, **25(OH)-dihydrotachysterol** and calcitriol). However, because these compounds are metabolized rapidly, the duration of hypercalcemia in comparison with vitamins D_3 and D_2 is shortened.

c. Management of vitamin D intoxication includes reduction of dietary calcium intake and discontinuation of the vitamin D preparation. In severe cases, the use of steroids (prednisone, 40 to 60 mg per day), which block intestinal and probably skeletal actions of vitamin D, may be required, sometimes for weeks or months.

6. Other endocrine causes of hypercalcemia

a. Hyperthyroidism. Hypercalcemia has been reported to occur in thyrotoxicosis in 15% to 50% of cases. The mechanism appears to be thyroid hormone–mediated increased osteoclastic bone resorption. PTH and calcitriol levels are suppressed and hypercalcemia is generally mild, possibly reflecting compensatory urinary calcium losses and reduced intestinal absorption of calcium.

(1) The diagnosis is usually not difficult unless hyperthyroidism is not recognized or is complicated by coexisting disorders such as PHP, in which case confirmation of hyperthyroidism as the cause of hypercalcemia occurs with effective treatment of the hyperthyroidism.

(2) A beta-blocker (e.g., propranolol, 20 to 40 mg four times a day) may be effective treatment for hypercalcemia while awaiting response to antithyroid therapy in disorders such as Graves disease or toxic multinodular goiter.

b. Pheochromocytoma. Hypercalcemia is frequently observed in patients with catecholamine-secreting adrenomedullary tumors. Although pheochromocytoma and PHP occur together in MEN2a, hypercalcemia may also be found in the absence of intrinsic parathyroid disease. Several mechanisms are involved in the development of hypercalcemia. These include catecholamine-induced volume contraction and hemoconcentration, epinephrine-induced PTH secretion, and, in some cases of malignant tumors, secretion of PTHrP. Rapid resolution of hypercalcemia usually follows removal of the tumor.

c. Adrenal insufficiency. Acute adrenal insufficiency **(addisonian crisis)** can present with moderate to severe hypercalcemia. Few well-studied cases have been reported. Factors that probably contribute to the development of hypercalcemia include volume depletion with hemoconcentration and reduction in GFR, which facilitates increased tubular reabsorption of calcium, and increased skeletal release of calcium, possibly because of increased sensitivity to vitamin D. Correction of volume depletion and treatment with corticosteroids rapidly correct hypercalcemia in this setting. The disorder should be considered in hypercalcemic patients with AIDS because of the possible presence of concomitant infectious agents, such as *Mycobacterium avium-intercellulare,* which can cause adrenal insufficiency.

d. Pancreatic islet cell tumors. Hypercalcemia in patients with pancreatic islet cell tumors can occur as the result of several different abnormalities. These tumors may develop as part of MEN1 syndrome and occur in association with PHP. In other cases, elevated circulating levels of PTHrP have been reported. However, the occurrence of hypercalcemia is particularly high in patients with tumors that secrete **vasoactive intestinal polypeptide (VIPomas).** The mechanism of hypercalcemia in this condition has not been established.

7. Miscellaneous causes of hypercalcemia

a. Milk–alkali syndrome. Ingestion of excessive amounts of milk (or calcium supplements) and soluble alkali (absorbable antacid) can cause hypercalcemia. Treatment with vitamin D can further potentiate the syndrome, as can the presence of disorders in which augmented intestinal absorption of calcium is part of the pathophysiologic disturbance (e.g., PHP). The usual implicated salts are sodium bicarbonate and calcium carbonate. Acute and chronic forms of milk–alkali syndrome are recognized.

(1) **Chronic milk–alkali syndrome (Burnett syndrome)** is associated with soft-tissue calcification in the kidneys and nephrocalcinosis. Progressive renal insufficiency can occur.

(2) Diagnosis of **acute milk–alkali syndrome** is recognized by the appropriate clinical history and laboratory profile: hypercalcemia, frequently with slightly elevated serum phosphorus, mild azotemia, and metabolic alkalosis.

(3) Factors that contribute to the development of the disorder include increased intestinal absorption of calcium and decreased urinary excretion of calcium as a result of the reduction in GFR and increased tubular reabsorption of calcium in the presence of metabolic alkalosis.

(4) The incidence of the disorder has declined because of the availability of nonabsorbable antacids and the use of H_2 secretion–blocking agents such as cimetidine and ranitidine. However, recent emphasis on the use of calcium carbonate as part of management regimens for osteoporosis has resulted in increased incidence.

(5) Treatment consists of discontinuation of calcium supplements and alkali, and rehydration. This usually results in a rapid correction of hypercalcemia. Exclusion of coexisting PHP (with peptic ulcer disease) in a setting consistent with development of milk–alkali syndrome may be required in some cases.

b. Drug-induced hypercalcemia. Treatment with a number of drugs can raise serum calcium levels and induce hypercalcemia *de novo* or by exacerbating the effects of other conditions or disorders in which hypercalcemia commonly

TABLE 25.5	Medications Associated with Development of Hypercalcemia

Thiazide diuretics
Vitamin D analogs (vitamin D, calderol, calcitriol, DHT, topical calcipotriol)
Vitamin A and analogs (*cis*-retinoic acid, all-*trans*-retinoic acid)
Human PTH I-34; recombinant human PTH I-84
Lithium
Estrogen and antiestrogen (Tamoxifen)
Growth hormone
Aminophylline, theophylline
Foscarnet
8-Chloro-cAMP

cAMP, cyclic adenosine 3′,5′-monophosphate; DHT, dehydrotestosterone; PTH, parathyroid hormone.

occurs (Table 25.5). The mechanism(s) of hypercalcemia associated with some of these drugs is currently not understood.

(1) **Vitamin D analogs.** The term **"vitamin D intoxication"** was previously used to describe a condition in which prolonged treatment with large doses of vitamin D_2 or D_3 or dihydrotachysterol was used in the management of a specific disorder (e.g., hypoparathyroidism). Formation of high levels of 25-hydroxy metabolites of these drugs resulted in the development of hypercalcemia. Excessive commercial dairy fortification of cows' milk has also been demonstrated to produce vitamin D intoxication and hypercalcemia. With the availability of more potent vitamin D analogs, such as $25(OH)D3,1\alpha(OH)D3$, and $1,25(OH)_2D_3$, and their use in treatment in a variety of clinical settings, hypercalcemia is frequently encountered. The contributing factors to development of hypercalcemia can be multiple but include hyperabsorption of calcium (in the presence of excessive calcium supplementation) and increased bone resorption. Treatment includes reduction in dose or discontinuation of the drug, reduction of dietary calcium intake, and treatment with glucocorticoids for variable periods.

(2) **Vitamin A analogs.** Treatment with doses of vitamin A >50 000 IU/d can result in hypercalcemia. Hypercalcemia is also occasionally observed in patients being treated with **cis-retinoic acid** and **all-trans-retinoic acid.** The mechanism of increased serum calcium appears to be enhanced vitamin A–mediated osteoclastic bone resorption.

(3) **Thiazide diuretics.** Treatment with thiazide diuretics is frequently associated with mild hypercalcemia. The finding of more severe elevation in serum calcium usually indicates the presence of an underlying disorder of calcium metabolism (e.g., PHP) or a bone disorder associated with high rates of bone remodeling, such as juvenile osteoporosis. The mechanism(s) of hypercalcemia include increased renal tubular reabsorption of calcium and diuretic-induced volume depletion.

(4) **Lithium carbonate.** The use of lithium carbonate in the management of bipolar disorders is associated with a rise in serum calcium in most patients and development of hypercalcemia in ~5% of cases. Enlargement of the parathyroids has been described, but the predominant mechanism appears to be a reset in the CSR. Increased lithium-induced renal tubular reabsorption of calcium has also been described. Hypercalcemia is usually seen with higher doses of lithium carbonate. Reduction in dosage or discontinuation usually results in lower serum calcium levels. However, surgically documented cases of primary hyperparathyroidism in lithium-treated patients have been reported. Whether or not the lithium caused the tumors is unclear, but either surgery or **cinacalcet** has been effective therapy.

C. General principles for management of hypercalcemia

1. Correction of dehydration and volume depletion.
2. Correction of electrolyte abnormalities (frequently hypokalemia).
3. Discontinuation or reduction in dosage of digitalis (hypercalcemia potentiates digitalis toxicity).
4. Discontinuation of treatment with medications that contribute to the development of hypercalcemia (e.g., vitamin D, vitamin A, estrogens, antiestrogens, thiazide diuretics, etc.).
5. Reduction of dietary intake of calcium in those disorders in which intestinal hyperabsorption of calcium can contribute to the development of hypercalcemia (e.g., vitamin D intoxication, milk–alkali syndrome).
6. Weight-bearing mobilization of patients confined to bed when possible. When the cause of disordered mineral homeostasis is known, it may be feasible to select a therapeutic agent or regimen that acts at the site of generation of hypercalcemia.

D. Management of hypercalcemia

1. **Agents that decrease the release of calcium from bone or increase the uptake of calcium into bone**

   a. **Calcitonin.** Parenteral administration of calcitonin has been shown to be effective in the acute management of hypercalcemia. Salmon calcitonin is the only species of calcitonin available for use.

   (1) The mechanisms of action are rapid inhibition of osteoclastic activity and reduction in tubular reabsorption of calcium (e.g., increased urinary calcium excretion). Onset of action is rapid, with calcium lowering apparent within 2 to 4 hours of administration, but duration of action with a single dose is brief.

   (2) Calcitonin is administered either by continuous infusion, or by intramuscular or subcutaneous injections at 6- to 12-hour intervals at a dose of 3 to 8 IU/kg. Frequently, a loss of response efficiency occurs after repeated dosing for longer than 3 to 4 days. There is evidence that this "escape" phenomenon may be blocked by glucocorticoid administration (prednisone, 30 to 60 mg per day). The latter may result in sustained reduction in calcium levels for several weeks. Nasal spray and rectal suppository preparations (not available in the United States) are generally not useful in the management of hypercalcemia.

   (3) Calcitonin usually produces a modest reduction in serum calcium levels, but its low toxicity profile makes it a useful agent in the appropriate clinical setting. It may be particularly useful in the treatment of hypercalcemia associated with vitamin D intoxication. With the advent of intravenous bisphosphonate therapy, calcitonin use has dropped substantially.

   b. **Bisphosphonates**

   (1) The bisphosphonates are structurally related to pyrophosphate, a natural metabolic product. These compounds bind to hydroxyapatite in bone matrix and thereby provide sufficient tissue drug levels to inhibit osteoclastic bone resorption.

   (2) Parenteral preparations for administration of both **pamidronate (Aredia)** and **zoledronic acid (Zometa)** are currently available in the United States. Because of its greater potency in lowering serum calcium and longer duration of action, zoledronic acid is more frequently used than etidronate for this indication. The only advantage of pamidronate is the lower cost of generic pamidronate. Pamidronate is generally infused as a single dose (60 to 90 mg) over a 4-hour period. Individualized treatment regimens with repeat dosing with pamidronate can achieve control of serum calcium for days to weeks. Side effects to parenteral therapy may include low-grade fever, myalgias, and leukopenia. Mild hypocalcemia and hypophosphatemia may occur in some cases, usually when multiple doses of drug have been administered. These alterations are usually mild and do not require corrective measures. Zoledronic acid is infused as a single dose of

4 mg over 15 minutes. Similar side effects to pamidronate may be encountered after zoledronic acid infusion. Patients should be given vitamin D_3 prior to use if there is evidence of vitamin D deficiency. Both pamidronate and zoledronic acid are approved for use in hypercalcemia of malignancy by the FDA but have been used off-label in patients with other causes of hypercalcemia.

(3) Oral bisphosphonate preparations have generally not been effective in the acute or long-term management of hypercalcemia. However, pamidronate and zoledronic acid have been used in the management of breast cancer, multiple myeloma, and other malignancies. In breast cancer, bisphosphonate therapy has been used to reduce the development of metastases, delay the development of hypercalcemia, control bone pain and possibly exert an anticancer effect on tumor cells in bone, and delay progression of established metastatic lesions. Similarly, treatment with a bisphosphonate can delay or reduce the expression of skeletal complications in multiple myeloma and other malignancies.

c. Plicamycin (mithramycin). This cytotoxic drug is an anticancer chemotherapeutic agent that inhibits RNA synthesis. At single daily doses of 15 to 25 μg/kg, it rapidly decreases osteoclastic activity. Calcium-lowering effects can occur within 12 to 24 hours. Responses are variable, sometimes occurring with a single dose or requiring several daily doses to achieve control of hypercalcemia. Sustained lowering of serum calcium can last for extended periods with intervals of 1 to 3 weeks between treatments. Thus, plicamycin can be useful in long-term management of hypercalcemia, particularly that associated with malignancy. However, potential or demonstrable side effects may limit its usefulness. These may include bone marrow effects (thrombocytopenia), renal dysfunction (rise in serum creatinine and proteinuria), and liver damage (elevation in transaminases). Availability of potent bisphosphonates has greatly reduced the use of plicamycin in the management of hypercalcemia.

d. Gallium nitrate (Ganite). This agent inhibits bone resorption by adsorbing to and reducing solubility of hydroxyapatite in bone matrix. A direct effect on osteoclast function is possible but not clearly established. Administration is by continuous infusion, usually for 5 to 10 days. Shorter courses of therapy are effective in normalizing serum calcium in some cases. For severe hypercalcemia, the usual dose is 200 mg/m^2 of body surface area. Onset of action is usually apparent within 24 to 48 hours, with calcium falling gradually, often not reaching a nadir for 5 to 8 days. Duration of normocalcemia, when achieved, is usually 6 to 10 days. An important side effect of gallium nitrate is nephrotoxicity. The drug should be used with caution in patients with renal insufficiency and never when serum creatinine levels are >2.5 mg/dL. Its main indication is for treatment of patients who fail to have a desired response to a bisphosphonate.

e. Phosphate. Both orally and intravenously administered phosphate salts have been effective in the management of hypercalcemia and were used mainly when other effective agents were not available. Mechanisms of action include inhibition of osteoclastic activity and probable increased skeletal mineral accretion. Treatment with these agents is usually contraindicated in patients with renal insufficiency, because rapid worsening of renal function attributed to intrarenal precipitation of calcium phosphate salts can occur in this setting. The usual oral dose ranges from 1 000 to 1 500 mg per day of elemental phosphorus in divided doses, not exceeding 3 000 mg per day. Parenteral administration of phosphorus should not exceed 1 000 mg per 24 hours, with infusion occurring over a 4- to 6-hour period. Electrolytes and renal function should be carefully monitored. Ectopic soft-tissue deposition of calcium–phosphorus complexes can occur when the calcium–phosphorus product is >40. For this reason, long-term treatment with phosphate salts is usually not employed when serum calcium levels are >12 to 13 mg/dL and should be monitored with periodic radiographs and assessment of renal function.

2. **Agents that increase urinary excretion of calcium:**
   a. **Loop diuretics and saline.** Intermittent infusion of normal saline with periodic doses of furosemide (or ethacrynic acid) to maintain maximum natriuresis and calciuresis was widely used in the initial management of hypercalcemia before other effective agents were available. **Urinary calcium excretion is directly proportional to sodium excretion.** Therapy usually consists of administration of 4 to 8 L per 24 hours, alternating saline and 5% dextrose and water at a ratio of 3:1 to 4:1. The usual dose of furosemide is 80 to 120 mg every 2 to 6 hours. Administration of diuretics should be preceded by correction of volume depletion. Because urinary potassium and magnesium losses are large with this regimen, replacement requirements of these electrolytes are determined by careful monitoring of serum levels. Electrocardiographic and central venous pressure monitoring may be required in a setting of extremely aggressive therapy. Additional potential complications include volume overload as a result of insufficient diuresis and volume depletion as a result of excessive diuresis. Even in its most aggressive forms, this therapeutic approach usually produces only a modest drop in serum calcium levels, and because of the success of bisphosphonate therapy, only hydration with saline of dehydrated patients is presently commonly used.
   b. **Hemodialysis or peritoneal dialysis.** In situations in which marked renal insufficiency or fulminant or incipient congestive heart failure is present or where life-threatening malignant hypercalcemia exists, hemodialysis or peritoneal dialysis can be considered. Dialysis using a calcium-free dialysate can rapidly lower serum calcium levels. Careful monitoring of cardiovascular parameters is required, because rapid lowering of calcium can result in hypotension, requiring volume expansion and administration of pressor agents.
3. **Agents that reduce intestinal absorption of calcium.** Enteral hyperabsorption of calcium contributes to the development and maintenance of hypercalcemia in a limited number of clinical settings.
   a. In **disorders of vitamin D excess** [iatrogenic vitamin D intoxication or ectopic $1,25(OH)_2D_3$ production], treatment with glucocorticoids (prednisone, 30 to 60 mg per day) is highly effective in reducing calcium absorption.
   b. Short-term **reduction of dietary intake of calcium** may be a useful maneuver in vitamin D–excess states as well as in the milk–alkali syndrome. Treatment with **cellulose phosphate,** which complexes with calcium in the intestine, has also been used to reduce effective net intestinal absorption of calcium.
   c. **Ketoconazole,** an antifungal agent, has been shown to reduce plasma levels of $1,25(OH)_2D_3$ in normal individuals as well as in patients with sarcoidosis and primary hyperparathyroidism.

III. HYPOCALCEMIC DISORDERS

A. **Clinical features of hypocalcemia.** The signs and symptoms of hypocalcemia are a function of the level of serum calcium, age at onset and duration, levels of serum magnesium and potassium, and accompanying disturbances in acid–base homeostasis. To some extent the clinical manifestations of hypocalcemia relate to the type of underlying disease process. Thus, absence or deficiency of PTH per se can be responsible for some signs and symptoms of hypocalcemia in hypoparathyroidism. In contrast, **secondary hyperparathyroidism** can contribute to some symptoms present in patients with vitamin D deficiency or PTH-resistant disorders associated with hypocalcemia. Most frequently recognized clinical features of hypocalcemia involve the CNS and the neuromuscular, ocular, and ectodermal systems.
   1. Increased neuromuscular irritability resulting in muscle cramping (tetany) is a common feature of hypocalcemia. The classic sign of tetany is carpopedal spasm **(Trousseau sign). Chvostek sign** is evidence of increased irritability of the fifth cranial nerve. Other neuromuscular signs include paresthesias, laryngospasm, bronchospasm, abdominal cramping, and generalized hyperreflexia. These can be induced or aggravated by hyperventilation, which causes a mild metabolic

alkalosis. CNS disturbances include seizure equivalents **(hypocalcemic seizures),** grand or petit mal seizures, syncope, impaired memory, psychosis, and disturbances of extrapyramidal system function, such as parkinsonism and choreoathetosis. Changes seen on the electroencephalogram are nonspecific and are mainly increases in bursts of high-voltage, slow-wave activity. In general, these abnormalities improve or slowly revert to normal with correction of hypocalcemia.

2. The most common ocular manifestation of chronic hypocalcemia is the development of **cataracts;** calcium deposits can be found in subcapsular, anterior, or posterior zonular locations. Both papilledema and **pseudotumor cerebri** can occur.

3. **Cardiovascular disturbances** include electrocardiographic abnormalities characterized by **prolongation of the QT interval** and by nonspecific T-wave changes. **Refractory congestive heart failure** with resistance to digitalis therapy has been reported in chronic hypocalcemia associated with hypoparathyroidism. Hypotension resistant to conventional doses of pressor agents or volume replacement has also been described.

4. Other features of chronic hypocalcemia resulting from hypoparathyroidism include **soft-tissue calcification** and exostoses. Periarticular deposition of calcium salts is common, with occasional presentation of chondrocalcinosis and pseudogout. Basal ganglion calcification is frequently present. The mechanism responsible for the ectopic calcification has yet to be determined.

5. Macrocytic megaloblastic anemia attributed to deficient binding of vitamin B_{12} to intrinsic factor in the presence of hypocalcemia has been reported. This abnormality (abnormal Schilling test) and the anemia are reversible with correction of the hypocalcemia.

B. **Disorders of the parathyroid glands** (Table 25.6)

1. **Surgical hypoparathyroidism.** Surgical damage to or removal of parathyroid tissue accounts for the majority of cases of loss of parathyroid function. **Partial or transient PTH insufficiency** is also a common occurrence, the latter becoming apparent during periods of stress when symptomatic hypocalcemia develops. A spectrum of PTH insufficiency can be demonstrated by infusion of ethylenediaminetetra-acetic acid (EDTA) or sodium citrate, both of which chelate calcium and stimulate PTH secretion. It is also possible to subgroup patients according to the degree of severity of hypocalcemia and hyperphosphatemia present in the untreated state.

2. **Idiopathic hypoparathyroidism.** This term encompasses several different disorders in which hypoparathyroidism occurs as an isolated condition or as part of a syndrome complex. The disorders may occur as both sporadic and familial conditions. Depending on the specific disorder, onset or clinical expression can occur during childhood or later in adult life. The diagnosis is established by demonstrating low or absent circulating levels of PTH and normal physiologic responses to exogenous administration of the hormone. Other biochemical features include hyperphosphatemia, reduced plasma levels of $1,25(OH)_2D$, but normal levels of $25(OH)D$. Bone remodeling markers are generally reduced (osteocalcin, deoxypyridinoline) or normal (alkaline phosphatase). Urinary calcium excretion is low in the untreated state.

a. Autoimmune hypoparathyroidism (*vide infra*) occurs both as part of autoimmune polyglandular syndrome (APS) type I and as an isolated autoimmune disorder. APS, also referred to as autoimmune polyglandular endocrinopathy–candidiasis–ectodermal dystrophy (APECED), is transmitted as an autosomal recessive condition linked to mutations of the autoimmune regulator gene (*AIRE*) located on chromosome 21q22.3. Circulating parathyroid antibodies have been reported to be detected in 40% of patients with APS. The most common associated conditions include Addison disease and mucocutaneous candidiasis. Parathyroid antibodies have been described in ~30% of patients with isolated hypoparathyroidism. Autoimmune hypoparathyroidism either as an isolated condition or as part of APS can be expressed clinically between

TABLE 25.6	Classification of Disorders of the Parathyroids (Structure or Function) Associated with Hypocalcemia

Disorders of parathyroid development (agenesis)
Isolated hypoparathyroidism
DiGeorge syndrome (DiGeorge sequence)
Kenny-Caffey syndrome
Mitochondrial neuromyopathies
Long-chain hydroxyacyl-CoA dehydrogenase deficiency

Disorders resulting from destruction of the parathyroids
Postsurgical hypoparathyroidism
Autoimmune hypoparathyroidism (polyglandular autoimmune deficiency)
Metastases to parathyroids
Granulomatous disease
Radiation
Metal overload disorders
    Iron—hemochromatosis, multiple transfusions
    Copper—Wilson disease
    Aluminum—chronic renal failure

PTH resistance disorders
Pseudohypoparathyroidism type Ia (Albright hereditary osteodystrophy)
Pseudohypoparathyroidism type Ib
Pseudohypoparathyroidism type II
Magnesium depletion
PTH antibodies (iatrogenic)
Isolated deficiency of $1,25(OH)_2D_3$

Disorders of parathyroid hormone processing or secretion
Calcium sensor-receptor–activating mutations
Defective prepro-PTH processing
Magnesium depletion

CoA, coenzyme A; PTH, parathyroid hormone.

early childhood and young adulthood. Less common associated features of APS include alopecia, steatorrhea, primary hypogonadism, primary hypothyroidism, chronic active hepatitis, pernicious anemia, and vitiligo.

  b. Hypoparathyroidism resulting from defective PTH synthesis. Hypoparathyroidism may also result from defective PTH synthesis. Several types of **mutations in exon 2 of the *PTH* gene located on chromosome 11** have been described in families with isolated hypoparathyroidism. This portion of the *PTH* gene contains the initiation codon for PTH synthesis and subsequent peptide processing and intracellular translocation. In one case, a single base substitution in exon 2 resulted in impaired conversion of **PTH precursor peptide (preproPTH)** to the mature active hormone (autosomal recessive inheritance). **Autosomal dominant** forms of inheritance associated with other mutations have also been described. In one family, the entire exon 2 was found to be deleted. In these families, clinical disease was expressed very early, with low to undetectable circulating levels of PTH.

  c. Hypoparathyroidism resulting from altered PTH regulation. Activating mutations (constitutive activation) of the CSR produce a **functional hypoparathyroid state** (e.g., a decrease in the PTH secretion set point) characterized by the development of hypocalcemia, hypercalciuria, and low to absent circulating levels of PTH. Both sporadic cases and autosomal dominant inheritance have been identified. In many instances, the hypocalcemia is mild and does not require treatment.

3. **Developmental abnormalities of the parathyroids.** See Chapter 27.
4. **Other forms of hypoparathyroidism**
   a. Individuals with idiopathic **hemochromatosis** or secondary iron overload syndrome as a result of long-term treatment with blood transfusions (e.g., **thalassemia**) have been shown to develop hypoparathyroidism. Examination of parathyroid tissue in such cases reveals iron deposition and fibrotic destruction.
   b. Hypoparathyroidism has also been described in **Wilson disease,** presumably because of copper deposition in the parathyroids.
   c. In patients with chronic renal insufficiency, **aluminum deposition in the parathyroids** may result in impaired PTH secretion and thus partial to complete parathyroid insufficiency.
   d. Transient (and infrequently permanent) parathyroid insufficiency has been reported following ^{131}**iodine therapy** for hyperthyroidism. This should be distinguished from transient hypocalcemia as a consequence of "hungry bone syndrome" following treatment for hypothyroidism.
   e. Destruction of the parathyroids by **tumor metastases** (breast carcinoma) or **granulomatous disease** is an uncommon cause of hypoparathyroidism.
   f. **Hypermagnesemia** causes suppression of PTH secretion and, when sustained, is an unusual cause of hypoparathyroidism.
C. **PTH resistance syndromes.** The term **pseudohypoparathyroidism (PsHP)** has been used to describe a group of disorders with biochemical and clinical features of hypoparathyroidism but with target-organ resistance to PTH as indicated by elevated levels of PTH. In the two major forms of this disorder (PsHP type Ia and PsHP type Ib), correction of hypocalcemia usually results in suppression of PTH levels but fails to correct target-organ resistance to the hormone.
1. **PsHP type Ia**
   a. This classic disorder, originally described by Fuller Albright, is recognized by the characteristic biochemical features of hypoparathyroidism in association with characteristic developmental and somatic features (short stature, round facies, obesity, **brachydactyly, pseudowebbing of the neck, subcutaneous calcifications, and ossifications**). Mental retardation is a variable feature. The term **Albright hereditary osteodystrophy (AHO)** has been used to describe the characteristic phenotypic features associated with PsHP type Ia.
   b. Individuals with PsHP type Ia share a sporadic or inherited defect in the function of **stimulatory guanine nucleotide coupling protein (Gs protein).** This heterotrimeric membrane-bound protein transmits a signal generated by binding of a hormone to a cell surface receptor to catalytic adenylate cyclase, which stimulates intracellular formation of cAMP as well as several other intracellular "second messengers." A number of different inactivating mutations have been identified in the *GNASI* **gene** (codes for α subunit of Gs protein [Gsα]) in patients with PsHP type Ia.
   c. In addition to PTH resistance, patients with PsHP type Ia may express other hormone-resistance syndromes and neurosensory defects attributable to a generalized defect in deficiency of Gsα protein. Most common of these disorders are **thyroid-stimulating hormone (TSH) resistance (hypothyroidism), glucagon resistance** (no clinical disorder), and **gonadotropin resistance (amenorrhea).** TSH and glucagon resistance can be demonstrated in 50% to 70% of patients, but gonadotropin resistance occurs less commonly.
   d. A **diagnosis** of PsHP type Ia is established by the presence of features of AHO, reduced Gsα protein activity (reduced by ~50% in red blood cell membranes), and evidence of target organ resistance to exogenous PTH. Evidence for the latter is implied by the finding of **hypocalcemia and elevated circulating PTH** or a blunted rise in urinary excretion of nephrogenous cAMP coupled with a blunted or absent phosphaturic response to exogenous PTH **(PTH infusion test).** Absent or blunted PTH stimulation of renal production of $1,25(OH)_2D$ and a calcemic response (skeletal resistance) can also be demonstrated.

e. Hypocalcemia is intermittent in some patients, although PTH levels are usually persistently elevated. Urinary calcium excretion is low, reflecting the action of PTH on distal nephron reabsorption of filtered calcium. Despite normocalcemia, these patients manifest blunted renal responses to exogenous PTH.

f. The term **pseudopseudohypoparathyroidism (pseudoPsHP)** has been used to describe a group of individuals who have the somatic features of AHO but who are normocalcemic and **lack evidence of PTH resistance.** PseudoPsHP is genetically related to PsHP in that both may occur in the same kindred and both demonstrate ~50% reduced Gsα protein activity in membrane isolates. Why individuals with pseudoPsHP do not express hormone resistance is currently unexplained.

g. Inheritance of PsHP type Ia and pseudoPsHP is by **autosomal dominant** transmission. There is strong evidence that maternal inheritance of Gsα protein deficiency results in PsHP type I, whereas paternal transmission results in pseudoPsHP, implicating the possible occurrence of **genomic imprinting** of the *GNASI* gene.

2. PsHP type Ib is characterized by the occurrence of isolated PTH resistance, normal Gsα protein activity, and absence of the features of AHO. The biochemical expression of PTH resistance is identical to that of PsHP type Ia, a blunted or absent rise in urinary cAMP, and phosphaturic response to exogenous PTH. It is likely that the diagnosis of PsHP type Ib encompasses more than one disorder. An imprinting defect of the *GNASI* gene has been described.

3. PsHP type Ic. Patients with this disorder have features of AHO, multiple forms of hormone resistance analogous to PsHP type Ia, but normal Gs protein activity. There is evidence that the metabolic defect in these patients resides in the catalytic adenylate cyclase. It is possible that the defect is in Gs protein activity, although it is not demonstrable with current assays.

4. PsHP type II. This type of PTH resistance appears to be rare, and several varieties have been reported. Affected individuals described lack the features of AHO. Administration of exogenous PTH produces a normal rise in urinary nephrogenous cAMP excretion but a blunted or absent phosphaturic response. Normalization of serum calcium can normalize the phosphaturic response to PTH. PsHP type II has been described in patients with osteomalacia secondary to vitamin D depletion.

5. Other forms of PsHP. Several other disorders with apparent resistance to both endogenous and exogenous PTH have been described. These are rare and appear to be unrelated to the previously described types of PsHP.

a. The term **pseudohypohyperparathyroidism** has also been applied to a disorder in which there appears to be renal resistance to PTH but a normal skeletal response. The latter is demonstrated by the presence of skeletal radiologic features of severe hyperparathyroidism (e.g., osteitis fibrosa, bone cysts, brown tumors).

b. Pseudoidiopathic hypoparathyroidism refers to a disorder in which a structurally abnormal form of PTH is present. These individuals fail to respond normally to their own PTH but respond in a normal manner to exogenous hormone.

c. A variant form of PsHP has been described in which skeletal resistance to exogenous PTH was attributed to a primary deficiency of 1,25(OH)$_2$D production. Short-term treatment with calcitriol restored skeletal responsiveness to exogenous PTH in a period too short to have allowed major healing of underlying metabolic bone disease.

D. Magnesium depletion. Magnesium depletion is a common cause of hypocalcemia in a public hospital setting.

1. Causes of development of magnesium depletion can be grouped into disorders of adequate dietary intake, excessive losses through the gastrointestinal tract, and excessive urinary excretion. In addition, magnesium deficiency and/or depletion may occur in several common endocrine and metabolic disorders. Gastrointestinal disorders or conditions associated with development of magnesium depletion include excessive loss of gastrointestinal fluids because of vomiting, nasogastric suction, diarrhea, malabsorption syndromes and steatorrhea of diverse etiologies, short-bowel syndrome because of surgical resection or ileojejunal bypass procedures, and acute pancreatitis. Rare cases of sporadic or familial defective intestinal magnesium transport have been described. Long-term treatment with magnesuric diuretics (thiazides or furosemide) is a common cause of magnesium deficiency that can result in depletion. Other conditions associated with increased urinary magnesium losses include acute and chronic alcoholism, hyperalimentation, chronic metabolic acidosis, and magnesium wasting associated with chronic renal diseases such as pyelonephritis and polycystic disease. Treatment with a number of medications can produce renal **magnesium wasting (magnesium wasting nephropathy).** These include **aminoglycoside antibiotics (gentamicin, tobramycin, amikacin),** other anti-infection agents **(amphotericin B, pentamidine),** the anticancer agent *cis*-**platinum,** and the immunosuppressive agent **cyclosporin.** Rare causes of magnesium depletion, including **familial or sporadic isolated magnesium wasting nephropathy,** have also been reported. Magnesium depletion is encountered frequently in patients with poorly controlled diabetes mellitus. Contributing factors include glycosuria-associated osmotic diuresis and enhanced urinary magnesium losses, metabolic acidosis, and relative malnutrition. Hypomagnesemia and magnesium depletion are frequently seen in patients with primary aldosteronism. The latter is attributed to both volume expansion and direct effects of aldosterone on magnesium excretion. Hypercalciuria is associated with decreased renal reabsorption of magnesium. Patients with vitamin D–managed hypoparathyroidism may develop magnesium depletion in the face of marked persistent hypercalciuria. Rapid skeletal remineralization (hungry-bone syndrome) following successful parathyroid surgery or, on rare occasion, thyroid surgery for Graves disease or other causes of thyrotoxicosis, can result in hypomagnesemia and clinical features of magnesium depletion.

2. The mechanism of hypocalcemia in magnesium depletion states is multifactorial.
   a. Impaired PTH secretion
   b. Target-organ resistance to PTH in both kidney and skeleton
3. In the untreated state, circulating levels of PTH are either low or reduced relative to the degree of magnesium depletion and hypocalcemia. Plasma levels of $1,25(OH)_2D$ are frequently low, and there may be resistance to the action of vitamin D at the intestine.
4. A diagnosis of magnesium depletion is accepted clinically with the demonstration of a low serum magnesium level (<1 mEq/L) and low urinary magnesium (<1 mEq per day, unless a renal magnesium wasting state exists) in an appropriate setting.
5. Replacement therapy with magnesium salts results in a rapid rise in circulating levels of PTH, within minutes to hours, initially reaching levels several times normal. However, restoration of the serum calcium levels to normal may require several days.

E. Diagnosis of hypoparathyroid and pseudohypoparathyroid disorders
   1. The diagnosis of idiopathic hypoparathyroidism is generally one of exclusion. Demonstration of little to no PTH in the presence of hypocalcemia, frequently with hyperphosphatemia and with no evidence for magnesium depletion, strongly supports this diagnosis.
   2. Magnesium depletion can develop in individuals with hypoparathyroidism, potentially complicating the diagnostic evaluation. Such individuals can manifest PTH resistance or fail to respond normally to vitamin D treatment on the basis of magnesium depletion; this is reversed with correction of the magnesium deficit.
   3. Demonstration of normal responsiveness to exogenous PTH through a standardized **PTH infusion test** excludes the diagnosis of some forms of PsHP, with the exception of the rare individual who has an abnormal circulating form of endogenous PTH (e.g., idiopathic hypoparathyroidism). The PTH infusion test is usually performed with a 5- to 10-minute infusion of 200 U of synthetic PTH 1-34 (human). The normal response is usually >10- to 20-fold increase in urinary cAMP and a doubling of the urinary fractional excretion of phosphorus.

4. Resistance to the action of PTH in stimulating renal formation of $1,25(OH)_2D$ has been demonstrated by measuring levels of calcitriol first on a control day and again the morning after administration of two separate doses of 200 U of PTH 1-34 injected IM at 12 and 24 hours before sampling. A normal response is an increase in calcitriol of $\sim 50\%$ or a rise from subnormal to normal levels.

5. Demonstration of <u>low tissue levels (red cells) of Gs protein</u> activity in the presence of secondary hyperparathyroidism with or without the presence of hypocalcemia supports the diagnosis of PsHP type Ia. If calcium and PTH levels are normalized as a consequence of vitamin D treatment, a PTH infusion test might be required to distinguish PsHP type Ia from pseudoPsHP, because Gs protein activity is also reduced in the latter condition.

6. Individuals with PsHP types Ib and Ic also have abnormal responses to PTH infusion but normal levels of Gs protein activity. Patients with PsHP type Ic thus far described have features of AHO.

7. Patients with PsHP type II in response to a PTH infusion test show a dissociation of the urinary cAMP response (normal) and the phosphaturic response (blunted). In some cases this is observed only under conditions of hypocalcemia, because normalization of calcium by vitamin therapy or calcium infusion can also normalize the phosphaturic response to PTH. Thus, it might not be possible to make a diagnosis of PsHP type II in a treated patient.

IV. DISORDERS OF VITAMIN D METABOLISM

Hypocalcemia may be present in a number of primary and secondary disorders of vitamin D metabolism. In this setting, hypocalcemia develops as a consequence of both selective malabsorption of calcium (and possibly phosphorus and magnesium) and emergence of vitamin D deficiency bone disease (e.g., **rickets** or **osteomalacia**). The latter is associated with acquired resistance to the calcemic actions of PTH. In addition, synergistic actions of vitamin D in promoting bone resorptive processes can be blunted or absent. In these disorders the development of hypocalcemia is associated with secondary hyperparathyroidism. Vitamin D deficiency bone disease is invariably associated with hypophosphatemia (in contrast to hypoparathyroidism or PTH-resistant disorders).

A. Disorders of 25(OH)D metabolism. Nutritional vitamin D deficiency is now a common condition throughout the world, particularly in elderly patients who are confined, with reduced dietary intake of vitamin D–fortified foods, inadequate vitamin supplementation, and reduced sunlight exposure. Development of vitamin D deficiency is also influenced by geographic location (reduced annual solar exposure) and culturally determined dress habits. Measurement of plasma levels of 25(OH)D can define clinical and physiologic **vitamin D status.** Alterations in 25(OH)D metabolism occur primarily as a consequence of hepatic or hepatobiliary disease, treatment with drugs that alter hepatic vitamin D metabolism, gastrointestinal disorders associated with malabsorption or disruption of enterohepatic circulation of vitamin D, and protein wasting disorders associated with massive loss of protein-bound vitamin D.

It should be emphasized that although 25(OH)D is low in these conditions, circulating levels of $1,25(OH)_2D$ can be low, normal, or elevated. Thus, normal to elevated levels of $1,25(OH)_2D$ do not exclude a diagnosis of vitamin D deficiency.

1. Hepatic and hepatobiliary disease. Circulating levels of 25(OH)D can be low in a number of parenchymal hepatic diseases because of impaired formation from vitamin D_3 or D_2. Disorders include alcoholic hepatitis, chronic active hepatitis, lupoid hepatitis, and alcoholic cirrhosis. However, clinically significant disease does not commonly occur unless severe malnutrition is present. A significant correlation has been described between circulating levels of 25(OH)D and results of the <u>aminopyrine breath test</u>, which provides a measure of hepatocellular function. In contrast, cholestatic hepatic disease, particularly biliary cirrhosis, is associated with a high incidence of metabolic bone disease, a significant component of which is osteomalacia. However, in these disorders, resistance to treatment with conventional doses of vitamin D has been reported, suggesting that factors other than vitamin D deficiency are involved in the associated bone disease.

2. **Gastrointestinal disorders.** Both intestinal <u>malabsorption</u> of fat-soluble vitamins and disruption of the enterohepatic circulation of vitamin D metabolites, particularly 25(OH)D, contribute to the development of vitamin D deficiency. Examples of conditions in which this occurs include primary small intestinal disease (regional enteritis, ulcerative enteritis) and surgical procedures such as total and subtotal gastrectomy and intestinal bypass surgery for weight reduction in the morbidly obese.

3. **Protein wasting disorders.** Vitamin D metabolites circulate predominantly in a protein-bound state. Disorders associated with protein wasting, such as various enteropathies and conditions in which the nephrotic syndrome develops, frequently manifest low plasma levels of 25(OH)D. The incidence of metabolic bone disease in this setting because of uncomplicated vitamin D deficiency remains unclear.

4. **Drug-induced alteration of 25(OH)D metabolism.** Anticonvulsant agents such as <u>phenobarbital</u> and phenytoin (<u>Dilantin</u>) have been shown to increase hepatic conversion of 25(OH)D to inactive metabolites. This results in low circulating levels of 25(OH)D and can cause rickets or osteomalacia in patients on long-term treatment. Adequate direct sunlight exposure or modestly increased vitamin D intake (1 000 to 3 000 U per day) is usually effective in preventing development of or managing the condition.

B. **Disorders of 1,25(OH)$_2$D metabolism**

1. Recognition of factors involved in the regulation of renal production of 1,25(OH)$_2$D has provided important insights into the pathophysiology of a number of disorders. Circulating levels of 1,25(OH)$_2$D are increased in $\sim$50% of patients with primary hyperparathyroidism, correlating closely with the degree of hypercalciuria and the prevalence of nephrolithiasis. In contrast, in patients with hypoparathyroidism and various forms of PsHP, levels of 1,25(OH)$_2$D are decreased in association with decreased intestinal absorption of calcium, providing a basis for hormone replacement therapy in these conditions. Similarly, in chronic renal insufficiency, an inverse correlation can be shown between renal function (creatinine clearance) and circulating levels of calcitriol. This observation, along with the knowledge that the kidney is the sole site of physiologic production of calcitriol (except for the placenta during pregnancy), has provided considerable understanding of a number of pathophysiologic features of renal osteodystrophy. Currently, recognition of the role of primary alterations in the metabolism of 1,25(OH)$_2$D has provided further information concerning the pathogenesis of several previously poorly understood disorders.

2. **Tumor-induced osteomalacia (TIO).** Although it is uncommon, TIO, also referred to as **oncogenic osteomalacia,** is being recognized with increasing frequency. This paraneoplastic syndrome was initially recognized by the association of a malignant or benign tumor and the presence of clinical, biochemical, and radiologic features of osteomalacia or, in some cases, rickets. Surgical cure, when possible, was followed by improvement or resolution of osteomalacia/rickets. Initial cases, mesenchymal in origin, involved ossifying and nonossifying mesenchymomas, hemangiomas, and giant-cell tumors of bone. Subsequently, a much greater diversity of tumor type has been recognized, including prostate carcinoma, breast carcinoma, small-cell and oat-cell carcinomas, multiple myeloma, and hematogenous malignancies such as chronic lymphocytic leukemia.

   a. **Clinical features** of TIO may initially be subtle and nonspecific but generally evolve to include bone pain, muscle weakness, recurrent pathologic fractures, and pseudofractures. Biochemical abnormalities include hypophosphatemia, serum calcium levels that vary from normal to overt hypocalcemia, PTH levels varying with the serum calcium, and elevated levels of alkaline phosphatase. Serum levels of 25(OH)D are normal, whereas levels of 1,25(OH)$_2$D are either low or inappropriately reduced for the degree of hypophosphatemia. Urinary phosphate wasting is present with a reduced threshold for phosphorus reabsorption (TmP/GFR). Aminoaciduria may be present in some cases.

b. Studies of the **pathogenesis** of TIO have demonstrated that the tumors produce FGF23 and that high levels are found in the circulation.

c. Complete surgical removal of the tumor reduces high levels of FGF23 and invariably results in a cure. Prior to surgery, affected individuals are characteristically resistant to treatment with pharmacologic doses of vitamin D or dihydrotachysterol. However, for patients who are not cured by surgery, treatment with phosphorus supplements and near-physiologic doses of $1,25(OH)_2D_3$ (1 to 3 μg per day) may result in clinical improvement of bone pain with healing of osteomalacia.

V. MANAGEMENT OF HYPOCALCEMIC DISORDERS

Administration of oral calcium supplements and vitamin D analogs is central to the management of hypocalcemic disorders. In treating hypoparathyroid disorders, the goal is to correct symptomatic hypocalcemia without inducing the development of hypercalcemia. In general, the therapeutic endpoint is to maintain serum calcium levels in the range of 8.5 to 9.5 mg/dL, with urinary calcium levels below ~400 mg per day. This endpoint is not always achievable in every patient.

A. Oral calcium supplements administered alone (3 to 7 g per day of elemental calcium) in multiple divided doses can be effective in correcting even moderately severe hypocalcemia unless a malabsorption syndrome is present. This form of treatment is usually effective on a short-term basis but may be the form of management chosen by some patients for prolonged therapy. Choice of the form of calcium supplement is often a matter of personal preference (Table 25.7).

B. Doses of various forms of vitamin D analogs required to correct hypocalcemia vary with the underlying disorder.

1. In disorders associated with underlying skeletal mineralization defects (e.g., osteomalacia), a higher dose of vitamin D might be tolerated or required early in the course of therapy. With progressive remineralization, dose reduction might be required to prevent development of hypercalcemia.

2. With the use of more potent forms of vitamin D, such as $1,25(OH)_2D_3$, the requirement for calcium supplementation is reduced. Some individuals who ingest diets that are high in calcium content might not require additional calcium. In contrast, treatment with vitamin D_2 or D_3 usually requires concomitant administration of larger amounts of calcium supplements.

3. Similarly, simultaneous adjustment of calcium intake and doses of $1,25(OH)_2D_3$ can be difficult because of the extreme potency of this form of vitamin D. Thus, either calcium intake or the dose of calcitriol should be adjusted.

The major considerations involved in choosing a particular form of vitamin D include potency, time of onset and offset of action, and the interval for returning serum calcium levels to normal, either on an inpatient or an outpatient basis. These

TABLE 25.7 Oral and Parenteral Calcium Preparations Available for Management of Acute and Chronic Hypocalcemic Disorders

Calcium salt	Percent elemental calcium	Calcium content
Oral preparations		
Calcium carbonate	40	400 mg/1 g (1 g/5 mL)
Calcium glubionate	7	64 mg/1 g (1.8 g/5 mL)
Calcium gluconate	9	90 mg/1 g
Calcium lactate	13	130 mg/1 g
Calcium citrate	21	211 mg/1 g
Tricalcium phosphate	39	390 mg/1 g
Intravenous preparations		
Calcium chloride	36	360 mg/1 g (1 g/10 mL)
Calcium gluconate	9	90 mg/1 g (1 g/10 mL)

TABLE 25.8 | **Commercially Available Vitamin D Preparations**

Compound	Trade name	Potency relative to vitamin D_3	Onset of action (d)	Offset of action
Vitamin D_3 (cholecalciferol)	Delta D_3	1	10–14	Weeks to months
Vitamin D_2 (ergocalciferol)	Drisdol	1	10–14	Weeks to months
Dihydrotachysterol	Hytakerol	5–10	4–7	7–21 d
Calcifediol (25-hydroxyvitamin D_3)	Calderol	10–15	7–10	Weeks
Alfacalcidiol[a,b] (1α-hydroxyvitamin D_3)	One-alpha	1 000	1–2	2–3 d
Calcitriol (1,25-dihydroxyvitamin D_3)	Rocaltrol, Calcijex+	1 000	1–2	2–3 d

[a]Not approved for clinical use in the United States.
[b]Available for parenteral administration.

properties, as applicable to treatment with various forms of vitamin D sterols or their analogs, are summarized in Table 25.8.

Selected References

Bilezikian JP, Raisz LG, ed. *Principles of Bone Biology.* 3rd ed. San Diego: Academic Press; 2007.

Favus MJ, ed. *Primer on the Metabolic Bone Diseases and Disorders of Mineral Metabolism.* 6th ed. Washington, DC: American Society for Bone and Mineral Research, 2006.

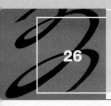

METABOLIC BONE DISEASE
Theodore J. Hahn

I. INTRODUCTION

A. Bone physiology. Bone is in a constant state of change. Its shape and strength are continually regulated by the balance between formation and resorption (breakdown). When resorption exceeds formation, decreased bone mass results. Bone is composed of three major elements: cells, protein matrix, and minerals. Bone cells occupy about 3% of bone volume and are of three main types: osteoblasts, osteocytes, and osteoclasts. **Osteoblasts,** the bone-forming cells, are derived from mesenchymal stem cell precursors. They are found in continuous layers on the surfaces of forming bone, are rich in alkaline phosphatase, and produce the protein matrix on which bone mineral is deposited. **Osteoclasts** are large, multinucleated cells responsible for bone resorption and are derived from cells of the monocyte macrophage series. **Osteocytes** are derived from mature osteoblasts, are found in lacunae created by the newly formed layers of bone, and appear to play a mechanosensing role in regulating bone formation. The cellular content of bone is higher in predominately trabecular bone (e.g., the vertebrae) than in predominately cortical bone (e.g., the hip). Hence, changes in bone mass and strength usually occur earlier and more markedly in the vertebrae than in the hip.

B. Basis of metabolic bone disorders. The chemical composition, mass, and mechanical properties of bone are largely controlled by external regulatory mechanisms. Factors that can disrupt normal bone homeostasis include: decreased mineral intake or absorption; defects in vitamin D absorption or activation; decreased production of estrogen, testosterone, or insulin; increased endogenous production of parathyroid hormone (PTH), thyroid hormone, cortisol, or other bone-regulatory hormones; increased levels of inflammatory cytokines; chronic treatment with supraphysiologic doses of glucocorticoids or thyroid hormone, or standard doses of certain drugs (e.g., anticonvulsants, chemotherapeutic agents); decreased physical activity leading to reduced osteoblastic bone formation; age-related declines in osteoblast generation from mesenchymal stem cells; and congenital disorders of bone collagen formation.

II. DIAGNOSTIC TESTS

A. Serum determinations. Serum total calcium, ionized calcium, phosphate, intact PTH, and bone gla protein (osteocalin) concentrations are best measured on a morning fasting blood sample because of considerable diurnal and/or postprandial variation.

B. Urinary determinations

1. Measurements of **24-hour urinary calcium** should be performed with the patient on a customary dietary intake. Reduced urinary calcium excretion is defined as <1.5 mg calcium per kilogram ideal body weight (IBW) every 24 hours; hypercalciuria corresponds to calcium excretion of >4 mg calcium per kilogram IBW every 24 hours. Creatinine should be measured simultaneously to assure completeness of collection. **Note:** Thiazide diuretic administration reduces 24-hour urinary calcium excretion by 24% to 40%, and furosemide administration may increase calcium excretion.

2. **N-Telopeptide (NTx)** excretion, an indicator of bone-loss (resorption) activity, should be determined on the second-morning voiding. Normal values vary with sex and age, but in general, values >65 nm BCE/mmol creatinine indicate increased bone loss activity, and values <35 nm BCE/mmol indicate satisfactory suppression of bone resorption.

C. Radiologic detection of decreased bone mass

1. **Standard radiographs** are unreliable in assessing bone mass. They can detect decreased bone mass only after a 30% to 50% decline and are subject to significant technical variation. The most generally useful standard radiographs for assessing the degree of bone loss are lateral views of the thoracic and lumbar vertebrae. Early changes with osteoporosis include concave indentation of the upper and lower vertebral cortex as a result of pressure from the intervertebral disks (codfish vertebrae). Later, multiple full or partial vertebral compression fractures occur. Vertebral fractures may be asymptomatic in up to two thirds of patients. Their presence indicates a high risk of subsequent fractures in the spine and elsewhere, and warrants further assessment. In addition, in cases of severe, long-standing osteomalacia, radiographs of the femur, tibia, pelvis, and scapulae may reveal asymptomatic pseudofractures that confirm the diagnosis and can occasionally evolve into overt clinical fractures if treatment is not instituted.

2. **Spine and total hip bone mass measurement** by dual-beam x-ray–based photon absorptiometry (DEXA) is the most sensitive and reproducible routine method of detecting and quantitating bone loss. A 1.5% or greater change in bone mass can usually be detected reliably, with good reproducibility and a minimal dose of radiation (2 to 4 mrem). Quantitative computed tomography (QCT) measurement of spine bone density may have a similar accuracy in experienced hands but imparts a higher radiation dose (~300 mrem).

III. DECREASED BONE MASS

A. Definition. Decreased bone mass is a clinical and radiologic diagnosis indicating a deficiency in bone mass relative to normal values for sex and race. Bone histologic changes in this situation are of three main types: **osteoporosis,** a parallel loss of bone mineral and matrix because of deceased bone formation and often increased resorption; **osteomalacia,** deficient bone mineralization with an accumulation of unmineralized, newly formed matrix (osteoid) because of vitamin D and/or phosphate deficiency; and **osteitis fibrosa,** the result of increased PTH-mediated bone resorption, with replacement by fibrous tissue. In many situations, these histologic patterns can occur in combination, with one type predominating.

B. Evaluation

1. **Radiographs.** Standard lateral radiographs of the spine are useful for detecting vertebral compression fractures, which indicate increased fracture risk. Also, if chronic osteomalacia is suspected, the pelvis, femurs, tibias, and fibulas can be surveyed for pseudofractures.

2. **DEXA or QCT bone mass measurements** are the appropriate technique for precise quantitation of bone mass. DEXA bone mineral density **(BMD)** measurement of the spine and hip is the most commonly used method.

   a. Individual BMD measurements are commonly expressed in terms of a **T value,** which is the number of standard deviations (SD) by which the individual's value differs from the population mean peak BMD value at age 20. For example, a T value of -2.0 indicates a BMD value lying 2.0 SD below the mean peak value. The **Z value** indicates the number of SD difference from the mean age/gender-normal value. The T value is the most useful and most commonly used indicator of BMD status.

   b. The commonly used World Health Organization (WHO) criteria for the **severity of bone loss** as measured by DEXA are as follows:

   (1) Normal: T = -0.9 or above

   (2) Osteopenia: T = -1.0 to -2.4

   (3) Osteoporosis: T = -2.5 or lower

   (4) Severe osteoporosis: T = -2.5 or lower, with a history of one or more minimal trauma fractures

   Note: The term "osteoporosis" as used in BMD measurement reports does not imply a histologic diagnosis of osteoporosis but merely indicates the degree of bone loss as measured by DEXA. For each 1 SD of decrease in BMD, the current (5-year) fracture risk increases by about twofold. Thirty percent or more of postmenopausal women are classified as having "osteoporosis" or "severe osteoporosis" by BMD measurement.

c. When to measure DEXA bone density

(1) By current criteria, in order to determine whether treatment for decreased bone mass is indicated, spine and hip BMD should be determined in:

(a) All women over age 65 and men over age 75

(b) Women younger than age 65 and men younger than 75, who have one or more **risk factors** (see below)

(c) All women and men who have had a vertebral, hip, or other significant fracture with minimal trauma, regardless of age

(2) Risk factors for osteoporotic fractures include:

(a) Genetic factors, including history of osteoporosis in a first-degree relative and Caucasian and Asian ethnic status (lower peak adult bone mass)

(b) Endocrine disorders associated with bone loss (hyperparathyroidism, hyperthyroidism, premature menopause, Cushing disease, hypogonadism, type 1 diabetes mellitus)

(c) Gonadal hormone ablation therapy, including aromatase therapy for breast cancer and androgen deprivation therapy for prostate cancer

(d) Previous history of fracture as an adult, especially low-trauma fractures

(e) Treatment with supraphysiologic doses of glucocorticoids or thyroid hormone, or other agents known to cause bone loss (anticonvulsants, chemotherapeutic agents, transplant medications, high-dose heparin, etc.)

(f) Vertebral deformity on standard radiographs suggesting decreased bone mass

(g) Age $\geq$65 years in women and $\geq$75 in men

(h) Increased falls risk because of advanced age, frailty, peripheral neuropathy, etc.

(i) Chronic liver or renal disease

(j) Chronic obstructive pulmonary disease

(k) Elevated levels of inflammatory cytokines, as in rheumatoid arthritis

(l) Lifestyle risk factors, including smoking, excessive alcohol intake, chronic low calcium intake, and low level of physical activity

(m) Body mass index <19

3. Biochemical studies. A minimal baseline evaluation for a patient with established osteoporosis includes a complete blood count and erythrocyte sedimentation rate; fasting blood chemistry panel for calcium, phosphate, liver, and renal function, ultrasensitive thyroid-stimulating hormone level, serum 25-hydroxyvitamin D (25-OHD) level, bone gla protein/osteocalcin or bone-specific alkaline phosphatase (to measure osteoblastic activity); and a morning second-void spot urinary NTx level (or other bone resorption index) to assess current bone-loss rate. Serum iPTH, gonadal hormone measurements, cortisol levels, serum protein electrophoresis, or other disease-specific indices may be useful in individual cases.

IV. SPECIFIC DISORDERS ASSOCIATED WITH DECREASED BONE MASS

A. Osteoporosis. Osteoporosis increases fracture risk as a result of **(1)** a decrease in bone mass and **(2)** disruptions of the microarchitecture of bone (decreased **bone quality**), leading to decreased bone strength. A major factor in the decreased bone quality is a disruption of the supporting trabecular "cross-struts" in the interior of long bones and vertebrae that provide major structural stability. Trabecular integrity is disrupted early in osteoporosis and improves soon after treatment because of its high cellular content. In addition, decreased bone formation rate (as occurs in glucocorticoid and age-related osteoporosis) can lead to inadequate repair of the multiple microscopic subclinical bone "microfractures" that occur in normal daily life, resulting in increased risk of clinical fractures.

Increased fracture risk particularly involves the spine, hips, wrists, humerus, and pelvis. Hip fractures are associated with a 10% to 25% or greater 1-year mortality and loss of independent functioning in at least a third of the survivors, whereas vertebral fractures result in height loss, deformity, chronic pain, and difficulty with daily activities. With the exception of various disease-specific approaches as noted later, the management of all varieties of osteoporosis is similar.

1. **Postmenopausal and age-related osteoporosis.** More than 80% of osteo-porosis in women, and 50% in men, is primarily the result of **(a)** inherited low peak bone mass combined with **(b)** aging-related decreases in bone formation and increased resorption. This is often referred to as "primary" osteoporosis. The process can be further accelerated by a decline in gonadal hormone levels, especially menopause in women.

    a. **Pathogenesis**

    (1) In women, acute **estrogen deficiency** after menopause (or at any age) results in accelerated bone loss at a rate of ~3% per year for a period of 5 to 6 years, as a result of loss of the estrogen inhibition of osteoclas-tic bone resorption. Up to 20% of vertebral bone mass can be lost over this interval. Similarly, acute **testosterone deficiency** and the gradual decline in testosterone levels with age are associated with bone loss in men.

    (2) With **aging**, bone mass in all individuals tends to decrease by ~0.7% per year after age 35 to 40. This aging loss is a result in part of a decrease in bone formation rate as a result of reduced osteoblast generation from mesenchymal stem calls, and an increase in osteoclastic bone resorption caused by secondary increases in PTH levels because of decreased vitamin D levels and decreased calcium intake and absorption.

    (3) **Gender** is an important determinant of bone mass. After adolescence, women have consistently lower bone mass values than men. As a result, the incidence of osteoporosis in women is greater than that in men of corresponding age. In addition, larger bone size in men confers a lesser tendency to fracture at any BMD level.

    (4) **Ethnic factors** are also important. Caucasians and Asians have a lower peak adult bone mass and therefore a higher incidence of clinical osteo-porosis.

    b. **Diagnosis.** The diagnosis of primary/postmenopausal/age-related osteoporo-sis is essentially that of exclusion of other metabolic bone disorders, such as osteomalacia, as well as endocrine disorders (exogenous and endogenous glucocorticoid excess, hyperparathyroidism, hyperthyroidism, severe type 1 diabetes) and other secondary causes of osteoporosis. In addition, multiple myeloma should always be considered, because it may present as generalized osteopenia.

    c. **Treatment**

    (1) **General measures. Prevention** is an important approach, because es-tablished osteoporosis may be difficult to reverse.

        (a) Achieving **maximal peak adult bone mass** is an important measure, especially when there is a family history of osteoporosis. This is best accomplished by ensuring a total calcium intake of 1 200–1 500 mg per day, regular exercise, and maintenance of normal menses in women in the teen and early adult years.

        (b) **Diet.** From young adulthood through middle age, all adults should have a daily total **calcium** intake of at least 1 000 mg per day in order to maintain calcium balance. An average diet generally contains 400 to 700 g of calcium per day, depending on dairy intake. In women af-ter menopause, a total daily calcium intake of 1 200 to 1 500 mg per day (diet plus supplements) is recommended. Calcium supplementa-tion is most conveniently given as calcium carbonate in divided doses with meals. Calcium citrate provides better calcium absorption in older patients with reduced gastric acid secretion.

Vitamin D intake in both men and women should be sufficient to maintain the serum 25-OHD level in the range of 30 to 70 ng/mL at which intestinal calcium absorption is optimal, thereby reducing secondary increases in PTH activity that can stimulate bone resorption. This can usually be achieved by supplementation with 400 to 1 000 IU of vitamin D per day through middle age, whereas 1 500 to 2 000 IU per day of vitamin D may be required in older adults. Vitamin D supplementation also reduces falls in older persons, possibly by improving muscle strength.

- **(c) Exercise.** Regular weight-bearing exercise should be encouraged at all ages to stimulate osteoblastic bone formation and improve gait and balance. A brisk 20- to 30-minute daily walk is a convenient minimal regimen.
- **(d) Avoidance of smoking and excessive alcohol intake,** both of which are risk factors for osteoporosis.

(2) Specific treatment
- **(a) General measures.** Optimal dietary calcium and vitamin D intake should be maintained (see **Diet,** above), and attempts made to modify harmful lifestyle factors (physical inactivity, smoking, alcohol excess).
- **(b) Treatment indications** for the management of osteoporosis in both women and men are based on BMD and risk factors, as follows (WHO criteria):
    - **(1) Normal BMD** (T = −1.0): Optimize dietary intake and lifestyle factors, and perform a follow-up BMD measurement in 3 to 5 years.
    - **(2) Osteopenia** (T < −1.0 to T = −2.4): If the patient strongly prefers to take antiresorptive therapy, or two or more risk factors are present (especially age and falls risk) and the BMD is in the lower osteopenic range (T −1.5 to −2.4), bisphosphonate treatment plus vitamin D and calcium supplementation can be initiated. Otherwise, it is appropriate to optimize serum vitamin D levels (to 30 to 70 ng/mL), implement calcium supplementation and modification of lifestyle factors, and repeat the BMD in 2 to 3 years.
    - **(3) Osteoporosis** (T < −2.5 at either spine or hip) or **severe osteoporosis** (T < −2.5 with one or more minimal trauma fractures) should always be treated at any age.
    - **(4)** All patients being started on **glucocorticoid therapy** at a dose of 5 mg of prednisone per day or greater for at least 3 months should have a baseline BMD performed and then be started on preventive treatment (usually bisphosphonates) for osteoporosis (see Section IV.3.A).
    - **(5)** Anyone with **a minimal-trauma ("fragility") fracture** of the vertebrae, hip, or long bones has a high risk for subsequent fractures and should be treated for osteoporosis regardless of BMD values.
    - **(6)** Women undergoing **premature menopause** (because of surgery, irradiation, or chemotherapy) should have a baseline BMD performed and then be started on standard hormone replacement therapy until at least age 52. Where estrogens are contraindicated, treatment with bisphosphonates or other antiresorptive agents will maintain bone mass (see Section IV.3.A).
- **(c) Evaluating the response to treatment**
    - **(1)** In patients undergoing treatment for osteoporosis, **BMD measurements** at least 12 months apart are needed to accurately detect a 1.5% or greater change in BMD. BMD measurements should be performed every 1 to 2 years during treatment to monitor progress.

(2) Bone biochemical markers provide a convenient means of assessing treatment response and medication compliance between BMD measurements. For example, a standard index of adequate response to antiresorptive agents is a decrease in the morning second-void urinary **NTx** value by 35% or more from baseline, and/or a fall to <35 BCE units mm/mm creatinine, by 3 months after initiation of therapy. Thereafter, the NTx value can be followed every 6 to 12 month to ensure continued compliance and efficacy.

(d) Treatment regimens. All patients receiving treatment for osteoporosis should be encouraged to maintain proper calcium and vitamin D intake and exercise levels (see above), and to modify adverse lifestyle habits, such as physical inactivity, smoking, and excessive alcohol intake. Most currently approved therapeutic agents for osteoporosis are antiresorptive agents that increase bone mass and strength by reducing osteoclastic bone resorption (bisphosphonates, selective estrogen-receptor modulators [SERMs], estrogen, and calcitonin), with the exception of teriparatide, which stimulates bone formation directly. Both types of agents can significantly increase bone mass and reduce fracture incidence.

(1) Bisphosphonates. The current **first-line agents** for the treatment of osteoporosis are those bisphosphonates that have been shown to reduce fractures at the spine, hip, and other nonvertebral sites. These include two oral bisphosphonates (alendronate [Fosamax] and risedronate [Actonel]) and one intravenous bisphosphonate (zoledronic acid [Reclast]).

a. Oral bisphosphonates. Bisphosphonates are nonhormonal chemical analogs of pyrophosphate that are adsorbed onto bone surfaces and inhibit bone resorption by blocking osteoclast activity. The primary side effect of oral bisphosphonates is gastrointestinal (GI) irritation, usually gastric upset or bloating. Severe esophagitis, ulcerations, and bleeding have occasionally been reported. Bisphosphonates must be taken fasting, usually first thing in the morning, with 6 to 8 ounces of water. Patients should sit upright (to prevent esophageal irritation) and fast (to optimize absorption) for 30 to 45 minutes after dosing. Oral bisphosphonates are **contraindicated** in patients with esophageal abnormalities that delay esophageal emptying (e.g., stricture or achalasia) and in patients who are unable to stand or sit upright for at least 30 minutes. These agents must be used with **caution** in patients with active upper GI disorders, such as dysphagia, esophageal diseases, gastritis, duodenitis, or ulcers.

Oral **alendronate** (Fosamax) and **risedronate** (Actonel) are approved for treatment of postmenopausal and glucocorticoid-induced osteoporosis, and alendronate is approved for osteoporosis in men. In standard practice, both agents are generally used for all common forms of osteoporosis. The dose of alendronate is 70 mg once weekly, whereas risedronate can be given either as 35 mg once a week or as 70 mg per day for 2 consecutive days per month. After a 3-year course of treatment, these bisphosphonates generally increase spine BMD by 4% to 8% and hip BMD by 3% to 4%, respectively, with a corresponding average 30% to 50% decrease in vertebral and hip fracture incidence. Oral **ibandronate** (Boniva) is generally used as a second-line agent, because it has been shown to decrease vertebral but not hip fracture incidence, and is given as 150 mg once per month.

b. Intravenous bisphosphonates. Intravenous **zoledronic acid** (Reclast) has recently been approved for postmenopausal osteoporosis. When given as a single 15-minute intravenous dose once yearly for 3 years, it increases spine and hip BMD by ~7% and ~6%, respectively, and decreases vertebral and hip fracture incidence by 70% and 40%, respectively, with a 33% decrease in all fracture incidence. In high-risk patients with previous hip fracture, a 3-year course of yearly zoledronic acid reduced recurrent hip fracture by 40% and decreased overall mortality by 28% because of a reduction in hip fracture incidence. Common side effects include transient mild fever in ~15% of patients, a 1-day flulike syndrome in 7%, and arthralgias in 6% after the first infusion, with a marked decrease in the incidence of side effects after subsequent yearly infusions. Intravenous **ibandronate**, a second-line agent, given as a 30-second, 3-mg infusion every 3 months, has been shown to produce an increase in spinal BMD similar to that produced by oral ibandronate.

Note: Prior to the administration of any intravenous bisphosphonate treatment for osteoporosis, it is **essential** to **(1)** ensure that the 25-OHD level is at least 20 ng/mL and **(2)** supplement with calcium, 1 000 to 1 500 mg per day plus 400 to 800 IU of vitamin D per day for 2 weeks before and 3 weeks after bisphosphonate infusion in order to reduce the risk of hypocalcemia because of a sudden decrease in osteoclast activity. Patients with low 25-OHD levels (<20 ng/mL) should be loaded with 50,000 to 150,000 U of vitamin D orally 2 to 3 weeks before infusion, as needed to bring serum 25-OHD levels to >20 ng/mL, after ensuring the absence of pre-existing hypercalcemia or hypercalciuria.

c. **Newly recognized bisphosphonate side effects. Osteonecrosis of the jaw** is an often severe, suppurative inflammatory process that occurs in the mandible or maxilla in certain bisphosphonate-treated patients, often following tooth extractions or implants. More than 95% of cases occur in patients being treated chronically for metastatic cancer to the bone with very high doses of intravenous bisphosphonates (zoledronate, 4 mg per month, or pamidronate, 60 mg per month), often in combination with other chemotherapeutic agents. The incidence of jaw osteonecrosis appears to be in the range of 1% to 10% in such patients. If possible, major dental procedures should be completed prior to starting high-dose bisphosphonate treatment for bone cancer. In contrast, jaw osteonecrosis occurs in only 1/10,0000- to 1/100,000 patient-years in patients on the standard oral or intravenous doses of bisphosphonates used for the treatment of osteoporosis, an incidence that may not exceed that in the normal population.

The etiology of jaw osteonecrosis remains uncertain, but may represent impaired bone healing leading to local infection as a result of "overlap" suppressive effect of very high doses of bisphosphonates on osteoblastic bone formation in addition to inhibition of bone resorption. Treatment consists of discontinuing the bisphosphonate and dental management of the infection. Prevention includes performing all required major dental procedures prior to high-dose intravenous bisphosphonate therapy for bone cancer and maintenance of good oral hygiene. The low risk for jaw osteonecrosis in patients on standard doses of bisphosphonates for osteoporosis may be further reduced by checking serum osteocalcin or bone alkaline phosphatase levels before major dental procedures to ensure that the bone formation rate is normal; and discontinuing bisphosphonates for several months before and after tooth extractions and implants.

Suppression of bone formation leading to often atypical bone fractures (e.g., mid-shaft of the femur, bilateral pelvic and sacral fractures) has been reported in a small subgroup of patients on chronic bisphosphonate therapy. The usual clinical picture is the sudden appearance of atypical low-trauma fractures in a patient on an oral bisphosphonate for 5 years or more. Chronic glucocorticoid therapy and advanced age appear to be risk factors. Bone formation rate as measured by serum markers is markedly suppressed. The etiology of this disorder is as yet undefined, but it may be caused by "overlap" bisphosphonate suppression of osteoblast function (as for jaw osteonecrosis, above) in a susceptible population. Treatment consists of discontinuing bisphosphonate therapy and instituting anabolic therapy with teriparatide (see later) to stimulate osteoblast activity. Older and glucocorticoid-treated patients who are at higher risk for bisphosphonate-induced osteoblast suppression should be followed with serum osteocalcin levels at 6- to 12-month intervals, and bisphosphonate treatment should be temporarily discontinued if the bone formation rate falls below the lower limit of normal.

(2) Second-line agents for osteoporosis

 a. Teriparatide (Forteo). Teriparatide, the 1-34 amino-terminal fragment of human <u>PTH</u>, is currently the only agent capable of directly stimulating osteoblast bone-forming activity. It is administered as a daily subcutaneous 20 μg microinjection using a 28-day dose pen unit. A 2-year course of teriparatide generally increases spine and hip BMD by 10% to 14% and by 4% to 6%, respectively, while significantly reducing vertebral and nonvertebral fracture rates, by ~60% and 50%, respectively. Teriparatide is not currently considered a first-line agent for osteoporosis because of its high cost (roughly 10 times that of weekly alendronate) and concerns regarding possible osteosarcoma risk based on animal studies. Current indications for teriparatide use include bisphosphonate failure (no increase in BMD or occurrence of fractures while on bisphosphonates), inability to tolerate oral or intravenous bisphosphonates, unusually severe osteoporosis (e.g., T < -3.0 with previous fragility fracture), or severe osteoblast suppression with bone fractures. <u>Contraindications</u> include primary hyperparathyroidism, Paget disease of bone, or a history of bone cancer or x-ray therapy to bone. Side effects are minimal and include occasional mild transient hypercalcemia that is responsive to discontinuing calcium supplements.

After initiating daily teriparatide treatment, serum osteoblast markers such as osteocalcin increase two- to fourfold within 2 months and remain elevated, while osteoclast markers (e.g., NTx) increase gradually, usually reaching maximal levels by 18 to 24 months. <u>Treatment is limited to 2 years</u>, by which point bone resorption and formation have usually increased to a comparable degree. It is **essential** to institute antiresorptive therapy, preferably with bisphosphonates, immediately at the end of teriparatide treatment in order to preserve the increase in BMD. However, <u>teriparatide and bisphosphonates should **not** be used concurrently</u>, because the effect of teriparatide is paradoxically decreased by combined therapy with bisphosphonates.

b. **Estrogen replacement therapy (ERT)** is no longer standard therapy for postmenopausal osteoporosis, because of observations of adverse cardiovascular effects of ERT in older postmenopausal women. However, bisphosphonates and other antiresorptive agents are effective in managing postmenopausal bone loss. In addition, low-dose estrogen used to reduce symptoms of estrogen deficiency (hot flushes, etc.) in older women, and standard ERT in younger women following premature menopause, also enhance maintenance of bone mass.

c. **Selective estrogen-receptor modulators (SERMs)** have differential effects on key target organs. Raloxifene (Evista) is the SERM currently approved for use in osteoporosis. Raloxifene, 60 mg per day for 3 years, produces ~3% and ~2% increases in vertebral and hip BMD, respectively, and reduces vertebral fracture risk by ~30%. Effects on hip fracture risk have not been demonstrated. Raloxifene has smaller positive effects on bone mass and lipid levels than do standard estrogens, but it reduces the risk of breast cancer and does not stimulate endometrial or breast tissue. Side effects include hot flushes, nocturnal leg cramps, and increased risk of thrombosis.

d. **Calcitonin** nasal spray (Miacalcin) at 200 IU (one puff) per day for 3 years has been reported to increase BMD at the spine and hip by ~1% and ~0.5%, respectively, and to slightly reduce vertebral (but not hip) fracture rate in postmenopausal osteoporosis. Side effects of nasal calcitonin are largely limited to occasional irritation of the nasal mucosa.

e. **Vitamin D and calcium** are commonly used to supplement other modes of treatment in osteoporosis. However, treatment with vitamin D (700 to 800 U per day) plus calcium (500 to 1 000 mg per day) alone can slightly increase spine and hip BMD and reduce vertebral fracture incidence in older persons. Current recommended preventive doses of vitamin D are 400 IU per day to age 50, 400 to 1000 U per day from age 50 to age 70, and 1 000 to 1 500 U per day after age 70.

(3) **Duration of treatment.** The optimal duration of treatment of osteoporosis remains undefined. Certainly, exercise, proper calcium and vitamin D intake, and avoidance of smoking and alcohol excess should continue throughout life. SERMs and calcitonin typically produce an increase in BMD for 3 to 5 years, after which BMD remains stable or may decline slowly, whereas bisphosphonate therapy produces a continual increase in BMD for at least 10 years. Discontinuation of hormonal treatment (SERMs, calcitonin) is associated with a rapid return to the previous rate of bone loss, whereas BMD may remain stable for a year of more after bisphosphonate treatment because bisphosphonate is retained in bone. It has been suggested that individuals in whom the spine or hip T value remains at -2.5 after 5 years of bisphosphonate treatment should be treated for a total of 10 years. Moreover, in patients with risk factors and a hip or spine T of -1.5 to -2.4, it seems reasonable to continue reduced-dose therapy (e.g., alendronate, 70 mg every 2weeks) for at least several years after the standard course of treatment in order to maintain BMD increases.

2. **Male osteoporosis**

a. **Incidence and etiologies.** With the increasing longevity of the population, the incidence of osteoporosis in men is rising. The age incidence of osteoporotic fractures in men lags roughly 10 years behind that in women because of their higher initial bone mass in early life, larger bone size, and absence of a sudden loss of gonadal hormones as occurs in menopause. Approximately

6% of men over age 50 have severe osteoporosis, and 30% of all osteoporotic hip fractures now occur in men. The overall causes of osteoporosis in men and women are similar. However, because of the current lower incidence of primary/age-related osteoporosis in men, ~30% of male osteoporosis is a result of **secondary causes,** particularly glucocorticoid therapy, hypogonadism, alcoholism, renal disease, and gastrointestinal/hepatic disorders. Hip fracture in men is associated with a higher mortality because of these coexisting morbidities. The criteria for measuring BMD in men are given in Section III.B.

b. Prevention. General measures for prevention of osteoporosis in men are as described previously for women in Section IV.A.1.c and include maintaining good calcium and vitamin D intake, regular physical exercise, and avoiding smoking and excessive alcohol intake.

c. Treatment approaches include the measures described previously and the management of any concurrent medical disorders that could accelerate bone loss. If there is evidence of hypogonadism, testosterone replacement therapy may increase bone mass somewhat; if not, testosterone is of little benefit. Bisphosphonates are more effective in this disorder and have been shown to increase BMD and reduce fracture incidence in men with osteoporosis of various causes.

3. Secondary osteoporosis

a. Glucocorticoid excess

(1) Pathogenesis. Supraphysiologic levels of glucocorticoids produce bone loss by two mechanisms: **(a)** suppressing bone forming by inhibiting osteoblast generation from mesenchymal stem cell precursors; and **(b)** increasing bone resorption by enhancing osteoclast generation. In addition, bone quality is decreased as a result of a low bone formation and repair rate.

(2) Exogenous (iatrogenic) glucocorticoid excess is the most common secondary cause of osteoporosis. The severity of the bone loss correlates roughly with total glucocorticoid dose and duration of therapy, and can be aggravated by the decreased physical activity often associated with the underlying disease.

(a) Diagnosis is based on the clinical situation and the exclusion of other causes of bone loss.

(b) Management

(1) Glucocorticoid dose should be reduced to the lowest possible level by use of nonsteroidal anti-inflammatory agents and other adjuvant drugs. Weight-bearing physical activity for at least 20 to 30 minutes per day should be encouraged, and appropriate calcium and vitamin D intake should be maintained.

(2) After the initiation of glucocorticoid therapy, there is often an **initial hypercalciuric phase,** which can last for 6 to 12 months and is presumably a result of severe depression of osteoblast function with urinary "spillover" of unassimilated calcium. Hydrochlorothiazide, 25 to 50 mg per day, plus potassium supplements should be given as needed to reduce urinary calcium levels to normal.

(3) When urinary calcium excretion falls to normal (1.5 to 4.0 mg/kg body weight in 24 hours) or subnormal levels after 6 to 12 months, patients should be supplemented with **(a)** vitamin D, 800 to 1 000 IU per day, or 50 000 IU once or twice per month, to maintain serum 25-OHD in the normal range (30–70 ng/mL) and **(b)** calcium, 1 200 to 1 500 mg per day, to promote calcium absorption.

(4) Standard **bisphosphonate therapy** to reduce fracture risk should be initiated in any patient being started on the equivalent of prednisone, 5 mg/day for 3 months or longer.

(3) Endogenous. Cushing disease is usually associated with severe osteoporosis resulting from glucocorticoid excess. Management is surgical or medical correction of the underlying hormonal disorder. Bone mass usually increases when glucocorticoid levels return to normal. The residual osteoporosis should be managed as described in Section IV.A.1.

b. Transplantation osteoporosis. Organ transplant patients are at high risk for marked bone loss because of the adverse effects on bone produced by both their primary disease and the effects of the glucocorticoids and other immunosuppressants used after transplantation. Rapid bone loss and increased fracture incidence occur very commonly following kidney, heart, lung, liver, and bone marrow transplants. Various recent studies have reported a 4% to 12% loss of spine and hip bone mass, and a 17% to 40% incidence of new fractures, within the first year after transplantation. Although established posttransplant bone loss responds to standard osteoporosis treatment regimens, prevention is an important approach to this problem.

Preoperatively, all candidates for organ transplantation should have a bone evaluation including BMD as soon as possible, and should be started on appropriate treatment for osteoporosis or other observed bone disorders immediately. **Postoperatively,** the rapid bone loss is produced by the effects of high-dose glucocorticoids, which suppress osteoblastic bone formation and stimulate resorption, combined with the effects of calcineurin inhibitors such as cyclosporin A and tacrolimus (Prograf), which appear to activate osteoclastic bone resorption directly. This results in a high-turnover bone-loss state, with the most rapid bone loss occurring during the first 6 to 18 months posttransplantation, followed by slower loss or stabilization. Both oral and intravenous bisphosphonates have been shown to be effective in preventing posttransplantation bone loss. In addition, general measures such as early ambulation, proper nutrition, and vitamin D and calcium supplementation should be encouraged. It has been suggested that all transplantation candidates can benefit from being started on bisphosphonate therapy prior to transplantation in order to have effective concentrations in bone immediately preoperatively. The one exception would be renal transplant candidates, who might require bone biopsy to rule out adynamic bone disease that could be aggravated by bisphosphonates.

c. Premature gonadal hormone deficiency

(1) Pathogenesis. Congenital absence or premature loss of gonadal function invariably leads to significant bone loss. Hypogonadism is a common cause of osteopenia in adult males. Commonly encountered clinical conditions include idiopathic testicular atrophy and primary hypogonadotropism in men, and premature radiation-, surgery-, or drug-induced menopause in women. Hypogonadism as a result of androgen ablation therapy for prostate cancer in men and estrogen ablation with aromatase therapy for breast cancer in postmenopausal women are increasingly common causes of accelerated bone loss in adults.

(2) Diagnosis. The diagnosis of hypogonadism is made by standard measures of testicular or ovarian function.

(3) Treatment. All individuals with gonadal hormone deficiency because of primary or acquired hypogonadotropism or gonadal failure are at risk for accelerated bone loss and fractures. Initial BMD should be quantitated, and treatment with bisphosphonates or other antiresorptive agents should be started as soon as the diagnosis of hypogonadal bone loss is established, with hormone replacement generally reserved for management of hormone deficiency symptoms.

d. Hyperthyroidism

(1) Pathogenesis. Thyroid hormone stimulates osteoclastic resorption in excess of osteoblastic bone formation activity, thus producing net bone loss. Bone loss is most rapid in younger individuals, who have higher basal bone turnover rates. In these patients, transient hypercalciuria and even mild hypercalcemia can occur, especially when osteoblast function is decreased by reduced physical activity. Prolonged treatment with supraphysiologic doses of thyroid hormone can also produce significant bone loss in postmenopausal women.

(2) Diagnosis and management. Hyperthyroidism is diagnosed by standard clinical and biochemical means. Routine weight-bearing exercise should be encouraged. Generally, only reversal of the hyperthyroid state is required, because the bone loss is generally not severe owing to the short duration of hyperthyroidism. In older individuals, residual osteoporosis should be managed as described in Section IV.A.1.

e. Diabetes mellitus

(1) Pathogenesis. An increased incidence of osteoporosis and fracture is seen in patients with long-standing type 1 diabetes mellitus, with impaired bone formation likely resulting from the decrease in the anabolic effects of insulin and amylin on bone. Bone loss appears to be slightly greater in males. In type 2 diabetes, bone fracture incidence is increased despite a higher mean BMD, the latter apparently in part a result of the increased stimulatory effects of obesity-related weight loading and adipokine effects on bone mass. In this population, the increase in fracture incidence results from increased risk of falling because of peripheral neuropathy, visual impairment, and decreased physical fitness.

(2) Management. In type 1 diabetes, good glycemic control, exercise, and optimum vitamin D (600 to 1 000 U per day) and calcium (1 000 to 1 500 mg per day) intake should be maintained to optimize bone status. Bisphosphonate therapy is also effective in increasing BMD. Patients with type 2 diabetes may also benefit from frequent visual assessment, treatment of neuropathy, and regular exercise to improve muscle strength and balance.

f. Immobilization

(1) Pathogenesis. Acute immobilization produces a rapid decline in bone formation rate as a result of decreased physical stimulation of osteoblast activity. Osteoclastic bone resorption initially remains unchanged. As a result, bone loss occurs. Loss is more rapid in younger individuals and others with high bone turnover rates (e.g., hyperparathyroidism, Paget disease). Total immobilization can produce hypercalciuria and hypercalcemia in such individuals.

(2) Management. Calcium, phosphate, and vitamin D supplementation are contraindicated in acute immobilization because of the tendency toward hypercalciuria and hypercalcemia. Passive exercise and mechanical compression therapy are of minimal benefit. The patient should be mobilized as soon as possible. Good hydration is required to promote calcium diuresis and reduce urinary calcium concentration. Bisphosphonates given intravenously (zoledronic acid, pamidronate) in standard doses for osteoporosis may be useful in controlling hypercalcemia and attenuating bone loss.

4. Osteogenesis imperfecta (OI) is a rare genetic disorder, the mildest variant of which (type I) exhibits autosomal dominant inheritance and can first appear as severe osteoporosis at ages ranging from early childhood to early middle age.

a. Pathogenesis. The basis of the osteoporosis is a congenital defect in bone formation because of defective bone collagen synthesis as a result of type I collagen gene mutations. The mid-shaft diameter and strength of affected long bones can be markedly reduced. Occasionally, the disorder may not become clinically apparent until the third or fourth decade.

b. Diagnosis. In the childhood-onset variant of type I OI, there is a history of multiple long-bone fractures dating from early childhood. Blue sclerae, a result of scleral thinning, are often but not always present. Hearing loss frequently appears in the third decade. Bone radiographs may demonstrate "flask deformities" of several long bones, especially the metacarpals and metatarsals. These deformities are the result of marked thinning of the mid-shaft. All other causes of osteoporosis must be excluded.

c. Management. There is currently no specific treatment for this disorder. However, bisphosphonate therapy can be effective in reducing vertebral fracture risk.

B. **Osteomalacia and rickets. Osteomalacia** is characterized by the accumulation of increased amounts of unmineralized bone matrix (osteoid). The bone formation rate is markedly reduced. In the growing child, this process results in defective mineralization of epiphysial cartilage, leading to fraying and thickening of the epiphyses, accompanied by bowing of the weight-bearing long bones because of deficient mineralization. These clinical features are characteristic of children with **rickets.** Although mild osteomalacia is characterized by a tendency to bone fracture, this condition is frequently asymptomatic in adults. In more severe forms, pain in the ribs, pelvis, and lower extremities is common. Radiographs may demonstrate a mild generalized decrease in bone mass and may occasionally reveal **pseudofractures** (Looser zones), which are painless linear radiolucencies extending perpendicularly from the cortex partway through the long bones, pelvis, and scapulae. Osteomalacia and rickets can be caused by vitamin D deficiency, defective vitamin D metabolism, chronic hypophosphatemia, and rare congenital or acquired defects of osteoblast function.

1. **Vitamin D deficiency** is characterized by low serum 25-OHD (<20 ng/mL), with desired normal being 30 to 60 ng/mL, reduced intestinal calcium absorption, reduced serum calcium and phosphate concentrations, reduced 24-hour urinary calcium excretion, mildly increased iPTH levels, and elevated serum bone alkaline phosphatase (often with a paradoxically normal serum osteocalcin level).

   a. **Gastrointestinal disorders**

   (1) **Pathogenesis.** Moderate to severe vitamin D deficiency occurs most commonly in disorders associated with fat malabsorption: gluten-sensitive enteropathies, pancreatic insufficiency, biliary obstruction, blind-loop syndromes, and following jejunoileal bypass for obesity. Binding of dietary calcium by fatty acids to form insoluble soaps may further decrease calcium absorption. In postgastrectomy patients, altered dietary habits may contribute to vitamin D deficiency. Osteoporosis frequently occurs concomitantly, probably because of chronic calcium and protein malnutrition and increased bone resorption due to secondary hyperparathyroidism.

   (2) **Treatment.** Management of the underlying disorder and correction of fat malabsorption are of primary importance. Vitamin D is given orally at a dose of 50 000 U or more 1 to 5 times weekly as needed to maintain the serum 25-OHD level at 30 to 70 ng/mL. Oral 25-OHD (Calderol), 50 to 150 μg per day, may be a useful alternative because of its increased water solubility and more rapid onset of action. Calcium supplementation (1 000 to 2 000 mg per day) is given as calcium carbonate. Serum calcium and 24-hour urinary calcium should be followed frequently, because improvement in the underlying disease can be associated with a marked reduction in vitamin D requirements.

   b. **Mild nutritional vitamin D deficiency** (serum 25-OHD ranging from 12 to 20 ng/mL) is occurring with increasing frequency in the United States. Mild vitamin D deficiency is usually associated with low dietary vitamin D intake, limited sunlight exposure and/or use of sunscreens, and older age, when cutaneous production of vitamin D is reduced. Administration of a loading dose of vitamin D (e.g., 50 000 U per day for 5 to 7 days), followed by maintenance of physiologic dose (400 to 1 000 U per day or 50 000 units once a month), is usually sufficient to normalize vitamin D status.

2. **Defective vitamin D metabolism and action**

   a. **Anticonvulsants and other liver oxidase enzyme–activating drugs.** Long-term use of certain anticonvulsant drugs, particularly phenobarbital and phenytoin and certain other mediations (e.g., rifampin) produces an increased incidence of vitamin D deficiency and osteomalacia in individuals with marginal vitamin D intake and sunlight exposure. The basis of the disorder is increased hepatic catabolism and biliary excretion of vitamin D and its biologically active metabolites. Serum 25-OHD levels and urinary calcium excretion are reduced, and other biochemical markers of vitamin D deficiency are present. Severe cases require 2 000 to 5 000 U of vitamin D plus 1 000 to 1 500 mg of calcium per day for 6 months or longer. Routine prophylaxis is 800 to 1 200 U of vitamin D per day or 50 000 U once or twice per month.

b. Pseudo-vitamin D deficiency rickets (vitamin D-dependent rickets) is a rare autosomal recessive disorder that mimics nutritional rickets but requires higher doses of vitamin D (10 000 to 30 000 U per day). The basis of the disorder appears to be congenitally defective renal 1,25-$(OH)_2$D production. The diagnosis is based on characteristic somatic abnormalities, normal serum 25-OHD and reduced 1,25-$(OH)_2$D levels, and failure to respond to physiologic doses of vitamin D (400–1 000 U per day). Another group of disorders characterized by partial vitamin D resistance and originally termed **vitamin D-dependent rickets type II** results from hereditary cellular resistance to 1,25-$(OH)_2$D. Clinical and biochemical features of osteomalacia, occasionally associated with alopecia, occur in the presence of normal serum 25-OHD and increased 1,25-$(OH)_2$D levels. Variable supraphysiologic doses of 1,25-$(OH)_2D_3$ are required for treatment.

3. Hypophosphatemia resulting from disorders of the PHEX/phosphatonin system. The recently described PHEX/phosphatonin endocrine system appears to play a major role in the regulation of serum phosphate levels. Disorders of this system can cause chronic severe hypophosphatemia, resulting in osteomalacia or rickets. Phosphatonin (primarily FGF-23 and possibly other phosphaturic factors) is an osteoblast- and osteocyte-derived circulating factor(s) that acts on the kidney to **(a)** reduce renal tubular phosphate resorption and **(b)** inhibit 1,25$(OH)_2$D production. The result is a decline in serum phosphate levels without the normal compensatory rise in serum 1,25$(OH)_2$D. The PHEX gene encodes a membrane-bound endopeptidase that is expressed in osteoblasts, osteocytes, muscle, lung, and other tissues, and serves to cleave and inactivate phosphatonin.

a. Tumor-associated osteomalacia. Certain slow-growing soft-tissue or bone tumors of mesenchymal origin produce high amounts of phosphatonin, resulting in chronic renal phosphate wasting and hypophosphatemia leading to osteomalacia, bone pain, and proximal muscle weakness and aching. Serum calcium, iPTH, and 25-OHD levels are normal, but the low to normal serum 1,25-$(OH)_2$D concentration is inappropriately reduced relative to the elevated levels expected in hypophosphatemia. Renal phosphate wasting is demonstrated by a reduced renal tubular threshold maximum for phosphate (TmP/GFR). Administration of nonsodium neutral phosphate (e.g., Neutra-Phos-K, K-Phos-Neutral), 2 to 4 g per day in four or five divided doses, calcium supplements (1 000 to 1 500 mg per day), plus 1,25-$(OH)_2D_3$ (calcitriol, 0.5 to 3.0 μg per day), can usually reverse the biochemical abnormalities and osteomalacia if maintained chronically. Removal of the tumor is curative. However, the tumors are often difficult to locate, and total-body magnetic resonance imaging may be useful in difficult cases.

b. Familial X-linked hypophosphatemia (XLH, hypophosphatemic vitamin D–resistant rickets)

(1) Clinical features. XLH is one of the most common etiologies of rickets and osteomalacia. Most cases are familial, with X-linked dominant transmission. The classic clinical triad is hypophosphatemia, lower-limb deformities, and stunted growth rate. Clinical manifestations range from asymptomatic mild hypophosphatemia to marked hypophosphatemia with severe bone disease. Males are more severely affected. The clinical picture is that of severe rickets with general demineralization, pseudofractures, bowing of the long bones, and increased incidence of fractures. Biochemical findings include normal serum calcium, reduced phosphate, increased alkaline phosphatase, and normal iPTH. There is marked renal phosphate wasting (reduced TmP/GFR), and urinary calcium excretion may be slightly decreased. The diagnosis can be established before the age of 2 years. The severity of bone symptoms decreases after closure of the epiphyses, but severe bone disease can occur in untreated older adults.

(2) Pathogenesis. The basis of the disorder appears to be an inactivating mutation in the *PHEX* gene on the X chromosome, resulting in decreased degradation of circulating phosphatonin, leading to renal phosphate wasting combined with inappropriately normal serum $1,25(OH)_2D$ levels. Serum calcium, iPTH and 25-OHD levels are normal. An autosomal dominant form of the disorder is caused by a mutation in the FGF-23 gene causing resistance to degradation by the PHEX endopeptidase.

(3) Treatment. Phosphate supplementation, 1.5 to 3.0 g of elemental phosphorus per day given as nonsodium neutral phosphate (e.g., Neutra-Phos-K, K-Phos-Neutral), 2 to 4 g per day in four or five doses, $1,25-(OH)_2D_3$ (calcitriol), 0.5 to 2.0 μg per day, and calcium, 1 000 to 1 500 mg per day, are given to stimulate calcium absorption, maintain serum phosphate levels, and prevent the secondary hyperparathyroidism that may be caused by the phosphate supplementation. This regimen can produce significant reversal of radiologic and biochemical changes, and improve growth rate in children. However, responses vary. Osteotomy may be required to correct lower-extremity bowing. Treatment should probably be maintained throughout life, but lower doses of phosphate are required in adults.

C. Primary hyperparathyroidism

1. Incidence and pathogenesis. Primary hyperparathyroidism occurs relatively commonly in the adult population ($\sim$1/500 to 1/1 000 individuals), with a 3:1 female/male ratio. At least 50% of cases occur in postmenopausal women. Only 20% of patients are symptomatic, with most cases being detected as hypercalcemia on a routine biochemical profile. Roughly 80% of cases are to the result of a single adenoma, with 15% to 20% being due to four-gland hyperplasia. Parathyroid cancer accounts for <0.5% of patients. Some degree of loss of bone mass can be demonstrated in most patients because of a PTH-stimulated increase in bone osteoclastic activity, and is usually more marked in areas that are rich in cortical bone (forearm, hip)

2. Diagnosis. The diagnosis is usually readily established by demonstrating fasting hypercalcemia, low or low-normal fasting serum phosphate, and increased serum iPTH. The presence of typical biochemical findings of hyperparathyroidism in association with suppressed serum iPTH levels suggests malignancy-associated hypercalcemia because of tumor production of PTH-related peptide (PTHrP). This latter diagnosis can be confirmed by serum PTHrP assay.

3. Management. Indications for surgical treatment of primary hyperparathyroidism include **(a)** symptomatic presentation (new kidney stones, symptomatic bone disease), **(b)** marked hypercalcemia (mean serum calcium >1.0 mg/dL above the upper limits of normal), **(c)** hypercalciuria (24-hour urine calcium >400 mg per day), **(d)** enlargement of existing kidney stones, **(e)** decreasing renal function (creatinine clearance >30% below age-sex normal values), or **(f)** marked bone loss as demonstrated by BMD with a T value below − 2.5 at any site. In addition, surgical intervention should be strongly considered in younger patients (<50 years of age) because of the increased risk of progression. Thus, by current criteria, $\sim$20% of patients are surgical candidates. Parathyroid surgery is increasingly being performed by minimally invasive parathyroidectomy when a single adenoma can be demonstrated by a preoperative ^{99m}Tc-sestamibi parathyroid scan.

Many patients can be managed medically by maintaining **normal** calcium and sodium intake, hydration, avoiding thiazide diuretics (which can increase serum calcium levels by reducing urinary calcium excretion), and increased weight-bearing exercise. Most nonsurgery candidates do quite well on this regimen, with only 25% showing progression of laboratory values and BMD changes over a 10-year period. Mild to moderate bone loss usually responds well to bisphosphonate treatment. Recently, the use of calcimimetic agents such as cinacalcet has been shown to reduce serum calcium and PTH levels and stabilize BMD for up to 3 years, and can be considered in surgical candidates who are poor operative risks.

V. RENAL OSTEODYSTROPHY

A. Renal osteodystrophy is the result of multiple disorders in bone and mineral metabolism that can occur in chronic kidney disease. These can include changes in serum calcium, phosphate, vitamin D, bone formation and resorption, and bone mass and quality, often in association with extraskeletal calcification. Bone pain may occur, and reduced BMD and bone quality with increased fracture risk is common.

B. Bone disorders range from an abnormally high turnover state to a condition of very low turnover. Defective mineralization and increased fracture risk can occur in both situations. The high-turnover state is driven by elevated PTH levels resulting from the hypocalcemia stimulus produced both by phosphate retention and by decreased renal production of $1,25(OH)_2D$ as renal function declines. The primary bone histologic change is osteitis fibrosa. Low-turnover renal bone disease is characterized by an extremely low rate of bone formation termed "adynamic bone disease," and it is often the result of an oversuppression of PTH secretion because of excessive vitamin D metabolite and calcium supplementation. Other contributing factors include diabetes, advanced age, poor nutrition, and glucocorticoid therapy. Previously, low-turnover renal bone disease accompanied by marked osteomalacia and bone pain was often caused by aluminum accumulation at the mineralization front. However, this disorder, termed "aluminum bone disease," has largely disappeared in recent years after the discontinuance of the use of aluminum-containing phosphate binders and dialysis solutions. Chronic acidosis in renal insufficiency can aggravate bone loss because of increased bone resorption. Extraskeletal cardiovascular system and other tissue calcification can be aggravated by an excessive calcium load provided by calcium-containing phosphate binders. The preceding histologic patterns generally occur in combination, with one form often predominating, in a disorder termed "mixed renal osteodystrophy."

C. Prevention and treatment. Primary goals are to: **(1)** maintain blood phosphate and calcium as close to normal as possible, with the calcium X phosphate product always <55; **(2)** prevent or reverse secondary hyperparathyroidism; **(3)** avoid extraskeletal calcifications; and **(4)** prevent or reverse aluminum or iron accumulation.

The five stages of chronic kidney disease are **stage 1,** normal or raised estimated GFR (eGFR) >90 mL/min; **stage 2,** mild, eGFR 60 to 90 mL/min; **stage 3,** moderate, eGFR 30 to 59 mL/min; **stage 4,** severe, eGFR 15 to 29 mL/min; and **stage 5,** kidney failure, eGFR <15 mL/min. Management goals by stage are as follows:

Stage 1. Ensure good calcium and vitamin D nutrition, maintaining serum 25-OHD in the normal range (30 to 70 ng/mL) and serum iPTH at 30 to 60 pg/mL.

Stage 2. As for stage 1, plus mild dietary phosphate restriction.

Stage 3. As for stage 2, plus moderate dietary phosphate restriction, and use of non–aluminum-containing calcium-based phosphate binders (calcium carbonate or acetate) or non–calcium-based phosphate binders such as sevelamer hydrochloride (Renagel) or lanthanum carbonate (Fosrenal) to keep serum phosphate at 2.7 to 4.6 mg/dL. Ensure total oral calcium supplementation of no more than 1.0 g per day, and use vitamin D metabolites, especially paricalcitol (Zemplar), to maintain serum iPTH at 35 to 70 pg/mL.

Stage 4. As for stage 3, plus increased phosphate restriction while maintaining protein intake, use of calcimimetics such as cinacalcet (Sensipar) as needed to maintain iPTH at 70 to 110 pg/mL.

Stage 5. As for stage 4, plus use of dialysate calcium concentration to control iPTH at 150 to 300 pg/mL and consideration of parathyroidectomy for uncontrollable secondary hyperparathyroidism.

Oral or intravenous bisphosphonates may be effective in increasing BMD in stage 1–3 patients, but are not recommended in patients with an eGFR <30 mL/min. To reduce the risk of adynamic bone disease, bone formation markers (osteocalcin, bone alkaline phosphatase) must be followed at 3- to 6-month intervals in renal disease patients treated with bisphosphonates and treatment discontinued if markers fall below normal limits.

VI. PAGET DISEASE
A. Clinical features
1. **Presentation.** Paget disease occurs in 1% of the population over age 40, and 15% to 30% of patients have a family history of the disorder. The disorder is frequently asymptomatic and is often detected via an <u>elevated serum alkaline phosphatase on</u> a routine blood panel. Usually, there is only local involvement of one or two bones, but extensive multifocal forms can produce marked pain, deformity, and disability. The process may "burn out," remain localized, wax and wane, or progress rapidly.

2. **Symptoms** are produced by the following (in approximate order of frequency): bone pain at a pagetic site, possibly caused by frequent microfractures; muscular strain and accelerated osteoarthritis caused by changes in posture and the weight-bearing axis as a result of bowing of the femur and tibia; joint deformity because of involvement of periarticular bone, especially in the hip; nerve root compression caused by vertebral enlargement; narrowing of cranial ostia with compression of cranial nerves; otosclerosis leading to progressive air-conduction hearing loss; involvement of the base of the skull, causing platybasia and long-track damage; high-output heart failure in older individuals with extensive disease, because of increased blood flow to bone; and development of osteogenic sarcoma in patients with extensive, long-standing disease. This rare (<1% of patients), lethal complication occurs most commonly in the proximal humerus and manifests itself as new pain at a pagetic site.

B. Pathogenesis.
The initiating lesion is a local increase in osteoclastic bone resorption activity, followed by a chaotic, overexuberant increase in osteoblastic bone formation. The basis of the increased osteoclastic activity is unknown, but it appears to be a combination of genetic susceptibility and unknown environmental factors, with a possible viral etiology postulated. In involved areas, bone turnover is markedly increased. Involved bones may gradually increase in size, and they are susceptible to deformity and fracture because of their disorganized structure.

C. Diagnosis.
Characteristic radiographic findings, increased serum bone alkaline phosphatase, and increased ^{99m}Tc bone scan activity in radiologically involved areas are sufficient for diagnosis. In long bones, Paget disease always begins at one end and progresses toward the mid-shaft. Bone scanning is particularly useful in detecting activity in unsuspected areas. Areas showing increased uptake on bone scan should be confirmed as pagetic by standard radiography. Occasionally, regions with a characteristic radiographic appearance of Paget disease do not show increased activity on bone scan. These areas represent "burned-out" disease. The earliest radiologic finding is a local radiolucency, corresponding to initial osteoclastic overactivity, and is most commonly seen as a broad lucency in one region of the skull (osteoporosis circumscripta). Serum and urinary calcium levels are usually normal but may become significantly elevated when a patient with widespread involvement is put on bed rest. Bone biopsy is indicated only in the rare patient in whom radiologic findings suggest malignancy. Sudden accentuation of bone pain in a specific area in a patient with extensive, long-standing disease should raise the possibility of the development of osteogenic sarcoma. A characteristic "sunburst" pattern with periosteal elevation may be seen on a radiograph.

D. Treatment
is directed toward arresting the disease and is indicated to relieve symptoms and/or prevent complications. The **symptoms** most likely to be relieved by treatment include bone aches or pain at pagetic sites, excessive warmth over involved bones, headache resulting from skull involvement, and back pain because of vertebral involvement with neural compression syndromes (radiculopathy, slowly progressive spinal cord compression). **Preventive** treatment is indicated in patients with involvement of weight-bearing long bones or joints (especially the hip), extensive osteolytic areas, widespread involvement of the skull (to prevent foraminal compressions). Treatment for at least 6 months before elective surgery on pagetic bones (e.g., hip replacement) is indicated to increase bone strength.

1. **General measures.** Adequate hydration and mobilization should be maintained in all patients. In patients acutely confined to bed rest, extreme care should be

taken to ensure abundant fluid intake to avoid hypercalcemia. Early ambulation should be encouraged. Most patients with mild disease who manifest only musculoskeletal and osteoarthritic symptoms, and who are not candidates for specific treatment, can receive satisfactory symptomatic relief from mild analgesic therapy such as ibuprofen or acetaminophen.

2. **Specific treatment.** Bisphosphonates are the mainstays of therapy and inhibit osteoclastic bone-resorption, with the osteoblastic response subsiding secondarily. Significant reversal of neural compressive symptoms may occur after prolonged treatment. However, long-bone deformities cannot be reversed. Response is monitored by following serum alkaline phosphatase and clinical symptoms. With extensive involvement, bone scans at 12-month intervals may be useful in following disease activity. After treatment, the serum alkaline phosphatase should be followed at 6 month intervals and treatment reinstituted with disease recurrence.

   a. **Bisphosphonates** approved for use in Paget disease in the United States include oral risedronate and alendronate, and intravenous zoledronic acid and pamidronate. Currently, intravenous **zoledronic acid** appears to be the treatment of choice. Comparisons of the effects of a single 15-minute intravenous infusion of 5 mg of zoledronic acid versus risedronate, 30 mg per day orally for 2 months, have shown zoledronic acid to be superior to risedronate in median time to initial response (64 vs. 89 days), 6-month response rate assessed by alkaline phosphatase normalization (89% vs. 58%), and maintenance of remission in initial responders at 24 months (97% vs. 60%). Side effects of zoledronic acid include occasional mild flulike illness and arthralgias. A less potent alternative is intravenous **pamidronate** (Aredia) given as a 30-mg infusion for 2 consecutive days every 3 months (45% 6-month response). Oral bisphosphonates are also effective, but less so than IV zoledronate, and require prolonged administration. Oral **risedronate,** 30 mg per day for 2 months, and oral **alendronate,** 40 mg per day for 6 months, both produce a 50% to 70% initial 6-month response rate. Injectable **calcitonin** is rarely used because of its relatively low effectiveness, the inconvenience of injections, and bothersome side effects. Nasal spray calcitonin (Miacalcin) is not effective in Paget disease.

Selected References

Black DM, Bilezikian JP, Ensrud KE, et al. One year of alendronate after one year of parathyroid hormone (1-84) for osteoporosis. *N Engl J Med* 2005;353:555–565.

Black DM, Schwartz AV, Ensrud KE, et al. Effects of continuing or stopping alendronate after 5 years of treatment: the Fracture Intervention Trial Long-term Extension (FLEX): a randomized trial. *JAMA* 2006;296:2927–2938.

Campion JM, Maricic MJ. Osteoporosis in men. *Am Fam Phys* 2003;67:1521–1526.

Canalis E, Giustina A, Bilezekian JP. Mechanisms of anabolic therapies for osteoporosis. *N Engl J Med* 2007;357:905–916.

Cummings SR, Bates D, Black DM. Clinical use of bone densitometry: scientific review. *JAMA* 2002;16:1889–1897.

de Menezes Filho H, de Castro LC, Damiani D. Hypophosphatemic rickets and osteomalacia. *Arq Bras Endocrinol Metabol* 2006;50:802–813.

Farford B, Presutti J, Moraghan TJ. Nonsurgical management of primary hyperparathyroidism. *Mayo Clin Proc* 2007;82:351–355.

Gal-Moscovici, Sprague SM. Osteoporosis and chronic kidney disease. *Semin Dialysis* 2007;20:423–430.

Greenspan SL, Schneider DL, McClung MR, et al. Alendronate improves bone mineral density in elderly women with osteoporosis residing in long-term care facilities. *Ann Intern Med* 2002;136:742–746.

Hodsman AB, Bauer DC, Dempster DW, et al. Parathyroid hormone and teriparatide for the treatment of osteoporosis: a review of the evidence and suggested guidelines for its use. *Endocrine Rev* 2005;26:688–703.

Hofbauer LC, Brueck CC, Singh SK, et al. Osteoporosis in patients with diabetes mellitus. *J Bone Miner Res* 2007;1317–1328.

Holick MF. Resurrection of vitamin D deficiency and rickets. *J Clin Invest* 2006;116:2062–2072.

Holick MF. Vitamin D deficiency. *N Engl J Med* 2007;357:266–281.

Hosking D, Lyles K, Brown JP, et al. Long-term control of bone turnover in Paget's disease with zoledronic acid and risedronate. *J Bone Miner Res* 2007;22:142–148.

Hruska KA, Saab G, Mathew S, et al. Renal osteodystrophy, phosphate homeostasis, and vascular calcification. *Semin Dialysis* 2007;20:309–315.

Jackson C, Caugris S, Sen SS, et al. The effect of cholecalciferol (vitamin D3) on the risk of falls and fracture: a meta-analysis. *Q J Med* 2007;100:185–192.

Jan de Beur S. Tumor induced osteomalacia. *JAMA* 2005;294;1260–1267.

Khosla S, Burr D, Cauley J, et al. Bisphosphonate-associated osteonecrosis of the jaw: report of a task force of the American Society for Bone and Mineral Research. *J Bone Miner Res* 2007;22:1479–1491.

Khosla S, Melton J. Osteopenia. *N Engl J Med* 2007;356:2293–2300.

Levine JP. Effective strategies to identify postmenopausal women at risk of osteoporosis. *Geriatrics* 2007;62:22–30.

Lyles KW, Colon-Emeric CS, Magaziner JS, et al. Zoledronic acid and clinical fractures and mortality after hip fracture. *N Engl J Med* 2007;357:1–11.

Merlotti D, Gennari L, Martini G, et al. Comparison of different intravenous bisphosphonate regimens for Paget's disease of bone. *J Bone Miner Res* 2007;22:1510–1517.

Nagano N. Pharmacological and clinical properties of calcimimetics: calcium receptor activators that afford an innovative approach to controlling hyperparathyroidism. *Pharmacol Ther* 2006;109:339–365.

Poole KS, Compston JE. Osteoporosis and its management. *Br J Med* 2006;333:1251–1256.

Raisz LG. Pathogenesis of osteoporosis: concepts, conflicts, and prospects. *J Clin Invest* 2005;115:3318–3325.

Raisz LG. Screening for osteoporosis. *N Engl J Med* 2005;353:164–171.

Rauch F, Travers R, Glorieux F. Pamidronate in children with osteogenesis imperfecta: histomorphometric effects of long-term therapy. *J Clin Endocrinol Metab* 2006;91:511–516.

Rosen CJ. Postmenopausal osteoporosis. *N Engl J Med* 2007;353:595–603.

Rossouw JE, Prentice RL, Manson JE, et al. Postmenopausal hormone therapy and risk of cardiovascular disease by age and years since menopause. *JAMA* 2007;297:1465–1477.

Sambrook PN. How to prevent steroid induced osteoporosis. *Ann Rheum Dis* 2005;64:176–178.

Schiavi SC, Kumar R. The phosphatonin pathway: new insights in phosphate homeostasis. *Kidney Int* 2004;65:1–14.

Seibel MJ. Clinical application of biochemical markers of bone turnover. *Arq Bras Endocrinol Metab* 2006;50:603–620.

Simmons J, Zeitler P, Steelman J, et al. Advances in the diagnosis and treatment of osteoporosis. *Adv Pediatr* 2007;54:85–114.

Suliburk JW, Perrier ND. Primary hyperparathyroidism. *Oncologist* 2007;12:644–653.

Whyte MP. Paget's disease of bone. *N Engl J Med* 2006;355:593–600.

Woo S-B, Hellstrom JW, Kalmar JR. Systemic review: bisphosphonates and osteonecrosis of the jaws. *Ann Intern Med* 2006;144:753–761.

COMMON BONE AND MINERAL DISORDERS OF CHILDHOOD

Michael A. Levine

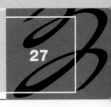

27

*A*t all ages, ~99% of total body calcium is in the skeleton, where, in combination with 89% of total body phosphorus, it constitutes the major inorganic matrix of bone. Therefore, metabolic disorders involving these two elements and the hormones that regulate them, as well as disorders of skeletal development and mineralization, can conveniently be considered together. This chapter describes childhood disorders of mineral metabolism as well as other specific skeletal disorders that affect children.

I. CALCIUM HOMEOSTASIS

Approximately 50% of total serum calcium is in the ionized form (i.e., Ca^{2+}) at normal serum protein concentrations, and it represents the biologically active component of the total serum calcium concentration. Another 8% to 10% is complexed to organic and inorganic acids (e.g., citrate, sulfate, and phosphate); together, the ionized and complexed calcium fractions represent the diffusible portion of circulating calcium. Approximately 40% of serum calcium is protein-bound, primarily to albumin (80%) but also to globulins (20%). The protein-bound calcium provides a reserve of available calcium that can respond immediately to an acute need for increased ionized calcium. The extracellular Ca^{2+} concentration must be maintained within narrow limits (Fig. 27.1).

A. Physiology. See Chapter 25.

B. Normal values. Normal serum calcium and phosphate levels for infants and older children are indicated in Table 27.1. Levels tend to be marginally higher (by ~0.2 mg) in growing children compared with adults. The physiologically active component of serum calcium is the ionized calcium (Ca^{2+}). Increases in the extracellular fluid concentration of anions, such as phosphate, citrate, bicarbonate, or edetic acid, will increase the proportion of bound calcium and decrease ionized calcium. Extracellular fluid pH also affects the distribution of calcium between ionized and bound fractions. Alkalosis increases the affinity of albumin for calcium and thereby decreases the concentration of ionized calcium. By contrast, acidosis increases the ionized calcium concentration by decreasing the binding of calcium to albumin. When it is not possible, or practical, to determine the ionized calcium concentration directly, a "corrected" total calcium concentration can be calculated using one of several proposed algorithms that are based on albumin or total protein concentrations. None of these formulas is absolutely accurate, but they often provide useful estimates of the true concentration of calcium in serum. One widely used algorithm estimates that total serum calcium declines by ~0.8 mg/dL for each 1 g/dL decrease in albumin concentration, without a change in ionized calcium. The unique pattern of serum proteins in neonates can lead to inaccurate calculation of ionized calcium using formulas based on calcium–protein relationships derived from adult data.

II. DISORDERS OF CALCIUM HOMEOSTASIS

A. Hypocalcemia. Clinically important categories of hypocalcemia and some features associated with the failure of calcium control are listed in Table 27.2. Hypocalcemia is usually defined as a total serum calcium concentration of <8.5 g/dL (2.1 mmol/L) in children, <8 mg/dL (2 mmol/L) in term neonates, and <7 mg/dL (1.75 mmol/L) in preterm neonates. The symptoms and signs of hypocalcemia are largely explained by the disturbance in neuromuscular excitability attributable to a reduction in extracellular fluid Ca^{2+} concentration. Common features include neuromuscular

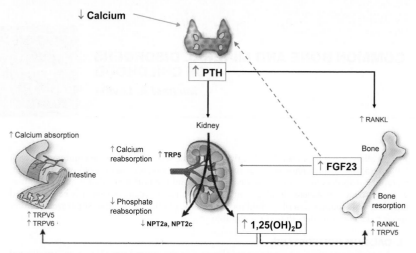

Figure 27.1. Central role of parathyroid glands in regulating extracellular ionized calcium concentration (Ca^{2+}). Parathyroid hormone (PTH) mobilizes Ca^{2+} from bone and reduces fractional renal clearance of Ca^{2+}. In turn, Ca^{2+} acts on parathyroids to inhibit PTH secretion. By stimulating renal 25-hydroxycalciferol 1α-hydroxylase, PTH enhances calcitriol formation and hence intestinal Ca^{2+} absorption. Calcitriol increases expression of TRPV5 and TRPV6, increasing calcium absorption in the intestine, calcium reabsorption in the distal tubule, and osteoclastic bone resorption. Calcitriol and PTH both increase secretion of RANKL from osteoblasts, which enhances the number and function of osteoclasts. PTH and FGF23 decrease expression of renal tubule sodium–phosphate cotransporters Npt2a and Npt2c, thereby reducing phosphate reabsorption. FGF23 also decreases expression of renal 25-hydroxycalciferol 1α-hydroxylase. *Dashed line* indicates a direct inhibitory effect of FGF23 on PTH secretion.

irritability in the form of myoclonic jerks, "twitching," exaggerated startle responses, or seizures. Apnea, cyanosis, tachypnea, tachycardia, vomiting, laryngospasm, or heart failure may also be seen. Markedly reduced ionized calcium concentrations may be associated with prolongation of the Q_o-T_c interval on the electrocardiogram and decreased cardiac contractility. Often, however, hypocalcemia is clinically silent and detected only by routine blood chemistry panels. Neuromuscular tetany and distressing paresthesias are more common in older children and adults, whereas bronchospasm and epileptic seizures are more common manifestations of hypocalcemia in babies and young children.

1. **Neonatal hypocalcemia.** Neonatal hypocalcemia is the most prevalent type of hypocalcemia encountered by the pediatrician. It can be divided into early

TABLE 27.1	Normal Values of Serum Calcium and Phosphorus in Infancy and Childhood

Age category	Total calcium (mg/dL)	Ionized calcium (mM)	Phosphorus (mg/dL)
Newborn (0–3 mo)	8.8–11.3	1.22–1.40	4.8–7.4
Boys and girls 1–5 y	9.4–10.8	1.22–1.32	4.5–6.5
Boys and girls 6–12 y	9.4–10.3	1.15–1.32	3.6–5.8
Boys 15–17 y	9.5–10.5	1.12–1.30	2.3–4.5
Boys 17–19 y and girls 12–15 y	9.5–10.4	1.12–1.30	2.3–4.5
Girls 15–19 y	9.1–10.3	1.12–1.30	2.3–4.5

TABLE 27.2 Clinically Important Categories of Hypocalcemia

| | Serum level | | | |
Category	Phosphorus	25-OHD	1,25(OH)$_2$D	PTH
Neonate				
Early hypocalcemia	N	N	N or L	N or L
Late hypocalcemia				
Hypoparathyroidism	H	N	N or L	L
Transient hypocalcemia	H	N	N	N or H
Older child				
Critical illness	N	N	N	L
Hypoparathyroidism	H	N	L	L
Pseudohypoparathyroidism	H	N	L	H
Vitamin D deficiency	L, N, or H	L	L, N, or H	H
Vitamin D dependency type 1	L	N	L	H
Vitamin D dependency type 2	L	N	H	H
Acute phosphorus overload	H	N	?	H

H, high; L, low; N, normal; PTH, parathyroid hormone.

hypocalcemia, which occurs within the first 3 days of life, and late neonatal hypocalcemia, which begins at the end of the first week of life. Hypocalcemia is relatively common in the neonatal intensive care unit and may occur in as many as 30% of infants with very low birth weight (<1 500 g) and in as many as 89% of infants whose gestational age at birth was <32 weeks. A high incidence is also reported in infants of mothers with diabetes mellitus and in infants with birth asphyxia. Infants with low calcium levels may lack specific symptoms or signs.

In the newborn, as well as in the older child, intestinal absorption of calcium occurs both passively and through a vitamin D–dependent active transport mechanism. At birth, the newborn's vitamin D status is related directly to maternal vitamin D status and to materno-fetal transfer of vitamin D and its metabolites. Serum levels of both 25-hydroxyvitamin D and calcitriol are lower than maternal values, and babies whose mothers have marked vitamin D deficiency will have compromised vitamin D status. Circulating calcitriol concentrations rise over the first 2 days of life, and calcitriol stimulates calcium absorption in the intestine. In premature infants, passive calcium absorption accounts for most of the intestinal calcium; however, neonates, even very-low-birth-weight infants, can absorb and metabolize vitamin D, and supplementation with vitamin D can increase calcium absorption within 4 weeks of birth. Serum levels of 25-hydroxyvitamin D in breast-fed infants do not correlate with concentrations of vitamin D and its metabolites in human milk. Under usual circumstances, human milk is not an adequate source of vitamin D, and the predominant sources of vitamin D in the breast-fed infant are endogenous synthesis after exposure to sunlight or supplementation.

Because the maternal calcium concentration and vitamin D status during pregnancy influences parathyroid function in the developing fetus, a thorough evaluation of the newborn with hypocalcemia or hypercalcemia must include analysis of mineral metabolism in the infant's mother. Moreover, the association of neonatal hyperparathyroidism with inherited defects in the gene encoding the calcium-sensing receptor (CaR) provides strong justification to determine the serum calcium levels in the child's biologic father and siblings as well.

Hypomagnesemia predisposes to neonatal hypocalcemia and can exacerbate its symptoms. The basis for these effects is not well understood but may relate to the association of hypomagnesemia with impaired parathyroid hormone (PTH) release or action.

a. Early neonatal hypocalcemia

(1) Clinical features. In the neonate, jittery movements, convulsions, and occasionally apnea and myocardial dysfunction may all represent the clinical consequences of hypocalcemia. Although the prognosis for hypocalcemic seizures in the newborn is good, it is quite possible that the consequences of hypocalcemia can contribute to decreased chances of survival in otherwise very sick infants. Any newborn with these signs should have the serum calcium level determined, preferably by direct measurement of ionized calcium. A Ca^{2+} concentration <2.5 mg/dL (0.63 mmol/L) can be clinically significant and is often accompanied by a prolonged Q–T_c interval on the electrocardiogram. Similarly, a value >0.4 for $Q_0T/\sqrt{t}$ (where Q_0T is the time from the Q wave to the origin of the T wave and t is the length of the cardiac cycle) has been proposed as evidence of hypocalcemia, but the accuracy of such estimates is low.

(2) Etiology and pathophysiology. This disorder commonly affects low-birth-weight and sick neonates between 1 and 4 days of age. It is often considered an <u>exaggeration of the physiologic fall</u> in the plasma calcium concentration that occurs in all newborn infants during the first 2 to 3 days of life. Early neonatal hypocalcemia apparently results from insufficient release of PTH by immature parathyroid glands or inadequate responsiveness of the renal tubule cells to PTH. An exaggerated rise in calcitonin secretion in premature infants may play a contributory role. <u>Maternal diabetes mellitus</u> is a significant risk factor and is commonly associated with hypomagnesemia, birth asphyxia, and prematurity. Prematurity, low birth weight, hypoglycemia, difficult delivery, and respiratory distress syndrome are other findings in infants with early-onset hypocalcemia.

In the premature, small, or sick neonate, maintenance of a normal Ca^{2+} concentration is further jeopardized by the lack of substantial food (and hence calcium) intake by mouth. It is also possible that stress hormones such as calcitonin and cortisol act to stabilize bone, diminishing PTH-induced calcium release. In addition to these risk factors for hypocalcemia, the transfusion of large volumes of citrate- or phosphate-containing whole blood can lower ionized calcium by the formation of nonionizable calcium phosphates or citrates. The overly rapid correction of acidosis with bicarbonate or by hyperventilation can also lead to a rapid fall in Ca^{2+} by increasing the fraction of circulating calcium bound to protein. A more severe form of transient neonatal hypoparathyroidism and tetany occurs in infants who were exposed to maternal hypercalcemia in utero. Intrauterine hypercalcemia suppresses parathyroid activity in the developing fetus and apparently leads to impaired responsiveness of the parathyroid glands to hypocalcemia after birth

b. Late neonatal hypocalcemia. This term describes hypocalcemia that occurs at 5 to 10 days of age in full-term and apparently healthy neonates, but that may occur as late as 6 weeks after birth. Late-onset hypocalcemia is invariably associated with **elevations in serum phosphorus levels.** Hyperphosphatemia, and consequent hypocalcemia, generally reflects a high intake of phosphate, which typically occurs through diet but may also occur by enema. Late-onset hypoparathyroidism usually is associated with serum levels of PTH that are low or insufficiently elevated relative to the degree of hypocalcemia. This may reflect an inability of the parathyroid gland to secrete adequate amounts of PTH or partial resistance of the immature kidney to PTH. Rarely, late-onset hypocalcemia may occur as a manifestation of maternal hypercalcemia. Hyperphosphatemia tends to shift the equilibrium in calcium flow between bone and the extracellular fluid toward bone. It also diminishes calcitriol synthesis.

Both of these changes act to reduce the plasma calcium level. Rarely, late-onset hypocalcemia may occur as a manifestation of maternal hypercalcemia or hypoparathyroidism.

(1) Hypoparathyroidism. Congenital hypoparathyroidism may present in the neonatal period but is less common than transient hypoparathyroidism associated with maternal hypercalcemia. The mother's serum levels of calcium and 25-hydroxyvitamin D should always be checked in cases where infantile hypocalcemia is of late onset or prolonged duration, particularly if accompanied by hyperphosphatemia.

(2) Phosphorus overload. Cows' milk contains six times as much phosphorus as human milk (950 vs. 162 mg/L). Ingestion of a calorically adequate volume of cows' milk overwhelms the capacity of the neonatal kidney to excrete phosphate, with consequent hyperphosphatemia. This phenomenon was also observed with early infant feeding formulas that still had a much higher phosphorus content than human milk. However, even in modern "humanized" cows' milk–based formulas, the calcium/phosphorus ratio is lower than in breast milk. Because human milk is low in phosphate, breast-fed infants rarely, if ever, develop late hypocalcemia. Compared with breast-fed babies, infants receiving these formulas have slightly but significantly lower serum Ca^{2+} levels during the first 2 weeks of life.

(3) Uremia. Renal failure can present in the first week or two of life with seizures or tetany. These signs might be due to hypocalcemia secondary to renal phosphate retention. The blood urea nitrogen and creatinine should be measured in all cases of neonatal hypocalcemia with hyperphosphatemia.

(4) Transient pseudohypoparathyroidism of the newborn. Although most newborns with late-onset hypocalcemia have low levels of PTH, ~25% of affected babies have elevated levels of PTH. Hypocalcemia is associated with hyperphosphatemia, which is due to a high transport maximum of the phosphate/glomerular filtration rate despite elevated PTH levels. Serum levels of magnesium and vitamin D metabolites are typically normal. These biochemical features strongly resemble those of pseudohypoparathyroidism, but, in contrast to genetic forms of pseudohypoparathyroidism that are associated with defects in the *GNAS* gene, infants with this transient form of PTH resistance show normal nephrogenous cyclic adenosine monophosphate (cAMP) responses to administered PTH. By contrast, the phosphaturic response to the PTH infusion is typically impaired. Affected newborns respond to treatment with calcium and/or active (i.e., 1α-hydroxylated) metabolites of vitamin D. The condition appears to be transient, and normal serum levels of calcium, phosphorus, and PTH are achieved by age 6 months. These features are suggestive of delayed maturation of the post-cAMP signaling pathway in the proximal renal tubule.

(5) Defects in vitamin D supply or action. Vitamin D deficiency can cause hypocalcemia at any age (see later). Congenital vitamin D deficiency can manifest as late-onset neonatal hypocalcemia when intestinal absorption of calcium begins to rely on vitamin D–dependent transport. Because neonatal stores of vitamin D are derived entirely from maternal sources in utero, it is not surprising that maternal vitamin D insufficiency is usually associated with this disorder.

Vitamin D insufficiency can occur as a consequence of either decreased supply of vitamin D or accelerated metabolism as a result of drugs that activate the vitamin D catabolic pathway (e.g., the anticonvulsants phenytoin and phenobarbital). Although nutritional vitamin D deficiency is the most common cause of congenital vitamin D deficiency and rickets, these conditions can also be caused by genetic defects that impair activation of vitamin D or reduce target-tissue responsiveness to $1,25(OH)_2D$ (see later).

TABLE 27.3 Hypoparathyroidism and Related Disorders in Childhood

Type	Parathyroid	Age of onset[a]	Associated features
Transient neonatal	Physiologic suppression	2–10 d	Maternal hypercalcemia
Di George sequence	Parathyroid dysgenesis	0–1 mo	Del22q11; *TBX1* mutation Cardiac and thymic (immune) deficits
Type 1 polyglandular autoimmune syndrome	Autoimmune destruction or activating antibodies	3+ y	Mutation of *AIRE* gene Mucocutaneous candidiasis, adrenal failure
Autosomal dominant hypocalcemia	Reduced: "set point" for Ca^{2+}	Infancy and childhood	Mutation of *CaSR* gene; positive family history; hypercalciuria
Thalassemia/iron overload	Iron deposition	Adolescence and beyond	Cardiac, liver, and endocrine dysfunction
Postsurgical	Removal or damage	Any	Following thyroidectomy
Pseudohypoparathyroidism	Resistance to PTH	Infancy to 10 y	
Hypomagnesemia	Reduced PTH production and/or resistance to PTH	Any	Specific intestinal defect or generalized malabsorption

PTH, parathyroid hormone.
[a]Most typical ages given. Individual cases may vary widely.

2. **Critical illness.** Hypocalcemia has long been known to occur in infants and children who are critically ill or who have sustained a significant burn injury. Often such hypocalcemia is noted after cardiac surgery or major injury. There are conflicting views as to whether hypocalcemia in these cases is a result of relative hypoparathyroidism or of some other factor such as hypercalcitoninemia.

3. **Hypoparathyroidism.** The causes of PTH deficiency, together with some of the clinical features associated with these syndromes, are listed in Table 27.3. Hypoparathyroidism can be classified as disorders of parathyroid gland formation, destruction of the parathyroid glands, or reduced parathyroid gland function.

   a. **DiGeorge sequence (DGS)** results from dysmerogenesis of the third and fourth pharyngeal pouches, and it is associated with hypoplasia of the thymus and parathyroid glands. Patients also often manifest conotruncal cardiac abnormalities, cleft palate, and dysmorphic facies. Hypoparathyroidism is present in up to 60% of patients with DGS. DGS is the leading cause of persistent hypocalcemia of the newborn, but hypoparathyroidism may resolve during childhood. Primary hypothyroidism and growth-hormone deficiency have also been described in children with DGS, albeit far less frequently than hypoparathyroidism. Thymic defects are associated with impaired T-cell–mediated immunity and frequent infections.

   Molecular mapping has attributed most (70% to 80%) cases of DGS to hemizygous microdeletions within a critical 250-kb region of 22q11.21-q11.23. Although many genes are located within this region, the presence in some patients with DGS of point mutations that inactivate the *TBX1* gene suggests that this may be the critically important gene.

   DGS most commonly arises from *de novo* mutations, but autosomal dominant inheritance can occur. Microdeletions of 22q11 are the most common cause of contiguous gene deletion syndromes in humans, and occur in ~1:3 000 newborns. In addition to DGS, deletions within 22q11 can cause the conotruncal anomaly face syndrome and the **velocardiofacial syndrome (VCFS).** VCFS is typically diagnosed later in childhood, and hypocalcemia has been found to be present in up to 20% of cases. Because of the phenotypic variability of the various overlapping syndromes, these conditions are all included within the acronym "CATCH-22," representing a syndrome of **C**ardiac abnormality, **A**bnormal facies, **T**hymic hypoplasia, **C**left palate, and **H**ypocalcemia with deletion or chromosome **22**q11.

DGS has also been reported to arise in patients with deletions of 10p13, 17p13, and 18q21. Gestational diabetes, as well as exposure to alcohol and other toxins (e.g., retinoids) in the intrauterine stage, can also cause similar phenotypic syndromes. Deletions within two nonoverlapping regions of 10p have been found to contribute to a phenotype similar to DGS, namely, the **hypoparathyroidism, sensorineural deafness, and renal dysplasia syndrome (HDR,** MIM146255). Unlike DGS/CATCH-22, individuals with HDR do not exhibit cardiac, palatal, or immunologic abnormalities. The HDR disorder is a result of haploinsufficiency of the GATA-binding protein-3 (*GATA3*) gene.

b. Hypoparathyroidism-retardation-dysmorphism and Kenny-Caffey syndromes. The **hypoparathyroidism-retardation-dysmorphism syndrome (HRD,** MIM241410), also known as the **Sanjad-Sakati syndrome,** is a rare form of autosomal recessive hypoparathyroidism that is associated with other developmental anomalies. In addition to parathyroid dysgenesis, affected patients have severe growth and mental retardation, microcephaly, microphthalmia, small hands and feet, and abnormal teeth. This disorder is seen almost exclusively in individuals of Arab descent. **Kenny-Caffey syndrome** (MIM244460) is an allelic disorder that is characterized by hypoparathyroidism, dwarfism, medullary stenosis of the long bones, and eye abnormalities. Both disorders result from mutations in the tubulin-specific chaperone E (*TBCE*) gene on chromosome 1q42-43, which encodes a protein required for folding of α-tubulin and its heterodimerization with β-tubulin, although a second gene locus for this disorder is also probable.

c. Isolated hypoparathyroidism. The leading cause of isolated hypoparathyroidism is inactivation of the *GCM2* (*GCMB*) gene at 6p23-24 (MIM146200). Parathyroid aplasia or dysplasia is associated with severe hypocalcemia and low or undetectable levels of plasma PTH.

Isolated hypoparathyroidism can also be inherited as an X-linked recessive trait (MIM307700). Affected males present with infantile hypocalcemic seizures, whereas hemizygous females are unaffected. Autopsy of an affected individual revealed complete agenesis of the parathyroid glands as the cause of hypoparathyroidism. Linkage analysis has localized the underlying mutation to a 1.5-Mb region on Xq26-q27, and recent molecular studies have identified a deletion-insertion involving chromosomes Xq27 and 2p25 as the basis for the defect.

d. Autoimmune polyendocrinopathy-candidiasis-ectodermal dystrophy (APECED). See Chapters 25 and 57.

The syndrome's classic triad constitutes the "HAM" complex of **H**ypoparathyroidism, **A**drenal insufficiency, and **M**ucocutaneous candidiasis. Recent studies indicate that patients with APS1 and hypoparathyroidism have circulating antibodies that react with the NALP5 protein and that damage or destroy the parathyroid glands. An alternative pathophysiology implicates the presence of circulating antibodies that bind and activate the calcium-sensing receptor (CaSR), thereby reducing PTH secretion from parathyroid cells (and increasing calcium excretion from the kidney).

The natural history of APS1 is quite predictable, with the appearance of mucocutaneous candidiasis and hypoparathyroidism in the first decade of life, followed by primary adrenal insufficiency before 15 years of age. The candidiasis may affect the skin, nails, and mucous membranes of the mouth and vagina and is often resistant to treatment. Addison disease can mask the presence of hypoparathyroidism, or may manifest only after improvement of the hypoparathyroidism, with a reduced requirement for calcium and vitamin D. By diminishing gastrointestinal absorption of calcium and increasing renal calcium excretion, glucocorticoid therapy for the adrenal insufficiency may exacerbate the hypocalcemia and could cause complications if introduced before the hypoparathyroidism is recognized.

Some patients do not manifest all three primary elements of the HAM complex, whereas other individuals may develop additional endocrinopathies such as hypogonadism, insulin-dependent diabetes, hypothyroidism, and hypophysitis. Nonendocrine components of the disorder that occur in some patients include malabsorption, pernicious anemia, vitiligo, alopecia, nail and dental dystrophy, autoimmune hepatitis, and biliary cirrhosis.

e. **Autosomal dominant hypocalcemia** (also autosomal dominant hypocalcemic hypercalciuria, MIM 146200) most commonly occurs as a result of an activating mutation of the gene encoding the CaSR at 3q13.3–21. Most mutations lower the set point for extracellular calcium sensing. The effect of the activating mutation on the parathyroid cell is to reduce PTH secretion and thereby produce a state of <u>functional hypoparathyroidism</u>. In the tubule cells of the thick ascending limb of the loop of Henle, activated CaSR stimulates calciuresis and increases the fractional excretion of calcium (FeCa), thus producing relative (or absolute) hypercalciuria relative to the filtered load of calcium. Nephrocalcinosis and nephrolithiasis are common complications of vitamin D therapy. Although in most cases the degree of hypocalcemia and hypercalciuria are mild and well tolerated, severe hypocalcemia occurs in some patients.

Autosomal dominant hypocalcemia may be sporadic, and it has been shown to arise from *de novo* activating mutations of the CASR.

f. **PTH gene mutations.** See Chapter 25.

g. **Anti-CaSR antibodies.** Autoimmune hypoparathyroidism had been previously thought to be caused by the binding of cytotoxic autoantibodies to parathyroid cells. However, many patients with late- or adult-onset primary hypoparathyroidism have circulating antibodies that activate the CaSR and impair release of PTH rather than produce irreversible destruction of the parathyroid glands. The ability of these antibodies to activate the CaSR in the distal nephron accounts for the increased urinary excretion of calcium in these patients, and thus affected patients resemble those with autosomal dominant hypocalcemia (see above) and activating mutations of the CaSR. It appears that there might be a specific autoimmune reaction against the CaSR on parathyroid cells.

h. **Mitochondrial disease.** Several syndromes caused by deletions in mitochondrial DNA have been associated with hypoparathyroidism. These include **Kearns-Sayre syndrome** (encephalomyopathy, ophthalmoplegia, retinitis pigmentosa, heart block), **Pearson marrow-pancreas** syndrome (sideroblastic anemia, neutropenia, thrombocytopenia, pancreatic dysfunction), and **maternally inherited diabetes and deafness syndrome**. Hypoparathyroidism has also been described in **MELAS** (**M**itochondrial myopathy, **E**ncephalopathy, **L**actic **A**cidosis, and **S**trokelike episodes) **syndrome**, a result of point mutations in mitochondrial tRNA. Because renal magnesium wasting is frequently seen in these conditions, a readily reversible form of hypoparathyroidism caused by <u>hypomagnesemia</u> should also be considered.

i. **Parathyroid gland destruction.** See Chapter 25.

4. **Pseudohypoparathyroidism (PHP).** See Chapter 25.

a. **Pseudohypoparathyroidism type 1a.** See Chapter 25.

b. **Pseudohypoparathyroidism type 1b.** See Chapter 25.

c. **Pseudohypoparathyroidism type 1c.** See Chapter 25.

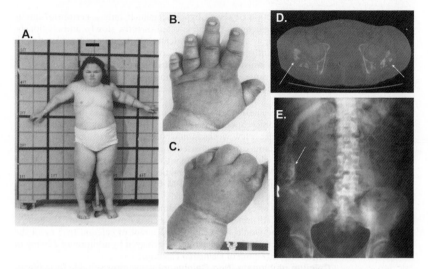

Figure 27.2. Young woman with typical features of Albright hereditary osteodystrophy (AHO) and PHP type 1a. Panel **A** shows short stature, round face, obesity, and sexual immaturity; panels **B** and **C** show brachydactyly, with Archibald dimples rather than knuckles visible when a fist is made; panel **D** shows CT scan of lower extremity with heterotopic ossification present in deep muscle *(arrows)*, whereas panel **E** shows superficial heterotopic ossification in the abdominal wall subcutaneous tissues *(arrow)*.

    d. Osteoma cutis and progressive osseous heteroplasia. Osteoma cutis and **progressive osseous heteroplasia (POH)** represent alternative manifestations of Albright hereditary osteodystrophy (AHO) in which only heterotopic ossification occurs. In osteoma cutis, ectopic ossification is limited to the superficial skin, whereas in POH, heterotopic ossification involves the skin, subcutaneous tissue, muscles, tendons, and ligaments (Fig. 27.2). POH can be disabling because extensive dermal ossification occurs during childhood, followed by widespread ossification of skeletal muscle and deep connective tissue. Nodules and lacelike webs of heterotopic bone extend from the skin into the subcutaneous fat and deep connective tissues and may cross joints, leading to stiffness, joint locking, and permanent immobility.

    Heterozygous inactivating *GNAS* mutations have been identified in most patients with osteoma cutis and POH, and in each case the defective allele was paternally inherited. Although patients with POH lack other features of AHO or PHP, maternal transmission of the defective *GNAS* allele leads to the complete PHP type 1a phenotype in affected children.

    e. Pseudohypoparathyroidism type 2. See Chapter 25.

  5. Management of hypocalcemia. Although mild hypocalcemia might not require therapy, any neonate with a serum calcium level <7.5 mg/dL (Ca^{2+} <2.8 mg/dL) or an older child with a serum calcium level <8 to 8.5 mg/dL should be treated to prevent tetany and other symptoms.

    a. Acute. In acute symptomatic hypocalcemia, intravenous therapy is required. This should not be undertaken lightly, because **(1)** rapid injection can cause serious cardiac dysrhythmias and **(2)** all calcium salts are locally toxic and can lead to tissue damage upon accidental extravasation. Rapid injections of calcium salts (0.1 mL/kg of 10% calcium chloride or 0.3 mL/kg of 10% calcium gluconate) should be given only in acute cardiac emergencies. Under other circumstances, an intravenous infusion of 1 to 3 mg/kg per hour of elemental calcium as the gluconate salt (10% solution of calcium gluconate) can be used for the correction of severe hypocalcemia. If only a peripheral line is available, calcium gluconate can be injected directly, slowly, and cautiously. When a central line is available, the calcium gluconate can be diluted with saline or dextrose infusion fluids and given continuously at the appropriate rate. A continuous infusion of elemental calcium is superior to intermittent bolus infusions, because it maintains a consistent serum calcium concentration and avoids excessive fluctuations that can intensify symptoms or signs of hypocalcemia.

b. Chronic. In the absence of tetany, seizures, and severe degrees of hypocalcemia, oral therapy will suffice. Spontaneous recovery of normal mineral homeostasis typically occurs after a few weeks in newborns, but the serum calcium levels of symptomatic infants can be increased within 1 to 2 days by supplementing artificial formulas with sufficient calcium to achieve a high (3:1 to 4:1) molar ratio of calcium to phosphorus. Our practice has been to supplement a low-phosphorus formula such as **Similac PM 60/40** (11.2 mg calcium and 5.5 mg phosphorus per ounce). For example, 5 oz of Similac PM 60/40 contains 1.4 mmol (56 mg) of calcium and 0.90 mmol (28 mg) of phosphorus, which corresponds to a Ca:P molar ratio of only 1.6:1. In order to achieve the desired 4:1 Ca:P ratio, one would have to add 2.2 mmol of calcium to 5 oz of the Similac PM 60/40 formula, which could be achieved by addition of 220 mg of calcium carbonate (88 mg of elemental calcium).

Calcium glubionate (Neo-Calglucon) is the most suitable form of calcium for babies and young children because it is available as a somewhat pleasant-tasting syrup. The usual dosage is 5 mL/kg per day (115 mg elemental calcium per kilogram per day) given in 4 to 6 divided doses. Higher doses can cause diarrhea because of the preparation's high sugar content.

In older children, oral therapy is often used as an adjunct during treatment for chronic hypocalcemia, both to provide a constant supply of dietary calcium and to reduce intestinal absorption of phosphorus. The supplemental calcium (~20 to 50 mg/kg per day) should be administered in divided doses and taken with meals. Tablets of calcium gluconate, carbonate, or lactate can be given as an alternative to the glubionate syrup. In clinical practice, all calcium salts perform similarly, and the choice may be guided by the number of tablets needed to deliver the desired dose of calcium. The gluconate consists of ~9% elemental calcium, the carbonate 40%, citrate 21%, and the lactate 13%.

c. Vitamin D

(1) Chronic hypocalcemia, except in the mildest cases, is managed by the administration of vitamin D or its metabolites. Because of their slow onset of action and persistence after the discontinuation of therapy, native vitamin D and its analog, dihydrotachysterol, are now rarely used in the management of hypocalcemia, and the most active metabolite of vitamin D, **calcitriol, has become the treatment of choice for patients with chronic hypocalcemia.** Calcitriol is favored over vitamin D because it is the most active metabolite and does not require either hepatic or renal hydroxylation in order to have full activity in vivo. Calcitriol has a very short half-life, and overall its duration of action is no more than 1 to 2 days, whereas the prohormone vitamin D may persist for weeks or months. Calcitriol provides a greater margin of therapeutic safety because hypercalcemia due to inadvertent overdosage is rapidly reversed once calcitriol is discontinued.

(2) The dosage of calcitriol in childhood (e.g., 50 to 90 ng/kg per day) is generally higher on a weight-adjusted basis than that in adults. Anything from 0.25 to 3.0 μg per day may be needed. The medication is administered once or twice daily and the dosage adjusted until normocalcemia is attained. Because hypoparathyroidism lowers the renal threshold for calcium, our practice is to maintain serum calcium at the lower end of the normal range in order to minimize hypercalciuria and the risk of urolithiasis. A low-salt diet, and occasionally a thiazide diuretic, such as chlorothiazide or

TABLE 27.4 Classification of Hypercalcemia in Childhood

| Type | Serum | | | | Urine | |
	Phos	Calcidiol	Calcitriol	PTH	Ca	Notes
Idiopathic (Williams syndrome)	N	N	N	N	H	Deletion in 17q11.23. Cognitive impairment. Elfin facies, aortic stenosis
Childhood hyperparathyroidism	L	N	H	H	H	Often genetic (multiple endocrine neoplasia)
Severe neonatal hyperparathyroidism	L	N	H	H	L/N	Loss-of-function mutation (generally homozygous) in CaSR
Familial hypocalciuria	N	N	N	N	L	Loss-of-function mutation (generally heterozygous) in CaSR
Immobilization	N	N	L	L	H	
Malignancy (metastatic)	N	N	L	L	H	
Malignancy (nonmetastatic)	L	N	L	L (PTHrP elevated)	H	Unregulated and excessive secretion of bone-resorbing substances; notably PTHrP, less frequently $1,25(OH)_2D$

CaSR, calcium-sensing receptor gene; PTH, parathyroid hormone; PTHrP, parathyroid hormone–related peptide.

hydrochlorothiazide, can be added to the regimen to reduce urinary calcium losses.

B. Hypercalcemia. Some of the causes of elevated serum calcium levels in childhood and associated biochemical findings are summarized in Table 27.4.

The clinical features of hypercalcemia are dependent on the underlying disorder, the age of the child, and the degree of hypercalcemia. Infants with mild increases in serum calcium (11 to 13 mg/dL or 2.75 to 3.25 mmol/L) often fail to manifest specific symptoms of hypercalcemia. Nonspecific signs and symptoms such as anorexia, vomiting, abdominal pain, and constipation (rarely diarrhea) may occur with moderate to severe hypercalcemia. Neurologic symptoms can range from drowsiness or irritability to confusion; in extreme cases, stupor and coma can ensue. Chronic hypercalcemia may cause only failure to thrive. The nonspecificity or absence of symptoms of hypercalcemia in young children is problematic, as unrecognized hypercalcemia in newborns or infants can cause significant morbidity or death. Polyuria as a result of renal resistance to vasopressin can lead rapidly to severe dehydration in infants. Elevated serum concentrations of calcium can cause hypertension and affect cardiac conduction, with shortening of the ST segment and heart block. Severe hypercalcemia can affect the nervous system and cause lethargy and seizures. Renal complications such as nephrocalcinosis, nephrolithiasis, or hematuria may be the earliest clinical manifestation of hypercalcemia and hypercalciuria.

The laboratory evaluation of hypercalcemia must include determination of the serum phosphorus concentration. Hypophosphatemia can cause hypercalcemia, particularly in the case of the premature or very-low-birth-weight infant who receives inadequate dietary phosphorus. Hypophosphatemia stimulates renal synthesis of calcitriol, which activates intestinal absorption and osteoclastic bone resorption, increasing transport of calcium (and phosphorus) into the circulation. Other causes of iatrogenic hypercalcemia include the use of extracorporeal membrane oxygenation, which can cause transient hypercalcemia in up to 30% of infants, and vitamin D intoxication, either from administration of excessive vitamin D supplements or infant formulas that contain very high concentrations of vitamin D.

1. **Familial hypocalciuria hypercalcemia (FHH).** FHH, also termed familial benign hypercalcemia, is genetically related to **neonatal severe primary hyperparathyroidism (NSHPT).**

   a. **Etiology.** Although adults and older children with FHH have moderate and asymptomatic hypercalcemia, infants with FHH may manifest NSPHT, a severe, life-threatening condition characterized by marked hypercalcemia during the first few days of life. NSHPT is associated with elevated PTH levels, normal to low serum phosphate, normal to high serum magnesium, elevated alkaline phosphatase, and inappropriately normal or low urinary calcium excretion. In addition, affected newborns may have osteopenia. Both FHH and NSHPT have been attributed to mutations in the *CASR* gene at 3q13.3-21 that inactivate the calcium-sensing receptor (CaSR) expressed on the surface of the parathyroid cell. In many families, NSHPT and FHH are the respective homozygous and heterozygous manifestations of the same genetic defect. NSHPT can also occur in heterozygous infants born to affected fathers but unaffected normocalcemic mothers, or in neonates with an apparent *de novo* heterozygous mutation in the *CASR* gene. Decreased receptor activity in the kidney is thought to account for relative hypocalciuria, the hallmark of the disorder. Children who survive NSHPT but who remain hypercalcemic can have poor feeding with failure to thrive, hypotonia, and developmental delay, and they may be at risk of subsequent neurodevelopmental deficits.

   The diagnosis of NSHPT is based on the presence of inappropriately normal or elevated PTH levels along with relative hypocalciuria in an infant with hypercalcemia. A family history of FHH or NSHPT in a sibling can provide strong confirmation of the diagnosis. Care must be taken to distinguish these disorders from the transient neonatal hyperparathyroidism associated with maternal hypocalcemia, as seen in mothers with pseudohypoparathyroidism or renal tubular acidosis. Genetic testing of the *CASR* gene is diagnostic for FHH and NSPHT, and is available in many commercial reference laboratories.

   b. **Clinical findings.** By comparison with equivalently hypercalcemic individuals with primary hyperparathyroidism, subjects with FHH have higher creatinine clearances and serum magnesium levels and lower values for PTH and nephrogenous cAMP excretion. A characteristic of FHH is the lower-than-expected (for the degree of hypercalcemia) urinary calcium excretion. The fractional excretion of calcium (FeCa) rather than the calcium-to-creatine ratio is the preferred method to analyze renal clearance of calcium, and it can be calculated using a spot urine sample or a 24-hour collection. The FeCa is <1% in patients with FHH or NSPHT, and it is increased in most patients with other causes of hypercalcemia. As a result of the mutation in *CASR*, it appears that various cells, including renal tubule and parathyroid cells, share a defect in divalent cation (Ca^{2+} and Mg^{2+}) transport. Because of the benign nature of the syndrome, treatment is not usually needed.

2. **Williams syndrome.** Williams syndrome is characterized by facial anomalies, cardiovascular and renal defects, hyperacusis, and visuospatial cognitive impairment, and it is often accompanied by hypercalciuria and transient infantile hypercalcemia. The cognitive impairment does not appear to be a consequence of high serum calcium levels in infancy. The facies are characteristic and the cardiovascular anomalies, e.g., supravalvular aortic stenosis, and peripheral pulmonary stenosis, also form an easily recognizable combination. The hypercalcemia may be severe and is exacerbated by dietary vitamin D supplementation.

   a. **Etiology.** Williams syndrome is classically associated with heterozygous microdeletions in the chromosomal region 7q11.2, which contains some 16 genes, including the elastin gene. The loss of the elastin gene may account for some of the morphologic and cardiac defects, but the molecular cause of the hypercalcemia remains mysterious. Serum concentrations of calcitriol have been found to be elevated in many, but not all, subjects with Williams syndrome and hypercalcemia. A disturbance in vitamin D metabolism has been proposed as the basis of the hypercalcemia and has been tentatively attributed to loss of the Williams syndrome transcription factor (WSTF) gene within the common Williams syndrome microdeletion. A similar sensitivity to vitamin D occurs in some children who lack the typical clinical and molecular features of Williams syndrome; this has been termed "idiopathic infantile hypercalcemia."

b. Treatment. Patients with Williams syndrome and idiopathic infantile hypercalcemia often respond to a low-calcium (<400 mg calcium per day) and low–vitamin D diet. Severe hypercalcemia can be treated effectively by administration of corticosteroids (hydrocortisone, 10/mg/kg per day) or bisphosphonates. The hypercalcemia usually remits between 9 and 18 months of age. Because the hypercalcemia is self-limiting, the need for continued therapy should be reassessed regularly.

3. Hyperparathyroidism

a. Pathophysiology. Primary hyperparathyroidism is very rare in childhood, although childhood neck irradiation is a significant risk factor for the later development of parathyroid adenoma as an adult. Affected children are hypercalcemic because of increased bone resorption and increased calcium absorption, the latter being a consequence of enhanced PTH-mediated calcitriol synthesis. Serum phosphorus is low because PTH decreases the renal tubular reabsorption of phosphate. PTH and calcitriol levels are elevated. Children and adolescents with primary hyperparathyroidism tend to be far more symptomatic than adults at initial presentation, which may reflect earlier case ascertainment in affected adults because of the frequent and routine measurement of serum calcium levels. Low bone density and hypercalciuria, with nephrocalcinosis or nephrolithiasis, are more common in children and adolescents than in adults with primary hyperparathyroidism. In secondary hyperparathyroidism, overactivity of the parathyroids is an appropriate response to hypocalcemia. Secondary hyperparathyroidism is seen in vitamin D–deficiency rickets and in uremia and is discussed in Chapter 25.

Tertiary hyperparathyroidism is the term used to describe the development of autonomous hypersecretion in parathyroid glands subject to prolonged stimulation. It is very rare in childhood but can occur in uremia or during prolonged therapy for hypophosphatemic rickets.

b. Treatment. See Chapter 25.

4. Immobilization

a. Pathophysiology. Prolonged immobilization or even the weightlessness of space travel can lead to rapid loss of skeletal mineral and an increased risk of fracture. Children and young adults are particularly susceptible to extensive bone loss when immobilized, resulting in hypercalciuria and often hypercalcemia. Hypercalcemia can be observed after immobilization following burns or the application of extensive lower-body casts. However, most of the time, hypercalcemia follows high spinal cord injuries that result in traumatic quadriplegia. The hypercalcemia may be severe, with impairment of renal glomerular function. The hypercalcemia appears to be almost entirely attributable to increased bone resorption. Parathyroid function and the production of calcitriol are suppressed.

b. Treatment. Early mobilization, where possible, and effective hydration can prevent the manifestations of immobilization hypercalcemia. Hydration with saline (up to 4 L per day in a fully grown adolescent, proportionately less for younger children) can increase renal calcium excretion. Under extreme conditions it may be necessary to administer furosemide (1 mg/kg, 1 to 4 times daily) to further increase the calciuresis, but loop diuretics should be used cautiously to avoid dehydration. Agents that inhibit bone resorption, such as calcitonin or bisphosphonates, may be needed when hypercalcemia or hypercalciuria is intractable or when bone loss is associated with an increased risk of fracture (see General Principles for Treatment of Hypercalcemia).

5. **Vitamin D–dependent hypercalcemia.** See Chapter 25.
6. **Malignancy.** See Chapter 25.
7. **Other causes of hypercalcemia.** A variety of unusual disorders can also cause hypercalcemia. **Neonatal transient hyperparathyroidism** may occur in infants born to mothers with poorly treated hypoparathyroidism or pseudohypoparathyroidism. The birth weights of these infants are frequently <2 500 g, but otherwise they usually appear clinically normal at birth. The pathogenetic mechanism probably involves fetal hyperparathyroidism secondary to decreased calcium transport from the hypocalcemic mother to the fetus, leading to fetal hypocalcemia. The secondary increased secretion of fetal PTH mobilizes calcium from the fetal skeleton, causing generalized skeletal demineralization and subperiosteal resorption. The hyperfunction of the parathyroid glands may persist after birth, resulting in moderate transient hypercalcemia, although most neonates have been normocalcemic and have had somewhat elevated rather than depressed plasma phosphate concentrations. Following birth, the skeleton avidly takes up calcium, and the bone lesions heal spontaneously within 4 to 6 months.

Blue diaper syndrome is caused by a defect in tryptophan metabolism that leads to urinary excretion of excessive amounts of indole derivatives, including a derivative called "indican" that gives the urine-soaked diaper a blue tint. The mechanism of hypercalcemia in this disorder is unknown. **Congenital lactase and disaccharidase deficiency** can cause hypercalcemia and hypercalciuria during the first few months of life. The etiology of the hypercalcemia is unclear but is thought to be related to metabolic acidosis and/or an increase in intestinal calcium absorption secondary to increased gut lactose.

Hypercalcemia can also occur in children with the **IMAGe** syndrome, which consists of **I**ntrauterine growth retardation, **M**etaphyseal dysplasia, **A**drenal hypoplasia congenital, and **Ge**nital defects.

Hypercalcemia and hypercalciuria are frequent findings in the **infantile form of hypophosphatasia** and reflect the imbalance between intestinal calcium absorption and skeletal deposition. The plasma concentrations of vitamin D metabolites are appropriate for the high plasma calcium with normal $25(OH)D_3$, low calcitriol, and relatively high plasma $24,25(OH)_2D$ concentration. Serum PTH levels are low or suppressed in hypercalcemic patients. Infantile hypophosphatasia presents before 6 months of age when failure to thrive and hypotonia become apparent. The characteristic radiologic findings are severe demineralization of the skeleton but less pronounced than in the perinatal form. The fontanels appear widely open because of hypomineralized areas of calvarium, but in fact functional craniosynostosis can occur with raised intracranial pressure. The patients develop hypercalcemia, hypercalciuria, and some nephrocalcinosis with renal failure. Rachitic skeletal deformities, including flail chest, predispose to pneumonia, and >50% of patients die during the first year of life. Those children who survive beyond infancy seem to show some improvement.

Chronic hypervitaminosis A appears after ingestion of excessive doses for several weeks or months. The child develops anorexia, pruritus, irritability, bone pain, and tender swellings of bone. Roentgenograms might show osteopenia, signs of increased osteoclastic bone resorption, hyperostosis of the shafts of the long bones, and osteophyte formation, particularly in the thoracic spine. Spontaneous recovery with alleviation of hypercalcemia follows discontinuation of vitamin A intake. Neonates and children who have impaired renal function appear to be at particular risk of vitamin A–induced hypercalcemia. More recently, severe hypercalcemia has been associated with administration of the vitamin D analog all-*trans*-retinoic acid (ATRA) during therapy for acute promyelocytic leukemia.

Children with **Jansen metaphyseal chondrodysplasia** have hyperkalemia and bone lesions that are typical of primary hyperparathyroidism but have suppressed PTH levels. This unusual disorder is a result of mutations in the

PTH1R gene that lead to ligand-independent activation of the receptor. This causes increased bone resorption, metaphyseal defects, elevated serum levels of $1,25(OH)_2D$, and growth delay

Hypercalcemia may also occur in patients with **severe hyperthyroidism** or **acute adrenal insufficiency.**

8. **General Principles for Treatment of Hypercalcemia.** Specific approaches that apply to distinct causes of hypercalcemia have been described previously. The general approach to the medical treatment of severe or symptomatic hypercalcemia is to **increase the urinary excretion of sodium,** because sodium clearance and calcium clearance are very closely linked during water or osmotic diuresis. Infants are frequently dehydrated, and two-thirds to full-strength saline containing 30 mEq of potassium chloride per liter should be infused to correct dehydration and maximize glomerular filtration rate. Furosemide in a dose of 1 mg/kg may be given intravenously at 6- to 8-hour intervals once hydration has been optimized to inhibit tubular reabsorption of calcium as well as sodium and water.

In most cases, hypercalcemia is a result of excessive release of calcium (and phosphorus) from the skeleton, and treatment will require an agent that can directly reduce osteoclastic bone resorption. **Calcitonin** (4 U/kg q12h) given by subcutaneous injection is effective at first, but resistance to the hormone occurs quite rapidly. Direct inhibition of bone resorption can be achieved with bisphosphonates (see Chapter 25).

III. METABOLIC BONE DISEASE

A large number of skeletal disorders in childhood are directly or indirectly attributable to systemic metabolic derangements or to metabolic disorders confined to the tissues of the skeleton.

A. Rickets

1. **General principles.** Rickets results from defects that affect cellular proliferation and mineralization of the cartilaginous epiphysial growth plate. It follows that rickets is confined to childhood, when the skeleton is growing, and affects only the growth plate. The equivalent in adults is a generalized softening of the skeleton as a result of reduction in mineralization, known as **osteomalacia.** Children with rickets often also suffer from osteomalacia, so that the shafts of the long bone as well as the growth plates are affected (Fig. 27.3). Although some characteristics of rickets vary with the cause, the widening and flaring of the epiphyses is seen with all forms. The osseous manifestations depend on the age of onset and the relative growth rate of different bones. In the first year of life the skull, upper limbs, and ribs are the fastest-growing bones and thus most prone to be affected. Accordingly, in the youngest infants, craniotabes, frontal bossing, thickening of the wrist, visible enlargement, or palpable swelling of the costochondral junction (rachitic rosary) are the characteristic skeletal manifestations. Late ambulation and delayed eruption of teeth are additional clinical findings. Because of the softening of the ribs, a depression corresponding to the costal insertion of the diaphragm (Harrison sulci) may also be visible. Craniotabes is a result of thinning of the skull and is particularly found in prematurely born infants. When pressing firmly over the occiput or posterior parietal bones, a "ping-pong" ball sensation will be felt.

The severity of involvement of particular epiphyses depends on the relative growth rate, which varies with age. Deformity because of uneven epiphysial growth and softening of the long bones is common in severe cases. The nature of the deformity is age-dependent. The typical lower-limb deformity is genu varum ("bow legs") when the age of onset is less than 3 or 4 years and genu valgum ("knock knees") when rickets starts in school-aged children. These differences are possibly a result of the changing relative rates of growth at various epiphyses.

Although vitamin D deficiency is the most common cause of rickets and osteomalacia, these conditions can also result from nutritional deficiency of calcium or genetic defects that impair activation of vitamin D, reduce target-tissue

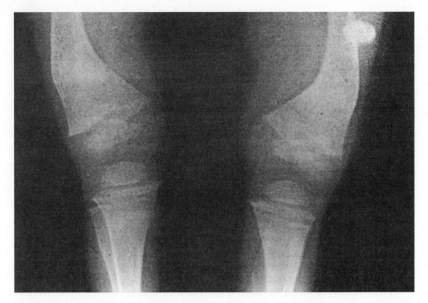

Figure 27.3. Long-standing rickets in a 5-year-old child. Note flared lower femoral and upper tibial epiphyses as well as marked angulation of lower femoral as a result of osteomalacia.

responsiveness to $1,25(OH)_2D$, or impair phosphorus reabsorption in the kidney. Regardless of the etiology, a common feature of rickets and osteomalacia is a low-normal or low serum phosphorus level. Without an adequate calcium–phosphorus product, mineralization of newly synthesized collagen matrix in the skeleton is diminished, resulting in the development of rickets in children and osteomalacia in adults.

2. **Nomenclature.** As the underlying causes of the varieties of rickets are discovered, more rational names, based on the molecular pathophysiology, have been applied to describe the specific conditions. The names of the various kinds of rickets given in this chapter have been selected because they are the least ambiguous and most informative with regard to etiology.

3. **Causes of rickets**

   a. **Vitamin D deficiency rickets.** The sources and metabolism of vitamin D are outlined in Figure 27.4, and a summary of the salient biochemical findings is presented in Table 27.5. Vitamin D and its metabolites are not only essential components in the process of bone mineralization, they also participate in the more ubiquitous "osteoimmune" system that controls cellular immune defenses. Therefore vitamin D deficiency can impair not only mineral metabolism but also immune function.

   The efficiency of the intestinal absorption and renal reabsorption of calcium and phosphorus is increased by $1,25(OH)_2D$, and vitamin D deficiency leads to hypocalcemia and secondary hyperparathyroidism.

   The early manifestations of rickets are biochemical rather than clinically recognizable or radiographic signs. The important finding at this stage is slight hypocalcemia with some or only moderate elevation of alkaline phosphatase activity (Table 27.5). The fall in plasma calcium leads to increased PTH secretion, which, in turn, normalizes the plasma calcium level. However, if the rickets proceed to a moderate stage, the compensatory secondary hyperparathyroidism leads to increased urinary excretion of cAMP, aminoaciduria, phosphaturia with subsequent fall in plasma phosphate, and rise of alkaline

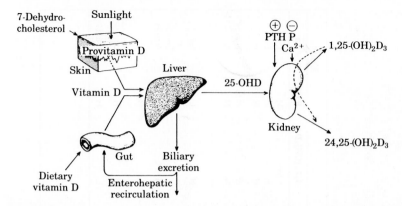

Figure 27.4. Sources and metabolic fate of vitamin D in humans. Factors promoting or antagonizing renal 1α-hydroxylation of calcidiol are indicated by + and −, respectively. 24-Hydroxylation is stimulated by calcitriol as shown by *dotted line*. (From Gertner JM. Disorders of bone and mineral metabolism. In: Clayton BE, Round JM, eds. *Chemical Pathology and the Sick Child*. Oxford, UK: Blackwell Scientific; 1984.)

phosphatase. In the florid forms of rickets, increased PTH secretion and calcium mobilization from bone can no longer compensate for the deficient calcium absorption from the intestine, and the plasma calcium concentration may drop sufficiently to induce symptoms of tetany (Table 27.5).

The plasma concentration of 25(OH)D is a sensitive index of vitamin D nutritional status, and is typically found at the lower limit or slightly below the normal range. Many published normal ranges for plasma 25(OH)D are incorrect, and a normal lower limit for plasma 25(OH)D is likely closer to 30 ng/mL than 10 ng/mL. There is no apparent relationship between the 25(OH)D concentration and the severity of the rickets. Even more perplexing, perhaps, the plasma concentration of calcitriol can be low, normal, or elevated in nutritional vitamin D deficiency, and thus can be more confusing than illuminating.

Elevated levels of circulating PTH induce phosphaturia and result in a low-normal or low serum phosphorus level. Without an adequate calcium–phosphorus product, mineralization of newly synthesized collagen matrix in the skeleton is diminished. Vitamin D metabolites are not only required for maintenance of adequate extracellular fluid calcium and phosphorus concentrations but also play important roles in skeletal growth and development. Children with vitamin D deficiency rickets often manifest bone pain and myopathy, the combination of which can lead to a loss of the skill of walking in affected toddlers. Hypocalcemia is common and can lead to tetany and even convulsions.

(1) Risk factors

   (a) Once considered to be limited to poorer children in the northern industrialized countries, vitamin D deficiency is now recognized to be common throughout the world, particularly in countries where milk is not fortified with vitamin D. Because vitamin D is obtainable from the diet or is synthesized in the skin on exposure to sunlight, most affected children suffer from a combination of inadequate nutrition and lack of exposure to direct sunlight. Infants who are exclusively breast-fed for more than 6 months and do not receive recommended supplementation with vitamin D are at particular risk, as under usual circumstances human milk is an inadequate source of vitamin D. Congenital rickets may occur in infants who are born with inadequate vitamin D stores

TABLE 27.5 Biochemical Features of Rickets

Type of rickets		Serum					Urine	
		P	Ca	HCO$_3$	25-OHD	1,25(OH)$_2$D	PTH	Ca
Nutritional	Vitamin D deficiency	L to H	L	N	L	L to H	H	L
	Ca deficiency	L	L	N	N	H	H	L
	Prematurity[a]	L	N	N	N	H	H	H
Hypophosphatemic	X-linked (PHEX)	L	N	N	N	N	N to H[a]	N to H[b]
	Autosomal dominant (FGF23)/autosomal recessive (DMP1)	L	N	N	N	N	N	N
	Hereditary hypophosphatemic rickets with hypercalciuria (SLC34A3)	L	N	N	N	H	L	H
	Fanconi syndrome	L	N	L	N	N to L	N to H	N to H
Vitamin D–dependent rickets	Type 1 (1α-hydroxylase deficiency; CYP27B)	L to N	L	N	N	L	H	L
	Type 2 (calcitriol resistance, VDR)	L to N	L	N	N	H	H	L
Uremic	Osteodystrophy	H	L to H	L	N	L	H	L to H

H, high; L, low; N, normal; PTH, parathyroid hormone.
[a]Most commonly due to relative phosphorus deprivation.
[b]Elevated PTH and urine Ca seen as consequences of treatment.
Note: Alkaline phosphatase and other markers of bone turnover are increased in all forms.

because their mothers have marginal vitamin D nutrition. Most cases involve black or darkly pigmented children, as the increased melanin in the skin absorbs ultraviolet light before it can reach the cells that synthesize vitamin D.

(b) Vitamin D deficiency rickets is common in children (and adults) who have gastrointestinal disorders that affect absorption of fats. These conditions include biliary atresia, cystic fibrosis, inflammatory bowel disease, and celiac disease. The vitamin D deficiency probably results from complex causes involving reduced exposure to sunlight, reduced dietary intake of vitamin D, and malabsorption in patients with steatorrhea. In most types of chronic liver disease, mean plasma levels of 25(OH)D are usually low normal, and in patients with rickets and osteomalacia they are usually subnormal. Reduced production of vitamin D–binding protein in the liver may contribute to the reduction of serum concentration of 25(OH)D, and also the plasma concentration of calcitriol, without reducing the biologically active free fraction. True vitamin D deficiency should be associated with elevated plasma levels of PTH. The finding of subnormal plasma concentrations of vitamin D metabolites in these patients should therefore be interpreted with caution.

(c) Vitamin D deficiency rickets is seen in children on long-term anticonvulsant therapy with specific agents that induce CYP450 drug-metabolizing enzymes (e.g., CYP3A4 and CYP24) that are present in the liver and other sites. These drugs increase the demand for vitamin D by accelerating its elimination. Phenobarbital, carbamazine, and diphenylhydantoin have been incriminated in the pathogenesis of anticonvulsant osteopathy and rickets. The doses and duration of therapy that can lead to the development of rickets have not been defined clearly. However, it is evident that only modest supplementation with vitamin D can prevent anticonvulsant rickets and that this condition affects epileptic children who are already receiving inadequate vitamin D from the diet and inadequate exposure to sunlight. A variety of other drugs that can similarly induce specific CYP enzymes, such as rifampin, have also been implicated in this pathophysiology.

(2) Medical treatment

(a) Prevention. Rickets can be prevented by sufficient exposure to ultraviolet (UV) light and/or by oral supplementation of vitamin D. For most of the children and adolescents of the world, exposure to sunlight is the principal source of vitamin D. However, because there is insufficient sunlight-derived UV light during the winter in the temperate zones for skin to produce adequate vitamin D, vitamin D supplements (200 to 400 IU per day) will protect children from rickets during these months. Because human milk contains inadequate amounts of vitamin D, all infants who are exclusively breast-fed should receive 200 to 400 IU of vitamin D daily by 6 weeks of age.

(b) Vitamin D treatment. Vitamin D deficiency rickets can be safely and effectively healed by daily doses of 50 to 100 μg or 2 000 to 4 000 IU of vitamin D. Supplemental calcium (25 to 50 mg/kg per day of elemental calcium, not to exceed 1 to 2 g per day) is also recommended. Radiologic signs of healing will usually be evident within 2 to 4 weeks, and the vitamin D dose may then be reduced to 400 IU (10 μg) daily. More protracted therapy for 6 to 8 weeks with daily doses of 2 000 IU of vitamin D may be beneficial in long-standing rickets to replenish vitamin D fat stores. In some cases, it may be more practical to administer a large dose of vitamin D (150 000 to 300 000 IU) at one time, so-called **stoss** therapy. However, the incidence of hypercalcemia after large-dose vitamin D treatment is significant, and this form of treatment should be reserved for those children who have failed more usual treatment regimens because of poor compliance. If no healing occurs, the rickets is probably resistant to vitamin D.

Anticonvulsant-induced rickets can be prevented by the daily administration of supplemental doses (e.g., 400 to 2 000 IU) of vitamin D per day. The precise dose of vitamin D needed will depend on the amount of anticonvulsant used, specific genotypes for the CYP enzymes involved, and the child's usual intake of vitamin D from exposure to sunshine and other sources. The treatment of established vitamin D deficiency consists of the administration of 1 600 to 4 000 IU daily unless intestinal malabsorption is present. This dosage can be reduced to 400 IU per day when the rickets heals. In cases of malabsorption, the optimum replacement dose may be as high as 10 000 IU per day.

Patients with vitamin D deficiency have elevated levels of PTH, which induces the expression of the 1α-hydroxylase enzyme. Therefore, treatment with vitamin D is associated with rapid increases in the plasma level of calcitriol, which can rise well above the upper limit of the normal range, often with transient hypercalcemia.

(3) Orthopedic treatment. Surgery may be needed in severe cases.

b. Calcium deficiency rickets. In recent years it has become clear that typical rickets of young children, attributed entirely to vitamin D deficiency, may be due wholly or in part to calcium deficiency. This condition has been described as endemic in parts of Africa (Nigeria and South Africa) and Asia but also occurs sporadically in other regions, including the United States. Affected patients tend to have a reduced period of breast-feeding in comparison with controls. Plasma concentrations of 25(OH)D and 1,25(OH)$_2$D are typically normal, but patients develop secondary hyperparathyroidism because of the lack of dietary calcium. Urinary excretion of calcium is very low. The reasons why some children on low calcium intake develop rickets whereas others, on the same low intake, do not, remain unclear.

(1) Treatment. In a 24-week controlled trial carried out in Nigeria, calcium supplementation (1 000 mg per day) with or without vitamin D was more effective in the management of childhood rickets than vitamin D alone.

c. Rickets of prematurity

(1) Etiology. Premature babies can develop rickets, particularly when they require parenteral hyperalimentation. Recent evidence suggests that some otherwise healthy very-low-birth-weight infants can develop rickets. This has been attributed to phosphorus deficiency in infants fed exclusively on breast milk. It has been pointed out that not only the phosphorus but also the calcium content of human milk is inadequate for the needs of the rapidly growing low-birth-weight baby.

(2) Therapy. Appropriate therapy lies in supplementing these infant's diet with calcium and phosphorus. It has been suggested that early supplementation of the feed of very-low-birth-weight infants can **prevent** rickets. Vitamin D supplements are not sufficient to prevent the rickets of prematurity and, indeed, the concentration of calcitriol is elevated, as might be expected under conditions of dietary phosphorus deprivation. With appropriate mineral supplementation, no more than the recommended daily allowance for vitamin D (400 IU per day) need be given to these infants.

d. Vitamin D–dependent rickets 1

(1) Etiology and genetics. Vitamin D–dependent rickets type 1 (VDDR1) was first termed pseudovitamin D deficiency, because the clinical findings of this condition are similar to those of ordinary vitamin D deficiency rickets, but rickets develops despite a history of adequate vitamin D intake. The complete response of the original index cases to vitamin D suggested simple vitamin D deficiency, but the continuing requirement for doses of vitamin D that are ~100 times the normal daily intake to sustain the remission indicated an unusual form of vitamin D dependency. Thus, this condition is also known as "selective and simple deficiency of calcitriol," "hereditary vitamin D-pseudodeficiency type 1," and "hereditary 25D, 1α-hydroxylase deficiency rickets."

The plasma concentration of calcitriol is low in patients with VDDR1, and it does not increase in response to parathyroid hormone administration. The observation that rickets in one patient was corrected with physiologic doses of calcitriol first suggested that this disorder represented a defect in the renal 1∼-hydroxylase (CYP27B1) that converts 25(OH)D to calcitriol. Subsequently, a wide variety of mutations in the *CYP27B1* gene at 12q13.3 has been described in affected subjects. VDDR1 is a rare cause of autosomal recessive rickets, but the disorder occurs with unusual frequency in the French Canadian population.

(2) Treatment. The drugs of choice in treatment are **calcitriol** or its synthetic analog, 1α-hydroxyvitamin D (1α-OHD) Both compounds have much shorter biological half-life than the parent vitamin D, which is an advantage in the event of inadvertent overtreatment. The biological activity of 1α-OHD is about 1/2one half to 2/3two thirds that of calcitriol. The recommended doses for treatment of active rickets are 2- to 8 μg/ per day of 1α-OHD, or 1- to 4 μg/ per day of calcitriol. Following radiologically evident healing of the rickets, the life-long substitution therapy will require 1- to 3 μg/ per day of 1α-OHD or 0.5- to 2 μg/ per day of calcitriol. To avoid overtreatment, the plasma concentration of calcium and phosphate, as well as urinary calcium excretion, should be measured periodically.

e. Vitamin D–dependent rickets 2

(1) Etiology and genetics. Vitamin D–dependent rickets 2 (VDDR2) is a rare autosomal recessive form of rickets in which target-organ resistance to calcitriol is a result of a defect in the *VDR* gene encoding the vitamin D receptor. The hallmarks of the disorder include early-onset rickets, hypocalcemia, secondary hyperparathyroidism, and very high plasma concentrations of calcitriol. The clinical features are almost identical to those that occur in patients with VDDR1, but in VDDR2 alopecia (head and body) is found in about half of the patients. In most cases alopecia develops during the first year of life, but it has also been present at birth. Patients with VDDR2 appear normal at birth and develop features of calciferol deficiency over the first 2 to 8 months of life. Alopecia, generally developing at 2 to 12 months of age, may be total or incomplete. Sometimes there is selective sparing of the eyelashes. Alopecia seems to be a marker of the more severe forms of the disease, as judged by earlier onset of hypocalcemia, more marked clinical presentation, and poor response to therapy. Other ectodermal defects have been reported in small numbers of cases and have an uncertain relation to the syndrome; these include oligodontia, epidermal cysts, and multiple milia. In several cases, neonatal development was apparently normal, and dysfunction was not evident until late in childhood or even in adulthood.

(2) Treatment. Patients with VDDR2 are usually responsive to high doses of calcitriol, or 1α-OHD, with or without calcium supplementation. Such treatment can often heal the rickets and normalize calcium homeostasis, but alopecia never improves. Cases with mild-to-moderate resistance respond to very high doses of vitamin D, which should then be of the order of 0.5 to 5 mg per day, i.e., 200 000 to 2 million IU per day. By increasing substrate in this way, these patients can sustain very high plasma levels of calcitriol in part because of deficient receptor-mediated feedback inhibition.

In cases of intermediate severity, endogenous production of calcitriol cannot be sufficiently increased with vitamin D therapy, and therapy may require extremely high doses of calcitriol or 1α-OHD, which then should be of the order of 5- to 60 μg/day. A supplementation dose of about 2 g of calcium per day is an important adjunct to avoid fluctuations of the plasma concentration of calcium due to variable dietary calcium content.

In the most severely affected patients there is complete refractoriness to the action of calcitriol on intestinal calcium absorption, even to calcitriol doses that achieve sustained plasma concentrations of the order of 2 000 pg/mL, i.e., 3 to 400 times above normal. In such cases the only effective therapy is high doses of oral or intravenous calcium.

f. Hypophosphatemic rickets

(1) Etiology and genetics. Hypophosphatemia is a characteristic of the various forms of vitamin D deficiency and dependency rickets and osteomalacia, and in these conditions reflects the decrease in TmP/GFR induced by secondary hyperparathyroidism. By contrast, hypophosphatemia also occurs in the absence of vitamin D deficiency, and with minimal, if any, hyperparathyroidism and without significant net changes in serum concentrations of PTH or calcium (Table 27.5). These diseases include genetic forms of hypophosphatemic rickets, tumor-induced osteomalacia, nutritional phosphorus deficiency, and primary renal tubular disorders. It is believed that in such cases the extracellular phosphate concentration is lower than that needed for optimal skeletal mineralization.

By far the most common cause of hypophosphatemic rickets, particularly in children, is **X-linked hypophosphatemia** (XLH, formerly termed hypophosphatemic vitamin D–resistant rickets, MIM 307800), which occurs with a prevalence of ~1 in 20 000. Serum levels of phosphate are reduced and serum calcitriol levels are reduced or inappropriately normal, while serum calcium and PTH levels are normal. Hypophosphatemia results from decreased renal tubular reabsorption of phosphorus, but in children with active rickets there is also a variable degree of reduced intestinal absorption of both phosphate and calcium. There is no evidence of a gene dosage effect, imprinting, or genetic anticipation, and there is little, if any, difference in the severity or extent of the disorder in affected males and females In its fullest expression, XLH is associated with rickets (osteomalacia in adults), lower-extremity deformities, short stature, bone pain, enthesopathy, and dental abscesses.

XLH is caused by mutations in the *PHEX* gene (phosphate-regulating gene with homologies to endopeptidases on the X chromosome) that lead to a loss of enzymatic function. *PHEX* defects have been identified throughout the gene in patients with XLH, and invariably lead to a loss of function (see http://data.mch.mcgill.ca/phexdb for Phexdatabase). Although the genetic defect is highly penetrant, the severity of disease and specific clinical manifestations are variable, even among members of the same family. Commercial laboratories now provide clinical testing for mutations in the *PHEX* gene, and defects can be identified in 80% of patients with suspected XLH. However, the presence of the trait may be readily ascertained in most patients by 6 months of age by documentation of a reduced age-corrected concentration of plasma phosphate.

Patients with XLH, and *Hyp* mice, have elevated plasma levels of FGF23, a phosphate-regulating hormone that is the principal circulating "phosphatonin." FGF23 acts directly on the kidney to alter phosphate transport and renal parameters of vitamin D metabolism. FGF23 reduces expression of the renal tubular sodium phosphate cotransporters Npt2a and Npt2c, thus impairing phosphate reabsorption in the proximal renal tubule and leading to hypophosphatemia. In addition, FGF23 suppresses activity of the renal 1α-hydroxylase while inducing activity of the renal 24-hydroxylase, which may in part explain the inappropriately normal (or low) circulating concentrations of $1,25(OH)_2D$ despite hypophosphatemia.

In addition to XLH, at least three additional forms of inherited hypophosphatemic rickets have now been described. **Autosomal dominant hypophosphatemic rickets** (MIM 193100) is caused by mutations in the *FGF23* gene that encodes the phosphatonin FGF23; **autosomal**

recessive hypophosphatemic rickets (MIM 600980) is caused by loss-of-function mutations in the *DMP1* gene that encodes dentin matrix protein 1, a noncollagenous bone matrix protein expressed in osteoblasts and osteocytes; and **hereditary hypophosphatemic rickets with hypercalciuria** (HHRH, see later) is caused by homozygous mutations in the *SLC34A3* gene encoding the renal Npt2c sodium phosphate cotransporter. Circulating levels of FGF23 are normal or elevated in subjects with XLH, ADHR, and *DMP1* mutations, but the mechanisms differ. Patients with XLH appear to be unable to degrade FGF23 normally.

(2) **Pathogenesis.** Hypophosphatemia appears in the first year of life. The biochemical findings (Table 27.5) are dominated by hypophosphatemia with normocalcemia. The ratio of renal tubular threshold maximum for phosphate to glomerular filtration rate (TmP/GFR) is always subnormal in hypophosphatemic rickets. The normal calcitriol concentration in the face of hypophosphatemia (which generally stimulates calcitriol formation) reflects the elevated circulating concentrations of FGF23 in these disorders.

(3) **Clinical findings.** The primary clinical manifestations of hypophosphatemic rickets are skeletal pain and deformity, bone fractures, slipped epiphyses, and abnormalities of growth. Classic skeletal features of rickets, such as frontal bossing, may appear as early as 6 months of age in untreated infants. Boys with XLH have early severe deformities, viz., shortness of stature and skeletal disproportions, which become apparent during childhood with the legs short relative to the trunk. The deformities include bilateral coxa vara, anterior and lateral femoral bowing, genu valgum or varum, and medial deviation and torsion of the lower third of the tibia. Unlike the findings in infants with vitamin D deficiency rickets, craniotabes and rachitic rosary are not seen. In addition to the mineralization defect induced by hypophosphatemia, an intrinsic osteoblast defect also contributes to the bone disease and does not appear to respond to conventional treatment (see below).

Proximal myopathy is absent, in contrast to the findings in hypophosphatemia that occurs in patients with tumor-induced osteomalacia or antacid-induced hypophosphatemia. Thus, the waddling gait seen in boys and severely affected girls is probably due to coxa vara. Poor dental development and spontaneous tooth abscesses may occur. There is considerable variation in the severity of the disease, particularly among girls and between families.

In middle age, other clinical problems begin to appear, with mineralization of the spinal ligaments and thickening of the neural arches. There is loss of mobility of the spine, shoulders, elbows, and hips. The lumbar spine is flat and rigid, and reduction in the diameter of spinal canal can lead to cord compression at more than one level. Painful secondary osteoarthritis in the hips and knees is common, as is a unique disorder of the entheses (tendons, ligaments, and joint capsules), with exuberant calcification of tendon and ligament insertions and of joint capsules, particularly in the hand and sacroiliac joints.

Radiologic manifestations are evident by 1 to 2 years of age and include widening, splaying, and cupping of the metaphyses and coarse trabeculation of the whole skeleton. These findings are most pronounced in the lower extremities. The characteristic wedge-shaped defect of the medial surface of the proximal tibia in patients with genu varum deformity is probably the result of the increased weight on the medial side of the knee.

Although the primary renal lesion consists of isolated proximal tubular phosphate wasting, renal glycosuria can also be seen in some older patients.

In contrast to XLH, there seems to be greater variability in the age of onset and expression of the biochemical and clinical features of ADHR. Those with childhood onset look phenotypically like XLH, but some patients present with an apparent adult-onset form of the disorder, with osteomalacia, bone pain, weakness, and fractures, but no skeletal deformity. Thus, ADHR is a phenotypically variable disorder with incomplete penetrance, delayed onset, and, in several kindreds, postpubertal spontaneous resolution of the biochemical defect.

(4) Therapy. A combination of vitamin D and oral phosphorus is the most effective therapy.

The main role of vitamin D is to raise plasma calcium, thus countering the tendency of phosphate therapy to lead to secondary hyperparathyroidism. Calcitriol is the preferred vitamin D metabolite in the management of FHR because its short half-life greatly lessens the risk and severity of iatrogenic hypercalcemia. Current practice is to use calcitriol together with a soluble phosphate preparation, giving up to 1 000 mg of phosphorus daily, divided into four doses. The dosage of calcitriol is adjusted to avoid causing hypercalciuria or hypercalcemia (usually 1 to 2 μg per day). Recent observations suggest that renal sonography is an effective way of guarding against potential renal damage from nephrocalcinosis. Hyperparathyroidism can still be troublesome in some patients treated with this type of combination therapy. It has been suggested that treatment with the metabolite 24,25-dihydroxyvitamin D can reduce PTH secretion and improve bone histology during treatment for FHR.

g. Hereditary hypophosphatemic rickets with hypercalciuria (HRHH)

(1) Etiology and genetics. HHRH is an autosomal recessive disorder that can be distinguished from other forms of inherited hypophosphatemic rickets (described previously) by the presence of elevated levels of urinary calcium and plasma calcitriol and suppressed concentrations of plasma FGF23. HHRH is caused by mutations in *SLC34A3* that reduce expression or activity of the NaPi-IIc renal sodium phosphate cotransporter.

(2) Pathogenesis. PTH and FGF23, in response to elevated levels of dietary and serum phosphorus, decrease the abundance of cotransporters at the cell membrane and thereby reduce the tubular reabsorption of phosphorus from the glomerular filtrate. Plasma levels of FGF23 are appropriately suppressed in the presence of low serum phosphate levels in HHRH, and as a result, activity of the renal 25-hydroxyvitamin D 1α-hydroxylase (CYP27B1), the rate-limiting enzyme in the two-step activation process of vitamin D, is stimulated, leading to increased production of 1,25(OH)$_2$D. This increased synthesis of 1,25(OH)$_2$D acts to normalize the serum phosphorus but also leads to increased absorption of dietary calcium and excessive bone resorption, with resultant hypercalciuria and osteopenia.

(3) Treatment. Patients with HHRH have very high serum levels of calcitriol. Such high levels of calcitriol may lead to a higher than usual efficiency of calcium absorption from the gastrointestinal tract and reduced synthesis and secretion of PTH. Together, such physiologic changes in calcium homeostasis favor hypercalciuria and thus may promote kidney stone formation. Treatment with phosphate salts without vitamin D has resulted in improvement of clinical and roentgenologic abnormalities, and decreases the urinary calcium excretion and plasma concentration of calcitriol. Thus, **vitamin D treatment is contraindicated** in this condition because it may further increase intestinal absorption of calcium and increase the risk of nephrolithiasis.

B. Osteoporosis

1. Definition. In osteoporosis, bone mass is reduced but mineralization is generally normal (see Chapter 26). This definition cannot be applied to children, who have not yet achieved peak bone mass. Although there is no generally accepted clinical definition of osteoporosis in children, it is reasonable to consider a diagnosis of osteoporosis in a child with low bone mass for age, gender, and race who has sustained a fragility fracture or skeletal deformity. A summary of some causes of osteoporosis in childhood is given in Table 27.6.

TABLE 27.6   A Classification of Osteoporosis in Childhood

Category	Diagnosis	Comment
Genetic disorders of connective tissue matrix	Osteogenesis imperfecta, Ehlers-Danlos syndrome Osteoporosis-pseudoganglioma syndrome	
Locally mediated bone resorption	Malignancies incl. leukemia Thalassemia and other causes of myeloid expansion or proliferation	Skeletal pain may be severe May be exacerbated by chelating agents used to manage iron overload
Cytokine-mediated catabolic states affecting connective tissue matrix	Inflammatory bowel disease Inflammatory arthritis	May be worsened by corticosteroid use May be worsened by corticosteroid use
Endocrine and metabolic	Hypercortisolism, iatrogenic or due to pituitary or adrenal disease Thyrotoxicosis Hypogonadism	Includes failure to convert androgens to estrogens (i.e., aromatase deficiency) and rare estrogen-receptor defects
	Anorexia nervosa	
Disuse and underuse	Congenital and acquired paraplegia Muscular dystrophy	
Unclassified	Idiopathic juvenile osteoporosis	Usually remits at puberty; heritable disorders of collagen identified in some cases

2. **Assessment of bone mass.** There is no generally accepted method for determination of bone mass in children and adolescents. Techniques to measure bone density in adults have assumed that bone mass is reflective of the extent and breadth of bone remodeling rates at specific sites, such as the spine, and portions of the hip. In children, bone modeling occurs at many sites that are not measured by these machines, and alterations in modeling may account for much more of the lack of bone mass accretion than changes in remodeling. As a result, assessment of distinct trabecular and cortical bone compartments is more critical for understanding the bone mass dynamics in children than in adults.

   Dual-energy x-ray absorptiometry (DXA) is the preferred technique to assess bone mineral density (BMD). Although DXA can accurately measure bone density in adults, several critical characteristics of DXA affect the reliability of this technique in the assessment of BMD in growing children. For example, because DXA provides an analysis of areal bone mineral density (aBMD) rather than a true determination of volumetric bone mineral density (vBMD), the size (i.e., area) of the bone assessed will have a disproportionate impact on the derived measurements for BMD. Thus the reliability of DXA to identify young patients with reduced BMD is limited by the lack of appropriate reference databases that allow for adjustments, if any, for bone size or height, weight, maturity, pubertal status, and other clinical variables. Not surprisingly, given these unique characteristics of growing children, interpretation of their DXA results is often incorrect or inadequate.

Quantitative computed tomography (qCT) is an exact method to determine vBMD in children, with adequate separation of cortical and trabecular compartments. However, enthusiasm for qCT is reduced by the relatively high radiation dose delivered.

At present, ultrasound technology remains an attractive research tool that shows promise for future clinical use in children.

An important general limitation to the use of bone densitometry in children is that the clinical implications of low BMD are less certain than in adults. In children, upper-extremity fractures, particularly forearm fractures, appear to be associated with reduced BMD. However, it is likely that BMD alone does not explain fracture risk in children (or adults), and bone quality, bone turnover, and the nature of trauma are also likely to be important contributors to the risk of fractures. Thus it has not been possible to establish BMD criteria for "fracture threshold" in children. By contrast, the proven association between low BMD and fractures in older adults led the World Health Organization (WHO) to propose quantitative criteria for "osteopenia" and "osteoporosis" that are based solely on BMD T scores, which reflect the number of standard deviation's above or below peak bone mass. It is inappropriate to express BMD in children using T scores, as children and adolescents have not yet achieved peak bone mass, and they will normally have negative T scores. The use of T scores, rather than age-adjusted Z scores, to express BMD in children and adolescents is a leading cause of misinterpretation of bone densitometry and often leads to an inappropriate diagnosis of osteoporosis. Bone densitometry by itself should not be relied on to provide a clinical diagnosis.

3. **Etiology of osteoporosis**
    a. **Specific causes.** Osteoporosis is probably the most common manifestation of metabolic bone disease in adults, but it is rare in childhood. Table 27.6 provides a general classification of osteoporosis in children and adolescents. Bone mass is determined both by modeling and remodeling. Bone begins to form (modeling) during early fetal life, and the skeleton continues to enlarge by replacement and expansion of existing bone (remodeling) well into the early third decade of life (early 20s), a bit after cessation of statural growth has occurred (see Chapter 26). Pubertal gain in bone mass represents the largest percentage increase after that seen in the first year of life, and it may respond to different sets of genes but similar environmental stressors than prior to puberty. During the pubertal growth spurt, a lag in mineralization of rapidly growing bone may lead to a transient reduction in BMD that is accompanied by temporary bone fragility that promotes fractures.

    In children, osteopenia is often a consequence of disuse atrophy of the skeleton (e.g., after immobilization for severe trauma), neuromuscular disease (e.g., Duchenne muscular dystrophy), or a consequence of glucocorticoid therapy. Osteoporosis is also seen in association with malignancy (e.g., leukemia or neuroblastoma) and in cancer survivors, and after bone marrow and solid-organ transplantation. Low bone density is also present in many children with celiac disease or cystic fibrosis as well as in many chronic inflammatory diseases (e.g., inflammatory bowel disease and juvenile idiopathic arthritis). In addition, low bone mass is a characteristic of Klinefelter, Ehlers-Danlos, Marfan, and Turner syndromes, in which osteoporosis may be present in >50% of untreated patients older than 18 years. Reduced bone density is also common in children with delayed puberty, hypogonadism, anorexia nervosa, and the female athlete triad (amenorrhea, disordered eating, and osteoporosis). Osteoporosis occurs in ~40% of children with idiopathic hypercalciuria. Osteoporosis is also a feature of many rare inherited disorders such as homocystinuria, galactosemia, as well as osteoporosis pseudoglioma (OPPG) syndrome.

b. Idiopathic osteoporosis. When these conditions and osteogenesis imperfecta (see below) have been excluded, there remain a small number of children with idiopathic osteoporosis. Recently, molecular analysis of some cases has suggested the presence of heterozygous loss-of-function mutations in the *LRP5* gene that encodes the low-density lipoprotein receptor–related protein 5. *LRP5* mutations that prevent Wnt from binding to LRP5 lead to pathway inactivation and autosomal recessive OPPG, a disorder characterized by severely reduced bone mass and neovascularization of the retina, which in turn leads <u>to retinal detachment</u> and blindness. Patients who are heterozygous for loss-of-function LRP5 mutations have moderately reduced bone mass but no eye pathology.

By contrast, mutations that prevent LRP5 from binding to cofactor Dikkopf lead to pathway activation and excessive bone formation. These activating mutations in *LRP5* cause **familial high bone mass syndrome,** an autosomal dominant form of osteopetrosis that is associated with nonpathologic high bone mass. The Wnt signaling pathway is also regulated by sclerostin, which is expressed exclusively by osteocytes in bone. Slerotosin, a product of the *SOST* gene, acts in a paracrine manner to inhibit bone formation by binding to the LRP5 and LRP6, thereby antagonizing Wnt actions. Loss of sclerostin expression in humans results in the high-bone-mass disorders Van Buchem disease and sclerosteosis, providing compelling evidence that osteocytes can control bone mass. Thus, osteocytes exert negative feedback control of osteoblast number and bone formation via production of sclerostin.

Idiopathic juvenile osteoporosis (IJO) is a rare condition that follows a rather predictable clinical pattern. IJO occurs in previously apparently healthy children of either sex in the years immediately preceding puberty. Patients present with osteoporotic collapse of one or more (usually lumbar) spinal vertebrae or with fractures of long bones, mostly at metaphyseal sites, upon minor trauma. Radiologic evidence of osteoporotic new bone is characteristic. A waddling gait is common. Bone histology sometimes shows an excess of osteocytes associated with woven bone and normal mineralization. There are no extraskeletal biochemical abnormalities.

Although disability and deformity can be severe during the active phase of the disease, IJO tends to remit spontaneously soon after the onset of puberty, although skeletal deformity may persist. The recovery presumably occurs under the influence of gonadal steroid secretion. The cause of the disease is unknown, and no satisfactory methods of therapy have been described. In severe cases, orthopedic maneuvers (splinting, casting) might be needed, but it should be remembered that the consequent local immobilization can make the degree of bone loss even worse.

c. Osteogenesis imperfecta (OI) describes several inherited conditions characterized by low bone mass and an increased incidence of bone fractures in connection with minimal trauma. Of the various forms of OI, type I is the most common, and overall OI occurs with an incidence at birth of ~1 in 5 000, with a population prevalence of about 1 in 20 000. All ethnic and racial groups seem to have a similarly affected frequency.

(1) Etiology. The various types of OI are caused by mutations that affect the nature or synthetic rate of the peptide chains that constitute type I collagen, the major collagen of the skeleton. Although some of these affect nonosseous connective tissue, the effect of most falls particularly heavily on the skeleton.

(2) Taxonomy. OI is divided into subtypes that are genetically, pathologically, and clinically distinct from one another. The taxonomy was initially clarified by Sillence and has been expanded by the description of additional new forms of OI (Table 27.7). The expanded Sillence classification is useful for clinical purposes and has superseded the formerly used terms OI congenita and OI tarda as well as other descriptive and eponymous terms.

(3) Inheritance. Types I, IV, and V are inherited as autosomal dominant conditions, whereas the other forms of OI are usually inherited in an

TABLE 27.7 Expanded Sillence Classification of Osteogenesis Imperfecta[a]

Type	Fragility	Sclerae	Teeth	Inheritance	Typically associated mutations	OMIM	Comments
IA	Present	Blue	Abnormal	Autosomal dominant	Premature stop codon in COL1A1	166240	Relatively common; normal height or mild short stature
IB	Present	Blue	Normal	Autosomal dominant	Premature stop codon in COL1A1	166200	Variable severity
IIa	Extreme	Blue[a]	—	? Dominant (germ cell)	Glycine substitutions in COL1A1 or COL1A2	166210	Perinatal lethal; multiple rib and long-bone fractures at birth; low density of skull bones
IIb	Extreme	Blue	—	Autosomal recessive	CRTAP		As above
III	Severe	Grayish	Abnormal	? Dominant (germ cell)	Glycine substitutions in COL1A1 or COL1A2	259420	Severe deformity; very short with triangular face
IVA	Present	Normal	Abnormal	Autosomal dominant	Glycine substitutions in COL1A1 or COL1A2	166220	Uncommon
IVB	Present	Normal	Normal	Autosomal dominant	Glycine substitutions in COL1A1 or COL1A2		Variable severity; moderately short, mild to moderate scoliosis
V	Present	Normal	Normal	Autosomal dominant	?	610967	Moderately deforming; mild to moderate short stature; dislocation of radial head; mineralized interosseous membrane; hyperplastic callus; meshlike bone lamellation
VI	Present	Faintly blue	Normal	Autosomal recessive	?	610968	Moderately short; excess osteoid and fish-scale pattern of bone lamellation
VII	Present	Normal	Normal	Autosomal recessive	CRTAP	610682	Mild short stature; short humeri and femora; coxa vara
VIII	Present	Normal	Normal	Autosomal recessive	LEPRE1	610915	Similar to VII

[a]Sclerae are often blue in normal infants.

autosomal recessive manner. The autosomal dominant forms of OI are sustained through the occurrence of new, spontaneous mutations. Germline mosaic in one of two healthy parents has been proposed as an explanation for the occurrence of more than one affected child with a dominant form of OI.

(4) Clinical features. The clinical features of OI depend on the genetic type of the disorder, the age of onset, and the severity of the skeletal effects. Table 27.7 summarizes the typical and distinguishing features of the various forms of OI. In general, babies affected at birth have a poor prognosis. Individuals with milder forms of OI, for example, some patients with type I, may have normal stature, no deformities, and no fractures, and the condition may be diagnosed only when a radiograph is taken for other reasons. Those with Sillence type II are born with multiple fractures that have arisen in utero, some healing with shortening and broadening of the long bones. Stillbirth or early death usually results from respiratory failure or brain damage. In type III the fractures are less widespread, and shortening and deformity of the limbs can be absent at birth. These children often survive for several years with progressive severe deformities of the long bones (Fig. 27.5). Once again, respiratory failure is often the terminal event. Respiratory complications may occur in patients with all forms of OI, particularly when there are significant thoracic deformities or kyphoscoliosis.

Basilar invagination is an uncommon but potentially fatal complication of OI. Other neurologic manifestations of OI include idiopathic seizures, macrocephaly and benign communicating hydrocephalus, and cerebral atrophy. Hearing problems may be present in ~50% of individuals after the third decade, but mild hypoacusis may be detected by careful hearing examination during childhood and adolescence. Because bone remodeling rates are increased, hypercalciuria is common and may occur in ~40% of individuals. Some patients with OI have an apparent hypermetabolic state, with increased diaphoresis and increased oxygen consumption.

Types I and IV of Sillence are milder conditions in which the mode of inheritance is dominant. The skeletal tendency to excess fracturing is accompanied by lax jointedness, easy bruisability, and conductive deafness. Joint laxity can lead to dislocation of hips and radial heads. Constipation, sprains, flat feet, and hernias may occur. The teeth can be affected by dentinogenesis imperfecta (so-called subtypes Ia and IVa), whereas subtypes Ib and IVb sufferers have normal teeth. Permanent teeth seem less affected than primary dentition. The distinguishing characteristic of type I is a persistent blueness of the sclerae (blue sclerae are normal in infancy) and in most cases normal stature. Bone mineral density can be normal at birth but fails to increase appropriately. The first fracture typically occurs in preschool children, and fractures may be present at birth. Cardiovascular problems, particularly aortic valve disease and mitral valve prolapse, can be present. Type I OI is often a consideration during the evaluation of a child with nonaccidental fractures who is suspected to be the victim of abuse. Type IV patients present a very similar clinical picture, but the sclerae are a normal white.

Type V OI is moderately deforming, and patients exhibit moderate to severe bone fragility of long bones and vertebral bodies. Patients experience fractures in the first year of life but do not have blue sclerae or dentinogenesis imperfecta. Type V OI is characterized by three distinctive radiographic features: hyperplastic callus formation at fracture sites; calcification of the interosseous membrane between the radius and ulna; and radio-opaque metaphyseal bands adjacent to the growth plates, particularly in the metaphyses of the distal femora, proximal tibias, and the distal radii. Other radiologic findings include flattened, wedge-shaped, or biconcave vertebrae and Wormian bones of the skull. Iliac biopsy specimens

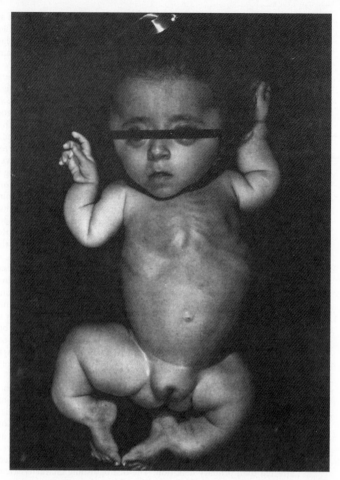

Figure 27.5. Severe deformities of long bones and ribs in a 5-year-old child with osteogenesis imperfecta. (From Gertner JM, Root L. Osteogenesis imperfecta. *Orthop Clin N Am* 1990;20:151–162.)

show lamellae that are arranged in an irregular meshlike pattern distinct from normal lamellar organization. Levels of biochemical bone markers are generally within the reference range, but serum alkaline phosphatase and urinary collagen type I N-telopeptide excretion (NTx) increase during periods of active hyperplastic callus formation

Type VI OI is a rare, moderate to severe form of the disease that has been described in the small First Nations community in northern Quebec. Multiple fractures have been noted at birth in all children. Fracture frequency decreases after puberty.

Type VII and type VIII OI share similar phenotypes. Type VII OI is caused by homozygous mutation of the *CRTAP* gene encoding cartilage-associated protein, a protein that is required for prolyl 3-hydroxylation of fibrillar type I and II collagens. Type VIII OI is a lethal/severe form of osteogenesis imperfecta that is caused by mutation in the *LEPRE1* gene, which encodes prolyl 3-hydroxylase 1 (P3H1). Accordingly, type VIII OI closely resembles type VII OI clinically. The phenotype of this form of OI overlaps Sillence lethal type II/severe type III osteogenesis imperfecta. Affected patients have severe osteoporosis, shortened long bones, and a soft skull with wide open fontanels. Several features distinguish type VIII from other lethal forms of OI, including white sclerae, a round face, and a short barrel-shaped chest.

4. **Treatment of osteoporosis.** Although there is little evidence that calcium and vitamin D supplementation is of benefit in childhood osteoporosis, it is recommended that such children maintain an adequate calcium intake and receive sufficient supplemental vitamin D to sustain normal serum levels of 25(OH)D (i.e., >32 ng/mL).

To prevent immobilization bone loss, weight-bearing activity should be maximized, which in healthy children and adolescents has been shown to increase bone mineral accrual and bone size. For children with extreme bone fragility, swimming and hydrotherapy may be beneficial. In nonambulant children with cerebral palsy, a standing frame to facilitate an upright position has been shown to improve BMD, with the gains in BMD being proportional to the duration of standing.

Bisphosphonates have been shown to increase bone density and reduce fractures in children and adolescents with a variety of forms of osteoporosis, but these agents must still be considered investigational and experimental in children. Bisphosphonates are potent antiresorptive agents that disrupt osteoclastic activity by preventing the attachment of osteoclast precursor cells to both. Histomorphometric studies in OI have shown that pamidronate increases bone mass by increasing cortical thickness and trabecular number. Pamidronate, a powerful nitrogen-containing bisphosphonate, suppresses bone turnover in children with OI to well below that of normal age-matched controls. This can interfere with bone modeling and result in undertubularization of long bones. In the growing skeleton, a reduction in bone remodeling results in the accumulation of mineralized cartilage within the bone. The mineralized cartilage has a high density, which contributes to the increase in bone density seen with pamidronate treatment. Further, acute reductions in remodeling and persistence in calcified cartilage account for the characteristic sclerotic metaphyseal lines seen on long-bone radiographs of children receiving cyclic pamidronate therapy. Suppressed bone remodeling can also interfere with the repair of microdamage and may account for the delay in osteotomy and possibly fracture repair seen in children with OI who receive pamidronate. Oral bisphosphonates may result in chemical esophagitis.

Bisphosphonates are contraindicated during pregnancy, and all females of reproductive age should have a negative pregnancy test before each treatment cycle or before commencing oral bisphosphonates. Because bisphosphonates persist in mineralized bone for many years, there is theoretical concern that bisphosphonates administered before conception could be released from the maternal skeleton during the pregnancy and affect the fetus.

Many studies, most of which have been uncontrolled, have shown that administration of bisphosphonates, particularly cyclical intravenous pamidronate (mean dose 6.8 mg/kg IV every 4 to 6 months) to children with severe OI can alleviate bone pain, reduce the incidence of fractures, enhance growth, and improve overall quality of life. It appears that the best response to pamidronate therapy occurs in children who are first treated in infancy. These findings highlight the importance of prompt diagnosis and initiation of medical and supportive therapy during early life. The mean incidence of radiologically confirmed fractures decreased by 1.7 per year ($p < 0.001$), but treatment did not alter the rate of fracture healing, the growth rate, or the appearance of growth plates. Mobility and ambulation improved in 16 children and remained unchanged in the other 14. All children reported substantial relief of chronic pain and fatigue. Twenty-six children experienced an "acute-phase reaction" on the second day of the first infusion cycle; this was controlled with acetaminophen and did not recur during subsequent treatment cycles.

Both intravenous and oral bisphosphonates have been used successfully in children and adolescents with other forms of osteoporosis. No new fractures were observed after alendronate therapy was initiated. Intravenous pamidronate also appears to be a useful therapeutic option in childhood osteoporosis. Treated children have reported rapid pain relief following the first treatment, followed by large increments in lumbar spine bone density over 1 year (increments of 26% to 54% compared to the expected increases due to growth of 3% to 15%).

C. Uremic osteodystrophy (UOD)

  1. Pathogenesis

  a. Growth failure, skeletal deformity, and severe orthopedic problems, especially in the weight-bearing lower limbs, can all result from UOD. Growth failure and biochemical and histologic abnormalities can occur in children with mild renal impairment (GFR 25 to 50 mL/min per 1.73 m^2), but the most severe forms are confined to children with more pronounced renal failure.

  b. The bony disorder arises principally from a combination of inadequate vitamin D activation and hyperparathyroidism. The latter is itself a result of compensation for the calcium-lowering effects of low levels of calcitriol and high plasma phosphate concentrations. Histologically and radiologically, the bones show a combination, to varying degrees, of osteomalacia with rickets and hyperparathyroid bone disease. The hyperparathyroidism contributes to bone resorption, which can be observed on radiographs as subperiosteal erosions of the phalanges and erosions of the metaphysial corners of the long bones. Histologically, the picture is one of fibrosis and high osteoclast activity. Severe destruction and lysis of epiphysial areas, particularly the hips, can occur, giving rise to the so-called rotting stump appearance or to necrosis of the femoral heads.

  c. The biochemical features accompanying UOD are given in Table 27.5. It should be noted that uremic children are generally acidotic and that the acidosis may contribute to the severity of the skeletal problem.

  2. Treatment. Considerable importance is attached to the management of childhood UOD during conservative treatment for chronic renal failure. Adequate nutrition, including an adequate calcium intake, should be maintained and acidosis corrected. The tendency to hyperphosphatemia can be reduced by dietary restriction and the administration of phosphorus-binding substances. Several different calcium salts (e.g., calcium carbonate and calcium acetate) as well as nonabsorbable calcium- and aluminum-free agents (e.g., lanthanum carbonate and sevelamer hydrochloride) are now preferred over aluminum hydroxide gel for this purpose. These agents work by binding to phosphate in the gastrointestinal tract, thereby making it unavailable to the body for absorption. Therefore, for optimal efficacy these drugs must be taken with meals to bind any phosphate that may be present in the ingested food.

  Active vitamin D metabolites, usually calcitriol, are given to maintain the serum calcium, to improve skeletal mineralization, and to suppress secretion and synthesis of PTH. PTH secretion can also be directly inhibited using calcimimetics that modulate activity of CaSRs that are expressed on the surface of parathyroid cells. Patients with end-stage renal disease tend to have fewer and/or less sensitive CaSRs. Thus Cinacalcet, a type II calcimimetic agent that binds to the transmembrane region of the CaSR, induces a structural configuration that increases the sensitivity of CaSRs to ambient Ca^{2+} concentrations and thereby reduces PTH secretion.

Selected References

Arikoski P, Silverwood B, Tillmann V, et al. Intravenous pamidronate treatment in children with moderate to severe osteogenesis imperfecta: assessment of indices of dual-energy

X-ray absorptiometry and bone metabolic markers during the first year of therapy. *Bone* 2004;34:539–546.

Astrom E, Jorulf H, Soderhall S. Intravenous pamidronate treatment of infants with severe osteogenesis imperfecta. *Arch Dis Child* 2007;92:332–338.

Cheng JB, Levine MA, Bell NH, et al. Genetic evidence that the human CYP2R1 enzyme is a key vitamin D 25-hydroxylase. *Proc Natl Acad Sci U S A* 2004;101:7711–7715.

Colletti RB, Pan MW, Smith EWP, et al. Detection of hypocalcemia in susceptible neonates. The Q–oTc interval. *N Engl J Med* 1974;April 25:290(17):931–935.

Dent CE, Friedman M. Idiopathic juvenile osteoporosis. *Q J Med* 1966;34:177–210.

DiMeglio LA, Peacock M. Two-year clinical trial of oral alendronate versus intravenous pamidronate in children with osteogenesis imperfecta. *J Bone Miner Res* 2006;21:132–140.

Forman DT, Lorenzo L. Ionized calcium: its significance and clinical usefulness. *Ann Clin Lab Sci* 1991;21:297–304.

Henrich LM, Rogol AD, D'Amour P, et al. Persistent hypercalcemia after parathyroidectomy in an adolescent and effect of treatment with cinacalcet HCl. *Clin Chem* 2006;52:2286–2293.

Hochberg Z, Bereket A, Davenport M, et al. Consensus development for the supplementation of vitamin D in childhood and adolescence. *Horm Res* 2002;58:39–51.

Juppner H, Schipani E, Bastepe M, et al. The gene responsible for pseudohypoparathyroidism type Ib is paternally imprinted and maps in four unrelated kindreds to chromosome 20q13.3. *Proc Natl Acad Sci U S A* 1998;95:11798–11803.

Kollars J, Zarroug AE, van Heerden J, et al. Primary hyperparathyroidism in pediatric patients. *Pediatrics* 2005;115:974–980.

Land C, Rauch F, Travers R, et al. Osteogenesis imperfecta type VI in childhood and adolescence: effects of cyclical intravenous pamidronate treatment. *Bone* 2007;40:638–644.

Letocha AD, Cintas HL, Troendle JF, et al. Controlled trial of pamidronate in children with types III and IV osteogenesis imperfecta confirms vertebral gains but not short-term functional improvement. *J Bone Miner Res* 2005;20:977–986.

Lowery MC, Morris CA, Ewart A, et al. Strong correlation of elastin deletions, detected by FISH, with Williams syndrome: evaluation of 235 patients. *Am J Hum Genet* 1995;57:49–53.

Misra M, Pacaud D, Petryk A, et al. Vitamin D deficiency in children and its management: review of current knowledge and recommendations. *Pediatrics* 2008;122:398–417.

Rizzoli R, Bonjour JP. Determinants of peak bone mass and mechanisms of bone loss. *Osteoporos Int* 1999;9(suppl 2):S17–S23.

Schwaderer AL, Cronin R, Mahan JD, et al. Low bone density in children with hypercalciuria and/or nephrolithiasis. *Pediatr Nephrol* 2008;Dec 23(12):2209–2214.

Semler O, Fricke O, Vezyroglou K, et al. Results of a prospective pilot trial on mobility after whole body vibration in children and adolescents with osteogenesis imperfecta. *Clin Rehabil* 2008;22:387–394.

Specker BL, Tsang RC, Ho ML, et al. Low serum calcium and high parathyroid hormone levels in neonates fed "humanized" cow's milk-based formula. *Am J Dis Child* 1991;145:941–945.

Stewart AF, Adler M, Byers CM, et al. Calcium homeostasis in immobilization: an example of resorptive hypercalciuria. *N Engl J Med* 1982;306:1136–1140.

Strom TM, Juppner H. PHEX, FGF23, DMP1 and beyond. *Curr Opin Nephrol Hypertens* 2008;17:357–362.

Troughton O, Singh SP. Heart failure and neonatal hypocalcemia. *Br Med J* 1972;4:76–79.

Verge CF, Silink M, Howard NJ, et al. Effects of therapy in X-linked hypophosphatemic rickets. *N Engl J Med* 1991;325:1843–1848.

Zaloga GP. Hypocalcemia in critically ill patients. *Crit Care Med* 1992;20:251–262.

Zeitlin L, Rauch F, Plotkin H, et al. Height and weight development during four years of therapy with cyclical intravenous pamidronate in children and adolescents with osteogenesis imperfecta types I, III, and IV. *Pediatrics* 2003;111:1030–1036.

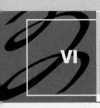

VI   *Thyroid Disorders*

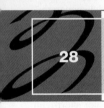

28   **EVALUATION OF THYROID FUNCTION**
Peter A. Singer

**I. GENERAL PRINCIPLES OF THYROID HORMONE SECRETION AND METAB-
OLISM**

A. Hypothalamic–pituitary–thyroid axis. The thyroid hormones thyroxine (T_4) and
tri-iodothyronine (T_3) are secreted under the stimulatory influence of pituitary thyrotropin (thyroid-stimulating hormone, or TSH). TSH secretion is primarily regulated by a dual mechanism.

   1. Thyrotropin-releasing hormone (TRH), a hypothalamic tripeptide, traverses a
   venous plexus connecting the stalk median eminence and the anterior pituitary
   and stimulates the synthesis and release of TSH.

   2. The thyroid hormones T_4 and T_3 directly inhibit pituitary TSH secretion. T_4
   has more of an inhibitory effect than T_3, and exerts its effect on the thyrotroph
   via intracellular conversion to T_3. Thyroid hormone also exerts a lesser negative
   feedback effect on the hypothalamus.

   Figure 28.1 depicts the hypothalamic-pituitary-thyroid axis. (Note that a
   number of other factors alter TSH secretion, either directly or indirectly, although
   the role of any of these agents as a physiologic regulator of TSH secretion is most
   likely minor.)

B. Thyroid-binding proteins and free hormone. Thyroid hormone exists in circulation in both free (or unbound) and bound forms. The amount of free hormone,
which is the metabolically active component of thyroid hormone, is extremely small,
accounting for ~0.03% of total circulating T_4 and ~0.3% of total circulating T_3,
respectively. The majority of hormone is avidly bound to thyroid-binding proteins,
the most important of which is thyroxine-binding globulin (TBG), which accounts
for 75% of thyroid hormone binding. The other binding proteins, thyroid-binding
prealbumin (TBPA), also termed transthyretin, and albumin, account for ~15% and
~10% of binding of T_4, respectively. T_3 is not bound to TBPA or albumin.

   1. Alterations in the concentrations of the thyroid-binding proteins, mainly TBG,
   result in changes in the concentrations of T_4 and T_3. An increase in TBG results

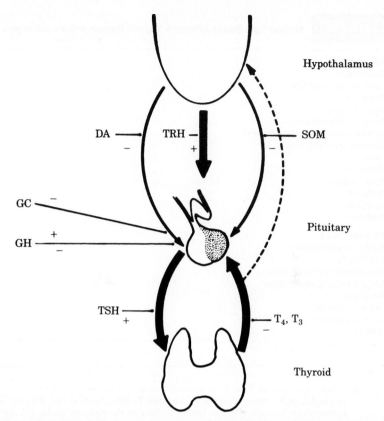

Figure 28.1. Hypothalamic–pituitary–thyroid axis. Dopamine (DA) and somatostatin (SOM) may be minor physiologic regulators of thyroid-stimulating hormone (TSH) secretion. The possible inhibitory effects of growth hormone (GH) may be via stimulating hypothalamic SOM synthesis. Glucocorticoids (GC) may have effects on both the thyrotrope and the hypothalamus. TRH, thyrotropin-releasing hormone; T_3, tri-iodothyronine; T_4, thyroxine.

in increased thyroid hormone levels, and TBG deficiency results in lower total T4 and T3 concentrations. However, the amounts of free hormone *do not change,* so that thyrometabolic status remains unchanged, despite alterations in TBG concentrations. The states of altered TBG concentrations are shown in Table 28.1.

2. Changes in the concentrations of either TBPA or albumin lead to less significant alterations in serum T_4 levels because of the significantly smaller binding affinity of T_4 for these proteins. There is, however, a syndrome of familial euthyroid T_4 excess, in which abnormal binding of T_4 (but not of T_3) to serum albumin occurs. In this disorder, free T_4 (FT_4) remains normal. Also, there is a rare disorder of increased serum levels of TBPA, in which total T_4 is elevated and FT_4 is normal.

C. Peripheral metabolism of thyroid hormone

1. The thyroid gland is the sole source of circulating T_4. Approximately 80% of circulating T_3, however, is derived from peripheral tissue (mainly hepatic and renal) deiodination of T_4 to T_3. Therefore, only 20% of the daily production of T_3 is derived from thyroid gland secretion. Approximately 80 to 90 μg of T_4 is secreted by the thyroid gland daily, and the average daily production of T_3 is ~20 to 30 μg.

TABLE 28.1	Altered TBG States Affecting Thyroid Hormone Concentrations

TBG excess
Pregnancy
Estrogen administration
Tamoxifen
Acute hepatitis
Chronic active hepatitis
Acute intermittent hepatic porphyria
Estrogen-producing tumors
Heroin
Methadone
Perphenazine
Clofibrate
Idiopathic
Heredity

TBG deficiency
Androgen administration
Acromegaly
Testosterone-producing tumors
Large doses of glucocorticoids
Nephrosis
Hypoproteinemia
Chronic liver disease (e.g., cirrhosis)
Heredity

TBG, thyroxine-binding globulin.

2. When conversion of T_4 to T_3 is impaired, an alternative deiodinative pathway is employed, and a stereoisomer of T_3, **reverse T_3 (RT$_3$)**, is produced. RT_3 has no known tissue biologic effect or feedback effect on the pituitary gland. The daily production rate of RT_3 is ~30 μg, the majority of which is derived from T_4. Factors that impair T_4 to T_3 conversion are listed in Table 28.2.

II. THYROID FUNCTION TESTS
A. In vitro tests
1. Serum T_4 (average reference range 5–12 μg/dL). Serum T_4 is measured by immunochemiluminometric assay (ICMA) methods and usually reflects the

TABLE 28.2	Factors That Inhibit T_4-to-T_3 Metabolism

Systemic illness (acute or chronic)
Caloric deprivation: fasting, anorexia nervosa, protein-calorie malnutrition
Surgery
Newborn status
Aging
Glucocorticoids
Propranolol
Amiodarone
Ipodate, iopanoic acid
Propylthiouracil

T_3, tri-iodothyronine; T_4, thyroxine.

functional state of the thyroid. However, changes in the concentration of thyroid-binding proteins, usually secondary to estrogen therapy or pregnancy, alter the concentration of T_4 without affecting thyrometabolic status (see Section I.B.1). Other factors that may alter the concentration of total T_4 without changing metabolism include nonthyroidal illness, peripheral resistance to thyroid hormone, endogenous antibodies to T_4, and certain drugs (see later). Thus, in some circumstances, the serum T_4 may not accurately reflect the metabolic status of the individual. Nonthyroidal systemic illnesses may also be associated with abnormal total T4 levels, with low concentrations of T4 in $\sim25\%$ of seriously ill individuals, and mildly elevated T4 levels in $\sim2\%$ of ill patients.

2. **Free thyroxine (FT$_4$)** (average reference range 0.8 to 2.0 ng/mL). The serum FT_4 most accurately reflects metabolic status and should not be affected by alterations in serum proteins or nonthyroidal illness. The "gold standard" is measurement of FT_4 by equilibrium dialysis, which separates free T4 from T4 bound to plasma proteins; however, the dialysis method is time-consuming and relatively expensive, so its clinical usefulness is limited. Most commercial FT_4 assays are not dialysis methods; they are immuno (ICMA) assays, and they may be affected by changes in binding proteins. To overcome this limitation, a reasonably accurate estimate of FT_4 may be calculated. This is done by multiplying the serum total T_4 by an indirect assessment of TBG capacity. Indirect TBG methods vary; they include the T_3 uptake test, the thyroid uptake test, and the thyroid uptake ratio. Whatever method is used, an estimate of FT_4 (also termed free T_4 index, FT_4I) generally correlates closely with FT_4. Many laboratories nowadays have abandoned doing T3 uptake tests, so clinicians need to rely on FT4 measurements rather than on estimates of free T4.

3. **Serum T$_3$** (average reference range 80 to 180 ng/dL). T_3 is measured by ICMA methods. Because T_3 is bound to TBG, it is subject to the same changes as T_4 because of alterations of binding proteins. Therefore, a free T_3 index (FT_3I) can be obtained using the same method as that used in calculating an FT_4I. Because the principal source of circulating T_3 is T_4, the conditions that affect the metabolism of T_4 also affect T_3 levels (see Table 28.2). Alternatively, free T3 may be measured, either by radioimmunoassay (RIA), or by dialysis. Clinically, illness is the most common nonthyroidal condition associated with low serum T_3.

4. **Serum TSH** (average reference range 0.3 to 3.0 mU/L). Methodological advances in the measurement of TSH have resulted in this test being ideally suited for detecting very mild thyroid dysfunction. Most commercial assays have a functional sensitivity of 0.01 mIU/L and enable clinicians to detect even the mildest forms of hyperthyroidism. TSH is typically measured by ICMA methods. Although TSH assays are highly sensitive and reproducible, the TSH test has limitations, especially in hospitalized patients (see Section III).

B. **In vivo tests**
   1. **Radioactive iodine uptake (RAIU) test.** The RAIU test is performed by administering ^{123}I orally and measuring the percent uptake of the radionuclide dose from 4 to 24 hours later. The test is most useful for differentiating between high- and low-uptake types of hyperthyroidism and should be performed in hyperthyroid patients in whom a diagnosis of Graves disease is not evident. The average normal range for the 24-hour RAIU test in the United States is 8% to 25%. Table 28.3 classifies hyperthyroidism according to the RAIU test.
   2. **TRH test.** This test historically was used to assess pituitary TSH reserve, as well as the degree of TSH suppression. As a result of the widespread availability of sensitive TSH assays, this test is rarely used in the United States today, although it's still used occasionally in other countries, especially in Latin America.
   3. **T$_3$ suppression test.** This is also a test of historical interest, and was designed to test autonomous thyroid function. The widespread availability of accurate biochemical tests and thyroid imaging techniques has rendered this test obsolete.
C. **Other serologic tests.** A number of tests associated with thyroid autoimmunity, such as measurement of antithyroglobulin and antimicrosomal antibodies, antibodies to T_4 and T_3, and thyroid-stimulating and -blocking antibodies, are discussed in

TABLE 28.3	RAIU in Hyperthyroid States

High RAIU	Low RAIU
Graves disease	Subacute thyroiditis
Toxic multinodular goiter	Painless thyroiditis
Toxic adenoma	Graves disease with acute iodine load
Hashitoxicosis	Iodine-induced hyperthyroidism
Choriocarcinoma	Thyroid hormone therapy
Hydatidiform mole	Metastatic functioning thyroid carcinoma
TSH-producing pituitary tumor	Struma ovarii

RAIU, radioactive iodine uptake; TSH, thyroid-stimulating hormone.

Chapter 30. The usefulness of serologic tests for thyroid cancer, such as measurement of thyroglobulin and calcitonin, is discussed in Chapter 31.

III. EVALUATION OF SUSPECTED THYROID DYSFUNCTION
A. Hypothyroidism
1. **Primary hypothyroidism.** The laboratory diagnosis of primary hypothyroidism is established by the presence of a low serum T4 (or free T4) and an elevated serum TSH. The serum TSH is the most sensitive test in the diagnosis of primary hypothyroidism. In mild hypothyroidism, the T_4 level may be within normal limits in the presence of TSH elevation. This is termed **subclinical hypothyroidism.** A suggested algorithm for evaluation of suspected hypothyroidism employing the serum TSH is shown in Figure 28.2.
2. **Secondary hypothyroidism.** A low serum T_4 and a normal or low serum TSH suggest the diagnosis of secondary (pituitary) or tertiary (hypothalamic)

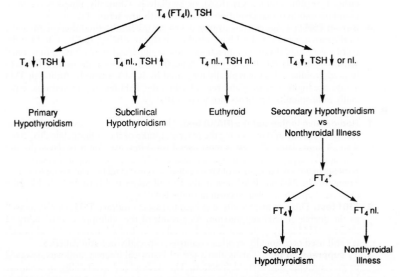

Figure 28.2. Laboratory evaluation of suspected hypothyroidism. FT$_4$, free T$_4$; FT$_4$I, free T$_4$ index; nl, normal; TSH, thyroid-stimulating hormone; T$_4$, thyroxine; (*Where there is uncertainty about the clinical diagnosis, FT$_4$ should be measured by equilibrium dialysis to avoid changes induced by binding proteins.)

hypothyroidism. Such patients must be further evaluated for suspected pituitary or hypothalamic disease. Patients with low serum T_4 and normal or low serum TSH levels secondary to nonthyroidal illness must also be differentiated from patients with secondary and tertiary hypothyroidism (see Chapter 30).

   3. **Serum T_3.** The serum T_3 is not useful in the evaluation of suspected hypothyroidism, because it may be normal in up to one third of hypothyroid individuals. Therefore, this test is not recommended for patients with suspected hypothyroidism.

B. Hyperthyroidism

   1. Figure 28.3 outlines a strategy for evaluating patients with suspected hyperthyroidism. Note that the serum TSH is important in this strategy, in part because rare types of hyperthyroidism, including TSH-producing pituitary tumors and central thyroid hormone resistance, are associated with inappropriately normal or only mildly elevated TSH concentrations.

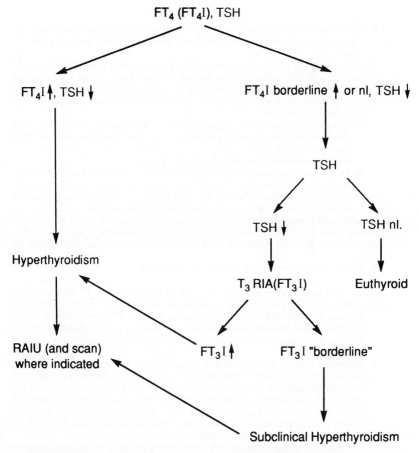

Figure 28.3. Laboratory evaluation of suspected hyperthyroidism. This approach can be used for evaluation of obvious hyperthyroidism. Otherwise, serum TSH should be used as a first-line test (see text). FT_3, free T_3; FT_3I, free T_3 index; FT_4I, free T_4 index; nl, normal; RIAU, radioactive iodine uptake; T_3, tri-iodothyronine; TSH, thyroid-stimulating hormone; T_4, thyroxine.

	Test				
State	**T₄**	**T₃**	**FT₄I**	**Free T₄**	**TSH**
TBG excess	↑	↑	N	N	N
Abnormal albumin binding	↑	N	↑	N	N
Increased TBPA	↑	N	↑	N	N
Peripheral thyroid hormone resistance	↑	↑	↑	↑	N or ↑
Nonthyroidal illness (mild)	↑	↓	↑	N, ↑, or ↓	N
Amiodarone therapy	↑	N	↑	↑	N

TABLE 28.4 Thyroid Function Tests in Hyperthyroxinemia without Hyperthyroidism

FT₄I, free T₄ index; N, normal; TBG, thyroxine-binding globulin; TBPA, thyroxine-binding prealbumin; TSH, thyroid-stimulating hormone; T₃, tri-iodothyronine; T₄, thyroxine; ↑, elevated; ↓, lowered.

2. The serum T4 (or FT4) is elevated with all types of hyperthyroidism except for "T₃ toxicosis," in which serum T₃ levels are elevated and serum T₄ may be normal.

3. Serum T₃ levels are elevated in virtually all patients with hyperthyroidism, and patients with Graves disease have disproportionate T₃ elevations in comparison with other types of hyperthyroidism. It is not necessary to obtain T₃ levels to make a diagnosis of hyperthyroidism. However, a T₃ measurement is helpful in the following situations:

  a. In patients with symptoms suggestive of hyperthyroidism in whom serum TSH levels are suppressed and FT₄ levels are normal or borderline elevated. Such patients may include those being treated for thyrotoxic Graves disease, or those with autonomously functioning thyroid adenomas.

  b. In patients with hyperthyroxinemia who have normal TSH concentrations. Such individuals may have the inherited defect of peripheral resistance to thyroid hormone, or an inherited defect in binding-carrier proteins. Table 28.4 outlines hyperthyroxinemic states without hyperthyroidism.

C. Pitfalls of TSH measurements. It should be stressed that the serum TSH is most reliable if measured in otherwise healthy, ambulatory individuals. There are a number of conditions in which the serum TSH does not accurately reflect thyrometabolic status.

  1. Nonthyroidal illness (sick euthyroid syndrome). The serum TSH may be low or even suppressed in hospitalized patients with severe illness. During recovery, the TSH may become elevated, although usually not above 10 mU/L. Despite alterations in TSH concentrations during illness, FT₄ levels remain normal, and patients are euthyroid. A pitfall in the measurement of FT₄ levels, though, is that commercial and hospital laboratories do not routinely employ dialysis methods, so FT₄ measurements may also be affected by illness, or by significant changes in binding proteins.

  2. Changing thyroid status. Thyroid status must be stable to allow reliable interpretation of the serum TSH. Although a suppressed TSH level is indicative of hyperthyroidism in the untreated thyrotoxic individual, patients who are being treated with antithyroid drugs or who have undergone thyroid ablation with radioactive iodine for hyperthyroidism may exhibit suppressed TSH levels for several months after serum T₄ and T₃ have reached normal levels. This reflects prolonged suppression of the hypothalamic–pituitary–thyroid axis.

  Hypothyroid patients recently begun on thyroid hormone therapy also may have discordant serum TSH and T₄ levels because of the lag in fall of TSH after initiation of thyroid hormone therapy. Thus, normal serum T₄ and elevated TSH levels after a month or so of therapy may not necessarily reflect underreplacement with levothyroxine (L-T4). This underscores the recommendation that dose changes should be made no more frequently than every 6 to 8 weeks, unless the clinical situation dictates otherwise.

Variable compliance L-T4 therapy may also give misleading results. Patients who take medication intermittently, or who take it consistently for only a few weeks prior to an office visit, may have relatively normal serum T4 and elevated serum TSH levels.

3. **Central hypothyroidism.** As mentioned previously, hypothyroidism due to either hypothalamic or pituitary disease is characterized by low serum T4 and normal TSH levels. Therefore, relying on the serum TSH to screen for possible hypothyroidism in such patients will result in a failure to make the correct diagnosis. Fortunately, most individuals with central hypothyroidism exhibit additional hormone deficiencies or have symptoms of a mass effect (such as visual abnormalities), thus decreasing the likelihood that the correct diagnosis may be overlooked.

4. **Hyperthyroidism associated with inappropriate TSH secretion**
   a. **TSH-secreting pituitary tumor.** Serum TSH levels are elevated or inappropriately normal in patients with hyperthyroidism due to TSH-producing tumors. Such lesions are rare, comprising only ~0.5% of all pituitary tumors, and are typically macroadenomas.
   b. **Central resistance to thyroid hormone.** This rare genetic disorder is characterized by elevated serum T4 and T3 levels and inappropriately normal or mildly elevated TSH concentrations. As with patients with TSH-producing pituitary tumors, awareness of this disorder will prevent inappropriate therapy for hyperthyroidism.

D. **Other uses for serum TSH.** In addition to screening for thyroid dysfunction, measurement of serum TSH is useful for **(1)** assessing adequacy of thyroid hormone replacement in patients with hypothyroidism; **(2)** assessing adequacy of thyroid hormone–suppressive therapy in patients with differentiated thyroid cancer; and **(3)** assessing TSH-suppressive therapy in patients with nodular goiter. It should be mentioned that the use of L-T4 for goiter or benign nodules is being used much less nowadays.

IV. **EFFECTS OF DRUGS ON THYROID FUNCTION** (Table 28.5)
Many pharmacologic agents can significantly affect thyroid function by **(1)** altering central regulation of TSH secretion, **(2)** altering thyroid hormone synthesis or release, **(3)** affecting the concentration of thyroid-binding proteins and binding affinity of thyroid hormones for proteins, **(4)** altering peripheral thyroid hormone metabolism or thyroid hormone uptake into cells, and **(5)** impairing gastrointestinal absorption of administered hormones.

A. **Drugs that affect central regulation of TSH secretion**
   1. **Dopamine,** an agent that is commonly used in the intensive care unit, causes central inhibition of TSH secretion; therefore, a low TSH in a patient receiving dopamine is often not reliable. The degree of TSH inhibition with dopamine is insufficient to result in central hypothyroidism, however.
   2. **Glucocorticoids,** when given in pharmacologic amounts, inhibit TSH secretion. Hospitalized patients receiving steroids frequently have low TSH levels. As with dopamine, patients receiving glucocorticoids do not become hypothyroid because of inhibition of TSH.
   3. **Octreotide,** a synthetic analog of somatostatin used in the management of acromegaly, decreases TSH levels but does not cause hypothyroidism because the effects on TSH secretion are minor.
   4. **Bexarotene,** a retinoid x-receptor ligand, is currently approved for the treatment of cutaneous T-cell lymphoma. It affects thyroid function by inhibiting TSH production and results in secondary hypothyroidism.

B. **Drugs that affect thyroid hormone synthesis or release**
   1. **Decreased thyroid function**
      a. **Iodides** may cause hypothyroidism by inhibiting thyroid hormone release. Hypothyroidism secondary to iodides most often occurs in individuals with

TABLE 28.5 Effects of Pharmacologic Agents on Thyroid Function

Site of action and drug	Serum T$_4$	Free T$_4$	T$_3$	TSH	Comments
Hypothalamic–pituitary axis					
Dopamine	↓	↓	↓	↓	
Levodopa	N	N	N	↓	Clinical hypothyroidism not seen in normals
Glucocorticoids	↓	↓	↓	↓	
Amphetamines	↑	↑	↑	N or ↑	Clinical effects minor
Metoclopramide	N	N	N	↑	TSH increase transient
Baroxetane	↓	↓	↓	↓	Clinical effects—hypothyroidism
Thyroid synthesis/release					
Sulfonamides, sulfonylureas, PAS, phenylbutazone, aminoglutethimide, 6-mercaptopurine	↓	↓	↓	↑	Effects minor and usually with underlying thyroid abnormality
Lithium carbonate	↓	↓	↓	↑	Synergistic with iodides producing hypothyroidism
Iodides	↓	↓	↓	↑	
Sunitinib	↓	↓	↓	↑	
Altered protein binding					
Estrogens, perphenazine, clofibrate, heroin, methadone	↑	N	↑	N	Increased TBG concentrations; normal FT$_4$, FT$_3$
Androgens, danazol, glucocorticoids, L-asparaginase,	↓	N	↓	N	Decreased TBG concentrations; normal FT$_4$
Phenytoin	↓	↓	N	N	Inhibits T$_4$, T$_3$ binding to TBG; additional effects on metabolism (see text)
Salsalate, salicylates, fenclofenac	↓	N		N	Inhibits T$_4$, T$_3$ binding to TBG
Altered thyroid hormone metabolism					
Propranolol, propylthiouracil, glucocorticoids	N	N	↓	N	Inhibits peripheral T$_4$-to-T$_3$ conversion
Ipodate, iopanoic acid, amiodarone	↑	↑	↑	↓	Inhibits intrapituitary as well as peripheral T$_4$-to-T$_3$ conversion; also iodide effects with amiodarone
Phenytoin	↓	↓	N	N	Accelerates cell uptake and disposal of T$_4$ clinical changes observed in T$_4$-treated patients with hypothyroidism
Phenobarbital	↓	↓		↑	Accelerates disposal; changes noted only in T$_4$-treated patients
Heparin	N	↑	N	N	Decreased cell uptake of T$_4$
Ipodate	↑	↑	↓	↑	Decreased cell uptake of T$_4$
Inhibits gastrointestinal absorption of thyroid hormone					
Cholestyramine, colestipol, ferrous sulfate, calcium carbonate, aluminum hydroxide, sucralfate, proton pump inhibitors	↓	↓	↓	↑	Take L-T$_4$ at least 4 h apart

FT$_3$, free tri-iodothyronine; FT$_4$, free thyroxine; N, normal; TBG, thyroxine-binding globulin; TSH, thyroid-stimulating hormone; T$_3$, tri-iodothyronine; T$_4$, thyroxine.

underlying thyroid disease, especially chronic autoimmune (Hashimoto) thyroiditis or previously treated Graves disease. Common over-the-counter cold preparations contain sufficient amounts of iodides to result in thyroid hormone **inhibition.**

Amiodarone, an antiarrhythmic drug, contains 37% iodine by weight and has been shown to produce primary hypothyroidism in ~10% of patients treated with this agent in the United States, particularly those individuals with underlying chronic autoimmune thyroiditis.

b. **Lithium carbonate,** an agent used in the management of manic depression, inhibits thyroid hormone release, resulting in decreased T4 and increased TSH concentrations in 15% to 40% of patients, most with underlying autoimmune thyroid disease. If used in conjunction with iodides, the effects tend to be significant.

c. **Ketoconazole,** an antifungal agent known to inhibit adrenal steroidogenesis, also has been reported to cause hypothyroidism, probably by impairing thyroid hormone synthesis. The clinical effects of ketoconazole are minor.

d. **Cytokines** (see Chapter 29), especially interferon-α and interleukin-2, may cause hypothyroidism, usually in individuals with underlying chronic autoimmune thyroiditis.

e. **Thionamides** (methimazole, propylthiouracil), used in the treatment of thyrotoxicosis, decrease thyroid hormone synthesis.

f. **Sunitinib,** a tyrosine kinase inhibitor used for the treatment of advanced renal cell cancer and refractory gastrointestinal stromal tumors, causes hypothyroidism in up to 40% of patients. The mechanism is not completely known, but it may relate to a form of thyroiditis, because a significant number of patients have suppressed TSH levels prior to developing primary hypothyroidism (with elevated TSH levels).

2. **Increased thyroid function**

a. In addition to **inhibiting** thyroid function, iodides can also **increase** thyroid function. Patients with nodular goiter who have autonomously functioning thyroid tissue may develop hyperthyroidism following exogenous iodide ingestion or intravenous administration, usually within 2 to 3 weeks.

b. **Amiodarone** may also cause hyperthyroidism, either because of iodide excess in patients with underlying goiter or because of induction of a painless thyroiditis-type syndrome in patients without a history of thyroid disease (see Chapter 29).

c. **Cytokines** may result in hyperthyroidism by producing a thyroiditis-typical response (see Chapter 29).

C. **Drugs that affect thyroid-binding proteins**

1. **Alterations in thyroid-binding protein concentrations**

a. **Increased TBG** concentration is usually caused by pregnancy or estrogen-containing compounds but may also be increased by other drugs (see Table 28.1).

b. **Decreased TBG** concentrations are produced by androgens, such as danazol (an agent used in the treatment of endometriosis) and L-asparaginase (an anticancer drug).

c. The net effect of altering TBG concentrations is to produce corresponding increases in total T_4 and T_3 when TBG is increased, or, when TBG levels are lowered, a decrease in T_4 and T_3 levels. Free hormone concentrations remain unaltered, and patients are euthyroid.

2. **Alterations in thyroid-binding protein affinity.** Several drugs inhibit binding of thyroid hormone to TBG. Clinically, the most frequently observed changes occur with phenytoin, where the effect is to lower total T_4 levels without changing TSH. Fenclofenac and salsalate may also cause similar changes.

D. **Drugs that alter metabolism of thyroid hormone**

1. **Peripheral T_4 deiodination.** A number of pharmacologic agents inhibit T_4-to-T_3 deiodination, with a resultant decrease in T_3. Propranolol, propylthiouracil, and glucocorticoids exert their effects primarily via hepatic and renal deiodinative

pathways. Iodate, iopanoic acid, and amiodarone, in addition to decreasing peripheral T_4-to-T_3 conversion, also inhibit intrapituitary T_4-to-T_3 conversion. This may result in a mild increase in TSH secretion, with a secondary mild increase in serum T_4 and free T_4 levels. Increased T_4 levels have also been observed in patients taking large doses of propranolol.

2. **Agents that affect cellular uptake of thyroid hormone.** Phenytoin appears to increase the cellular uptake of T_4 into tissues; in addition, it accelerates T4 metabolism, by increased liver activity of cytochrome P450. This is important to recognize because patients taking thyroid hormone for hypothyroidism who also take phenytoin will require greater doses of thyroid replacement. Similarly, **phenobarbital,** as well as the antituberculosis drug rifampin, appears to accelerate T_4 metabolism, and hypothyroid patients receiving replacement therapy also may require increased doses of T_4.

E. **Agents that affect absorption of administered thyroid hormone.** The hypolipidemic agents cholestyramine and colestipol, as well as soybean flour, inhibit absorption of exogenous thyroid hormone by binding T_4 and T_3 in the gut. The antiinflammatory agent sucralfate may also have similar effects, as does ferrous sulfate, especially when taken with thyroid hormone. Calcium carbonate, when ingested along with levothyroxine, has also been shown to cause mild inhibition of thyroxine absorption. Therefore, patients taking thyroid hormone should be instructed to take their medication several hours apart from drugs that interfere with thyroid hormone absorption.

Selected References

Arafah BM. Increased need for thyroxine in women with hypothyroidism during estrogen therapy. *N Engl J Med* 2001;344:1743–1749.

Basaria S, Cooper DS. Amiodarone and the thyroid. *Am J Med* 2005;118:706–714.

Bocchetta A, Bernardi F, Pedditzi M, et al. Thyroid abnormalities during lithium treatment. *Acta Psychiatr Scand* 1991;83:193–198.

Borst GC, Eil C, Burman KD. Euthyroid hyperthyroxinemia. *Ann Intern Med* 1983;98:366.

Casko G, et al. Direct and indirect techniques for free thyroxin compared in patients with nonthyroidal illness: effect of prealbumin and thyroxin-binding globulin. *Clin Chem* 1989;35:1655.

Chopra IJ, et al. Thyroid function in nonthyroidal illnesses. *Ann Intern Med* 1983;98:946.

Cooper DS. Thyroxine suppression therapy for benign nodular disease. *J Clin Endocrinol Metab* 1995;80:331–334.

Demers LM, Spencer CA. The National Academy of Clinical Biochemistry Laboratory Medicine Practice Guidelines: laboratory support for the diagnosis and monitoring of thyroid disease. www.nacb.org/Impg/thyroid_Impg_pub.stm.

Emerson CH, Dyson WL, Utiger RD. Serum thyrotropin and thyroxine concentrations in patients receiving lithium carbonate. *J Clin Endocrinol Metab* 1973;36:338.

Faber J, Kirkegaard C, Rasmussen B, et al. Pituitary-thyroid axis in critical illness. *J Clin Endocrinol Metab* 1987;65:315–320.

Fradkin JE, Wolff J. Iodide-induced thyrotoxicosis. *Medicine* 1983;62:1.

Hamblin PS, Dyer SA, Mohr VS, et al. Relationship between thyrotropin and thyroxine changes during recovery from severe hypothyroxinemia or critical illness. *J Clin Endocrinol Metab* 1986;62:717–722.

Klee GG, Hay ID. Biochemical thyroid function testing. *Mayo Clin Proc* 1994;69:469–470.

Larsen PR. Feedback regulation of thyrotropin secretion by thyroid hormones. *N Engl J Med* 1982;306:23.

Larsen PR, Alexander NM, Chopra IJ, et al. Revised nomenclature for tests of thyroid hormones and thyroid related proteins in serum. *J Clin Endocrinol Metab* 1987;64:1089.

Moses AC, Lawler J, Haddow J, et al. Familial euthyroid hyperthyroxinemia resulting from increased thyroxine-binding to thyroxine-binding prealbumin. *N Engl J Med* 1982;306:966–969.

Refetoff S, Weiss RE, Usala SJ. The syndromes of resistance to thyroid hormone. *Endocr Rev* 1993;14:348–399.

Ross DS. Hyperthyroidism, thyroid hormone therapy and bone. *Thyroid* 1994;4:319–326.

Samuels MH, Pillote K, Asher D, et al. Variable effects of nonsteroidal anti-inflammatory agents on thyroid test results. *J Clin Endocrinol Metab* 2003;88:5710–5716.

Sawin CT, Geller A, Wolfe PA, et al. Low serum thyrotropin concentrations as a risk factor for atrial fibrillation in older persons. *N Engl J Med* 1993;77:334–338.

Schimmel M, Utiger RD. Thyroidal and peripheral production of thyroid hormones. *Ann Intern Med* 1977;87:760.

Silva JE. Effects of iodine and iodine-containing compounds on thyroid function. *Med Clin North Am* 1985;69:881.

Simons RJ, et al. Thyroid dysfunction in elderly hospitalized patients: effect of age and severity of illness. *Arch Intern Med* 1990;150:1249.

Singer PA, Cooper DS, Levy EG, et al. Treatment guidelines for patients with hyperthyroidism and hypothyroidism. *JAMA* 1995;273:808–812.

Smallridge RC. Thyrotropin secreting tumors. *Endocrinol Metab Clin North Am* 1987;16:765–792.

Wartofsky L. Does replacement thyroxine therapy cause osteoporosis? *Adv Endocrinol Metab* 1993;4:157–175.

Wartofsky L, Burman KD. Alterations in thyroid function in patients with systemic illness: the "euthyroid sick syndrome." *Endocr Rev* 1982;3:164.

Weiss R, Wu SY, Refetoff S. Diagnostic tests of the thyroid. In: DeGroot LJ, Jameson JL, eds. *Endocrinology.* 5th ed. Philadelphia: Elsevier-Saunders; 2006:1899–1961.

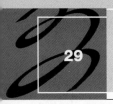

29

THYROIDITIS
Peter A. Singer

$\mathcal{T}$he various types of thyroiditides encompass a heterogeneous group of inflammatory disorders of diverse etiologies and clinical features. With all forms of thyroiditis, destruction of the normal follicular architecture occurs, yet each disorder has distinctive histologic characteristics. Varying classifications of thyroid inflammatory disorders have been proposed. For the purpose of this chapter, thyroiditis is subdivided into painful and painless types (Table 29.1).

PAINFUL THYROIDITIS

I. ACUTE THYROIDITIS (SUPPURATIVE THYROIDITIS, ACUTE BACTERIAL THYROIDITIS, PYOGENIC THYROIDITIS)

   A. Etiology. This rare disorder generally occurs only in immunocompromised hosts, although before the advent of antimicrobial therapy it was typically associated with mastoiditis or severe pharyngeal infections. It is usually caused by a bacterial pathogen, most commonly *Staphylococcus aureus, Streptococcus hemolytica, Streptococcus pneumoniae,* or anaerobic streptococcal organisms. Infection due to other bacterial pathogens, such as *Meningococcus, Salmonella,* and *Escherichia coli,* has been reported, as well as fungal infections such as coccidioidomycosis. Infection occurs either secondarily to hematogenous or lymphatic spread, or as a result of direct introduction of an infective agent by direct trauma. Persistent thyroglossal duct abnormalities have also been associated with acute thyroiditis.

   B. Clinical features. Fever, chills, and other systemic signs or symptoms of abscess formation are present. Rapid onset of anterior neck pain and swelling are usual, with pain occasionally radiating to the ear or mandible. The physical examination is notable for the presence of a tender, fluctuant mass, with erythema of the overlying skin.

   C. Laboratory tests. Leukocytosis with a left shift is usually present. Thyroid hormone concentrations in blood are usually normal, although hyperthyroxinemia has been reported, probably as a result of discharge of preformed hormone. The thyroid scan (which is indicated in any patient with a tender anterior neck mass) reveals an absence of isotope uptake in the involved area. If acute thyroiditis is suspected, fine-needle aspiration should be performed, and appropriate smears and cultures obtained.

   D. Differential diagnosis. The differential diagnosis includes any disorder associated with an acutely tender, painful anterior neck mass, including subacute thyroiditis, cellulitis of the anterior neck, acute hemorrhage into a thyroid cyst, adenoma or carcinoma, anterior deep neck space infection, infected thyroglossal duct cyst, and infected branchial cleft cyst (Table 29.2).

   E. Treatment. Parenteral antibiotics should be administered according to the specific pathogen identified. If fluctuance is present, incision and drainage are required. Bacterial thyroiditis must be managed early and aggressively because abscess formation can occasionally dissect downward into the mediastinum. Recurrences of the disorder are very rare, as is permanent thyroid dysfunction. If recurrence of acute thyroiditis occurs, an examination is indicated to facilitate discovery of an undiagnosed defect, such as an internal fistula or thyroglossal duct cyst.

| **TABLE 29.1** | Classification of Inflammatory Thyroid Disorders |

Painful thyroiditis
Infectious agents
   Pyogenic (bacterial) thyroiditis
   Subacute viral thyroiditis
   Opportunistic agents (e.g., *Pneumocystis carinii, Mycobacteriae, Aspergillus*)
Trauma
   Radiation thyroiditis
   Direct trauma (e.g., fine-needle aspiration, surgery, palpation)

Painless thyroiditis
Spontaneous disorders
   Chronic autoimmune (Hashimoto) thyroiditis
   Subacute lymphocytic (postpartum) thyroiditis
   Subacute lymphocytic (sporadic) thyroiditis
Pharmacologic agents
   Cytokines (interferon-α, interleukin-2)
   Amiodarone-induced thyroiditis
   Lithium carbonate
Invasive fibrous (Riedel) thyroiditis

II. SUBACUTE THYROIDITIS (VIRAL THYROIDITIS, SUBACUTE GRANULOMATOUS THYROIDITIS, DE QUERVAIN THYROIDITIS, GIANT CELL THYROIDITIS)

  A. Etiology. Subacute thyroiditis (SAT) is most likely <u>viral</u> in origin. Viruses implicated to be responsible for the disorder include coxsackie virus, adenovirus, mumps virus, echovirus, influenza, and the Epstein-Barr virus. Clinical evidence suggesting a viral cause includes reports of outbreaks of infection, the common presence of a viral-like prodrome, and a summer and fall seasonal distribution of the illness. In addition, convalescent sera to viral antibodies are present in patients with SAT.

  B. Clinical features. The most common symptom is unilateral <u>anterior neck pain</u>, often associated with radiation of pain to the ear or mandible. The pain is often preceded by a few weeks of myalgias, low-grade fever, malaise, and sore throat.

| **TABLE 29.2** | Differential Diagnosis of the Painful Neck Mass |

Subacute viral thyroiditis
Hemorrhage into thyroid cyst or nodule
Acute bacterial thyroiditis
Infected thyroglossal duct cyst
Infected branchial cleft cyst
Rapidly enlarging thyroid cancer
Painful Hashimoto thyroiditis
Radioactive thyroiditis
Trauma-induced thyroiditis
Cellulitis of the anterior neck

Note that subacute viral thyroiditis and hemorrhage into a cyst or nodule constitute the overwhelming majority of painful thyroid lesions.

Dysphagia is also common. Symptoms of thyrotoxicosis are common and include tachycardia, palpitations, weight loss, nervousness, and diaphoresis. As the disorder progresses, pain often migrates to the contralateral side.

Physical examination reveals a very tender, hard, ill-defined mass that is usually unilateral, although tenderness of the opposite lobe may be present. Tenderness is often so extreme that palpation is limited. Tachycardia, warm skin, and a fine tremor of the hands are also observed when hyperthyroidism is present.

C. Laboratory tests

1. The complete blood count usually reveals a mild normochromic-normocytic anemia and a normal total white blood cell count. However, mild leukocytosis may occur. The erythrocyte sedimentation rate is usually >50 mm per hour. The serum thyroxine (T_4) or free thyroxine (FT4) and tri-iodothyronine (T_3) levels are often elevated, and the serum thyrotropin (thyroid-stimulating hormone, TSH) is suppressed. The severity of the thyrotoxicosis correlates with the degree of the destructive process. There tends to be a disproportionate elevation of serum T_4 relative to serum T_3, because the blood levels reflect proportional amounts of preformed hormones released into the circulation during the active inflammatory phase.

2. Thyroid autoantibodies (antimicrosomal [TPO] and antithyroglobulin) may be mildly elevated several weeks after the onset of symptoms and then return to normal, usually within a few months. The transient antibody elevation is probably a response to the release of thyroglobulin into the circulation and not an autoimmune response. The serum thyroglobulin is significantly elevated during active inflammation.

3. The thyroid radioactive iodine uptake (RAIU) is always suppressed during the acute phase of the illness, usually to <2% at 24 hours. The suppressed uptake is a result of disruption of the iodine-trapping mechanism from the inflammation and cell destruction. The RAIU test is necessary to confirm the clinical diagnosis of SAT and is essential in excluding other disorders associated with a painful anterior neck mass.

D. Differential diagnosis. Subacute thyroiditis must be differentiated from both euthyroid and hyperthyroid states associated with pain in the anterior neck (Table 29.2).

E. Clinical course and treatment. Subacute thyroiditis typically consists of four phases.

1. The initial, or acute, phase is associated with pain, tenderness, a suppressed RAIU, and hyperthyroidism. This phase lasts for anywhere from 4 to 12 weeks, during which treatment is directed to relief of pain, inflammation, and symptoms of hyperthyroidism. Prednisone, 10 to 20 mg orally, 2 to 4 times a day, is virtually always effective in reducing pain, often within several hours of the initial dose. Indeed, if the pain does not abate quickly, the clinician should question the diagnosis of SAT. After 1 to 2 weeks, the prednisone can be tapered by 5 mg every 2 to 3 days. An increase in pain may occur during steroid tapering, at which time the prednisone dosage can be increased again and the tapering process resumed.

   Very mild bouts of SAT may be treated with nonsteroidal anti-inflammatory agents.

   Symptoms of thyrotoxicosis may be controlled with the use of β-adrenergic–blocking agents. Antithyroid drugs are not indicated, nor would they be of any benefit.

2. Following the acute painful thyrotoxic phase, euthyroidism is restored, as the thyroid becomes depleted of stored hormone. Patients may either remain euthyroid or, in more severe cases, progress to a hypothyroid phase, characterized by biochemical and at times symptomatic hypothyroidism. The hypothyroid phase rarely lasts longer than 2 to 3 months, and during this interval, thyroid hormone replacement, in the form of sodium levothyroxine (LT_4), 0.10 to 0.15 mg per day, should be given. After several months of treatment, LT_4 can be discontinued and a serum TSH repeated in 6 to 8 weeks.

3. Following the hypothyroid phase, _recovery_ occurs, and the normal histologic features and secretory capacity of the thyroid are restored. During this phase, plasma thyroid hormone levels are normal, but the RAIU can be temporarily elevated because of avid iodine trapping by the recovering thyroid. It should be emphasized that it is unnecessary to perform RAIU tests during the course of SAT, except initially to confirm the diagnosis. Although permanent hypothyroidism has been reported following subacute thyroiditis, it is uncommon, and patients almost always return to euthyroidism. However, it has been shown that administration of exogenous iodides in patients with prior episodes of SAT may result in hypothyroidism. Thus, even though SAT is nearly always self-limiting, patients with a history of SAT who receive iodides should be evaluated for hypothyroidism with a serum TSH.

III. RADIATION THYROIDITIS

Radiation thyroiditis is usually characterized by mild to moderate anterior neck pain and thyroid tenderness, and may occur approximately a week after receiving ^{131}I for thyrotoxic Graves disease. Symptoms may last for up to a month after ^{131}I administration.

Patients treated with ^{131}I for thyroid cancer may also develop radiation thyroiditis, especially if a significant amount of normal thyroid tissue was left remaining after thyroidectomy. If pain and tenderness is significant, short-term prednisone (20 to 40 mg per day) may be used.

IV. _PNEUMOCYSTIS CARINII_ (PCC) THYROIDITIS

Pneumocystis carinii thyroiditis has been reported by several authors, and its clinical characteristics are similar to those of SAT, including neck pain, either hyperthyroidism or hypothyroidism, and a suppressed RAIU. **_Pneumocystis carinii_** should be considered in immunocompromised patients with neck pain. The diagnosis can be established only by performing a fine-needle aspiration and staining for **_P. carinii_** organisms with Gomori silver methenamine. This form of thyroiditis has become extremely rare, because aerosolized pentamidine is no longer used for PCC prophylaxis.

PAINLESS THYROIDITIS

Spontaneous Disorders

I. SUBACUTE LYMPHOCYTIC THYROIDITIS (PAINLESS THYROIDITIS, SUBACUTE LYMPHOCYTIC THYROIDITIS, SILENT THYROIDITIS)

   A. Background. This disorder is characterized by symptoms of thyrotoxicosis, elevated serum T_4 and T_3 levels, a suppressed serum TSH, a low RAIU, and a painless nontender goiter. Subacute lymphocytic thyroiditis (PT or LT) usually occurs in women, and most patients are seen postpartum. Sporadic cases are uncommon. The disorder is reported to occur in ~8% of postpartum women in North America.

   B. Etiology. The subacute lymphocytic variant of painless thyroiditis is most likely autoimmune in origin and is probably a variant of chronic autoimmune (Hashimoto) thyroiditis (see later). Approximately 80% of patients have elevated levels of thyroid microsomal (TPO) antibodies. A genetic predisposition is also likely because there is a significant prevalence of HLA-DRw3 and HLA-DRw5 histocompatibility antigens. Because of the similar clinical course that LT shares with SAT, a viral cause has also been suggested.

   C. Clinical features

   1. Hyperthyroid symptoms, such as nervousness, palpitations, anxiety, diaphoresis, heat intolerance, and weight loss, are common, varying from mild to marked, depending on the severity of the disorder. Postpartum cases occur anywhere from 6 weeks to 3 months after delivery.

TABLE 29.3	Differentiation between Painless Lymphocytic Thyroiditis and Graves Hyperthyroidism	

Clinical feature	Lymphocytic thyroiditis	Graves thyroiditis
Onset	Abrupt	Gradual
Severity of symptoms	Mild to moderate	Moderate to marked
Duration of symptoms (usual)	<3 mo	>3 mo
Goiter	Firm, diffuse, mildly enlarged, or absent	Mildly to moderately firm, diffuse, large
Thyroid bruit	Absent	Often present
Exophthalmos, dermopathy	Absent	May be present
T_4/T_3 ratio	<20:1	>20:1
RAIU	Suppressed	Elevated

RAIU, radioactive iodine uptake; T_3, tri-iodothyronine; T_4, thyroxine.

2. Physical examination often discloses a mildly enlarged, nontender goiter, although up to 50% of patients have been reported to have absence of palpable goiter.
3. The clinical features of PT may also be very difficult to distinguish from those of Graves disease. Clinical and laboratory findings that may be helpful in differentiating the two disorders are listed in Table 29.3.

D. Laboratory tests
1. Serum total and free T_4 and T_3 levels are mildly to moderately elevated, and the serum TSH is suppressed. Serum T_3 levels are less elevated proportional to T_4 levels than is observed with Graves disease. The ratio of T_3 to T_4 has been suggested as being helpful in distinguishing LT from Graves thyrotoxicosis, in which T_3 levels are considerably higher because of preferential secretion of T_3 by thyroid-stimulating immunoglobulin.
2. The RAIU is suppressed, usually to <3% at 24 hours, during the hyperthyroid phase of LT. It is essential to obtain a RAIU test unless the diagnosis of Graves disease is clinically evident on clinical grounds.

E. Differential diagnosis. Once Graves disease has been excluded, the differential diagnosis of painless hyperthyroidism associated with a low RAIU must be considered (see Chapter 30). Most of the disorders can be readily distinguished from each other based on a careful history and physical examination.

F. Clinical course and treatment. The clinical course of PT is similar to that of SAT:
1. There is an initial hyperthyroid phase lasting from ~6 weeks to 3 or 4 months (rarely longer). Treatment during this phase is directed to relief of hyperthyroid symptoms, using beta-blockers. Antithyroid drugs, such as methimazole and propylthiouracil, are ineffective and should be avoided.
2. Following the hyperthyroid phase there is a euthyroid interval of ~3 to 6 weeks, during which the thyroid becomes depleted of hormone.
3. This is followed in 25% to 40% of patients by a hypothyroid period, during which symptomatic and biochemical hypothyroidism may occur. Hypothyroidism usually lasts no longer than 2 to 3 months, and thyroid hormone supplementation with LT_4 may be required.
4. Following the hypothyroid phase, patients usually remain clinically euthyroid. Persistent thyroid abnormalities, such as goiter and/or frank hypothyroidism occur in up to one third of patients. Thus, long-term follow-up of patients who have had an episode of PT is necessary. Patients who have had postpartum PT are at significant risk of experiencing a recurrence following a subsequent pregnancy. Postpartum thyroiditis occurs in ~25% of women with type 1 diabetes mellitus.

| **TABLE 29.4** | Differentiating Features of Amiodarone-Induced Hyperthyroidism |

	Type 1 (iodine excess)	Type 2 (thyroiditis)
History of thyroid disease	Often	No
Goiter	Nodular	Small or absent
FT_4	↑, ↑↑	↑, ↑↑
FT_3	↑	↑
TSH	↓	↓
IL-6	N or slightly ↑	↑
Thyroid RAIU	↓, N, occasionally ↓	↓
Color Doppler ultrasound	Increased flow	Decreased flow

FT_3, free tri-iodothonine; FT_4, free thyroxine; IL-6, interleukin-6; N, normal; RAIU, radioactive iodine uptake.

II. HASHIMOTO THYROIDITIS (HT; ALSO KNOWN AS CHRONIC AUTOIMMUNE THYROIDITIS, CHRONIC LYMPHOCYTIC THYROIDITIS, CHRONIC THYROIDITIS)

A. Etiology. HT is an organ-specific autoimmune disorder that is the most common thyroid inflammatory disease. The basic defect underlying this disorder likely is due to an abnormality in suppressor T lymphocytes that allows helper T lymphocytes to interact with specific antigens directed against the thyroid cell. A genetic predisposition is suggested because of the frequent occurrence of HLA-DR5 and HLA-B8 histocompatibility antigens in patients with HT. The disorder may be associated with other organ-specific autoimmune disorders (Table 29.4).

B. Clinical manifestations

1. HT may exhibit a wide spectrum of clinical features, ranging from an asymptomatic euthyroid individual with a goiter to frank myxedema. It is the principal cause of hypothyroidism in the iodine-sufficient world. The most common presentation is that of a middle-aged woman with a small, asymptomatic goiter. Approximately 95% of patients are women. Occasionally, patients may complain of mild anterior neck discomfort, especially if the thyroid is enlarging rapidly, although this is uncommon. In general, thyroid enlargement is insidious and asymptomatic. Symptoms of hypothyroidism may be present, depending on the degree of hypothyroidism, if present. Hypothyroidism is the presenting manifestation in ~20% of patients.

2. Physical examination usually discloses a symmetrically enlarged, very firm goiter; a pebbly or knobby consistency is common. Occasionally, patients present with a single thyroid nodule.

3. Although hypothyroidism is the typical form of thyroid dysfunction associated with HT, a smaller subset of patients (probably 2% to 4%) present with hyperthyroidism and have "hashitoxicosis." Thyroid-stimulating immunoglobulin has been detected in the sera of some of these patients, suggesting commonality with Graves disease.

C. Laboratory tests

1. Approximately 80% of patients with HT have normal circulating T_4 and TSH levels at the time of diagnosis. Antimicrosomal (TPO) antibodies are elevated in >90% of patients. Although antithyroglobulin antibodies also are generally elevated, performing both tests is unnecessary.

2. The presence of a rapidly enlarging, firm to hard goiter and strikingly elevated thyroid TPO antibodies, especially in elderly patients, should alert the clinician to the possibility of primary thyroid lymphoma. However, HT is not felt to be etiologic in the development of lymphoma.

3. The thyroid ultrasound (not recommended in routine evaluation) reveals a heterogenous, micronodular pattern, often with increased blood flow on Doppler exam.

D. Treatment

1. Levothyroxine (L-T$_4$) is the treatment of choice for HT when hypothyroidism is present. Goiters tend to shrink with normalization of TSH levels. Thyroid hormone should be continued indefinitely in hypothyroid patients with HT. Patients with mild thyroid failure (i.e., normal serum T$_4$ levels and elevated TSH concentrations) have an ~5% per year likelihood of becoming overtly hypothyroid, so L-T$_4$ administration may be warranted in such patients.

2. Pharmacologic doses of glucocorticoids have been reported to be effective in HT when there is a rapidly enlarging goiter associated with pressure symptoms. Such a presentation is rare, though, and if glucocorticoids are employed, their use should be brief.

3. Surgery is indicated in HT only if persistent significant symptoms of obstruction are present. Such a scenario is rare.

III. RIEDEL THYROIDITIS (RIEDEL STRUMA)

Riedel thyroiditis is an extremely rare inflammatory disorder of uncertain etiology, and earlier suggestions that it might be a fibroid variant of HT have not been substantiated. Clinically, Riedel thyroiditis presents with pressure symptoms, and on examination an extremely hard, "woody," immobile thyroid gland is palpated. Riedel thyroiditis has a female-to-male prevalence of 3:1 and usually occurs between the ages of 30 and 60 years. The disorder may be associated with other focal sclerosing syndromes, including retroperitoneal and mediastinal fibrosis, and ascending cholangitis, so patients with Riedel thyroiditis should be evaluated for the possibility of other sclerosing conditions. Thyroid function tests reveal hypothyroidism in ~30% of patients. Thyroid antibody tests are usually negative. Ultrasound of the thyroid reveals an "invasive"-type picture, with obliteration of the normal thyroid margins.

Management of Riedel thyroiditis is surgical for patients in whom symptoms of obstruction occur. Recently, **tamoxifen** has been shown to be helpful in some patients, because of its inhibitory effects on growth factors. Glucocorticoids are rarely effective. L-T$_4$ is required for management of hypothyroidism but is not effective for goiter shrinkage.

IV. PAINLESS THYROIDITIS DUE TO PHARMACOLOGIC AGENTS

A. Cytokines

1. **Interferon-α (IFN-α)**, which is used in the management of chronic hepatitis C (HCV), may be associated with a lymphocytic thyroiditis type of syndrome. Patients with IFN-α–induced thyroid dysfunction may present with hypo- or hyperthyroidism.

   Predisposing factors for the development of IFN-α–associated thyroid dysfunction include female sex, older age, longer duration of IFN treatment, and the pre-existence of anti-TPO antibodies. Thyroid abnormalities may occur in up to 60% of patients receiving IFN-α who have positive TPO antibodies prior to treatment, whereas only ~3% of patients who develop thyroid dysfunction have negative TPO antibodies.

   The mechanism for IFN-α–induced thyroid dysfunction is likely related to the enhancement of the autoimmune process. Also, IFN-α therapy has been shown to induce TPO antibody production in patients with HCV.

   a. **Clinical features.** IFN-α–induced thyroid dysfunction may present with either hypothyroidism or hyperthyroidism. Differentiating hypothyroidism from the fatigue normally associated with IFN-α therapy may be difficult, underscoring the importance of monitoring all patients receiving IFN-α with periodic serum TSH levels.

   A small, painless, firm goiter may be present, especially in patients with underlying HT, although goiter may be absent.

   b. **Laboratory findings.** Thyroid function test results of IFN-α–associated thyroid dysfunction are similar to those noted with painless LT. Patients who present with hyperthyroidism should be evaluated with a RAIU test to exclude the possibility of Graves thyrotoxicosis.

c. Treatment. Management of IFN-α–induced thyroid dysfunction depends on the severity of clinical manifestations and the degree of the biochemical abnormality. Hypothyroidism should be treated with L-T$_4$ for the duration of IFN-α treatment, and patients should be monitored with periodic serum TSH levels. After IFN-α is discontinued, L-T$_4$ may be stopped and a serum TSH checked 4 to 6 weeks later. Hypothyroidism may persist for a number of months (or even permanently) in some patients.

The symptoms of hyperthyroidism associated with IFN-α therapy may be managed with beta-blockers. Patients who have Graves disease (infrequent) should be treated with radioactive iodine rather than thionamide drugs because of the potential, albeit small, risk of liver damage from antithyroid drugs.

2. Interleukin-2 (IL-2) is used as an adjunctive therapy in the treatment of various malignancies, including metastatic solid tumors and leukemias, and may be associated with a painless lymphocytic thyroiditis type of syndrome. Prevalence rates have varied from 2% to 39% of IL-2–treated patients, and, as with IFN-α, female gender and pre-existence of thyroid autoantibodies are risk factors for developing thyroid dysfunction. Like IFN-α, IL-2 probably activates the autoimmune process, because its administration is associated with the development of thyroid antibodies as well as an increase in titers of pre-existing TPO antibodies. Of note is that combination immunotherapy with IFN-α and IL-2 results in an even greater prevalence of thyroid dysfunction than occurs with either agent alone.

The laboratory assessment, clinical features, and management of IL-2–associated thyroid dysfunction are the same as those associated with IFN-α therapy.

B. Amiodarone-induced thyroiditis

1. Amiodarone, a potent antiarrhythmic agent containing 37% iodine, causes hyperthyroidism in ~3% of patients in the United States who take the medication. This contrasts with the ~10% of patients who develop amiodarone-associated hyperthyroidism who reside in iodine-deficient areas. Hyperthyroidism generally occurs within a few months after beginning the drug but may have its onset at any time after initiation of treatment. Symptoms of hyperthyroidism are often lacking, probably because of the beta-blocker activity of amiodarone. However, patients are not protected from the tissue effects of thyrotoxicosis and may experience weight loss, worsening of arrhythmia, or development of congestive heart failure.

2. There are two types of amiodarone-induced hyperthyroidism: Type 1 results from iodine excess and increased thyroid hormone synthesis, and type 2 is an inflammatory thyrodestructive process. It is important for the clinician to differentiate between the two types of amiodarone-induced hyperthyroidism because the treatment is different for each. The presence of a nodular goiter suggests iodine-induced hyperthyroidism, whereas absence of thyroid enlargement suggests inflammatory thyroiditis. Table 29.4 outlines some diagnostic features of both types of disorders. The measurement of serum IL-6 levels may occasionally allow for differentiating between the two types of amiodarone-induced hyperthyroidism, although the amount of overlap limits its usefulness. Perhaps the most useful study is color flow on Doppler thyroid ultrasound; flow is increased in patients with type 1 and decreased in patients with type 2 amiodarone-induced thyrotoxicosis.

3. Treatment of type 2 amiodarone-induced hyperthyroidism consists of pharmacologic doses of glucocorticoids (e.g., as prednisone, 40 mg per day) in divided doses. Thionamide agents are not helpful, although if the diagnosis is in question, a combination of glucocorticoids and thionamide drugs (which are usually reserved for type 1) may be indicated. Type 2 amiodarone-induced hyperthyroidism follows a course similar to that observed with other forms of painless or lymphocytic thyroiditis.

ACKNOWLEDGMENT

The author gratefully acknowledges the expert secretarial assistance of Elsa C. Ahumada.

Selected References

Barsaria S, Cooper DS. Amiodarone and the thyroid. *Am J Med* 2005;118:706–714.

Berger SA, Zonsein J, Villamena P, et al. Infectious diseases of the thyroid gland. *Rev Infect Dis* 1983;5:108–122.

Bogazzi F, Dell'Unto E, Tanda ML, et al. Long-term outcome of thyroid function after amiodarone-induced thyrotoxicosis, as compared to subacute thyroiditis. *J Endocrinol Invest* 2006;29:694–699.

Dayan CM, Daniels GH. Chronic autoimmune thyroiditis. *N Engl J Med* 1996;335:99–107.

Farid NR, Hawe BS, Walfish PG. Increased frequency of HLA-DR3 and 5 in the syndromes of painless thyroiditis with transient thyrotoxicosis: evidence for an autoimmune etiology. *Clin Endocrinol* 1983;19:699.

Farwell AP, Braverman LE. Inflammatory thyroid disorders. *Otolaryngol Clin N Am* 1996; 29:541–556.

Fatourechi V, Aniszewski JP, Fatourechi GZ, et al. Clinical features and outcome of subacute thyroiditis in an incidence cohort: Olmsted County, Minnesota, study. *J Clin Endocrinol Metab* 2003;88:2100–2105.

Gerstein HC. How common is postpartum thyroiditis? A methodologic overview of the literature. *Arch Intern Med* 1990;150:1397–4000.

Guttler R, Singer PA, Axline SG, et al. *Pneumocystis carinii* thyroiditis: report of three cases and review of the literature. *Arch Intern Med* 1993;153:393–396.

Lazarus JH, Hall R, Othman S, et al. The clinical spectrum of postpartum thyroid disease. *Q J Med* 1996;89:429–435.

Lucas A, Pizarro E, Granada ML, et al. Postpartum thyroiditis: Long-term follow-up. *Thyroid* 2005;15:1177–1181.

Nikolai TF, Turney SL, Roberts RC. Postpartum lymphocytic thyroiditis: prevalence, clinical course, and long term follow up. *Arch Intern Med* 1987;147:221.

Ohsako N, Tamai H, Sudo T, et al. Clinical characteristics of subacute thyroiditis classified according to human leukocyte antigen typing. *J Clin Endocrinol Metab* 1995;80:3653–3656.

Pearce EN, Farwell AP, Braverman LE. Thyroiditis. *N Engl J Med* 2003;348:2846–2850.

Roti E, Minelli R, Gardini E, et al. Iodine induced hypothyroidism in euthyroid subjects with a previous episode of subacute thyroiditis. *J Clin Endocrinol Metab* 1990;70:1581.

Singer PA. Thyroiditis, acute, subacute and chronic. *Med Clin North Am* 1991;75:1–77.

Stagnaro-Green A. Clinical review 152: postpartum thyroiditis. *J Clin Endocrinol Metab* 2002;87:4042–4050.

Stagnaro-Green A, Roman SH, Cobin RH, et al. A prospective study of lymphocytic-initiated immunosuppression in normal pregnancy: evidence of T cell etiology for postpartum thyroid dysfunction. *J Clin Endocrinol Metab* 1992;74:645–653.

Volpe R. The management of subacute (DeQuervain's) thyroiditis. *Thyroid* 1993;3:253–255.

Weetman AP. Chronic autoimmune thyroiditis. In: Braverman LE, Utiger RD, eds. *The Thyroid: A Fundamental and Clinical Text.* 8th ed. Philadelphia: Lippincott–Raven; 2000:738–748.

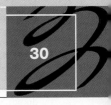

HYPOTHYROIDISM AND HYPERTHYROIDISM

Jerome M. Hershman

30

 HYPOTHYROIDISM

I. DEFINITION

Hypothyroidism is a condition resulting from a lack of the effects of thyroid hormone on body tissues. Because thyroid hormone affects growth and development and regulates many cellular processes, the absence or deficiency of thyroid hormone has many detrimental consequences.

II. CAUSES OF HYPOTHYROIDISM

A. Infancy or childhood
1. Maldevelopment—hypoplasia or aplasia
2. Inborn deficiencies of biosynthesis or action of thyroid hormone
3. Hashimoto thyroiditis
4. Hypopituitarism or hypothalamic disease
5. Severe iodine deficiency

B. Adults
1. Hashimoto thyroiditis
2. Lymphocytic thyroiditis following transient hyperthyroidism
3. Thyroid ablation
   a. Surgery
   b. Following ^{131}I therapy for hyperthyroidism
   c. Radiation of cervical neoplasms
4. Hypopituitarism or hypothalamic disease
5. Drugs
   a. Iodine, inorganic or organic (e.g., amiodarone)
   b. Antithyroid: thionamides (propylthiouracil, methimazole), potassium perchlorate, thiocyanate
   c. Lithium
   d. Interferon-α
   e. Sunitinib

III. INCIDENCE

Hypothyroidism is a common condition. Congenital hypothyroidism is diagnosed by screening methods in 1 of every 3 000 newborns. In adults >65 years of age, the incidence is ~10%. The overall incidence in the population is 4.6%; 4.3% is subclinical and 0.3% is overt.

IV. SYMPTOMS, SIGNS, AND PATHOPHYSIOLOGY

A. **Nervous system.** Patients with hypothyroidism may complain of forgetfulness, reduced memory, mental slowing, depression, paresthesia (sometimes associated with compression of nerves, such as carpal tunnel syndrome), ataxia, and reduced hearing. Tendon jerks show slowed or "hung-up" relaxation.

B. **Cardiovascular system.** There may be bradycardia, diastolic hypertension, reduced cardiac output, quiet heart sounds, a flabby myocardium, pericardial effusion, reduced voltage on the electrocardiogram and flat T waves, endothelial

435

dysfunction, arterial stiffness, and dependent edema. Cardiomegaly seen on plain film is usually shown by echocardiography to be attributable to effusion.

C. **Gastrointestinal system.** Constipation is common in hypothyroidism. Achlorhydria occurs, often associated with pernicious anemia. Ascitic fluid, like other serous effusions in myxedema, has a high protein content.

D. **Renal system.** Reduced excretion of a water load may be associated with hyponatremia. Renal blood flow and glomerular filtration rate (GFR) are reduced, but serum creatinine is normal.

E. **Pulmonary system.** Ventilatory responses to hypoxia and hypercapnia are reduced. Severe hypothyroidism may cause carbon dioxide retention. Pleural effusions have a high protein content.

F. **Musculoskeletal system.** Arthralgia, joint effusions, muscle cramps, and stiff muscles occur. Serum creatinine phosphokinase may be very high.

G. **Hemopoiesis.** Anemia may occur, usually of the normocytic type. Megaloblastic anemia suggests coexisting pernicious anemia.

H. **Skin and hair.** The presence of dry, cool skin is common. Glycosaminoglycans, mainly hyaluronic acid, accumulate in skin and subcutaneous tissues, causing retention of sodium and water. The face is puffy and features are coarse. The skin has a sallow appearance and can be flaky. Skin also may be orange because of accumulation of carotene. The hair lacks luster. Lateral eyebrows thin out and body hair is scanty.

I. **Reproductive system.** Menorrhagia from anovulatory cycles may occur, or the menses may become scanty and even cease completely because of deficient secretion of gonadotropins. In adolescents, there may be primary amenorrhea. Hyperprolactinemia occurs because of the absence of the inhibitory effect of thyroid hormone on prolactin secretion, resulting in galactorrhea and amenorrhea.

J. **Development.** Growth and development of children are retarded. Epiphyses remain open. Secretion of growth hormone is deficient because thyroid hormone is needed for synthesis of growth hormone. Untreated hypothyroidism in pregnant women can result in reduced intellectual function of the progeny.

K. **Metabolic system.** Hypothermia is common. Intolerance of cold temperature is a specific finding. Hypercholesterolemia with increase of serum low-density lipoprotein (LDL)-cholesterol occurs because of reduced number of LDL receptors. Hypertriglyceridemia may occur because of reduced degradation of lipoproteins and reduced lipoprotein lipase activity. Hereditary hyperlipidemic conditions are exacerbated by hypothyroidism. Weight gain is common despite reduced food intake, but severe obesity is rarely caused by hypothyroidism.

L. **Thyroid gland.** Enlargement of the thyroid gland in young children with hypothyroidism suggests a biosynthetic defect. Goitrous hypothyroidism in adults is caused by Hashimoto thyroiditis.

V. DIAGNOSTIC TESTS

A. Serum thyrotropin (thyroid-stimulating hormone, TSH) concentration and serum free thyroxine (T_4) concentration or free T_4 index are an excellent battery for diagnosis of hypothyroidism.

B. Serum **TSH** concentration (normal range, 0.4 to 4.0 mU/L) may be modestly elevated in the range of 4 to 10 mU/L in patients with normal free T_4 concentration and indicates subclinical hypothyroidism. Serum TSH values of 10 to 20 mU/L indicate more severe impairment of thyroid function although the serum T_4 may still be normal. When serum TSH concentration exceeds 20 mU/L, it is likely that frank hypothyroidism is present. Because of the sensitivity of the serum TSH level as an indicator of primary hypothyroidism, serum TSH is the best method to screen for the disorder.

C. **Central hypothyroidism** is usually associated with other evidence of pituitary or hypothalamic dysfunction. Serum free T_4 and TSH concentrations are low. In some patients, especially those with hypothalamic lesions, serum TSH is in the normal range but the TSH probably has reduced biologic activity. Magnetic resonance imaging (MRI) may show the lesion, most commonly a pituitary tumor. Enlargement of the pituitary also occurs in primary hypothyroidism as a result of hyperplasia of the thyrotropes. In response to thyroid hormone therapy, restoration of normal pituitary size occurs.

VI. DIAGNOSIS OF HYPOTHYROIDISM IN PATIENTS TAKING THYROID HORMONE

Many patients take thyroid hormone without an adequate diagnosis of hypothyroidism having been established. Typical faulty indications include fatigue, weight gain, and irregular menses. If both the patient and the doctor agree that the diagnosis was never adequately established, then the best approach to diagnosis involves stopping the replacement therapy for 5 weeks. At this time, the serum T_4 and TSH concentrations will indicate either a euthyroid state or primary hypothyroidism. If the tests are carried out 10 to 14 days after withdrawal of therapy, they may reflect physiologic hypothyroidism from the suppression of the pituitary–thyroid axis by the exogenous hormone. An alternative approach is reduction of the thyroxine dose by half and then assessing thyroid function after 5 weeks. If the TSH is elevated above normal on the reduced dose, the patient has primary hypothyroidism.

VII. THYROID FUNCTION AND NONTHYROID ILLNESS

A. Tri-iodothyronine (T_3). Severe systemic illness will reduce serum T_3 concentrations by blocking the extrathyroidal production of T_3 from T_4. Inhibition of $5'$-monodeiodination occurs in many illnesses, including liver disease, uremia, severe infections, diabetic ketoacidosis, general surgery, starvation, burns, and severe myocardial infarction.

B. Thyroxine (T_4). With more severe illness, serum T_4 concentration falls to subnormal levels and free T_4 concentration may be normal or low. Serum TSH is usually normal, or sometimes low. This condition may be interpreted as a transient form of central hypothyroidism that is an adaptation to severe catabolic illness. During recovery, serum TSH rises, sometimes to levels of 10 to 20 mU/mL, and T_3 and T_4 concentrations return to normal.

VIII. THERAPY

A. Preparations

1. **Sodium levothyroxine.** The preparation of choice is synthetic sodium levothyroxine because it produces stable serum levels of both T_4 and T_3. The absorption is ~75%.

2. **Desiccated thyroid extract, USP** is an extract of pig thyroid glands, which is standardized based on its iodine content, although assays of the hormone content are also performed by the leading pharmaceutical manufacturers. It contains a T_4/T_3 ratio of about 4:1. Approximately 4 to 8 hours after ingestion, T_3 levels may rise to the supranormal range. The relative potency of desiccated thyroid to T_4 is 1:1 000 (1 mg desiccated thyroid is equivalent to 1 μg of synthetic thyroxine).

3. **Synthetic T_3 (liothyronine, Cytomel).** There are really no indications for chronic therapy with synthetic T_3. It is used only when rapid withdrawal of thyroid hormone therapy is planned and for some diagnostic tests. Absorption is ~90%. Patients taking T_3 therapy have elevated T_3 concentrations for several hours after ingestion, which gradually fall to much lower levels 24 hours later. Substitution of 12.5 μg of T_3 for 50 μg of T_4 as a component of therapy was reported to improve mood and psychometric parameters. However, several carefully performed studies could not confirm any psychological or metabolic benefit from using T_3 together with T_4 for therapy of hypothyroidism.

4. **Synthetic T_4–T_3 combination (Liotrix).** This preparation was developed before it was appreciated that T_4 is converted to T_3 outside the thyroid. It has a synthetic T_4/T_3 molar ratio of 4:1 and is available in various doses.

B. Young adults. The usual replacement dose of thyroxine is 1.5 to 1.7 μg/kg ideal body weight. The full replacement dose may be prescribed from the inception of therapy. In following patients, it is important to explain to the patient that clinical improvement occurs gradually over several weeks and that the full effect of therapy in restoring the euthyroid state is likely to take 2 to 3 months. Laboratory indices of response show a rise in serum free T_4 to the normal range within 2 weeks, but serum <u>TSH concentrations require about 6 weeks to fall to normal.</u> After this time, adjustment of the dose by 12.5 to 25 μg of T_4 is made to optimize the clinical response and bring the serum TSH into the mid-normal range. There are no worthwhile laboratory indices of the action of thyroid hormone, so reliance is placed mainly on serum TSH because it is more sensitive than clinical evaluation.

C. **Middle-aged patients.** Hypothyroid individuals in this age group who are otherwise healthy may be treated with ~1.5 μg T_4 per kilogram. If there is coexisting ischemic heart disease or chronic pulmonary disease, then it is best to initiate therapy with a small dose of T_4, such as 25 μg a day, and increase the dose by 25 μg each subsequent month depending on the clinical response. The basis for this "low and slow" approach is the fear that **(1)** restoration of the euthyroid state will increase demands and worsen angina, and **(2)** the heart is particularly susceptible to the chronotropic action of thyroid hormone, so fatal tachycardia may be induced in susceptible patients. This fear tends to be exaggerated and overemphasized. The "low and slow" approach leads to prolongation of the hypothyroid state, so the justification for it must be clearly apparent.

D. **Elderly patients.** In the elderly, it is best to assume that ischemic heart disease may exist, possibly subclinically, and to initiate replacement therapy with a low dose of T_4, such as 12.5 to 25 μg/d. The dose may be increased every 4 to 6 weeks by 25 μg until the serum TSH is in the normal range.

E. **Pregnancy.** In pregnant women with pre-existing hypothyroidism, the dose of thyroid hormone must be increased by 25% to 50% in pregnancy to maintain a normal serum TSH, preferably in the range of 0.5 to 2.5 mU/L. <u>The increased requirement for thyroid hormone,</u> based on elevation of serum TSH above normal, occurs early in pregnancy, usually by 8 weeks. After delivery, the patient may return to the prepregnancy dose of thyroxine.

IX. SUBCLINICAL HYPOTHYROIDISM

Subclinical hypothyroidism is usually defined as an asymptomatic state in which free T_4 is normal but serum TSH is elevated. If serum TSH is >10 mU/L, there is consensus that the patient should be treated with thyroxine because of the likelihood that the patient will develop overt hypothyroidism with subnormal free T_4 and because this degree of subclinical hypothyroidism <u>predisposes to cardiovascular disease.</u> When the serum TSH is in the range of 4.5 to 10 mU/L, there is controversy about the efficacy of T_4 therapy. Many endocrinologists will treat such patients with T_4, especially if hypercholesterolemia or depression is present. Even in the absence of hyperlipidemia, a trial of therapy may be warranted to determine whether the patient experiences improvement (i.e., the therapy may provide the patient with more energy, a feeling of well-being, desirable weight reduction, improved bowel function, or other signs of better health even though the patient is not aware of these symptoms before therapy). Presumably, the normal serum free T_4 concentration before therapy did not reflect adequate tissue effects of thyroid hormone in such a patient. Unfortunately, it is difficult to differentiate this type of response from a placebo effect. Therefore, it is also reasonable to follow these patients without T_4 therapy by surveying thyroid function at 6-month intervals to determine whether thyroid failure has occurred, as indicated by further increase of serum TSH and fall of the serum T_4 to subnormal level along with the appearance of clear-cut symptomatology. However, I prefer to treat anyone in whom the serum TSH is persistently and clearly elevated, because even minimal hypothyroidism is a risk factor for atherosclerosis.

X. CORONARY ARTERY DISEASE, ELECTIVE SURGERY, AND HYPOTHYROIDISM

Occasionally, patients have both severe coronary artery disease and coexisting untreated hypothyroidism. In such patients, arteriography and coronary artery bypass procedures should be performed, if indicated, prior to initiation of therapy with thyroid hormone. Afterward, the patient will have better tolerance of the inotropic and chronotropic effects of thyroid hormone. Untreated hypothyroidism is probably not a major risk factor for general surgery, as was once believed. Nevertheless, in the absence of severe coronary artery disease, it is preferable to restore a euthyroid state before elective surgery. Urgent surgery need not be postponed because of hypothyroidism.

XI. MYXEDEMA COMA AS THE END RESULT OF LONG-STANDING UNTREATED HYPOTHYROIDISM

These patients have hypothermia, bradycardia, alveolar hypoventilation, typical myxedematous facies and skin, and severe obtundation or coma. Usually the condition is precipitated by an intercurrent illness, such as an infection or stroke, or a sedative drug state from which the patient does not awaken. If untreated, mortality approaches 100%. This mortality is prevented with aggressive therapy, which consists of giving 300 to 500 μg sodium levothyroxine IV. Subsequent parenteral dosages may be about 100 μg T_4 daily. Some authorities prefer to use IV tri-iodothyronine in a dose of 10 to 20 μg every 4 to 8 hours for the first few days because of reduced conversion of T_4 to T_3 in myxedema. Therapy consisting of both T_4 and T_3 IV has also been advocated. The initial therapy is 250 μg T_4 plus 25 μg T_3 IV, followed by 10 μg T_3 every 8 hours until the patient responds. Supportive therapy and treatment of underlying diseases are essential. Rewarming the patient can be harmful because it can cause peripheral vasodilatation and consequent hypotension.

HYPERTHYROIDISM

I. DEFINITION

Hyperthyroidism is the condition resulting from the effect of excessive amounts of thyroid hormones on body tissues. Thyrotoxicosis is a synonym. Some prefer to use the term "hyperthyroidism" in a narrower sense to denote the state in which the thyroid gland is producing too much thyroid hormone, in contrast to excessive ingestion of thyroid hormone medication or release of thyroid hormone in thyroiditis.

II. CAUSES (Table 30.1)

A. **Graves disease** is the most common cause of hyperthyroidism. **Toxic multinodular** goiter is found mainly in the elderly and the middle-aged.

B. Administration of inorganic iodine, such as potassium iodide, or organic iodine compounds, such as amiodarone, to patients with multinodular goiter or a tendency for Graves disease may cause iodine-induced hyperthyroidism. Amiodarone also causes thyroiditis, resulting in thyrotoxicosis.

C. Iodine-induced thyrotoxicosis (the Jod-Basedow phenomenon) may also occur in <1% of those receiving iodine supplementation in regions of endemic goiter.

D. Most autonomous hyperfunctioning adenomas do not produce hyperthyroidism, but when the adenoma ("hot" nodule) exceeds 3 cm in diameter, this outcome is more likely. Activating mutations of the TSH receptor have been found in many of these adenomas.

E. The TSH-secreting pituitary adenoma is rare and usually relatively large, but TSH-secreting microadenomas have also been reported in 15% of the cases. The condition may be a part of another functioning pituitary tumor, such as one causing acromegaly or hyperprolactinemia; the serum TSH is elevated or inappropriately normal and does not suppress with administration of T_3.

F. The *pituitary may be resistant* to the suppressive effect of thyroid hormone, whereas other tissues are more sensitive to thyroid hormone; serum T_4 and T_3 concentrations in these patients are elevated, whereas serum TSH is inappropriately normal. The patients do not have neuroradiologic evidence of a pituitary tumor. These patients usually have <u>mutations of the T_3 β-receptor</u> that are responsible for the pituitary resistance.

G. Hydatidiform moles and choriocarcinomas secrete large amounts of human chorionic gonadotropin (HCG). When serum HCG concentrations exceed 200 IU/mL

TABLE 30.1	Causes of Hyperthyroidism

Cause	Thyroid activator
Overproduction of thyroid hormone	
Graves disease	TSI
Toxic multinodular goiter	Autonomy or TSI
Autonomous hyperfunctioning adenoma	Activating TSH-R mutation
TSH-secreting pituitary adenoma	TSH
TSH overproduction due to pituitary resistance to the suppressive effect of thyroid hormone	TSH
Hydatidiform mole or choriocarcinoma	HCG
Hyperemesis gravidarum	HCG
Thyroid destruction resulting in leakage of thyroid hormone	None
Lymphocytic thyroiditis	
Granulomatous (subacute) thyroiditis	
Other	
Thyrotoxicosis medicamentosa (or factitia)	
Struma ovarii	
Metastatic thyroid carcinoma	

HCG, human chorionic gonadotropin; TSH, thyroid-stimulating hormone; TSI, thyroid-stimulating immunoglobulin.

(several times the peak levels of normal pregnancy), hyperthyroidism may be present. HCG is a weak thyroid stimulator, triggers the TSH receptor, and causes hyperthyroidism in these patients. Removal of the mole or effective chemotherapy of the choriocarcinoma is curative. In hyperemesis gravidarum, HCG secretion is increased and hyperthyroidism (gestational thyrotoxicosis) may occur.

H. Thyroiditis. See Sections VII.B and VII.C.

I. Excessive ingestion of thyroid hormone may cause thyrotoxicosis. Some patients are given excessive doses of thyroid hormone by their physicians, with poor rationale. Other patients take excessive amounts surreptitiously, sometimes to achieve weight loss. These patients have small thyroid glands, low thyroid uptake of radioiodine, and low serum thyroglobulin levels, whereas patients with thyroiditis and low thyroid uptake have elevated serum thyroglobulin levels.

J. Ovarian teratomas with thyroid elements (struma ovarii) and large metastatic functioning follicular thyroid carcinomas are very rare causes of hyperthyroidism.

III. FREQUENCY

Graves disease is the most common cause of hyperthyroidism and is fairly common in the population. Based on the NHANES 3 survey, ~1% of the population suffers from hyperthyroidism, either overt or subclinical.

IV. SYMPTOMS, SIGNS, AND PATHOPHYSIOLOGY

The manifestations depend on the duration and severity of the disorder.

A. Nervous system. Nervousness and a feeling of inner tension are common symptoms in hyperthyroid patients. Inability to get along with others, depression, emotional lability, poor concentration, and reduced performance in school and work may also occur. Tremor is common and reflexes are brisk.

B. Cardiac system. There is tachycardia, usually supraventricular, because of direct effects of thyroid hormone on the conduction system. Atrial fibrillation may be superimposed on the underlying heart disease or may be due to hyperthyroidism alone. Long-standing thyrotoxicosis can cause cardiomegaly and result in heart failure despite a high cardiac output. Flow murmurs are common. Extracardiac sounds are due to the banging hyperdynamic heart.

C. **Musculoskeletal system.** Muscles become atrophic and weak because of excessive muscle catabolism. There is reduced muscle performance in walking, climbing, rising from a knee bend, or weight lifting. **Myasthenia gravis** or **hypokalemic periodic paralysis** may accompany hyperthyroidism. The patient appears gaunt. Bone resorption exceeds bone formation, resulting in hypercalciuria and sometimes hypercalcemia. Long-standing hyperthyroidism may cause osteopenia.

D. **Gastrointestinal system.** Food intake increases, and some patients have insatiable appetites. Despite this, weight loss is common. Hyperdefecation occurs because of more rapid motility, but diarrhea is uncommon. Abnormal liver function tests reflect the malnutrition of far-advanced hyperthyroidism.

E. **Eyes.** Retraction of the upper lid as a result of increased sympathetic tone gives some patients a wide-eyed stare. Infiltrative ophthalmopathy is part of Graves disease, but only a minority of Graves patients have clinical evidence of ophthalmopathy. There may be proptosis, extraocular muscle swelling, and fibrosis causing restriction of ocular motility and diplopia. The exposed eyes become red. Pressure on the optic nerve or keratitis can cause blindness. Graves eye disease usually parallels hyperthyroidism but may run an independent course. The disorder is attributed to an autoimmune retro-orbital inflammation. Rarely, this ophthalmopathy occurs in patients with Hashimoto thyroiditis and in euthyroid patients without any history or evidence of thyroid disease (euthyroid Graves disease).

F. **Skin.** The patient's skin is warm, moist, and velvety, giving it a youthful appearance. The sweaty palms are hot rather than cool. Onycholysis (retraction of the nail from its bed) indicates a long duration of hyperthyroidism. Dermopathy of Graves disease, an orange-peel thickening of the pretibial areas, is rare.

G. **Reproductive system.** Hyperthyroidism impairs fertility in women and may cause oligomenorrhea. In men, the sperm count is reduced and impotence may occur. Gynecomastia occurs because of increased peripheral conversion of androgen to estrogen despite high testosterone levels. Thyroid hormone increases sex hormone–binding globulin and thus raises total testosterone and estradiol levels, whereas serum luteinizing hormone and follicle-stimulating hormone may be increased or normal.

H. **Metabolic system.** Weight loss is a common finding, especially in older patients who develop anorexia. Some teenagers and young adults lose control of their appetite, "pig out," and gain weight. The increased heat production caused by thyroid hormones is dissipated by increased sweating accompanied by mild polydipsia. Many patients describe an aversion to heat and a preference for cold temperatures. The insulin requirement of diabetic patients usually increases.

I. **Thyroid gland.** The thyroid is usually enlarged. Its size and consistency depend on the underlying pathology. The enlarged hyperfunctioning gland has increased blood flow causing a thyroid bruit.

V. GRAVES DISEASE

Graves disease is an **autoimmune disorder** responsible for >80% of cases of hyperthyroidism. In this condition, there is an antibody to the thyrotropin receptor on the thyroid follicular cell that results in stimulation of this receptor and is thus given the name thyroid-stimulating immunoglobulin (TSI) or TSH receptor antibody. The concentration of TSI in the serum bears a rough correlation with severity of the hyperthyroidism. The cause of production of TSI is unclear. Antibodies to other thyroid constituents, especially antiperoxidase antibody, are also present.

Graves disease is familial, but the genetics are not well-established. HLA-DR3 confers a fivefold increased risk for developing the disease.

VI. THYROID FUNCTION TESTS

Thyroid function tests may be categorized into **(a)** those needed to establish whether there is hyperthyroidism and **(b)** those that show the cause of hyperthyroidism.

A. Tests of thyroid function

1. Serum free T_4 concentration or free T_4 index are increased in nearly all hyperthyroid patients.
2. Serum T_3 concentration, free T_3 concentration, and free T_3 index are also elevated. In a small fraction of patients ($<5\%$), serum T_3 concentration or free T_3 is elevated when serum free T_4 is not; this entity is termed $\underline{T_3 \text{ thyrotoxicosis}}$.
3. Serum TSH, measured by the sensitive methods now commonly available, is undetectable or subnormal. About 2% of euthyroid elderly individuals will have a suppressed serum TSH. A normal or elevated TSH in a hyperthyroid patient indicates TSH-induced hyperthyroidism, which is rare (see Table 30.1).
4. Thyroid uptake of radioiodine (^{123}I or ^{131}I) at 4, 6, or 24 hours is increased in patients with increased production of thyroid hormone and reduced when the gland is leaking thyroid hormone (granulomatous or lymphocytic thyroiditis).

B. Tests for etiology

1. TSI (TSIgG) is now available commercially as a marker for active Graves disease. If positive, it confirms that the hyperthyroidism is a result of Graves disease.
2. TSH receptor antibody measures the binding of the patient's IgG to a TSH receptor. It is positive in $\sim$90% of patients with active Graves disease and is technically easier to measure than TSIgG.
3. The antiperoxidase (antimicrosomal) antibody test is positive in Graves disease (and in Hashimoto lymphocytic thyroiditis), thus helping to differentiate Graves disease from other causes of hyperthyroidism.
4. Thyroid scans are useful in patients with nodular goiter and hyperthyroidism to determine **(a)** whether there is an autonomous hyperfunctioning nodule that concentrates all the radioiodine and suppresses the normal glandular tissue, **(b)** whether multiple nodules concentrate radioiodine, or **(c)** whether the nodules are cold and the hyperfunctioning tissue is between the palpable nodules. This differentiation may be important with regard to therapy (see Section VII).

VII. DIFFERENTIAL DIAGNOSIS

A. Establishment of diagnosis of hyperthyroidism.
In patients with weight loss and features of hypermetabolism, the thyroid function tests are very sensitive, so the diagnosis of hyperthyroidism is straightforward. Milder cases may be difficult to diagnose. The serum TSH is subnormal in patients with minimal hyperthyroidism. Therefore, a discussion of differential diagnosis based on subtle clinical features is superfluous.

B. Thyroiditis.
Subacute granulomatous thyroiditis is an uncommon disorder in which there are signs of an inflammatory viral illness with fever and malaise associated with thyroid pain and tenderness. The sore throat is unusually severe; there is pain on swallowing that radiates to the ears. The thyroid gland is irregular and very firm. The process may begin in one lobe and progress to involve the other lobe in a few days. The sedimentation rate is elevated; antithyroid antibodies are usually negative, and the thyroid uptake of radioiodine is very low. A **hyperthyroid phase** lasts for several weeks, followed by a transition to a hypothyroid phase of several weeks and then recovery. $\underline{\text{Thyroid tenderness}}$ is the hallmark of the disorder. Cases of "silent subacute thyroiditis" in which thyroid tenderness is absent probably represent lymphocytic thyroiditis.

The features of hyperthyroidism usually respond well to β-adrenergic blockers. Propranolol may be used to reduce the tachycardia. Nonsteroidal anti-inflammatory drugs or aspirin may be sufficient for the pain and discomfort and will reduce the inflammation and fever. In patients who do not improve in a few days, prednisone is given, 30 to 40 mg per day for 10 to 14 days, then tapered and discontinued in 2 to 3 weeks.

C. Lymphocytic thyroiditis.
Lymphocytic thyroiditis is currently responsible for a small percentage of new cases. It is a variant of Hashimoto thyroiditis. Usually, a small firm goiter is present, but the thyroid may not be enlarged or may be up to three times the normal size. There is usually no thyroid tenderness. The differentiation

from Graves disease is based on the low thyroid uptake in lymphocytic thyroiditis. The increased T_4 blood levels occur because the gland is "leaking" thyroid hormone. The T_3/T_4 ratio is lower than in Graves disease because the stimulated Graves thyroid secretes more T_3, but this is not invariable. Thyroid antiperoxidase antibodies are positive.

Lymphocytic thyroiditis with hyperthyroidism occurs commonly in the postpartum state. The hyperthyroid phase may last 4 to 12 weeks and is followed by a hypothyroid phase that lasts for several months. A mild subclinical form occurs in 8% of postpartum women. Recovery, rather than persistent hypothyroidism, is the rule. Nearly three fourths of postpartum women with the disorder will have a recurrence after a subsequent pregnancy.

For the hyperthyroid phase, β-adrenergic blockers may be given to control symptoms. The use of antithyroid drugs that block the synthesis of thyroid hormone is not appropriate.

D. Acute psychosis. In many patients hospitalized with acute psychosis, transient elevation of serum T_4 and free T_4 index has been reported. About half of these patients also have elevation of serum T_3 concentration. The abnormality is self-limiting. Tests repeated 2 weeks later are generally normal. Whether this is due to central release of TSH by the process underlying the psychosis is unclear. Measurements of serum TSH performed after recognition of the disorder have usually shown suppressed rather than elevated levels, but in an earlier phase of the disorder, serum TSH levels may be elevated or inappropriately normal rather than suppressed. A few patients with amphetamine abuse have had inappropriately normal serum TSH levels when the serum T_4 was elevated.

E. Hyperthyroidism in the elderly. Elderly patients with hyperthyroidism may not have typical clinical features. The presenting features of their "apathetic" hyperthyroidism may be weight loss, weakness, and depression or apathy. In one study, 20% of elderly hyperthyroid patients did not have a goiter. Atrial fibrillation and heart failure are more common than in the young. Proptosis and Graves ophthalmopathy are unusual in the elderly.

VIII. THERAPY
A. Drugs
1. **Antithyroid drugs of the thionamide series** remain the backbone of therapy. The effectiveness of the therapy has been established by >60 years of experience with propylthiouracil (PTU) and methimazole (Tapazole). They block the biosynthesis of thyroid hormones by inhibiting thyroid peroxidase. In addition, propylthiouracil (but not methimazole) blocks the peripheral production of T_3 from T_4 by inhibiting the type 1 deiodinase.
   a. **Dosage.** The usual daily therapeutic dose is 300 to 600 mg of propylthiouracil or 20 to 60 mg of methimazole given in divided doses every 8 hours. Both drugs are concentrated in the thyroid gland. The experience with once-a-day therapy using propylthiouracil suggests that divided doses are much more effective. For the forgetful patient, methimazole may be given once daily, if necessary, because it has a longer action than propylthiouracil, but initiation of therapy with twice-daily dosing is probably more effective.
   b. **Follow-up.** Patients should be followed at monthly intervals initially to assess the response to therapy and to adjust the dose of drug. When the patient responds well, the dose can be reduced to one half to two thirds of the initial dose. I prefer to maintain the therapy for 1.5 to 2 years because there is evidence that long-term remission is more likely to occur in patients who receive the therapy for at least 18 months, in contrast to patients treated for only the few months necessary to control the hyperthyroidism.
   c. **Adverse effects.** Side effects of these drugs include skin rash, urticaria, arthralgia, serum sickness, abnormal liver function tests, vasculitis, and, rarely, agranulocytosis. I warn patients to contact me if an unusual infection occurs, but I do not perform routine white cell counts and differentials unless there is an infection.

    d. Prognosis. In my experience, about one third of patients undergo long-term remission when the course of therapy is completed. Relapses usually occur within the first year after stopping therapy. Long-term follow-up of patients treated with antithyroid drugs 20 to 25 years earlier showed that some had become hypothyroid, suggesting that thyroid destruction occurs spontaneously in Graves patients, probably as a result of autoimmune thyroiditis.

2. β-Adrenergic blockers

    a. Propranolol causes rapid improvement by blocking the excessive adrenergic activity of hyperthyroidism. It also causes a modest reduction in serum T_3 concentration by blocking T_4-to-T_3 conversion, which is probably independent of its effect on $β$ receptors. The usual dose is 20 to 40 mg every 4 to 6 hours. The dose is adjusted to lower resting heart rate to about 70 to 80 beats per minute. As the hyperthyroidism is controlled, the dose is tapered and the drug is discontinued when a euthyroid state is achieved.

    b. Effective $β$-adrenergic blockade will eliminate the tachycardia, tremor, anxiety, nervousness, and sweating, thus masking the condition and making clinical evaluation more difficult.

    c. Other $β$-adrenergic blockers are equally effective. Atenolol is longer-acting and less likely to cause depression. Reduction of serum T_3 concentration does not occur with the more selective $β_1$ agents.

    d. $β$-Adrenergic blockers are especially indicated for tachycardia, even in the presence of heart failure, if the tachycardia is a result of thyrotoxicosis and if the cardiac failure is due to the tachycardia. Asthma and obstructive pulmonary disease are relative contraindications to the use of $β$-adrenergic blockers.

    e. Hyperthyroid patients should not be treated with beta-blockers alone, because these agents have no direct effect on the thyroid.

3. Other agents

    a. Inorganic iodine. Saturated solution of potassium iodine (SSKI), 250 mg (5 drops) twice a day, is effective for most patients, but escape from its effect usually occurs in about 10 days. Its principal use is to prepare patients for surgery, because iodine firms up the thyroid and reduces its vascularity. Nowadays it is seldom used for definitive therapy. Sodium iodide may be given intravenously if necessary.

    b. Sodium ipodate (Oragrafin) and iopanoic acid (Telepaque). The radiographic contrast agents sodium ipodate and iopanoic acid are very potent inhibitors of peripheral conversion of T_4 to T_3. In addition, the iodine in these drugs is deiodinated, taken up by the thyroid, and inhibits the release of hormone from the gland. A dose of 1 g of sodium ipodate daily usually results in a dramatic fall of serum T_3 within 24 to 48 hours and may be continued for 7 to 14 days. Unfortunately, these drugs are not currently available.

    c. Corticosteroids. Large doses of corticosteroids, such as 8 mg per day of dexamethasone, reduce the secretion of thyroid hormone by an unknown mechanism and also inhibit peripheral conversion of T_4 to T_3. Thus, steroid therapy for 2 to 3 weeks may be indicated for severe hyperthyroidism.

B. Radioiodine-131. [131]I has been used for >60 years for definitive therapy of hyperthyroidism. It is efficacious and simple to administer. The usual doses are 5 to 15 mCi (185 to 555 MBq) to deliver ~80 to 120 mCi/g thyroid estimated weight, corrected for the 24-hour thyroid uptake. Such doses deliver 5 000 to 15 000 rad (50 to 150 Gy) to the thyroid. There has been a trend in recent years to use doses at the upper end of this range to achieve greater certainty that the hyperthyroidism is eliminated. [131]I therapy results in gradual restoration of a euthyroid state in most patients over a period of 6 months. Doses should be increased by ~25% in patients who have taken antithyroid drugs within the previous 10 days.

1. In some patients, ^{131}I causes little improvement, and in others, permanent hypothyroidism may develop. The hypothyroidism is transient in some who become hypothyroid in the first few months after therapy. Because the patients are usually very symptomatic when they undergo a rapid transition from hyperthyroidism to hypothyroidism, I prescribe T_4 therapy for all hypothyroid patients in the usual replacement dose for about 1 year, and then give a short trial of a reduced dose in this group to determine whether the hypothyroidism is permanent. Hypothyroidism that develops >6 months after therapy is nearly always permanent. The incidence of hypothyroidism with current doses exceeds 50% after 1 year and increases at a rate of 2% to 4% each year. Patients receiving ^{131}I therapy require permanent annual evaluations for hypothyroidism. Approximately one fourth of patients require more than one dose of ^{131}I, but only a few require three or more doses. Such patients have resistance to the radiation for reasons that are not clear.

2. ^{131}I therapy may cause an acute release of hormone from the gland, resulting in significantly increased serum concentrations of T_4 and T_3 in about one fifth of patients, usually about 5 to 10 days after the ^{131}I is given. This may be associated with exacerbation of symptoms. Because of the potential for worsening of the condition by ^{131}I, I do not administer it to severely hyperthyroid patients until the disease has been controlled with antithyroid drugs. The thionamide must be stopped for 1 to 2 days before giving ^{131}I so that it will not interfere with the retention of the therapeutic dose; it can be restarted 2 or 3 days later.

3. Because of the uncertain control of the hyperthyroidism with ^{131}I, I prefer to administer antithyroid drugs afterward for a period of 3 to 12 months to control the condition with greater certainty in most middle-aged and elderly patients. I discontinue the thionamide when the patient is hypothyroid or euthyroid on a small daily dose of the drug, such as 50 mg of propylthiouracil or 5 mg of methimazole. In younger patients, I do not give a second dose of ^{131}I until 1 year after the first dose in order to allow the full effect of the ^{131}I to occur and to reduce the possibility of hypothyroidism from unnecessary administration of a second dose of ^{131}I. However, others will retreat patients after 3 months if the hyperthyroidism persists. In older patients with complicating illnesses, I recommend additional doses of ^{131}I, 4 months or more after the first dose, if the hyperthyroidism has not been cured. There is reluctance to use ^{131}I in young adults and children because of the potential carcinogenic effect of the radiation. Careful follow-up of patients for >30 years has shown no increase of thyroid carcinoma, leukemia, or birth defects in the progeny of those who received this therapy for hyperthyroidism, so skepticism regarding treatment of patients <25 years of age does not appear to be justified. Radioiodine-131 is now used as the treatment of choice for children with hyperthyroidism in some referral centers.

C. Surgical thyroidectomy

1. Preparation for surgery. Subtotal thyroidectomy has been used for >80 years as effective therapy of hyperthyroidism. It is preferable to perform it after patients have regained their weight and are in good condition. Thus, these patients should be treated with thionamide drugs for several months. Inorganic iodine is added for 7 to 10 days prior to surgery to reduce the vascularity of the gland. Alternatively, patients may be treated for a short period with high doses of beta-blockers alone as preparation for surgery. This controls some symptoms and cardiovascular effects of hyperthyroidism but does not reverse the catabolic state. It may be justifiable under circumstances in which patients cannot take thionamide drugs or have mild hyperthyroidism.

2. Complications. Subtotal thyroidectomy has an appreciable incidence of complications. These include hypothyroidism in ~25%, persistent or recurrent hyperthyroidism in 10%, hypoparathyroidism in 1%, recurrent laryngeal nerve palsy in 1%, wound infections, and keloids. Because of these complications, surgical therapy should be reserved for special situations, such as side effects to antithyroid drugs, a patient's unwillingness to take ^{131}I, multinodular toxic goiter that is also causing obstruction of the airway or esophagus, or coexisting hyperparathyroidism. In addition, the financial cost is probably greater than that of definitive drug therapy or ^{131}I at the present time.

D. Choice of therapy. I prefer to use antithyroid drugs as the definitive therapy for most patients, especially young and middle-aged adults. Its main advantage is that the therapy is reversible and does not destroy the thyroid gland. For older patients and those with cardiovascular disease or complicating disorders, ^{131}I is the preferred therapy because it is more likely to produce a permanent cure of hyperthyroidism; its main drawback is that it causes a high incidence of hypothyroidism. [131]I administration has become the most commonly used treatment for hyperthyroidism in the United States. Surgery is reserved for special situations as stated previously.

IX. HYPERTHYROIDISM IN PREGNANCY

A. Incidence. Graves disease occurs commonly in women of child-bearing age, complicating ~0.1% of pregnancies. Because severe hyperthyroidism tends to reduce fertility, it is unusual to have this combination. More commonly, drug treatment of patients with hyperthyroidism improves fertility, and a pregnancy may then ensue. To avoid this complication, hyperthyroid young women on thionamide drugs should be urged to practice contraception. Hyperemesis gravidarum is associated with mild hyperthyroidism in a high proportion of cases. This is a result of high HCG concentrations; the disorder is self-limiting and disappears when the hyperemesis remits.

B. Management. Antithyroid drugs and surgery are the alternatives.
   1. [131]I is never used in women known to be pregnant because it crosses the placenta and is concentrated in the fetal thyroid after 10 weeks of gestation, resulting in cretinism.
   2. Propylthiouracil (PTU) crosses the placenta to a smaller extent than methimazole, so it is the preferable drug. In addition, methimazole has been associated rarely with aplasia cutis and more severe embryopathy. To avoid fetal hypothyroidism, the dose of PTU should be adjusted to the smallest necessary to maintain a near-euthyroid state, with serum T_4 in the upper-normal to slightly elevated range for pregnancy. Young pregnant women tolerate mild hyperthyroidism very well.
   3. If necessary, surgical thyroidectomy is best performed in the first or second trimester because general surgery in the third trimester may induce premature labor.

C. Outcome. About 80% to 90% of adequately treated hyperthyroid women have a normal outcome of pregnancy. The incidence of prematurity and spontaneous abortion is no greater than that found in pregnancies without hyperthyroidism.

D. Newborn. Hyperthyroidism may occur in the newborn as a result of transmission of the Graves TSI across the placenta to the fetus. The antithyroid drug given to the mother may control the hyperthyroidism in utero, but it may also cause goiter and hypothyroidism. Therefore, the newborn of a Graves mother requires special attention for these possibilities. Measurement of TSH receptor antibody in the pregnant woman with Graves disease is currently recommended as an indicator of the need for therapy of hyperthyroidism in the newborn (see Chapter 32).

X. THYROID STORM

A. Clinical. Thyroid storm is a dangerous condition of decompensated thyrotoxicosis. The patient has tachycardia, fever, agitation, restlessness or psychosis, nausea, vomiting, and/or diarrhea. It usually results from long-neglected severe hyperthyroidism to which there is added a complicating intercurrent illness, such as gastroenteritis or pneumonia, or emergency surgery.

B. Treatment. Therapy is multifactorial and includes appropriate supportive measures such as fluids and electrolytes, and management of an underlying infection with appropriate antibiotics. Specific treatment directed at the hyperthyroidism includes:
   1. Antithyroid drugs in large doses (600 mg of propylthiouracil or 60 mg of methimazole stat and half this dose q6h) given by gavage if necessary.
   2. Sodium ipodate, 1 g per day for 2 weeks, or iodine orally (0.5 mL saturated solution of potassium iodide twice a day) or intravenously (1 g sodium iodide).

3. Propranolol in large oral doses (40 to 80 mg every 4 to 6 hours) or small doses IV ~1 mg every 5 minutes, up to 10 mg) to reduce heart rate based on cardiac monitoring, or esmolol IV ~250 to 500 μg/kg per minute loading dose followed by 50 μg/kg per minute for 4 minutes with cardiac monitoring. A maintenance infusion at this dose can be used with cardiac monitoring.
4. Dexamethasone, 4 to 8 mg per day, unless contraindicated by a severe infection. As a result of receiving all or several of the preceding drug therapies concurrently, patients usually experience significant improvement in a few days.

XI. GRAVES EYE DISEASE
A. Clinical. Graves eye disease (ophthalmopathy) affects ~25% of patients with Graves hyperthyroidism and also occurs rarely in patients with Hashimoto thyroiditis or in those without overt autoimmune thyroid disease. Only 1% to 5% of patients with Graves disease have significant eye disease. The main findings are proptosis, redness of the conjunctiva, ocular discomfort, diplopia, and periorbital edema. Computed tomography CTs0 scans of the orbit show thickened eye muscles that may impinge on the optic nerve and impair vision. The pathogenesis is a result of retro-orbital inflammation induced by cytokines. There is evidence that the TSH receptor may be the orbital antigen that has a role in triggering the disorder.
B. Treatment. There is no entirely satisfactory therapy. Fortunately, the condition improves spontaneously in the majority of patients, even though complete resolution does not occur. In patients with severe manifestations, corticosteroid therapy in high doses is sometimes effective in reducing the inflammation. Patients should be followed in consultation with an ophthalmologist. Orbital decompression by an experienced eye surgeon can be performed after the condition stabilizes, which may take 6 to 24 months. Complete thyroidectomy may improve the condition. [131]I therapy may worsen Graves eye disease, so it should not be used until the eye condition is stable.

Selected References

Alexander EK, Marqusee E, Lawrence J, et al. Timing and magnitude of increases in levothyroxine requirements during pregnancy in women with hypothyroidism. *N Engl J Med.* 2004;351:241–249.

Allannic H, et al. Antithyroid drugs and Graves' disease: a prospective randomized evaluation of the efficacy of treatment duration. *J Clin Endocrinol Metab* 1990;70:675–679.

Bartalena L, Pinchera A, Marcocci C, et al. Management of Graves ophthalmopathy: reality and perspectives. *Endocr Rev* 2000;21:168–199.

Braverman LE, Utiger RD, eds. *Werner and Ingbar's The Thyroid.* 9th ed. Philadelphia: Lippincott Williams & Wilkins; 2005.

Cappola AR, Fried LP, Arnold AM, et al. Thyroid status, cardiovascular risk, and mortality in older adults. *JAMA* 2006;295:1033–1041.

Cooper DS. Clinical practice. Subclinical hypothyroidism. *N Engl J Med* 2001;345:260–265.

Degroot L, ed. Thyroid Disease Manager. www.thyroidmanager.org.

Escobar-Morreale HF, Botella-Carretero JI, Gómez-Bueno M, et al. Thyroid hormone replacement therapy in primary hypothyroidism: a randomized trial comparing L-thyroxine plus liothyronine with L-thyroxine alone. *Ann Intern Med* 2005;142:412–424.

Haddow JE, Palomaki GE, Allen WC, et al. Maternal thyroid deficiency during pregnancy and subsequent neuropsychological development of the child. *N Engl J Med* 1999;341:549–555.

Hershman JM. Physiological and pathological aspects of the effect of human chorionic gonadotropin on the thyroid. *Best Pract Res Clin Endocrinol Metab* 2004;18:249–265.

Iagaru A, McDougall IR. Treatment of thyrotoxicosis. *J Nucl Med* 2007;48:379–389.

Klein I, Becker DV, Levey GS. Treatment of hyperthyroid disease. *Ann Intern Med* 1994;121:281–288.

Martino E, Bartalena L, Bogazzi F, Braverman LE. The effects of amiodarone on the thyroid. *Endocr Rev* 2001;22:240–254.

Menconi F, Marinò M, Pinchera A, et al. Effects of total thyroid ablation versus near-total thyroidectomy alone on mild to moderate Graves' orbitopathy treated with intravenous glucocorticoids. *J Clin Endocrinol Metab* 2007;92:1653–1658.

Mestman JH. Hyperthyroidism in pregnancy. *Best Pract Res Clin Endocrinol Metab* 2004; 18:267–288.

Razvi S, Ingoe L, Keeka G, et al. The beneficial effect of L-thyroxine on cardiovascular risk factors, endothelial function, and quality of life in subclinical hypothyroidism: randomized, crossover trial. *J Clin Endocrinol Metab* 2007;92:1715–1723.

Robuschi G, Safran M, Braverman LE, et al. Hypothyroidism in the elderly. *Endocr Rev* 1987;8:142–153.

Samuels MH. Subclinical thyroid disease in the elderly. *Thyroid* 1998;8:803–813.

Singer PA, Cooper DS, Levy EG, et al. Treatment guidelines for patients with hyperthyroidism and hypothyroidism. Standards of Care Committee, American Thyroid Association. *JAMA* 1995;273:808–812.

Surks MI, Ortiz E, Daniels GH, et al. Subclinical thyroid disease: scientific review and guidelines for diagnosis and management. *JAMA* 2004;291:228–238.

Weetman AP. Graves' disease. *N Engl J Med* 2000;343:1236–1248.

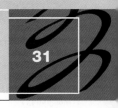
THYROID TUMORS IN ADULTS*
Jerome M. Hershman

I. GENERAL PRINCIPLES
A. Prevalence of thyroid nodules
1. In the Framingham population study, the lifetime risk of developing a palpable thyroid nodule was estimated to be 5% to 10% based on prospective follow-up of >5 000 patients with a female/male ratio of 5/1. In an ultrasound survey of people in Italy without apparent thyroid disease, nodules were detected in ∼40% of those over age 60 years and in 25% of those under age 60. Three fourths of the nodules were <10 mm in size, only 7% were 20 mm or larger, and the female/male ratio of those with nodules was 1.4/1. In a large autopsy series in the United States, 50% of the population with no known history of thyroid disease had discrete nodules, 35% of whom had nodules >2 cm in diameter. Older studies reported a higher incidence of thyroid cancer in single nodules than in multinodular goiter. However, a recent study of almost 2 000 patients in Boston found the <u>same thyroid cancer incidence of 15% in patients with a single nodule and in those with multinodular goiter</u> when all nodules >1 cm were biopsied.
2. There are ∼30 000 new cases of thyroid cancer in the United States each year, accounting for 2.2% of all new cancers. Mortality from thyroid cancer is 0.3% of all cancer deaths. The increased incidence of thyroid cancer during the last two decades is attributed to improved diagnosis.
B. Classification. Almost any pathologic process involving the thyroid gland (benign and malignant neoplasms, colloid goiter, inflammatory processes, developmental abnormalities, intrinsic metabolic defects, or hemorrhage) can present as a thyroid nodule. Table 31.1 lists the pathologic classification of thyroid tumors.

II. EVALUATION OF THYROID NODULES
A. Clinical evaluation. Although thyroid nodules are found more frequently in women, the likelihood of a thyroid nodule being malignant is higher in men than in women. A history of radiation exposure during childhood is important, because a thyroid adenoma or carcinoma can develop many years later in those who received radiation therapy for treatment of benign conditions such as tonsillitis, acne, tinea capitis, impetigo, sinusitis, or an enlarged thymus.

A family history of thyroid cancer suggests familial papillary thyroid cancer or familial medullary thyroid cancer as a component of multiple endocrine neoplasia (MEN) type 2. Familial papillary thyroid cancer is much more common than familial medullary thyroid cancer. A history of goiter in the family suggests a benign disorder.

The distinction between solitary and multiple nodules by neck examination may be limited. In ∼50% of patients with a clinically solitary nodule on palpation, the lesion subsequently was found to be a dominant nodule in a multinodular goiter on ultrasound or pathologic examination.

Most thyroid nodules do not cause symptoms. Pain may occur with a hemorrhage into a pre-existing colloid nodule or a benign adenoma. Currently, a large majority of nodules are found incidentally during carotid ultrasonography, computed tomography (CT) scan, or magnetic resonance imaging (MRI) of the neck.

---

*Updated from Van Herle AJ. In: Lavin N. *Manual of Endocrinology and Metabolism.* 3rd ed. Philadelphia: Lippincott Williams & Wilkins; 2002:410–421.

TABLE 31.1	Pathologic Classification of Thyroid Tumors

Epithelial tumors
Benign
  Follicular adenoma
  Hürthle cell adenoma
  Adenomatous hyperplasia in colloid goiter
Malignant
  Papillary carcinoma
  Follicular carcinoma
  Hürthle cell carcinoma
  Undifferentiated (anaplastic) carcinoma
  Medullary carcinoma

Malignant nonepithelial tumors
Lymphoma
Metastatic carcinoma
Squamous cell carcinoma

The following clinical features are highly suggestive of the presence of a malignant thyroid lesion:
1. Rapid expansion of an existing nodule
2. Firm texture of the lesion
3. Pressure on adjacent structures
4. Fixation of the nodule to surrounding structures
5. Obstructive symptoms
6. Dysphagia
7. Vocal cord paralysis manifested as hoarseness
8. Presence of enlarged cervical lymph nodes (especially suspicious in children)
   Nearly all these symptoms or signs have also been associated with proven benign lesions, so they are only suggestive but indicate the need for a pathologic diagnosis.
B. Diagnostic procedures. Laboratory evaluation of thyroid function is useful to assist in determining whether a nodule is benign or malignant. Figure 31.1 illustrates a recommended approach to management of a thyroid nodule.

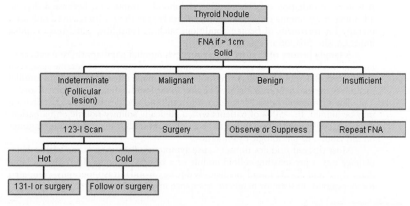

Figure 31.1. Decision tree for the management of a thyroid nodule based on fine-needle aspiration (FNA).

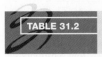

TABLE 31.2	Serum Thyroglobulin (Tg) Levels in Normal Subjects and in Patients with Various Benign Pathologic Conditions of the Thyroid Gland	

	Serum Tg level mean	
Condition	± SEM (ng/mL)	No. of subjects
Control subjects (blood donors)	5.1 ± 0.49	95
Active Graves disease	176.0 ± 30.0	33
Non–Graves disease thyrotoxicosis[a]	145.0 ± 27.0	7
Subacute thyroiditis (acute phase)	136.8 ± 74.5	12
Thyroid adenoma	424.6 ± 189.4	27
Endemic goiter	108.1 ± 19.8	77

SEM, standard error of the mean.
[a]Multinodular toxic goiter and toxic adenomas.
From Van Herle AJ. Thyroid nodules and thyroid cancer. In: Carlson HE, ed. *Endocrinology*. New York: Copyright © 1983, John Wiley and Sons. Reprinted by permission.

1. **Thyroid function tests.** Nearly all patients with either thyroid carcinoma or benign nodules are euthyroid. An abnormal thyroid function test in a patient with a thyroid nodule does not rule out thyroid cancer but may make thyroid carcinoma a less likely possibility. Low serum thyroid-stimulating hormone (TSH) concentration in the setting of a nodular goiter suggests the presence of either an autonomously functioning adenoma or a toxic multinodular goiter. Elevated antiperoxidase and antithyroglobulin antibody titers indicate lymphocytic thyroiditis that may present as a nodule. The serum thyroglobulin level is not a useful test to distinguish benign from malignant nodules because it is increased with any goitrous process (Table 31.2).
2. **Thyroid ultrasound** is a noninvasive test that distinguishes cystic from solid lesions. It is routinely used to guide fine-needle aspiration biopsy. Thyroid ultrasonography is capable of identifying impalpable solid and cystic nodules as small as 0.2 mm. The ultrasonographic features that suggest the diagnosis of malignancy are hypoechogenicity in a solid nodule, fine stippled calcifications, and intranodular vascularity.
3. **Fine-needle aspiration (FNA) biopsy.** FNA biopsy is the most important diagnostic technique. This technique consists of removal of cells from the thyroid gland via a fine needle (23 to 27 gauge). There are many variations of this technique. It is usually performed under ultrasound guidance. FNA reliably identifies thyroid nodule cytology and is the most effective method to diagnose malignancy. In experienced hands, the procedure is safe, with accuracy, sensitivity, and specificity of ~90%. With common use of FNA, the number of patients requiring surgery has declined by >40%. FNA biopsy should be performed on solid nodules >1 cm, on nodules with both a solid and cystic component >2.0 cm, on the solid component of large cystic nodules, and on nodules with evidence of recent growth.

   FNA biopsy results are divided into four categories: **(a)** benign, **(b)** suspicious (includes aspirates with some features of thyroid carcinoma but not conclusive), **(c)** malignant, and **(d)** insufficient. In a large series of FNA biopsy of thyroid nodules, benign cytology was found in 69% (mainly colloid goiter), malignant cytology in 3.5%, suspicious cytology in 10%, and insufficient result in 17%. The suspicious category consists of variants of follicular neoplasm, but follicular adenomas are about 10-fold more common than follicular carcinomas. The finding of nuclear atypia in a follicular lesion gives a 44% prevalence of malignancy, and absence of nuclear atypia suggests a benign lesion. Those patients with a nondiagnostic or "insufficient" cytologic diagnosis should have a repeat biopsy. An adequate specimen is obtained in a majority of repeat FNA of nodules.

4. **Radioiodine scans with^{123}I or ^{131}I.** Nodules may be classified into hyperfunctional ("hot") nodules, nonfunctional ("cold") nodules, or normal functioning ("warm") nodules by radioiodine scan. Most studies show that a hot nodule is rarely malignant. The finding of a cold nodule has relatively low sensitivity because the majority of both benign and malignant solitary thyroid nodules appear hypofunctional relative to adjacent normal thyroid tissue. Therefore, a radioiodine scan is not recommended in the initial evaluation of a thyroid nodule. In patients with nodules that are follicular lesions by FNA, radioiodine scan should be performed; hot or functional nodules are rarely malignant.

5. **Serum calcitonin** measurement represents an excellent marker in the preoperative diagnosis of medullary carcinoma of the thyroid, especially if a calcitonin rise can be demonstrated 3 to 5 minutes after the administration of pentagastrin (not currently available in the United States), $0.5\mu g$/kg IV push, or after a calcium infusion. Serum calcitonin should be ordered in all subjects belonging to a kindred with familial multiple endocrine neoplasia type 2 (MEN2). However, calcitonin levels may be elevated in patients with Hashimoto thyroiditis and other benign thyroid conditions; neuroendocrine tumors; lung, colon, breast, and prostate cancers; sepsis; and generalized inflammation. In several studies of the routine measurement of serum calcitonin in patients with nodular thyroid disease, medullary carcinoma was found in 0.3% to 1.4%. False positives occur in about one half of those with an elevated baseline calcitonin. Currently the test is not routinely performed in the evaluation of a thyroid nodule.

6. **Positron emission tomography (PET) Scan.** PET scans with fluorodeoxyglucose are useful to localize recurrent thyroid cancers but are probably not useful to differentiate between benign and malignant thyroid nodules.

III. MANAGEMENT OF THYROID NODULES

A. **Nonsurgical management.** The vast majority of thyroid nodules are benign and can be followed with observation alone or with thyroxine suppression therapy in selected patients. Spontaneous regression of thyroid nodules may occur. Thyroid hormone suppression therapy is based on the assumption that TSH is a growth factor for the nodule. The aim of therapy is to reduce serum TSH to the low-normal range. L-Thyroxine suppression therapy may be used for nodules that do not decrease in size over several months of observation. This therapy for the treatment of benign thyroid nodules has been challenged by failure of some studies to show a significant decrease in nodule size and concern about decreasing mineral bone density or triggering atrial fibrillation, especially in the elderly. Several controlled studies showed >50% reduction in nodule size in one fourth of patients with a single nodule. Generally, patients are followed by palpation at intervals of 3 to 6 months. Ultrasonographic examination can be performed to assess growth or shrinkage of a nodule annually. Unfortunately, the therapy has to be continued for years to prevent regrowth of the nodule.

B. **Operative management**
   1. The extent of thyroidectomy varies from a lobectomy to a near-total thyroidectomy. Indications for thyroid nodule removal are
      a. The presence of a malignant or suspicious lesion (follicular neoplasms and Hürthle cell neoplasms should be considered suspicious)
      b. When the nodule or goiter causes compression of the surrounding structures, causing dysphagia, dysphonia, or breathing problems
      c. Cosmetic reasons

C. **Postoperative management of benign nodules.** In the postoperative period, thyroxine (T$_4$) is usually given to the patients to prevent recurrent nodule or goiter formation. I prescribe a dose of levothyroxine that brings the serum TSH to the low-normal range.

IV. THYROID CANCER

A. **Classification and features.** Thyroid carcinoma is classified into five major types: papillary, follicular, medullary, anaplastic, and thyroid lymphoma (Table 31.1). Most

TABLE 31.3	Staging of Differentiated Thyroid Cancer Using the TNM Classification

Tumor (T)

TX	Primary tumor size unknown but without extrathyroidal extension
T1	Tumor diameter 2 cm or less
T2	Tumor diameter 2–4 cm
T3	Tumor >4 cm in greatest dimension limited to the thyroid or with minimal extrathyroid extension
T4a	Tumor of any size extending beyond the thyroid capsule to invade subcutaneous tissue, larynx, trachea, esophagus, recurrent laryngeal nerve
T4b	Tumor invades prevertebral fascia or encases carotid artery or mediastinal vessels

Regional lymph nodes (N)
(Regional lymph nodes are the cervical and upper mediastinal lymph nodes.)

NX	Regional lymph nodes not assessed at surgery
N0	No regional lymph node metastasis
N1	Regional lymph node metastasis
N1a	Metastasis to level VI (pretracheal, paratracheal, and prelaryngeal lymph nodes)
N1b	Metastasis to unilateral, bilateral, contralateral cervical, or mediastinal lymph nodes

Distant metastasis (M)

MX	Presence of distant metastasis cannot be assessed
M0	No distant metastasis
M1	Distant metastasis

Stage grouping

	Papillary or follicular	
	<45 years old	45 years and older
Stage I	Any T, any N, M0	T1, N0, M0
Stage II	Any T, any N, M1	T2, N0, M0
Stage III		T3, N0, M0; T1-3, N1a, M0
Stage IVA		Any T, any N, M0
Stage IVB		T4b, any MN, M0
Stage IVC		Any T, any N, M1

Used with the permission of the American Joint Committee on Cancer (AJCC), Chicago, Illinois. The original source for this material is the AJCC Cancer Staging Manual, Sixth Edition (2002) published by Springer-Verlag New York, www.springer-ny.com.

thyroid cancers grow slowly over years, but a few are more aggressive and have high mortality rates. Thyroid carcinomas tend to be more aggressive clinically in older patients compared with younger individuals. This is reflected in the TNM classification of differentiated thyroid cancers (papillary and follicular) (Table 31.3).

1. **Papillary thyroid carcinoma** accounts for >80% of all thyroid cancers. The stage depends on the age of the patient at the time of initial diagnosis, the size of the primary lesion, local invasion, and the degree of metastases, as noted in Table 31.3. The tumor tends to invade lymphatics and metastasize to the regional lymph nodes and lungs. Most papillary thyroid cancers contain one of two activating oncogenes: the BRAF V600E mutation or the RET/PTC1 rearrangement. BRAF V600E is associated with a worse prognosis.

2. **Follicular thyroid carcinoma** accounts for ~10% of all thyroid cancers in the United States and is relatively more common in countries with iodine deficiency. Follicular thyroid carcinoma is slightly more aggressive than papillary carcinoma. Cervical lymph node involvement is less common, but distant metastasis is more frequent compared to papillary thyroid cancer. Hürthle cell carcinoma is a more lethal variant of follicular carcinoma.

3. **Medullary thyroid carcinoma** accounts for 2% to 4% of thyroid cancers and is derived from the calcitonin-secreting cells or parafollicular cells. Elevated serum calcitonin levels establish the diagnosis and correlate with tumor mass. Approximately 20% are familial tumors and are associated with other endocrine neoplasias (MEN type 2A or 2B). The recognition of point mutations in the *ret* proto-oncogene on chromosome 10 has enhanced the ability to detect these neoplasms at an early and potentially curable stage in suspected family members. The treatment is total thyroidectomy with dissection of central compartment nodes.

4. **Anaplastic thyroid carcinoma,** the most aggressive and lethal neoplasm, makes up only 2% of all thyroid cancers. Anaplastic thyroid cancer is often derived from a well-differentiated thyroid carcinoma. Three quarters of patients are >60 years of age. Examination of the neck usually reveals a fixed, large, firm mass. Surgical resection is usually contraindicated unless the tumor is in its initial stage. A tracheostomy can be performed to prevent suffocation by these rapidly growing tumors. The patient is usually treated with external irradiation beam therapy or chemotherapy or both. The mortality exceeds 80% at 12 months.

5. **Thyroid lymphoma** accounts for ~1% of thyroid malignancies and is often engrafted on a background of chronic lymphocytic thyroiditis. The tumor arises from B-cell lymphocytes. Patients are usually women >60 years of age with a long history of Hashimoto thyroiditis and present with a rapidly enlarging thyroid mass. The patient may complain of neck pressure, local swelling of the thyroid gland, hoarseness, and dysphagia. Fine-needle aspiration may suggest the diagnosis, but definitive diagnosis generally requires an open biopsy. Treatment with external radiation and four to six courses of chemotherapy usually produces a permanent remission.

B. **Management of Papillary and Follicular Thyroid Cancer**
1. **Surgical resection.** For differentiated carcinoma, a near-total or total thyroidectomy is performed. Total thyroidectomy is associated with more complications, such as recurrent laryngeal nerve damage and hypoparathyroidism. Lymph node dissection is based on surgical findings.

2. **Radioiodine-131 remnant ablation.** Ablation of thyroid remnants following surgery improves the prognosis in patients with more extensive disease. However, there is no benefit in patients with minimal disease such as 1-cm papillary carcinomas confined to the thyroid. The treatment is given 1.5 to 3 months postoperatively, after the patient has been withdrawn from thyroid hormone. The patient is treated with tri-iodothyronine (T_3) (Cytomel, 25 μg twice a day) for 4 to 8 weeks; then T_3 is discontinued for 2 weeks during which the patient follows a low-iodine diet. The routine use of a diagnostic scan before an ablative dose has been discontinued because the large diagnostic dose can impair the uptake of the therapy dose. The ablative dose varies from 30 to 100 mCi. Seven to 10 days after the ablative dose, the patient undergoes a posttherapy scan, which sometimes reveals extrathyroid disease.

3. **Levothyroxine suppression of TSH.** A suppressive dose of thyroid hormone is given after thyroidectomy to reduce thyroid cancer recurrence rates. TSH stimulates thyroid tumors that contain TSH receptors. The dose of thyroxine should be adjusted to keep the TSH suppressed without causing clinical thyrotoxicosis. The degree of suppression should be based on the stage of the patient. In patients with a good prognosis, TSH should be suppressed to the slightly subnormal range. In patients with poor prognosis, TSH should be suppressed to <0.1 mU/L without causing clinical thyrotoxicosis, provided that this can be done safely.

4. **Metastatic or recurrent tumors.** Surgical removal is preferable for metastases or recurrence that is accessible to surgery. Radioiodine-131 is the principal treatment of distant metastatic tumors. If the tumor does not concentrate the isotope, external radiation may be effective.

5. **Routine follow-up**
a. **Serum thyroglobulin.** Patients are followed at intervals of 3 to 6 months by clinical evaluation, measurements of TSH and serum thyroglobulin, occasional radioiodine scans, and neck ultrasonography. In the absence of the thyroid

gland, thyroglobulin should be undetectable in serum; measurable thyroglobulin signifies persistent thyroid tissue, either differentiated thyroid cancer or persistent normal tissue. On levothyroxine suppression therapy, a thyroglobulin level >1 to 2 ng/mL is regarded as abnormal. TSH-stimulated serum thyroglobulin is a more sensitive assessment of recurrence than the radioiodine scan. Unfortunately, antibodies to thyroglobulin, found in 10% to 20% of patients, interfere with the measurement and make it uninterpretable.

b. ^{131}**I scanning with recombinant TSH injection.** Recombinant TSH (Thyrogen) permits performance of ^{131}I scans while patients remain on their levothyroxine therapy. The current protocol consists of the intramuscular injection of 0.9 mg of Thyrogen on Monday and Tuesday; on Wednesday the patient is given 4 mCi of ^{131}I; and on Friday the patient's serum Tg level is obtained and a total body scan is performed. If the scan is negative and the patient's serum Tg level remains low after Thyrogen stimulation, the patient is considered free of disease. The cost of Thyrogen is substantial, but its use avoids symptoms of hypothyroidism.

c. Ultrasound. Annual ultrasound of the neck is very useful for detection of metastases to lymph nodes. Abnormal nodes or masses can be biopsied by FNA under ultrasound. Measurement of thyroglobulin in the aspirate is a useful addition to histologic evaluation.

Selected References

Ashcraft MW, Van Herle AJ. The comparative value of serum thyroglobulin measurements and iodine 131 total body scans in the follow up study of patients with treated differentiated thyroid cancer. *Am J Med* 1981;71:806–814.

Bartolotta TV, et al. Incidentally discovered thyroid nodules: incidence, and greyscale and colour Doppler pattern in an adult population screened by real-time compound spatial sonography. *Radiol Med (Torino)* 2006;111:989–998.

Bucci A, Shore-Freedman E, Gierlowski T, et al. Behavior of small thyroid cancers found by screening radiation-exposed individuals. *J Clin Endocrinol Metab* 2001;86:3711–3716.

Carmeci C, Jeffrey RB, McDougall IR, et al. Ultrasound-guided fine-needle aspiration biopsy of thyroid masses. *Thyroid* 1998;8:283–289.

Caron NR, Clark OH. Papillary thyroid cancer. *Curr Treat Options Oncol* 2006;7:309–319.

Ciampi R, Nikiforov YE. RET/PTC rearrangements and BRAF mutations in thyroid tumorigenesis. *Endocrinology* 2007;148:936–941.

Cooper DS, et al. Management guidelines for patients with thyroid nodules and differentiated thyroid cancer. *Thyroid* 2006;16:109.

Costante G, Meringolo D, Durante C, et al. Predictive value of serum calcitonin levels for preoperative diagnosis of medullary thyroid carcinoma in a cohort of 5817 consecutive patients with thyroid nodules. *J Clin Endocrinol Metab* 2007;92:450–455.

Davies L, Welch HG. Increasing incidence of thyroid cancer in the United States, 1973–2002. *JAMA* 2006;95:2164–2167.

Dulgeroff A, Hershman JM. Medical therapy for differentiated thyroid carcinoma. *Endocrine Rev* 1994;15:500–515.

Durante C, Haddy N, Baudin E, et al. Long-term outcome of 444 patients with distant metastases from papillary and follicular thyroid carcinoma: benefits and limits of radioiodine therapy. *J Clin Endocrinol Metab* 2006;91:2892–2899.

Frates MC, Benson CB, Charboneau JW, et al: Management of thyroid nodules detected at US: Society of Radiologists in Ultrasound consensus conference statement. *Radiology* 2005;237:794–800.

Frates MC, Benson CB, Doubilet PML. Prevalence and distribution of carcinoma in patients with solitary and multiple thyroid nodules on sonography. *J Clin Endocrinol Metab* 2006;91:3411–3417.

Gharib H, Goellner JR. Fine-needle aspiration biopsy of the thyroid: an appraisal. *Ann Intern Med* 1993;118:282–289.

Jonklaas J, Sarlis NJ, Litofsky D, et al. Outcomes of patients with differentiated thyroid carcinoma following initial therapy. *Thyroid* 2006;16:1229–1242.

Matsuzuka F, Miyauchi A, Katayama S, et al. Clinical aspects of primary thyroid lymphoma: diagnosis and treatment based on our experience of 119 cases. *Thyroid* 1993;3:93–99.

Mazzaferri EL, Jhiang SM. Long-term impact of initial surgical and medical therapy on papillary and follicular thyroid cancer. *Am J Med* 1994;97:418–428.

Mazzaferri EL, Robbins RJ, Spencer CA, et al. A consensus report of the role of serum thyroglobulin as a monitoring method for low-risk patients with papillary thyroid carcinoma. *J Clin Endocrinol Metab* 2003;88:1433–1441.

Pacini F, Molinaro E, Lippi F, et al. Prediction of disease status by recombinant human TSH-stimulated serum Tg in the postsurgical follow-up of differentiated thyroid carcinoma. *J Clin Endocrinol Metab* 2001;86:5686–5690.

Smallridge RC, Meek SE, Morgan MA, et al. Monitoring thyroglobulin in a sensitive immunoassay has comparable sensitivity to recombinant human TSH-stimulated thyroglobulin in follow-up of thyroid cancer patients. *J Clin Endocrinol Metab* 2007;92:82–87.

Torlontano M, Crocetti U, D'Aloiso L, et al. Serum thyroglobulin and ^{131}I whole body scan after recombinant human TSH stimulation in the follow-up of low-risk patients with differentiated thyroid cancer. *Eur J Endocrinol* 2003;148:19–24.

Vander JB, Gaston EA, Dawber TR. The significance of nontoxic thyroid nodules: final report of a 15 year study of the incidence of thyroid malignancy. *Ann Intern Med* 1968; 69:537–540.

Wartofsky L, Van Nostrand D, eds. *Thyroid Cancer.* 2nd ed. Totawa, NJ: Humana Press; 2006.

NEWBORN THYROID DISORDERS AND SCREENING

32

Stephen LaFranchi and Stephen A. Huang

*A*lthough thyroid hormone is important for regulating body metabolism throughout life, it is crucial for growth and development of the fetal central nervous system and during the first 3 years of life. Lack of sufficient thyroid hormone during this period results in mental retardation and other neurologic sequelae. For the most part, congenital hypothyroidism is not a heritable disorder because the majority of cases are sporadic. Thus, it is not possible to identify a population of high-risk pregnant women who might deliver an infant with congenital hypothyroidism, and to date no reliable prenatal test for fetal hypothyroidism short of fetal blood sampling (cordocentesis) has been developed. Furthermore, the clinical manifestations of congenital hypothyroidism are often subtle or nonspecific, or even absent, so that the condition is usually not suspected or diagnosed in the neonatal period. Yet few disorders respond so dramatically to treatment. For these reasons, newborn screening programs were developed for congenital hypothyroidism. These screening programs were made possible by the application of precise radioimmunoassays for thyroid hormones to mass screening techniques, allowing for the diagnosis and treatment of hypothyroidism in the first few weeks of life, before clinical manifestations are apparent. Screening programs permit detection of hypothyroidism at a rate of 1:3 000 to 1:4 000 newborns. The majority of cases of congenital hypothyroidism are the result of an embryologic defect.

I. FETAL THYROID PHYSIOLOGY

A. Fetal thyroid development. The fetal thyroid develops from an outpouching of the foregut at the base of the tongue and migrates to its normal location over the thyroid cartilage in the first 4 to 8 weeks of gestation. Its bilobed shape is recognizable at 7 weeks of gestation. The first sign of thyroid function, thyroglobulin production, is apparent by the eighth week of gestation, and at the tenth week, the thyroid is capable of trapping iodine. By the twelfth week of gestation, thyroid hormone production occurs and colloid storage is apparent histologically. Fetal thyroid-stimulating hormone (TSH), thyroxine-binding globulin (TBG), and total and free thyroxine (T_4) concentrations gradually rise from week 12 of gestation and reach mean adult levels by 36 weeks of gestation. The rise in fetal serum triiodothyronine (T_3) is smaller, most likely the result of placental and fetal deiodinases that convert T_4 to reverse T_3 (rT_3).

B. Maternal–fetal thyroid relationship

1. A portion of maternal thyroid hormones crosses the placenta, sufficient to result in serum T_4 concentrations that are 25% to 33% that of full-term infants. Thus, maternal thyroid hormones may have a role in normal fetal development prior to the maturation of the fetal hypothalamic–pituitary-thyroid axis. Evidence suggests that maternal thyroid hormones can partially protect a hypothyroid fetus until delivery but will not normalize fetal serum T_4 concentrations. Additional protection is afforded by more efficient fetal brain 5′-deiodinase activity, which increases T_4-to-T_3 conversion.

2. Hypothyroid women (0.3% of pregnancies) tend to be anovulatory, and if they conceive they have a spontaneous abortion rate approaching 50%; this can be prevented by T_4 replacement. Maternal hypothyroidism during pregnancy may adversely affect neurologic development in offspring. In one study, offspring born to mothers with TSH elevations (occurring at a frequency of 1 in 400) had an IQ of 103 compared with a control group at 107. In a second study, offspring born to mothers with T_4 concentrations in the lowest 5th percentile had a psychomotor developmental index 14 points lower (PDI = 86) compared to the remainder of the group (PDI = 100).

C. Treatment of fetal hypothyroidism. Rarely, a fetus is discovered to be hypothyroid during pregnancy. This can occur with familial dyshormonogenesis, maternal autoimmune thyroid disease with transfer of thyrotropin receptor–blocking antibodies (TRBAb), antithyroid drug treatment of Graves disease, or inadvertent radioactive iodine (RAI) treatment of a pregnant woman. Fetal hypothyroidism can be proven by fetal blood sampling. Fetal hypothyroidism resulting from treatment of a mother with Graves disease can be managed by reducing or discontinuing the dose of maternal antithyroid medication with or without enteral levothyroxine administration. In severe cases of other forms of fetal hypothyroidism, especially those detected late in gestation, intra-amniotic injections of levothyroxine, 250 to 500 μg weekly until term, have been shown to rapidly reduce fetal goiter size and normalize cord-blood T_4 and TSH concentrations.

II. NEONATAL THYROID PHYSIOLOGY

A. Term infant

1. **Thyroid changes at birth.** There are dramatic changes in thyroid function shortly after birth. Within 30 minutes of delivery, there is a sharp increase in the serum TSH concentration up to 80 μU/mL, most likely a result of the stresses of the birth process and clamping of the cord. The serum TSH concentration gradually falls to <10 μU/mL during the first week of life.

2. **Thyroid function over the next 6 weeks.** This sharp rise in TSH stimulates rapid increases in serum T_4, free T_4, and T_3 concentrations into the hyperthyroid range (see Table 32.7 for normal values with age). Serum T_4 and T_3 concentrations gradually decrease over several weeks.

B. Preterm infant

1. **Thyroid changes at birth.** Preterm infants have a reduced TSH surge, up to 50 mU/L. Cord-blood T_4, free T_4, and T_3 concentrations are reduced in comparison with term infants and directly proportional to gestational age and birth weight.

2. **Thyroid function after birth.** Thyroid changes in preterm infants after birth are qualitatively similar to but quantitatively smaller than that of term infants. In very-low-birth-weight infants, serum T_4 and T_3 concentrations may actually fall to below birth levels in the first week of life. This drop is a result of multiple factors, including immaturity of the hypothalamic–pituitary–thyroid axis, lack of the maternal contribution of thyroxine, and nonthyroidal illness–like changes.

3. **Hypothyroxinemia of prematurity, morbidity, and neurologic outcome.** Several studies correlate measures of morbidity and mortality with reduced serum T_4 concentrations, but they do not establish cause and effect. While some studies show improvement in some of these measures with thyroxine treatment, most controlled trials show no effect. Overall, thyroxine treatment does not appear to affect IQ, although evidence from a Dutch study suggested that the subgroup of premature infants younger than 27 weeks may benefit from thyroxine treatment.

C. Neurologic consequences of congenital hypothyroidism

1. **Pathophysiology.** Thyroid hormone stimulates fetal neuroblast proliferation and migration, axonal and dendritic outgrowth, oligodendrocyte differentiation, and myelination. Animal studies have shown nuclear thyroid receptors in both neuronal and glial components of the brain; hypothyroidism results in a delay in myelin protein gene expression.

2. **IQ.** Several studies indicate an inverse correlation between the age of diagnosis and treatment and intellectual prognosis (Table 32.1). Even when treatment was started in the first 3 months of life, the mean IQ was 89, somewhat reduced. Although there was individual variation, it usually held that the later the diagnosis, the lower the IQ. One study found the incidence of hypothyroidism in mentally handicapped institutionalized patients to be ~5%.

3. **Other neurologic sequelae.** Besides abnormal cognitive function, abnormalities of muscle tone, gait, coordination, speech, hearing, and vision can be present

TABLE 32.1	Age Treatment for Congenital Hypothyroidism Started and Intellectual Outcome prior to Newborn Screening[a]	

Age (mo)	IQ ($\bar{X}$)	Range
0–3	89	64–107
3–6	71	35–96
>6	54	25–80

$\bar{X}$, mean.
[a]Other neurologic sequelae include the following: (1) ataxia, (2) gross and fine motor incoordination, (3) hypotonia and spasticity, (4) speech disorder, (5) sensorineural hearing loss, (6) strabismus, and (7) short attention span.
Adapted from Klein AH, et al. Improved prognosis in congenital hypothyroidism treated before age 3 months. *J Pediatr* 1972;81:912.

(Table 32.1). In an attempt to prevent mental retardation and neurologic sequelae, screening programs were developed to diagnose and treat infants with congenital hypothyroidism in the first weeks of life.

III. SCREENING PROGRAMS FOR CONGENITAL HYPOTHYROIDISM

Screening for hypothyroidism has become routine throughout the United States and in Canada, Western Europe, Israel, Japan, Australia, and New Zealand, and it is under development or established in Mexico, and several countries in Eastern Europe, Latin and South America, Asia, and Africa. Worldwide, out of a total birth population of 130 million, it is estimated that 20% to 25% (25 to 30 million infants) are screened yearly for congenital hypothyroidism.

A. Approaches to screening

1. Primary T$_4$-follow-up TSH. About half the screening programs in the United States use this approach.

  a. A filter-paper T$_4$ measurement is carried out on all infants; in those infants with a T$_4$ level below a prescribed cutoff, usually 10%, a TSH determination is performed. In a report from California, 80% of affected infants had serum T$_4$ values <7 μg/dL (<90 nmol/L), and 20% fell in the 7- to 12-μg/dL (90- to 154-nmol) range. About 67% had TSH values >100 μU/mL, 88% were over 50 μU/mL, but 12% had TSH values of 20 to 50 μU/mL. The incidence of primary hypothyroidism detected in these programs is around 1 in 3 000 to 1 in 4 000.

  b. If low T$_4$ nonelevated TSH screening tests are followed up, this approach also has the potential to detect infants with hypothyroidism and a delayed TSH rise, hypothalamic–pituitary hypothyroidism, and TBG deficiency; it will miss infants with subclinical hypothyroidism (normal T$_4$, elevated TSH). Primary T$_4$-follow-up TSH tends to have a higher recall rate, ~0.2%. This means that eight infants will be retested for every one in whom hypothyroidism is detected. Although programs would like to switch to a primary TSH test approach to reduce this recall rate, early discharge of infants <24 hours old when the normal TSH level can extend above 50 μU/mL makes this problematic. Programs that have gone to a primary TSH screen have done so successfully by developing a TSH cutoff adjusted for the age at which the specimen is obtained.

2. Primary TSH. Most screening programs in Canada, Europe, Japan, and Australia use the primary TSH approach, and about half the screening programs in the United States have switched to a primary TSH test. This approach has a slightly higher detection rate, around 1 in 3 000, perhaps because it identifies infants with subclinical hypothyroidism and transient hyperthyrotropinemia. A primary TSH screening approach will not identify infants with primary hypothyroidism and a delayed TSH rise, hypothalamic-pituitary hypothyroidism,

TABLE 32.2	Potential Indications for a Second or Discretionary Screening Test

A. Very-low-birth-weight infants: <1 500 g

B. Perinatal complications, including the following:
   1. NICU admission
   2. Transfusion
   3. Congenital heart disease
   4. Other severe congenital anomalies
   5. Same-sex twins
   6. Dopamine administration
   7. Steroid administration
   8. Iodine exposure

NICU, neonatal intensive care unit.

or TBG deficiency. The recall rate tends to be slightly lower, ~0.05%, with two infants retested for every one with congenital hypothyroidism.

3. Simultaneous T$_4$ and TSH. As of 2000, five states and Puerto Rico carry out simultaneous T$_4$ and TSH testing. This screening approach has the potential to pick up all the thyroid disorders described above. One would expect the detection rate to be highest with this testing approach.

4. Specimen collection at two time periods. Approximately 10 states, representing 20% of newborns in the United States, perform newborn screening on specimens collected at two time periods, initially in the first 5 days of life and then later at the first return visit, usually between 2 and 6 weeks of age. In general, these programs use a primary T$_4$-follow-up TSH approach. Approximately 10% of cases (1 in 30 000) are detected by the second screening test. These programs tend to pick up more infants with subclinical hypothyroidism plus those with delayed TSH rise. Several screening programs have instituted "discretionary" second specimen collection in newborns at high risk for delayed TSH rise; potential indications for such an approach are presented in Table 32.2.

B. Screening program results. A summary of worldwide screening for congenital hypothyroidism is presented in Table 32.3.

1. Thyroid scanning shows that aplasia/hypoplasia is present in 30%, ectopic glands in 60%, and large glands with increased uptake, most likely representing dyshormonogenesis, are present in 10%. Transient primary hypothyroidism is rare in the United States, occurring in ~1 in 50 000; it is more common in

TABLE 32.3	Summary of Worldwide Screening for Congenital Hypothyroidism

Type	Incidence
Permanent primary hypothyroidism Aplasia (30%) Ectopia (60%) Dyshormonogenesis (10%)	1:3,000–4,000
Transient primary hypothyroidism	1:50 000 (North America) 1:200–1:8 000 (Europe)
Hypothalamic-pituitary hypothyroidism	1:30,000–100,000

Adapted from Fisher DA. Second international conference on neonatal thyroid screening: progress report. *J Pediatr* 1983;102:653.

Europe, varying in incidence from 1 in 200 to 1 in 8 000. The higher incidence results from maternal and therefore fetal iodine deficiency in areas of endemic iodine deficiency. The transient cases in the United States may be the result of transplacental passage of TRBAb in mothers with autoimmune thyroid disease, fetal exposure to antithyroid drugs in mothers treated for Graves disease, or fetal or neonatal exposure to excess iodine, as in amniofetography or the use of iodine antiseptics.

  2. The incidence of hypothalamic-pituitary hypothyroidism is ~1 in 50 000, accounting for 5% of all cases, although the screening experience in the northwestern United States indicates the incidence might be closer to 1 in 25 000.

C. Atypical screening results

  1. Low T_4–nonelevated TSH. In primary T_4-follow-up TSH screening programs, by definition, a certain percentage of infants will have low T_4-nonelevated TSH results. The vast majority of these infants are normal, so most programs choose to follow-up only infants with low T_4-elevated TSH screening results. In programs that attempt to investigate the low T_4-normal TSH results further, the following conditions have been described.

   a. Premature and other low-birth-weight infants, who make up ~5% of the normal birth population, tend to have lower total T_4 concentrations while maintaining a normal serum TSH level; free T_4 levels are often normal (see Section II.B). With time, the total T_4 concentrations tend to rise to the normal range without therapy. For premature and low-birth-weight infants who have low T_4 and elevated TSH concentrations indicative of primary hypothyroidism, thyroxine treatment is indicated.

   b. Nonthyroidal illness. Acute or chronic illness can result in <u>reduced thyroid hormone</u> concentrations; this nonthyroidal illness syndrome is characterized by low T_4 or T_3 concentrations; low, normal, or high free T_4 concentrations; <u>increased rT_3 levels</u>; and normal TSH concentrations. With resolution of the nonthyroidal illness, thyroid function studies revert to normal. In sick, premature, or other low-birth-weight infants, this can explain the low serum total T_4 and even free T_4 levels.

   c. Delayed TSH rise. Some infants initially have a low T_4 and nonelevated TSH concentration, but on a second screening test have a low T_4 and elevated TSH concentration, confirmed by serum studies. These cases are uncommon, occurring in ~1 in 30 000 newborns; they are more common in preterm or acutely ill infants and appear to be the result of late maturation of the hypothalamic-pituitary-thyroid axis.

   d. Hypothalamic-pituitary hypothyroidism. See Section V.C.

   e. TBG deficiency

  2. Normal T_4-elevated TSH

   a. Subclinical hypothyroidism. Infants with a normal T_4 and elevated TSH concentration are most commonly detected by primary TSH screening programs. They can also be detected by a primary T_4-follow-up TSH program when the initial filter paper T_4 is low and the TSH is elevated, yet the confirmatory serum test shows a normal T_4 and elevated TSH concentration. In these cases, thyroid scanning usually shows residual thyroid tissue.

   b. Transient hyperthyrotropinemia. In Japan, ~1 in 18 000 infants has a syndrome of transient hyperthyrotropinemia with normal T_4 and T_3 concentrations, which resolves after several months to years. The mechanism to explain these findings is unknown.

IV. EPIDEMIOLOGY

  A. Incidence. Newborn screening programs detect hypothyroidism at a rate of 1 in 3 000 to 1 in 4 000.

  B. Inheritance. Approximately 85% of cases of congenital hypothyroidism are sporadic and 15% are hereditary. Hereditary forms most commonly are secondary to one of the inborn errors of thyroid hormone synthesis, secretion, or utilization, but they may also occur as a result of the rare mutations for the transcription factors that regulate thyroid gland development. Familial cases occur in infants born to mothers with autoimmune thyroid disease and passage of TRBAb.

1. Nearly all screening programs report a **female preponderance, with a 2:1 female-to-male ratio.** A recent study reported a nearly 3:1 female-to-male ratio in infants with ectopic glands, whereas the sex ratio in infants with athyrosis was nearly equal, suggesting that different genetic and nongenetic mechanisms are responsible for ectopia and athyrosis.

2. Although there are a **few reports of thyroid dysgenesis** occurring in both monozygous twins, most studies report discordance for congenital hypothyroidism in twins.

3. **Some racial differences** have been reported in the prevalence of congenital hypothyroidism. In the Georgia state screening program the incidence of congenital hypothyroidism in the white population was 1 in 5 526, whereas in the black population it was much lower, 1 in 32 378; yet the incidence of TBG deficiency was approximately the same in both groups. A study from California similarly reported a <u>lower incidence of congenital hypothyroidism in the black</u> population than in the white population and also found a higher incidence in the Hispanic and Asian populations.

4. **Hypothalamic or pituitary** hypothyroidism also tends to be sporadic in nature, although there are occasional reports of familial pituitary hypothyroidism. Perhaps the most common recognizable cause of congenital hypothalamic–pituitary hypothyroidism involves congenital midline brain developmental defects, such as **septo-optic dysplasia;** this syndrome has a female preponderance and tends to occur in infants born to teenage mothers. Genetic mutations in the genes for the thyrotropin-releasing hormone (TRH) receptor or for TSH or its receptor are rare causes of hypothalamic or pituitary hypothyroidism.

C. **Prenatal diagnosis.** Studies of amniotic fluid levels of T_4, T_3, rT_3, and TSH do not show any correlation between maternal and fetal or neonatal thyroid function. However, the prenatal diagnosis of hypothyroidism can be made by fetal blood sampling by cordocentesis.

V. ETIOLOGY

Congenital hypothyroidism is not the result of a single disorder; rather there is a spectrum of thyroid dysfunction, as listed in Table 32.4.

A. **Permanent primary hypothyroidism**

1. **Thyroid dysgenesis,** which includes aplasia, hypoplasia, and ectopic glands, accounts for 80% to 90% of permanent primary hypothyroidism. Ectopic thyroid glands are the cause of two thirds of all cases of thyroid dysgenesis. The etiologic factors involved in thyroid dysgenesis are mostly unknown. Investigation of the transcription factors **TTF-1, TTF-2, and PAX-8**, which have a role in thyroid gland morphogenesis and differentiation, show that rare familial (and sporadic) cases of thyroid dysgenesis are the result of mutations in these genes. Both dyskinesia and hypothyroidism have been reported in individuals who are heterozygous for mutations in TTF-1. In one report, two siblings with a TTF-2 mutation and thyroid dysgenesis also had a cleft palate and choanal atresia. As most cases of thyroid dysgenesis do not appear to be hereditary, it is not surprising that germline mutations in these genes are not found more commonly.

Some studies suggest that an **intrauterine autoimmune thyroiditis,** as evidenced by antibody-dependent cell-mediated cytotoxicity, may have a role in thyroid dysgenesis. Evidence of a **linkage** with certain human leukocyte antigen (HLA) haplotypes—Bw44, Aw24, and B18—lends indirect support to the autoimmune hypothesis.

2. **Dyshormonogenesis,** or the inborn errors of thyroid hormone synthesis, secretion, and utilization, comprises the hereditary autosomal recessive enzyme deficiencies that account for ~10% of permanent primary hypothyroidism. Hereditary defects in virtually all of these steps have now been described.

TABLE 32.4	**Causes of Congenital Hypothyroidism**

A. Permanent primary hypothyroidism
  1. Thyroid dysgenesis
    a. Aplasia
    b. Hypoplasia
    c. Ectopic gland
  2. Dyshormonogenesis
  3. Maternal radioactive iodine treatment
  4. Associated with the nephrotic syndrome
B. Transient primary hypothyroidism
  1. Maternal transfer of thyrotropin receptor–blocking antibodies
  2. Maternal Graves disease and transplacental passage of antithyroid drug
  3. Maternal iodine deficiency
  4. Iodine exposure of fetus or newborn
C. Permanent hypothalamic-pituitary hypothyroidism
  1. Congenital midline brain developmental defects
  2. Birth trauma or asphyxia with pituitary stalk transection
  3. Congenital pituitary aplasia
  4. Genetic mutations in TRH receptor, TSH, or TSH receptor
D. Transient hypothalamic-pituitary hypothyroidism

TRH, thyrotropin-releasing hormone; TSH, thyroid-stimulating hormone.

   a. **TSH receptor or postreceptor defect** (rare). Loss-of-function mutations in the TSH-binding receptor located on the thyroid cell membrane are recognized as a cause of thyroid hypoplasia. In rare situations, the TSH receptor is normal but there is failure to activate the adenylate cyclase system.
   b. **Iodide transport defects** (uncommon). Mutations in the sodium/iodide symporter result in failure of the iodide pump to concentrate blood iodide across the thyroid cell membrane.
   c. **Peroxidase system defects** (most common). Mutations in the thyroid peroxidase gene results in failure to oxidize iodide to iodine so that it can bind to the tyrosine residue of thyroglobulin (organification). A peroxidase enzyme defect can also result in failure to couple monoiodotyrosine (MIT) and di-iodotyrosine (DIT) to form T_3, or DIT and DIT to form T_4. Mutations in the THOX2 gene that encodes a thyroid oxidase involved in the generation of thyroidal hydrogen peroxide can cause either transient (monoallelic mutation) or permanent (biallelic mutation) congenital hypothyroidism.
   d. **Thyroglobulin defects** (uncommon). Mutations leading to an abnormal thyroglobulin protein result in failure to release T_4 and T_3 into the circulation properly.
   e. **Iodotyrosine deiodinase defects** (uncommon). Defects in the deiodinase enzymes result in failure of deiodination of the iodotyrosines MIT and DIT, and recycling of iodine does not occur.
  3. **Maternal radioactive iodine treatment.** If a woman inadvertently receives radioactive iodine as treatment for Graves disease or thyroid cancer beyond the eighth to tenth week of gestation, the radioactive iodine will cross the placenta, be trapped by the fetal thyroid, and result in thyroid ablation. This can also produce other problems, such as tracheal stenosis and hypoparathyroidism.
  4. **Associated with nephrotic syndrome.** Congenital hypothyroidism has been reported in association with congenital nephrotic syndrome. The pathogenesis of this situation most likely involves increased urinary loss of iodine and iodotyrosines, along with malnutrition and inadequate iodine intake.

B. Transient primary hypothyroidism
1. **Maternal transfer of TRBAb.** Maternal antibody-mediated congenital hypothyroidism resulting from transplacental passage of TRBAb is reported to occur in ~1 in 100 000 newborns. These mothers have some form of autoimmune thyroiditis and produce an IgG TRBAb that crosses the placenta and blocks fetal TSH binding to the thyroid receptor. At birth, these infants have a low T_4 and elevated TSH concentration, and a thyroid scan may show aplasia, but an ultrasound exam may show some thyroid tissue in the normal location. With disappearance of the IgG antibody over the first several months of life, the infant's thyroid gland develops and begins to function. When there is a history of maternal autoimmune thyroid disease or in cases of congenital hypothyroidism in subsequent siblings, it is recommended that mothers and infants be tested for TRBAb. If present, thyroxine replacement can be discontinued when the infant's thyroid function returns to normal.
2. **Maternal Graves disease** and transplacental passage of antithyroid drug. The thiouracil drugs used to treat maternal Graves disease cross the placenta and block fetal thyroid hormone production. Propylthiouracil, in doses as low as 200 to 400 mg per day, is associated with neonatal hypothyroidism. This form of hypothyroidism is transient, because the thiouracil drug is metabolized and excreted by the neonate, and usually resolves in 1 to 2 weeks.
3. **Maternal iodine deficiency.** In geographic areas of iodine deficiency, associated with endemic goiter, maternal and therefore fetal iodine deficiency is the most common cause of congenital hypothyroidism. The main areas of endemic goiter are the South Pacific, China, and Africa, but parts of Europe are also affected. The hypothyroidism can be transient if the neonate receives adequate iodine intake, or longer-lasting if iodine deficiency persists. Two forms of endemic cretinism have been described.
   a. **Neurologic cretinism** is associated with a gait disorder, pyramidal signs, and hearing and speech problems; growth is less affected, and subjects are in a euthyroid state.
   b. **Myxedematous cretinism** is characterized by goiter, growth failure, neurologic sequelae, and persistent hypothyroidism.
      The differences between the two clinical types of endemic cretinism may be the length and severity of postnatal hypothyroidism owing to ongoing iodine deficiency.
4. **Iodine exposure of fetus or newborn.** Excess iodine inadvertently taken by the pregnant mother or received through painting the cervix with iodine-containing antiseptics, as is sometimes done after antepartum rupture of the amniotic membranes, via amniofetography, or through painting the umbilical stump postpartum, or preparation of the skin for intravenous lines or surgical procedures, can produce transient neonatal hypothyroidism. This practice should be avoided and another antiseptic solution used if necessary. Premature infants are more susceptible to iodine-induced or iodine-deficient hypothyroidism.
C. Permanent hypothalamic–pituitary hypothyroidism accounts for ~5% of cases of congenital hypothyroidism detected by screening programs. These defects are usually at the hypothalamic level (TRH deficiency) and are commonly associated with other pituitary hormone deficiencies.
1. **Congenital midline brain developmental defects.** Hypopituitarism associated with other midline developmental defects now appears to be the most common recognizable cause of congenital TSH deficiency. These midline defects can involve hypoplasia of the optic nerve, include absence of the septum pellucidum or corpus callosum (septo-optic dysplasia), or be associated with midline clefting of the lip or palate. Rare cases of sepo-optic dysplasia are caused by mutations in the HES-X gene.
2. **Birth trauma or asphyxia with pituitary stalk transection.** An association between sporadic cases of congenital hypopituitarism and birth trauma or asphyxia has been noted in the past. Imaging techniques, such as magnetic resonance imaging (MRI), now reveal that some cases are the result of

pituitary stalk transection. An associated finding is an ectopic posterior pituitary gland.

3. **Congenital pituitary aplasia,** sometimes familial, is an uncommon cause of hypopituitarism. Increasingly recognized are mutations in the Pit-1, Prop-1, and LHX3 genes, which function as transcription factors important in pituitary gland morphology and differentiation. Prop-1 gene defects may also be associated with large pituitary glands.

4. **TRH receptor and TSH mutations** have been described and are relatively rare causes of congenital hypothalamic–hypopituitary hypothyroidism.

D. **Transient hypothalamic–pituitary hypothyroidism.** Infants with low total and free T_4 concentrations but normal TSH can have hypopituitary hypothyroidism of a transient nature. This disorder appears to occur more frequently in premature infants, where immaturity of the hypothalamic–pituitary axis might have a role in its development. It can be difficult to separate transient hypopituitary hypothyroidism from nonthyroidal illness in sick full-term or premature infants. Measurement of serum free T_4 by equilibrium dialysis is the most accurate method to make this distinction. In premature infants, the serum T_4 and T_3 levels rise with age and usually reach the normal range for term infants by 1 to 2 months of age (see Section II.B.1–3).

VI. CLINICAL MANIFESTATIONS

At the time infants with hypothyroidism are detected by newborn screening programs, the clinical manifestations are subtle, nonspecific, or absent in the majority of infants. Fewer than 5% of the infants detected by screening programs are suspected of having hypothyroidism on clinical grounds prior to notification by the screening laboratory. The absence of initial clinical features can be the result of the partially protective effects of maternal thyroid hormones, but they also most likely depend on the cause of the hypothyroidism, the age of onset in utero, its severity, and duration. Given that an ectopic thyroid is the most common etiology, most infants will have some residual thyroid hormone production. In the few infants who are so affected that they have obvious clinical manifestations in the first week of life, one can surmise that they have had more severe, long-lasting hypothyroidism in utero. In general, mean birth weight and length are near the 50th percentile; head circumference is slightly increased, approximately at the 70th percentile, owing to **cerebral myxedema.** Despite normal somatic growth, there is evidence of in utero hypothyroidism based on retarded skeletal maturation at birth. Although serum T_4 concentrations are low, serum T_3 levels are often maintained in the normal range, and this can also help explain the lack of clinical manifestations in at least some cases. There is also a tendency to prolonged gestation, with one third of the pregnancies lasting 42 weeks or longer. The most common symptoms and signs of congenital hypothyroidism are listed in Table 32.5.

A. **Symptoms.** Common symptoms include lethargy, delayed stooling and constipation, poor suck and feeding problems, and hypothermia. Fewer than a third of infants with congenital hypothyroidism detected by screening programs manifest any of these symptoms at the time of detection.

B. **Signs**

1. **On physical examination** at the time of detection, the majority of infants have few if any of the signs listed in Table 32.5. A small number of infants present with the classic physical appearance, including puffy, myxedematous facies, depressed nasal bridge with pseudohypertelorism, large fontanels (particularly the posterior fontanel), wide sutures, a large protruding tongue with an open mouth (macroglossia), a hoarse cry, an umbilical hernia with distended abdomen, cold mottled skin (cutis marmorata), jaundice (secondary to delayed maturation of the hepatic enzyme glucuronyl transferase), hypotonia, and delayed deep tendon reflexes. Galactorrhea associated with elevated prolactin levels has also been reported. Although it is unusual, a goiter may be palpable in infants with one of the inborn errors of thyroid hormone biosynthesis. However, in infants born to mothers with Graves disease treated with thiouracils, large goiters that can produce airway obstruction have been reported.

TABLE 32.5	Clinical Manifestations of Congenital Hypothyroidism

Symptoms	Signs
Prolonged jaundice	Skin mottling
Lethargy	Umbilical hernia
Constipation	Jaundice
Feeding problems	Macroglossia
Cold to touch	Large fontanels, wide sutures
	Distended abdomen
	Hoarse cry
	Hypotonia
	Dry skin
	Slow reflexes
	Goiter

Adapted from LaFranchi SH, et al. Neonatal hypothyroidism detected by the Northwest Regional Screening Program. *Pediatrics* 1979;63:180.

2. **If the diagnosis is delayed** or not made, infants manifest a subnormal growth rate and delayed development. These can be apparent by 3 to 6 months of age. Mental retardation along with neurologic damage, including incoordination, ataxia, hyper- or hypotonia, neurosensory hearing loss, and strabismus, is also likely to develop.

3. **Hypothalamic–pituitary hypothyroidism.** In these infants, TSH deficiency in general produces <u>milder</u> hypothyroidism, so that clinical manifestations are less obvious than with primary hypothyroidism. However, one should be suspicious of secondary hypothyroidism in infants with midline defects such as cleft lip or palate, infants with ocular signs such as wandering eye movements or nystagmus, and infants with signs of other pituitary hormone deficiencies. These include hypoglycemia, which can be secondary to growth hormone (GH) and/or adrenocorticotropic hormone (and cortisol) deficiency, and males with microgenitalia, including micropenis, hypoplastic scrotum, and undescended testes, which can be due to GH and gonadotropin deficiencies. Diabetes insipidus resulting from antidiuretic hormone deficiency is seen uncommonly with congenital hypopituitarism.

C. **Associated congenital anomalies.** Infants with congenital hypothyroidism appear to be at increased risk for other congenital anomalies. One study showed a fourfold higher prevalence of congenital anomalies (8.4%) compared to a control infant population (2%). Cardiovascular anomalies are the most commonly associated, including pulmonary stenosis, atrial septal defect, and ventricular septal defect. It is unclear whether these anomalies are secondary to an underlying genetic abnormality or teratogen, or whether in utero hypothyroidism contributes to their development, although the former seems more likely. Congenital hypothyroidism occurs more commonly with trisomy 21 and trisomy 18. Infants with congenital hypothyroidism and cleft palate may have a TTF-2 (FOXE1) gene mutation. Infants with associated, persistent neurologic problems, including ataxia, are suspect for a NKX2 gene mutation.

VII. DIAGNOSTIC TESTS

Although screening tests identify infants who are likely to have congenital hypothyroidism, laboratory tests should be obtained to confirm the diagnosis before treatment is started (Table 32.6).

A. **Routine tests.** The simplest tests to confirm the diagnosis of primary hypothyroidism are serum free T_4 and TSH measurements. A serum total T_4 and some measure of thyroxine-binding proteins, such as T_3 resin uptake (T_3RU), can be

TABLE 32.6	**Diagnostic Tests in Congenital Hypothyroidism**

A. Routine (required to confirm diagnosis)
   1. Serum free T_4, or total T_4 and T_3 resin uptake
   2. Serum TSH
B. Optional
   1. Thyroid uptake and scan using ^{123}I or ^{99m}Tc
   2. Thyroid ultrasound
   3. Maternal (and infant) thyrotropin receptor–blocking antibody[a]
   4. Serum thyroglobulin
   5. Urinary iodine
   6. Radiograph of knee and foot for bone age

T_3, tri-iodothyronine; T_4, thyroxine; TSH, thyroid-stimulating hormone.
[a]Commercial assays currently available measure thyrotropin-binding inhibitor immunoglobulin.

substituted for a free T_4. Serum T_3 is not useful in the diagnosis, as it is often in the normal range in hypothyroidism. It is important to keep in mind that the normal range of serum thyroid hormone concentrations is higher in the first few weeks and months of life, so that abnormal results can be determined only by comparison to age-related normals. The normal ranges for serum free T_4, T_4, free T_3, T_3, TBG, and TSH through infancy and childhood are presented in Table 32.7. Measurement of serum free T_4, total T_4, T_3RU, and TSH separates out the common neonatal thyroid disorders, as summarized in Table 32.8.

1. **The biochemical hallmarks** of primary hypothyroidism are a low serum free T_4 (or T_4) and elevated TSH levels; infants with subclinical hypothyroidism have normal free T_4 (or T_4) and elevated TSH levels. Infants with transient hypothyroidism have abnormal screening results that revert to normal, usually in the first few months of life, depending on the underlying etiologic factor (see Section V.B).

2. **With hypothalamic–pituitary hypothyroidism,** the serum free T_4 (or T_4) is low, whereas the TSH can be low but it is usually in the normal range. This likely results from altered glycosylation of the TSH molecule, leading to reduced bioactivity. TSH determination by the usual laboratory assays, with binding to an antibody (e.g., radioimmunoassay) is normal, as the immunologic properties of TSH are not altered, but the biologic activity of TSH is reduced by altered glycosylation, as measured by a functional assay (e.g., generation of cyclic AMP). TRH stimulation fails to produce a TSH rise in pituitary disorders, although the separation of pituitary from hypothalamic dysfunction is usually not clinically important.

3. **Infants with TBG deficiency** have a low T_4 and normal TSH on screening; on follow-up, serum testing shows a low T_4 but a normal free T_4 with a normal TSH concentration. T_3RU, inversely proportioned to TBG levels, is elevated. TBG deficiency, usually inherited in an X-linked manner, occurs in ~1 in 5 000 infants. No treatment is indicated in infants with TBG deficiency because thyroid function itself is normal.

B. **Optional studies.** We do not recommend these tests routinely, as generally their results do not alter management. They do provide useful information and, in cases of equivocal diagnosis, they do help in management decisions.

1. **Thyroid uptake and scan** using radioactive iodine (^{123}I) or sodium pertechnetate (^{99m}Tc). Thyroid uptake and scanning are best done before treatment is started; exogenous thyroxine replacement blocks uptake of ^{123}I and ^{99m}Tc. ^{131}I delivers a higher dose of radioactivity to the thyroid and body and should not be used in infants. If thyroid uptake and scan show an ectopic gland, the cause of the hypothyroidism is established and no additional tests are necessary. In

TABLE 32.7 Normal Mean and Range (± SD) for Total Thyroxine, Free Thyroxine, Tri-iodothyronine, Free Tri-iodothyronine, Thyroxine-Binding Globulin, and Thyroid-Stimulating Hormone in Infancy and Childhood

Age	T$_4$ (μg/dL)[a]	Free T$_4$ (ng/dL)[a]	T$_3$ (ng/dL)[a]	Free T$_3$ (pg/dL)[a]	TBG (mg/dL)[a]	TSH (μU/mL)[a]
Premature infant	4.0 (2.0–6.5)	1.2 (0.5–1.6)	32 (14–50)	—	—	2.0 (0.8–5.2)
Cord blood	10.2 (7.4–13.0)	1.5 (0.9–2.2)	45 (15–75)	—	5.6	9.0 (1.0–17.4)
1–3 d	17.2 (11.8–22.6)	3.7 (2.2–5.3)	124 (32–216)	470 (180–760)	5.0	8.0 (1.0–17.4)
1–2 wk	13.2 (9.8–16.6)	2.7 (1.6–3.8)	250 —	—	—	4.0 (1.7–9.1)
2 wk–4 mo	10.7 (7.0–15.0)	1.5 (0.9–2.2)	180 (120–240)	480 (185–770)	—	2.3 (1.7–9.1)
4–12 mo	11.0 (0.7–1.9)	1.3 (0.7–1.9)	176 (110–280)	465 (215–720)	4.4 (3.1–5.6)	2.0 (0.8–8.2)
1–5 y	10.5 (7.3–15.0)	1.5 (0.8–2.3)	168 (105–269)	460 (215–700)	4.2 (2.9–5.4)	2.0 (0.8–8.2)
5–10 y	9.3 (6.4–13.3)	1.4 (0.7–2.1)	150 (94–241)	440 (230–650)	3.8 (2.5–5.0)	2.0 (0.7–7.0)
10–15 y	8.1 (5.6–11.7)	1.3 (0.6–2.0)	113 (83–213)	440 (230–650)	3.3 (2.1–4.6)	1.9 (0.7–5.7)

SD, standard deviation; T$_3$, tri-iodothyronine; T$_4$, thyroxine; TBG, thyroxine-binding globulin; TSH, thyroid-stimulating hormone.

[a]Conversion factors:

T$_4$: 1 ng/dL = 12.87 pmol/L
Free T$_4$: 1 μg/dL = 12.87 nmol/L
T$_3$: 1 ng/dL = 15.36 pmol/L
Free T$_3$: 1 pg/dL = 0.1563 pmol/L
TBG: 1 mg/dL = 10 mg/L
TSH: 1 μU/mL = 1 mU/L

Adapted from LaFranchi SH. Hypothyroidism, congenital and acquired. In: Kaplan SA, ed. *Clinical Pediatric and Adolescent Endocrinology*. Philadelphia: WB Saunders; 1982:87; and Nichol's Institute and Esoterix normal reference range.

Disorder	Screening		Confirmatory			
	T_4	TSH	Free T_4	T_4	T_3RU	TSH
Primary hypothyroidism	↓	↑	↓	↓	↓–N	↑
Subclinical hypothyroidism	↓–N	↑	N	N	N	↑
Transient hypothyroidism	↓	↑	N	N	N	N
Hypothalamic-pituitary hypothyroidism	↓	"N"	↓	↓	↓–N	↓–N
TBG deficiency	↓	N	N	↓	↑	N

TABLE 32.8 — Interpretation of Screening and Confirmatory Thyroid Blood Tests

N, normal; "N," below the level of sensitivity of the screening assay (i.e., <25 μU/mL); T_4, thyroxine; T_3RU, tri-iodothyronine resin uptake; TSH, thyroid-stimulating hormone; ↓, decreased; ↑, increased.

cases in which uptake is elevated and an inborn error of thyroxine biosynthesis is suspected, ^{123}I uptake can be followed by a perchlorate discharge test, which will be abnormal in cases of defective iodine oxidation or organification.

a. If no uptake is found, this usually indicates thyroid aplasia. This should be confirmed by an ultrasound examination (see Section VII.B.2).

b. In a situation in which uptake is absent but ultrasound reveals a normal gland, a TSH receptor defect, iodine transport defect, or maternal transfer of TRBAb may be present. Measurement of TRBAb (see Section VII.B.3) in mother and infant will diagnose this disorder.

c. Exposure to excess iodine blocks ^{123}I uptake, which masquerades as an iodine transport defect; measurement of urinary iodine (see Section VII.B.5) in the infant pinpoints this etiologic factor.

d. If thyroid uptake and scan are normal or appear to be increased with a large gland, one of the inborn errors beyond a trapping defect is most likely present. Measurement of serum thyroglobulin (see Section VII.B.4) will help separate out the thyroglobulin synthetic defects from the peroxidase or deiodinase defects. Exposure to an exogenous goitrogen other than iodine, such as antithyroid drugs, produces a similar picture. If an inborn error of thyroid hormone biosynthesis is suspected, DNA testing for mutations in the genes regulating iodine uptake (sodium iodide symporter), oxidation, organification or coupling (thyroid peroxidase), iodine recycling (deiodinase), or the thyroglobulin protein may lead to a diagnosis of the exact defect.

e. Last, some infants with TRBAb can have a normal scan if their hypothyroidism is partially compensated (subclinical hypothyroidism).

2. Thyroid ultrasound examination is generally a more convenient first-line imaging test than radionuclide uptake and scan to search for an underlying etiology. If radionuclide uptake is found to be absent, an ultrasound examination can confirm thyroid aplasia. These findings can also be seen with a TSH receptor defect, iodine transport defect, or maternal transfer of TRBAb (see Section VII.B.1.b). A large gland suggests one of the dyshormonogeneses. Ultrasound examination is less accurate in localizing ectopic thyroid glands.

3. TRBAb. Measurement of TRBAb in infants and mothers is recommended in cases of congenital hypothyroidism with maternal autoimmune thyroid disease and in cases of recurrent transient hypothyroidism in siblings. In the situation of absent radionuclide uptake but a normal gland by ultrasound examination, the presence of TRBAb by testing in infants and mothers separates these cases of transient hypothyroidism from other causes. The presence of TRBAb can also explain hypothyroidism in infants with a normal radionuclide uptake if they are partially compensated (subclinical hypothyroidism) (see Section VII.B.1).

4. **Serum thyroglobulin concentrations** roughly correlate with the amount of functioning thyroid tissue. Thyroglobulin levels are low in aplasia, intermediate in ectopic glands, and elevated in dyshormonogeneses, with the exception of thyroglobulin synthetic defects. However, there is overlap in the thyroglobulin levels among these groups, so this test cannot distinguish the underlying disorder in individual cases. In the setting of a normal radioiodine uptake where TRBAb problems have been excluded, this test is useful in diagnosing thyroglobulin synthetic defects. In some cases of absent radioiodine uptake, serum thyroglobulin concentrations have been normal, indicating some functioning thyroid tissue. In these instances, serum thyroglobulin is more sensitive than scanning.

5. **Urinary iodine.** When there is a history of excess iodine exposure either in utero or postnatally or in areas of endemic goiter as a result of iodine deficiency, measurements of urinary iodine can help pinpoint these causes of transient congenital hypothyroidism.

6. **Bone age evaluation.** An evaluation of skeletal maturation through radiography of the <u>knee and foot</u> is useful in indirectly dating the onset of hypothyroidism. Most newborn infants show ossification of the distal femur, proximal tibia, and cuboid bone of the foot. Whether these centers of ossification are present or absent and whether they are smaller than normal can indicate roughly the duration of hypothyroidism prior to birth.

VIII. TREATMENT

It is important to start thyroid hormone at as early an age as possible and to pick a starting dose that will raise the serum T_4 level up into the target range as rapidly as possible to prevent (or minimize) the untoward effects of hypothyroidism on the developing nervous system. Once this is accomplished, the long-term goal is to maintain serum T_4 concentrations in the upper half of the normal range along with a normalized TSH to ensure normal growth and development, including maximal intellectual potential without neurologic sequelae. Because central nervous system development is dependent on normal thyroid levels for at least the first 2 or 3 years of life, this is a crucial treatment period.

A. **T_4 dosage.** Sodium levothyroxine is the treatment of choice; only tablets should be used, as there are no FDA-approved liquid preparations. We instruct parents to crush the tablets between two spoons (or they can use a mortar and pestle), then dissolve the powder in expressed breast milk or water. This mixture, prepared daily, can be placed in the cheek pad using a spoon, or drawn up in a syringe and squirted in, or it can be placed in an open nipple and given before a feeding. It should not be placed in a full bottle.

The recommended L-T_4 starting dose is <u>10 to 15 μg/kg per day</u> (see Table 32.9). The dose can be tailored to the severity of hypothyroidism, such that patients judged to have severe hypothyroidism (serum T4 <5 μg/dL [<65 nmol/L]) should be started at the higher end of this dosage range. Some studies report better outcomes using starting doses of 12 to 17 μg/kg per day. The total dose is gradually increased

TABLE 32.9	**Recommended Daily Dose of Sodium Levothyroxine (Na L-T$_4$) in the Management of Hypothyroidism**

Age	Na L-T$_4$ (μg/kg/d)
Initial starting dose	10–15
0–3 mo	8–12
3–6 mo	7–10
6–12 mo	6–8
1–5 y	4–6
6–12 y	3–5
>12 y	2–4

with age, but the dose expressed as micrograms per kilogram body weight gradually decreases with age. Levothyroxine should not be given with any food or nutrient supplement that contains soy protein, iron, or concentrated calcium preparations, as these have the potential to bind thyroxine and interfere with its absorption. Increasing the levothyroxine dose might be acceptable, but the concern is that the binding and inhibition of absorption is variable, so one might see variable serum T_4 levels. If soy protein formula must be used, the more common recommendation is to space the thyroid hormone treatment halfway between feedings.

B. Serum T_4. The serum T_4 treatment target range for infants is 10 to 16 μg/dL (130 to 206 nmol/L); for free T_4 it is 1.4 to 2.3 ng/dL (18 to 30 pmol/L), i.e., in the upper half of the normal range. The recommended initial starting dosage of T_4 of 10 to 15 μg/kg per day, generally 37.5 to 50 μg daily for a 3- to 4-kg infant, has been shown to raise the serum T_4 concentration above 10 μg/dL by the third day of treatment. This starting dose has been shown to be safe, with no obvious thyrotoxic side effects. To minimize any delays, treatment should be started after confirmatory serum studies have been obtained but pending results.

C. Serum TSH. Whereas serum T_4 or free T_4 concentrations should reach the target range quickly, serum TSH concentrations take somewhat longer to fall into the normal range. Using the higher L-T_4 starting doses described earlier, serum TSH will normalize by 2 to 4 weeks of treatment. However, some infants, usually those with aplasia or severe hypothyroidism, have serum TSH concentrations in the 10- to 20-μU/mL range despite T_4 or free T_4 levels in the upper half of the normal range. Raising the treatment dose lowers the serum TSH, but this often results in T_4 or free T_4 levels above normal and thyrotoxic symptoms and signs—features that should be avoided. This apparent resistance to thyroid hormone appears to be a result of in utero hypothyroidism producing a resetting of the pituitary–thyroid feedback threshold level. It may be present in up to 30% of infants with congenital hypothyroidism in the first year of life, but it drops to 10% by 10 years of age.

IX. FOLLOW-UP MANAGEMENT

Careful follow-up management with proper adjustments of T_4 dose is crucial in ensuring normal growth and neurocognitive development. The New England Collaborative Group has shown an association between a serum T_4 level <8 μg/dL (103 nmol/L) in the first year of life and a lower IQ outcome. A Norwegian study reported that children with a mean serum T_4 level >14 μg/dL (180 nmol/L) in the first year of life had a significantly higher mental developmental index at 2 years and verbal IQ at 6 years than did children with serum T_4 levels <10 μg/dL (129 nmol/L). On the other hand, a Toronto study reported that treated hypothyroid infants with higher serum T_4 levels, ~15 μg/dL (193 nmol/L), had a "difficult" temperament in the first year, indicating that overtreatment should be avoided. Guidelines from the American Academy of Pediatrics for follow-up monitoring and treatment are presented in Table 32.10; it should be emphasized that management must be individualized in each case.

A. Clinical follow-up. The aim of treatment is to achieve normal growth and development within the context of the family's genetic potential. At each visit, the child's length, weight, and head circumference should be measured and plotted. Developmental milestones, including gross and fine motor skills, language, and social development, may be assessed at each visit, using a tool such as the Denver Developmental Screen.

B. Laboratory follow-up. Serum thyroid function tests should be determined approximately 2 and 4 weeks after onset of therapy, every 1 to 2 months in the first year, and every 3 to 4 months in the second and third years of life.

　　1. Serum T_4 concentrations should be maintained in the upper half of the normal range, 10 to 16 μg/dL (130 to 206 nmol/L). If serum free T4 is used instead of T4, the target range is 1.4 to 2.3 ng/dL (18 to 30 pmol/L).

　　2. Serum TSH is generally suppressed into the normal range, although this can take 2 to 4 weeks. Once the serum TSH concentration falls below 10 μU/mL, it can be relied on as a sensitive indicator of appropriate therapy. On stable dosing, the serum TSH is often <2 mU/L. A subsequent abnormal elevation generally

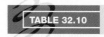

TABLE 32.10	Follow-up Monitoring and Management of Congenital Hypothyroidism

A. Biochemical (T_4 or free T_4 and TSH) evaluation
   1. 2 and 4 weeks after starting treatment
   2. Every 1–2 mo in first year
   3. Every 3–4 mo in second and third years
   4. Goals
      a. Serum T_4, 10–16 μg/dL (130–206 nmol/L)
      b. Serum TSH generally <10 U/L without elevated T_4 or thyrotoxic features
B. Clinical evaluation of growth and development at less frequent intervals
C. Bone age radiograph at 1- to 2-y intervals
D. Psychometric testing: initial testing at 12–18 mo and repeat at 5 y; earlier if necessary

is a sign of a need to increase the T_4 dose, although compliance problems or coadministration with soy protein, iron, or concentrated calcium are potential causes to be explored.

3. T_4 overtreatment. Overtreatment is undesirable because it has been associated with craniosynostosis. Overtreatment may adversely affect the tempo of brain development, and it has been associated with disorders of temperament and attention span.

4. Skeletal maturation can be evaluated by use of a hemiskeleton radiograph in the first 2 years and hand and wrist radiographs roughly every 2 years after that.

C. Psychometric follow-up. Formal psychometric testing is recommended initially at 12 to 18 months of life and again at age 5 years, just prior to starting school. The exact test instrument does not appear to be critical, and the consultant may use whichever test is most familiar. The results from the psychometric testing are important in identifying any infant with decreased IQ or those with specific neurologic problems; identification allows early intervention to help these infants achieve maximum intellectual and neurologic potential. Given that **up to 20%** of infants with congenital hypothyroidism may have **a hearing problem,** it is recommended that infants undergo formal hearing tests.

D. Documentation of permanent hypothyroidism. If imaging studies were carried out, it may be clear that an infant has permanent hypothyroidism (i.e., an ectopic gland documented by scan or aplasia documented by scan and ultrasound exam). In cases in which the exact etiology was not determined based on studies performed, it may be unclear whether an infant has a transient or permanent form of hypothyroidism. In such cases, if an infant has a "secondary rise" of TSH above 10 μU/mL after 6 months of age while on therapy, it can be assumed that he or she has permanent hypothyroidism. If this does not occur by age 3 years, it is recommended that treatment be discontinued for 1 month and repeat diagnostic studies undertaken. Measurements of T_4 or free T_4 and TSH will determine whether hypothyroidism is present. Again, other studies, such as a thyroid scanning or ultrasound examination, are optional.

X. PROGNOSIS

   A. Growth and pubertal development. Essentially all programs report that infants detected by screening and adequately treated grow at normal percentiles. Onset and progression of puberty are normal, although one study showed that girls started on higher L-T_4 doses entered puberty at a slightly younger age. Adult heights are within the range expected for genetic potential.

   B. Intellectual and neurologic outcome. In general, screening programs report that infants started on early treatment (2 to 6 weeks of life) and treated appropriately through the first 3 years of life have IQs similar to those in control groups. The New England Collaborative Group reported a mean verbal IQ of 109, a performance

IQ of 107, and a full-scale IQ of 109 at 6 years, essentially identical to sibling and classmate control groups. With further follow-up, now out to adult age in some cases, many programs report small differences in IQ (5 to 15 points) between children with congenital hypothyroidism and control children. Even when there are no differences in global IQ scores, there may be differences in subtest components, such as verbal skills, arithmetic skills, reading comprehension, visual-spatial skills, memory, or executive function.

C. **Factors affecting neurocognitive outcome.** Factors that have been shown to affect neurocognitive outcome in children with congenital hypothyroidism include age of onset of treatment, severity of hypothyroidism (as judged by pretreatment T_4 level, scan or ultrasound findings, or skeletal maturation), starting L-T_4 dose, and serum T_4 in the first year of life.

1. **Age of onset of treatment.** It is important to start infants on thyroid hormone treatment at as early an age as possible, after detection by newborn screening tests. In a review of studies comparing starting treatment at an earlier age (range, 12 to 30 days of life) versus at a later age, infants starting at the earlier age averaged 15.7 IQ points higher than those started at a later age.

2. **Severity of hypothyroidism**

   a. **Low pretreatment serum T_4.** The Quebec Screening Network reported that children with a pretreatment serum T_4 <2 μg/dL (<26 nmol/L), along with a smaller epiphysial area as shown on radiographic film of the knee, had a lower IQ (89 $\pm$ 17) in comparison with the group with serum T_4 >2 μg/dL (>26 nmol/L) and larger epiphysial area (IQ of 104 $\pm$ 12) at age 12 years. The lower serum T_4 presumably reflects a more severe form of hypothyroidism.

   b. **Aplasia verus ectopia/hypoplasia or dyshormonogenesis.** Some studies find no difference in IQ in infants with aplasia as compared to other etiologies. However, in a review of studies comparing IQ outcome to severity by etiology, most found a difference, ranging from 5- to 12-point decrease in IQ in infants with aplasia.

   c. **Delayed pretreatment bone age.** The Toronto group reported that infants with bone ages <36 weeks' gestation had lower IQ scores (98 $\pm$ 15) compared to the group with bone age of 37 weeks to term (IQ of 109 $\pm$ 13). The retarded bone ages are thought to reflect a greater degree of fetal hypothyroidism.

3. **L-T_4 starting dose:** Studies find that children started on the currently recommended L-T_4 dose of 10 to 15 μg/kg per day have a better neurocognitive outcome than children started on the dose used when newborn screening programs were initiated, 6 to 8 μg/kg per day. In a review of studies comparing outcomes and starting doses, children started on the lower doses averaged a 12-point lower IQ compared to children started on the higher doses.

4. **Low serum T_4 in the first year.** The New England Collaborative Group reported that four infants who received inadequate treatment in the first year of life, as judged by a history of poor compliance, with serum T_4 concentrations <8 μg/dL and serum TSH levels that did not suppress into the normal range until 18 to 24 months of age, had IQs of 62, 67, 76, and 83 (mean = 72).

5. **Other neurologic sequelae.** A small proportion of infants, including those with normal IQs, can have other neurologic problems. These include gross and fine motor incoordination, ataxia, increased or decreased muscle tone, short attention span, and speech defects. A sensorineural hearing loss can also be present; this has been diagnosed in up to 20% of children with congenital hypothyroidism detected before newborn screening was initiated.

XI. MISSED CASES

As a public health measure, newborn screening was initiated to identify infants with primary hypothyroidism. After >30 years of experience, it is apparent that newborn screening has been extremely successful; approximately one case is missed for every 120 cases detected. Factors responsible for cases being missed include the following: no specimen collected (a concern with home deliveries and infants transferred from one hospital to another), collection of an inadequate specimen, failure to transport the specimen to the screening laboratory, errors in laboratory procedures, which include technical assay errors or human errors in recording abnormal results, and lack of follow-up of infants with abnormal screening results (especially when families transfer care to another physician or relocate). Finally, some infants with milder forms of hypothyroidism pass an initial screen yet develop more overt hypothyroidism in the first months of life (see Sections III.A.4 and III.C.1.c). Thus, physicians caring for infants should not assume that in cases with compatible clinical features, hypothyroidism has been excluded on the basis of a normal newborn screening test. Physicians need to stay alert to the possibility of undiagnosed congenital hypothyroidism and should perform their own serum thyroid function test when infants manifest suspicious symptoms and signs.

XII. NEONATAL HYPERTHYROIDISM

Neonatal hyperthyroidism (neonatal Graves disease) is an uncommon, usually transient disorder in infants born to mothers who had Graves disease either during the pregnancy or in the past. Neonatal Graves disease occurs in <3% of infants born to mothers with Graves disease, which is evidence that only mothers with very high thyrotropin receptor–stimulating antibody (TRSAb) concentrations have affected newborns. Because the transient form of the disease is the result of transplacental passage of maternal TRSAb, neonatal Graves disease occurs equally in female and male infants.

A. Pathogenesis. The transient form of neonatal Graves disease results from transplacental passage of TRSAb. It is usually associated with active maternal Graves hyperthyroidism during pregnancy, but it also occurs in infants whose mothers are euthyroid but still have high circulating TRSAb. In most infants, neonatal Graves disease resolves spontaneously in 3 to 12 weeks as the maternal TRSAb disappears from the infant's blood. A rarer form of neonatal hyperthyroidism is not necessarily associated with maternal autoimmune thyroid disease and persists for a longer time than can be explained by transplacental passage of TRSAb. Thyrotoxicosis can persist for years and has long-term sequelae. In the past, it was thought that these infants developed true Graves disease and produced their own TRSAb. It is now clear that many of these infants have an **activating mutation of the TSH receptor** causing hyperthyroidism. These may be inherited as an autosomal dominant trait or occur sporadically as a new mutation. They may present in the neonatal period or later in infancy or childhood. Neonatal hyperthyroidism has also been reported in association with **McCune-Albright syndrome.** This is caused by an **activating mutation in the α subunit of the G protein.** These latter forms of hyperthyroidism persist indefinitely and so require more definitive treatment, such as thyroidectomy or radioiodine ablation.

B. Clinical manifestations

1. **Fetal tachycardia** exceeding 160 beats/min after midgestation is a sign of fetal thyrotoxicosis in the at-risk fetus.

2. **Infants with neonatal hyperthyroidism** can be born prematurely (although the thyrotoxic state can influence estimates of fetal maturity), and there is often intrauterine growth retardation with birth weights of 2.0 to 2.5 kg in full-term infants.

3. **Microcephaly and ventricular enlargement** may be present.

4. **Exophthalmos** is often present.

5. **A goiter is palpable** in about half the cases, and this can enlarge and cause upper airway obstruction.

6. The **infants are irritable**, sweaty, hyperactive, and tend to have an increased appetite (although some feed poorly). Nevertheless, they manifest poor weight gain or even weight loss, which can be exacerbated by vomiting and diarrhea.

7. **Hepatosplenomegaly and jaundice** may be present.

8. **Tachycardia** is usually present, and arrhythmias and cardiac failure have been described.

9. The **onset, severity, and duration** of symptoms are variable. Symptoms and signs might not be apparent for 10 days or so after birth as maternal antithyroid

medication disappears. Rarely, both maternal TRBAb and TRSAb are transplacentally acquired, and the type of disease and time course depends on which antibody is dominant or persists.

C. **Diagnosis**

1. **Maternal screening during pregnancy should include measurement of maternal** thyrotropin-receptor antibodies, as a **TRSAb** level >500% of control values is predictive of neonatal Graves disease. Thyrotropin-receptor antibody levels should be measured at 26 to 28 weeks of gestation in all women with active Graves disease and also in those with levothyroxine-replaced hypothyroidism after ^{131}I-mediated thyroid ablation or surgical thyroidectomy. If antibody levels are elevated or if the mother is taking antithyroid drugs, **fetal sonography** at 28 to 32 weeks of gestation is indicated to screen for evidence of fetal thyroid dysfunction, including fetal goiter and tachycardia.

2. **Measurement of serum** T_4 or free T_4, and TSH determines thyroid status; one must keep in mind the higher range of normal thyroid function tests during infancy (Table 32.7). Infants with neonatal Graves disease manifest abnormally elevated serum T_4 or free T_4 and T_3 for age with a suppressed TSH concentration. These indices can be measured in fetal cord blood upon delivery. Because the appearance of neonatal thyrotoxicosis can be delayed by the presence of maternal thionamide drugs, serum thyroid function tests should be repeated at 1 week of age if antithyroid medications were administered during the last month of pregnancy. Similarly, because cotransfer of maternal TRBAb can delay the presentation of neonatal thyrotoxicosis for weeks, the possibility of late hyperthyroidism should be considered in high-risk infants.

3. **Thyroid uptake or scanning** is usually not necessary and may not be helpful in equivocal cases, because radioactive iodine uptake is elevated in newborns.

4. **Radiographic films of the skeleton** show accelerated bony maturation. Later on, they may show craniosynostosis.

5. **Serial serum T_4 and T_3** concentrations are an indication of the effectiveness of treatment.

D. **Treatment.** In moderate or severe cases, treatment should be immediate and vigorous because this disease can be life-threatening. Medical therapy consists of a thionamide drug and beta-blocker; some specialists also add iodides.

1. **Propylthiouracil,** 5 to 10 mg/kg per day, or methimazole, 0.5 to 1.0 mg/kg per day, is given in divided doses every 8 hours.

2. **Propranolol, 2 mg/kg per day,** is an important adjunct in reducing sympathetic overstimulation. If no clinical improvement is seen in 2 to 4 days, the dose can be increased by 50% to 100%.

3. **Iodides** inhibit thyroid hormone synthesis and release; an iodide solution, such as Lugol's (5% iodide and 10% potassium iodide, equivalent to 37.7 mg and 75.5 mg, respectively, of iodide per milliliter), is given as one drop (~1.9 mg or 3.8 mg, respectively) every 8 hours. Once a euthyroid state is reached, iodides should be discontinued.

4. **Adjunctive therapy.** If heart failure develops, digitalis is indicated. Should an enlarged goiter produce airway obstruction, extension of the neck on a pillow can be tried in mild cases, whereas endotracheal intubation is indicated in more severe cases. In severe cases, adding corticosteroids can acutely inhibit thyroid hormone secretion.

5. **In mild cases,** in which the infant manifests minimal clinical problems, observation alone or short-term propranolol treatment may be all that is necessary. Overtreatment and hypothyroidism should be avoided.

E. **Prognosis**

1. **Improvement** is often seen in 7 to 10 days, with remission by 3 to 6 weeks. However, 20% of cases are prolonged up to 3 to 6 months. Mortality in the range of 15% to 20% has been reported in the past and usually is the result of complications of prematurity, but it can be associated with cardiac decompensation or airway obstruction.

2. **Craniosynostosis** can be a long-term sequela.
3. **Intellectual impairment** is a common sequela in many infants. This can occur even when antithyroid therapy is started early, suggesting that intrauterine thyrotoxicosis affects the developing brain and skeleton.
4. **Pituitary hypothyroidism,** which can be secondary to prenatal exposure of the pituitary to excessive thyroid hormone levels during a critical stage of development, has been reported to follow neonatal thyrotoxicosis.

Selected References

Adams LM, et al. Reference range for newer thyroid function tests in premature infants. *J Pediatr* 1995;126:122.

Bellman SC, et al. Mild impairment of neuro-otological function in early treated congenital hypothyroidism. *Arch Dis Child* 1996;74:215.

Black EG, et al. Serum thyroglobulin in normal and hypothyroid neonates. *Clin Endocrinol* 1982;16:267.

Bongers-Schokking JJ, deMuinck Keizer-Schrama SM. Influence of timing and dose of thyroid hormone replacement on mental, psychomotor, and behavioral development in children with congenital hypothyroidism. *J Pediatr* 2005; 147:768.

Brown RS, et al. Incidence of transient congenital hypothyroidism due to maternal thyrotropin antibodies in over one million babies. *J Clin Endocrinol Metab* 1996;81:1147.

Chan GW, Mandel SJ. Therapy insight: management of Graves' disease during pregnancy. *Nat Clin Pract Endocrinol Metab* 2007;3:470.

Davidson KM, et al. Successful in utero treatment of fetal goiter and hypothyroidism. *N Engl J Med* 1991;324:543.

Delange F, et al. Increased risk of primary hypothyroidism in preterm infants. *J Pediatr* 1984;105:402.

Eugster EA, LeMay D, Zerin JM, Pescovitz OH. Definitive diagnosis in children with congenital hypothyroidism. *J Pediatr* 2004;144:643.

Fisher DA. Euthyroid low thyroxine (T_4) and triiodothyronine (T_3) states in prematures and sick neonates. *Pediatr Clin North Am* 1990;37:1297.

Fisher DA, Foley BL. Early treatment of congenital hypothyroidism. *Pediatrics* 1989;83:785.

Fisher DA, Schoen EJ, La Franchi S, et al. The hypothalamic-pituitary-thyroid negative feedback control axis in children with treated congenital hypothyroidism. *J Clin Endocrinol Metab* 2000;85:2722.

Frank JE, et al. Thyroid function in very low birth weight infants: effects on neonatal hypothyroid screening. *J Pediatr* 1996;128:548.

Glorieux J, Dussault J, Van Vliet G. Intellectual development at age 12 years of children with congenital hypothyroidism diagnosed by newborn screening. *J Pediatr* 1992;121:581.

Haddow JE, et al. Maternal thyroid deficiency during pregnancy and subsequent neuropsychological development of the child. *N Engl J Med* 1999;341:549.

Hanna CE, et al. Detection of congenital hypopituitary hypothyroidism: ten years experience in the Northwest Regional Screening 91 Program. *J Pediatr* 1986;109:959.

Hunter MK, et al. Follow-up of newborns with low T_4 and "non-elevated" TSH concentrations: results of the 20 year experience in the Northwest Regional Newborn Screening Program. *J Pediatr* 1998;132:70.

Klein AH, Meltzer S, Kenny FM. Improved prognosis in congenital hypothyroidism treated before age three months. *J Pediatr* 1972;81:912.

Kopp P. Perspective: genetic defects in the etiology of congenital hypothyroidism. *Endocrinology* 2002;143:2019.

LaFranchi SH, et al. Neonatal hypothyroidism detected by the Northwest Regional Screening Program. *Pediatrics* 1979;63:180.

LaFranchi SH, et al. Screening program for congenital hypothyroidism with specimen collection at two time periods: results of the Northwest Regional Screening Program. *Pediatrics* 1985;76:734.

LaFranchi SH, Austin J. How should we be treating children with congenital hypothyroidism? *J Pediatr Endocrinol Metab* 2007;May 20(5):559–578.

Larson C, Hermos R, Delaney A, et al. Risk factors associated with delayed thyrotropin elevations in congenital hypothyroidism. *J Pediatr* 2003;143:587.

Madison LD, LaFranchi S. Screening for congenital hypothyroidism: current controversies. *Curr Opin Endocrinol Metab* 2005;12:36.

Maniatis AK, Taylor L, Letson W, et al. Congenital hypothyroidism and the second newborn metabolic screening in Colorado, USA. *J Pediatr Endocrinol Metab* 2006;19:31.

Moreno JC, de Vijlder JJ, Vulsma T, et al. Genetic basis of hypothyroidism: recent advances, gaps and strategies for future research. *Trends Endocrinol Metab* 2003;14:318.

Oerbeck B, Sundet K, Kase BF, Heyerdahl S. Congenital hypothyroidism: influence of disease severity and L-thyroxine treatment on intellectual, motor, and school-associated outcomes in young adults. *Pediatrics* 2003;112:923.

Polak M. Hyperthyroidism in early infancy: pathogenesis, clinical features and diagnosis with a focus on neonatal hyperthyroidism. *Thyroid* 1998;8:1171.

Pop VJ, et al. Low maternal free thyroxine concentrations during early pregnancy are associated with impaired psychomotor development in infancy. *Clin Endocrinol* 1999;50:149.

Rose SR, Brown RS, Foley T, et al. Update of newborn screening and therapy for congenital hypothyroidism. *Pediatrics* 2006;117:2290.

Selva KA, Harper A, Downs A, et al. Neurodevelopmental outcomes in congenital hypothyroidism: comparison of initial T4 dose and time to reach target T4 and TSH. *J Pediatr* 2005;147:775.

Simpson J, Williams FL, Delahunty C, et al. Serum thyroid hormones in preterm infants and relationships to indices of severity of intercurrent illness. *J Clin Endocrinol Metab* 2005;90:1271.

Takashima S, et al. Congenital hypothyroidism: assessment with ultrasound. *Am J Neuroradiol* 1995;16:1117.

Van Wassenaer AG, et al. Effects of thyroxine supplementation on neurologic development in infants born at less than 30 week's gestation. *N Engl J Med* 1997;336:21.

Zakarija M, McKenzie JM, Eidson MS. Transient neonatal hypothyroidism: characterization of maternal antibodies to the thyrotropin receptor. *J Clin Endocrinol Metab* 1990;70:1239.

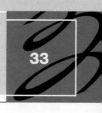

THYROID DISORDERS IN CHILDREN AND ADOLESCENTS

33

Norman Lavin

GOITER

A goiter is an enlargement of the thyroid gland that may result from several different pathogenic mechanisms. The incidence of goiter (4% to 5%) increases with advancing age and is more common in girls at all ages. The presence of goiter does not correlate with thyroid function; patients may be euthyroid, hypothyroid, or hyperthyroid, although most children are clinically euthyroid. Goiters may be classified in many ways; one such classification is given in Table 33.1.

I. TYPES OF GOITERS (Fig. 33.1)

- **A. Simple goiter** is an acquired enlargement of the thyroid gland with normal function that is not caused by an inflammatory process or a tumor. (Other names given to this entity include colloid goiter, adolescent goiter, simple colloid goiter, and nontoxic goiter.) At least 25% of all children with thyroid enlargement have a "simple goiter." It affects females three to five times more frequently than males. Recent evidence suggests that some cases result from a thyroid-stimulating immunoglobulin (TSI).

  - **1. Physical examination.** The gland tends to be symmetric, smooth, and of normal texture.
  - **2. Diagnosis**
    - **a.** Diagnosis is commonly one of exclusion.
    - **b.** Normal function tests.
    - **c.** Negative thyroid antibodies.
    - **d.** Normal radioactive iodine uptake (RAIU) scan (not usually indicated).
  - **3. Treatment.** Thyroxine (T_4) is usually not advocated when the gland is cosmetically insignificant. No other treatment is recommended except for periodic reassessment.
  - **4. Prognosis.** The goiter usually regresses gradually.

- **B. Hashimoto thyroiditis.** See Thyroiditis, Section III.

- **C. Graves disease.** See Hyperthyroidism, Section II.A.

- **D. Congenital goiters** may be present at birth or may develop over the first few years of life (see Chapter 32). Dyshormonogenesis should be considered in any patient with a goiter who tests negative for thyroid antibodies.

  - **1.** Iodine deficiency in the mother was once a major cause of congenital goiter (insufficient substrate for thyroid hormone synthesis).
  - **2.** Currently, the most common cause of congenital goiter is a defect in hormone formation. For example, an enzyme deficiency along the pathway of thyroid hormone synthesis leads to decreased levels of thyroid hormone, increased secretion of thyroid-stimulating hormone (TSH), and development of a goiter. If enough hormone is produced as a result of this mechanism, the patient may develop euthyroid goiter. If the compensatory process is incomplete, the patient can manifest goitrous cretinism (sporadic or familial).

TABLE 33.1	Classification of Goiter in Children

1. Simple goiter (idiopathic, colloid, or adolescent)
   a. Found in adolescent girls (possibly caused by an increase in iodine demand in puberty)
   b. Iodine-induced
   c. Idiopathic
2. Thyroiditis
   a. Acute
   b. Subacute
   c. Chronic
3. Graves disease
4. Congenital goiter
5. Thyroid tumor
   a. Benign
   b. Malignant
6. Endemic goiter

E. Thyroid tumor

F. Endemic goiter occurs predominantly in iodine-deficient areas. Iodine deficiency is the most common cause of goiter in the world. Extreme deficiency occurs when daily urine contains <25 μg of iodine; moderate deficiency occurs when it is 25 to 50 μg; and adequate intake is reflected by an excretion of 100 to 200 μg per day. Iodine supplementation, therefore, has led to eradication of endemic goiter in many countries. The diagnosis of iodine-deficient goiter can be confirmed if urinary iodide excretion is <50 μg/g of creatinine. Iodine-induced thyrotoxicosis is more common in iodine-deficient areas and affects patients with multinodular goiters, as well as those with Graves disease who are iodine-deficient and who do not express the disease until exposed to adequate amounts of iodine. It also occurs in these areas after ingestion of amiodarone.

The most serious consequence of iodine deficiency is <u>endemic cretinism</u>. There are two types: **(1)** The **neurologic syndrome** includes mental retardation, deafness, abnormal gait, foot clonus, Babinski sign, euthyroid goiter, and normal thyroid function. It is believed that the pathogenesis may be iodine deficiency and low T_4 in pregnancy, leading to fetal and postnatal hypothyroidism. **(2)** The **myxedematous syndrome** is characterized by mental retardation, deafness, neurologic symptoms, absence of goiter, myxedema, delayed growth, low T_4, and high TSH levels. The ultrasound scan shows thyroid atrophy but the pathogenesis is not clear.

1. **Laboratory findings.** The T_4 level is slightly low, the tri-iodothyronine (T_3) level is normal or mildly high, and the TSH level is elevated, but these patients are clinically euthyroid. T_3 is secreted preferentially in greater amounts than normal in the iodine-deficient gland because T_3 requires only 75% as much iodine for synthesis. This adaptive mechanism for the more efficient use of iodine can occur only at the expense of goiter formation and TSH elevation.
2. **Treatment**
   a. Iodine. In many iodine-deficient countries, a single intramuscular injection of iodinated poppy seed oil is administered to women. Oral iodized peanut oil is better than iodized poppy seed oil containing the same amount of iodine. It prevents iodine deficiency during future pregnancies for $\sim$5 years. This treatment can also be used in children <4 years of age who have myxedematous cretinism.
   b. **T_4.** (For dosage, see Hypothyroidism, Section V.B). Either iodine or T_4 interrupts the cycle, leading to a decrease in TSH secretion and regression of the

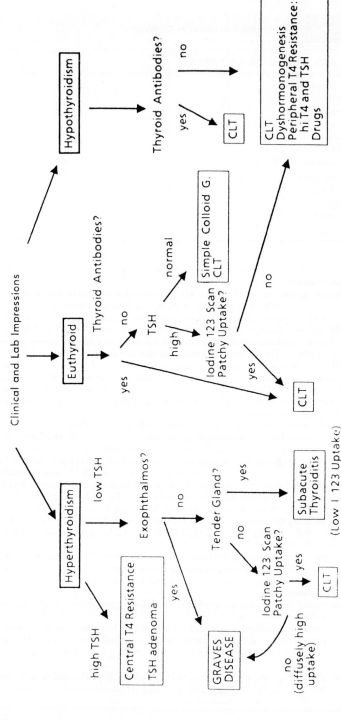

Figure 33.1. Evaluation of a diffuse goiter. (Reproduced with permission from Alter C, Moshang T. Diagnostic dilemma—the goiter. *Pediatr Clin North Am* 1991;38:3.)

goiter. Because most of these goiters grow by mechanisms other than TSH stimulation, T_4 may not always be helpful when used alone.

G. Goitrogens. The goiter-inducing drugs, such as iodides (saturated solution of potassium iodide [SSKI]), amiodarone, aminoglutethimide, di-iodoquinone, cobalt, ethionamide, and *p*-aminosalicylic acid, interfere with thyroid hormone synthesis and release.

Large doses of iodine inhibit the organification of iodine; therefore, it also inhibits the synthesis of thyroid hormone (Wolff-Chaikoff effect). It is short-lived, and hypothyroidism does not occur. If iodine continues to be administered, an autoregulatory mechanism limits iodine trapping, causing intrathyroidal iodine to decrease and organification to proceed normally in normal people. In patients (lymphocytic thyroiditis, inborn errors) with iodine-induced goiter, this escape does not occur because of an underlying defect of the biosynthesis of thyroid hormone.

II. MIDLINE CERVICAL MASSES IN CHILDREN
A. Ectopic thyroid gland
B. Pyramidal lobe of thyroid
C. Nodule of thyroid
D. Thyroglossal duct cyst. As the thyroid gland migrates caudad to its normal anatomic site, it forms an epithelial-lined duct behind its path (the thyroglossal duct). Failure of the duct to atrophy in utero may give rise to a thyroglossal duct cyst later in life. These may rise anywhere from the base of the tongue to the suprasternal notch, usually in the midline. The incidence of carcinoma within these cysts is 1% (*Int. Surg.* 2006;91:141–146). Ultrasonography of the thyroid gland and the neck mass is the initial screening procedure. Iodine-123 (^{123}I) or technetium-99m (^{99m}Tc) pertechnetate scintigraphy will eliminate the possibility of an ectopic thyroid gland masquerading as a thyroglossal duct cyst. Excision of a misdiagnosed ectopic thyroid gland may result in hypothyroidism, because 75% of patients with an ectopic thyroid gland have no other functioning thyroid tissue.
E. Cystic hygroma
F. Lipoma
G. Dermoid cyst
H. Lymph node
I. Brachial anomalies

THYROIDITIS

Thyroiditis and diabetes mellitus are two of the most common endocrine disorders in childhood, and inflammatory processes are the most common causes of thyroid disorders (Tables 33.2 and 33.3).

I. ACUTE BACTERIAL THYROIDITIS (SUPPURATIVE THYROIDITIS)
This disorder is rarely seen today. It is usually caused by gram-positive bacteria, such as *β*-hemolytic streptococci, staphylococci, or pneumococci, and is amenable to

TABLE 33.2   **Classification of Thyroiditis in Children**

Type	Etiology	Frequency
Hashimoto	Autoimmune	Very common, 10–20% of all thyroid disorders
Subacute	Viral	1.5% of all thyroid disorders
Acute (bacterial) suppurative	Bacterial	Rare

TABLE 33.3 Differential Diagnosis of Thyroiditis

Type	Fever	Goiter	WBC	T₄, T₃	Thyroid antibodies	RAIU
Acute bacterial thyroiditis	High	Tender, may be fluctuant	Elevated	Normal	Negative	Normal
Subacute thyroiditis	Usually present	Firm, tender	Normal	Elevated initially, then may be low	Low titers early, absent later	Low
Hashimoto thyroiditis	Absent	Firm, lobular, or pebbly	Normal	Normal or low (high in 5%)	Moderate to high titers	Low, normal, or high

RAIU, radioactive iodine uptake; T₃, tri-iodothyronine; T₄, thyroxine; WBC, white blood count.

appropriate antibiotic therapy after incision, drainage, and culture for aerobes and anaerobes. The gland is enlarged, tender, red, hot, and often fluctuant, with the left lobe affected predominantly in children.

The low incidence of bacterial infection in childhood exists because of the thyroid capsule, which impedes spread of infection, and because of the high intrathyroidal iodine content, which inhibits bacterial growth.

A. Clinical findings. The patient typically complains of chills, fever, and anterior neck pain and swelling; pain may radiate to the ears or mandible. An abscess over the thyroid region is evident as described earlier.

B. Laboratory findings. The white blood cell count (WBC) is elevated, with a shift to the left. Thyroid function tests are usually normal, and a thyroid scan will show a "cold" or nonfunctioning area corresponding to the abscess. The RAIU is normal, in contrast to the markedly decreased uptake in subacute thyroiditis. A search for anatomic defects that predispose to infection must be initiated in children, such as a barium esophagram to rule out a left pyriform sinus fistula, which should be removed to prevent recurrent infection.

C. Differential diagnosis
1. Subacute thyroiditis
2. Cellulitis
3. Thyroid cyst hemorrhage
4. Infected thyroglossal duct cyst
5. Infected branchial cleft cyst

D. Treatment
1. Antibiotics, preferably parenteral
2. Incision and drainage

II. SUBACUTE THYROIDITIS

Subacute thyroiditis (SAT; also termed de Quervain disease) is rare in childhood; it is most common in women between the ages of 20 and 50 years.

A. Etiology. SAT is probably caused by a virus (mumps or cat-scratch fever) or a local sensitivity reaction to the virus, and it occurs more often in colder climates. In addition, it can be preceded by an upper respiratory infection, emotional crisis, dental work, or streptococcal infection.

B. Signs and symptoms. Patients usually complain of anterior neck pain with occasional radiation to the ear, mandible, skull, or chest. Dysphagia can occur in up to 50% of patients. Signs and symptoms of hyperthyroidism (tachycardia, weight loss, nervousness, diaphoresis) can occur. On examination, the gland is tender, nodular, and often unilaterally enlarged.

C. Laboratory findings. The WBC is normal, but a normochromic normocytic anemia is frequently present. T_4 and T_3 levels may be mild to moderately elevated because of discharge of these hormones into the circulation. Thyroid antibodies may be found in mildly elevated titers and usually disappear as the process resolves. The RAIU is low because of the impairment of follicular function caused by the disorder, and because of the TSH suppression resulting from the elevated levels of thyroid hormone in the circulation. Thus, the RAIU is very helpful in distinguishing these patients from those with other hyperthyroid syndromes, such as Graves disease (or toxic nodular goiter), in which the RAIU is increased.

D. Clinical course
1. The acute phase of SAT usually lasts 4 to 8 weeks, but it may last longer and can be associated with hyperthyroidism. The RAIU is suppressed.
2. Patients become euthyroid during the second phase, but occasionally hypothyroidism ensues that lasts 2 to 3 months. The RAIU gradually increases to normal. Low to normal T_4 and T_3 levels with elevated TSH can be seen at this time.
3. During the recovery phase, thyroid function tests are normal, but the RAIU may be higher than normal as a result of greater trapping of iodine by the recovering thyroid gland.

E. Prognosis. Relapses may occasionally occur, but generally, the disease is self-limiting. Permanent hypothyroidism has rarely occurred.

F. Management of SAT in children

1. Acute phase

 a. Aspirin (1 grain for each year of age q3–4h).

 b. Prednisone, 0.5 to 1.0 mg/kg per day in 3 or 4 divided doses (if no response to aspirin) for 1 week, then taper over next 2 to 3 weeks.

 c. Propranolol, if hyperthyroidism is manifested.

 d. Not indicated are thionamides, thyroidectomy, radioactive iodine, or antibiotics.

2. Recovery phase. If the patient is hypothyroid, treat with T4 (0.1 to 0.15 mg) for 3 to 6 months, then taper and discontinue. Continue to follow for the rare case of permanent hypothyroidism.

III. HASHIMOTO THYROIDITIS (HT; AUTOIMMUNE THYROIDITIS, CHRONIC LYMPHO-CYTIC THYROIDITIS)

Hashimoto thyroiditis is the most common thyroid disorder in children; it is the most common cause of euthyroid goiter as well as hypothyroidism.

A. Incidence. Females predominate in a ratio of 2:1, with a peak age in mid-puberty; HT is rare in children <4 years of age. The specific mode of inheritance is not yet known, but there is a high familial incidence (up to 25%).

B. Etiology. Autoantibodies formed against thyroid tissue produce disorders that result in both stimulation (as in Graves disease) and suppression and destruction of the gland (as in HT). Usually one or the other is expressed, but occasionally HT and Graves disease may coexist within the same gland. Altered cellular and humoral immunity occurs in HT from either **(1)** defective suppression of thyroid-directed T lymphocytes that act against the host thyroid or **(2)** liberation of an antigen after thyroid damage, such as by a viral infection (mumps, rubella) that initiates an autoimmune reaction.

 Microsomal (thyroid antiperoxidase, TPO) and thyroglobulin antithyroid antibodies are usually positive; higher titers are seen in the later stages of the disease. The microsomal antibody has been found to be specific against thyroid peroxidase, the enzyme that oxidizes iodide to iodine, and is felt to be cytotoxic to thyroid follicular cells. Other antibodies have been described, including TSI, which might contribute to the enlargement of the gland.

 The haplotypes HLA-DR4 and HLA-DR5 are associated with an increased risk of goiter and thyroiditis, whereas the atrophic variant of thyroiditis is found with HLA-DR3.

C. Pathogenesis. There is a block in the organification of iodine that causes impairment of thyroid hormone synthesis. Thus, newly acquired thyroid iodine is readily discharged by perchlorate. With decreasing thyroid hormone levels, TSH increases, resulting in compensatory hyperplasia of the thyroid gland, which may prevent hypothyroidism for many months or years. Goiter results from both hyperplasia and lymphocytic infiltration. The child more commonly manifests a **hyperplastic form,** with some lymphocytes, minimal fibrosis, and, rarely, Hürthle cells.

D. Clinical findings. The patient may present in one of three ways.

1. The most common presentation initially is an **enlarged thyroid gland** with euthyroidism. This gland may be symmetrically or asymmetrically enlarged with a granular surface; it may be firm and lumpy, lobulated, irregular, or nodular in the later stages. Sometimes a midline pea-sized lymph node (delphian node) may be present above the isthmus. The goiter may shrink in size, disappear, or remain unchanged even without treatment.

2. Toxic thyroiditis (hashitoxicosis) is a transient, self-limited form of hyperthyroidism that occurs in <5% of patients, with manifestations of nervousness, irritability, sweating, hyperactivity, and tachycardia.

3. Hypothyroidism can occur with or without thyromegaly (5% to 10%). Children who present with hypothyroidism may remain permanently hypothyroid. At least 10% to 20% of patients who are euthyroid will become hypothyroid within 5 years from the time of diagnosis. Most cases of atrophic (nongoitrous) hypothyroidism are caused by autoimmune thyroiditis.

E. Diagnostic evaluation

1. Thyroid function tests will reflect the metabolic state of the gland (low, normal, or elevated).

    Most children are euthyroid initially. The incidence of hypothyroidism is 3% to 13%, and subclinical hypothyroidism (high TSH, normal T_4) occurs in up to 35%; a small number of patients present with transient thyrotoxicosis at the time of diagnosis.

2. **Autoantibodies** (e.g., thyroglobulin, microsomal). The microsomal complement fixation test is positive more often than the thyroglobulin test. If both microsomal and thyroglobulin antibody tests are performed, the incidence of positivity with biopsy-proven HT is 90% to 95% (less with only one antibody ordered). Thyrotropin receptor–blocking antibodies are often found, which may relate to the development of hypothyroidism and thyroid atrophy in patients with autoimmune thyroiditis. Other antibodies have been described (against sodium/iodide symporter protein and against thyroid nuclei).

    a. These thyroid antibodies are thought not to be toxic to the thyroid gland but rather reflect the presence of lymphocytic infiltration. Recent studies now show that TPO antibodies inhibit enzyme activity and stimulate killer-cell cytotoxicity.

    b. Positive antibodies are not specific for HT, as slightly elevated titers may be present in other thyroid disorders (e.g., Graves disease). The differentiation of the toxic phase of HT, Graves disease, and the coexistence of Graves disease with HT may be difficult. The presence of exophthalmos favors Graves disease. Laboratory tests may be needed, such as thyrotropin-releasing hormone (TRH) stimulation (or the ultrasensitive TSH assay), TSI, and RAIU tests (high in Graves disease; low or normal in HT). In a rare case with the presence of TSI in HT, the uptake will be increased.

3. Needle biopsy is diagnostic but not necessary.

4. RAI scan reveals patchy distribution. Also, the RAIU scan (and the perchlorate discharge test) may be used in suspect patients with negative antibodies.

5. One study found that the result of ultrasonography was abnormal in 100% of patients who tested positive on cytology; but only 90% of such patients had positive antibodies.

6. Positive **perchlorate discharge test.** This test is used to confirm the presence of a congenital or an acquired oxidation-organification defect such as found in HT.

    a. Give potassium perchlorate, 10 mg/kg (or potassium thiocyanate) PO. After 2 to 4 hours, measure RAIU.

    b. If a defect is present, >20% of the accumulated iodide leaves the thyroid gland. (Normally, iodide is not lost following perchlorate administration.)

F. Treatment

1. If a patient is hypothyroid, treat with L thyroxine (L-T_4), 3 to 4 μg/kg in children and 1 to 2 mg in adolescents. Treatment is continued until adult height is attained, and then a trial without medication can be considered to determine whether thyroid function has returned to normal.

2. If a patient has "impending hypothyroidism" (normal T_4 but elevated TSH), L-T_4 administration is also recommended.

3. If a patient has positive antibodies but is euthyroid, L-T_4 administration is not necessary. However, the child should be followed at regular intervals (e.g., every 6 to 12 months) to monitor the T_4 and TSH levels. According to Foley (1983), L-T_4 does not influence the thyroid antibody titer or the progression of the disease. In one study, 50% of HT patients resolved spontaneously in a 6-year period with no treatment. In a more recent study, the combination of goiter plus progressive increases in antibody levels may be predictive of future hypothyroidism (*J Pediatr* 2006;149:827–832).

4. If the patient is hyperthyroid (hashitoxicosis), propranolol may be prescribed (10 mg tid–qid).

G. Associated disorders
  1. Thyroid malignancy and HT
  a. There is some question whether there is an increase in the incidence of carcinoma; but recent evidence is not confirmatory.
  b. Very few HT patients have lymphoma, but many patients with lymphoma of the thyroid have HT.
  2. Graves disease and HT
  a. Familial diseases.
  b. Relatives of patients with Graves disease often have HT and vice versa.
  3. Cytogenetic disorders and syndromes. There is a higher association of HT in patients with:
  a. Chromosomal abnormalities (e.g., Down, Turner [41% positive antibodies], and Klinefelter syndromes).
  b. Syndromes (e.g., Noonan and congenital rubella syndrome [23% positive antibodies]).
  c. Other autoimmune diseases (e.g., diabetes mellitus type I [20% positive antibodies]). Early treatment with thyroxine reduces the size of the thyroid gland in euthyroid children and adolescents with autoimmune thyroiditis and type I diabetes mellitus utilizing a non-TSH–suppressant dose for the treatment even in the absence of latent or overt hypothyroidism. The dose was 1.5 μg/kg daily.
      Children with juvenile idiopathic arthritis have a higher-than-normal incidence of antithyroid antibodies and subclinical hypothyroidism and should be routinely screened for these variables.
  4. Autoimmune polyglandular syndromes
  a. Type I: hypoparathyroidism, Addison disease, type 1 diabetes mellitus, gonadal failure, moniliasis, alopecia, pernicious anemia, vitiligo, malabsorption, chronic active hepatitis, HT
  b. Type II: Addison disease, type 1 diabetes mellitus, HT
  c. Type IIIa: type 1 diabetes mellitus, HT
  d. Type IIIb: Graves disease or HT, pernicious anemia
  e. Type IIIc: Graves disease or HT, alopecia, vitiligo, myasthenia gravis, idiopathic thrombocytopenic purpura

HYPOTHYROIDISM

I. GENERAL PRINCIPLES
Hypothyroidism is a thyroid disorder in which there is an inadequate amount of thyroid hormone to meet the body's metabolic requirements. In children, the earlier the age of onset of hypothyroidism, the greater is the chance of irreversible brain damage (see Chapter 30). If the onset is after age 2 or 3 years, however, most of the adverse effects are reversible.

II. CAUSES OF ACQUIRED HYPOTHYROIDISM IN CHILDREN
A. Primary
  1. HT is the most common cause of hypothyroidism in children. Studies of young students revealed that 1.2% had positive antithyroid antibodies and 10% to 20% of those with positive antibodies eventually became hypothyroid.
  2. Subacute thyroiditis (de Quervain) is rare in children and seldom results in hypothyroidism.
  3. Iodide ingestion may result in a hypothyroid state.
  a. Underlying thyroid disease may predispose the patient to iodide-induced hypothyroidism.
  b. Other goitrogens (e.g., sulfadiazine, lithium, and sulfonylureas) in combination with iodide may lead to hypothyroidism.
  c. The fetus may become hypothyroid secondary to the transplacental passage of iodides.

4. **Management of antecedent hyperthyroidism with radioactive iodine** may result in hypothyroidism. If it occurs in the first year following treatment, it is considered to be dose-related. Subsequently, there may be a 2% to 4% incidence of new cases of hypothyroidism each year that are not dose-related.

5. **Thyroidectomy** for hyperthyroidism or a thyroid nodule can cause hypothyroidism if excessive tissue is removed.

6. **Surgical removal of a thyroglossal duct cyst** may result in hypothyroidism; therefore, either **(a)** obtain an RAIU scan before surgery to determine if all of the thyroid tissue is found in the cyst wall or **(b)** obtain a T_4 and TSH 6 to 8 weeks postoperatively to determine thyroid function.

7. **Infiltrative disease** of the thyroid gland with cystinosis or histiocytosis X may occasionally involve enough tissue to prevent normal hormonal production.

8. **"Sick euthyroid" syndrome or low T_3 syndrome.** The thyroid gland in "sick euthyroid" syndrome is functioning normally, but there is an abnormality in the peripheral metabolism of the thyroid hormones secondary to a severe nonthyroid illness that results in low T_3, elevated reverse T_3 (rT_3), low or normal T_4, low or normal free T_4, normal TSH, and low or normal thyroxine-binding globulin (TBG).
   a. This condition is found in:
      (1) Infants with prematurity and respiratory distress syndrome
      (2) Children with acute leukemia or renal failure (free T_4 and total T_4 correlate inversely with the degree of renal failure)
   b. Treatment. Thyroid hormone replacement is not indicated for this condition.

9. Subclinical hypothyroidism has been described in several cases of **cystic fibrosis.**

10. **Iodide deficiency** may lead to hypothyroidism with a compensatory TSH-stimulated goiter.

11. **Late-onset congenital thyroid disorders,** such as ectopia (cryptothyroid) and organification defects, may occur. Thyroid gland function may not fail until late childhood even though the disorder was present at birth.
   a. Lingual thyroid. Most patients have inadequate functional thyroid tissue and ultimately require T_4 replacement. If the gland is enlarged or causes pressure symptoms and does not shrink with hormone treatment, then surgical removal may be considered. There is no evidence that lingual thyroid glands have an increased incidence of malignancy in children.
   b. Enzymatic defects. In the typical child with hypothyroidism, the gland is small or not palpable, but in disorders associated with deficiencies of enzymes, the thyroid gland may be enlarged. To assist in diagnosing the specific defect, the following tests may be ordered:
      (1) 24-hour RAIU.
         (a) Low value = iodine-trapping defect.
         (b) High value = other enzymatic defects.
      (2) Perchlorate discharge test is positive in peroxidase deficiency, such as **Pendred syndrome,** in which the child manifests a goiter and nerve deafness associated with euthyroidism or mild hypothyroidism.

B. **Central hypothyroidism (secondary [TSH] or tertiary [TRH]).** Deficiency of TSH or TRH occurs in <5% of hypothyroid pediatric patients and may be secondary to pituitary or hypothalamic disorders, such as tumors (adenoma or craniopharyngioma), trauma, infection, and congenital anomalies (e.g., septo-optic dysplasia), and irradiation or chemotherapy.

   If hypoadrenalism secondary to hypopituitarism is suspected, T_4 administration given alone before correcting the hypoadrenalism may result in adrenal crisis. Therefore, it is important to <u>evaluate adrenal function if the patient has a low T_4</u> **and low TSH** prior to initiating T_4 replacement.

III. CLINICAL MANIFESTATIONS

The clinical manifestations of childhood hypothyroidism vary and depend largely on the age of onset (Table 33.4; see Chapter 30 and 32). Typically, the child is short and mildly overweight rather than very obese. (The euthyroid child with marked

TABLE 33.4 Clinical Manifestations of Childhood Hypothyroidism

Symptoms
Slow growth
Poor appetite
Constipation
Lethargy
Poor school performance
Cold intolerance
Weakness, fatigue
Dry, coarse skin
Weight gain

Signs
General
  Short stature
  Mildly overweight
  Dull, placid expression
  Goiter (occasional)
  Pale, cool skin
  Delayed dentition
  Slow, hoarse, low-pitched speech
  Constipation
Hematologic: anemia (three types)
  Normochromic normocytic
  Hypochromic-microcytic (iron deficiency secondary to menorrhagia or achlorhydria)
  Macrocytic (secondary to vitamin B_{12} or folic acid deficiency)
Cardiologic
  Bradycardia
  Pericardial effusions
  Flat T waves on ECG
Neuromuscular
  Delayed reflex return
  Acute encephalopathy (rare)
  Weakness and lethargy
  Occasionally hypertrophied muscles, e.g., Kocher-Debré-Sémélaigne syndrome
    ("herculean" appearance of unknown pathogenesis)
  Increased cerebrospinal fluid protein
  Mental retardation (if untreated newborn)
  Memory loss
  Neurosensory hearing loss
  Ataxia
  Myopathy (creatine phosphokinase elevation)
  Entrapment neuropathies
Hypothalamic–pituitary–gonadal axis
  Delayed puberty
  Overlap syndrome (precocious puberty)
  Amenorrhea/scant menses
Skeletal
  Delayed bone age
  Epiphysial dysgenesis (epiphysial stippling)
  Slipped capital femoral epiphysis
  Enlarged sella turcica (in long-term primary hypothyroidism secondary to hypertrophy
    of thyrotropes)

exogenous obesity manifests accelerated growth with advanced bone age and advanced pubertal development.) If the hypothyroid state is prolonged before treatment, catch-up growth may be incomplete. Also, excess dosage may advance bone age disproportionately.

Commonly, the hypothyroid adolescent presents with delayed puberty, but occasionally precocious puberty **(overlap syndrome)** is evident. The low T_4 feeds back to stimulate TRH and TSH as well as prolactin secretion, which can produce breast development, galactorrhea, pubic hair, and other features of precocious puberty. The TSH as well as luteinizing hormone (LH) and follicle-stimulating hormone (FSH) have the same a chains; therefore, TRH may also stimulate TSH and LH secretion. In a study of 12 girls with severe and long-standing hypothyroidism, 9 were found on ultrasound to have multicystic ovaries along with high LH levels, which resolved on T_4 therapy. The pathogenesis of the cysts is not well understood. Restoration of the euthyroid state has been associated with resolution of these cysts; long-term follow-up of these patients is lacking, however. Hypothyroidism should be excluded in young girls with ovarian cysts.

IV. DIAGNOSIS OF HYPOTHYROIDISM (Fig. 33.2 and Table 33.5)
The following laboratory tests may be useful in the diagnosis of hypothyroidism:
- T_4—low.
- T_3 resin uptake (T_3RU)—low.
- Free T_4 index (FT_4I)—low (useful in pregnancy and TBG deficiency).
- TSH—high.
- T_3 (radioimmunoassay, RIA) (not usually needed)—low.
- Free T_4 (useful in hypothalamic/pituitary hypothyroidism)—low.
- Antithyroid antibodies (positive in thyroiditis).
- TBG (see Table 26.1).
- Thyroid scan (thyroiditis).
- RAIU (enzyme deficiencies).
- Other laboratory tests may be abnormal:
  - Serum cholesterol may be elevated.
  - Muscle enzymes (creatine phosphokinase [MM fraction], aspartate aminotransferase, alanine aminotransferase, lactate dehydrogenase) may be elevated.

A. Primary hypothyroidism
1. Low T_4, low free T_4, low T_3RU (low FT_4I), high TSH.
2. Borderline low T_4, low free T_4, and elevated TSH may be seen in early primary hypothyroidism.

B. Secondary hypothyroidism
1. Low T_4, low free T_4, normal or low TSH.
2. TRH test (failure of TSH to respond). (Note that pituitary-hypothalamic lesions may cause variable responses to TRH.)

C. Tertiary hypothyroidism
1. **TRH test.** In patients with hypothalamic lesions, the TSH peak is **delayed** but reaches a **normal** level.
2. **Computed tomography (CT)** of the head may be indicated to rule out a tumor.
3. In some patients, serum TSH is in the normal range but the TSH probably has reduced biologic activity (TRH is probably necessary to confer full biologic activity to TSH).

V. TREATMENT
A. The **goals** of treatment are normal growth and development. These are accomplished by:
1. **Maintaining** the serum T_4 in the upper half of the normal range
2. **Suppressing** TSH into the normal level (except for infant hypothyroidism) (see Chapter 30)

B. Thyroid replacement
1. L-T_4 is the most recommended drug for treatment of hypothyroidism.
   a. 102 $\mu g/m^2$ per day or 3.0 to 5.0 $\mu g/kg$ per day (higher in infants) (see Table 30.8).

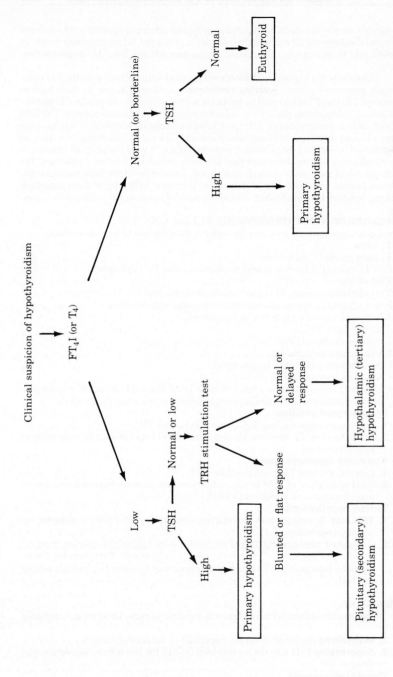

Figure 33.2. Evaluation of hypothyroidism in children. FT_4I, free thyroxine index; TSH, thyroid-stimulating hormone; TRH, thyroid-releasing hormone. (From *Endocr Pract* 1999;5:191–192.)

TABLE 33.5 Thyroid Function Tests in Various Thyroid Disorders

	T_4	Free T_4	T_3 (RIA)	FT_4I	TSH	TSH response to TRH	RT_3	T_3
Primary hypothyroidism	↓	↓	↓	↓	↑	Exaggerated ↑	↓	↓ or N
Secondary hypothyroidism	↓	↓	↓	↓	↓ or N	↓	↓	↓ or N
Tertiary hypothyroidism	↓	↓	↓	↓	↓ or N	Delayed or N	↓	↓ or N
Low TBG	↓	N	↓	N	N	N		↓ or N
High TBG	↑	N	↑	N	N	N	↑ or N	↑ or N
Hyperthyroid	↑	↑	↑	↑	N or ↓	↓	N	↑
Sick-euthyroid syndrome (low T_3 syndrome)	↓ or N	↓ or N	↓ or N	↓ or N	↓ or N	N	↑ or N	↓

FT_4I, free thyroxine index; N, normal; RIA, radioimmunoassay; RT_3, reverse T_3; T_3, tri-iodothyronine; T_4, thyroxine; TRH, thyrotropin-releasing hormone; TSH, thyroid-stimulating hormone; ↑, high; ↓, low.

    b. Adjustment in dosage is based on the clinical and laboratory response of the child, who should be evaluated at least every 6 to 12 months, at which time:

        (1) Growth rate is determined.

        (2) T_4 and TSH levels are measured.

        In addition, bone age should be evaluated every 1 to 2 years to determine if accelerated epiphysial fusion has occurred from excessive L-T_4 administration.

  2. Desiccated thyroid is extracted from animal thyroid glands. Potency may vary from batch to batch, which may result in an elevated T_3 despite a normal T_4. Therefore, endocrinologists generally do not recommend the use of desiccated thyroid.

  3. Liotrix is a 4:1 mixture of L-T_4 and L-T_3 that can cause elevated T_3 and normal or low T_4 values.

  4. L-T_3 is generally not used in the treatment of hypothyroidism.

C. Adverse effects with appropriate dosage. Pseudotumor cerebri associated with initiation of T_4 has been described in children.

D. Adverse effects with excessive dosage

  1. Nervousness

  2. Tremors

  3. Tachycardia

  4. Hypertension

  5. Delayed neurologic development

  6. Premature craniosynostosis

  7. Early closure of epiphysis

VI. PROGNOSIS

A. The signs and symptoms listed in Table 33.4 should be eliminated with adequate thyroid replacement therapy. If the age at onset of hypothyroidism is later than 2 to 3 years, there should be no permanent brain damage or impairment of central nervous system function.

B. The growth rate will accelerate and the bone age will advance to normal. Weight loss occurs because of increased metabolic rate and mobilization and excretion of myxedematous fluid.

C. The child's behavior may change from being quiet or placid to more aggressive; therefore, the parents should be made aware of this possible transition.

D. Hypothyroid patients with HT who recover thyroid function do not require life-long T_4 therapy. They can be identified during T_4 treatment by a normal thyroid response to TSH in a TRH stimulation test, obviating the need to stop thyroid hormone for 6 to 8 weeks.

 HYPERTHYROIDISM

I. GENERAL PRINCIPLES

Hyperthyroidism is a disorder of an excessive secretion of thyroid hormone resulting in a hypermetabolic state of virtually all body organs. It is caused by a variety of conditions, the most common of which is Graves disease. Typically, hyperthyroidism requires antithyroid medication, radioactive iodine, or surgical therapy for treatment and is associated with an elevated radioactive uptake. Conversely, thyrotoxicosis may also be associated with a low thyroid RAIU, which is found in self-limited disorders that are not usually treated with antithyroid therapy (see Chapter 30), such as SAT or iodine-induced hyperthyroidism (Jod-Basedow phenomenon).

II. ETIOLOGY OF HYPERTHYROIDISM (Table 33.6)

A. Graves disease is the autonomous production of excessive thyroid hormones by a usually enlarged thyroid gland that is not under pituitary control. It is the most

TABLE 33.6	Etiology of Hyperthyroidism in Childhood

Graves disease
Functioning adenoma (toxic adenoma)
Excessive ingestion of thyroid hormones (factitious hyperthyroidism)
Inappropriate TSH hypersecretion
Subacute thyroiditis
Hashitoxicosis (transient hyperthyroidism due to Hashimoto thyroiditis)
Acute psychosis
Iodine-induced thyrotoxicosis (rare in United States)

TSH, thyroid-stimulating hormone.

common cause of hyperthyroidism in children. This disease may rarely consist of a triad of goiter, exophthalmos, and pretibial myxedema in addition to the thyrotoxicosis; however, dermopathy in children is virtually nonexistent, and exophthalmos is less severe than in adults. Graves disease arises from autoimmune processes, which include production of immunoglobulins against antigens in thyroid, orbital tissues, and dermis. Rarely, Graves disease can occur in children without a goiter.

1. **Etiology**
   a. There is a high familial incidence, and females predominate in a 3:1 to 5:1 ratio.
   b. Some studies have shown an increased association with HLA-B8 and BW-35; in whites, a higher incidence of HLA-B8 and HLA-DR3 has been reported.
   c. Thyrotoxicosis is occasionally precipitated by an emotional crisis.
   d. A defect in autoimmunity (alteration of suppressor T lymphocytes) has been postulated as a cause of Graves disease.
      (1) **TSIs** (also known as TRSAb, thyrotropin receptor–stimulating antibody) have been demonstrated in virtually 100% of patients and are responsible for causing the increased synthesis of thyroid hormone in Graves disease. TSI preferentially occupies the TSH receptor on the thyroid gland and initiates the synthesis of the hormones in the same way it would if TSH were present. The first TSI described was long-acting thyroid stimulator. There are now several more TSIs involving different assay systems, but it is not certain whether they are all the same antibodies assayed differently or actually different antibodies. Measurement of TSI is not needed for the diagnosis and management of Graves disease but may be used to help determine remission status.
      (2) **Microsomal and thyroglobulin** antibodies are also found in many patients, but in lower levels than in HT. If very high levels are found, consider both disorders in the same patient. Some investigators believe that Graves disease and HT may be part of a spectrum of the same disease process.
            Spontaneous development of hypothyroidism after antithyroid drug therapy for Graves disease (up to one third of patients) can be secondary to autoimmune thyroiditis or TSH-blocking antibodies.
2. **Associated disorders.** Down syndrome, diabetes mellitus, hypoadrenalism, collagen disease, HT, McCune-Albright syndrome, myasthenia gravis, rubella syndrome, pernicious anemia, idiopathic thrombocytopenia purpura, and systemic lupus erythematosus have been reported in association with Graves disease.
3. **Variant types of Graves disease**
   a. **Euthyroid Graves disease.** The patient presents with the clinical picture of true Graves disease, but the T_4 and T_3 are normal. The diagnosis is made by a blunted response of TSH to TRH infusion (or an exaggerated response if HT is also present).

TABLE 33.7 Clinical Features of Graves Disease in Childhood

Organ		Signs	Symptoms
Eyes	Less severe than in adults	Lid retraction Lid lag Proptosis Chemosis Ophthalmoplegia	Blurring of vision Diplopia
Thyroid		Enlarged Burit/thrill Cervical/venous hum	
Skin		Soft, warm (vitiligo) Smooth, moist	Flushing Excessive sweating
	Very rare in children	Dermopathy Pretibial myxedema Clubbing	Swelling in legs
Heart		Increased heart rate Forceful apical beat Flow murmurs Arrhythmias Increased pulse pressure (mitral regurgitation)	Palpitations Rapid heart rate
Gastrointestinal		Hyperperistalsis	Diarrhea Increased thirst Increased appetite
Central nervous system		Fine tremor Hyperreflexia	Nervousness
Muscle		Muscle atrophy Myasthenia gravis Periodic paralysis	Muscle weakness Easy fatigability
Respiratory		Increased respiratory rate	Exertional dyspnea

Metabolic		Accelerated growth rate
		Hypercalciuria
		  (hypercalcemia)
			Heat intolerance
			Weight loss
			Occasional weight gain
			  from overeating

Mental			Nervousness Irritability Emotional lability School problems Poor attention span
Reproductive		Amenorrhea Delayed menarche Gynecomastia in boys	

    b. T_4 toxicosis is a condition in which untreated hyperthyroidism coexists with severe nonthyroidal illness. The T_4 and free T_4 are elevated while the T_3 is normal.

    c. T_3 toxicosis occurs with a normal T_4 and elevated T_3 (see Section A.6.b).

  4. Clinical features of Graves disease (Table 33.7)

  5. Graves ophthalmopathy. Even though up to 50% of children with Graves disease manifest ophthalmopathy, this problem is not as severe as in adults. Lid retraction and stare are the most common, whereas chemosis, lid eversion, and paresis of extraocular muscles are found predominantly in adults.

The ophthalmopathy is believed to be related to the altered immunity as described in Section II.A.1.d. It is generally believed that the responsible antigen may be molecules expressed by thyroid epithelial cells and orbital tissues or antigens released from the thyroid together with autoreactive T lymphocytes that reach the orbit. Therefore, removal of thyroid antigens has been shown to attenuate the autoimmune response. However, the severity of the eye changes is unrelated to the severity of thyroid dysfunction. It appears to be caused by antibodies against antigens shared by thyroid and eye muscle.

6. Diagnosis

   a. Elevated FT_4I (or T_4).

   b. If FT_4I is normal or borderline high, then get a T_3 (RIA). If only T_3 is elevated, this condition is called **T_3 toxicosis** (15% to 20% of patients). This actually represents an early stage of thyrotoxicosis, prior to the elevation of T_4.

   c. If FT_4I is normal and T_3 (RIA) is borderline, then a TRH stimulation test may help make a definitive diagnosis; for example:

   (1) Normal TSH response—euthyroid.

   (2) Absent or depressed TSH response—hyperthyroid. TRH stimulation test: Give 7 $\mu g/kg$ or 250 $\mu g/m^2$ TRH IV (over 1 to 2 minutes) or IM. Obtain prolactin and TSH levels at 0, 30, and 60 minutes. The recently developed immunoradiometric assay (IRMA) for TSH can be sufficiently sensitive at low levels to detect hyperthyroidism, <u>obviating the need for the TRH stimulation test</u>.

   d. A radioactive iodine scan can be used to differentiate a toxic nodule from Graves disease if clinically indicated.

   e. Radioactive uptake is not generally used to diagnose Graves disease (high uptake in children) but may be used to differentiate "silent" or painless thyroiditis (low uptake) from Graves disease (see Chapter 29; 30). It may also be used to distinguish the toxic phase of subacute thyroiditis (low uptake). Rarely, a patient is so hyperthyroid that an early uptake at 2 to 4 hours is very high, but by 24 hours, the uptake is normal.

   f. The ultrasensitive TSH will be normal or low unless the hyperthyroidism is caused by a rare TSH-producing tumor.

   g. Thyroglobulin is frequently increased in hyperthyroidism but is not needed for diagnosis or management.

   h. In the majority of patients, microsomal antibodies are mildly elevated.

   i. The electrocardiogram typically reveals an increased heart rate and left axial deviation.

   j. TSI may be used to confirm the diagnosis of Graves disease.

B. Toxic adenoma (hyperfunctioning solitary nodule). Thyroid hormone from an adenoma is secreted independent of TSH stimulation. The excessive release of thyroid hormone suppresses the pituitary release of TSH, resulting in diminished activity in the remainder of the gland. On thyroid scan, the toxic adenoma appears as a "hot nodule" surrounded by little or no thyroid tissue. T_3 may be preferentially elevated.

C. Factitious hyperthyroidism (ingestion of excess thyroid hormone). The gland is not enlarged because of TSH suppression by exogenous hormone, and there is little or no RAIU. Free T_4 and TSH are the same as in Graves, but the <u>thyroglobulin is low whereas in Graves it is high</u>.

D. Inappropriate TSH hypersecretion. This condition of high TSH along with an elevated T_4 is secondary to either a TSH-secreting pituitary tumor or an abnormal set point in the negative feedback interaction of thyroid hormone and TSH. There are three types.

   1. TSH-secreting pituitary tumors. These rare tumors secrete TSH alone or multiple pituitary hormones along with TSH. Elevated levels of TSH α chain help distinguish this tumor from pituitary resistance.

   2. Isolated pituitary resistance to thyroid hormone. The patient presents with an elevated TSH and T_4 but a normal T_3 level. There is also an exaggerated TSH response to TRH stimulation. The administration of T_3 or an analog of T_3 will decrease TSH and control hyperthyroidism within a few months.

3. **Generalized resistance to thyroid hormone.** This disorder does not cause hyperthyroidism but may be confused with it (see Section III.F).
E. **SAT**—hyperthyroid phase.
F. **Lymphocytic thyroiditis with hyperthyroidism (hashitoxicosis).**
G. **Acute psychosis (see Chapter 30).**
H. **Iodine-induced thyrotoxicosis** is also known as the Jod-Basedow phenomenon.

III. EUTHYROID HYPERTHYROXINEMIA

There are many conditions that cause hyperthyroxinemia but *not* hyperthyroidism (total T_4 is elevated, but free T_4 and TSH are normal):
A. Elevated TBG
B. Dysproteinemia (e.g., familial dysalbuminemic hyperthyroxinemia)
C. Organic illness
D. Psychiatric illness
E. Drug-induced (e.g., propranolol)
F. **A generalized resistance to thyroid hormone** can be confused with Graves disease because there are elevated thyroid hormones associated with a goiter, but there are no other signs or symptoms of hyperthyroidism. Elevated levels of T_4, free T_4, and T_3 are needed to maintain a **eumetabolic** state because resistance to the effects of thyroid hormone occurs. The TSH is inappropriately elevated and the TRH stimulation test is normal (it is blunted in Graves disease). The prolactin response to TRH is normal (it is blunted in thyrotoxicosis; increased in hypothyroidism). Delayed bone age and learning problems have been reported. Some cases exhibited goiter, sensorineural deafness, and stippled epiphyses along with delayed bone age and learning problems. These features are consistent with hypothyroidism in the peripheral tissues. The diagnosis is one of exclusion. No therapy is indicated, and the elevated hormone levels should not be lowered.
G. Laboratory error

IV. MANAGEMENT OF HYPERTHYROIDISM

A. **Antithyroid medication,** such as propylthiouracil **(PTU)** or methimazole **(MMI),** renders the patient <u>euthyroid within 6 weeks</u> with a remission rate of 36% to 61% within 18 months. Because there is no effect on the release of thyroid hormone, there will be little improvement for the initial 1 to 3 weeks. If a relapse occurs, it usually appears within 3 to 6 months after cessation of medication.
1. **Dosage**
   a. **PTU.** Initially, 6 to 8 mg/kg per day (or 150 mg/m² per day) in 3 divided doses.
   b. **MMI.** One tenth of PTU dose (0.6 to 0.8 mg/kg per day) may be given once a day.
2. **Complications**
   a. **Mild.** Pruritus, skin rash, urticaria, arthralgia, benign leukopenia, lymphadenopathy, and hepatitis. Hypothyroidism and increasing gland size secondary to increased TSH may occur, which are caused by decreased T_4 synthesis. (To treat hypothyroidism, reduce the dosage of antithyroid drug and add T_4. If you only reduce the antithyroid medication without adding T_4, the hypothyroidism may get worse.) In addition, up to 5% to 10% of patients develop permanent hypothyroidism after discontinuing antithyroid therapy.
   b. **Severe**
      (1) **Agranulocytosis** or bone marrow depression (incidence 0.2%) is most common during the first 4 months after diagnosis but can occur at any time. It is more common in children than in adults. A periodic WBC in an asymptomatic child is probably not useful, but if the patient develops a sore throat and fever, a WBC should be obtained immediately. This is usually reversible by stopping the thionamides (PTU or MMI) if the total WBC is <2 500/μL. Unfortunately, there is some cross-reactivity between MMI and PTU; therefore, other drugs or forms of therapy should be used.
      (2) **Aplastic anemia.** Rare occurrence.

B. Mechanism of action of agents used for hyperthyroidism. Drugs and other agents used in the management of hyperthyroidism act as inhibitors at many different points in the chain of thyroid hormone synthesis, secretion, and metabolism. Recent studies suggest that antithyroid drugs decrease production of TSI with an increase in suppressor T lymphocytes.

1. Hormone synthesis inhibition
   a. PTU. Blocks organification and coupling of iodine.
   b. MMI. Blocks only organification of iodine.
2. Inhibition of hormone release
   a. Iodide
   b. Lithium carbonate
3. All thyroid gland functions inhibited
   a. Complete thyroidectomy
   b. ^{131}I and ^{125}I
4. Impaired conversion of T$_4$ to T$_3$ (drugs act extrathyroidally)
   a. PTU
   b. Dexamethasone
   c. Propranolol
   d. Ipodate (Oragrafin)
5. β-Adrenergic blockers. All of the β-adrenergic blockers effectively neutralize many symptoms of autonomic hyperactivity, but there is no inhibition of thyroid hormone synthesis or release. However, propranolol impairs conversion of T$_4$ to T$_3$ by ~30%.
   a. Propranolol (Inderal)
      (1) Dosage. 2.5 to 10.5 mg/kg per day given q6–8h.
      (2) Indications
         (a) Can be used alone in mild hyperthyroidism.
         (b) Can be used in combination with thionamides for moderate or severe hyperthyroidism.
         (c) May be used to control hyperthyroidism in SAT or HT.
         (d) Has been used alone instead of iodine prior to thyroidectomy or radioactive iodine therapy.
         (e) A thyrotoxic patient may be prepared for surgery, if necessary, by IV propranolol in 1 hour or by oral route in 24 hours.
      (3) Action. Rapidly controls tremors, agitation, tachycardia, and cardiac arrhythmias.
      (4) Side effects. Bradycardia, hypoglycemia.
      (5) Contraindications
         (a) Asthma
         (b) Emphysema
         (c) Congestive heart failure
         (d) Complete heart block
         (e) Raynaud phenomenon
         (f) Should be used with caution in patients with diabetes mellitus
   b. Metoprolol (Lopressor). A β$_1$ blocker.
   c. Nadolol (Corgard). A long-acting β blocker.
6. Other antithyroid drugs
   a. Lithium
      (1) Mechanism of action. Lithium inhibits hormone release.
      (2) Indications for use. It is used primarily in place of stable iodine for severe hyperthyroidism or preoperatively for Graves thyroidectomy. Prior to radioactive iodine treatment, it is preferred by some over stable iodine because it does not block RAIU.
   b. Stable iodine (inorganic iodine). Physiologic amounts of iodine are essential in the synthesis of thyroid hormones, but pharmacologic amounts temporarily inhibit this synthesis (Wolff-Chaikoff effect) as well as retard hormone release from the gland. Improvement of hyperthyroidism may occur within 24 to 48 hours.

(1) Indications for use
    (a) It is used primarily preoperatively to decrease hormone levels and vascularity of the gland, but it *may be used* initially in the treatment of hyperthyroidism until the thionamide takes effect.
    (b) It should *not be used* preoperatively for patients with toxic adenomas or multinodular goiter because it can exacerbate the hyperthyroidism.
(2) Stable iodine is *not used* routinely to correct hyperthyroidism because of the following:
    (a) High incidence of toxicity (edema, serum sickness, skin lesions).
    (b) Not always effective.
    (c) High incidence of recurrence of thyrotoxicosis.
(3) The **dose** of SSKI is 250 mg (5 drops) twice a day for not more than 10 days.

  c. Oral cholecystographic agents, such as ipodate (Oragrafin)
    (1) Mechanism of action. Blocks peripheral conversion of T_4 to T_3.
    (2) Indications. Thyroid storm, because it has a rapid onset of action.
    (3) Adverse effects. No toxic effects have yet been reported.
    (4) Dosage. A dose of 1 g sodium ipodate daily is effective within 48 hours and is not usually used for more than 3 to 4 weeks.

C. Treatment with RAI. In children, RAI therapy is used primarily if antithyroid medication results in serious side effects, if there is a recurrence after thyroidectomy, or occasionally because of noncompliance. Even though many clinicians are still concerned about the virtually negligible risks of leukemia, thyroid carcinoma, and genetic mutation, several medical centers are now using this modality. According to recent studies, properly administered radioactive iodine remains an ideal form of treatment for Graves disease in the pediatric population. Because of the increased risk of thyroid cancer associated with low-dose thyroid irradiation in children, larger, rather than smaller, doses of ^{131}I should be given.

  1. Advantages. Easy administration and effectiveness.
  2. Contraindications. Pregnancy and gross enlargement.
  3. Complications
    a. Hypothyroidism is very common (more so after RAI therapy than after thyroidectomy). Early hypothyroidism is dose-related, whereas late hypothyroidism is not dose-related. It occurs in 10% to 20% after a year and in 3% in the year after.
    b. Hypoparathyroidism or hyperparathyroidism is a rare complication that can occur 3 to 45 years after RAI therapy. The incidence of **hyperparathyroidism in children is higher** than in adults. Therefore, it is important to follow children with calcium and parathormone levels.
  4. Techniques of administration of ^{131}I
    a. Do a pregnancy test in adolescent females.
    b. Discontinue antithyroid medication for several days (at least 3 days) before the administration of the RAIU.
    c. Propranolol may be given during this time, if necessary, which will not interfere with the RAIU.
    d. The dose of ^{131}I is based on the estimated weight of the gland and the uptake of a tracer dose of the iodine. ^{131}I is measured at 6 hours and 24 hours. Use the larger value in calculation. A dose of ^{131}I is chosen that will deliver 100 to 200 μCi/g (average 150).

$$\text{Dose} = \frac{\text{thyroid weight} \times 150\,\mu\text{Ci/g}}{\text{RAIU}}$$

    e. An RAI tracer dose is given to ensure that the uptake is not blocked.
    f. On day 4 (if thionamides have been discontinued for 4 days), the ^{131}I is given.
      (1) A **high dose** (8 to 12 mCi) will probably induce hypothyroidism; therefore, thyroid hormone may be added after treatment. Evaluate thyroid

function tests frequently (e.g., in 4 to 6 weeks) and begin sodium L-T_4 (100 μg/m^2 or 2.0 to 2.5 μg/kg per day) as soon as hypothyroidism occurs. This higher dose causes no increase in overall cancer risk, no decrease in fertility, and no increase in congenital abnormalities in the offspring of treated patients.

   (2) A **smaller dose** (3 to 5 mCi) is given in an attempt to render the patient euthyroid. Follow the child with thyroid function tests for hypothyroidism or recurrence of hyperthyroidism (e.g., every 2 to 4 weeks).

g. Three to 7 days after treatment, if the patient is still hyperthyroid:

   (1) Thionamide may be given again and tapered within a few weeks to months to determine if the patient is euthyroid.

   (2) Propranolol may be used instead of or in addition to thionamides.

   (3) ^{131}I treatment may be repeated at 4-month intervals until euthyroidism is achieved.

D. Surgery for hyperthyroidism

1. Advantage. Rapid control of hyperthyroidism.

2. Indications
   a. Graves disease
   b. Toxic adenoma

3. Indications in children
   a. Severe drug reactions
   b. Relapse or failure to be cured after 2 to 3 years on antithyroid medication
   c. Noncompliance in taking medication
   d. Enlarging gland; failure of medication to decrease size
   e. Toxic adenoma (rare)

4. To prepare a patient for surgery:
   a. Continue antithyroid medication until euthyroid, if possible.
   b. Approximately 2 weeks before surgery, add iodides (e.g., Lugol's solution 5 drops b.i.d., or potassium iodide 10% solution 5 drops t.i.d. for 7 to 10 days) until the day before surgery. This drug reduces vascularity and reduces thyroid function by blocking secretion of thyroid hormone.
   c. If T_3 is still elevated after antithyroid medication and Lugol's solution, then add **corticosteroid,** such as prednisone, 1 mg/kg per day, in 3 divided doses, or propranolol, 2 mg/kg per day, in 3 or 4 divided doses. If propranolol is used preoperatively, it should be continued for 7 to 10 days postoperatively.

5. Possible complications of surgery for hyperthyroidism
   a. Transient hypocalcemia (up to 18% of patients). This probably occurs as a result of mild injury to the parathyroid glands during surgery or secondary to hyperthyroid osteodystrophy or transient parathormone insensitivity in bone tissue.
   b. Permanent hypoparathyroidism.
   c. Recurrent laryngeal nerve damage.
   d. Recurrence of thyrotoxicosis.
   e. Short term: 80% euthyroid; 15% hypothyroid; 5% hyperthyroid.
   f. Permanent hypothyroidism (30% to 66% of patients) within 1 year postoperatively.
   g. Wound infections.

E. Treatment plan for hyperthyroidism in children and adolescents. Not all therapeutic modalities are suitable for every child. The specific treatment depends on many factors, including the severity of the hyperthyroidism, age, associated illness, and the patient's or parent's preference.

1. Begin antithyroid medication when diagnosis is confirmed. Although MMI and PTU are essentially interchangeable, there may be situations in which one is preferred.
   a. If medication is to be given once daily, then MMI is preferred because of longer half-life.
   b. PTU may be more potent for severe hyperthyroidism because of the additional action of blocking T_4 conversion to T_3.

    c. PTU may be preferred in pregnancy because less may cross the placenta than MMI.

  2. If symptoms are severe, add propranolol immediately (2 to 3 mg/kg per day) in 3 or 4 equal doses.

  3. As symptoms subside, taper propranolol dosage and then discontinue it in 2 to 6 weeks as antithyroid medication takes full effect. Follow with serial T_4 and T_3 levels (initially at monthly intervals, then less frequently depending on the clinical course). If the patient is on PTU, a T_4 especially should be obtained because PTU, unlike MMI, blocks peripheral conversion of T_4 to T_3.

  4. If the patient remains euthyroid for 2 to 3 months, plan to continue medication for up to 2 to 3 years.

    a. If after 2 to 3 years the gland has decreased in size, one may opt to test for remission by discontinuing PTU or MMI, and then performing a TRH stimulation test (or T_3 suppression test) in 30 days.

      (1) If the test is normal, permanent remission is probable.

      (2) If the test is abnormal, follow thyroid function tests to determine whether there is a recurrence of hyperthyroidism. Surgery or RAI therapy may now be indicated.

    b. If the gland has not decreased in size, then remission is less likely. Surgery or RAI therapy may now be indicated.

  5. If the child remains hyperthyroid 1 to 3 months after the onset, gradually increase the dose of PTU or MMI. Propranolol may also be added or continued from onset, if indicated, to control severe symptoms. If a euthyroid state is not obtained in 6 to 8 months, consider surgery or RAI ablation.

  6. If aplastic anemia, agranulocytosis, or other serious drug reactions occur, opt for subtotal thyroidectomy. If hypothyroidism occurs, reduce the dose of antithyroid medication and add thyroxine.

V. PROGNOSIS FOR HYPERTHYROIDISM

A remission rate of 30% to 50% occurs after treatment for 6 to 12 months. However, up to 50% of patients in remission will eventually manifest recurrence. The predictability of which patients will go into remission is not very accurate.

A. The short (20 minutes or 1 hour) radioactive uptake may be used to determine remission.

B. TSI assay as a predictor of remission may prove useful, because most remissions are accompanied by a disappearance of TSI.

C. Remissions are more likely with a gland smaller than normal, and less likely with a gland larger than normal.

D. There is little evidence that antithyroid drugs alter the course of the disease.

E. Remission is more likely if thyroglobulin falls to low levels during therapy.

F. Patients who are positive for HLA-Dr3 almost never go into remission. Those who are negative have a **60% chance of remission.**

G. Adding L-T_4 to PTU or MMI in 3 to 6 months and continuing after stopping the antithyroid agent may decrease recurrence of hyperthyroidism. This is also true for decreasing the recurrence of postpartum thyrotoxicosis when T_4 (Synthroid) is started in the third trimester.

THYROID NODULES

I. MANAGEMENT OF THE SOLITARY THYROID NODULE

A. General approach. Opinions vary regarding the appropriate management of the solitary thyroid nodule in children. The clinician should individualize specific treatment after analysis of relevant historical, clinical, and laboratory data.

  1. History

    a. Radiation exposure directed to the head and neck in early childhood can subsequently result in a significant number of thyroid tumors (up to 7% incidence of thyroid carcinoma in young adults). The thyroid gland in children is particularly sensitive to radiation, with a dose–response effect. Recent studies have revealed that doses of 300 to 1 500 rad may cause thyroid cancer in up to 30% of patients. Higher dosages (10 000 rad) cause cell death prior to malignant degeneration and are therefore not a risk factor.

b. Rapid growth of a nodule suggests malignancy.

c. Pain within the nodule is usually *not* consistent with a malignant process.

d. Thyroid carcinoma is more common in **Graves** patients than in the general population.

2. **Physical examination**

   a. Lymphadenopathy suggests malignancy, but this is not diagnostic because an occasional benign tumor may be associated with lymph node enlargement.

   b. Even though most malignant tumors are very **firm,** the consistency of a nodule has limited diagnostic value because benign calcified lesions are hard, whereas some softer nodules may be malignant.

   c. Fixation of a nodule to adjacent tissue usually indicates malignancy.

   d. Tenderness suggests an inflammatory process.

3. **Laboratory findings**

   a. Almost all patients with solitary nodules are euthyroid, but elevated thyroid hormones may occur (autonomous hyperfunctioning nodules), suggesting a benign process. These patients have "hot" nodules on scintiscan.

   b. Calcitonin elevation is a useful diagnostic marker for medullary carcinoma.

   c. Serum thyroglobulin (Tg) may be elevated in patients with papillary and follicular carcinoma, but unfortunately, it can be high in benign conditions (e.g., thyroiditis); therefore, it is of **little diagnostic value.** However, it should be used postoperatively to detect recurrence and/or metastases (see Chapter 31) in patients previously treated with total thyroidectomy followed by RAI ablation.

4. **Thyroid imaging**

   a. Thyroid scintiscanning using radioiodine or technetium is very useful in the evaluation of a thyroid nodule. A "cold" area (hypofunctioning) on scan increases suspicion of malignancy but is not diagnostic, because most cold nodules are benign. In some studies, 17% to 36% may be malignant. Tumors that are "hot" or hyperfunctioning are even less likely to be malignant. These hyperfunctioning nodules have increased RAIU in comparison with the remainder of the gland. Some hot nodules can be suppressed with thyroid hormone, but many will not diminish in size and occasionally the patient may become hyperthyroid on attempts at thyroxine suppression. If the area surrounding the nodule is not visible on the scintiscan, TSH administration may be given to reveal this thyroid tissue in order to distinguish the nodule from nontumorous abnormalities, such as hemiagenesis. Occasionally, a nodule that would be cold on an iodine scan is hot using technetium. It may be prudent, therefore, to follow up a hot nodule on a technetium scan with a ^{123}I scan. (This is one disadvantage of ^{99m}Tc.)

   b. Ultrasound of the thyroid

   (1) Ultrasound of the thyroid is useful in differentiating cystic from solid tumors but cannot distinguish between hot and cold nodules. Cystic lesions are more often benign than solid lesions. Nodules that are cold on scan and solid on ultrasound increase the suspicion of malignancy, but these tests are not diagnostic because most solid lesions are benign. Lesions that are mixed with cystic and solid components should be evaluated in the same way as lesions that are purely solid.

   (2) Another use for ultrasound is to **monitor the size** of the nodule during suppressive therapy with thyroxine. (Echography is nonionizing and therefore harmless to tissue.)

   (3) Occasionally, there may be a question as to the existence of a nodule on clinical examination. Ultrasound may be used to affirm or deny the presence of the "questionable" nodule.

5. Needle biopsy

   a. Rationale. Needle biopsy is the most simple and direct method to help determine the architecture of a thyroid nodule. In addition, surgery can be avoided if the diagnosis of anaplastic or metastatic cancer is determined histologically. Ultrasound-guided fine-needle aspiration biopsy (US-FNAB) improved the cytologic diagnostic accuracy, sensitivity, and positive predictive value and reduced the false-negative rate in comparison with palpation-guided fine-needle aspiration biopsy (P-FNAB). The malignancy rate for nonpalpable thyroid nodules was similar to that for palpable nodules.

   b. Fine-needle biopsy technique. Lidocaine is injected into cleansed skin overlying the nodule. A 22-gauge needle is then inserted into the target area. Once the mass is penetrated, firm suction is applied to the aspiration syringe (20-mL disposable syringe with Leur-Lok tip). The needle is then moved back and forth briskly and rotated in different directions. The aspirated material should be placed on a slide and prepared in cell blocks. If one obtains fluid on aspirating a thyroid nodule and the fluid is clear and light in color, consider a parathyroid cyst in the differential diagnosis and therefore measure parahormone levels in the aspirate.

   c. Limitations. The major limitation is the requirement for an experienced and knowledgeable cytologist to interpret the aspirate. In addition, because of poor technique, the aspirate may be inadequate, providing insufficient thyroid tissue for diagnosis. Another limitation is the histologic overlap of some benign and malignant tumors. Fifteen percent of all aspirations are consistent with a follicular tumor, but both fine-needle aspiration and frozen sections are often inconclusive. Because a child <8 years old has an increased risk of mortality from thyroid carcinoma, many feel that open biopsy is preferred over fine-needle aspiration.

6. Radiography

   a. Radiographs of the neck may reveal punctate calcifications that correlate with psammoma bodies found frequently in papillary thyroid carcinomas.

   b. Chest radiographs may reveal pulmonary metastases.

7. Treatment. There are several possible approaches:

   a. Observation, if the nodule is believed to be almost certainly benign.

   b. Thyroid hormone suppression

   (1) Allegedly, thyroid tumors thrive under the influence of TSH and may diminish in size when TSH is decreased to low normal or subnormal levels. Therefore, some investigators suggest that TSH suppression should be the initial mode of therapy. If the nodule does not shrink in size, malignancy is a possibility and the nodule should be excised.

   (2) The usual dose of thyroid hormone for suppression is slightly more than the replacement dose for hypothyroidism (see **Hypothyroidism**) to keep the TSH at a low level.

   (3) Suppression is maintained for at least 3 months and is considered **successful if the tumor is reduced in size by 50% or more.** If at the end of 3 months the nodule is not decreased by more than 50% or has enlarged, then surgical excision is recommended. If the nodule is <50%, then L-T$_4$ is continued.

   (4) One can follow nodular size by ruler or ultrasound. During suppressive therapy, the T$_4$ and TSH values should be measured to evaluate the completeness of suppression. A good endpoint for measuring TSH suppression is the inability of TRH to stimulate TSH.

   c. Surgical excision

   (1) Removal of the nodule surgically is often recommended if the nodule is solid and cold on scintiscan and with one or more of the following (Table 33.8):

   (a) History of radiation therapy in early childhood.

   (b) Patient is younger than 20 years.

   (c) Recent and/or rapid growth of a hard nodule.

TABLE 33.8	High Index of Suspicion for Cancer in Thyroid Nodules

Male child
Recent onset
Prior history of irradiation
Solitary nodule
"Cold" nodule on scan
Solid nodule on ultrasound
Does not regress with thyroid hormone
Pressure symptoms
Regional lymphadenopathy

(2) Many clinicians are now performing fine-needle biopsy first to determine if the nodule is malignant (see Chapter 31). In a young child, we are more inclined to remove most solid cold nodules and many hot nodules without prior biopsy, because general anesthesia may be necessary to perform the biopsy.

(3) Once surgery is contemplated, opinions differ regarding how much thyroid tissue should be excised. There are several arguments for **total or near-total thyroidectomy:**

   (a) As many as 87.5% of patients have microscopic cancer in the contralateral lobe.

   (b) In as many as 10% of patients, clinical cancer develops in the remaining lobe.

   (c) Follow-up with RAI scanning is easier to assess for disseminated disease.

   (d) Thyroglobulin can be used as a tumor marker for metastatic differentiated thyroid cancer because serum levels should be negligible in patients after total thyroidectomy (see Chapter 31).

(4) However, the extent of lymph node surgery has no significant influence on recurrence or survival. The surgeon should remove any lymph nodes that appear to contain metastases, but a radical neck dissection is not indicated because it would confer no advantage.

d. Postoperative management

   (1) There are fewer recurrences of cancer when both ^{131}I and thyroid hormone are given postoperatively than when radiation or thyroid hormone is administered alone.

   (2) L-T$_4$ is given daily as replacement for the surgically removed thyroid tissue and also to prevent recurrence of the TSH-responsive cancer. A maximally suppressive effect can be verified by demonstrating complete inhibition of the TSH response to TRH stimulation or by measuring ultrasensitive TSH.

   (3) To determine whether metastases (especially to the lung) are present, I recommend total-body ^{131}I scanning (5 to 10 mCi) 4 to 6 weeks after thyroidectomy. In Winship's series, pulmonary metastases were present soon after surgery in 14.4% of children, and an additional 5.2% of the same study group manifested metastatic lung disease several years later. Obtaining a chest radiograph alone to determine the presence of lung metastases is not sufficient, because in my experience several children presented at the time of diagnosis with pulmonary metastases that were evident on scans but not on radiographs.

   Because normal thyroid tissue traps ^{131}I with greater avidity than does cancerous tissue, a radionuclide scan may be misleading if a significant amount of thyroid tissue remains. However, the visibility of metastatic tissue can be enhanced by increasing the serum TSH level, which in turn increases tumor uptake of ^{131}I. Endogenous TSH levels may be raised by substituting the patient's usual dose of Synthroid (T_4) with an equivalent dose of Cytomel (T_3) (25 μg of T_3 is equivalent to ~0.1 mg of T_4) 4 weeks before the scan is performed. T_3 is given t.i.d. for 2 weeks and then discontinued for the 2-week period prior to initiation of scanning. TSH should ascend to levels of ~50 μU/mL before radioiodine is given.

(4) The Tg level should be measured at this time and subsequently at regular intervals. If there is absence of normal thyroid remnant and tumor tissue, the Tg level should be low (<10 ng/mL). If the level is high, tumor tissue is probably present. This may even occur in the absence of cancerous tissue detectable by external scanning for ^{131}I.

However, recent studies suggest that total-body scanning is superior to Tg for detection of residual or recurrent disease in the thyroid bed and local neck structures, whereas Tg is helpful in patients with metastatic disease. The presence of anti-Tg antibodies can prevent the use of Tg in a subset of patients with thyroid cancer.

(5) Alternatively, giving no medication (discontinuing T_4) for 4 to 6 weeks before the scan will result in an elevated TSH level. Some clinicians recommend administration of intramuscular TSH (10 U per day for 3 days) to stimulate incorporation of ^{131}I, but a few patients may be allergic to this hormone. Recombinant TSH is now used.

(6) If residual tissue is present but there is no evidence of metastases, an ablative dose of 30 to 50 mCi is administered followed by repeat scanning in 1 week to determine if metastatic tissue is now visible under this higher dose. If metastases are evident on either of the two scans, a dose of 100 to 150 mCi of ^{131}I is given. Repeat doses are usually given at about 6- to 12-month intervals, if necessary, and should not be administered before the bone marrow has fully recovered from the previous dose. Leukemia may infrequently occur in patients who receive multiple large doses of ^{131}I given at frequent intervals.

(7) Pulmonary fibrosis rarely occurs. Following initial therapy, if the patient is shown by total-body scan to be free of disease, scans can usually be repeated at 3- to 5-year intervals.

e. Summary: **Treatment for thyroid carcinoma**

(1) Perform total (or near-total) thyroidectomy.

(2) Remove affected lymph nodes.

(3) Ablate remaining thyroid tissue with ^{131}I.

(4) Obtain Tg after surgery.

(5) Institute thyroid hormone suppression postoperatively.

(6) Postoperative RAI treatment should be considered in children with larger tumor size, local or regional disease, extrathyroidal extension, and distant metastases.

(7) Follow-up

(a) Serial Tg (every 6 to 12 months).

(b) Chest radiography (yearly).

(c) ^{131}I total-body scanning (3- to 5-year intervals or more often if Tg is elevated).

f. Treatment of a patient with previous exposure to external radiation of the head and neck

(1) Overall approach

(a) If a thyroid nodule is present, then remove surgically and treat postoperatively with thyroxine (see Table 33.9 for classifications of thyroid nodules).

(b) Obtain a thyroid scintiscan or ultrasound (or both) if a nodule is not palpable or if confirmation is desired.

(c) If no nodule is present, suppress potential tumor formation with T_4.

TABLE 33.9	Classification of Thyroid Nodules

A. Non-neoplasm
  (1) Cyst
  (2) Abscess
  (3) Subacute thyroiditis (in one lobe)
  (4) Hashimoto thyroiditis
  (5) Hemithyroid
  (6) Parathyroid cyst
B. Benign neoplasm
  (1) Adenoma
    (a) Follicular
    (b) Embryonal
    (c) Fetal
    (d) Hürthle cell
  (2) Teratoma (found mostly in newborns)
C. Malignant neoplasm
  (1) Well differentiated
    (a) Papillary
    (b) Follicular
    (c) Papillary-follicular (most common)
  (2) Medullary carcinoma
  (3) Anaplastic carcinoma
  (4) Primary lymphoma
  (5) Metastatic (to thyroid) carcinoma

(2) Aggressive treatment should be instituted because of the following:
  (a) There is an incidence of up to 7% of thyroid carcinoma in adult patients with a history of irradiation to the head and neck during infancy or childhood.
  (b) The incidence of thyroid carcinoma appears to be 50 to 300 times greater in patients with radiation exposure in comparison with controls.
  (c) The incidence of parathyroid adenomas appears to be increased particularly in children. However, the latent period is longer than for the formation of thyroid tumors.

Selected References

Amrikachi M, Ponder TB, Wheeler TM, et al. Thyroid fine-needle aspiration biopsy in children and adolescents: experience with 218 aspirates. *Diagn Cytopathol* 2005 Apr;32(4): 189–192.

Sharma Y, Bajpai A, Mittal S, et al. Ovarian cysts in young girls with hypothyroidism: follow-up and effect of treatment. *J Pediatr Endocrinol Metab* 2006 Jul;19(7):895–900.

Hasanhodzić M, Tahirović H, Lukinac L. Down syndrome and thyroid gland. *Bosn J Basic Med Sci* 2006 Aug;6(3):38–42.

Izquierdo R, Arekat MR, Knudson PE, et al. Comparison of palpation-guided versus ultrasound-guided versus ultrasound-guided fine-needle aspiration biopsies of thyroid nodules in an outpatient endocrinology practice. *Endocr Pract* 2006 Nov-Dec;12(6): 609–614.

La Franchi S. Thyroid hormone in hypopituitarism, graves' disease, congenital hypothyroidism and maternal thyroid disease during pregnancy. *Growth Hormone IGF Res* 2006 Jul;16(suppl A):520–524.

Karges B, Muche R, Knerr I, et al. Thyroid replacement in euthyroid autoimmune thyroiditis in type i diabetes. *J Clin Endocrinol Metab* 2007;92:1647.

Menconi F, Marinò M, Pinchera A, et al. Effects of total thyroid ablation versus near-total thyroidectomy alone on mild to moderate graves orbitopathy treated with intravenous glucocorticoids. *J Clin Endocrinol Metab* 2007 May;92(5):1653–1658.

Mihailescu DV, Collins BJ, Millour A, et al. Ultrasound-detected thyroid nodules in radiation exposed patients: changes over time *Thyroid* 2005 Feb;15(2):127–133.

Radetti G, Gottardi E, Bona G, et al. The natural history of euthyroid hashimotos thyroiditis in children. *J Pediatr* 2006 Dec;149(6):827–832.

Rivkees SA, Dinauer C. An optional treatment for pediatric graves disease is radioiodine. *J Clin Endocrinol Metab* 2007 Mar;92(3):797–800.

Untero J, Schultink W, West CE, et al. Efficacy of oral iodized peanut oil is greater than that of iodized poppy seed oil among Indonesian school children. *Am J Clin Nutr* 2006 Nov;84(5):1208–1214.

34

THYROID CANCER IN CHILDREN
Kuk-Wha Lee

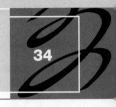

$\mathcal{T}$hyroid cancer is uncommon during childhood. Older children and adolescents are more likely to be diagnosed. Despite this fact, incidence is increasing. This could be a result of increased surveillance (sequelae of treatment for childhood cancer); improved detection methods; effects of radiation or other pollutants in the environment; incidental detection of nodules during imaging for other reasons; and previous radiation exposure. Because of the lack of prospective research, differentiated thyroid cancer in children and adolescents generally is managed similarly to that in adults. The clinician should individualize specific treatment after careful analysis of the history, physical examination, and pathologic diagnosis. Papillary and follicular cell tumors (differentiated thyroid cancer) account for the majority of thyroid neoplasms (especially papillary) and will be the main focus of this chapter. Medullary thyroid cancer will be addressed briefly later in the chapter.

I. OVERVIEW
   A. Thyroid cancer, the most common pediatric endocrine neoplasm, represents 1% to 1.5% of all pediatric malignancies and 5% to 5.7% of malignancies in the head and neck.
   B. The risk of malignancy is greater in pediatric than adult patients. Pediatric thyroid nodules are four times more likely to carry a diagnosis of thyroid cancer than adult nodules.
   C. There is a strong tendency for regional and distant spread and recurrence. The lungs are the most common sites of metastasis.
   D. In spite of this, there is excellent overall survival and prognosis with appropriate treatment.
   E. Risk factors
      1. Female sex
      2. Pubertal age
      3. Family history of thyroid disease
      4. Previous or coexisting thyroid disease
      5. History of steroid- or endocrine-related condition
      6. Radiation exposure
         a. Especially for children under age 10
         b. Childhood cancer survivors
         c. Chernobyl nuclear accident exposure

II. PATHOGENESIS
   A. Most thyroid cancers (papillary, follicular, anaplastic) originate from follicular cells, but all histologic types have been observed (e.g., anaplastic, Hürthle; these tend to have a less favorable prognosis).
   B. Papillary carcinoma lesions, the majority subclass, are irregular, solid, or cystic masses that arise from follicular epithelium.
   C. Follicular thyroid cancers are related to iodine deficiency, whereas the opposite is true of papillary thyroid cancers.
   D. From a genetic standpoint, papillary thyroid cancers are characterized by RET, TRK, and BRAF gene alterations, while follicular cancers feature RAS mutations.

III. CLINICAL PRESENTATION

A. A painless noninflammatory metastatic cervical mass is the presenting symptom in the majority of children and is found during routine examination.

B. Reported incidence of cervical lymphadenopathy ranges from 35% to 83%.

C. Patients who have lung metastases usually do not report pulmonary symptoms.

IV. DIAGNOSIS

A. History, including the prior existence and treatment of a benign thyroid disease

1. A history of Graves disease, hypothyroidism, or goiter should suggest a benign thyroid disease process. Long-term suppression of Graves disease with antithyroid drugs may lead to increased risk of malignant thyroid transformation, especially when associated with a nodule. Incidence of papillary thyroid cancer detected post–surgical thyroidectomy for Graves in various series ranges from 10% to 35%, especially when associated with a palpable nodule.

2. Autoimmune disease, which often results in rapidly enlarging thyroid glands, confounds any associated glandular nodularity for which malignancy must be excluded.

3. Thyroid cancer may be one feature of a group of dominantly inherited tumor syndromes including Gardner syndrome, Cowden syndrome, and the Carney complex.

B. Physical

1. One or more painless firm neck or thyroid nodules.

2. Tenderness of the nodule suggests hemorrhage into a nodule, a cyst, or an inflammatory process.

3. Lymphadenopathy increases the likelihood of malignancy.

4. Diffuse thyroid enlargement or multiple nodules are more suggestive of a benign process.

C. Lab studies

1. Total **tri-iodothyronine** (T_3), total thyroxine (T_4), and thyroid-stimulating hormone (TSH) are usually normal in malignancy. They help shape the differential diagnosis of a child's thyroid mass.

2. Antithyroid antibodies are helpful in diagnosing chronic lymphocytic thyroiditis. Although controversial, positive studies that link thyroiditis and differentiated thyroid cancer state a two- to threefold elevated risk for developing thyroid cancer if antibody-positive.

D. Imaging studies

1. **Ultrasonography**

   a. First-line imaging test in all pediatric patients with thyroid nodules.

   b. Children with a history of radiation exposure should be observed with yearly serial ultrasonography. Nodules that enlarge even a few millimeters should undergo fine-needle aspiration and biopsy.

   c. A solid nodule is more likely to be malignant; however, up to 50% of malignant lesions may have a cystic component, and approximately 8% of cystic lesions represent malignancies.

   d. May help guide fine needle aspiration and biopsy. Success is operator dependent.

2. **Computed tomography (CT) scan**

   a. Noncontrast CT scans can be helpful in patients with substernal extension, local invasion, or lymph node metastasis.

   b. At initial evaluation, ~20% of children have pulmonary metastasis that can be revealed by either chest radiography or CT scan.

   c. Children have a much higher incidence of pulmonary involvement than adults.

3. **Radionucleotide scan (scintigraphy)**

   a. Thyroid scintigraphy is most useful in revealing tissue function in thyroglossal duct cysts (e.g., ensuring that thyroid tissue in the normal location is functioning) and in diagnosing ectopic thyroid. However, thyroid scintigraphy has not proven worthwhile in distinguishing malignant from benign disease.

V. TREATMENT

The goals of treatment are to eliminate the disease and to reduce the chance of recurrence. Sometimes the disease cannot be entirely eradicated, and therefore, another therapeutic goal is to achieve stability and no symptoms of disease.

A. Surgical care

1. Because of the unusual combination of an excellent prognosis and an advanced-stage disease presentation, the initial extent of surgery is controversial. Some recommend that the initial surgical approach should be conservative, whereas others advocate aggressive management with total thyroidectomy and radioactive iodine (RAI) for all patients. The relative infrequency of thyroid malignancy makes this controversy difficult to resolve. There are several arguments for total or near-total thyroidectomy.

    a. Some argue that almost 90% of patients have microscopic cancer in the contralateral lobe.

    b. In as many as 10% of patients, clinical cancer develops in the remaining lobe.

    c. Thyroidectomy makes follow-up RAI scanning easier.

    d. Thyroglobulin (TG) can be used as a tumor marker after surgical removal and ablation with RAI postsurgery.

2. Benign tumors such as follicular adenomas should be considered at risk for tumor progression toward follicular thyroid carcinoma, and they must be surgically addressed.

3. Selective ipsilateral neck dissection in pediatric thyroid surgery is indicated for proven or suspected regional lymph node metastasis. During the dissection, lymph nodes in the paratracheal region, tracheoesophageal groove, and lateral areas can be inspected.

4. Risks include parathyroid damage and recurrent laryngeal nerve injury.

5. Serum calcium levels are measured daily for the first 2 to 4 postoperative days in all patients who have undergone a total or subtotal thyroidectomy. The calcium level usually drops slightly (to about 7 mg/dL) as the remaining parathyroid tissue recovers from surgical trauma. Mild hypocalcemia of this level requires treatment only if symptomatic. Mild symptoms include a positive Trousseau or Chvostek sign, mild cardiac arrhythmia, or perioral tingling. Treatment of these mild symptoms requires only oral calcium combined with vitamin D. Intravenous calcium gluconate is used for a more rapid replacement for severe arrhythmia or impending tetany.

B. Medical Care

1. **Postsurgical**

    a. **Radioactive therapy** with iodine-131 (^{131}I), RAI, is indicated to ablate residual normal thyroid and to treat functioning metastases in differentiated thyroid tumors. Doses in the range of 50 mCi (localized to thyroid only) to 100 mCi (local lymph node involvement) are commonly used as therapy for thyroid cancer. Higher doses of RAI may be indicated.

        (1) Fluid intake is encouraged, and antiemetics can be given.

        (2) Sour hard candies are encouraged to stimulate salivary flow and reduce risk of sialadenitis.

        (3) A 7- to 10-day post-therapy scan is indicated to assess extent of disease and assess iodine avidity.

        (4) Total-body RAI scans often reveal pulmonary nodal metastases, which are often missed by other imaging modalities.

        (5) Dosimetry to calculate delivery of a maximum of 80 mCi to the lungs is indicated in known pulmonary metastasis to avoid pulmonary fibrosis.

        (6) Gonadal function is usually preserved, but testes are more sensitive.

    b. Postoperative suppression of TSH with thyroid hormone. Degree of suppression is debated, but most authors recommend levothyroxine (LT$_4$) administration to maintain TSH levels near zero without clinical symptoms of hyperthyroidism.

    c. External beam radiation is not recommended in children.

VI. FOLLOW-UP AND SURVEILLANCE

A. Recurrence is common in children, especially during the immediate years following therapy. Risk factors include
1. Younger age
2. Male gender
3. Large tumors (>2 cm in diameter)
4. Multifocal disease
5. Regional lymph node involvement
6. Distant metastasis

B. Serial neck exams

C. Annual thyroid hormone withdrawal recombinant human TSH (rhTSH)–stimulated whole-body RAI scan until free of disease. RAI treatment as indicated.
1. Withdrawal from LT$_4$ for 14 days along with a low-iodine diet for the last 7 days is usually sufficient to achieve a serum TSH level >25 μIU/mL for RAI administration (either diagnosis or treatment) and may be used instead of rhTSH as preparation.
2. Serum thyroglobulin (Tg) levels during thyroid hormone suppression and in response to rhTSH stimulation is a reliable marker of tumor burden. Tg levels are not reliable if patient is positive for anti-Tg antibodies, so serial imaging must be used (RAI scans/ultrasound). Disappearance of anti-Tg antibodies in a previously positive patient is a good prognostic sign in adults.

D. ^{18}F-fluorodeoxyglucose positron emission tomography (PET) scanning has assumed a more central role in the follow-up of adult differentiated thyroid cancer (DTC) patients over the past several years. It is well established that the DTCs most likely to be visible on PET scan are those that are not iodine-avid.

E. Several algorithms exist for follow-up (which include serial TG measurements and RAI scans(ultrasounds) and should be individualized to the patient.

F. Serial pulmonary function testing is indicated when pulmonary metastasis is present in children.

G. Life-long follow-up is required.

H. Thyroid cancer persists, despite treatment, in many affected children. This is more common in children who present with distant metastasis.

VII. MEDULLARY THYROID CANCER (MTC)

A. MTC constitutes 5% to 10% of all thyroid cancers. In children and adolescents, it is a very rare but very aggressive disease with regional metastases, affecting less than one child per million per year.

B. MTC arises from the thyroid parafollicular or C cells, which secrete calcitonin. Hyperplasia of the C cells is thought to represent a precancerous state. Calcitonin is measured at baseline and as a tumor marker.

C. MTC is almost always the familial form, due to a specific mutation (defect) in the RET proto-oncogene. The inheritance pattern occurs either sporadically or as familial MTC without other associated endocrine abnormalities.

D. MTC is associated with multiple endocrine neoplasia type 2 (MEN2). MEN2 consists of MTC and pheochromocytoma and either hyperparathyroidism (type 2A) or mucosal neuromas (type 2B) of the tongue, palpebral conjunctiva, and lips with marfanoid body habitus. Both are inherited in an autosomal dominant fashion. MTC associated with MEN2B is more virulent and may occur and metastasize early in infancy. All family members should be genetically screened for this mutation in the RET proto-oncogene.
1. Obtain a 24-hour urine collection to screen for catecholamine metabolites, as a pheochromocytoma or paraganglioma should be surgically removed before thyroidectomy to avoid a hypertension crisis during surgery.
2. Obtain serum calcium to screen for hyperparathyroidism.

E. Serum carcinoembryonic antigen (CEA) should be measured in those in whom MTC is suspected.

F. Total thyroidectomy and aggressive central neck dissection with laparoscopic examination of the liver are indicated for biopsy-proven medullary carcinoma.

Prophylactic total thyroidectomy may be indicated in children with a family history of the multiple endocrine neoplasia (MEN) syndrome. Genetic screening is now possible for the MEN2 gene, and prophylactic surgery must be performed to prevent the occurrence of C-cell hyperplasia or carcinoma.

G. Thyroid hormone replacement but not suppression is indicated postsurgery, because C cells are not responsive to TSH. There is no role for RAI in MTC.

Selected References

Bauer AJ, Tuttle RM, Francis GL. Thyroid nodules and thyroid cancer in children and adolescents. In: Pescovitz OH, Eugster EA, eds. *Pediatric Endocrinology: Mechanisms, Manifestations, and Management.* Philadelphia: Lippincott, Williams & Wilkins; 2004:522–547.

Chaukar DA, Rangarajan V, Nair N, Dcruz AK. Pediatric thyroid cancer. *J Surg Oncol* 2005; 92:130–133.

Cooper DS, Doherty GM, Haugen BR, Kloos RT. Management guidelines for patients with thyroid nodules and differentiated thyroid cancer. *Thyroid* 2006;16:109–142.

Davies SM. Subsequent malignant neoplasms in survivors of childhood cancer: Childhood Cancer Survivor Study (CCSS) studies. *Pediatr Blood Cancer* 2007;June 15;48(7):727–730.

Halac I, Zimmerman D. Thyroid nodules and cancers in children. *Endocrinol Metab Clin North Am* 2005;34:725–744.

Holt E. Controversies in the surveillance of patients with well differentiated thyroid cancer. *Curr Opin Oncol* 2007;19:6–10.

Kuijt WJ, Huang SA. Children with differentiated thyroid cancer achieve adequate hyperthyrotropinemia within 14 days of levothyroxine withdrawal. *J Clin Endocrinol Metab* 2005;90:6123–6125.

Luboshitzky R, Lavi I, Ishay A. Serum thyroglobulin levels after fine-needle aspiration of thyroid nodules. *Endocr Pract* 2006;12:264–269.

Niedziela M. Pathogenesis, diagnosis and management of thyroid nodules in children. *Endocr Relat Cancer* 2006;13:427–453.

Rachmiel M, Charron M, Gupta A, Hamilton J. Evidence-based review of treatment and follow up of pediatric patients with differentiated thyroid carcinoma. *J Pediatr Endocrinol Metab* 2006;19:1377–1393.

Yoskovitch A, Laberge JM, Rodd C, et al. Cystic thyroid lesions in children. *J Pediatr Surg* 1998;33:866–870.

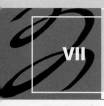

VII | Metabolic Disorders

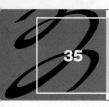

35 | HYPOGLYCEMIA IN INFANTS AND CHILDREN
Cem S. Demirci, Shadi Tabba, and Mark A. Sperling

I. GENERAL PRINCIPLES
  A. **Perspective.** The hypoglycemias of infancy and childhood are a group of disorders that collectively reflect failure to maintain normal glucose homeostasis because of defects in available substrate, enzymes, or hormones. Hypoglycemia of infants and children can be classified as occurring at two times:
    1. In the **immediate newborn period,** when hypoglycemia is due to prematurity or dysmaturity, reflecting inadequate substrate stores, genetic defects in enzymes, hyperinsulinemia, and hormone deficiencies. These defects are relatively common and are an important cause of neonatal morbidity. The most common of these entities is hyperinsulinemic hypoglycemia, either transient and usually associated with stressful delivery/hypoxia/prematurity/intrauterine growth retardation (IUGR), or permanent as a result of defects in the adenosine triphosphate (ATP)–regulated potassium channel that governs insulin secretion.
    2. In **infancy and childhood,** when hypoglycemia is less common and is usually a result of an acquired lesion of the endocrine system, environmental insults, and, occasionally, persistence of congenital or developmental abnormalities such as hyperinsulinemic hypoglycemia or glycogen storage disease.
  B. **Significance of hypoglycemia.** The major impetus for recognition and treatment of neonatal hypoglycemia is to permit normal brain development; the larger proportion of glucose turnover is utilized by brain metabolism. Controversy remains as to the degree and duration as well as associated conditions, such as seizures or asphyxia, that lead to neurointellectual impairment. Although a threshold of 60 mg/dL or less was suggested as important for newborns, there is evidence that the neonatal brain is more resistant than adult brain to hypoglycemia, especially in its ability to use lactate (and ketones) as alternate fuel. However, the duration of hypoglycemia determines the outcome: Duration of more than 24 hours or multiple episodes over a period of days are more likely to be associated with poorer outcome. Worse

neurodevelopmental outcomes are more likely if symptoms of hypoglycemia, especially seizures, accompany the low glucose measurement.

C. Definition. Clinically significant hypoglycemia in the immediate newborn, whether symptomatic or not, is considered to be present when whole-blood glucose is <40 to 45 mg/dL (<50 mg/dL in serum or plasma) in full-term neonates and <40 mg/dL in low-birth-weight or premature infants (<45 mg/dL in serum or plasma). Many authorities view with suspicion any blood glucose values <50 mg/dL in a neonate; beyond 3 to 5 days of life, such values are considered to be definitely abnormal and require treatment.

D. Symptoms and signs

   1. Symptoms and signs in **older children** are similar to those in adults and include features associated with activation of counterregulatory sympathetic response, including sweating, trembling, tachycardia, anxiety, weakness, hunger, nausea, and vomiting; and those reflecting cerebral glucopenia, including headache, mental confusion, somnolence, personality changes, inability to concentrate, convulsions, and loss of consciousness.

   2. In **infants,** these features may be subtler and predominantly reflect the impairment of neurologic function, including cyanotic episodes, apnea, refusal to feed, wilting spells or myoclonic jerks, somnolence, subnormal temperatures, and convulsions. Because these symptoms are nonspecific and can occur in other conditions, such as sepsis, asphyxia, intraventricular bleeds, congenital heart disease, and maternal drug therapy, it is important to demonstrate that the blood glucose is low at the time of the occurrence of symptoms and that symptoms disappear when parenteral glucose is given in amounts adequate to elevate blood glucose concentrations. (Whipple triad: low glucose at time of symptoms; disappearance of symptoms and signs when glucose is elevated; reappearance of signs and symptoms when glucose is lowered.) Moreover, obtaining blood at the time of symptoms provides the unique opportunity of the "critical sample," in which, once hypoglycemia is confirmed, insulin, growth hormone, cortisol, free fatty acids, and ketones can be measured in order to arrive at a likely diagnosis.

II. CLASSIFICATION AND INCIDENCE OF HYPOGLYCEMIA IN INFANTS AND CHILDREN

A. Classification. A classification based on a developmental approach is outlined in Table 35.1. In the neonatal transient form, it is important to emphasize that hypoglycemia can be asymptomatic and that there are certain high-risk groups, as outlined in the table.

B. Incidence. The overall reported incidence of hypoglycemia in the newborn varies from 1.5 to 3 in 1 000 live births and can be several-fold higher in certain vulnerable groups. The premature or small-for-gestational-age (SGA) infant is especially vulnerable to hypoglycemia. Two thirds of infants who are both premature and SGA develop clinically significant hypoglycemia that usually is transient, lasting only several days. Hypoglycemia in these infants is a result of immaturity in the glucoregulatory mechanisms that involve hormones, receptors, their signaling cascades, enzymatic effectors, and substrate availability to sustain glucose production. The majority of infants (80% to 90%) born to insulin-dependent or gestational diabetic mothers are included in this group of neonatal transient hypoglycemias. Only a minority (<20%) have severe persistent hypoglycemia. When hypoglycemia persists, some form of hyperinsulinism is most likely, especially those presenting as newborns. Some asphyxiated infants display more persistent hypoglycemia that is associated with hyperinsulinism and responds well to diazoxide.

III. MANAGEMENT

A. Neonatal transient. Newborns with symptoms suggestive of hypoglycemia and all newborns in high-risk groups (Table 35.1) should be screened for hypoglycemia via a test strip (Chemstrips; Dextrostix) and have low values confirmed by formal laboratory glucose determination. If low glucose values are confirmed, start treatment with

TABLE 35.1 Classification of Hypoglycemia in Infants and Children

Neonatal—Transient
Associated with inadequate substrate or enzyme function
  Prematurity
  Small for gestational age
  Smaller of twins
  Infants with severe respiratory distress
  Infants of toxemic mother
Associated with hyperinsulinemia
  Infants of diabetic mothers
  Infants with erythroblastosis fetalis

Neonatal, Infantile, or Childhood—Persistent
Hyperinsulinemic states
  Hyperinsulinemic hypoglycemia of infancy (HHI)
  KATP channel defects
    SUR1 mutations
    Kir6.2 mutations
  Glucokinase-activating mutations
  Glutamate dehydrogenase–activating mutation (leucine sensitivity)
  β-Cell hyperplasia
  β-Cell adenoma: multiple endocrine neoplasia type I
  Beckwith-Wiedemann syndrome
  Congenital disorders of glycosylation (CDGs)
    DG-1a
    CDG-1b (phosphomannose isomerase deficiency)
    CDG-1d
  Short-chain L-3-hydroxyacyl-CoA dehydrogenase mutation
  Insulin administration (Münchhausen by proxy)
  *Most of these are associated with specific genetic defects in insulin secretion

Hormone deficiency
  Panhypopituitarism
  Isolated growth hormone deficiency
  ACTH deficiency
  Addison disease
  Glucagon deficiency
  Epinephrine deficiency
Substrate-limited
  Ketotic hypoglycemia
  Branched-chain ketonuria (maple syrup urine disease)
Glycogen storage disease
  Glucose 6-phosphatase deficiency
  Amylo-1,6-glucosidase deficiency
  Liver phosphorylase deficiency
  Glycogen synthetase deficiency
Disorders of gluconeogenesis
  Carnitine deficiency
  Medium-chain and long-chain acyl-CoA dehydrogenase deficiency
  Acute alcohol intoxication
  Valproic acid ingestion
  Salicylate intoxication
  Fructose 1,6-diphosphatase deficiency
  Pyruvate carboxylase deficiency
  Phosphoenol pyruvate carboxykinase deficiency
Other enzyme defects
  Galactosemia: galactose 1-phosphate uridyltransferase deficiency
  Fructose intolerance: fructose 1-phosphate aldolase deficiency

ACTH, adrenocorticotropic hormone; CoA, coenzyme A.

an intravenous infusion of glucose at 6 to 8 mg/kg per minute. Low glucose values tend to occur during the first 6 to 10 hours, especially if feeding is delayed, if there is associated illness such as respiratory distress, or if the mother is diabetic. Hypoglycemia usually resolves over 2 to 3 days, when intravenous glucose can be gradually tapered and then discontinued. Three important caveats are as follows:

1. Oral glucose supplementation may not of itself be adequate, but oral feedings should be given as tolerated.
2. Sudden interruption of hypertonic glucose (10% to 15%) that has been infused can itself trigger hypoglycemia, so all management strategies require gradual tapering of the intravenous glucose delivery rate. The prognosis for this group is very good. Although minimal impairment of intellectual function can occur, severe neurologic handicaps do not.
3. During labor and delivery, intravenous infusion of glucose to the mother should not produce maternal hyperglycemia in excess of ~100 mg/dL. Because this glucose may be transferred to the fetus, its sudden curtailment after separation of the umbilical cord may lead to a precipitous fall in the neonate's glucose concentration.

In infants of diabetic mothers, it is becoming increasingly apparent that strict antepartum metabolic control minimizes or eliminates newborn hypoglycemia as well as the other characteristics traditionally associated with these infants: macrosomia, respiratory distress, polycythemia, hyperbilirubinemia, hypocalcemia, and congenital malformation. In diabetic mothers who have not been aggressively managed antepartum, these neonatal problems require therapy in addition to management of hypoglycemia.

B. Neonatal persistent (Table 35.1). When hypoglycemia and symptoms persist or recur despite increasing the rates of glucose infusion from 6 to 8 mg/kg per minute to 12 to 16 mg/kg per minute, hormone excess (hyperinsulinemia), hormone deficiency (cortisol, growth hormone, glucagon), or an inborn error of glycogen synthesis or gluconeogenesis is most likely. Rates of glucose infusion of up to 20 to 25 mg/kg per minute may be necessary to maintain euglycemia, and this requirement signifies that the patient likely has hyperinsulinism. Clinical clues to the existence of one of these syndromes are often present: perinatal asphyxia or large size (macrosomia) in hyperinsulinemia; microphallus, midline facial defects (cleft palate), or holoprosencephaly and cholestatic jaundice in hypopituitarism; and hepatomegaly in glycogen storage disease. At the time of hypoglycemic symptoms, the critical step in determining cause is a blood sample before and 30 minutes after an intravenous or intramuscular injection of glucagon at 30 μg/kg. Prior to the glucagon test, glucose infusion should be discontinued for 30 to 60 minutes. While these samples are analyzed for substrates and hormones as outlined in Table 35.2, therapy is begun in a sequential manner. Neonatal persistent hypoglycemia can almost always be precipitated by a period of fasting. A fast of 6 hours or less that provokes hypoglycemia is almost always due to excessive insulin.

TABLE 35.2	Analysis of Blood Sample before and 30 min after Glucagon Administration[a]	

Substrates	Hormones
Glucose	Insulin
Free fatty acids	Cortisol
Ketones	Growth hormone
Lactate	T_4, TSH[b]
Uric acid	Glucagon

T_4, thyroxine; TSH, thyroid-stimulating hormone.
[a]Glucagon, 30 μg/kg IV or IM.
[b]Measure once only before or after glucagon.

1. **Hyperinsulinemic states**
   a. **Evaluation.** If the infant requires >12 to 15mg/kg per minute to maintain euglycemia, is large, the *increment* in glucose after glucagon exceeds 40 mg/dL, ketones are absent or low, and free fatty acids (FFAs) are low, then hyperinsulinemia is most likely. An insulin level >5 μU/mL at the time when glucose is <40 mg/dL confirms this diagnosis. Commonly, levels of insulin are >20 μU/mL, but any level >5 μU/mL at the time of hypoglycemia is strongly suggestive of hyperinsulinemia. An elevated level of ammonia in the serum (>80 μM/L) suggests glutamate dehydrogenase deficiency. Patients with activating mutations of glucokinase (Fig. 35.1) often have a family history consistent with autosomal dominant inheritance. Such patients respond favorably to medical measures such as diazoxide (at a modest dose of 5 to 15 mg/kg per day) or long-acting somatostatin. When these measures fail after 2 or 3 days, when there is a strong family history consistent with autosomal recessive inheritance, or if the infant was macrosomic at birth, one of the severe forms of defects in the potassium channel (K_{ATP}) governing insulin secretion with variable diffuse or focal islet hyperplasia is likely.
   b. **Etiology.** Whether the infant has some form of diffuse islet cell hyperplasia or focal adenoma can be definitely confirmed only by histologic examination of biopsied tissue. Positron emission tomography (PET) with ^{18}F-L-DOPA imaging is a highly promising diagnostic tool in the evaluation of hypoglycemic hyperinsulinemia of infancy. It appears likely that PET scanning with ^{18}F-L-DOPA will obviate the need for more invasive procedures, such as ASVS (arterial stimulation with hepatic venous sampling for detection of a step-up gradient in insulin secretion). All of these approaches are available at only a limited number of medical centers around the world for the preoperative localization of the lesion as focal or diffuse. These techniques help to determine whether partial or near-total pancreatectomy is indicated. Hyperinsulinemia and hypoglycemia also occur in ~50% of infants with Beckwith-Wiedemann syndrome, which is characterized by gigantism, exomphalos, macroglossia, visceromegaly, distinctive earlobe fissures, and hyperplasia of the kidneys, pancreas, and gonads. Other features include macrocephaly, hemihypertrophy, and, occasionally, flame nevus of the face. Affected individuals have a predilection for future development of tumors such as Wilms tumor, hepatoblastoma, and rhabdomyosarcoma.
   c. **Management.** Appropriate treatment of hypoglycemic hyperinsulinism of infancy (HHI) is exceedingly important to prevent serious brain damage. Usually, diazoxide is the first-line drug, which is used at a dose of 10 to 20 mg/kg per day divided into 2 to 3 doses. Side effects include hypertrichosis, hyperglycemia, and salt and water retention. Octreotide (somatotropin release inhibitory factor analog) can be effective in the short-term treatment of HHI, but the development of tachyphylaxis may limit its efficacy with chronic use. The starting dose is 2 to 5 μg/kg per day, subcutaneously, divided into 3 to 4 doses (with a subsequent increase to 20 μg/kg per day). It also can be administered by continuous IV infusion at a dose of 10 μg/kg per day. Side effects include diarrhea, gallstones, and suppression of growth hormone. In the short term, an infusion of glucagon at 5 to 1.0 μg per minute, not to exceed 1.5 mg per day, may increase blood glucose levels temporarily by promoting glycogen breakdown. If medical treatment fails, surgical pancreatectomy is required. The distinction between diffuse and local lesion is a crucial step in defining the extent of pancreatectomy and the long-term prognosis. A near-total pancreatectomy is required for the diffuse form, whereas only partial pancreatectomy with only local excision is needed for the localized form.

   It is important not to delay local, subtotal (80%), or near-total (95%) pancreatectomy when the diagnosis of hyperinsulinemia is confirmed and hypoglycemia persists despite administration of intravenous glucose in excess of 10 mg/kg per minute in addition to ongoing treatment with diazoxide, as indicated previously. This group of patients is most likely to suffer permanent

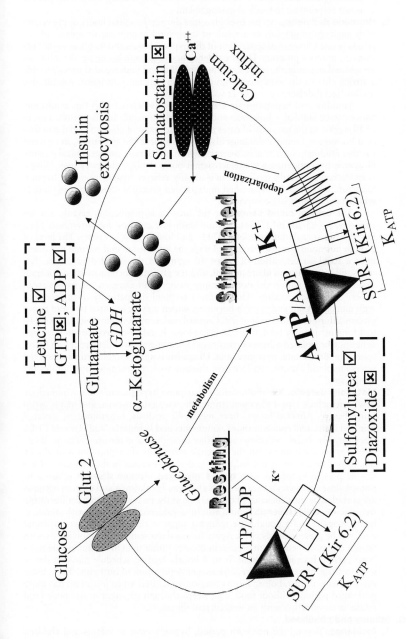

Figure 35.1. Model of insulin secretion and its regulation in the pancreatic β cell. (See *Endocrinol Metab Clin North Am* 1999;28:695–708.)

neurologic deficits if definitive treatment by surgery is delayed when the patient is not responding to medical management.

2. **Hormone deficiency.** Severe hypoglycemia during the initial hours of life occurs with <u>panhypopituitarism</u> as a result of congenital hypoplasia or aplasia of the pituitary or of functional separation of the hypothalamus and its releasing factors from the anterior pituitary. Despite a <u>deficiency of growth hormone</u>, these infants are normal size at birth. In males, a microphallus and undescended testes provide a strong clue to the existence of gonadotropin deficiency in utero. An anterior midline facial defect may occur in some patients.

Jaundice and hepatomegaly are frequently associated with this syndrome, which can be familial. Cholestasis and hepatosplenomegaly resolve within a mean of 10 weeks, in the majority of cases after replacement of glucocorticoid and thyroid hormones. Frequent feedings also help to relieve the symptoms, in contrast to other etiologies such as galactosemia, which may have a similar clinical picture. However, hypoglycemia with galactosemia occurs only with severe liver failure, is exacerbated by milk feeding which usually relieves hypoglycemia in hypopituitarism, and should be identified in expanded neonatal screening programs in which galactosemia is a component.

The **critical blood sample** at the time of hypoglycemia reveals low insulin levels (<5 μU/mL) in association with low cortisol, low thyroxine (T_4), low thyroid-stimulating hormone (TSH), and low growth hormone. The level of growth hormone must be interpreted with the knowledge that normal newborns have a basal concentration of 20 to 40 ng/mL in the initial days of life. Ketones, FFAs, and uric acid are normal, and the glycemic increment after glucagon is subnormal or within the normal range rather than exaggerated, as occurs in hyperinsulinemic neonates. These infants respond dramatically to <u>replacement with glucocorticoid and growth hormone</u>, which may be essential to avoid hypoglycemia during the first year of life. Cortisol replacement in physiologic doses (10 to 15 mg/m^2 per day b.i.d. or t.i.d.) is life-long. Rarely, isolated growth hormone deficiency or isolated adrenocorticotropic hormone/cortisol deficiency can be responsible for neonatal hypoglycemia. Diagnosis is again established based on the screening blood sample. Replacement therapy with the hormone ameliorates the symptoms.

3. **Metabolic defects.** Metabolic defects that cause hypoglycemia in the immediate newborn include type 1 glycogen storage disease, galactosemia, and <u>maple syrup urine disease</u>. Affected infants have metabolic acidosis, hepatomegaly, elevated uric and lactic acid concentrations, ketonemia and ketonuria, and elevated FFAs. They may also have a reducing sugar other than glucose in the urine. Plasma levels of hormones are normal, but the glycemic increment after glucagon is markedly diminished or absent. If not fed, profound hypoglycemia in the first days of life can be present in infants with **type 1 glycogen storage disease** (glucose 6-phosphatase deficiency), because both glycogen breakdown and gluconeogenesis are curtailed by the deficiency of this enzyme at the final critical step for liberating free glucose. **Galactosemia** should also be considered in an infant with jaundice, hepatomegaly, and a nonglucose reducing sugar in the urine, but hypoglycemia need not be present consistently. Apart from galactosemia, most individuals with inborn errors of metabolism present in infancy rather than in the immediate newborn period, because the usual 3- to 4-hourly feeding schedule masks a defect in gluconeogenesis that may require longer deprivation of nutrients. Thus, these inborn errors of metabolism more commonly manifest when the infant has more prolonged periods without food, e.g., sleeps through the night or has poor food intake in conjunction with an intercurrent illness.

C. **Infancy and childhood**

1. **Incidence.** Beyond the newborn period, hypoglycemia in infants and children is distinctly uncommon. An inability to maintain euglycemia during fasting and acquired deficiency of hormones predominates during late infancy and childhood.

2. **Age at presentation:** A common time for presentation of milder hyperinsulinemia and defects in gluconeogenesis is between age 3 and 6 months of age, when

infants are sleeping at night for progressively longer periods. Feedings are no longer given at 3- to 4-hour intervals, and the infant is progressively "fasting" for up to 8 hours during the nighttime sleep.

3. **Signs and symptoms.** Symptoms can result from neuroglycopenia and include seizures activity and coma or may be due to activation of counterregulatory hormones, such as irritability, anxiety, tachycardia, and sweating. A high index of suspicion is required, especially if symptoms recur at regular times of day in relation to feeding and its intervals.

4. **Evaluation.** An adequate blood sample at the time of symptoms can document hypoglycemia and can be used for measurement of substrates or hormones. This "critical sample" needs to be drawn when the serum glucose level is <50 mg/dL. If the critical blood sample is not obtained at the time of symptoms, it is necessary to admit the child for a 10- to 20-hour fast under observation. A urine sample is also sent to dipstick for ketones. Glucagon is given after the critical sample is drawn, and the glucose level is checked at 15 and 30 minutes after glucagon to assess for the rise in glucose; a rise of >40 mg/dL is consistent with hyperinsulinism. Worth noting is the importance of making sure that the glucose level is truly hypoglycemic before glucagon is given, because once it is administered, the fasting test cannot continue. Therefore, if the child is *symptomatic* and/or the meter reading is well below 50 mg/dL, the critical sample is drawn and glucagon is given. However, if the glucose level is in the 40's mg/dL, or less, it is prudent to draw the critical sample, including immediate laboratory glucose measurement, *even if the patient is asymptomatic,* and await the result to confirm hypoglycemia before giving glucagon.

5. **Differential diagnosis**
   a. **Hyperinsulinemia**

   (1) Hyperinsulinemia is the most common cause of hypoglycemia in the first 6 months of life. The findings in the initial blood sample at the time of symptoms demonstrate low glucose, low FFAs, and low ketones, whereas insulin values are inappropriately high (>5 to 10 μU/mL) when glucose is inappropriately low (<50 mg/dL). Cortisol and growth hormone levels are normally elevated in response to hypoglycemia, and there is no metabolic acidosis. Leucine sensitivity, formerly considered a distinct identity, is now regarded as a variant of hyperinsulinemia provoked by the amino acid content of milk and a result of activating mutations of glutamate dehydrogenase (Fig. 35.1). At the time of spontaneous symptoms, or if provoked by fasting, glucagon challenge results in an exaggerated response of blood glucose.

   (2) **Management** differs from that for the neonate in that affected infants do not require continuous infusion with glucose. A more prolonged trial of diazoxide, at a dose of 5 to 15 mg/kg per day (up to 25 mg/kg per day in some instances) PO in three divided doses, is warranted. Frequently, diazoxide in these dosages can maintain euglycemia in these patients so that, if successful, diazoxide therapy can be continued for months to years. Octreotide can be of benefit in this circumstance. However, if hypoglycemia recurs despite adequate doses of diazoxide, or if side effects such as hirsutism, edema, hypertension, and hyperuricemia become intolerable, partial pancreatectomy may be indicated.

   Endogenous insulin production may come from a focal insulin-producing lesion or diffuse pancreatic excessive, nonregulated insulin production. Finding a focal lesion in cases planned for pancreatectomy may be helpful, thus allowing for a partial resection to be therapeutic. Distinguishing focal and diffuse types may be done using PET scanning with ^{18}F-L-DOPA.

   Factitious or **exogenous hyperinsulinemia** resulting from deliberate injection of insulin as a form of child abuse or Münchhausen by proxy can mimic spontaneous hypoglycemia due to endogenous hyperinsulinemia and lead to repeated episodes of symptomatic hypoglycemia. Suspicion is raised by the presence of inappropriately high insulin levels (>100 μU/mL), requiring measurement of **C-peptide** concentration in the same sample. Because C-peptide concentrations reflect endogenous insulin secretion, they are low while insulin levels are high in factitious hypoglycemia.

b. Hormone deficiency. Deficiency of **growth hormone** or **cortisol** can *rarely* cause hypoglycemia after the first months of life, but if it does occur, it is likely to occur during prolonged fasting. The diagnosis is established on the basis of the results of the critical sample at the time of symptoms; the glycemic increment following glucagon administration is diminished or near normal. During fasting, glucose also declines while FFAs and ketones increase, thereby simulating so-called **ketotic hypoglycemia**. In older children, there may be clinical clues of deficiency of either hormone, such as short stature, poor growth velocity, or symptoms associated with a space-occupying intracranial lesion indicative of pituitary pathology; there also may be hyperpigmentation, salt craving, hyponatremia, and hyperkalemia in progressive adrenal failure or Addison disease. Treatment involves supplying the deficient hormone as needed. Investigations will be needed to assess for other possible associated deficiencies that may be present.

c. Ketotic hypoglycemia. This is the **most common cause** of hypoglycemia in infants and children aged 6 months to 6 years.

(1) Etiology. The cause appears to be an inability to adapt to fasting. Apart from the nonidiopathic ketotic hypoglycemia associated with hormone deficiency, specific mechanisms are not understood. Hypoglycemia, occasionally with severe symptoms such as seizures, may occur after limited glucose (food) intake during intercurrent infection or gastrointestinal disturbances combined with a relatively long fast after prolonged sleep, and occurs after resources for glycogenolysis and gluconeogenesis have been consumed.

(2) Evaluation. In the critical diagnostic blood sample, glucose and insulin are low whereas ketones are high, and there may be ketonuria. There is a subnormal glycemic increment with glucagon challenge, and the syndrome can be produced by a fast of 14 to 24 hours. Because the syndrome can be simulated by hormone deficiency, the levels of growth hormone and cortisol should always be measured as outlined in Table 35.2.

(3) Management. Management consists of a high-carbohydrate, high-protein diet, with frequent daily feedings. During intercurrent illness, high glucose–containing drinks are encouraged and the urine is checked for ketones. The appearance of ketonuria despite high-carbohydrate feeding or administration of high carbohydrate–containing liquids warrants admission for temporary intravenous glucose at a rate of 6 to 8 mg/kg per minute to avoid a serious hypoglycemic reaction. Most patients spontaneously resolve the tendency for hypoglycemia by age 7 to 8 years.

d. Carnitine deficiency. Systemic **carnitine deficiency** and **acylcarnitine transferase deficiency** are rare causes of hypoglycemia provoked by fasting and are sometimes associated with muscle hypotonia and cardiomyopathy. Carnitine and its enzyme transferase are essential for the transport of FFAs across the mitochondrial membrane, where metabolism of FFAs produces energy for gluconeogenesis and where ketogenesis occurs. Hypoglycemia in these conditions is characterized by low to absent blood ketones, low insulin and growth hormone levels, and a normal cortisol level; there is negligible glycemic response to glucagon. Definitive diagnosis can require measurement of carnitine levels in liver and blood.

(1) A similar clinical situation results from the ingestion of hypoglycin, the active principle of the unripe akee fruit that is responsible for hypoglycemia in **Jamaican vomiting sickness.**

(2) Nonketotic hypoglycemia and low carnitine levels sometimes associated with hypotonia are also features of the increasingly recognized syndromes of **medium-chain acyl coenzyme A (acyl-CoA) dehydrogenase deficiency (MCADD) and long-chain acyl-CoA dehydrogenase deficiency.**

MCADD is not an uncommon entity, with an incidence as high as 1 in 10 000 births. Hence, this entity should be considered in a child presenting with seizure and hypoglycemia during an intercurrent illness with vomiting and inability to retain ingested food. Dicarboxylic acids in the urine and other special tests are necessary to confirm the diagnosis. *Note that these conditions and all forms of hyperinsulinemia are associated with low ketones and can easily be distinguished from each other on the basis of the insulin level and the glycemic response to glucagon, which is high in hyperinsulinemia and low in carnitine deficiency. In all other forms of hypoglycemia, ketones are high. Because of the relative frequency of MCADD, this condition forms part of the expanded neonatal screening programs of many states. Knowledge of this fact permits checking with relevant state offices whether the entity has been excluded or diagnosed by neonatal screening.*

e. **Enzyme deficiencies**
   (1) **Glycogen storage disease** (see Chapter 39)
      (a) Glucose 6-phosphatase deficiency (G6PD; type 1 glycogen storage disease) rarely presents in the first days or weeks of life. This is because babies are fed every 3 to 4 hours, hence masking the defect in glucose production during fasting. More typically, G6PD presents in infancy and childhood with poor growth, protuberant abdomen, hepatomegaly, eruptive xanthomas, chronic acidosis, and hyperlipidemia; levels of FFAs, triglycerides, lactate, pyruvate, and uric acid are high, and insulin levels are low. Bleeding tendencies are caused by abnormal platelet function but not abnormal platelet numbers. In response to glucagon injection, lactate levels rise but the glycemic response is absent. Definitive diagnosis requires a liver biopsy for histologic examination together with in vitro measurement of enzyme activity. Molecular testing is now available. Continuous intragastric nighttime feeding of glucose, glucose polymer (4 to 6 mg/kg per minute), or cornstarch (so as to provide approximately one third of total daily calories) together with frequent high-carbohydrate feedings during the day will markedly ameliorate the biochemical abnormalities and result in catch-up growth as well as marked reduction of liver size. In the untreated child, symptoms of hypoglycemia spontaneously improve with age. However, with institution of intensive therapy by intragastric feeding and normalization of several of the abnormal biochemical indices, the sensitivity to hypoglycemic symptoms and signs, including seizures, returns. Meticulous monitoring is therefore necessary once intensive therapy is started.
      (b) The clinical features of fasting hypoglycemia and hepatomegaly (but usually without acidosis) occur in a much milder degree in type 3 glycogen storage disease (amylo-1,6-glucosidase deficiency; debrancher deficiency) and in type 6 glycogen storage disease (liver phosphorylase deficiency). Both require tissue biopsy and enzyme measurement for definitive diagnosis, and both types respond to frequent high-carbohydrate feeding, although continuous intragastric nocturnal feeding can be beneficial in some cases of type 3 glycogen storage disease.
      (c) Glycogen synthase deficiency, a rare enzyme deficiency, causes severe hypoglycemia with fasting because no accumulation of glycogen is possible. Paradoxically, affected children have **hyperglycemia** after meals, because the ingested glucose cannot be deposited as glycogen in the liver. **Fasting produces a "ketotic" hypoglycemia** and can be distinguished from the usual ketotic hypoglycemia described earlier by the presence of hyperglycemia after meals in the case of glycogen synthase deficiency.
   (2) **Disorders of gluconeogenesis**
      (a) **Fructose 1,6-diphosphatase deficiency** is associated with severe hypoglycemia during prolonged fasting or with infections. Hepatomegaly

is present, as is chronic acidosis exaggerated by fasting. Episodes of hypoglycemia can be treated acutely with glucose and bicarbonate; **fructose should be avoided** at all times because it, as well as various metabolic intermediates (alanine, glycerol, lactate), acutely inhibits glucose production, and hence provokes hypoglycemia. Definitive diagnosis requires enzyme assay in liver biopsy or in leukocytes.

(b) With **hereditary fructose intolerance (fructose 1-phosphate aldolase deficiency),** hypoglycemic episodes are provoked only after ingestion of fructose. Symptoms can be severe and associated with acute vomiting; poor feeding and failure to thrive are present at other times. Affected infants learn to avoid fructose-containing foods and sweets. *A fructose-free diet must be instituted.*

(c) In **phosphoenolpyruvic acid carboxykinase deficiency** (PEPCK deficiency), fasting hypoglycemia results from an inability to initiate gluconeogenesis at the key entry point of several intermediates. Diagnosis requires a demonstration that infusion of lactate or alanine has no glycemic effect because they require PEPCK to enter gluconeogenesis, whereas glycerol infusion results in a normal glycemic response because PEPCK is bypassed. This cause is extremely rare. Molecular diagnostic techniques are becoming available for the glycogen storage diseases and may eliminate the need for liver biopsy or other tissue enzymatic assays.

f. Alcohol and other drugs. An important cause of hypoglycemia due to acute interruption of gluconeogenesis in infants and children is alcohol ingestion.

| **TABLE 35.3** | **Diagnosis of Acute Hypoglycemia in Infants and Children** |

Acute symptoms present

1. Obtain blood sample before and 30 min after glucagon administration.
2. Obtain urine as soon as possible. Examine for ketones; if not present and hypoglycemia confirmed, suspect hyperinsulinemia or carnitine deficiency; if present, suspect ketotic, hormone deficiency, inborn error of glycogen metabolism, or gluconeogenesis.
3. Measure glucose in original blood sample. If hypoglycemia confirmed, proceed with substrate-hormone measurement as in Table 35.2.
4. If glycemic increment after glucagon exceeds 40 mg/dL above basal, suspect hyperinsulinemia.
5. If insulin level at time of confirmed hypoglycemia is >100 μU/mL, suspect factitious hyperinsulinemia (exogenous insulin injection). Admit to hospital for provocative testing.
6. If cortisol is <10 μg/dL and growth hormone is <5 ng/mL, suspect adrenal insufficiency or pituitary disease. Admit to hospital for provocative testing.

History suggestive: acute symptoms not present

1. Careful history for relation of symptoms to time and type of food intake, bearing in mind age of patient (Table 32.1); exclude possibility of alcohol or drug ingestion; assess possibility of insulin injection; salt craving; growth velocity; intracranial pathology.
2. Careful examination for hepatomegaly (glycogen storage disease; defect in gluconeogenesis); pigmentation (adrenal failure); stature and neurologic status (pituitary disease).
3. Admit to hospital for provocative testing via:
   a. 24-hour fast under careful observation; when symptom provoked, proceed with steps 1 through 4 as when acute symptoms present.
   b. Pituitary-adrenal function via arginine-insulin stimulation test if indicated.
4. Liver biopsy for histology and enzyme determination if indicated.
5. Oral glucose tolerance test (1.75 g/kg; max 75 g) if reactive hypoglycemia suspected in an adolescent.

TABLE 35.4 Clinical and Differential Diagnoses in Childhood Hypoglycemia

Condition	Hypoglycemia	Urinary ketones (K) or reducing sugars (S)	Hepatomegaly	Serum Lipids	Serum Uric acid	Glycemic response to glucagon Fed	Glycemic response to glucagon Fasted	Effect of 24- to 36-h fast on plasma Glucose	Effect of 24- to 36-h fast on plasma Insulin	Effect of 24- to 36-h fast on plasma Ketones	Effect of 24- to 36-h fast on plasma Alanine	Effect of 24- to 36-h fast on plasma Lactate
Normal	0	0	0	N	N	↑↑	↑	↓	↓	↑	↓	N
Hyperinsulinemia	Recurrent severe	0	0	N or ↓	N	↑↑	↑↑	↓↓	↑↑	↓↓	N	N
Ketotic hypoglycemia	Severe with missed meals	K+++	0	N	N	↑	0–↑	↓↓	↓	↑↑	↓↓	N
Hypopituitarism	Moderate with missed meals	K++	0	N	N	↑	0–↑	↓↓	↓	↑↑	↓↓	N
Adrenal insufficiency	Severe with missed meals	K++	0	N	N	↑	0–↑	↓↓	↓	↑↑	↓↓	N
Enzyme deficiency												
Glucose 6-phosphatase	Severe constant	K+++	+++	↑↑	↑↑	0	0	↓↓	↓	↑↑	↑↑	↑↑
Debrancher	Moderate with fasting	K++	+	N	N	↑	0	↓↓	↓	↑↑	↓↓	N
Phosphorylase	Mild to moderate	K++	+	N	N	0–↑	0	↓	↓	↑↑	↓↓	N
Fructose 1,6-diphosphatase	Severe with fasting	K++++	+++	↑↑	↑↑	↑	0	↓↓	↓	↑↑	↑↑	↑↑
Galactosemia	After milk or milk products	0–S+++	+++	N	N	↑	0	↓	↓	↑	↓	N
Fructose intolerance	After fructose	0–S+++	+++	N	N	↑	0–↑	↓	↓	↑	↓	N
Carnitine deficiency	Moderate to severe with fasting	0	0–+	↓	N	↑	0	↓	↓	↓	N	N–↑

N, normal; 0, absent; ↑, low increase; ↑↑, great increase; ↓, some decrease; ↓↓, marked decrease; +, slight; ++, small; +++, moderate; ++++, large.

The metabolism of alcohol to acetaldehyde requires cofactors that are also essential for gluconeogenesis. However, hepatic alcohol metabolism seems to take preference, thereby depleting the cofactors essential for gluconeogenesis. Consequently, **alcohol-induced hypoglycemia** occurs only when liver glycogen stores are depleted after 6 to 8 hours of fasting. The inadvertent swallowing of alcohol left unattended (Sunday morning syndrome) or the deliberate feeding of alcohol such as wine or beer to infants and young children deprived of food (e.g., during a long car trip) can provoke a hypoglycemic reaction. The response to intravenous glucose is dramatic. No investigation for this isolated episode of hypoglycemia is necessary if the history of alcohol ingestion is elicited. Similarly, isolated episodes of hypoglycemia caused by inadvertent use of **oral hypoglycemic drugs** in children do not require investigation. **Valproic acid**, used for seizure disorders, interferes with fatty acid oxidation and, indirectly, gluconeogenesis. Hence, its toxic effects include nonketotic hypoglycemia, especially during fasting.

g. **Reactive hypoglycemia.** This form of postprandial hypoglycemia is frequently suspected in children and adolescents but is actually quite uncommon. Diagnosis requires demonstration of blood glucose levels <50 mg/dL between the third and fifth hour of an oral glucose tolerance test performed in the prescribed manner (1.75 g/kg with a maximum of 75 g after 3 days of normal carbohydrate intake). This may be preceded by hyperglycemia during the first 2 hours. Measurements in the critical sample during hypoglycemia will show results consistent with hyperinsulinism (as above). This is commonly seen in children who have had a <u>Nissen fundoplication</u>, as there is a rapid gastric emptying, and so a rapid absorption of glucose (hyperglycemia), followed by a rapid (excessive) release of insulin (hypoglycemia). Treatment involves changes in the feeding regimen to give feeds more slowly, or using lower-osmolarity feeds. Acarbose has been used as well, as it slows the conversion of oligosaccharides to monosaccharides, and so leads to a slower rise in glucose and slower insulin release as well.

IV. SUMMARY

An approach to the diagnosis of hypoglycemia in infants beyond the immediate newborn period and in children is outlined in Table 35.3. The clinical features and differential diagnosis of the most common forms of childhood hypoglycemia are outlined in Table 35.4. Management is discussed for each cause in the text.

Selected References

Burchell A, Bell JE, Busuttil A, et al. Hepatic microsomal glucose-6-phosphatase system and sudden infant death syndrome. *Lancet* 1989;2:291–294.

Clark W, O'Donovan D. Transient hyperinsulinism in an asphyxiated newborn infant with hypoglycemia. *Am J Perinatol* 2001;18:175–178.

Daly LP, Osterhoudt KC, Weinzimer SA. Presenting features of idiopathic ketotic hypoglycemia. *J Emerg Med* 2003;25:39–43.

Dekelbab BH, Sperling MA. Hypoglycemia in newborns and infants. *Adv Pediatr* 2006;53:5–22.

DeLonlay-Debeney P, Poggie-Travert F, Founet JC, et al. Clinical features of 52 neonates with hyperinsulinism. *N Engl J Med* 1999;340:1169–1175.

Glaser B, Kesavan P, Heyman M, et al. Familial hyperinsulinism caused by an activating glucokinase mutation. *N Engl J Med* 1998;328:226–230.

Hardy OT, Hernandez-Pampaloni M, Saffer JR, et al. Diagnosis and localization of fecal congenital hyperinsulinism by 18F-fluorodop PET scan. *J Pediatr* 2007;150:140–145.

Hoe FM, Thornton PS, Wanner LA, et al. Clinical features and insulin regulation in infants with a syndrome of prolonged neoanatal hyperinsulinism. *J Pediatr* 2006;148:207–212.

Karnsakul W, Sawathiparnich P, Nimkarn S, et al. Anterior pituitary hormone effects on hepatic functions in infants with congenital hypopituitarism. *Ann Hepatol* 2007;6:97–103.

Lteif AN, Schwenck WF. Hypoglycemia in infants and children. *Endocrinol Metab Clin North Am* 1999;28:619–646.

Menni F, de Lonlay P, Sevin C, et al. Neurologic outcomes of 90 neonates and infants with persistent hyperinsulinemic hypoglycemia. *Pediatrics* 2001;107:476–479.

Ng DD, Ferry RJ Jr, Kelly A, et al. Acarbose treatment of postprandial hypoglycemia in children after Nissen fundoplication. *J Pediatr* 2001;139:877–879.

Sperling MA. Hypoglycemia. In: Behrman R, ed. *Nelson Textbook of Pediatrics*. 16th ed. Philadelphia: WB Saunders; 2000:439–450.

Sperling MA, Menon RK. Differential diagnosis and management of neonatal hypoglycemia. *Pediatr Clin North Am* 2004;51:703–723.

Sperling MA, Menon RK. Hyperinsulinemic hypoglycemia of infancy. *Endocrinol Metab Clin North Am* 1999;28:695–708.

Stanley CA. Dissecting the spectrum of fatty acid oxidation disorders. *J Pediatr* 1998;132:384–386.

Stanley CA, Baker L. The causes of neonatal hypoglycemia. *N Engl J Med* 1999;340:1200–1201.

Stanley CA, Lieu YK, Hsu BY, et al. Hyperinsulinism and hyperammonemia in infants with regulatory mutations of the glutamate deydrogenase gene. *N Engl J Med* 1998;238:1352–1357.

Steinkrauss L, Lipman TH, Hendell CD, et al. Effects of hypoglycemia on developmental outcome in children with congenital hyperinsulinism. *J Pediatr Nurs* 2005;20:109–118.

Verkarre V, Fournet JC, deLonlay P, et al. Paternal mutation of the sulfonylurea receptor *(SUR1)* gene and maternal loss of 11p15 imprinted genes lead to persistent hyperinsulinism in focal adenomatous hyperplasia. *J Clin Invest* 1998;102:1286–1291.

Weinstein DA, Correia CE, Saunders AC, Wolfsdorf JI. Hepatic glycogen synthase deficiency: an infrequently recognized cause of ketotic hypoglycemia. *Mol Genet Metab* 2006;87:284–288.

Wolfsdorf JI, Holm IA, Weinstein DA. Glycogen storage diseases. Phenotypic, genetic, and biochemical characteristics, and therapy. *Endocrinol Metab Clin North Am* 1999;28:801–823.

Yager JY. Hypoglycemic injury to the immature brain. *Clin Perinatol* 2002;29:651–674.

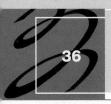

36 HYPOGLYCEMIA IN ADULTS
Mayer B. Davidson

*H*ypoglycemia is an abnormality, not a disease. An abnormally low glucose concentration can be caused by a number of factors, such as drugs, tumors, altered gastrointestinal anatomy, or failure of both endocrine and nonendocrine tissues. Hypoglycemia even occurs in association with impaired glucose tolerance, mild type 2 diabetes, and infection, situations that have classically been associated with elevated glucose levels. This chapter describes a practical approach in adults to the often-confusing subject of hypoglycemia.

I. DEFINITION
One major problem is how to define hypoglycemia, that is, what concentration of glucose is abnormally low? An important consideration is whether whole-blood or plasma glucose concentrations are being measured. The glucose concentration in plasma or serum is approximately 12% higher than in whole blood (*not* 12 mg/dL, sometimes written as 12 mg %). Although glucose meters measure concentrations in whole blood, recent models are now all calibrated to report out plasma values. The conditions under which the blood sample is drawn are also important. For instance, a plasma glucose concentration of 54 mg/dL is abnormal after an overnight fast but not 4 hours after a carbohydrate-rich meal or an oral challenge with dextrose. I define hypoglycemia by the criteria listed in Table 36.1.

II. GENERAL APPROACH
The clinical approach to a patient with possible hypoglycemia involves the documentation of a low glucose concentration and systematic efforts to determine what condition is responsible for the low concentration. In making this determination, it is important to ascertain whether hypoglycemia occurs in the fasting or the fed state. Do the symptoms develop when the patient misses breakfast (or other meals), or do they routinely occur after the patient has eaten (especially after ingestion of large amounts of simple carbohydrate)? This distinction is important because, with a few exceptions, fasting and fed (also termed reactive) hypoglycemias are caused by different conditions. Furthermore, the causes of fasting hypoglycemia are often more serious; consequently, a more diligent workup is usually required than with fed hypoglycemia. Therefore, the distinguishing of fed from fasting hypoglycemia considerably simplifies the differential diagnosis and alerts the physician to the potential gravity of the situation. So that the pathophysiology of the various types of hypoglycemia can be understood, normal fasting and fed glucose homeostasis are described.

III. NORMAL GLUCOSE HOMEOSTASIS
A. Fasting state
1. **Glucose utilization.** During a short fast, only a few tissues require glucose. The most important obligate glucose consumer is the brain, which in a 70-kg person uses approximately 100 g per day. The red blood cells and muscle are the next most avid consumers, utilizing approximately 35 g and 30 g per day, respectively. Most other tissues use predominantly free fatty acids (produced by the hydrolysis of adipose tissue triglycerides) or a small amount of ketone bodies (produced by hepatic catabolism of free fatty acids).
2. **Glucose production.** The liver is responsible for approximately 80% and the kidneys approximately 20% of glucose production during short fasts. Glucose is

| **TABLE 36.1** | **Criteria for Definition of Hypoglycemia** | |

| | **Condition of patient** | |
Glucose concentration (mg/dL)	**Fasted**	**Fed[a]**
Plasma	<60	<50
Whole blood	<50	<40

[a]After ingestion of glucose or meals.

produced through two separate pathways: glycogenolysis and gluconeogenesis. Only gluconeogenesis operates in the kidneys.

   a. Glycogenolysis is the breakdown of glycogen, the storage form of glucose. Hepatic glycogen is slowly hydrolyzed and released as glucose to maintain stable levels of plasma glucose during periods when an individual is not eating. During an overnight fast, approximately 75% of hepatic glucose is produced by glycogenolysis.

   b. Gluconeogenesis is the synthesis of new glucose from noncarbohydrate precursors. There are three major gluconeogenic substrates: **lactate,** derived from glucose metabolism by the peripheral tissues; **amino acids** (especially alanine), released by muscle; and **glycerol,** derived from the breakdown of triglycerides in adipose tissue. Although only 25% of hepatic glucose production derives from gluconeogenesis after an overnight fast, the contribution from glycogen decreases considerably soon thereafter, and gluconeogenesis becomes dominant as the period of fasting lengthens.

3. Response to fasting. Because powerful mechanisms defend the plasma glucose concentration (even during a prolonged fast), the obligate glucose consumers can continue to function normally. The glucose level decreases initially by 15 to 20 mg/dL during the first several days and then usually stabilizes. However, in some normal-weight individuals (especially females), glucose concentrations may fall to values as low as 35 to 40 mg/dL without the development of symptoms of hypoglycemia. **Insulin concentrations uniformly fall to low levels and remain there.** Therefore, with regard to the workup of a patient with fasting hypoglycemia, the important point is that glucose concentrations decrease modestly in association with a profound drop in insulin levels during total starvation.

B. Fed state. A normal diet includes both simple (mono- and disaccharide) and complex (polysaccharide) carbohydrates. There is little difference in the rate of appearance of glucose in the circulation derived from simple and complex carbohydrates as long as they are ingested with a meal rather than singly. The rising concentration of glucose in the bloodstream stimulates the β cells of the pancreas to release insulin into the portal vein. The newly secreted insulin first traverses the liver, where approximately 50% is degraded on each passage. The remainder escapes into the general circulation, where the hormone binds to specific receptors in the three insulin-sensitive tissues—liver, muscle, and adipose tissue. Approximately 10% of dietary carbohydrate is stored directly as hepatic glycogen. Another 10% to 15% is eventually stored in the liver, but only after being converted to gluconeogenic precursors in the peripheral tissues, returning to the liver, and being converted to glucose via gluconeogenesis.

   Postprandial changes in concentrations of glucose and insulin are shown in Figure 36.1. The normal pattern is one of peak values of both glucose and insulin at 1 hour with a return to baseline by 3 to 4 hours. Note the markedly higher insulin response and modestly elevated glucose concentrations in obese as opposed to lean subjects. However, a **peak value of insulin at 1 hour characterizes both groups.**

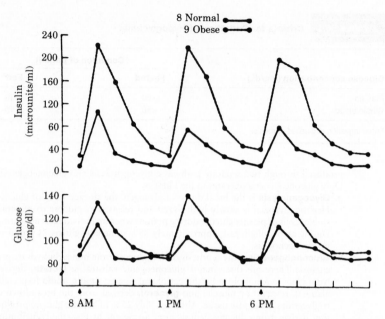

Figure 36.1. Concentrations of glucose and insulin throughout a 16-hour period in subjects who had normal carbohydrate tolerance and ate three identical meals. (Reproduced with permission from Genuth SM. Plasma insulin and glucose profiles in normal, obese, and diabetic persons. *Ann Intern Med* 1973;79:812.)

IV. HORMONAL RESPONSES TO HYPOGLYCEMIA

A. Normal. Glucoreceptors in the hypothalamus initiate certain hormonal responses either to low levels of glucose or to rapidly falling concentrations that are not yet in the hypoglycemic range. Thus, although the rate of fall from euglycemia to hypoglycemia does not seem to affect the release of these counterregulatory hormones, a rapid fall from marked hyperglycemia (300 to 400 mg/dL) to near-euglycemia (100 to 150 mg/dL) may. The released hormones (Table 36.2) stimulate potent metabolic mechanisms that prevent glucose concentrations from dropping to dangerously low levels. Concentrations of epinephrine, norepinephrine, and glucagon quickly increase, whereas those of cortisol and growth hormone increase more slowly. Thus, the response to hypoglycemia is finely orchestrated (Table 36.2). Antihypoglycemic factors start to exert their effects almost immediately after hypothalamic recognition of low or rapidly falling (from very high to near-normal) glucose concentrations, and continue to operate until 8 to 12 hours later.

B. Type 1 diabetes. Shortly after the onset of type 1 diabetes (1 to 5 years), the glucagon response to hypoglycemia decreases and eventually is lost. Later (>10 years), the epinephrine response also becomes attenuated, even in patients without clinical evidence of autonomic neuropathy. Although the other hormonal responses remain nearly normal, these patients sometimes lose the ability to recognize the autonomic symptoms of hypoglycemia (see hypoglycemia unawareness in Section V) and are at increased risk for hypoglycemic coma during intensive insulin therapy.

C. Type 2 diabetes. Hormonal responses to hypoglycemia remain mostly normal in type 2 diabetes, although after many years, when insulin secretion is markedly attenuated, glucagon concentrations are lower than normal. However, hypoglycemia unawareness does not seem to occur in patients with type 2 diabetes, probably because the catecholamine response is maintained.

| **TABLE 36.2** | Hormonal Responses to Hypoglycemia |

| | Onset of | | |
Hormone	Secretion	Action	Effects
Epinephrine, norepinephrine	Rapid	Rapid	Inhibits glucose utilization by muscle; increases hepatic gluconeogenesis; stimulates glucagon secretion; inhibits insulin secretion; stimulates hepatic glycogenolysis[a]
Glucagon	Rapid	Rapid	Increases hepatic glycogenolysis; increases hepatic gluconeogenesis
Cortisol	Delayed	Delayed	Increases hepatic gluconeogenesis; inhibits glucose utilization by muscle
Growth hormone	Delayed	Delayed	Inhibits glucose utilization by muscle; increases hepatic gluconeogenesis (?)

[a]Norepinephrine only.

V. SIGNS AND SYMPTOMS

The signs and symptoms of hypoglycemia (Table 36.3) fall into two categories: **autonomic** (those caused by increased activity of the autonomic nervous system) and **neuroglucopenic** (those caused by depressed activity of the central nervous system). In normal individuals, the counterregulatory hormones begin to be released and the autonomic nervous system discharged when the plasma glucose level declines to approximately 70 mg/dL (Fig. 36.2). If the initial response does not restore euglycemia, the magnitude of the catecholamines and acetylcholine (the latter not shown in Fig. 36.2) released usually produces the autonomic symptoms at a glucose level of approximately 55 mg/dL. Neuroglucopenic symptoms usually start at approximately 50 mg/dL. These relationships between the counterregulatory hormones and autonomic nervous system responses, glucose concentrations, and signs and symptoms of hypoglycemia may not hold in diabetic patients.

As discussed earlier, patients with type 1 diabetes may suffer from **hypoglycemia unawareness**, one cause of which is impaired glucagon, epinephrine, and autonomic

| **TABLE 36.3** | Signs and Symptoms of Hypoglycemia |

Adrenergic[a]	Neuroglucopenic[b]
Weakness	Headache
Sweating	Hypothermia
Tachycardia	Visual disturbances
Palpitations	Mental dullness
Tremor	Confusion
Nervousness	Amnesia
Irritability	Seizures
Tingling of mouth and fingers	Coma
Hunger	
Nausea[c]	
Vomiting[c]	

[a]Caused by increased activity of the autonomic nervous system; may be triggered by a rapid fall in the glucose concentration.
[b]Caused by decreased activity of the central nervous system; requires an absolutely low level of glucose.
[c]Unusual.

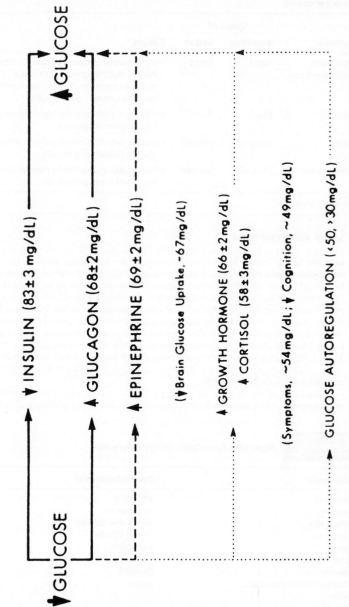

Figure 36.2. Normal glucose counterregulation. (Adapted from Cryer PE. Glucose counterregulation: the prevention and correction of hypoglycemia in humans. *Am J Physiol* 1993;264:E149.)

nervous system responses. They experience the neuroglucopenic symptoms but not the autonomic ones. In addition, the brain seems to accommodate to the prevailing glucose concentrations. Therefore, diabetic patients (type 1 or type 2) with marked chronic hyperglycemia may experience the autonomic (but not the neuroglucopenic) signs and symptoms at glucose levels that are not hypoglycemic but are much lower than the patient is usually at (e.g., 120 to 150 mg/dL). Readjustment to the brain's perception that these levels are not low may take several weeks. On the other hand, hypoglycemic unawareness can occur in tightly controlled diabetic patients (type 1 or type 2) whose prevailing glucose concentrations are usually normal and necessarily associated with many low values. These individuals might not experience any signs and symptoms of hypoglycemia until much lower glucose concentrations are reached (e.g., 40 to 50 mg/dL). This decreased sensitivity to hypoglycemia is associated with a lowered threshold for counterregulatory hormone release and autonomic nervous system activation (i.e., these do not start to occur until glucose levels reach approximately 50 mg/dL). Because chronic hypoglycemia from any cause is associated with this decreased sensitivity, patients with β-cell tumors (insulinoma) (see Section VI.G) often experience no symptoms until their glucose levels reach a very low point.

The other two causes of hypoglycemia unawareness (in addition to loss of glucagon and epinephrine responses in type 1 diabetes and maintaining below-normal glucose concentrations) are **antecedent hypoglycemia** and **autonomic neuropathy.** An episode of hypoglycemia the day before impairs the counterregulatory response to current hypoglycemia in both normal subjects and diabetic patients. Clinically, hypoglycemia unawareness occurs in type 1 diabetes patients who have frequent episodes of hypoglycemia and/or maintain below-normal glucose concentrations. Avoidance of hypoglycemia and/or maintenance of glucose concentrations in the normal or slightly elevated range often reverses hypoglycemia unawareness.

Autonomic neuropathy is an uncommon cause of hypoglycemia unawareness. As stated earlier, hypoglycemia unawareness is not a problem for type 2 diabetic patients. Finally, although the signs and symptoms of hypoglycemia vary widely among subjects, the pattern in an individual patient tends to be similar during each episode.

VI. FASTING HYPOGLYCEMIA

    A. General principles. Because the onset of fasting hypoglycemia is often gradual, the autonomic component of the signs and symptoms is minimal or absent in many cases. Fasting hypoglycemia is usually persistent and requires glucose administration for reversal. The **differential diagnosis** of hypoglycemia in adults is described in Table 36.4. Although hypoglycemia can occur both in the fasting state *and* after meals in three situations (adrenal insufficiency, with insulinomas, and in the

TABLE 36.4   **Differential Diagnosis of Hypoglycemia in Adults**

Fasting	Fed (reactive)
Drugs[a]	Hyperalimentation
Ethanol	Impaired glucose tolerance/mild type 2 diabetes mellitus
Non–β-cell tumors	Idiopathic reactive
Hepatic failure	Adrenal insufficiency[b]
Adrenal insufficiency	β-Cell tumors (insulinomas)[b]
β-Cell tumors (insulinomas)	Insulin autoantibodies[c]
Renal failure	
Insulin autoantibodies	
Insulin receptor autoantibodies	
Sepsis	

[a]Includes factitious hypoglycemia.
[b]Although fed hypoglycemia occasionally occurs, fasting hypoglycemia predominates.
[c]Experience is too limited to determine which form of hypoglycemia predominates.

presence of autoantibodies to insulin), the fasting component predominates. All of the other factors and conditions listed in Table 36.4 cause *either* fasting *or* postprandial hypoglycemia. This fact underscores the importance of determining whether the signs and symptoms occur in the fasted state or after a meal in a patient with suspected hypoglycemia.

B. Drugs

1. Specific drugs. Insulin is obviously the most common drug causing hypoglycemia, and sulfonylurea agents are the next most common. Several other medications may potentiate the hypoglycemic effect of the sulfonylurea agents by competing for their binding sites on albumin, thus increasing the free component. These include the sulfonamide antibiotics chloramphenicol (Chloromycetin), bishydroxycoumarin (Dicumarol), phenylbutazone (Butazolidin), oxyphenbutazone (Tandearil), clofibrate (Atromid-S), and clarithromycin. Salicylates and intravenous (IV) (but not inhaled) pentamidine (Lomidine) are the next most common drugs causing hypoglycemia when taken alone. Other drugs that occasionally cause hypoglycemia are propranolol (Inderal), monoamine oxidase inhibitors (only the hydrazine derivatives), oxytetracycline, disopyramide (Norpace), quinine, and fluoroquinolones (gitaloxin, levofloxacin). There are a number of isolated case reports of hypoglycemia secondary to various drugs acting either alone or in the presence of sulfonylurea agents or insulin, but often the circumstances do not support a bona-fide cause-and-effect relationship, and usually there are no confirming reports.

2. Treatment. With the exception of insulin-induced hypoglycemia, the treatment (by IV glucose) of hypoglycemia caused by other drugs should not be discontinued too soon. Hypoglycemia relapse can be difficult to prevent with oral carbohydrate ingestion, especially if the inciting drug was a sulfonylurea agent. Patients with sulfonylurea-induced hypoglycemia and altered mental status should be admitted to the hospital, because hypoglycemia can recur for days. Because IV glucose continues to stimulate insulin secretion in this situation, treatment with **octreotide** (the long-acting form of somatostatin) or oral **diazoxide** can be helpful.

Factitious hypoglycemia is an unusual form of drug-induced hypoglycemia in which emotionally disturbed patients surreptitiously take insulin or, occasionally, sulfonylurea agents. They are usually women in health-related occupations or female relatives of diabetic patients with access to these drugs. Because commercial insulin preparations do not contain connecting peptide (C-peptide), the diagnosis of hypoglycemia induced by **exogenously** administered insulin is made by finding low concentrations of C-peptide in association with low levels of glucose and high concentrations of insulin (Table 36.5). In patients harboring insulinomas with hypoglycemia induced by **endogenous** insulin, C-peptide levels are high because equimolar amounts of insulin and C-peptide are secreted by functioning pancreatic β cells. Because surreptitious ingestion of sulfonylurea agents also results in hypoglycemia associated with high levels of both insulin and C-peptide, measurement of these compounds or their degradation products in serum or urine is necessary to help diagnose this cause of factitious hypoglycemia. A high index of suspicion is necessary in these cases.

| TABLE 36.5 | Distinguishing among Patients with Insulinomas and Factitious Administration of Insulin or Sulfonylurea Agents |

Condition	Glucose	Insulin	C-Peptide	Proinsulin
Insulinoma	Low	High	High	High
Insulin[a]	Low	High	Low	Normal
Sulfonylurea[a]	Low	High	High	Normal

[a]Factitious administration.

C. Ethanol. Ethanol ingestion is a common cause of hypoglycemia. In addition, many drug-induced cases of hypoglycemia occur in association with ethanol intake.

1. **Pathogenesis.** The metabolism of ethanol in the liver inhibits gluconeogenesis. Thus, ethanol-induced hypoglycemia is seen when glycogen stores are no longer capable of sustaining glucose concentrations and gluconeogenesis is necessary. This obviously occurs in a <u>setting of restricted food intake</u>. This condition often takes place in malnourished chronic alcoholics but may also develop in heavy weekend drinkers or even in social drinkers who miss meals. It should be stressed that ethanol decreases glucose concentrations in patients with normal liver function. Children are particularly sensitive to this effect of alcohol.

2. **Clinical setting.** Clinically, the neuroglucopenic signs and symptoms predominate in alcohol-induced hypoglycemia. The autonomic response is inhibited by ethanol and is often diminished or absent. Because glucose utilization is not increased, glucose concentrations decrease gradually, which may contribute to a diminished autonomic response.

3. **Treatment.** Prompt diagnosis and treatment are important. Failure to recognize this syndrome may be responsible for the **high associated mortality** (approximately 25% in children and approximately 10% in adults). Glucagon therapy is usually not effective because glycogen stores are already depleted. In contrast to drug-induced hypoglycemia, alcohol-induced hypoglycemia may not require long-term continuous IV administration of glucose after the initial response to such therapy. Relapses can usually be prevented by the ingestion of modest amounts of carbohydrate.

D. Non–β-cell tumors. Many non–β-cell tumors can cause hypoglycemia. The types and relative frequency are listed in Table 36.6.

1. **Pathogenesis.** Only in very rare instances can production of insulin be proven. Excess glucose consumption by the large mesenchymal tumors is not responsible. Non–β-cell tumors secrete incompletely processed **insulinlike growth factor type II** (IGF-II). Normally, IGF-II is synthesized in the liver and released into the circulation. In the serum, normal IGF-II is complexed to a heterotrimeric 150-kDa IGF-binding protein (IGFBP), which consists of IGF-I, IGF-II, an acid-labile protein, and the IGFBP. This renders IGF-II not very biologically active. Incompletely processed IGF-II is larger than normal IGF-II (specialized assays can measure "big" IGF-II) and is sequestered into a smaller binary complex with IGFBP-3, which increases its bioavailability. Thus, although IGF-II levels are normal or only slightly elevated, there is more <u>free IGF-II to bind to insulin receptors</u>, which is the mechanism by which hypoglycemia is thought to occur. These levels of active IGF-II inhibit growth-hormone secretion, which not only limits the response to hypoglycemia but also causes low IGF-I levels, another growth factor synthesized in the liver. However, a recent patient has been described with metastatic large cell carcinoma of the lung that secreted IGF-I, not IGF-II.

2. **Differential diagnosis.** The diagnosis of tumor hypoglycemia can be difficult if hypoglycemia is the initial manifestation of the neoplasm. The differential usually

TABLE 36.6 **Non–β-Cell Tumors Associated with Hypoglycemia**

1. Large mesenchymal tumors (approximately 50%)—mesotheliomas, fibrosarcomas, neurofibromas, neurofibrosarcomas, spindle-cell sarcomas, leiomyosarcomas, rhabdomyosarcomas
2. Hepatocellular carcinomas (hepatomas) (approximately 25%)
3. Adrenal carcinomas (5–10%)
4. Gastrointestinal tumors (5–10%)
5. Lymphomas (5–10%)
6. Miscellaneous tumors (occasional)—most common: kidney, lung, anaplastic carcinomas, carcinoid

includes only β-cell tumors, adrenal insufficiency, and factitious hypoglycemia, because the other causes of fasting hypoglycemia (Table 36.4) are easily ruled out. Differentiation from β-cell tumors and factitious hypoglycemia requires a fast (usually only a short fast can be tolerated) with concomitant monitoring of glucose and insulin concentrations. Evaluation of the pituitary–adrenal axis is also simple and is described later. However, in many instances the tumor is already known to be present. This is usually the case with large mesenchymal tumors and often with many other types, because hypoglycemia is a relatively late manifestation. High or high-normal IGF-II levels and low or low-normal IGF-I levels are often seen in these patients. A **low IGF-I** level usually characterizes these patients and is very helpful in making the diagnosis of a non–β-cell tumor producing big IGF-II.

Adrenal carcinomas deserve special mention from a diagnostic standpoint. Although they are rare, they are commonly represented among neoplasms associated with hypoglycemia. In endocrine testing, many of these patients have increased serum dehydroepiandrosterone sulfate (DHEAS) concentrations. Therefore, adrenal carcinoma should be suspected in a patient with fasting **hypoglycemia** and elevated serum **DHEAS** concentrations.

3. **Treatment.** The treatment of patients with tumor hypoglycemia is often difficult. If large amounts of the tumor (especially large mesenchymal tumors) can be surgically removed, long-term remissions from hypoglycemia are likely. Effective radio- or chemotherapy may also increase glucose concentrations. However, in many cases, therapy directed at the tumor is not successful and specific treatment for hypoglycemia is necessary. Frequent feedings are the obvious first choice but are often not effective. Continuous IV administration of glucose is not practical for any length of time. Administration of glucocorticoids is sometimes helpful because they stimulate hepatic gluconeogenesis and to some extent inhibit peripheral glucose utilization. The initial dose should be the equivalent of 15 to 20 mg of prednisone, with fairly rapid increases if no effect is detectable. Although there are few published accounts of experience with this form of treatment for tumor hypoglycemia, if a dose equivalent to 60 to 80 mg of prednisone is reached and no effect is noted, the dose should probably be tapered off rapidly to avoid adrenal suppression and dependence on exogenous glucocorticoid. If the patient is given glucocorticoid therapy for less than a month, the hypothalamic–pituitary–adrenal axis usually returns to normal.

E. **Hepatic failure.** Death from hepatic failure is common, but associated hypoglycemia is distinctly unusual. This is because the liver has a tremendous capacity to produce glucose, and hypoglycemia ensues only when the liver is severely compromised. The diagnosis is obvious because the patient has all of the clinical and laboratory stigmata of hepatic failure. Although treatment is simple (i.e., support of the glucose concentration with IV dextrose until the liver regenerates the capacity to maintain appropriate levels itself), hypoglycemia in this situation is a serious prognostic sign indicating that there is little functioning hepatic tissue left. Indeed, the capacity of the liver to produce glucose may be restored, but the patient still succumbs to the other complications of hepatic failure.

F. **Adrenal insufficiency**

1. **Pathogenesis.** The mechanism whereby either primary or secondary adrenal insufficiency leads to fasting hypoglycemia is straightforward. **Cortisol** is necessary to support gluconeogenesis; in its absence, hepatic glucose production is significantly impaired. Although a deficiency of growth hormone sometimes causes hypoglycemia in children, the absence of this hormone in adults is not associated with hypoglycemia. Patients with pituitary destruction who are receiving adequate replacement doses of glucocorticoids do not experience difficulties maintaining normal glucose concentrations.

2. The **diagnosis** of adrenal insufficiency usually is also straightforward once it is considered. There are at least three stimulation tests with blood sampling. None of these tests differentiates between primary and secondary adrenal insufficiency, which must be distinguished by other means (see Chapter 12).

a. **Cortrosyn stimulation test.** This test can be done routinely. Alternatively, if treatment with glucocorticoids is deemed imperative, the **Cortrosyn** (the 1–24 amino acid sequence of ACTH; cosyntropin) **stimulation test** should be performed before administration of the steroid. This is important because a reliable assessment of the pituitary–adrenal axis is extremely difficult after treatment is begun. The test, which can be completed within 1 hour, involves intravenous or intramuscular injection of 0.25 mg of Cortrosyn; blood samples for measurement of plasma cortisol levels are obtained before injection as well as 30 and 60 minutes afterward. A normal response is classically defined as a baseline value of at least 5 μg/dL *and* an increase of greater than 7 μg/dL *and* a maximal level of greater than 18 μg/dL. Some endocrinologists feel that any increase of greater than 10 μg/dL constitutes a normal response regardless of baseline and maximal levels. However, in some patients, plasma cortisol levels may increase by less than 7 μg/dL over a relatively high baseline value. Therefore, if any value is greater than 20 μg/dL, adrenal insufficiency is essentially ruled out.

An abnormal Cortrosyn stimulation test in secondary adrenal insufficiency depends on atrophy of the adrenal cortex because of a normal lack of stimulation by ACTH. The test can be normal in 10% to 15% of patients with secondary adrenal insufficiency, especially if it is carried out soon after pituitary insufficiency occurs. The Cortrosyn stimulation test is the test of choice if primary adrenal insufficiency is suspected.

A low-dose (1-μg) Cortrosyn stimulation test is sometimes used to identify mild adrenal insufficiency, but because hypoglycemia is very unlikely to be part of this picture, the low-dose test is not helpful in this situation.

b. The **insulin tolerance test** is considered the "gold standard" for the diagnosis of adrenal insufficiency. However, it is very labor-intensive (in many institutions, physician presence is required throughout the test), unpleasant for patients, occasionally dangerous, and sometimes must be repeated. Contraindications to the test are a fasting serum cortisol of less than 5 μg/dL (already suggestive of adrenal insufficiency), a seizure disorder, altered mental status, and ischemic heart disease. Symptoms of hypoglycemia should be explained to the patient before the test, and a "crash cart" should be available. After an overnight fast, a baseline sample is drawn and 0.15 U/kg of insulin is given as an intravenous bolus. Blood samples are taken 30 and 60 minutes later. Blood glucose monitoring at the bedside should be performed on each of these samples to determine if adequate hypoglycemia (<40 mg/dL) has been achieved. If adequate hypoglycemia has not been achieved, the dose of insulin is repeated with timings of the subsequent samples 30 and 60 minutes later. A peak cortisol concentration of more than 18 μg/dL indicates adequate hypothalamic–pituitary–adrenal function. A meal should be given at the conclusion of the test. If adrenal insufficiency is strongly suspected, the initial dose of insulin should be 0.1 U/kg. Because most patients have moderate to marked symptoms of hypoglycemia during the test and because of the potential dangers of the test, I rarely use it.

c. **Metyrapone stimulation test.** Metyrapone (Metopirone) blocks 11-hydroxylation in the adrenal cortex, which is the final step in the synthesis of cortisol (compound F). The release of ACTH is not inhibited by its immediate precursor, 11-deoxycortisol (compound S). Therefore, the brain senses a low cortisol level and secretes more ACTH, which stimulates the adrenal cortex to synthesize more compound S. Compound S can be measured separately in the plasma, and its accumulation signals a normal pituitary–adrenal response to metyrapone.

Metyrapone (0.25-mg tablets) is given by mouth at about 11 P.M. and a plasma sample is collected at 8 A.M. the next day. For patients who weigh more than 50 kg, the dose is 3.0 g; for those who weigh less than 50 kg, the dose is 2.0 g. A normal response consists of a concentration of compound S of greater than 7 to 8 μg/dL (regardless of the concomitant compound F value).

A valid abnormal response of less than 7 to 8 μg/dL **requires** that the cortisol level be less than 5 μg/dL. This latter value proves that the 11-hydroxylation step was adequately blocked and therefore the patient was unable to mount a satisfactory compound-S response. A concentration of compound S that is below normal in the presence of a compound F level of greater than 5 μg/dL signifies that the blockade was not complete. In this instance, either the test must be repeated (with a higher dose of metyrapone if a 2-g dose was used) or an alternative diagnostic approach used.

Some patients may experience nausea and occasionally vomiting secondary to metyrapone administration. These symptoms are recognized adverse reactions to the drug and do not represent acute adrenal insufficiency, which, although theoretically possible, has not, to my knowledge, been reported under these circumstances.

3. The **management** of the hypoglycemia associated with adrenal insufficiency is straightforward. In addition to the bolus of IV glucose, the patient should be given 100 mg of <u>cortisol</u> over an 8-hour period and started on maintenance doses thereafter.

G. **β-Cell tumors**

1. **Clinical findings.** Although **insulinomas** are rare tumors, the correct diagnosis is extremely important. Not only are they usually curable, patients who remain undiagnosed for long periods may develop permanent neuropsychiatric sequelae. Because the glucose level usually drifts down slowly in affected patients, autonomic signs and symptoms (Table 36.3) are often lacking, and the presence of hypoglycemia may not be evident. Patients with insulinomas tend to present with the more confusing neuroglucopenic signs and symptoms, which can include visual difficulties, transient neurologic syndromes, mental confusion, convulsions, and personality changes. Weight gain is common in these patients because chronic hyperinsulinemia and hypoglycemia lead to excessive caloric intake and fat deposition.

2. **Diagnosis** of a β-cell tumor is usually not difficult once it is considered. The <u>cardinal rule</u> in the evaluation of glandular function is to stimulate the gland if hypofunction is suspected and to suppress it if hyperfunction is suspected.

a. The most physiologic way to suppress insulin secretion is by **fasting.** Characteristic changes in the relationship between glucose and insulin concentrations during total caloric deprivation are the most reliable diagnostic criteria for insulinomas and are found in almost every patient who is tested appropriately. In normal subjects, levels of both glucose and insulin fall during starvation. In some women, as mentioned previously, plasma glucose concentrations can decrease asymptomatically to values as low as 30 to 35 mg/dL after 24 to 72 hours without food. However, insulin levels usually fall proportionally more, so that the insulin/glucose (I/G) ratio decreases (Fig. 36.3). In patients with insulinomas, insulin concentrations are either not suppressed or increased somewhat during fasting, so that I/G increases.

Therefore, the most reliable way to diagnose a β-cell tumor is simply to extend the overnight fast until the patient becomes symptomatic. Blood samples for glucose and insulin determinations are drawn after the overnight fast and then every 2 to 4 hours after that. If the history reveals that the patient must get up and eat overnight to avoid hypoglycemia, the fast must necessarily start in the morning when the patient is under medical supervision. Glucose levels can be measured from a fingerstick sample. A separate sample of blood should also be collected for insulin and plasma glucose if fingerstick values are less than 50 mg/dL (or when symptoms of hypoglycemia occur). The test should be extended until symptoms of hypoglycemia preclude continuing. Approximately two thirds of the patients will experience hypoglycemic symptoms within the first 24 hours of food deprivation. Another one fourth or so will become symptomatic during the second 24 hours of starvation. A third day of fasting is required in only approximately 5% of patients who harbor insulinomas. I/G ratios above 0.3 are abnormal and make the diagnosis, assuming that factitious hypoglycemia is excluded (see Table 36.5).

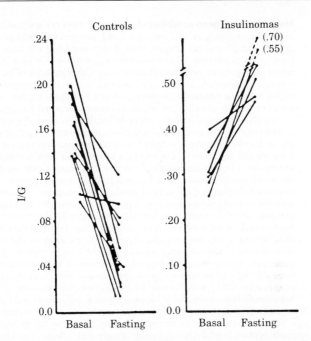

Figure 36.3. Plasma insulin (uU/mL)-to-glucose (mg/dL) ratios (I/G) at the beginning of a fast (basal) and at the nadir of the glucose concentration. (From Merimee TJ, Tyson JE. Hypoglycemia in man: pathologic and physiologic variants. *Diabetes* 1977;26:161. Reproduced with permission from the American Diabetes Association, Inc.)

b. **Stimulatory tests** with tolbutamide, glucagon, calcium (IV), or leucine produce too many <u>false negatives and false positives</u> to be relied on. An oral <u>glucose tolerance test is worthless</u> in making the diagnosis of an insulinoma because it may be normal, flat (which occurs in 20% of the normal population), or show impaired glucose tolerance.

c. Measurement of the **proinsulin content** of the fasting plasma is very helpful. Normally, proinsulin (which is measured along with insulin in the older radioimmunoassays) is less than 20% of the total immunoassayable insulin. In the large majority of patients with insulinomas, proinsulin constitutes more than 20% of total immunoassayable insulin. Current assays can measure proinsulin directly. When these assays are used, almost all patients with insulinomas have elevated levels of proinsulin. Recently, two patients have been described whose tumors produced proinsulin, not insulin. The diagnosis was made using an older assay for insulin that cross-reacted with proinsulin; insulin levels measured by a newer assay specific for insulin did not support the diagnosis of a β-cell tumor during the fast. Very high levels of proinsulin alerted the physicians to the diagnosis, emphasizing the importance of measuring this prohormone in the workup for a β-cell tumor.

d. Finally, in the extremely rare situation in which an insulinoma develops in an insulin-requiring type 2 diabetes patient, the secretion of endogenous insulin can be monitored by measurement of the levels of **C-peptide** because, as mentioned above, this polypeptide is not contained in commercial insulin preparations.

e. **Preoperative localization** of a diagnosed insulinoma is extremely helpful to the surgeon because of the small size of this type of lesion. **Localization should only be undertaken after the biochemical diagnosis of an**

insulinoma has been established. Otherwise, false positive results will lead to unnecessary surgery. On the other hand, patients with a biochemical diagnosis should undergo surgery even if the tumor has not been found by localization procedures. Pancreatic arteriography correctly identifies a β-cell tumor in only approximately half of the cases. Other methods of localizing the tumor (abdominal ultrasonography, radionuclide scanning, computed tomography, magnetic resonance imaging) may not be helpful because the tumors are often smaller than 2.0 cm in size. However, computed tomography with contrast has been used with success in the localization of small insulinomas in several patients. The most sensitive methods may be endoscopic ultrasonography or ultrasonography at surgery (i.e., with the pancreas exposed). Selective intra-arterial injections of calcium as a secretagogue with subsequent measurements of insulin concentrations in the right hepatic vein are frequently successful and often used after an unsuccessful previous surgery. A positive response is a doubling or more of insulin concentrations 30 to 60 seconds after the arterial calcium injection. A positive response after injection into the gastroduodenal or superior mesenteric artery helps localize the tumor to the head or neck of the pancreas. A response after injection into the proximal or distal splenic artery helps localize the tumor to the body or tail of the pancreas. A positive response after injection into the hepatic arteries suggests liver metastases. If pancreatic arteriography is performed, this method of localization adds only a few minutes to the time needed. Finally, positron emission tomography (PET) with fluorine-18-L-dihydroxyphenylalanine (^{18}F-DOPA) has recently been successful in localizing both β-cell tumors and hyperplasia.

3. **Treatment.** If surgery does not cure the patient because of the presence of multiple tumors, hyperplasia, or metastatic spread, drug therapy to block insulin secretion is often helpful. Oral diazoxide (Proglycem), 100 mg 3 to 4 times a day, is used most often, conferring benefit in approximately half of the patients. A few patients will respond to phenytoin (Dilantin), chlorpromazine, propranolol, or verapamil. The drug of choice for metastatic islet cell carcinoma is streptozotocin. Patients whose carcinoma is refractory to streptozotocin occasionally respond to L-asparaginase, doxorubicin (Adriamycin), or mithramycin.

H. **Renal failure.** Hypoglycemia accompanying renal failure is being increasingly recognized. Although poor dietary intake has been associated with many of the reported cases, some patients have clearly been well fed. Impairment of gluconeogenesis is probably involved, although a few patients remain hypoglycemic despite the IV administration of large amounts of glucose, suggesting enhanced glucose utilization in these circumstances. When it occurs, hypoglycemia may be a problem for several weeks to months and then spontaneously remit for no apparent reason. Because it tends to be intermittent in those patients in whom it occurs, frequent feedings should be used to prevent it. If that is ineffective, glucocorticoid therapy (15 to 20 mg of prednisone) may be needed, but such therapy should be tapered and eventually discontinued as soon as feasible. There is a clinical impression that hypoglycemia in patients with end-stage renal disease is a poor prognostic sign. Many of these patients die within a year or so, although usually not from hypoglycemia.

I. **Miscellaneous causes**

1. **Insulin autoantibodies.** Occasionally, a patient spontaneously develops antibodies to insulin despite never having received insulin injections. The mechanism involved in the hypoglycemia is probably related to the binding of large amounts of endogenous insulin with subsequent release of free insulin at inappropriate times. This unusual cause of hypoglycemia may be part of the autoimmune endocrine syndrome, as evidenced by its occurrence in patients with Graves disease, rheumatoid arthritis, and lupus erythematosus. The majority of cases have been reported in Japanese patients, many of whom had been taking sulfhydryl compounds (e.g., thionamides).

2. **Insulin-receptor autoantibodies.** A rare patient (usually female) has a syndrome of insulin resistance and acanthosis nigricans associated with certain immunologic features, such as elevated erythrocyte sedimentation rates, high

titers of antinuclear and anti-DNA antibodies, hypergammaglobulinemia, and decreased complement levels (see Chapters 2 and 57). Affected patients also have autoantibodies to the insulin receptor (not to the insulin molecule as described above). The presence of these antibodies accounts for insulin resistance in these patients because insulin is unable to exert its action at the critical initial step of binding. A few of these patients manifest recurrent hypoglycemia because the antibody bound to two adjacent receptors is able to exert an insulinlike effect under certain circumstances.

3. **Sepsis.** Hypoglycemia is not considered to be clinically associated with infection. Classically, in fact, insulin resistance and hyperglycemia have been described in conjunction with infection. However, hypoglycemia is occasionally seen in patients with septicemia with both gram-positive and gram-negative organisms.

4. **Falciparum malaria.** Hypoglycemia has been reported in severe falciparum malaria. The mechanism may involve increased glucose utilization by parasitized red blood cells. Although quinine (see Section B.1) may have contributed to it, hypoglycemia was still seen in patients with low or absent quinine levels. Pregnant patients and those with cerebral involvement seem to be particularly prone. However, some feel that hypoglycemia is not a specific complication of cerebral malaria but occurs in severely ill, fasted patients, especially children.

VII. FED (REACTIVE) HYPOGLYCEMIAS

A. **General principles.** In contrast to the signs and symptoms of fasting hypoglycemia, those of fed (reactive) hypoglycemia are predominantly **autonomic** (Table 36.3). Their onset is characteristically rapid. The neuroglucopenic component is unusual in reactive hypoglycemia. This type of hypoglycemia is transient and is usually reversed by the normal counterregulatory hormonal responses (Table 36.2). Administration of exogenous glucose will hasten, but is usually not needed for, abatement of the autonomic signs and symptoms.

The differential diagnosis of fed hypoglycemia is described in Table 36.4. As discussed earlier, two of the six causes listed (adrenal insufficiency and insulinomas) lead to predominantly fasting hypoglycemia. This may also be true for a third cause, the presence of autoantibodies to insulin, although there are too few reported cases on which to base a firm conclusion. The remaining three diagnoses listed—**hyperalimentation, impaired glucose tolerance/mild type 2 diabetes mellitus,** and **idiopathic reactive hypoglycemia**—must be considered when a patient gives a history suggestive of postprandial hypoglycemia only.

B. **Oral glucose tolerance test.** The patterns of glucose and insulin concentrations in these three conditions after an oral challenge with dextrose are depicted in Figure 36.4. "Alimentary hyperglycemia" is an older name for what is now called hyperalimentation. "Diabetes" in this figure represents people with impaired glucose tolerance or mild type 2 diabetes; and "functional hypoglycemia" has been renamed idiopathic reactive hypoglycemia. Each curve in the figure represents data from a different patient. The characteristic pattern for hyperalimentation hypoglycemia consists of very high initial glucose concentrations and relatively early hypoglycemia (after 2 to 3 hours). Both impaired glucose tolerance/mild type 2 diabetes and idiopathic reactive hypoglycemia are associated with later hypoglycemia (after 3 to 5 hours). Abnormally high glucose levels in the early part of the oral glucose tolerance test obviously define impaired glucose tolerance and mild type 2 diabetes, whereas normal early concentrations characterize idiopathic reactive hypoglycemia.

C. **Hyperalimentation.** The conventional setting for reactive hypoglycemia caused by hyperalimentation is in a patient who has undergone gastric surgery. The normal relationship between the stomach and the small intestine is altered, so that entry of the gastric contents into the duodenum is not delayed by the pyloric sphincter. This rapid entry into the duodenum increases the rate of absorption of glucose from the small intestine into the systemic circulation and accounts for the early hyperglycemia.

These high glucose levels trigger an enhanced insulin response (Fig. 36.4), which subsequently causes hypoglycemia. However, rapid gastric emptying may

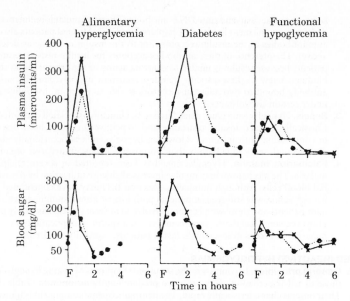

Figure 36.4. Hypoglycemia following an oral glucose load (100 g). Characteristic glucose and insulin concentrations in the three common types of fed (reactive) hypoglycemia. Data from two patients with each condition are shown. (From Yalow RS, Berson SA. Dynamics of insulin secretion in hypoglycemia. *Diabetes* 1965;14:341. Reproduced with permission from the American Diabetes Association, Inc.)

not be the sole explanation. Patients who have undergone antrectomy (removal of the lower part of the stomach) are much less likely to become hypoglycemic despite the fact that food enters the duodenum quickly. This observation suggests a role for one or more of the gastrointestinal hormones that amplify glucose-stimulated insulin secretion. The situation is further complicated by the occasional patient who has all of the characteristics of reactive hypoglycemia secondary to hyperalimentation but who has not had gastrointestinal surgery. Thus, reactive hypoglycemia secondary to hyperalimentation probably represents more than one disorder.

D. Impaired glucose tolerance/mild type 2 diabetes mellitus. The normal response in an oral glucose tolerance test is peak values of both glucose and insulin at 1 hour, just as occurs after a meal (depicted in Fig. 36.1). This normal pattern contrasts with the insulin response in patients with reactive hypoglycemia caused by impaired glucose tolerance/mild type 2 diabetes, as shown in the middle panel of Figure 36.4. In the two patients depicted, insulin concentrations were maximal at 2 hours or later. The conventional explanation for the late hypoglycemia is that high levels of insulin several hours after a meal cause glucose concentrations to become abnormally low because the influx of enough glucose from the intestinal tract is not available at this time to buffer the effect of the hormone. Although insulin secretion in patients with impaired glucose tolerance or mild type 2 diabetes and reactive hypoglycemia is delayed in comparison with that in normal subjects, many individuals with abnormal glucose tolerance have delayed insulin responses without late hypoglycemia. Therefore, other unidentified factors may also have a role.

E. Idiopathic reactive hypoglycemia

    1. Definition. Idiopathic reactive hypoglycemia is not a well-defined entity. The characteristic glucose pattern, as depicted in the right panel of Figure 36.4, consists of normal early concentrations and later low levels. The two subjects described in the figure had a normal insulin response, although other patients may have delayed or excessive responses.

2. **Controversial classification.** The classification of idiopathic reactive hypoglycemia as a discrete, bona-fide clinical entity is beset by a number of problems. Because the results of an oral glucose tolerance test in a single individual are not reliably reproducible, is the diagnosis legitimate one week but not the next? The large amount of simple carbohydrate used in the oral glucose tolerance test is certainly not physiologic. Thus, the question arises as to whether a diagnosis based on the results of this test is a valid explanation for symptoms occurring under different conditions. In addition, a disparity often exists between the numbers generated in glucose tolerance tests and the symptoms or lack thereof experienced during the tests. Of more serious concern in the establishment of a clinically relevant entity is that many patients who show the pattern of idiopathic reactive hypoglycemia during the oral glucose tolerance test according to biochemical criteria do not experience symptoms compatible with this diagnosis in their daily lives.

3. **Diagnostic criteria.** In spite of these considerations, there seem to be a few patients who have idiopathic reactive hypoglycemia and who routinely have symptoms when they ingest large amounts of simple carbohydrates. In my view, **four criteria** must be satisfied before this diagnosis can legitimately be made:

   a. Decreased glucose concentrations must be documented (Table 36.1).

   b. Signs and symptoms must occur at the time of hypoglycemia.

   c. Signs and symptoms must improve markedly **shortly** after the patient eats.

   d. The pattern just described must occur regularly.

   The first point raises the additional question of what value defines postprandial hypoglycemia. During oral glucose tolerance testing in asymptomatic normal people, a large proportion of those tested routinely have low glucose values. Therefore, the mere presence of a suitably low glucose concentration during a glucose tolerance test is not a sufficient basis on which to make the diagnosis of idiopathic reactive hypoglycemia. Only if all of these criteria are fulfilled in the patient's usual lifestyle setting is a diagnosis of idiopathic reactive hypoglycemia justified.

   Few individuals meet these criteria. Typically, a patient gives a vague history that includes some of the following: tiredness, lethargy, anxiety, weakness, depression, mental dullness, headache, paresthesias, loss of vitality, irritability, and a tremulous feeling. It is usually difficult to obtain a clear description of these symptoms; rather, the history is characterized by its vagueness. There is no clear relationship between food intake and either the onset or the relief of symptoms. Patients often have these symptoms on awakening, which improve only slowly (several hours) after eating. Other patients complain of the onset of symptoms within 30 to 60 minutes of eating. Unfortunately, these individuals are usually convinced that they are "hypoglycemic" and that their condition will improve if only the correct diet, vitamin, mineral, or other nostrum is prescribed.

4. **Nonhypoglycemia.** The syndrome of nonhypoglycemia is the result of: **(a)** the superficial similarity between the symptoms of anxiety and those of hypoglycemia; **(b)** the high prevalence of low glucose values during an oral glucose tolerance test; **(c)** the high incidence of anxiety in our society; and **(d)** misattribution. The last term refers to the patient's (and sometimes the physician's) desire to attribute functional complaints to a biochemical abnormality rather than confront the social or personal situation that is usually the basis for the symptoms. The fact that a high percentage of patients with the syndrome of nonhypoglycemia have abnormal profiles on the Minnesota Multiphasic Personality Inventory (MMPI) test or have had psychiatric disorders supports the link between emotional disturbances and the syndrome of nonhypoglycemia. However, a few individuals seem to have recurring symptoms following meals that are consistent with those of hypoglycemia in the absence of low glucose concentrations. This has been termed the **"postprandial syndrome."**

5. **Flat glucose tolerance test.** One other situation should be mentioned with regard to the diagnosis of idiopathic reactive hypoglycemia. Patients whose oral

TABLE 36.7	Menu for approximately 75-g–Carbohydrate Meal (Half Simple and Half Complex)

Breakfast

1. 2.5- to 3-oz bagel (1 medium) (or 3 slices toast): 35 g complex CHO
   10 oz fruit juice (apple, orange): 37 g simple CHO

   or

2. 1½ cup unprocessed, unrefined cold cereal (bran type; no raisins, etc.): 30–40 g complex CHO
   4 oz low-fat milk: 6 g simple CHO
   10 oz fruit juice (apple, orange): 37 g simple CHO

   or

3. 1 cup unsweetened hot cereal (oatmeal, cream of wheat, etc.): 30 g complex CHO
   4 oz low-fat milk: 6 g simple CHO
   10 oz fruit juice (apple, orange): 37 g simple CHO

Lunch

1. Sandwich with 2 slices bread: 30 g complex CHO
   3 saltine crackers: 8 g complex CHO
   10 oz juice or regular cola: 37 g simple CHO

   or

2. 1 cup cooked pasta: 30 g complex CHO
   ½ cup tomato sauce: 5 g complex/simple CHO
   10 oz juice or regular cola: 37 g simple CHO

   or

3. 6 oz baked potato: 30 g complex CHO
   1 cup raw vegetables (broccoli, carrots, etc.): 5 g complex CHO
   10 oz juice or regular cola: 37 g simple CHO

CHO, carbohydrate.

glucose tolerance tests give "flat" results are sometimes considered to have fed hypoglycemia. However, a flat glucose tolerance test result is seen in ~20% of the normal population and simply reflects the efficiency of the physiologic mechanisms in disposing of an oral glucose load.

6. **Diagnosis.** The usual task facing the physician is to persuade the patient that he or she does not have hypoglycemia and that the low glucose values during the oral glucose tolerance test have no clinical meaning. The most specific way to accomplish this is to teach patients blood glucose self-monitoring and have them measure and record their blood glucose levels when symptoms are experienced. Only a very few will have bona-fide hypoglycemia at these times. If that approach is not feasible, I perform a **meal tolerance test** consisting of 37.5 g of simple and 37.8 g of complex carbohydrate (Table 36.7), and sample every 30 minutes for 5 hours. When patients realize that they do not become hypoglycemic when they experience symptoms or after a heavy-carbohydrate meal, some of them are more willing to consider the possibility of an emotional basis for their symptoms.

F. Management of reactive hypoglycemia

1. **Diet.** The mainstay of treatment for persons with fed hypoglycemia is diet. The most important element in the dietary prescription is the **avoidance of simple or refined carbohydrates.** Patients who truly suffer from reactive hypoglycemia usually make this discovery for themselves. Because approximately 50% or more of the calories in the typical American diet are derived from carbohydrate and half of the carbohydrate calories are in the simple form, there is much potential for decreasing simple carbohydrate intake. For obese individuals, a weight-reduction diet is important. If the reduction of simple carbohydrate intake is not entirely effective, the next step is to limit carbohydrate intake to 35% to 40% of the total number of calories ingested. Should this dietary change not alleviate the symptoms, food intake should be divided into multiple smaller feedings

(e.g., three meals a day interspersed with three snacks). Placing limits on the intake of simple carbohydrates is effective in the majority of patients. A reduction in total carbohydrate intake takes care of the problem in most of the remaining cases. Multiple small feedings are usually not needed except in patients with hyperalimentation, in whom this dietary approach is often used.

2. **Drugs.** If dietary changes are not effective, several drugs may be tried. Propantheline bromide (Pro-Banthine), 7.5 mg taken 30 minutes before meals, has been helpful, although anticholinergic symptoms (dry mouth, blurred vision, and urinary retention) may limit its usefulness. Phenytoin, 100 to 200 mg 3 times a day, may be effective and probably works by inhibiting insulin secretion. Propranolol (10 mg given 30 minutes before meals) was effective in abolishing symptoms in patients with hyperalimentation, although the low glucose levels were not changed much. Finally, calcium-channel blockers and α-glucosidase inhibitors (acarbose and miglitol) may be helpful. The latter seem particularly appropriate because they inhibit the breakdown of complex carbohydrates to glucose in the small intestine.

3. **Surgery.** Finally, in patients with hyperalimentation with severe symptoms that are refractory to other therapy, placement of a reversed jejunal segment near the gastric outlet resulted in antiperistaltic inhibition of rapid entry of glucose into the circulation and uniformly corrected the hypoglycemia as well as alleviating the disabling symptoms in a small group of patients.

Selected References

General

Boyle PJ, Kempers SF, O'Connor A, et al. Brain glucose uptake and unawareness of hypoglycemia in patients with insulin-dependent diabetes mellitus. *N Engl J Med* 1995; 333:1726.

Cersosimo E, Molina PE, Abumrad NN. Renal glucose production during insulin-induced hypoglycemia. *Diabetes* 1997 Apr;46(4):643–646.

Cryer PE, Davis SN, Shamoon H. Hypoglycemia in diabetes. *Diabetes Care* 2003;26:1902.

Gerich JE, et al. Hypoglycemia unawareness. *Endocr Rev* 1991;12:356.

Drugs

Burge MR, Schmitz-Fiorentino K, Fischette C, et al. A prospective trial of risk factors for sulfonylurea-induced hypoglycemia in type 2 diabetes mellitus. *JAMA* 1998;279:137.

Krentz AJ, Boyle PJ, Justice KM, et al. Successful treatment of severe refractory sulfonylurea-induced hypoglycemia with octreotide. *Diabetes Care* 1993;16:184.

Limburg PJ, Katz H, Grant CS, et al. Quinine-induced hypoglycemia. *Ann Intern Med* 1993;119:218.

Marks V, Teale JD. Drug-induced hypoglycemia. *Endocrinol Metab Clin North Am* 1999; 28:555.

Seltzer HS. Severe drug-induced hypoglycemia: a review. *Compr Ther* 1979;5:21.

Non-β-Cell Tumors

Daughaday WH. The pathophysiology of IGF-II hypersecretion in non-islet cell tumor hypoglycemia. *Diabetes Rev* 1995;3:62.

Le Roith D. Tumor hypoglycemia. *N Engl J Med* 1999;341:757.

Adrenal Insufficiency

Courtney CH, McAllister AS, Bell PM, et al. Low- and standard-dose corticotropin and insulin hypoglycemia testing in the assessment of hypothalamic-pituitary-adrenal function after pituitary surgery. *J Clin Endocrinol Metab* 2004;89:1712.

Kong WM, Alaghband-Zadeh J, Jones J, et al. The midnight to morning urinary cortisol increment is an accurate, noninvasive method for assessment of the hypothalamic-pituitary-adrenal axis. *J Clin Endocrinol Metab* 1999;84:3093.

β-Cell Tumors

Chia CW, Saudek CD. The diagnosis of fasting hypoglycemia due to an islet-cell tumor obscured by a highly specific insulin assay. *J Clin Endocrinol Metab* 2003;88:1464.

Cohen RM, et al. Proinsulin radioimmunoassay in the evaluation of insulinomas and familial hyperproinsulinemia. *Metabolism* 1986;35:1137.

Gorman B, Charboneau JW. Sonographic detection of insulinoma. *The Endocrinologist* 1992;2:29.

Grant CS, et al. Insulinoma: the value of intraoperative ultrasonography. *Arch Surg* 1988; 23:843.

Kauhanen S, Seppanen M, Minn H, et al. Fluorine-18-L-dihydroxyphenylalanine (^{18}F-DOPA) positron emission tomography as a tool to localize an insulinoma or β-cell hyperplasia in adult patients. *J Clin Endocrinol Metab* 2007;92:1237.

Rosch T, Lightdale CJ, Botet JF, et al. Localization of pancreatic endocrine tumors by endoscopic ultrasonography. *N Engl J Med* 1992;326:1721.

Sherman BM, et al. Plasma proinsulin in patients with functioning pancreatic islet cell tumors. *J Clin Endocrinol Metab* 1972;35:271.

Miscellaneous Causes of Fasting Hypoglycemia

Flier JS, et al. The evolving clinical course of patients with insulin receptor antoantibodies: spontaneous remission or receptor proliferation with hypoglycemia. *J Clin Endocrinol Metab* 1978;47:985.

Uchigata Y, Eguchi Y, Takayama-Hasumi S, et al. Insulin autoimmune syndrome (Hirata disease): clinical features and epidemiology in Japan. *Diab Res Clin Pract* 1994;22:89.

Fed (Reactive) Hypoglycemias

Charles MA, Hofeldt F, Shackelford A, et al. Comparison of oral glucose tolerance tests and mixed meals in patients with apparent idiopathic postabsorptive hypoglycemia: absence of hypoglycemia after meals. *Diabetes* 1981;30:465.

Johnson DD, et al. Reactive hypoglycemia. *JAMA* 1980;243:1151.

Jung Y, et al. Reactive hypoglycemia in women: results of a health survey. *Diabetes* 1971; 20:428.

Lev-Ran A, Anderson RW. The diagnosis of postprandial hypoglycemia. *Diabetes* 1981; 30:996.

Palardy J, et al. Blood glucose measurements during symptomatic episodes in patients with suspected postprandial hypoglycemia. *N Engl J Med* 1989;321:1421.

Yager J, Young RT. Non-hypoglycemia is an epidemic condition. *N Engl J Med* 1974; 291:907.

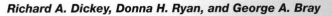

OBESITY

Richard A. Dickey, Donna H. Ryan, and George A. Bray

37

I. GENERAL PRINCIPLES

Obesity and overweight now affect 100 million Americans (more than 64% of the adult population). The presence of obesity or overweight should suggest the possibility of associated diseases such as diabetes mellitus, hypertension, heart disease, or gallbladder disease. Whether the associated disorders are present or not, the obese patient should be encouraged to lose weight by appropriate methods. As first steps, these include diet, nutritional education, self-help groups, and behavioral change. Under some circumstances, pharmacologic and/or surgical intervention may be considered for selected patients.

II. DEFINITION AND MEASUREMENT OF OBESITY

A. Obesity and overweight. The body mass index (BMI), which is the weight in kilograms divided by the square of the height in meters, provides the most widely accepted estimate of overweight and obesity. It is a valid estimate for assessing overweight and obesity in populations.

From the clinical point of view, when assessing individual patients, considering waist circumference along with BMI improves the assessment of an individual's health risk. A BMI of greater than 25 kg/m^2 is defined as overweight, and a BMI of 30 kg/m^2 or more is defined as obesity (Table 37.1). Adding information on waist circumference, as indicated in Table 37.1, refines health-risk estimation.

B. Visceral fat. An increase in visceral fat reflects central adiposity and increases risk for heart disease and diabetes. The waist circumference is used as a surrogate to assess the amount of visceral obesity. A waist circumference greater than 40 in (102 cm) in men or greater than 35 in (88 cm) in women is the current threshold for increased metabolic risk (Table 37.1) for Americans, but others have suggested that a waist circumference >80 cm for women and >94 cm for men may be more appropriate.

III. PREVALENCE OF OVERWEIGHT

The frequency of overweight increases with age, to a peak at 45 to 54 years in men and at 55 to 64 years in women. The National Health and Nutrition Examination Surveys (NHANES) 1999–2004 noted a BMI of ≥25 was present in 64.5% of men 20 years or older and in 50.7% of women 20 years or older. The prevalence of obesity (BMI ≥30) was 27% in men and 33.0% in women. Although the prevalence of overweight is higher in men, the prevalence of obesity is higher in women. Females at any age are disproportionately at greater risk for obesity, and especially extreme obesity (BMI ≥40). The prevalence of obesity continues to increase dramatically in the United States and is rising worldwide.

At birth, the human infant has about 12% body fat. During the first years of life, body fat increases rapidly to reach a peak of about 25% by age 6 months, and decreases over the next 10 years to about 18%. At puberty, there is a significant increase in the percentage of fat in females and a decrease in males. By age 18, males have about 15% to 18% body fat, and females about 25% to 28%. Between ages 20 and 50, the fat content of males approximately doubles and that of females rises by about 50%. However, total body weight rises by only 10% to 15%. The increased fat is accounted for in part by the rise in body weight and in part by a reduction in lean body mass.

545

TABLE 37.1 Classification of Overweight and Obesity by Body Mass Index, Waist Circumference, and Associated Disease Risk

| | BMI (kg/m²) | Obesity class | Disease risk relative to normal weight and waist circumference | |
			Men <102 cm (<40 in) Women <88 cm (<35 in)	>102 cm (>40 in) >88 cm (>35 in)
Underweight	<18.5		—	—
Normal	18.5–24.9		—	—
Overweight	25.0–29.9		Increased	High
Obesity	30.0–34.9	I	High	Very high
	35.0–39.9	II	Very high	Very high
Extreme obesity	≥40	III	Extremely high	Extremely high

BMI, body mass index.
Reprinted from National Institutes of Health/National Heart, Lung, and Blood Institute. *Clinical Guidelines on the Identification, Evaluation, and Treatment of Overweight and Obesity in Adults.* Publication No. 98-4083. Washington, DC: U.S. Government Printing Office; 1998.

IV. RISKS RELATED TO OBESITY

A. Obesity and excess mortality. As the BMI increases, there is a curvilinear rise in excess mortality. This excess mortality rises more rapidly when the BMI is above 30 kg/m². A BMI greater than 40 kg/m² is associated with a further increase in risk to overall health. Obesity has an impact on life expectancy that is equivalent to the impact of smoking; compared to those of normal BMI, for obese, nonsmoking 40-year-olds, about 7 years of life are lost; for obese smokers, about 13 years of life are lost. The principal causes of the excess mortality associated with overweight include hypertension, stroke and other cardiovascular diseases, diabetes mellitus, cancers (obesity increases risk for almost all types of cancer), sleep apnea, and sudden death. Obesity is also associated with reproductive disorders, gallbladder disease, and increased risk of cognitive dysfunction with aging.

B. The insulin-resistant or dysmetabolic state is strongly associated with excess visceral adiposity and may include consequences such as glucose intolerance or type 2 diabetes mellitus, hypertension, polycystic ovarian syndrome, dyslipidemia, and other disorders. These manifestations often improve with weight loss, especially when it is achieved early and the loss is maintained.

V. DEVELOPMENT OF OBESITY

There are multiple contributory etiologic pathways to obesity. We find the classification in Table 37.2 helpful in conceptualizing obesity mechanisms.

A. Neuroendocrine obesity

1. Hypothalamic obesity can follow damage to the ventromedial hypothalamus caused by tumors (i.e., craniopharyngioma), inflammatory lesions, trauma, or other hypothalamic conditions. Treatment is both symptomatic and specific when the underlying disease can be identified.

TABLE 37.2 An Etiologic Classification of Obesity

1. Neuroendocrine diseases associated with obesity
2. Drug-induced obesity
3. Dietary obesity
4. Reduced energy expenditure
5. Genetic factors in obesity

2. Cushing disease may present with obesity, and treatment should be directed at the cause of the increased production of corticosteroids, usually from a pituitary adenoma.

B. Drug-induced weight gain. Treatment of diabetics with insulin, sulfonylureas, or thiazolidinediones may increase hunger and food intake, resulting in weight gain. Metformin, exenatide, and gliptins do not cause weight gain, and the first two may cause weight loss. Treatment with some antidepressants, antiepileptics, neuroleptics, and glucocorticoids can increase body weight, as can cyproheptadine, probably through effects on the monoamines in the central nervous system.

C. Dietary obesity

1. Food intake. A high-fat diet, larger portion sizes, inexpensive food, and reduced physical activity of most Americans are among the causes of the increase of corpulence during the past century. Excessive consumption of sugar- or high-fructose corn syrup–sweetened beverages and the prevalence of abundant varieties of food in cafeterias or supermarkets may also be dietary factors contributing to the development of obesity. Estimates show that calorie intake has risen ~200 to 300 kcal per day over the past 30 years.

D. Reduced energy expenditure relative to energy intake is an important contributor to obesity in modern society. Energy expenditure can be divided into four parts.

1. Resting metabolism ranges from 800 to 900 kcal/m^2 (1 350 to 1 750 kcal) per 24 hours. It is lower in females than in males and declines with age. This decline with age could account for much of the increase in fat stores if food intake does not decline similarly.

2. Physical exercise is variable but on average is responsible for about one third of the daily energy expenditure. From a therapeutic point of view, this component of energy expenditure is the one most easily manipulated.

3. Dietary thermogenesis is the energy expenditure, measured as oxygen uptake, which follows the ingestion of a meal. This thermic effect of food may dissipate up to 10% of the ingested calories. Protein appears to have the greatest effect. The thermic effect of food is one type of metabolic "inefficiency" in the body, that is, where dietary calories are not available for "useful" work. In the obese, the thermic effect of food is reduced, particularly in individuals with impaired glucose tolerance or diabetes.

4. Adaptive thermogenesis. Acute over- or underfeeding produces corresponding shifts in overall metabolism, which can be as large as 15% to 20%.

E. Genetic factors in obesity

1. Dysmorphic or syndromic obesity. In some types of obesity, genetic factors are primary. Dysmorphic individuals usually have distinctive features, including **(a)** Bardet-Biedl syndrome, characterized by retinal degeneration, mental retardation, obesity, polydactyly, and hypogonadism; **(b)** Alström syndrome, characterized by pigmentary retinopathy, nerve deafness, obesity, and diabetes mellitus; **(c)** Carpenter syndrome, characterized by acrocephaly, mental retardation, hypogonadism, obesity, and preaxial syndactyly; **(d)** Cohen syndrome, characterized by mental retardation, obesity, hypotonia, and characteristic facies; and **(e)** Prader-Willi syndrome, characterized by hypotonia, mental retardation, hypogonadism, and obesity.

2. Genetic susceptibility to obesity. If both parents are obese, ~80% of the offspring will be obese. If only one parent is obese, the likelihood of obesity in the offspring falls to <10%. Studies with identical twins suggest that hereditary factors account for up to 70% of the variance in weight gain. Family studies suggest a lower genetic contribution of ~30% to 50%. Environmental factors (dietary composition, physical inactivity, reduced sleep time, among others) account for the remainder of the variation in body weight. Recent observations in human populations have supported the role of epigenetic events in programming the risk for obesity, with intrauterine and early childhood nutritional factors seeming to play a key role. Thus, there is increased interest in weight gain and nutrition during pregnancy, with guidelines limiting weight gain in obese women (see Table 37.3, later).

3. Single-gene causes of obesity. Genetic variation in the melanocortin-4 receptor is the most common single-gene defect associated with obesity and can account for up to 5% of severe obesity in children. Several families with either leptin deficiency or deficiency of the leptin receptor have been reported and are associated with massive obesity. Deficiency of pro-opiomelanocortin, the precursor for melanocyte-stimulating hormone and adrenocorticotropic hormone, is also associated with massive obesity, red hair, and adrenal insufficiency. Absence of proconvertase I has also been associated with obesity in one family.

VI. EVALUATION OF THE OBESE PATIENT
A. A thorough medical evaluation, including:
1. A comprehensive history incorporating the history of the illness (obesity and weight gain, family history, personal and social history, past medical history, system review, and medication history).
2. A psychological and mental-health status assessment, including questions targeting night eating, binge eating, and bulimia.
3. A comprehensive physical examination, including assessment of the patient's height, weight, waist circumference, blood pressure, and level of health risk due to obesity.
4. Appropriate laboratory testing, including lipid panel, glucose level and, if indicated, an OGTT, chemistry panel for hepatic function and uric acid, thyroid-function testing, and cortisol level, where indicated by the clinical findings.

B. The evaluation of the patient is directed to:
1. Establishing the degree of the patient's obesity and estimating visceral fat.
2. Determining the level of the patient's risk for obesity-related conditions, including hypertension, dyslipidemia, glucose intolerance, diabetes mellitus or insulin-resistant state, hyperandrogenism, and polycystic ovary syndrome.
3. Discovering underlying psychological disorders, such as eating disorders, sexual abuse, substance abuse, depression, or use of drugs that cause weight gain.
4. Identifying the rare genetic syndromes that are associated with obesity or neurologic disorders contributing to weight gain.

VII. RISK–BENEFIT CLASSIFICATION OF OBESITY (Table 37.3)
Individuals with a normal BMI (20 to 24.9 kg/m^2) have little or no risk associated with their weight status (Table 37.3). Any individual in this weight range who wishes to lose weight for cosmetic reasons should do so only by conservative methods.

A. Overweight individuals with a BMI of 25 to 29.9 kg/m^2 are in the low-risk group for developing disease associated with obesity. They too should be encouraged to

TABLE 37.3 A Risk–Benefit Classification of Obesity

Risk class	Body mass index (kg/m^2)	Recommended weight gain in pregnancy (kg)	Obesity classification relating risk to choices of treatment					
			Caloric intake (kcal/d)			Exercise	Drugs	Surgery
			<200	200–800	>800			
I	<25	10–12	NA	3	2	1	NA	NA
II	25–29.9	10–12	NA	2	1–2	1	3	NA
III	30–39.9	8–10	NA	1	2	3	2	NA
IV	40+	6–8	2	1	1	3	2	1–2

NA, not applicable; 1, first choice; 2, second choice; 3, third choice.

use low-risk treatments, such as caloric restriction and exercise. Individuals with a BMI of 27 to 30 kg/m² or more who have associated comorbid conditions are at higher risk; therefore, use of adjunctive pharmacotherapy for weight loss and control may be appropriate for them.

B. Individuals with a BMI of 30 to 39.9 kg/m² have moderate to high risk for developing diseases associated with obesity. This risk is enhanced even further in men and in individuals younger than 40 years. For those in the moderate-risk category of obesity, caloric restriction, drugs, and exercise all appear to be appropriate forms of treatment. Individuals with significant excess weight often find exercise a difficult method for losing weight; however, exercise is very useful in helping to maintain weight loss. The use of antiobesity medications as an adjunct to treatment may also be beneficial in this group.

C. Individuals who have a BMI of at least 40 kg/m² have a high to very high risk of developing diseases associated with their obesity. Moderate to severe restriction of calories is the first line of treatment, but for many of these patients, antiobesity medications or surgery may be advisable.

VIII. MANAGEMENT OF OBESITY

A. Dietary modification

1. **Calorie restriction.** Any diet must reduce caloric intake below daily caloric expenditure. This requires an assessment of caloric requirements, which can be done in two ways.

   a. The first way is a simple, but practical, rule of thumb: 10 calories per pound of current weight will generally equate to a safe weight-reduction diet.

   b. The second method involves assessing caloric requirements by use of a more complex calculation, as shown in Table 37.4. After the caloric requirement is determined, a reasonable calorie deficit can be prescribed. A caloric deficit of 500 kcal per day (3 500 kcal per week) will produce the loss of ~0.45 kg (1 lb) of fat tissue each week. Table 37.5 gives a list of diets divided into different levels of energy.

2. **Fasting** is not recommended as a form of therapy because of protein loss and hypotension. There is also a small increased risk of death. Total fasting should be done only in the hospital, where fluid losses and blood pressure can be monitored. The rise in <u>ketones with fasting inhibits uric acid excretion</u> and may precipitate development of urate renal stones if the patient is not appropriately treated.

3. **Very-low-calorie liquid diets (<800 kcal) and low-calorie (800 to 1 000 kcal) liquid diets.** Very-low-calorie diets (<800 kcal per day) will reduce the

---

 TABLE 37.4 | **Estimating Energy Needs: Revised WHO Equations for Estimating Basal Metabolic Rate**

Men
18–30 y = (0.0630 × actual weight in kg + 2.8957) × 240 kcal/d
31–60 y = (0.0484 × actual weight in kg + 3.6534) × 240 kcal/d

Women
18–30 y = (0.0621 × actual weight in kg + 2.0357) × 240 kcal/d
31–60 y = (0.0342 × actual weight in kg + 3.5377) × 240 kcal/d

Estimated total energy expenditure = BMR × activity factor

Activity level	Activity factor
Low (sedentary)	1.3
Intermediate (some regular exercise)	1.5
High (regular activity or demanding job)	1.7

BMR, basal metabolic rate; WHO, World Health Organization.

TABLE 37.5 Different Types of Diets

Type of diet	Examples
I. Low-calorie diet (>1 000 cal)	
A. Low-carbohydrate diet	Dr. Atkin's New Diet Revolution; Sugar Busters Diet
B. Low-fat/high-carbohydrate diet	Dr. Ornish's Diet
C. Balanced-deficit diet	Prudent Diet; Weight Watchers Diet
D. Portion-controlled diet	Frozen meals and liquid meals
E. Emphasizing single foods	Grapefruit diet; candy diet
II. Very-low-calorie diet (400–800)	Optifast; Modifast; HMR
III. Starvation (<400 kcal/d)	

net loss of nitrogen to <1 g per day from levels of 4 to 6 g per day found during starvation, and are used rarely and in limited clinical situations because loss of protein is not completely stopped. Protein from egg, casein, or soy comprises 33% to 70% of the energy in these diets. However, it is advisable that these diets should contain at least 25% of the calories as carbohydrate. Supplements of electrolytes, including potassium and other inorganic salts, as well as vitamins, including folate, pyridoxine, and thiamine, should be given. Very-low-calorie diets should be monitored with medical supervision. Low-calorie liquid diets (generally 800 to 1 000 kcal per day) can be used to achieve rapid weight loss safely, provided a high-quality protein source is used and similar supplementation is given. One of the advantages of this approach is the relatively good effect on appetite control; however, weight regain will occur unless there is a strong behavioral program when refeeding occurs.

  4. Reduced-calorie diets

    a. Types of diets. Diets with >1 000 kcal per day can be divided into several categories. These categories are based on the relative proportion of macronutrients included in the diet and whether it involves special foods (Table 37.5). All diets must reduce the caloric intake to produce a negative energy balance.

      (1) The **low-carbohydrate diet** that allows you to eat all of the protein and fat you want ends up reducing total calorie intake to ~1 500 kcal per day. These diets, which generally have carbohydrate levels <50 g per day, are thus **ketogenic** and can be monitored clinically by the appearance of ketones in the urine. These diets have been popular for nearly 150 years. They vary in the level of fiber that is used. The Atkins diet has low fiber levels; the Sugar Busters diet has higher fiber levels. Head-to-head comparisons with other macronutrient approaches suggest that very-low-carbohydrate diets may produce somewhat more weight loss.

      (2) Low-fat or high-carbohydrate diets can be associated with either low or very low levels of fat. The very-low-fat diets (in the range of 10% to 20% of total calories) have increased fiber intake. These diets were developed in a setting designed to reverse the atherosclerotic plaques associated with the risk for heart disease, but because of the high fiber content, they were often associated with weight loss. Hedonic issues limit their popularity.

      (3) Moderate fat levels with higher carbohydrate are characteristic of the widely recommended "healthy diets." For weight loss, the New York Department of Health diet that was adopted as the "Prudent Diet" and used by Weight Watchers has stood the test of time.

      (4) The **portion-controlled diet** makes use of prepared foods that have a narrow range of calories. These include liquid or powdered drinks as well as frozen or canned entrees that contain about 100 to 300 kcal per unit.

These can be combined conveniently, thus removing for the individual the problem of counting calories.

(5) Diets emphasizing **single foods.** A number of popular diets focus on a single food. Although nutritionally unbalanced, these diets have two features. They are simple to follow, and the monotony of single items tends to limit food intake.

5. Counting calories. There are at least two ways to determine energy or calorie intake.

   a. The first is to "count calories." Patients can weigh or measure the foods they eat and obtain the caloric values from various tables or popular free Web sites such as calorieking.com.

   b. A second way is to use the information that is published on the nutrition labels of packaged foods. A typical nutrition label shows the serving size, the number of servings per container, the calories per serving, the protein, carbohydrate, and fat in each serving, and the percentage of eight selected nutrients in each serving. This is followed by the ingredients listed in order of weight from highest to lowest.

6. MyPyramid—the USDA Plan for Nutrition. The MyPyramid Web site (www.mypyramid.gov) provides an approach to evaluating the quality of a person's diet. The pyramid includes the major food groups: Grains and pasta, beans, and starchy vegetables, which provide vitamins, minerals, fiber, and energy (6 or more servings are recommended); the Vegetable group (3 to 5 servings); the Fruit group (3 to 4 servings); the Meats, fish, poultry, and nuts group (2 to 3 servings); and the Milk and yogurt group (2 to 3 servings). Fats, sweets, and alcohol should be used sparingly. Reducing the number of servings proportionally will provide a calorie-reduced diet. Most important for the dieter, however, is to sharply reduce the fats and sugar and to reduce or eliminate alcoholic beverages. Not only do alcoholic beverages have calories, they tend to reduce the patient's control in selecting the quality and quantity of foods to eat.

7. Stepwise plan. This plan progresses from diet, through nutrition, to behavior and exercise, and finally to menu planning. The components of this stepwise plan are **(a)** a 1 000- to 1 500-calorie diet that uses portion-controlled food, such as formula drinks and frozen foods; **(b)** nutritional education, aimed primarily at the fat content of food; **(c)** exercise; **(d)** behavioral changes; and **(e)** menu planning.

8. Changing behavioral patterns of eating. The techniques used in behavioral modification include self-monitoring, problem solving, stimulus control, stress management, social support, cognitive restructuring, and contingency management.

B. Exercise and physical activity. The only part of energy expenditure that is amenable to significant manipulation is physical activity. During sleep, energy expenditure is ~0.8 kcal/min, the lowest of the day. Thus, if an individual sleeps for an entire 24 hours, ~1 150 calories will be expended. Reclining increases this level to ~1.0 kcal/min. Obese and diabetic patients should be encouraged to increase their physical activity for two reasons: First, exercise consumes calories; but second, and more important, exercise increases glucose utilization and may enhance insulin sensitivity.

C. Pharmacologic therapy. The antiobesity drugs currently marketed to treat obesity are listed in Table 37.6. Abuse of amphetamines, methamphetamine, and phenmetrazine is well established, and these agents should not be used in the management of obesity. Table 37.6 lists the drugs that are currently available for use in treating obesity. The use of these drugs should be reserved for patients with moderate- or high-risk obesity (BMI >30 kg/m^2 or a BMI >27 kg/m^2 if comorbidities are present). They should only be considered after the patient has completed a program such as the stepwise plan described in Section VIII.A.7.

D. Surgery

   1. Gastric operations reduce the size of, or bypass, the stomach. Several different operations are currently done. The gastric bypass consists of creating a small

TABLE 37.6 Drugs Approved by the U.S. Food and Drug Administration That Produce Weight Loss

Generic name	Trade names	Usual dose	Comments
Drugs approved by the U.S. FDA for long-term treatment of obesity			
Orlistat	Xenical	120 mg 3 times a day	May have gastrointestinal side effects
Sibutramine[a]	Meridia (U.S.) Reductil (rest of world)	5–15 mg once daily	Norepinephrine–serotonin reuptake inhibitor; May raise blood pressure
Rimonabant (approved in Europe; for U.S. FDA review in June 2007)	Accomplia (Europe)	20 mg once daily	May cause gastrointestinal distress; associated with mood change at greater rates than placebo
Drugs approved by the U.S. FDA for short-term treatment of obesity			
Diethylpropion[a]			Sympathomimetic drugs; Approved for only a short time
Tablets	Tenuate	25 mg, 3 times a day	
Extended release	Tenuate	75 mg in morning	
Phentermine HCl[a]			
Capsules	Phentridol Teramine Adipex-P	15–37.5 mg in the morning	
Tablets	Tetramine Adipex-P		
Extended release	Ionamin	15 or 30 mg/d in the morning	
Benzphetamine[b]	Didrex	25 to 150 mg/d in single or divided doses	
Phendimetrazine[b]			
Capsules—extended release	Adipost Bontril Melfial Prelu-2 X-trozine	105 mg once daily	
Tablets	Bontril Obezine	35 mg, 2–3 times a day	
Drugs approved by the U.S. FDA for purposes other than weight loss			
Bupropion			
Tablets and extended release	Wellbutrin Zyban (antismoking)	300–400 mg/d	Antidepressant and smoking-cessation indications
Topiramate	Topamax	25 mg/d titrated up to clinical effect	Anticonvulsant indication
Zonisamide	Zonegran	200 mg/d titrated up	Anticonvulsant indication
Metformin	Glucophage	500 mg, twice daily up to maximal dose of 2 500 mg	Antidiabetic drug used alone or in combination with other antidiabetic drugs

[a]Scheduled by the U.S. Drug Enforcement Agency as Schedule IV.
[b]Scheduled by the U.S. Drug Enforcement Agency as Schedule III.
Data from AHFS Drug Information 2005. Bethesda, MD: American Society of Health-System Pharmacists.

(50-mL) upper stomach pouch with a staple line. The pouch is drained into a loop of jejunum using a Roux-en-Y design. The second type of operation is a vertically banded gastroplasty, which extends along the length of the esophagus with a vertical staple line along the fundus of the stomach. The esophageal contents enter the stomach through a reinforced narrow entry. The third type of operation consists of placement of a plastic inflatable ring around the upper stomach, along with a reservoir of saline under the skin that can be used to constrict the opening between the upper and lower stomach. In the Swedish Obese Subjects study, the weight loss with the gastric bypass was superior to gastroplasty or gastric-banding, although there were only a limited number of patients in the gastric bypass group. Mortality rates and postoperative complications are now at very low levels, provided the surgical team is experienced and the patients are appropriately selected. There is emerging evidence that gastric bypass and gastric banding may reduce appetite through signals that originate in the gut. Bariatric operations are particularly beneficial in the amelioration of diabetes.

2. Scopinaro or biliopancreatic bypass. In this operation, the stomach is separated and the contents entering the upper stomach are bypassed into a loop of jejunum that is anastomosed to the upper stomach. The gastric juices from the lower stomach join the duodenal contents and flow downstream, where they are anastomosed to the ileum where these digestive enzymes and food from the stomach connected for a short part of the intestine. The operation is technically difficult, and protein malnutrition has been a reported side effect.

IX. THE OBESE CHILD
The obese child is discussed in Chapter 44.

Selected References

Adams KF, Schatzkin A, Harris TB, et al. Overweight, obesity and mortality in a large prospective cohort of persons 50 to 71 years old. *N Engl J Med* 2006;355:763–778.

Bray GA. *Obesity and the Metabolic Syndrome*. Totawa, NJ: Humana Press; 2007.

Bray GA, Greenway FL. Pharmacological treatment of obesity. *Pharmacol Rev* 2007.

Buchwald H, Avidor Y, Braunwald E, et al. Bariatric surgery: a systematic review and meta-analysis. *JAMA* 2004;292:1724–1737.

Clinical Guidelines on the Identification, Evaluation, and Treatment of Overweight and Obesity in Adults. National Heart, Lung, and Blood Institute (NHLBI), Clinical Guidelines for Obesity, Sept. 1998.

Dickey RA, Bartuska DG, Bray GA, et al. AACE/ACE position statement on the prevention, diagnosis, and treatment of obesity, 1998 revision. *Endocr Pract* 1998;4:299–350.

Gardner CD, Kiazand A, Alhassan S, et al. Comparison of the Atkins, Zone, Ornish, and LEARN diets for change in weight and related risk factors among overweight premenopausal women: The A to Z Weight Loss Study: a randomized trial. *JAMA* 2007;297: 969–977.

Ogden CL, Carroll MD, Curtin LR, et al. Prevalence of overweight and obesity in the United States, 1999–2004. *JAMA* 2006;295:1549–1555.

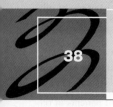

38 DISORDERS OF LIPID METABOLISM
Stanley H. Hsia

I. PHYSIOLOGY
Cholesterol and triglycerides (TG) are poorly soluble in the aqueous plasma. Lipoprotein particles are aggregates of phospholipids and free cholesterol that create a lipophilic environment in its core to transport lipid-soluble TG and cholesterol esters through an aqueous environment. Apolipoproteins are peptide constituents of lipoproteins that serve critical functions. The major lipoprotein classes differ widely in their size and composition (Table 38.1). The pathways and metabolic fates of exogenous (diet-derived) and endogenous (liver-derived) lipoproteins, as well as the intrahepatic fates of free cholesterol, are shown in Figure 38.1.

II. CLASSIFICATION OF LIPID DISORDERS
   A. Fredrickson classification. Historically, lipid disorders were classified according to their lipoprotein electrophoresis patterns (see Table 44.4). This scheme has limited clinical value, but is still occasionally used in the literature.
   B. Primary lipid disorders. Lipid disorders not attributable to coexisting factors are most likely genetically inherited (listed in Table 38.2).
   C. Secondary lipid abnormalities. Lipid and lipoprotein abnormalities may be manifestations of other coexisting conditions or concurrent medications (Table 38.3). First-line management should control the underlying disorder or eliminate the offending agent, if possible. Primary disorders sometimes cannot be definitively diagnosed unless these conditions have been controlled or ruled out.

III. DIAGNOSIS OF LIPID DISORDERS
   A. Clinical features. In extreme hypertriglyceridemia, **lipemia retinalis** may be seen on fundoscopy as a whitish discoloration of the retinal vessels, a result of turbidity from chylomicron accumulation, and cutaneous **eruptive xanthomata** may be seen on extensor surfaces as multiple small, raised, papular lesions. Nonspecific signs of chronic severe hypercholesterolemia include **xanthelasmas** that appear as yellow, well-demarcated, irregular plaques of cholesterol in the periorbital skin, a **corneal arcus** on the iris, and **tuberous xanthomata** that appear as larger, globular cutaneous deposits on extensor surfaces. **Palmar xanthomata** are yellowish discolorations in the palmar creases, and are more specific for familial dysbetalipoproteinemia. **Tendon xanthomata** usually affect extensor tendons (e.g., Achilles, knuckles), and are more specific for familial hypercholesterolemia.
   B. Measurements. Because TG levels increase postprandially, *TG must be measured only after an adequate (10- to 12-hour) fast. Cholesterol measurements are not affected by meals prior to the time of blood draw.* Low-density lipoprotein cholesterol (LDL-C) values are usually calculated based on the measurement of other fractions, using the Friedewald equation (in mg/dL):

$$LDL\text{-}C = (TC) - [(HDL\text{-}C) + (TG \div 5)]$$

This relationship applies *so long as the TG level is <400 mg/dL and familial dysbetalipoproteinemia is absent*; otherwise, LDL-C cannot be calculated with certainty. *Severe illnesses* (e.g., myocardial infarction, severe trauma, sepsis) will *falsely lower serum lipids* by as much as 50% as an acute-phase response, beginning within

TABLE 38.1 Characteristics of the Major Classes of Lipoproteins

	Chylomicrons and chylomicron remnants	Very-low-density lipoprotein (VLDL)	Intermediate-density lipoprotein (IDL)	Low-density lipoprotein (LDL)	High-density lipoprotein (HDL)
Particle diameter (nm)	70–600	30–70	10–30	20–25	7–10
Density (g/mL)	<0.94	<1.006	1.006–1.019	1.019–1.063	1.063–1.21
Composition:					
Cholesterol	~5%	~20%	~40%	~50%	~20%
Triglyceride	~90%	~60%	~35%	~10%	~5%
Phospholipid	~4%	~15%	~20%	~20%	~30%
Protein	~1%	~5%	~5%	~20%	~45%
Major core component	TG	TG	TG, CE	CE	CE
Major apolipoproteins	B48, CII, CIII, E, AI, AII	B100, CII, CIII, E	B100, E	B100	AI, AII, CII, CIII, E

CE, cholesterol esters; TG, triglycerides.

555

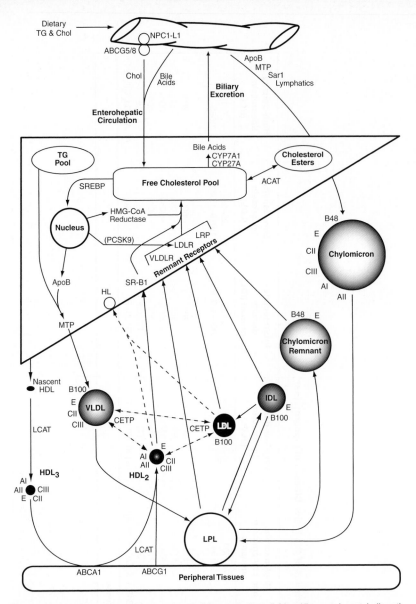

Figure 38.1. Metabolic fates of lipoproteins. *Solid arrows* indicate lipid and lipoprotein metabolic pathways; *dashed arrows* indicate pathways related to neutral lipid transfers among lipoprotein particles. AI, apolipoprotein AI; AII, apolipoprotein AII; ABCA1, ATP-binding cassette A1; ABCG1, ATP-binding cassette G1; ABCG5/8, ATP-binding cassettes G5 and G8; ACAT, acylCoA-cholesterol acyltransferase; ApoB, apolipoprotein B; B48, apolipoprotein B48; B100, apolipoprotein B100; CII, apolipoprotein CII; CIII, apolipoprotein CIII; CETP, cholesterol ester transfer protein; Chol, cholesterol; CYP7A1, cholesterol 7α-hydroxylase; CYP27A, cholesterol 27-hydroxylase; E, apolipoprotein E; HDL, high-density lipoprotein; HL, hepatic lipase; IDL, intermediate-density lipoprotein; LCAT, lecithin-cholesterol acyltransferase; LDL, low-density lipoprotein; LDLR, LDL receptor; LRP, LDL receptorlike protein; LPL, lipoprotein lipase; MTP, microsomal triglyceride transfer protein; NPC1-L1, Niemann-Pick C1-like-1 protein; PCSK9, Proprotein convertase subtilisin/kexin-9; Sar1, Sar1-GTPase; SR-B1, scavenger receptor-B1; SREBP, sterol response element–binding protein; TG, triglyceride; VLDL, very-low-density lipoprotein; VLDLR, VLDL receptor.

TABLE 38.2 Primary Lipid and Lipoprotein Disorders

Primary disorder	Molecular defect	Lipoproteins	Chol	TG
Familial LPL deficiency	LPL	↑↑ Chylomicrons	↔	↑↑↑
Familial apoCII deficiency	ApoCII	↑↑ Chylomicrons	↔	↑↑↑
Familial HL deficiency	HL	↑ VLDL, ↑ LDL, ↑ HDL	↑	↑
Familial hypertriglyceridemia	???	↑ VLDL, Chylomicrons	↔	↑↑
Familial apoAV deficiency	ApoAV	↑↑ Chylomicrons	↑	↑↑↑
Familial dysbetalipoproteinemia	ApoE	↑ IDL, ↑ remnants	↑↑↑	↑
Familial hypercholesterolemia	LDLR	↑↑ LDL, (↓ HDL)	↑↑	↔↓
Familial defective apoB	ApoB100	↑↑ LDL, (↓ HDL)	↑↑	↔↓
Proprotein convertase subtilisin/kexin-9	PCSK9	↑↑ LDL	↑↑	↔↓
Autosomal recessive hypercholesterolemia	LDLR adaptor protein	↑↑ LDL	↑↑	(↑)
Cholesterol ester storage disease	Lysosomal acid lipase	↑↑ LDL, (↓ HDL)	↑↑	(↑)
β-Sitosterolemia	ABCG-5 or ABCG-8	↑↑ LDL (phytosterols)	↑↑ Phytosterols	(↑)
Familial combined hyperlipidemia	???	↑ VLDL, ↑ LDL, ↓ HDL	(↑)	↔
Polygenic hypercholesterolemia	???	↑ LDL	↑	↔
Familial apoAI deficiency	ApoAI	↓↓ HDL	↔	↔
Familial hypoalphalipoproteinemia	???	↓ HDL	(↑)	(↑)
Familial hyperalphalipoproteinemia	???	↑ HDL	↑	↔
Tangier disease	ABCA-1	↓↓ HDL	↓	↑/↓
Familial LCAT deficiency	LCAT	↓↓ HDL	↑/↓	↑/↓
Fish-eye disease	LCAT	↓ HDL	↔	↑
Familial CETP deficiency	CETP	↑↑ HDL	↑/↓	↑/↓
Familial LDL deficiency (Abetalipoproteinemia)	MTP	↓↓ VLDL, ↓↓ LDL	↓↓	↓↓
Familial hypobetalipoproteinemia	ApoB	↓↓ LDL	↓↓	↓↓
Chylomicron retention disease	Sar-1	↓↓ LDL, ↓ HDL	↓↓	↔

???, unknown; (), possible increase/decrease; ABCA-1, ATP-binding cassette A-1; ABCG-5, ATP-binding cassette G-5; ABCG-8, ATP-binding cassette G-8; Apo, apolipoprotein; CETP, cholesterol ester transfer protein; Chol, cholesterol; HDL, high-density lipoproteins; HL, hepatic lipase; LCAT, lecithin cholesterol acyltransferase; LDL, low-density lipoproteins; LDLR, low-density lipoprotein receptor; LPL, lipoprotein lipase; MTP, microsomal triglyceride transfer protein, PCSK9, proprotein convertase subtilisin/kexin-9; Sar-1, Sar-1-GTPase; TG, triglycerides; VLDL, very low-density lipoproteins.

TABLE 38.3	Secondary Lipid and Lipoprotein Abnormalities		
Underlying disorder	**Lipoproteins**	**Chol**	**TG**
Obesity	↑ VLDL, ↓ HDL, (↑ LDL)	(↑)	↑
Insulin resistance/type 2 diabetes	↑ VLDL, ↓ HDL, (↑ LDL)	(↑)	↑
Uncontrolled type 1 diabetes	↑ VLDL, ↓ HDL	(↑)	↑↑
Alcohol	↑ VLDL, ↑ HDL	↔	↑↑
Hypothyroidism	↑ LDL, (↑ VLDL)	↑	(↑)
Pregnancy	↑ VLDL, ↑ HDL	↑/↓	↑
Nephrotic syndrome	↑ VLDL, ↑ LDL	↑	(↑)
Chronic renal failure	↑ VLDL, ↑ LDL	(↑)	↑
Obstructive liver disease	↑ Lp-X	↑	↔
Acromegaly	↑ VLDL, ↓ HDL, (↑ LDL)	(↑)	↑
Growth-hormone deficiency	↑ VLDL, ↑ LDL	↑	↑
Cushing syndrome	↑ VLDL, ↓ HDL, (↑ LDL)	(↑)	↑
Dysglobulinemia	↑ VLDL, ↑ LDL	↑	↑
Glycogen storage disease	↑ VLDL	(↑)	↑
Sphingomyelinase deficiency	↑ LDL	↑	↔
Anorexia nervosa	↑ LDL	↑	↔
Lipodystrophies	↑ VLDL, (↓ HDL, ↑ LDL)	(↑)	↑
Acute intermittent porphyria	↑ LDL	↑	↔
Estrogens	↑ VLDL, ↑ HDL, ↓ LDL	↓	↑
Raloxifene	↓ LDL	↓	↔
Tamoxifen	↑ VLDL, ↓ LDL	↓	↑
Progestins	↓ VLDL, ↓ HDL, ↑ LDL	↑	↓
Aromatase inhibitors	↓ VLDL, ↑ HDL	↔	↓
Androgens	↓ VLDL, ↓ HDL, ↑ LDL	↑	↓
Glucocorticoids	↑ VLDL, ↓ HDL, (↑ LDL)	(↑)	↑
Thiazides, beta-blockers	↑ VLDL, (↑ LDL)	(↑)	↑
Isotretinoin	↑ VLDL, (↓ HDL)	↔	↑
Cyclosporin	↑ LDL, (↑ VLDL)	↑	↔
Interferon-α	↑ VLDL, ↓ HDL	↔	↑
HIV protease inhibitors	↑ VLDL, ↓ HDL, (↑ LDL)	(↑)	↑
Atypical antipsychotics	↑ VLDL, ↓ HDL, (↑ LDL)	(↑)	↑

( ), possible increase/decrease; Chol, cholesterol; HDL, high-density lipoproteins; LDL, low-density lipoproteins; TG, triglycerides; VLDL, very-low-density lipoproteins.

24 hours after onset and lasting for up to 4 to 6 weeks afterward. Optimal lipid levels obtained during such hospitalizations do not rule out hyperlipidemia, and should be repeated after the patient has recovered.

C. NCEP ATP-III risk assessment and therapeutic targets. The National Cholesterol Education Program (NCEP) has published recommendations for the management of lipid disorders for all adults in the United States in its Third Adult Treatment Panel (ATP-III), published in 2001 and revised in 2004. It should be stressed that these guidelines are not intended to substitute for individualized clinical judgment.

  1. Population screening. ATP-III recommends a full fasting lipoprotein profile for all adults age 20 years and older, at least once every 5 years. Any results that are less than optimal for the patient's risk profile warrant more frequent assessments as treatment is instituted.

  2. Risk-factor assessment. LDL-C is recognized as the primary target of therapy because it bears the strongest evidence as an atherogenic lipoprotein. Therapy is targeted more aggressively for higher-risk patients while minimizing unnecessary therapy and cost for lower-risk patients. First, patients should be distinguished

TABLE 38.4	**Major Risk Factors for the Determination of LDL-C Goals**

- Cigarette smoking
- Hypertension (BP ≥140/90 mm Hg or on antihypertensive medications)
- Low HDL-C (<40 mg/dL)
- Family history of premature CHD
  - (CHD in a male first-degree relative <55 years of age)
  - (CHD in a female first-degree relative <65 years of age)
- Age (men ≥45 years of age; women ≥55 years of age)
- High HDL-C is a "negative" risk factor (If ≥60 mg/dL, subtract one of the risk factors above)

BP, blood pressure; CHD, coronary heart disease; HDL-C, high-density lipoprotein cholesterol; LDL-C, low-density lipoprotein cholesterol.

based on the presence of CHD or **CHD equivalents,** which are defined by ATP-III as:
- Atherosclerotic disease other than CHD (e.g., peripheral arterial disease, symptomatic carotid artery disease or carotid stenoses >50%, or abdominal aortic aneurysm)
- Diabetes mellitus
- The presence of multiple risk factors that confer a 10-year CHD risk >20% (by the Framingham risk assessment tables)

Second, six major risk factors are used to determine the LDL-C goal for patients without CHD or CHD equivalents (Table 38.4).

3. **Framingham risk assessment tables.** Third, patients in the moderate risk (≥2 risk factors) category may be more accurately classified according to their 10-year CHD risk using the point-based Framingham risk assessment (Table 38.5). Software versions of these tables are also available as computer- and PDA–based applications.

4. **NCEP 2004 revision.** Based on evidence from recent clinical trials, the following **very high-risk patients** may optionally intensify their treatment to an LDL-C goal of <70 mg/dL:
- Acute coronary syndrome
- Established CHD *plus*:
  - Multiple major risk factors, especially diabetes mellitus, or
  - Severe or uncontrolled risk factors, especially smoking, or
  - Multiple features of the metabolic syndrome, especially TG ≥200 mg/dL with high-density lipoprotein cholesterol (HDL-C) <40 mg/dL and non-HDL cholesterol (non–HDL-C) ≥130 mg/dL

Moderate-risk patients (with ≥2 risk factors) may also optionally target their LDL-C to <100 mg/dL if they have:
- Advanced age
- More than 2 risk factors
- Particularly severe or uncontrolled risk factors
- Multiple features of the metabolic syndrome, especially TG ≥200 mg/dL with HDL-C <40 mg/dL and non–HDL-C ≥160 mg/dL
- A highly-sensitive C-reactive protein (hsCRP) level >3 mg/L

5. **Recommended treatment targets.** The preceding assessments (Sections III.C.2–III.C.4) categorize the patient into the broad risk categories (and their corresponding treatment targets) shown in Table 38.6.

6. **The metabolic syndrome and non-HDL cholesterol.** The **combined dyslipidemia** of the metabolic syndrome is a CHD risk factor independent of LDL-C, and it *should be a secondary target of therapy after achieving the LDL-C goal.* NCEP has defined five conditions that represent the metabolic syndrome; exceeding the cutoff levels of three or more satisfies NCEP's diagnostic definition (Table 38.7). ATP-III proposes that *non–HDL-C be used as the index of lipoprotein risk*

TABLE 38.5 Framingham Risk Assessment Tables

Men

Age (y)	Points
20-34	-9
35-39	-4
40-44	0
45-49	3
50-54	6
55-59	8
60-64	10
65-69	11
70-74	12
75-79	13

TC (mg/dL)	Points (based on age):				
	20-39	40-49	50-59	60-69	70-79
<160	0	0	0	0	0
160-199	4	3	2	1	0
200-239	7	5	3	1	0
240-279	9	6	4	2	1
≥280	11	8	5	3	1

Smoker	Points (based on age):				
	20-39	40-49	50-59	60-69	70-79
No	0	0	0	0	0
Yes	8	5	3	1	1

HDL-C (mg/dL)	Points
≥60	-1
50-59	0
40-49	1
<40	2

SBP (mm Hg)	Points (based on treatment):	
	Untreated	Treated
<120	0	0
120-129	0	1
130-139	1	2
140-159	1	2
≥160	2	3

Add points from age, TC, smoking, HDL-C, and SBP:

Point total	10-y risk (%)
<0	<1
0	1
1	1
2	1
3	1
4	1
5	2
6	2
7	3
8	4
9	5
10	6
11	8
12	10
13	12
14	16
15	20
16	25
≥17	≥30

Women

Age (y)	Points
20-34	-7
35-39	-3
40-44	0
45-49	3
50-54	6
55-59	8
60-64	10
65-69	12
70-74	14
75-79	16

TC (mg/dL)	Points (based on age):				
	20-39	40-49	50-59	60-69	70-79
<160	0	0	0	0	0
160-199	4	3	2	1	1
200-239	8	6	4	2	1
240-279	11	8	5	3	2
≥280	13	10	7	4	2

Smoker	Points (based on age):				
	20-39	40-49	50-59	60-69	70-79
No	0	0	0	0	0
Yes	9	7	4	2	1

HDL-C (mg/dL)	Points
≥60	-1
50-59	0
40-49	1
<40	2

SBP (mm Hg)	Points (based on treatment):	
	Untreated	Treated
<120	0	0
120-129	1	3
130-139	2	4
140-159	3	5
≥160	4	6

Add points from age, TC, smoking, HDL-C, and SBP:

Point total	10-y risk (%)
<9	<1
9	1
10	1
11	1
12	1
13	2
14	2
15	3
16	4
17	5
18	6
19	8
20	11
21	14
22	17
23	22
24	27
≥25	≥30

HDL-C, high-density lipoprotein cholesterol; SBP, systolic blood pressure; TC, total cholesterol.

TABLE 38.6 **ATP-III Risk Classifications and Treatment Goals**

Risk category	LDL-C goal (mg/dL)	LDL-C level for initiating or intensifying drug therapy (mg/dL)[a]	Non–HDL-C goal (mg/dL)
High risk: CHD or CHD equivalents (10-y risk >20%)	<100 <70 (optional)[b]	≥100 (optional if 70–99)	<130 *If LDL goal is <70:* <100[b]
Moderate risk: 2 or more risk factors (10-y risk 10–20%)	<130 <100 (optional)‡	*If LDL-C goal is <100: ≥100[c]* *If 10-y risk 10–20%: ≥130* *If 10-y risk <10%: ≥160*	<160 *If LDL goal is <100: <130[c]*
Low risk: 0–1 risk factor (10-y risk <10%)	<160	≥190 (optional if 160–189)	<190

[a]Initiation or intensification of Therapeutic Lifestyle Change (TLC) should be instituted for all patients who are above their treatment target.
[b]Recent evidence justifies a lower LDL-C and non–HDL-C goal for patients with acute coronary syndrome, or CHD plus multiple major risk factors (especially diabetes mellitus), severe or uncontrolled risk factors, or multiple components of the metabolic syndrome.
[c]Recent evidence justifies a lower LDL-C and non–HDL-C goal for moderate-risk patients with advanced age, more than 2 risk factors, severe or uncontrolled risk factors, multiple components of the metabolic syndrome, or highly sensitive C-reactive protein level >3 mg/L.
‡ATP-III, Third Adult Treatment Panel; CHD, coronary heart disease; HDL-C, high-density lipoprotein cholesterol; LDL-C, low-density lipoprotein cholesterol.

associated with the metabolic syndrome. Non–HDL-C is simply the difference between TC and HDL-C:

$$\text{Non} - \text{HDL-C} = (\text{TC}) - (\text{HDL-C})$$

Non–HDL-C correlates with TG but appears to be a more reliable CHD predictor, and it does not rely on a fasting blood sample. *For patients with TG ≥ 200 mg/dL, the non–HDL-C should be calculated* after LDL-C has been optimized, and if it is not optimal, therapy should be further intensified. *Optimal levels of non–HDL-C are 30 mg/dL above the corresponding LDL-C goal* (Table 38.6).

IV. MANAGEMENT

A. Supporting evidence. Randomized, double-blind studies examining changes in CHD events or plaque size demonstrate the efficacy of lipid-lowering therapies. Early studies established the efficacy of niacin, cholestyramine, gemfibrozil, and extremely low-fat dietary modifications without drugs. A subtle increase in non-CHD mortality was observed in some of these earlier studies, but this has not been seen in the larger, more recent statin trials. Statins were shown to reduce total mortality in both

TABLE 38.7 **ATP-III Criteria for the Identification of the Metabolic Syndrome[a]**

- Abdominal obesity (waist circumference >40 in men; >35 in women) (Some men with waist circumference 37–40 in may also be at risk.)
- Triglycerides (≥150 mg/dL)
- HDL-C (<40 mg/dL in men; <50 mg/dL in women)
- Blood pressure (≥130 mm Hg systolic/≥85 mm Hg diastolic)
- Fasting glucose (≥100 mg/dL)

[a]The metabolic syndrome is diagnosed by the presence of three or more of these features.
ATP-III, Third Adult Treatment Panel; HDL-C, high-density lipoprotein cholesterol.

TABLE 38.8	Therapeutic Lifestyle Change (TLC)
Saturated fat (including *trans* fats)	<7% of total daily calories
Polyunsaturated fats	≤10% of total daily calories
Monounsaturated fats	≤20% of total daily calories
Total fat	25–35% of total daily calories
Complex carbohydrates	50–60% of total daily calories
Fiber	20–30 g daily
Protein	~15% of total daily calories
Dietary cholesterol	<200 mg daily
Total calories	Balance intake/expenditure to maintain desirable weight/ prevent weight gain; physical activity to expend ≥200 kcal/d

secondary and primary prevention populations by the 4S and the West of Scotland trials, respectively. Subsequent statin studies demonstrated clinical benefit in subjects with progressively lower baseline LDL-C levels. It is still not known if there is a level of LDL-C below which CHD risk does not fall any further. The VA-HIT trial reduced CHD mortality with gemfibrozil in men with low HDL-C, without changing LDL-C. In general, women, older patients, and diabetic patients appear to benefit equally (if not more) than men, younger patients, and nondiabetic patients, respectively. Statins also benefit patients in the early post–myocardial infarction (MI) period.

B. Nutritional and lifestyle therapy. *Therapy for lipid disorders should always begin with modifications of nutrition and lifestyle.* However, such modifications alone may be insufficient, and patients may be realistically incapable of making the degree of changes that are needed. Nevertheless, even while on pharmacologic therapy, regular counseling and reinforcement of the patient's adherence to nutrition and lifestyle modifications are always important.

  1. Nutritional therapy. ATP-III recommends the Therapeutic Lifestyle Change (TLC) (Table 38.8) as first-line therapy for up to 12 weeks. The TLC is indicated whenever lipid levels are above target, as well as for high- or moderate-risk patients with lifestyle factors (e.g., obesity, inactivity, high TG, low HDL-C, or the metabolic syndrome) *regardless* of their LDL-C level. Ideally, this should be conducted as *medical nutrition therapy* by appropriately trained nutritionists. If targets have not been reached after 6 weeks, the TLC should be intensified using additional reinforcements, fiber intake, or plant sterols.

    a. Total calories. Meal portion sizes should be controlled to *facilitate weight loss in overweight individuals and to maintain weight in normal-weight individuals.* A small daily calorie surplus, integrated over months to years, can amount to a significant total weight gain; so a small daily deficit of calories, if maintained over months to years, can amount to a significant weight loss. Thus, to be most effective, the TLC should be taught as a longitudinal lifestyle improvement ("healthier eating habits"), and applied as a series of smaller changes that are more easily tolerated and accomplished; frequent counseling, education, food diary review, and follow-up are required to help patients acquire and adhere to these skills.

    b. Nutritional composition. *To achieve LDL-C targets,* **saturated fat** *is the single most important nutritional component to be avoided.* Dietary **trans fats** and dietary **cholesterol,** which usually make up a smaller percentage of daily calories, should also be avoided. Polyunsaturated fats are more favorable, but high intake of omega-6 fatty acids may reduce HDL-C. Monounsaturated fats are relatively neutral to lipids and may help to reduce LDL-C. The majority of daily calories should still come from carbohydrates, but the intake of vegetables, fruits, whole-grain breads and cereals, and other **complex carbohydrate** sources, should predominate. Soluble dietary fiber independently reduces

LDL-C further (~10%). Regular alcohol intake may increase TG and HDL-C levels; the latter effect may account for the epidemiologic associations whereby mortality is lowest at the equivalent of two standard drinks per day. In the absence of hypertriglyceridemia or other contraindications (e.g., liver disease, addiction history), this level of alcohol intake should not be discouraged.

   c. Plant sterols/stanols. Available in the form of margarinelike spreads, plant sterols/stanols lower LDL-C an additional 10% to 13% when taken in typical quantities (~2 g daily) and are *useful as a dietary adjunct* to intensify the TLC therapy, if needed.

   2. Physical activity. ATP-III recommends moderate physical activity to expend an average of 200 kcal per day, especially for the management of the metabolic syndrome. Like nutritional therapy, a physical activity program must be sustained long-term to be most effective, so the exact frequency, duration, and mode of exercise should be individualized based on patient preference and coexisting medical conditions. Extreme changes in activity level may be difficult to sustain, so gradual progression of the exercise prescription is needed as the patient becomes more accustomed to physical activity. Choosing activities that are enjoyable for the patient, using self-monitoring tools, and involving family and peer supports will facilitate long-term adherence.

C. Pharmacotherapy. If an adequate trial of TLC (12 weeks) has not achieved treatment targets, pharmacologic therapy is indicated, along with continued TLC therapy. Although dosages are typically titrated upward until the patient's targets are achieved, NCEP recommends using a dosage sufficient to <u>achieve at least 30% to 40% lowering of LDL-C</u> regardless of the baseline LDL-C value. Features of the available lipid-lowering agents in the United States are listed in Table 38.9.

   1. HMG-CoA reductase inhibitors (Statins). Statins are the *most potent LDL-C-lowering agents available,* and they are well supported by large-scale clinical evidence. They are generally very well tolerated; hepatic transaminase elevations and myositis are uncommon reactions. There are no fixed guidelines as to how best to monitor for transaminase elevations, so individual clinical judgment should be used. If transaminase levels increase to more than three times the upper limit of the normal range (ULN), the drug should be discontinued; transaminases will return to normal over several weeks with no lasting sequelae. Elevations of less than three times ULN warrant closer monitoring, but discontinuation is not immediately necessary. **Myalgia,** defined as muscle symptoms in the absence of creatine kinase (CK) elevations, is the most common muscle symptom (incidence ~2% to 5%), but its clinical significance is debatable. **Myositis,** defined as muscle symptoms in the presence of CK elevations to *>10 times the ULN,* occurs with a frequency of ~0.1%, and requires immediate discontinuation of the statin and close patient follow-up. In most cases, the myositis resolves, with no lasting sequelae. However, progression to **rhabdomyolysis** and renal failure may occur if it is left untreated. There is a high prevalence of nonspecific CK elevations in the general population, so screening all statin-treated patients is not recommended; CK levels should only be measured to confirm or rule out myositis if patients complain of suggestive symptoms. The typical presentation is that of generalized myalgias with no other identifiable cause (such as injury, vigorous exercise, or flulike illness) occurring within days to weeks of starting or escalating the dose of therapy. Other causes of myopathy (e.g., alcohol, thyroid, inflammatory, neurologic, or congenital disorders) should also be considered. If a patient presents with classic myalgias and a normal CK level, clinical judgment should be used to decide whether the statin should be discontinued. If symptoms resolve upon discontinuation, switching to an alternate statin may not precipitate a recurrence. <u>Caution</u> is also warranted if there is concurrent use of macrolide antibiotics (erythromycin, clarithromycin), imidazole antifungals, cyclosporin, HIV protease inhibitors, or other drugs that share the cytochrome P450 3A4 clearance pathway along with many statins, thus increasing the risk of statin toxicity. Pravastatin, fluvastatin, and rosuvastatin are the least dependent on the 3A4 pathway, but caution should still be exercised.

TABLE 38.9 Lipid-Lowering Drugs Available in the United States

Drug	Dose	Efficacy	Side effects
HMG-CoA reductase inhibitors (statins)			
Lovastatin (Altoprev, Mevacor)	20–80 mg/d	LDL-C ↓ 20–60%	Transaminase elevations
Pravastatin (Pravachol)	20–40 mg/d	HDL-C ↑ 5–15%	Myopathy
Simvastatin (Zocor)	10–80 mg/d	TG ↓ 5–30%	Possible drug interactions
Fluvastatin (Lescol)	20–80 mg/d		
Atorvastatin (Lipitor)	10–80 mg/d		
Rosuvastatin (Crestor)	10–40 mg/d		
Fibric acid derivatives (fibrates)			
Gemfibrozil (Lopid)	600 mg b.i.d.	TG ↓ 20–50%	Dyspepsia, cholelithiasis
Fenofibrate (Antara, Lofibra, Tricor, Triglide)	43–200 mg/d	HDL-C ↑ 10–20%	Transaminase elevations
		LDL-C ↓ 5–20% (or ↑)	Myopathy
Nicotinic acid (niacin)			
Niacin	1.5–3.0 g daily (b.i.d./t.i.d)	LDL-C ↓ 15–25%	Flushing, Transaminase elevations
Extended-release niacin (Niaspan)	1–2 g/d	HDL-C ↑ 15–35%	Hyperglycemia, hyperuricemia/gout
		TG ↓ 20–50%	Peptic ulcer disease, Pruritis, Headache
Bile acid sequestrants			
Colestipol (Colestid) (resin)	5–20 g daily (b.i.d./t.i.d.)	LDL-C ↓ 15–30%	Gastrointestinal distress, constipation
Cholestyramine (Questran) (resin)	4–16 g daily (b.i.d./t.i.d.)	HDL-C ↑ 3–5%	Hypertriglyceridemia
Colesevelam (Welchol) *(tablets)*	2.6–3.8 g daily (q.d/b.i.d.)	TG ↑ 15%	Medication absorption (less with colesevelam)
Cholesterol absorption inhibitors			
Ezetimibe (Zetia)	10 mg/d	LDL-C ↓ 10–20%	No significant side effects
Other agents			
Omega-3 fatty acids (Omacor, Lovaza)	2–4 g/d (q.d/b.i.d.)	TG ↓ 20–40%	No significant side effects
		HDL-C ↑ ~5%	
		LDL-C ↑ 5–10%	
Combination agents			
Extended-release niacin/lovastatin (Advicor)	500 mg/20 mg–1 000 mg/40 mg	See individual agents	See individual agents
Ezetimibe/simvastatin (Vytorin)	10 mg/10 mg–10 mg/80 mg		

HDL-C, high-density lipoprotein cholesterol; LDL-C, low-density lipoprotein cholesterol; TG, triglyceride.

2. **Fibric acid derivatives (Fibrates).** Fibrates favorably affect all lipoproteins, but may paradoxically *increase* LDL-C, especially in patients with very high TG levels. They are *indicated for the management of combined dyslipidemias,* and have been shown to reduce CHD events and cardiovascular mortality. They are generally well tolerated, with only minor side effects of GI intolerance as well as uncommon risks of hepatic transaminase elevation and myopathy. Like statins, periodic monitoring of transaminases and muscle symptoms is warranted, but there are no fixed guidelines for such monitoring; individual clinical judgment should be used. Caution should be used in patients with renal insufficiency, in whom clearance of fibrates may be impaired, as well as in patients at risk of cholelithiasis because of increased lithogenicity of bile.

3. **Nicotinic acid (niacin).** Niacin has beneficial effects on all lipoprotein fractions and is *indicated for patients with combined dyslipidemias.* Its major drawback is the common, dose-related **flushing** *reaction.* Treatment should start with a low dose (250 to 500 mg) and gradually titrate upward toward the therapeutic range. Patients should be advised to avoid hot liquids with each dose, and/or try aspirin (325 mg) prior to the dose if needed to reduce the flush. If the flushing becomes unbearable, the patient should *not* discontinue the drug (as is often done), but rather titrate down to the previous dose for a longer period, and later reattempt titrating upward; discontinuation would require restarting the titration from the beginning. Diabetic patients may notice worsened glucose control, but this can be easily controlled with adjustment of antidiabetic therapies.

4. **Bile acid sequestrants.** Older bile acid sequestrants (colestipol, cholestyramine) are powdered resins that must be mixed in water (or juice, to improve palatability), whereas colesevelam is a newer hydrogel available in tablet form (that should still be taken with a large glass of water). Their primary effect is to *lower LDL-C, but an increase in TG may occur,* more so with resins than with colesevelam. Dosing is usually started low and titrated upward until goals are achieved or gastrointestinal side effects (constipation, bloating, nausea, flatulence, epigastric pain) become intolerable. The resins may also bind and limit the absorption of medications such as L-thyroxine, warfarin, thiazides, propranolol, estrogens, progestins, digitalis, penicillin G, and phenobarbital, and potentially any oral medication; pills should be taken at least 1 hour before or up to 4 hours after taking the resin. Colesevelam, however, does not interfere with these medications.

5. **Cholesterol-absorption inhibitors.** Ezetimibe lowers LDL-C less effectively than statins but additively with the effects of any statin. Because there is only minimal systemic absorption of the drug, the side-effect profile of ezetimibe is excellent. However, there is little change in other lipoproteins, and as yet, there are no controlled studies showing that ezetimibe reduces clinical CHD events.

6. **Pharmacotherapy combinations.** Patients with severe or complex lipid profiles may need drug combinations for additive effects. A common drug combination is a fibrate added to a statin. Although this significantly increases the risk of elevated transaminases and myopathy, these reactions are still sufficiently uncommon that this combination may be considered in compliant patients who will maintain regular follow-up. Gemfibrozil uniquely interferes with statin excretion, while fenofibrate does not, so *fenofibrate is the preferred fibrate when used in combination with a statin. Niacin may also be combined with statins or fibrates,* if the same cautions regarding transaminases and myopathy are taken. *Bile acid sequestrants may be safely combined with statins, fibrates, or niacin.* Because they are not systemically absorbed, there is no increased transaminase or myopathy risk. The only caution is to separate the dosing of a resin to avoid interfering with the absorption of the pills; this interference is much less when colesevelam is added to a statin. *Ezetimibe may be safely combined with any statin* to provide additive LDL-C lowering, but experience in combining with other lipid drug classes is still limited.

7. **Marine omega-3 fatty acids.** Modest intake of eicosapentaenoic acid (EPA) and docosahexaenoic acid (DHA), the marine omega-3 fatty acids (fish oils), reduces CHD events in high-risk patients through cardioprotective mechanisms other than

lipoprotein changes. The current recommendation is 500 mg per day of combined EPA + DHA (or two servings of coldwater fish per week) for patients without CHD; or 1 g of combined EPA + DHA per day for patients with known CHD. However, when taken in *much higher doses (2 to 4 g per day of combined EPA + DHA), omega-3 fatty acids have TG-lowering properties*. However, *LDL-C may paradoxically rise*. At these high doses, their *cardioprotective effects remain unproven*, but they may be useful in patients with *hypertriglyceridemia that is refractory to other TG-lowering therapies*. Over-the-counter fish oil preparations that are sold as dietary supplements are not FDA-regulated, and so their contents, purity, and safety cannot be guaranteed. In contrast, <u>Omacor/Lovaza</u> is now available as an FDA-approved prescription formulation that contains 465 mg EPA and 375 mg DHA (840 mg total fish oil) per 1-g capsule, and may be a safer alternative.

D. Hyperchylomicronemic emergencies. When TG levels rise to well over 1 000 mg/dL and <u>acute pancreatitis</u> is diagnosed or suspected, hospitalizing and keeping the patient NPO with intravenous fluid support will stop chylomicron production and allow the TG load to clear over several days. Once the TG level falls to <1 000 mg/dL, a very-low-fat diet should be gradually introduced. Other potential causes of pancreatitis should also be addressed. Strict dietary adherence must be emphasized, because of the high mortality of pancreatitis; fibrates, niacin, or high doses of omega-3 fatty acids may be added. TG levels seldom normalize, but proper adherence should keep the TG level low enough to minimize the risk of recurrent pancreatitis.

Selected References

Brunzell JD, Bierman EL. Chylomicronemia syndrome. *Med Clin North Am* 1982;66:455–467.

Canner PL, Berge KG, Wenger NK, et al. Fifteen year mortality in Coronary Drug Project patients: long-term benefit with niacin. *J Am Coll Cardiol* 1986;8:1245–1255.

Cannon CP, Braunwald E, McCabe CH, et al. Comparison of intensive and moderate lipid lowering with statins after acute coronary syndromes. *N Engl J Med* 2004;350:1495–1504.

Expert Panel on Detection, Evaluation, and Treatment of High Blood Cholesterol in Adults. Executive summary of the third report of the National Cholesterol Education Program (NCEP) Expert Panel on detection, evaluation, and treatment of high blood cholesterol in adults (Adult Treatment Panel III). *JAMA* 2001;285:2486–2497.

Frick MH, Elo O, Haapa K, et al. Helsinki Heart Study: primary-prevention trial with gemfibrozil in middle-aged men with dyslipidemia. Safety of treatment, changes in risk factors, and incidence of coronary heart disease. *N Engl J Med* 1987;317:1237–1245.

Grundy SM, Cleeman JI, Merz CNB, et al. Implications of recent clinical trials for the National Cholesterol Education Program Adult Treatment Panel III guidelines. *Circulation* 2004;110:227–239.

Heart Protection Study Collaborative Group. MRC/BHF Heart Protection Study of cholesterol lowering with simvastatin in 20,536 high-risk individuals: a randomized, placebo-controlled trial. *Lancet* 2002;360:7–22.

Hsia SH, Leiter LA. Obesity and dyslipidemia: epidemiology, physiology and effects of weight loss. *Endocrinologist* 1995;5:118–131.

Hu FB, Willett WC. Optimal diets for prevention of coronary heart disease. *JAMA* 2002;288:2569–2578.

Katan MB, Grundy SM, Jones P, et al. Efficacy and safety of plant stanols and sterols in the management of blood cholesterol levels. *Mayo Clinic Proc* 2003;78:965–978.

Kris-Etherton PM, Harris WS, Appel LJ, et al. Fish consumption, fish oil, omega-3 fatty acids, and cardiovascular disease. *Circulation* 2002;106:2747–2757.

Lipid Research Clinics Program. The Lipid Research Clinics Coronary Primary Prevention Trial results. I. Reduction in incidence of coronary heart disease. *JAMA* 1984;251:351–364.

Lipid Research Clinics Program. The Lipid Research Clinics Coronary Primary Prevention Trial results. II. The relationship of reduction in incidence of coronary heart disease to cholesterol lowering. *JAMA* 1984;251:365–374.

Lipoprotein and lipid metabolism disorders. In: Scriver CR, Beaudet AL, Sly WS, et al., eds. *The Metabolic and Molecular Bases of Inherited Diseases.* 7th ed. New York: McGraw-Hill; 1995:1841–2099.

NHLBI Obesity Education Initiative Expert Panel on the Identification, Evaluation, and Treatment of Overweight and Obesity in Adults. The practical guide: identification, evaluation, and treatment of overweight and obesity in adults. NIH Publication No. 00–4084, October 2000.

Ornish D, Brown SE, Scherwitz LW, et al. Can lifestyle changes reverse coronary heart disease? The Lifestyle Heart Trial. *Lancet* 1990;336:624–626.

Ros E. Intestinal absorption of triglyceride and cholesterol. Dietary and pharmacological inhibition to reduce cardiovascular risk. *Atherosclerosis* 2000;151:357–379.

Rubins HB, Robins SJ, Collins D, et al. Gemfibrozil for the secondary prevention of coronary heart disease in men with low levels of high-density lipoprotein cholesterol: Veterans Affairs High-Density Lipoprotein Cholesterol Intervention Trial Study Group. *N Engl J Med* 1999;341:410–418.

Scandinavian Simvastatin Survival Study Group. Randomised trial of cholesterol lowering in 4444 patients with coronary heart disease: the Scandinavian Simvastatin Survival Study (4S). *Lancet* 1994;344:1383–1389.

Schwartz GG, Olsson AG, Ezekowitz MD, et al. Effects of atorvastatin on early recurrent ischemic events in acute coronary syndromes: the MIRACL Study: a randomized controlled trial. *JAMA* 2001;285:1711–1718.

Shepherd J, Cobbe SM, Ford I, et al. Prevention of coronary heart disease with pravastatin in men with hypercholesterolemia. *N Engl J Med* 1995;333:1301–1307.

U.S. Department of Health and Human Services. Physical activity and health: a report of the Surgeon General. Atlanta: U.S. Department of Health and Human Services, Centers for Disease Control and Prevention, National Center for Chronic Disease Prevention and Health Promotion; 1996.

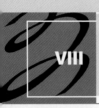

VIII Inborn Errors of Metabolism

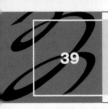

39

INTRODUCTION TO INBORN ERRORS OF METABOLISM
Stephen D. Cederbaum and Eric Vilain

I. GENERAL PRINCIPLES

Genetically determined inborn errors of metabolism are individually rare, but collectively they affect more than *1 in 500* individuals in the population. An abnormality in deoxyribonucleic acid (DNA) is expressed by the production of an enzyme that is deficient in its function of catalyzing and modulating the conversion of substrate to product. Each DNA abnormality results in a uniquely different protein product, some retaining full enzymatic potency, others retaining none, and others something in between. The resulting clinical picture ranges from normal to severely affected; the former can differ significantly in nature as well as severity from the most profound expression of the mutation. The severity of the clinical illness is influenced by other genetic characteristics and environmental circumstances of the patient.

A. Inheritance. Inborn errors of metabolism are generally inherited in an autosomal recessive or, less frequently, in a sex-linked recessive manner. Disorders of the electron-transport chain may be due to mutations in the mitochondrial genome and be inherited matrilineally. Instances of dominantly inherited inborn errors are rare, largely because 50% residual enzymatic activity appears to be sufficient for the retention of a normal phenotype. Some female carriers of sex-linked disorders can express the abnormal biochemical phenotype, probably because of the effect of X-chromosome inactivation. Most affected individuals have mental retardation and neurologic damage as cardinal features, but visceral organs may be affected, particularly in disorders of energy metabolism.

B. Categories. Inborn errors of metabolism can be divided into different categories (Table 39.1). The disorders of smaller, water-soluble substrates such as amino acids, organic acids, and sugars and disorders that impair energy generation in particular can cause acute disease, whereas those in the remaining categories cause more insidious disorders in which the onset of organ damage is slower and more indolent. Newer categories of disease are emerging as well; these are included in the list but are not discussed in detail. This discussion focuses on the first three categories, as they

568

TABLE 39.1	Classification of Inborn Errors of Metabolism

Small molecules
   Amino acids
   Organic acids
   Sugars
Lysosomal storage diseases
   Mucopolysaccharidoses
   Sphingolipidoses
   Mucolipidoses
Disorders of energy metabolism
   Oxidation defects
   Disorders of fatty acid mobilization and metabolism
   Glycogen storage diseases
Peroxisomal disorders
Disorders of cholesterol synthesis
Transport disorders
Carbohydrate-deficient glycoprotein disorders
Defects in purine and pyrimidine metabolism
Disorders of neurotransmitter metabolism
Receptor defects

are the most common, best understood, and most amenable to therapy. A number of inborn errors may present with hypoglycemia, but this is discussed elsewhere.

C. DNA. The explosion in the application of recombinant DNA methods to inborn errors of metabolism has altered our approach to these disorders in a number of diagnostic and therapeutic ways (e.g., utilizing DNA probes for prenatal diagnosis). This is especially true for newborn screening and will be discussed in the following.

II. DIAGNOSIS

A. Patient population. Except for a special category of disorders whose diagnosis is made, often pre-emptively, by population-wide newborn screening, the diagnosis of inborn errors of metabolism is established by recognizing a population of patients at higher risk, ascertained as a result of the presence of specific clinical features (Table 39.2). The clinical features can vary from neonatal collapse to a chemical abnormality lacking any clinical correlate. The early onset of symptoms or the profound metabolic derangements of later or intermittent occurrence are medical emergencies that require immediate therapeutic intervention. Examination of this list of clinical and laboratory findings in inborn errors clearly demonstrates that they are not unique to this group of diseases. The choice of patients to study further is based on one of three criteria:

1. A single sign or symptom persisting without adequate explanation

2. Several of the clinical findings coexisting without any other known basis

3. A clinical crisis compatible with an inborn error, making wholly rational and stepwise evaluation dangerously impractical

B. Diagnostic tests.

1. Inborn errors of small molecules and energy metabolism. Table 39.3 lists those tests that are part of the complete evaluation for inborn errors of intermediary metabolism. The routine tests listed are available in all but the smallest hospitals, whereas the specialized tests are sometimes available in tertiary centers for the study of inborn errors and, more prevalently, in some commercial clinical laboratories. The most commonly used specialized studies are the plasma amino

TABLE 39.2	Clinical and Laboratory Clues Suggesting the Presence of an Inborn Error of Metabolism

Signs and symptoms
  Neonatal catastrophe
  Developmental retardation
  Failure to thrive
  Gastrointestinal disorders
  Hyperpnea
  Neurologic and behavioral abnormalities
  Peculiar odors
  Organomegaly
  Ocular and/or hearing abnormalities
  Cutaneous changes
  Skeletal abnormalities
Laboratory clues
  Urine: ketones, reducing substances
  Blood: pancytopenia, acidosis, hypoglycemia, ketonemia
Course
  Developmental arrest or regression
Family history
  Consanguinity
  Similar illness

acid and urinary organic acid analyses. Urinary <u>organic acids</u> are most revealing in instances of acute, chronic, or intermittent metabolic acidosis. Spot specimens are usually adequate except in those instances in which the course is clearly intermittent. As we have become more aware of disorders of fatty acid oxidation as causes of inherited metabolic disease, plasma <u>acylcarnitine</u> analysis and plasma <u>carnitine</u> levels are more frequently obtained. With the advent of expanded newborn screening, virtually all children in developed countries will have been screened for disorders of amino acids, organic acids, fatty acid oxidation, and galactosemia. The previously used metabolic profile testing is most effectively deployed when reserved for children with a higher index of suspicion for an inborn error, and less as a routine procedure.

2. **Lysosomal storage diseases.** These disorders are characterized by relatively more normal levels of metabolites in the body fluids and more significant

TABLE 39.3	Laboratory Evaluation of Patients Suspected of Having an Inborn Error of Metabolism

Generally available studies
Blood sugar
Plasma and urine ketones
Blood pH and true bicarbonate
Blood lactate (and pyruvate)
Plasma ammonia

Specialized studies
Plasma amino acids
Urine organic acids
Plasma carnitine
Blood (or plasma) acylcarnitines
Mitochondrial DNA analysis

TABLE 39.4	Diagnosis of Lysosomal Diseases

Urinary mucopolysaccharide studies
Urinary oligosaccharide chromatography
Histologic examination of skin or conjunctival biopsy
Plasma "lysosomal enzyme screen"

abnormality within affected cells. The diagnosis is often suggested by the physical characteristics of the patients, which include coarsened physical features, abnormalities of the bones (described as dysostosis multiplex), and visceral enlargement. Standard laboratory approaches are listed in Table 39.4. Urine studies can indicate some lysosomal enzyme disorders through the detection of partially hydrolyzed, endogenous cellular constituents. Biopsy can expose abnormal material accumulation in cells. In centers with experience in reading conjunctival biopsies, this material is preferred to skin because of the wide variety of cell types represented and its diagnostic sensitivity. The plasma "lysosomal enzyme screen" is an ill-defined and variable battery of lysosomal enzyme assays that usually diagnose I-cell disease and the disorders whose enzymes are measured in a particular center. This approach carries a risk of misleading the clinician into believing, falsely, that lysosomal enzyme abnormalities have been ruled out.

C. Careful **neurologic and ophthalmologic evaluation** can be crucial to the diagnosis of a number of inborn errors of metabolism. Specialized tests might include auditory and somatosensory evoked responses, nerve conduction times, electromyograms, electroretinograms, and visual evoked responses. A lumbar puncture should be performed in any patient with undiagnosed neurologic disease, and glucose, amino acids, neurotransmitter, and lactate levels obtained. Nuclear magnetic resonance spectroscopy (MRS) is a powerful tool to measure brain levels of creatine, lactate, and glutamine, among others, and data for this analysis should be obtained whenever a neurologically handicapped child is having magnetic resonance imaging (MRI). If no diagnosis is made on MRI, then the MRS data should be analyzed.

D. **Enzymatic confirmation.** Some disorders of intermediary metabolism involve the only known enzyme responsible for the metabolism of a substrate, and enzyme assay in the face of substrate accumulation seems like an intellectual indulgence. In more instances the substrate accumulation can be due to a deficiency in one of several enzymes, so that appropriate therapy and an accurate prognosis depend on laboratory confirmation of the precise defect. Examples of incorrect inferences from substrate accumulation and current understanding of normal metabolism have been described repeatedly. It seems, then, that enzymatic or DNA confirmation of a putative defect should be the goal in every instance of an inborn error of intermediary metabolism and may be mandatory if prenatal diagnosis is contemplated.

E. **DNA studies.** The availability of DNA probes for many of the abnormal genes involved in inborn errors of metabolism has led to a definition of the primary genetic abnormality and to relatively simple means of diagnosis of those frequently seen in certain disorders. DNA studies might be preferable for those disorders in which the enzymatic diagnosis is difficult or not readily available, especially in prenatal diagnosis, where substrate accumulation can also fall short as a diagnostic indicator. Mitochondrial DNA studies are used frequently as a screen for disorders of the electron-transport chain, but the efficiency of this approach is open to question, particularly in patients in whom the prior probability is low. With advancing technology, the cost of sequencing DNA is falling and its ease is increasing. It is probable that DNA diagnosis will replace some enzyme assays as the confirmatory diagnostic method of choice, especially for those conditions that require invasive procedures, such as a liver biopsy, for diagnosis.

TABLE 39.5	Therapeutic Strategies for Inborn Errors of Intermediary Metabolism

Metabolite manipulation
  Substrate limitation
  Product supplementation
  Substrate diversion
  Inhibition of proximal enzyme
Enzyme augmentation
  Coenzyme (vitamin) supplementation
  Enzyme induction
  Enzyme replacement
    Allotransplantation
    Direct enzyme administration
      "Chaperone treatment"
    Enzyme reactor
Gene replacement

III. TREATMENT
A. General approaches.
1. **Small molecules and disorders of energy metabolism.** Management of these inborn errors is directed at alleviating the substrate accumulation or replacing the missing products of the reaction. There are two approaches to this: direct environmental manipulation of the metabolites, and augmentation or stabilization of the enzymatic levels. The different strategies for accomplishing these goals are given in Table 39.5.
   a. The most common treatment for disorders of intermediary metabolism is the **elimination diet** pioneered for galactosemia two generations ago and probably best associated with phenylketonuria (PKU). Whereas one can still constitute the galactose-poor diet for galactosemia from natural foods, that for PKU and for most other disorders is semisynthetic and derived from proprietary products. In the United States, a variety of dietary components are available from Mead-Johnson (Evansville, Indiana), Ross Laboratories (Columbus, Ohio), and Nutricia (Bethesda, Maryland), among others. These products can cause malnutrition if improperly used, and treatment is best carried out with the assistance of an expert in these disorders, at least until the pitfalls are clearly understood. Unlike in antibiotic therapy, the composition and amount of different components of the diet must be individualized for each patient because of the principles outlined at the beginning of this chapter. Therapy for an acute life-threatening episode is a unique instance in the application of these principles and is outlined in Section III.B.
   b. **Product supplementation** is well illustrated by the administration of glucose in glycogen storage diseases or excess lipid in pyruvate dehydrogenase deficiency. Several disorders, such as pyruvate dehydrogenase and pyruvate carboxylase deficiency, involve highly regulated enzymes in which moment-to-moment modulation of substrate-to-product transformation is mandatory. In these instances, external efforts to regulate metabolite levels are at best approximations of circumstances in the normal population, and only suboptimal results can be expected.
   c. More recently, a new approach has been brought to bear on the **control of substrate or precursor levels.** This involves augmenting precursor restriction with pharmacologic doses of chemicals that divert the poorly metabolized compounds into auxiliary pathways, diminishing the load on the defective enzymatic function. This is best illustrated by the use of **sodium benzoate and sodium phenylacetate** (or phenylbutyrate) in the management of

hyperammonemia. Benzoate is excreted as benzoylglycine (hippurate) and phenylacetate as phenylacetylglutamine, removing, respectively, 1 and 2 moles of nitrogen for each mole of organic acid added.

The two amino acids, when resynthesized in the body, divert ammonia that would have gone into the urea cycle. Similar approaches can prove useful with carnitine in an organic acid disorder such as methylmalonic acidemia and with betaine in homocystinuria.

2. **Vitamin or cofactor supplementation** is usually useful only for those disorders in which the deficient enzymatic phenotype is vitamin-responsive and refers only to the augmentation of the vitamin specifically involved in that reaction. Several types of inborn errors are involved.

   a. In the first, exemplified by vitamin B_{12}–responsive **methylmalonic acidemia,** the vitamin normally undergoes five or more genetically controlled processing steps prior to its function as cofactor in the enzymatic reaction converting methylmalonyl coenzyme A (methylmalonyl-CoA) to succinyl-CoA. Inherited deficiencies in these processing steps can be partially bypassed by administering huge doses of <u>vitamin B_{12}</u> (1 000 times the normal requirement, daily or several times a week).

   b. In the second type, the deficient enzyme is the catalytic one, which in some instances of specific mutations responds to augmented doses of its normal vitamin cofactor. This is best exemplified by <u>vitamin B_6</u> (pyridoxine)–responsive **homocystinuria.** The concordance of B_6 responsiveness in affected siblings in individual families confirms the site of the abnormality in the cystathionine synthase enzyme protein.

   c. In a third type, a vitamin cofactor or a compound mimicking a substrate or an inhibitor can act as a "chaperone" or stabilizing element for a mutant enzyme that has a shortened half-life in the cell. An example of this is <u>tetrahydro-biopterin (BH$_4$)</u>, a normal cofactor in the phenylalanine hydroxylase reaction. In some instances of missense mutations in the gene, it can stabilize the enzyme and allow better phenylalanine control and/or a more relaxed diet in patients with PKU.

   d. There are a number of proposals or protocols extant that suggest a cocktail of vitamins for treatment of disorders of the mitochondrial respiratory chain. Some of these are rational, but none has been proven efficacious.

3. Enzyme replacement with newer preparations of enzyme has proven to be effective for the palliation of **adenosine deaminase deficiency** and for **Gaucher disease** and an enlarging number of lysosomal storage disorders. The treatment costs are high, the response variable and dependent in part on the stage of the disease, the regimen arduous, but the approach represents a new and hopeful modality for patients who suffer from disorders that were previously untreatable.

   Bone marrow and renal transplantation seems to be effective in some cases of **lysosomal storage diseases,** whereas liver transplantation has been effective in disorders of intermediary metabolism, such as **hepato-renal tyrosinemia, Wilson disease, maple syrup urine disease,** and **urea cycle disorders,** in which activity of the missing enzyme is largely confined to the liver. Continued excitement and progress in this area are likely because all of the reagents and animal models are available for a number of disorders, including those caused by deficiencies of hypoxanthine-guanine phosphoribose transferase (Lesch-Nyhan syndrome), phenylalanine hydroxylase (PKU), ornithine transcarbamylase, and arginase, several lysosomal storage diseases, and many others.

4. Recently, [2-(nitro-4-trifluoromethylbenzoyl)-1,3-cyclohexanedione] (NT-BC), a specific inhibitor of 4-hydroxyphenylpyruvate dioxygenase, an enzyme proximal to fumarylacetoacetate hydrolase (the enzyme deficient in **hepatorenal tyrosinemia**), has proven to be miraculously efficacious in this disorder, presumably by starving the pathway of its toxic metabolite. Small-molecule inhibitors of glycosaminoglycan and sphingolipid biosynthesis are being studied as substitutes for or augmentors of enzyme replacement therapy in lysosomal storage disorders. Unlike the enzymes, they are usually accessible to the central nervous system.

Miglustat (Zavesca) has U.S. Food and Drug Administration (FDA) approval for the treatment of **Gaucher disease** and is being tried in others.

B. Therapy of acutely ill patients

1. **Diagnosis unknown.** The acute catastrophic presentation of an inborn error of metabolism requires **prompt** and decisive therapeutic **intervention,** even when the diagnosis is unknown. Therapy for these acutely ill infants must begin at once and then be modified when the diagnosis becomes known.

   a. At birth, the **signs and symptoms** are those of general multiorgan failure and cannot be distinguished from other neonatal emergencies, such as sepsis. They include lethargy, somnolence, irritability, rapid shallow respirations, jitteriness or seizures, poor temperature control, metabolic acidosis, hypoglycemia, and hypocalcemia. In older patients, the symptoms appear as an exaggerated response to minor infection or other stress and include neurologic signs, somnolence, acidosis, and, in some instances, hypoglycemia. The patients are often considered to have the postinfectious Reye syndrome, as a result of lethargy or coma, hepatomegaly with fat infiltration, hyperammonemia, hypoglycemia, and elevated plasma transaminase levels.

   b. Specimens for positive **diagnosis** must be obtained before the initiation of therapy, if possible. In case the patient's life cannot be saved, a rapid autopsy freezing liver, kidney, and brain at $-70°C$ is advisable.

   c. The principles of **therapy** at any age are similar, but the application requires modification according to the age and physiologic constraints of the patient.

      (1) **Elimination of protein** intake is mandatory in most instances and harmful in none. To minimize endogenous protein catabolism and gluconeogenesis, adequate calories in the form of carbohydrate and fat must be administered intravenously or intragastrically, with insulin if hyperglycemia occurs.

      (2) If metabolic acidosis is present, **blood lactate levels** must be ascertained, because at least one form of lactic acidosis is made worse by excessive glucose administration. In these instances, minimizing glucose intake to that needed to maintain blood glucose in the normal range and increasing fat is desirable.

      (3) **Bicarbonate** should be added to maintain plasma levels at 10 mEq/L or higher.

         If the situation is sufficiently serious and death or permanent brain damage seems imminent, peritoneal dialysis, at least, must be undertaken. Exchange transfusion is ineffective for disorders in which metabolite binding to plasma protein is not a problem. At least one exchange per hour of a twice-normal-osmolality dialysate should be used. However, peritoneal dialysis is less effective than hemodialysis or extracorporeal membrane oxygenation (ECMO). If deterioration continues and death seems possible, massive doses of all water-soluble vitamins (up to 1 000 times normal) are given. In cases of lactic acidosis, this vitamin mixture should include biotin. Once a definite or probable diagnosis has been made, more specific therapy can be instituted.

2. **Diagnosis known.** Although a protein-free diet is appropriate for the acute, short-term care of patients in virtually all metabolic catastrophes, soon plasma amino acid depletion causes protein breakdown and excessive levels of any amino acid whose catabolic pathway is impaired. Adequate regulation of plasma metabolite levels involves either intravenous or nasogastric repletion with an amino acid mixture properly constituted for the particular disorder.

   a. In **maple syrup urine disease,** a branched-chain-free amino acid mixture is used, with frequent plasma amino acid analyses to determine the appropriate amount of leucine, isoleucine, and valine added, usually from natural sources. In infants, the total amino acid intake should be no less than the amino nitrogen equivalent of 1.5 g protein per kilogram weight per day and at older ages no less than 1 g per kilogram per day.

   b. In **urea cycle defects** an essential amino acid mixture is used, and lower amounts may be required to keep ammonia levels near or in the normal range.

In most instances, specific or adaptable amino acid mixtures are unavailable for intravenous use, and enteral therapy with the amino acids alone is required. Fortunately, an adequate amino acid intake can be provided in extremely low volume. Amino acid preparations for a number of these disorders are available from commercial sources, but expect a delay of several days at least. These are not typically available in community hospitals.

    c. Hyperammonemia in which a primary organic acidemia is probably not the cause calls for special measures. In most instances, an <u>ammonia level of 500 μM</u> ($\sim$300 mg/dL) constitutes a serious threat to the central nervous system and, unless transient, should stimulate a heroic therapeutic response. The linchpin of this response, as noted, <u>is dialysis</u>. Because increased intracranial pressure is a common and threatening complication, efforts to ascertain and follow it are in order. Therapy consists of <u>mannitol</u>, extracellular volume depletion (difficult, but not impossible with dialysis), phenobarbital coma (efficacy not proven), and hyperventilation. <u>Sodium benzoate</u> and <u>sodium phenylacetate</u> in a combined preparation (Ammonul, Ucyclyd, Pheonix, AZ) is available and should be given at a dose of 500 mg (of each) per kilogram per day. A loading dose of 250 mg/kg over 90 minutes may be given. When the ammonia level abates, the infusion is reduced to 250 mg/kg per day.

    d. One product of the urea cycle is **arginine,** and this ordinarily semiessential amino acid can be <u>deficient in most of</u> these disorders. In all suspected urea cycle defects, it is supplemented at 2 mmol/kg per day, initially. In the case of **citrullinemia** and especially **argininosuccinic acidemia,** arginine, at dosages of up to 6 mmol/kg per day, can correct the hyperammonia. Fortunately, arginine hydrochloride is readily available as an intravenous preparation for growth-hormone studies. Its use can induce hyperchloremic acidosis, and patients must be closely monitored for this.

C. Long-term therapy. This form of treatment is the heart of the management of inborn errors of metabolism and embodies the same principles enumerated for the acute management of this class of disorders. Patients may require restriction of the substrate and provision of the product. They must be adequately nourished. Enzyme levels must be maximized, and catabolism is best avoided. In this circumstance, when immediate intervention is not required, therapy is best supervised by individuals trained in the management of these disorders.

1. The hyperphenylalaninemias

    a. No family of disorders better epitomizes the problems and principles in the approach to the inborn errors of metabolism than the hyperphenylalaninemias. They will be used to illustrate the principles of long term therapy in inborn errors. The majority of patients with hyperphenylalaninemia have a partial or complete <u>deficiency</u> of the apoenzyme <u>phenylalanine hydroxylase</u>. About 1% or fewer of patients are deficient in the ability to synthesize or reduce the cofactor dihydrobiopterin. The reduced form, tetrahydrobiopterin, also participates in the hydroxylation of tyrosine and tryptophan to L-DOPA and serotonin. The enzyme deficiency leads to deficiency of these neurotransmitters and a quite different and less readily treatable disorder. The primary enzyme defect in all hyperphenylalaninemic patients must be inferred from specific testing for cofactor abnormalities.

    b. The object of therapy is to bring phenylalanine levels to <350 μM if possible. Treatment consists of <u>reducing phenylalanine</u> intake from natural sources and supplementing the diet with amino acid products containing little or no phenylalanine. Practically speaking, the diet is a vegetarian one with focus on those fruits and vegetables that are particularly low in protein. Unlike a natural vegetarian diet, other essential amino acids are provided from synthetic products largely distributed through the commercial sources noted previously.

    c. Effective treatment has produced a population of intellectually normal affected women of child-bearing age. Such women, with various degrees of hyperphenylalaninemia, have heterozygote offspring that are at risk of having serious abnormalities, such as mental retardation, microcephaly, and cardiac malformations. **Dietary treatment during pregnancy** appears to improve the chances of delivery of a normal infant. And these woman should be placed on therapy before and during pregnancy, at least.

D. Newborn screening. Until recently, newborn screening was limited, at best, to a few disorders of amino acid metabolism, to hypothyroidism, and, on a more limited basis, congenital adrenal hyperplasia and hemoglobinopathies. With the advent of high-throughput, automated screening of newborn blood spots, particularly, the menu of disorders screened has expanded greatly, although it differs from state to state and internationally. Most disorders of amino acids, organic acids, and fatty acids and others can be diagnosed at birth with a high degree of probability using tandem mass spectrometry (MS/MS). In the near future it is likely that still more conditions, such as most lysosomal storage disorders, adrenoleukodystrophy, and immunodeficiencies, will prove amenable to screening as well. The list of primary and secondary screening targets currently recommended by the American College of Medical Genetics can be found on their web site, www.acmg.net. Although not apparent so far, once integrated into our diagnostic algorithms, newborn screening will alter the way that we approach symptomatic individuals.

Selected References

Blau N, et al., eds. *Physicians Guide to the Treatment and Followup of Metabolic Diseases.* New York: Springer-Verlag; 2006.

Fernandes J, ed. *Inborn Metabolic Diseases: Diagnosis and Treatment.* 4th ed. New York: Springer-Verlag; 2006.

McKusick VA. *Mendelian Inheritance in Man.* www3.ncbi.nlm.nih.gov/OMIM.

Scriver CR, Beaudet AL, Sly WS, et al., eds. *The Metabolic and Molecular Basis of Inherited Disease.* 8th ed. New York: McGraw-Hill; 2001. This book will no longer be published in a print edition. It is updated continually and available online at www.genetics.accessmed.com.

Joseph I. Wolfsdorf and Michael A. Dedekian

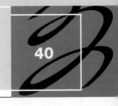

I. GENERAL PRINCIPLES

The glycogen storage diseases (GSDs) or glycogenoses comprise several inherited diseases caused by deficiencies of the enzymes that regulate the synthesis or degradation of glycogen. As a result, increased storage of glycogen occurs in several tissues, especially liver and muscle.

- **A. The structure of glycogen.** Glycogen is the only storage form of carbohydrate in humans and is likely present in all cells. It is a highly branched polymer of glucose residues, most of which form straight chains linked by α-1,4-glycosidic bonds. The branches are created by α-1,6-glycosidic bonds, which occur on the average of once in 10 residues. The two major sites of glycogen storage are the liver and skeletal muscle. During carbohydrate feeding the concentration of glycogen in the liver is 5 g/100 g wet weight; its concentration in muscle is 2 g/100 g wet weight. Because of the greater mass of skeletal muscle, more glycogen is stored in muscle than in the liver.
- **B. Glycogen synthesis, degradation, and conversion to glucose**
  - **1. Glycogen synthesis and degradation** in the liver follow distinct pathways that begin and end with glucose 1-phosphate (Fig. 40.1). The liver is freely permeable to glucose, which is first converted to glucose 6-phosphate (G6P) before it can enter one of several metabolic pathways. Glucose 6-phosphate can be reversibly converted to glucose 1-phosphate, which is the starting point for glycogen synthesis. Alternatively, glucose 6-phosphate can be hydrolyzed to glucose by glucose 6-phosphatase or it can be metabolized via the glycolytic pathway to pyruvate and lactate or, via the pentose phosphate pathway, to ribose 5-phosphate, a precursor of nucleotide synthesis. Glycogen synthase catalyzes the formation of α-1,4-linkages. A branching enzyme forms the α-1,6-linkages that make glycogen a branched polymer.
  - **2. Glycogen breakdown** requires the sequential interaction of several enzymes. First, phosphorylase successively cleaves the 1,4 links to within four glucosyl units of the branch point. Then 4-α-glucanotransferase exposes the 1,6-linked branch points by transferring three glucosyl residues elsewhere on the glycogen molecule. Amylo-1,6-glucosidase, the debranching enzyme, then splits the 1,6-linked glucosyl units. Thus, the sequential action of these enzymes liberates the stored glucose units; the action of phosphorylase yields glucose 1-phosphate, and the debranching enzyme liberates free glucose. Under normal conditions of fasting, some 8% of the glycogen is mobilized as free glucose by the debrancher enzyme. The remaining glucose mobilized in the fasted state requires hepatic glucose 6-phosphatase activity.
- **C. Clinical features of the hepatic glycogenoses.** The types of hepatic glycogenoses, the specific enzyme deficiencies, affected tissues, their modes of inheritance, and the chromosomal localization of the relevant genes are shown in Table 40.1. Table 40.2 lists the major biochemical characteristics of the hepatic glycogenoses (types 0, I, III, VI, and IX); their hallmark is **fasting hypoglycemia.**

II. GLYCOGEN STORAGE DISEASES

- **A. Glycogen synthase deficiency (type 0 GSD)**
  - **1. The nature of the defect.** Lack of liver glycogen synthase activity is a rare disorder that results in a marked decrease in liver glycogen content (0.5 g/100 g wet

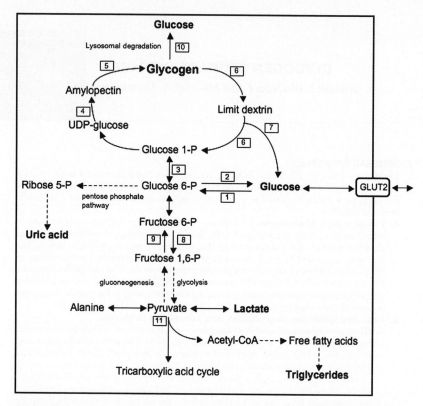

Figure 40.1. Simplified scheme of glycogen synthesis and degradation in the liver. UDP-glucose is uridine diphosphoglucose; 1, hexokinase/glucokinase; 2, glucose 6-phosphatase; 3, phosphoglucomutase; 4, glycogen synthase; 5, branching enzyme; 6, glycogen phosphorylase; 7, debranching enzyme; 8, phosphofructokinase; 9, fructose 1,6-bisphosphatase; 10, acid maltase; 11, pyruvate dehydrogenase.

weight 4 to 6 hours after a meal). Because dietary glucose cannot be stored as glycogen, glucose is preferentially converted to lactate.

2. **Clinical manifestations.** Symptoms of morning hypoglycemia appear with the cessation of nocturnal feeding. The disorder causes a unique metabolic disturbance characterized by <u>fasting hypoglycemia</u> and <u>hyperketonemia</u>, alternating with daytime hyperglycemia and hyperlacticacidemia after meals. Unlike the other GSDs that cause hypoglycemia, the <u>liver is not enlarged</u>. The disorder should be considered in the differential diagnosis of any child who presents with ketosis and hypoglycemia.

3. **Laboratory findings**
   a. **General laboratory tests.** Typical features are fasting hypoglycemia with ketosis and postprandial hyperglycemia and hyperlacticacidemia.
   b. **Provocative laboratory tests.** (See Section II.B.3.b for a general approach to defining the metabolic consequences of enzymatic deficiencies.) After an overnight fast, oral glucose (1.75 g/kg) causes hyperglycemia and hyperlacticacidemia, whereas glucagon (0.03 mg/kg IM) typically has no effect on the blood glucose level.
   c. **Specific laboratory tests.** Genetic testing for mutations in GYS2 is commercially available (refer to genetests.org for laboratory listing).

TABLE 40.1 Hepatic Glycogen Storage Diseases

Disorder	Affected tissue	Enzyme	Inheritance	Gene	Chromosome
Type 0 GSD	Liver	Glycogen synthase	AR	GYS2	12p12.2
Type Ia GSD	Liver, kidney, intestine	Glucose 6-phosphatase	AR	G6PC	17q21
Type Ib GSD	Liver	Glucose 6-phosphate transporter (T1)	AR	G6PT1	11q23
Type IIIa GSD	Liver, muscle, heart	Glycogen debranching enzyme	AR	AGL	1p21
Type IIIb GSD	Liver	Glycogen debranching enzyme	AR	AGL	1p21
Type VI GSD	Liver	Glycogen phosphorylase	AR	PYGL	14q21–22
Type IX GSD	Liver, erythrocytes, leukocytes	Liver isoform of α subunit of phosphorylase kinase	X-linked	PHKA2	Xp22.1–p22.2
	Liver muscle, erythrocytes, leukocytes	β subunit of liver and muscle phosphorylase kinase	AR	PHKB	16q12–q13
	Liver	Testis/liver isoform of γ subunit of phosphorylase kinase	AR	PHKG2	16p11–p12

AR, autosomal recessive.

579

TABLE 40.2 Biochemical Characteristics of the Hepatic Glycogenoses

Type	At time of hypoglycemia			Response to oral glucose		Response to glucagon 4–8 h after a meal[a]		Response to glucagon 2 h after a meal	
	Triglyceride	Uric acid	Lactate	Glucose	Lactate	Glucose	Lactate	Glucose	Lactate
GSD-0	N	N	N	↑↑	↑↑	0–↑	0	↑	→
GSD-I	↑↑↑	↑↑	↑↑↑	↑	↓↓	0	↑↑↑	0	↑↑
GSD-III	↑	N	N	↑	↑	0	0	↑	0
GSD-VI, IX	0–↑	N	N	↑	↑	0–↑	0	↑	0

N, normal; 0, no increase; 0–↑, variable increase; ↑, mild increase; ↑↑, moderate increase; ↑↑↑, marked increase; ↓, mild decrease; ↓↓, moderate decrease.
Subjects with suspected GSD-I should not be permitted to fast for more than 4 h.
[a]After a meal that provides glucose.

4. Treatment. The goal of treatment is to prevent hypoglycemia and ketosis during the night and hyperglycemia and hyperlacticacidemia during the day. Fasting hypoglycemia and ketosis are prevented by bedtime feedings of <u>uncooked cornstarch</u>, 1 to 1.5 g/kg. During illness, administration of a similar dose of cornstarch every 6 hours is used to prevent hypoglycemia. During the day, patients are fed frequently (e.g., every 4 hours). The diet should contain an increased amount of protein to provide substrate for gluconeogenesis, and a decreased amount of carbohydrate to minimize postprandial hyperglycemia and hyperlacticacidemia. The diet should contain predominantly complex, low-glycemic-index carbohydrates. Such a diet and feeding schedule relieves symptoms, reverses the biochemical abnormalities, and improves growth.

B. Glucose 6-phosphatase deficiency (<u>type I GSD</u>; von Gierke disease; hepatorenal glycogenosis)

1. The nature of the defect

  a. von Gierke first described this disorder in 1929; the enzyme defect was discovered by Cori and Cori in 1952. The disease results from lack of activity of the hepatic enzyme **glucose 6-phosphatase**, which catalyzes the final step in the production of glucose from glucose 6-phosphate. Deficiency of this enzyme, therefore, impairs glucose production both from glycogenolysis and gluconeogenesis. In its absence, there is decreased production of glucose, resulting in interprandial hypoglycemia and increased production of lactate, uric acid, and triglyceride. Glycogen and triglycerides accumulate in the liver, resulting in marked <u>hepatomegaly</u>.

  b. The **glucose 6-phosphatase enzyme** system comprises several subunits. The catalytic subunit catalyzes the terminal reaction of glycogenolysis and gluconeogenesis, conversion of glucose 6-phosphate to glucose. Glucose 6-phosphatase is located in the endoplasmic reticulum (ER) membrane; the active site faces into the ER lumen. Three transport systems transport the substrate, G6P, and the products, phosphate, inorganic orthophosphate, and glucose across the ER membrane. G6P transporter transports G6P into the ER. Current evidence suggests that the G6P transporter also transports phosphate out of the ER; glucose is transported out of the ER by GLUT2.

  c. Approximately 80% of patients with GSD-1 have deficient catalytic activity of the glucose 6-phosphatase system, which causes **type Ia GSD (GSD-Ia)**. Approximately 100 different mutations have been found in the gene that encodes G6Pase in patients with GSD-Ia.

  d. These mutations have not been found in patients **with type Ib**, which is caused by failure to transport G6P into the lumen of the ER owing to a mutation in the G6PT1 gene (about 80 mutations have been identified) that causes deficiency of the G6P transporter.

2. Clinical manifestations

  a. GSD-1 has an estimated incidence of 1 in 200 000 births. It affects the sexes equally and is transmitted as an autosomal recessive trait.

  b. The presenting **clinical symptoms** of this disease vary according to the patient's age. Symptomatic **hypoglycemia** may appear soon after birth; however, most patients are asymptomatic as long as they receive frequent feedings that contain sufficient glucose to prevent hypoglycemia. Symptoms of hypoglycemia typically appear only when the interval between feedings increases, such as when the infant starts to sleep through the night or when an intercurrent illness disrupts normal feeding.

  c. The condition may not be recognized until the child is several months old and an **enlarged liver and protuberant abdomen** are noted during a routine physical examination. Patients may present with hyperpnea from lactic acidosis and a low-grade fever without a demonstrable infection. Untreated patients may have a cushingoid appearance, failure to thrive, and delayed motor development. Social and cognitive development is not affected unless the infant suffers cerebral damage from recurrent hypoglycemic seizures.

(1) During infancy, the blood glucose concentration may fall to <40 mg/dL within 3 to 4 hours of a feeding. Longer intervals between feedings cause more severe hypoglycemia accompanied by **hyperlacticacidemia** and metabolic acidosis.

(2) The serum of untreated patients may be cloudy or milky, with very **high triglyceride concentrations** and moderately increased levels of phospholipids, total and low-density lipoprotein-cholesterol; high-density lipoprotein-cholesterol is low. High triglyceride concentrations result from increased hepatic synthesis (mobilization of fat from adipose tissue in response to hypoglycemia), impaired ketogenesis, and reduced clearance secondary to decreased lipoprotein lipase activity. The circulating concentration of free fatty acids is markedly increased. Eruptive xanthomata may appear on the extensor surfaces of the extremities and on the buttocks. Severe hypertriglyceridemia (>1 000 mg/dL) is associated with an increased risk of acute pancreatitis.

(3) A **bleeding tendency** manifested as recurrent epistaxis or oozing after dental or other surgery is caused by impaired platelet function. Reduced platelet adhesiveness, abnormal platelet aggregation, and impaired release of adenosine diphosphate (ADP) in response to collagen and epinephrine have been observed. The platelet defects are secondary to the systemic metabolic abnormalities and are corrected by improving the metabolic state.

(4) Although hypoglycemia becomes less severe with increasing age, inadequate therapy causes pronounced **impairment of growth and delayed onset of puberty.** However, when continuous glucose therapy is started early in life and long-term good metabolic control is maintained, patients can grow and develop normally.

(5) **Nephromegaly** is readily demonstrated by ultrasonography in GSD-1. Deficiency of glucose 6-phosphatase disturbs the metabolism of renal tubular cells, resulting in a relative energy deficiency. Increased renal blood flow and glomerular filtration rate may be a compensatory mechanism for the intracellular energy deficit. Proximal tubular dysfunction (glucosuria, phosphaturia, hypokalemia, and a generalized aminoaciduria) is reversible when biochemical control of the disease improves. Some patients have a distal renal tubular acidification defect associated with hypocitraturia and hypercalciuria, which predisposes to nephrocalcinosis and renal calculi. Increased urinary albumin excretion may be observed in adolescents. More severe renal injury with proteinuria, hypertension, and decreased creatinine clearance due to focal segmental glomerulosclerosis and interstitial fibrosis, which leads ultimately to end-stage renal disease, may be seen in young adults. Patients with persistently elevated blood lactate, serum lipids, and uric acid concentrations appear to be at increased risk of developing nephropathy. Normalization of metabolic parameters decreases proteinuria, and optimal therapy instituted at or before age 1 year may delay, prevent, or slow the progression of renal disease.

(6) Development of **hepatic adenomas** is a common complication occurring in a majority of patients by the time they reach adulthood. Whereas they are usually first observed in the second and third decades of life, they may appear before puberty. Adenomas may undergo malignant degeneration or hemorrhage. Ultrasonography is the preferred method of screening for hepatic adenomas. Magnetic resonance imaging provides greater definition when malignancy is suspected because of a change in appearance from a small, well-circumscribed lesion to one that is larger and poorly marginated. Serum α-fetoprotein levels are normal in patients with adenomas but have been elevated in some cases of hepatocellular carcinoma.

(7) Radiographic studies have demonstrated **osteopenia**, and pathologic studies reveal pure osteoporosis without evidence of abnormalities in calcium, phosphate, parathyroid, or vitamin D metabolism. Bone mineral content is decreased compared to normal children of the same age. Endocrine and metabolic disturbances, including lactic acidosis, elevated cortisol levels, resistance to growth hormone, and delayed pubertal development, may account for decreased bone mineralization.

(8) Menstrual irregularities and hirsutism are uncommon; however, in all types of hepatic GSDs, ultrasonography demonstrates a high prevalence of morphologically polycystic ovaries (even in prepubertal children), the clinical significance of which is still unclear.

(9) Pulmonary hypertension presenting in the second or third decade of life and leading to death from progressive heart failure has been described.

   d. Patients with **GSD-Ib** have similar symptoms, typically, with the addition of either constant or cyclic **neutropenia**, the severity of which ranges from mild to complete agranulocytosis and is associated with recurrent bacterial infections. Neutropenia is a consequence of disturbed myeloid maturation and is accompanied by functional defects of circulating neutrophils and monocytes. Patients frequently develop an **inflammatory bowel disease** resembling Crohn disease, which is responsive to treatment with granulocyte colony-stimulating factor (GCSF). Children with GSD-Ib are prone to **oral complications**, including recurrent mucosal ulceration, gingivitis, and rapidly progressive periodontal disease. Patients with GSD-Ib may have an increased prevalence of thyroid autoimmunity and primary hypothyroidism.

3. Laboratory findings

   a. General laboratory tests. During infancy, the blood glucose concentration typically falls to <40 mg/dL 3 to 4 hours after a feeding and is accompanied by hyperlacticacidemia and metabolic acidosis. The serum may be cloudy or milky, with very high triglyceride and moderately increased levels of cholesterol. Serum uric acid is increased and serum aspartate aminotransferase (AST) and alanine aminotransferase (ALT) levels are usually increased.

   b. Provocative laboratory tests

      (1) The simplest means of determining the probable nature of the enzymatic deficiency in a child suspected of having a glycogenosis is to obtain **serial blood samples for measurement of metabolites** (glucose, lactate, free fatty acids, ketones, and uric acid) for up to 6 hours (or until the plasma glucose concentration falls to ≤45 mg/dL) following oral glucose (1.75 g/kg) or 30 minutes after stopping a continuous overnight intravenous or intragastric infusion of glucose.

      (2) The plasma glucose and blood lactate responses to **glucagon** (30 μg/kg, maximum 1 mg, either IM or IV bolus), 4 to 6 hours after a meal or after the administration of oral glucose, is also a valuable functional test to evaluate a child with suspected GSD. Blood samples for measurement of glucose and lactate concentrations are obtained 1 minute before and then at 15, 30, 45, and 60 minutes after glucagon is injected. In GSD-I, glucagon causes little or no increase in the blood glucose concentration. In contrast, the blood lactate level, typically already markedly increased, increases further (Table 40.2).

   c. Specific laboratory tests. Mutational analysis is recommended to confirm type I GSD. A **liver biopsy** for measurement of glucose 6-phosphatase activity may be necessary in the small minority of patients who do not have an identifiable gene mutation. The glycogen itself has a normal appearance.

4. Treatment consists of providing a continuous dietary source of glucose to prevent the blood glucose concentration from falling below the threshold for glucose counterregulation or ~70 to 75 mg/dL. When hypoglycemia is prevented by providing an appropriate amount of glucose throughout the day and night, the biochemical abnormalities are ameliorated, liver size decreases, the bleeding tendency is reversed, and growth improves.

   a. Supply of glucose

      (1) Various methods may be used to provide a continuous source of glucose at a rate sufficient to satisfy glucose requirements in the intervals between meals: intravenously, via the gastrointestinal tract by intragastric infusion (either nasogastric or gastrostomy tube), or by use of low-glycemic-index foods. Of these, uncooked cornstarch has the most suitable properties described to date. The minimum amount of glucose required may be obtained by using the formula for calculating the basal glucose production rate:

$$y = 0.0014^3 - 0.214x^2 + 10.411x - 9.084$$

where y = mg glucose per minute and x = ideal body weight in kilograms. The amounts and/or schedule of glucose or uncooked cornstarch administered are modified, if necessary, based on the results of clinical and biochemical monitoring.

(2) In **infants**, we recommend feedings every 2 to 3 hours of a formula that does not contain either lactose or sucrose. The formula must contain a polymer of glucose (corn syrup solids, maltodextrins) that will yield, after digestion, an amount of glucose equal to the calculated glucose production rate. If nighttime feedings prove to be a problem, continuous overnight feedings using the same formula may be given via nasogastric or gastrostomy tube with the rate controlled by an infusion pump.

(3) Orally administered **uncooked cornstarch** acts as an intestinal reservoir of glucose that is slowly absorbed into the circulation. In many centers, uncooked cornstarch has replaced frequent daytime feedings of glucose or glucose polymers and overnight continuous intragastric infusion of glucose. It has been used successfully in infants as young as 8 months of age. The uncooked cornstarch is given in a slurry of water or artificially sweetened fluid (e.g., Kool-Aid) or in formula for infants, at 3- to 5-hour intervals during the day and at 4- to 6-hour intervals overnight. The amount given is determined by multiplying the time interval between feedings by the hourly glucose requirement for ideal body weight. One tablespoon (8 g) of cornstarch contains 7.3 g of carbohydrate. The optimum schedule and amounts of intermittent uncooked cornstarch feedings for patients of different ages is determined empirically by metabolic monitoring to ensure that the biochemical goals are being achieved.

b. When adequate exogenous glucose is provided in this manner, significant **hyperuricemia** and **hyperlipidemia** are usually restored to near normal. If severe hyperuricemia persists, allopurinol, a xanthine oxidase inhibitor (5 to 10 mg/kg per day as a single daily dose or divided q12 hours), effectively lowers serum uric acid to normal levels. Lipid-lowering agents (gemfibrozil or fenofibrate) are indicated when persistent severe hyperlipidemia despite optimal glucose therapy poses a significant risk of acute pancreatitis.

c. **Dietary fat** should be restricted to ~20% of the total energy intake, equally distributed among monounsaturated, polyunsaturated, and saturated fats. Dietary cholesterol is restricted to <300 mg per day. Carbohydrate typically provides ~60% to 65% of the daily calories. Of the total daily calories, ~30% to 45% is prescribed (both the amount and schedule) in the form of uncooked cornstarch. Most of the remaining dietary carbohydrate should, ideally, be low-glycemic-index starches. With the glucose requirements prescribed, the total caloric intake is determined largely by the child's appetite as long as the rate of weight gain is not excessive. The dietitian must ensure that the patient is consuming an adequate amount of protein, fat, minerals, and vitamins to support optimal growth. When adequate glucose is prescribed to maintain normoglycemia, milk products and fruit, despite their content of galactose and fructose, respectively, may be used sparingly to supply essential nutrients, minerals, and vitamins.

C. Amylo-1,6-glucosidase deficiency (type III GSD; debranching enzyme deficiency; limit dextrinosis; Cori disease; Forbes disease)

1. Nature of the defect

a. Two enzymes are involved in hydrolyzing the 1,6-linkages of glycogen. After phosphorylase has acted exhaustively on the outer branches, four glucosyl residues remain distal to the branch point. An oligo-1,4→1,4 glucan transferase transfers three glucosyl residues from the end of a branch to form an α-1,4-linkage with another chain, thus exposing the 1,6-linkage. The amylo-1,6-glucosidase can then hydrolyze the single glucose molecule linked α-1,6 to the main chain and produce free glucose. Absent debrancher activity permits breakdown of glycogen to proceed until the outermost branch points are reached, at which point further degradation is no longer possible. This leaves a limit dextrin, which consists of the core of the molecule bearing short branches of about four glucose units in length.

   b. There are four isoforms of the debranching enzyme. Isoform 1, the most widely distributed and the predominant form in the liver, is defective in GSD-IIIa. Isoforms 2, 3, and 4 are exclusively located in skeletal and cardiac muscle.

   c. The gene for all debranching enzyme isoforms is located on chromosome 1p21. Differential splicing of the 5'-untranslated region accounts for the various isoforms; all share the same translation initiation site. Mutations adjacent to the amino terminus are associated with a milder phenotype involving isolated deficiency of debranching enzyme activity in the liver only (GSD-IIIb).

   d. In the United States, 80% to 85% of patients with GSD-III lack debranching enzyme activity in both liver and muscle (GSD-IIIa). In contrast, the majority of Israeli patients lack enzyme activity only in the liver.

2. **Clinical manifestations**

   a. Clinical and enzymatic variability is a feature of glycogen debranching enzyme deficiency. During infancy and childhood, the disease may be indistinguishable from GSD-I. Hepatomegaly, fasting hypoglycemia with ketosis, hyperlipidemia, and growth retardation are the predominant features. About 70% of patients have muscle weakness, but this is usually not clinically significant in childhood.

   b. Biochemical distinctions between GSD-III and GSD-I

   (1) Because glucose can be produced from 1,4-segments beyond the outermost branch points and from gluconeogenesis, patients with debranching enzyme deficiency are usually able to tolerate longer periods of fasting, and **hypoglycemia usually is less severe** than in those with glucose 6-phosphatase deficiency. Indeed, hypoglycemia is common but not invariable. Infants with GSD-III may be asymptomatic on their usual frequent feeding schedules, and do not become as severely ill with infections and other stresses that disrupt feeding as do children with GSD-1.

   (2) Infants with GSD-III develop **fasting hyperketonemia** as a result of an accelerated transition to the starving state. **Blood levels of lactate and uric acid are normal** because the gluconeogenic pathway is intact and hepatic glycolysis is not increased.

   (3) Hyperlipidemia is less marked in GSD-III than in GSD-I.

   c. Physical characteristics. The presenting clinical finding may be hepatomegaly and growth failure. An **enlarged spleen** may be seen at 4 to 6 years of age in patients who have hepatic fibrosis. The kidneys are not enlarged; renal dysfunction does not occur. Untreated infants and children have a decreased rate of linear growth, and puberty is delayed. In patients who lack the enzyme in muscle, weakness is usually minimal and not clinically significant in childhood.

   d. Chronic conditions

   (1) Myopathy. With the exception of myopathy, symptoms and signs characteristically ameliorate with increasing age. Myopathy, however, usually becomes prominent in the third or fourth decade of life, manifesting as slowly progressive muscle weakness involving the proximal muscles. Some patients also have involvement of the small muscles of the hands.

   (2) Cardiac. Abnormal glycogen (limit dextrin) may accumulate in the heart, resulting in the development of a cardiomyopathy that resembles idiopathic hypertrophic cardiomyopathy. Significant concentric left ventricular hypertrophy usually develops after puberty. Subclinical evidence of cardiac involvement is common and manifests as ventricular hypertrophy on electrocardiogram (EKG) and echocardiographic abnormalities. Ventricular function, however, is usually relatively normal. Severe cardiac dysfunction and dysrhythmias are uncommon causes of cardiac mortality.

(3) Hepatic. The size of the liver tends to decrease to normal during puberty; however, biopsy usually shows hepatic fibrosis, and some adult patients develop cirrhosis. Hepatic <u>adenomas</u> have been found in 25% of patients. The development of hepatocellular carcinoma is rare but has recently been described in adult patients.

3. Laboratory findings

a. General laboratory tests. There is fasting hypoglycemia with ketosis and mild hypercholesterolemia and hypertriglyceridemia without elevation of blood lactate and serum uric acid concentrations. Liver transaminases are consistently elevated in children but decline at puberty and may be normal in adults.

b. Provocative laboratory tests. (See Section II.B.3.b for general approach.) After an overnight fast, blood glucose and lactate concentrations do not increase after administration of glucagon (30 μg/kg, maximum 1 mg IM or IV). When the test is repeated 2 hours after a high-carbohydrate meal (which lengthens the outer branches of glycogen), a glycemic response is elicited.

c. Specific assays. Definitive subtyping of GSD-III requires a <u>biopsy of both liver and muscle</u>. While muscle involvement can be inferred from the presence of high levels of serum creatine phosphokinase, a normal level does not rule out muscle enzyme deficiency. At the time of diagnosis, muscle biopsy is the only way to predict accurately whether skeletal muscle disease or heart muscle involvement is likely to develop in the future. Mutation analysis can be used to confirm clinical or enzymatic diagnosis.

4. Treatment. Because only a limited amount of glucose can be mobilized from glycogen, hypoglycemia develops during an overnight fast in infancy and early childhood. This occurs despite increased gluconeogenesis and enhanced hepatic uptake of gluconeogenic amino acids, which results in low levels of several plasma amino acids.

a. Thus, as in GSD-I, continuous provision of an adequate amount of glucose, using <u>uncooked cornstarch</u> (see Section II.B.4), combined with a normal intake of total calories, protein, and other nutrients, corrects the clinical and biochemical disorder and restores normal growth. Uncooked cornstarch, 1.75 g/kg at 6-hour intervals (e.g., at midnight, 6 A.M., etc.) maintains normoglycemia, increases growth velocity, and decreases serum aminotransferase concentrations.

b. For patients who have significant **growth retardation and myopathy**, continuous nocturnal feeding of a nutrient mixture composed of glucose, glucose oligosaccharides, and amino acids combined with intermittent feedings during the day of meals with a **high protein** content may be beneficial.

c. As in patients with GSD-I, annual measurement of **serum α-fetoprotein** and **hepatic ultrasound examinations** should be performed to screen for hepatic adenomas. Magnetic resonance imaging of the liver should be performed when an adenoma increases in size. Patients with muscle disease should have intermittent cardiac evaluations, including an EKG and echocardiogram.

D. Hepatic phosphorylase complex deficiency (<u>type VI GSD</u>, hepatic phosphorylase deficiency, Hers disease; type IX GSD, phosphorylase kinase deficiency)

1. Nature of the defect

a. Activation of hepatic phosphorylase, the rate-limiting enzyme of glycogenolysis, is activated by a cascade of enzymatic reactions. First, adenylate cyclase catalyzes the formation of cyclic adenosine monophosphate (cAMP), which then activates a cAMP-dependent protein kinase. Protein kinase then phosphorylates a phosphorylase kinase (PHK), which converts inactive hepatic phosphorylase to its active form. Active phosphorylase mobilizes glucose from glycogen. This cascade of reactions is triggered primarily by glucagon.

b. The GSDs caused by a reduction in liver phosphorylase activity are a heterogeneous group of disorders (Table 40.1). The most common disorder in this group is deficiency of hepatic PHK or type IX GSD. It occurs in approximately 1 in 100 000 births and accounts for ~25% of all cases of GSDs. Deficiency of hepatic phosphorylase itself is rare.

  c. PHK of liver and muscle is a complex enzyme consisting of four subunits: α, β, γ, δ. The enzyme is regulated by phosphorylation of specific serine residues of the α and β subunits and by calcium through the δ subunit, a member of the calmodulin family. The γ subunit is catalytically active. Mutations in three different genes of PHK subunits (PHKA2, PHKB, and PHKG2) can result in deficient activity of hepatic phosphorylase. Mutations of the gene for the hepatic isoform of the α subunit of PHK is the most common variant (Table 40.1).

  2. Clinical manifestations. These patients seldom have symptomatic hypoglycemia during infancy unless they fast for a prolonged period. They can then develop hyperketosis similar to, but usually milder than, that seen in type III GSD. Metabolic acidosis is rare. The disorder is usually discovered when an **enlarged liver** and protuberant abdomen are noted during a physical examination. Physical growth can be impaired, and motor development may be delayed as a consequence of muscular hypotonia. With increasing age, clinical and biochemical abnormalities gradually ameliorate, and most adult patients are asymptomatic.

  3. Laboratory features. Hypoglycemia is unusual, and blood lactate and uric acid levels are normal. Mild hypertriglyceridemia, hypercholesterolemia, and elevated transaminase levels may be present. Ketosis occurs with fasting. Functional tests are not especially useful in evaluating these patients. After an overnight fast, blood lactate level is normal and administration of glucagon elicits a brisk glycemic response without a rise in the blood lactate concentration. The glycemic response to glucagon cannot be used to distinguish between phosphorylase kinase deficiency and lack of phosphorylase itself. Thus, the definitive diagnosis of type IX GSD requires determination of phosphorylase kinase activity in erythrocytes or leukocytes. A liver biopsy is usually not necessary. The diagnosis of type VI GSD can be established by assaying the activity of phosphorylase in purified blood cell fractions and usually does not require a liver biopsy. Muscle phosphorylase activity is normal; muscle histology and glycogen content are normal.

  4. Treatment. Most patients do not require treatment; however, prolonged fasting should be avoided. For the minority of patients who are prone to fasting hypoglycemia during childhood, a late-night snack will suffice to prevent morning hypoglycemia. In the unusual patient who experiences overnight hypoglycemia and hyperketonemia, uncooked cornstarch, 2 g/kg, at bedtime prevents hypoglycemia and ketosis.

Selected References

Bandsma RH, Smit GP, Kuipers F. Disrupted lipid metabolism in glycogen storage disease type 1. *Eur J Pediatr* 2002;161:S65–S69.

Calderwood S, Kilpatrick L, Douglas SD, et al. Recombinant human granulocyte colony-stimulating factor therapy for patients with neutropenia and/or neutrophil dysfunction secondary to GSD type Ib. *Blood* 2001;97:376–382.

Chen YT. Glycogen storage diseases. In: Scriver C, Beaudet A, Sly W, Valle D, eds. *The Metabolic and Molecular Bases of Inherited Disease.* Vol. 1. 8th ed. New York: McGraw-Hill; 2001:1521–1555.

Chen Y-T, Coleman RA, Scheinman JI, et al. Renal disease in type 1 glycogen storage disease. *N Engl J Med* 1988;318:7–11.

Chen Y-T, Cornblath M, Sidbury JB. Cornstarch therapy in type 1 glycogen storage disease. *N Engl J Med* 1984;31:171–175.

Chou JY, Matern D, Mansfield BC, et al. Type 1 glycogen storage diseases: disorders of the glucose-6-phosphatase commplex. *Curr Mol Med* 2002;2:121–143.

Demo E, Frush D, Gottfried M, Koepke J. Glycogen storage disease type III—hepatocellular carcinoma a long term complication? *J Hepatol* 2007;46:492–498.

Franco LM, Krishnamurthy V, Bali D, Weinstein DA. Hepatocellular carcinoma in glycogen storage disease type Ia: a case series. *J Inherit Metab Dis* 2005;28:153–162.

Gremse DA, Bucuvalas JC, Balisteri WF. Efficacy of cornstarch therapy in type III glycogen-storage disease. *Am J Clin Nutr* 1990;52:671–674.

Labrune P, Trioche P, Duvaltier I, et al. Hepatocellular adenomas in glycogen storage disease type I and III: a series of 43 patients and review of the literature. *J Pediatr Gastroenterol Nutr* 1997;243:276–279.

Lee PJ, Dalton RN, Shah V, et al. Glomerular and tubular function in glycogen storage disease. *Pediatr Nephrol* 1995;9:705–710.

Melis D, Pivonello R, Parenti G, Della Casa R. Increased prevalence of thyroid autoimmunity and hypothyroidism in patients with glycogen storage disease type 1. *J Pediatr* 2007; 150:300–305.

Schwahn B, Rauch F, Wendel U, Schonau E. Low bone mass in glycogen storage disease type 1 is associated with reduced muscle force and poor metabolic control. *J Pediatr* 2002;141:350–356.

Visser G, Rake JP, Fernandes J, et al. Neutropenia, neutrophil dysfunction, and inflammatory bowel disease in glycogen storage disease type Ib: results of the European Study on Glycogen Storage Disease Type I. *J Pediatr* 2000;137:187–191.

Weinstein DA, Correia CE, Saunders AC, et al. Hepatic glycogen synthase deficiency: an infrequently recognized cause of ketotic hypoglycemia. *Mol Genet Metab* 2006;87:284–288.

Weinstein DA, Somers MJG, Wolfsdorf JI. Decreased urinary citrate excretion in type 1a glycogen storage disease. *J Pediatr* 2001;138:378–382.

Weinstein DA, Wolfsdorf JI. Effect of continuous glucose therapy with uncooked cornstarch on the long-term clinical course of type Ia glycogen storage disease. *Eur J Pediatr* 2002;161:S35–S39.

Willems PJ, Gerver WJ, Berger R, et al. The natural history of liver glycogenosis due to phosphorylase kinase deficiency: a longitudinal study of 41 patients. *Eur J Pediatr* 1990;149:268–271.

Wolfsdorf JI, Crigler JF Jr. Effect of continuous glucose therapy begun in infancy on the long-term clinical course of patients with type I glycogen storage disease. *J Pediatr Gastroenterol Nutr* 1999;29:136–143.

Wolfsdorf JI, Ehrlich S, Landy HS, et al. Optimal daytime feeding regimen to prevent postprandial hypoglycemia in type 1 glycogen storage disease. *Am J Clin Nutr* 1992;56:587–592.

Wolfsdorf JI, Keller RJ, Landy H, et al. Glucose therapy for glycogenosis type 1 in infants: comparison of intermittent uncooked cornstarch and continuous overnight glucose feedings. *J Pediatr* 1990;117:384–391.

Wolfsdorf JI, Laffel LMB, Crigler JF Jr. Metabolic control and renal dysfunction in type I glycogen storage disease. *J Inher Metab Dis* 1997;20:559–568.

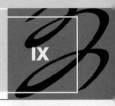
ETIOLOGY, PATHOGENESIS, AND THERAPY OF TYPE 1 DIABETES MELLITUS
Jay S. Skyler

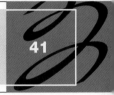

41

I. DEFINITION
Type 1 diabetes mellitus is characterized by pancreatic islet β-cell destruction and absolute insulinopenia. Thus, individuals are ketosis-prone under basal conditions. Onset of the disease is generally in youth (thus the former name **juvenile-onset diabetes**) but it can occur at any age. Patients are dependent on daily insulin administration for survival (thus the former name **insulin-dependent diabetes mellitus,** or IDDM).

II. OVERVIEW OF PATHOGENESIS
Current formulation of the pathogenesis of type 1 diabetes includes the following.
- **A.** A genetic predisposition, conferred by diabetogenic genes on the short arm of chromosome 6, either as part of or in close proximity to the major histocompatibility complex (MHC) region. There also are protective loci at the same location. When both susceptibility genes and protective genes are present, the protective genes usually confer dominant protection.
- **B.** Putative environmental triggers (possibly viral infections, chemical toxins, or exposure to cows' milk proteins in early infancy) that in genetically susceptible individuals might play a role in initiating the disease process.
- **C.** An immune mechanism gone awry, either initiation of immune destruction or loss of tolerance, leading to slow, progressive loss of pancreatic islet β cells and eventual clinical onset of type 1 diabetes. The immune destruction appears to be mediated by the TH1 subset of helper CD4 T lymphocytes and cytotoxic CD8 cells, whereas the TH2 subset of CD4 T lymphocytes and T-regulatory cells may confer protection.

III. GENETICS
- **A.** Evidence for genetic predisposition comes from demonstrations that the concordance rate for type 1 diabetes is higher in monozygotic than in dizygotic twins. Moreover, the empirical risk of developing type 1 diabetes is increased in

first-degree relatives of individuals with the disease. Among whites in the United States, the overall risk is 0.2% to 0.4%. On the other hand, siblings of probands with type 1 diabetes have a risk of ~5%, and offspring of diabetic parents have a 3% risk if the mother has the disease and a 6% risk if the father has the disease. The risk for an identical twin of a proband with type 1 diabetes is 30% to 50%.

B. The major genetic predisposition appears to be conferred by diabetogenic gene(s), at a locus called *IDDM1* on the short arm of chromosome 6, either within or in close proximity to the MHC region, that is, the human leukocyte antigen (HLA) region. A second locus—*IDDM2*—is on the short arm of chromosome 11 in the region flanking the insulin gene. There are a number of other diabetogenic genes on other chromosomes.

C. The relationship between type 1 diabetes and the HLA system is complex.

    1. Within families, there is clearly linkage between type 1 diabetes and the HLA system, regardless of what HLA alleles are manifest in any given family.

    2. Across populations, there is clearly an association between type 1 diabetes and certain HLA alleles. This is particularly true of the immune-response genes, also known as Class II MHC alleles. These include the HLA-DR, DQ, and DP loci.

        a. The HLA-DR3 and DR4 alleles of the DR locus occur more frequently in white subjects with type 1 diabetes, with the heterozygote HLA-DR3/DR4 being disproportionately increased (40% of subjects with type 1 diabetes, compared with only 3% of the general population). More than 95% of type 1 diabetic individuals are HLA-DR3, DR4, or DR3/DR4. On the other hand, HLA-DR2 confers protection against the development of type 1 diabetes.

        b. Alleles of HLA-DQ-β have a major role in determining relative disease susceptibility or resistance. DQB1*0602 (which is associated with DR2) confers disease protection. On the other hand, DQB1*0201 (which is associated with DR3) and DQB1*0302 (which is associated with DR4) confer increased risk.

        c. The structure of the DQ molecule, in particular residue 57 of the B chain, helps specify the immune response against the insulin-producing islet β cells. Alleles in which this residue is aspartic acid appear to have protection against the disease, whereas other amino acids at that site do not offer such protection.

    3. Debate exists as to how the immune-response genes alter disease susceptibility. Some could induce an immune response to islets, such as by having a high affinity for peptides that, when presented to the immune system, amplify the cellular immune response. Alternatively, the susceptibility genes could have a low affinity for peptides that establish and maintain tolerance.

    4. On the other hand, it should be noted that there are limitations with the HLA type 1 diabetes hypothesis. An all-or-none relationship between type 1 diabetes and the HLA system has not been defined, and diabetogenic gene(s) have not been clearly identified.

D. The search for diabetogenic genes continues. There has been much progress in the last several years in unraveling the genetics of type 1 diabetes, which could lead eventually to identification of specific diabetogenic genes and ultimately their gene products. Such identification might permit better genetic counseling, amniocentesis and fetal diagnosis, identification of susceptible individuals, and possibly even genetic manipulation either to alter susceptibility or to replace gene function.

IV. ENVIRONMENTAL TRIGGERS

A. The degree to which environmental events are important in the pathogenetic sequence is unresolved. There is compelling evidence that they can initiate the pathogenetic processes in genetically predisposed animals, but evidence for their role in type 1 diabetes in human beings is less secure. Although some have argued that the substantial discordance of type 1 diabetes in identical twins indicates that environmental factors must play a role in human type 1 diabetes, this view has been challenged by invoking the potential of genetic diversity between such "identical" twins, an argument that would eliminate the need to necessarily include environmental events in the disease sequence. Nevertheless, most investigators accept that, at the very least, environmental factors influence the probability of an individual developing type 1 diabetes.

B. Viral infections

1. A number of human viruses can infect and damage islet β cells in experimental animals, and some of them have the potential for contributing to the development of type 1 diabetes. In one case, a <u>coxsackie B</u> variant was isolated from the pancreatic tissue of a young boy who died 10 days after the onset of type 1 diabetes, and the isolate produced diabetes in experimental animals.

2. An unresolved question is whether many different viral infections, such as enteroviral infections, can cause type 1 diabetes in humans; or whether a single unknown diabetogenic virus is responsible for most cases of the disease; or whether viral infections merely serve to bring type 1 diabetes to clinical recognition, without playing any specific role in islet β-cell destruction.

3. Exposure can be remote in time from the onset of type 1 diabetes. This remoteness can even include exposure in utero; for example, <u>congenital rubella</u> can result in type 1 diabetes.

C. Chemical toxins

1. A variety of chemical toxins appear to have the potential of inducing islet β-cell damage. Among these are the <u>nitrosourea compounds</u>. These are ubiquitous in our environment and represent only one class of chemical compounds with the potential for leading to type 1 diabetes.

2. In one animal model of diabetes, a series of environmental insults (both viral and chemical) results in cumulative β-cell destruction, but only in genetically susceptible animals.

V. IMMUNOLOGIC FACTORS

A. Immune involvement. Abundant evidence suggests that islet β-cell destruction is immunologically mediated. The exact immunologic mechanisms involved in the pathogenetic pathway have not yet been defined, even in animal models. There may be several different pathogenetic sequences that eventuate in immune destruction of β cells. For example, the pathways involved in typical type 1 diabetes may be different from those involved when type 1 diabetes is only one component of a polyendocrine autoimmune syndrome. It appears that type 1 diabetes may be a group of clinically similar conditions that eventuate in β-cell failure.

1. It has been argued that the immune destruction is "autoimmune" in nature, which might be the case if environmental factors are not involved. Nevertheless, it must be emphasized that immune-mediated destruction does not necessarily imply spontaneous autoimmunity.

2. Initiating, or primary, events for the activation of immune destruction are not yet known. Once immune destruction commences, secondary and tertiary immune responses are activated, with virtually the whole immunologic army attacking β cells.

3. It is unclear whether immune activation occurs because of presentation of a diabetogenic peptide to the immune system and activation of an immune response, or because of failure to maintain tolerance to a diabetogenic peptide.

B. Insulitis. Important evidence of cell-mediated immune destruction of islet β cells is the finding of mononuclear cell infiltration of the islets (insulitis or isletitis) in pancreas examined near the time of clinical onset of type 1 diabetes. This lesion is consistent with an immune reaction and is similar to the lymphocytic infiltration encountered in other reputed autoimmune conditions, including endocrinopathies.

1. At diagnosis in human beings, the majority of infiltrating cells are lymphocytes, both activated CD8 T-cytotoxic cells and CD4 T-helper cells, with some B lymphocytes present as well. Macrophages and natural killer (NK) cells also are present.

2. In one series of pancreases obtained near time of onset of type 1 diabetes, there was aberrant expression of MHC molecules. The β cells showed expression

of Class II (HLA-DR) MHC, although at the electron microscopic level other workers have shown that Class II MHC expression can be on macrophages that have ingested β-cell material. Class I MHC was hyperexpressed by several islet cells, but only in those with some β cells. Islets with hyperexpression of Class I MHC also showed interferon-α, suggesting environmental stimulation of β cells and activation of interferon-α.

C. Cell-mediated immune processes are responsible for the destruction of islet β cells.

1. Lymphocytes, NK cells, and macrophages/monocytes appear to be involved. Cytokines produced by these cells may mediate damage to β cells. In vitro, several cytokines (e.g., interferon-γ, tumor necrosis factor, interleukin-1) can kill cultured islet cells. The β cells appear to be particularly vulnerable to tissue damage.

2. There is accelerated re-enactment of the pathogenetic sequence following pancreatic transplantation in identical twins (from a nondiabetic twin to a diabetic cotwin) in the absence of immunosuppression. The genetic identity precluded rejection (which was also excluded by virtue of the fact that the transplanted kidney from the same donor continued to function, and the histology was not consistent with rejection), yet insulitis (predominantly T lymphocytes) and pancreatic graft failure occurred in a rapid course.

D. Circulating antibodies. A variety of antibodies to islet cells and islet cell markers can be detected <u>at diagnosis</u> of type 1 diabetes, and even several years <u>prior to diagnosis</u>. These include antibodies to islet cells detected by immunofluorescence (islet cell antibodies, or ICAs); insulin (insulin autoantibodies, or IAAs); glutamic acid decarboxylase (GADs); an islet tyrosine phosphatase called IA2 or ICA-512; the zinc transporter ZnT8 (Slc30A8); islet-specific glucose 6-phosphatase catalytic subunit–related protein (IGRP); and others. These antibodies <u>only reflect β-cell damage</u> and are not responsible for mediating β-cell destruction. It is postulated that some may be directed against an antigen involved in initiating the immune process, particularly insulin, but more evidence is needed in this regard. These antibodies do serve as useful markers of immune activity and/or as markers of ongoing β-cell destruction in type 1 diabetes.

E. Evolution of immunopathology. The islet immunopathology can commence several years prior to clinical recognition of type 1 diabetes. The evidence is consistent with the notion that there is a slow, continuing immune process antedating the clinical diagnosis of type 1 diabetes.

1. In prospective studies of first-degree relatives (mostly parents and siblings, sometimes offspring) of probands with type 1 diabetes, there is an increased risk of developing type 1 diabetes. The clinical onset of disease is usually preceded by the appearance of various antibodies, often by many years.

2. In studies involving unaffected monozygotic twins and other first-degree relatives of type 1 diabetes probands, antibodies precede the development of clinical type 1 diabetes. Moreover, such subjects have a progressive decline in islet β-cell function, as measured by a decrease in early insulin release after an IV glucose load.

3. Not all islets are involved at the time of diagnosis. Histologically, a few show the classical pathognomonic insulitis lesion, but intact islets with β cells can be found, as well as an occasional hyperplastic islet. The majority of islets are pseudoatrophic (i.e., small islets without mononuclear infiltration and devoid of β cells, but with intact glucagon-secreting α cells and somatostatin-secreting δ cells). Presumably, the inflammatory process has abated, having occurred much earlier in those islets, with type 1 diabetes appearing only when sufficient β cells have been destroyed so that glucose tolerance can no longer be maintained.

F. Animal models

1. Spontaneous diabetes. There are two spontaneous animal models of type 1 diabetes, the BB rat and the NOD mouse. Both of these models have an MHC-related genetic predisposition, both have been shown to have immune-mediated

β-cell destruction, and both develop insulin deficiency, hyperglycemia, and ketosis.

2. **Induced diabetes.** Using repetitive low doses of <u>streptozotocin</u>, type 1 diabetes can be induced in genetically susceptible strains of mice. Destruction of β cells is immune-mediated. Thus, this is a model of immune-mediated, environmentally triggered disease.

3. **Immune intervention.** Immune intervention results in prevention or reversibility of disease in the BB rat, the NOD mouse, and in the low-dose streptozotocin mouse model.

G. **Immune intervention studies in humans**

1. If type 1 diabetes is an immunologically mediated disease, then immune intervention should alter the natural history of the disease and potentially abort the syndrome. This would be true whether the disease was due to spontaneous autoimmunity or was simply immune-mediated.

2. In human beings, immune intervention trials have been initiated for at least three reasons: to confirm that the immune system is involved in the pathogenesis of type 1 diabetes; to help clarify and define the immune mechanisms involved in the pathogenetic sequence; and to potentially lead to a clinically applicable intervention. Many of these studies have begun shortly after diagnosis, when there is still some residual β-cell function.

3. The earliest controlled trials used azathioprine, alone or with glucocorticoids, or cyclosporine. They demonstrated that immune intervention does indeed alter the natural history of the disease. This provided convincing support for the hypothesis that immune mechanisms are important in the etiopathogenesis of type 1 diabetes. Unfortunately, the data are too meager to permit conclusions about clinical utility of an early immune intervention strategy because of small sample sizes and short duration of follow-up of subjects. It is possible that intervention at this stage is effective in halting the destruction of β cells, resulting in milder disease.

4. Many new potential therapies are targeted to patients with new-onset type 1 diabetes. The hope is to find a strategy that permits specific intervention to abort the immune attack on pancreatic islet β cells while leaving the immune system otherwise intact. One of the more promising to date is the use of humanized <u>anti-CD3 monoclonal antibodies</u>, which in two trials (using two different anti-CD3 antibodies) have shown preservation of β-cell function and a milder course of disease. Ongoing are large confirmatory trials with these antibodies.

5. Treatment of the prediabetic state is the logical ultimate goal of immune intervention studies. Studies are currently under way in high-risk individuals (i.e., first-degree relatives of probands with type 1 diabetes, with antibodies and with diminished islet β-cell function, measured by decreased early insulin release after an IV glucose load, or in relatives who have dysglycemia but not yet diabetes).

6. Ultimately, it is possible to project the following sequence:

   a. At birth, routinely screen the population for diabetogenic genes or gene products.

   b. Having identified individuals with the potential of developing type 1 diabetes, follow them longitudinally, seeking evidence of initiation of immune damage to islet β cells.

   c. In such individuals, seek evidence of altered or diminishing β-cell function.

   d. If identified, such individuals become candidates for intervention therapy designed to abort the pathogenetic sequence.

VI. STRATEGIES FOR IMPROVING GLUCOSE CONTROL

A. **Contemporary management of type 1 diabetes mellitus** has vastly changed over the past three decades. Current management approaches emphasize patient self-direction of daily management under the guidance of the physician. Insulin regimens have multiple components, consisting of several daily injections or the use of an insulin pump. Diets are flexible and individually tailored to the patient's needs. Self-monitoring of blood glucose is an integral component of management, used to guide decision making in an attempt to achieve defined target blood glucose values. Continuous glucose monitoring is rapidly emerging as a therapeutic option. The goal of therapy is to incorporate diabetes management into the lifestyle of the patient by being flexible in approach while still striving for excellent glycemic control. This approach permits attainment of meticulous control in many educated, motivated patients.

B. Flexible intensive therapy of type 1 diabetes is a system that uses this contemporary approach. It consists of the following 10 elements.

1. Defined target blood glucose levels. Blood glucose targets must be individualized for each patient. They must be explicitly defined if they are to be achieved. For healthy young patients who readily recognize hypoglycemic symptoms and who spontaneously recover from hypoglycemia, such targets can nearly approximate the levels of glycemia seen in nondiabetic individuals, such as preprandial values of 70 to 130 mg/dL (3.9 to 7.2 mM). These targets need to be lower during pregnancy and should be raised in subjects who have difficulty perceiving hypoglycemic symptoms, who do not spontaneously recover from hypoglycemia, or in whom hypoglycemia might be particularly dangerous (e.g., patients with angina pectoris or transient ischemic attacks). In motivated patients, realistic targets are achievable at least 80% to 90% of the time.

2. A multiple-component insulin program tailored to the patient's lifestyle. Ideally, this program separates the insulin components providing basal insulinemia from those providing prandial insulinemia. This is accomplished by the following:

a. Preprandial injections (or pump boluses) of rapid-acting insulin analogs (insulin lispro, insulin aspart, or insulin glulisine) before meals (short-acting insulin [regular insulin] is no longer commonly used for this purpose). The doses should be dictated by planned carbohydrate intake with the meal and prevailing level of glycemia, with many individuals using both **(1)** insulin:carbohydrate ratios and **(2)** correction doses for hyperglycemia, to calculate preprandial insulin dosage.

b. Basal insulin provided by long-acting insulin (insulin glargine or insulin detemir) given at bedtime or twice daily; or by an insulin infusion pump (continuous subcutaneous insulin infusion, or CSII), providing continuous background delivery of insulin (intermediate-acting insulin [NPH] is no longer commonly used for this purpose).

In addition to insulin, it is often helpful to give preprandial pramlintide to better control glycemic excursions. Pramlintide is a synthetic version of the pancreatic β-cell hormone amylin, which, like insulin, is deficient in type 1 diabetes. Its use lowers postprandial glucose excursions, improves glycemic control, and often results in weight loss.

3. Careful balance of food intake, activity, and insulin dose. For this purpose, patients (and their families) learn a system of keeping track of food intake, such as carbohydrate counting, Exchange Lists for Meal Planning, or a similar system. This permits them to vary their food intake ad lib and to adapt their insulin dose accordingly. By learning general principles of the influence of various foods and of activity on glycemia, and how to balance these components with activity, patients can achieve their desired glycemic control.

4. Monitoring of blood glucose. This is accomplished either by self-monitoring of blood glucose (SMBG) or by the use of continuous glucose monitoring (CGM). SMBG involves patient measurement of blood glucose on capillary samples (obtained by using an automated device for pricking the finger) four times per day on most days (before meals and at bedtime), with additional samples obtained in the middle of the night (2 A.M. to 4 A.M.) once every 1 to 2 weeks and anytime the overnight insulin dosage is to be altered. Additional samples are obtained anytime hypoglycemia is suspected. Periodically, postprandial samples are obtained as well. Alternatively, as noted, the use of CGM is growing, and this greatly improves understanding of glucose fluctuations, as well as providing alarms when glucose levels are outside of a patient-determined window, to alert the patient to both hyperglycemia and impending hypoglycemia.

5. **Patient adjustments of food intake and insulin dose and timing, and the use of insulin supplements according to a predetermined plan.** Patients are provided with an action plan to alter their therapy and achieve individual blood glucose targets. These actions are guided by SMBG or CGM determinations and daily records, and are dictated by prevailing blood glucose, meal size, anticipated activity, and previous experience in similar circumstances. Actions dictated by the plan can include altering the size or content of food intake, activity, insulin dose, and timing of injections in relation to meals.

6. **Patient education.** Patients must be carefully instructed in all aspects of diabetes management, including the details of meal planning (particularly carbohydrate content), insulin dose adjustment, activity planning, monitoring, recognition and treatment of hypoglycemia, and adapting to other intercurrent events.

7. **Frequent contact between patient and staff.** The patient should have 24-hour access to the diabetes management team and should contact them when there is a question about how to achieve the desired level of glycemia, if an intercurrent illness develops, or when any problem arises that requires consultation.

8. **Motivation.** Successful participation in a flexible but demanding management program requires a committed, motivated patient. The management team often must make extra efforts to help maintain motivation. This is often the most difficult component of treatment.

9. **Psychologic support.** Patients with new-onset type 1 diabetes and their families need psychologic support to adjust to the diabetes as well as to aid in implementing and maintaining the management program. Regular attendance at diabetes support group meetings may be helpful.

10. **Assessment.** An independent measure of integrated glycemic control, glycated hemoglobin (A1c), is used for metabolic assessment. Thus, SMBG values are part of treatment, not assessment (but should be compared with the A1c value). In addition, patient understanding, commitment, and responsibility for diabetes management should be assessed regularly.

VII. FUTURE DIRECTIONS IN IMPROVING GLYCEMIC CONTROL

A. **External insulin infusion pumps.** Already in use, there should be increased use of these devices because of their pharmacokinetic advantages over insulin injections. These include greater reproducibility of insulin absorption and the absence of a subcutaneous insulin depot, which increases the risk of exercise-related hypoglycemia.

B. **Glucose sensor–controlled insulin infusion systems.** Rapid technical advances are facilitating the integration of CGM systems with insulin pumps, providing the potential of developing a miniaturized closed-loop insulin-delivery system.

C. **Pancreatic transplantation.** This is now being used in clinical practice in individuals undergoing simultaneous kidney transplantation. Graft survival, with the patient free from insulin therapy, now exceeds 80% up to 10 years after transplantation. Patient survival now exceeds 90%.

D. **Islet replacement therapy.** Islet isolation and implantation offers the hope of reversing diabetes. Recent human islet implantation experiments have been promising. However, the problem of islet availability probably will limit wide-scale application using human islet tissue per se. Protecting islets from rejection by encapsulation or by growing islets on hollow-fiber artificial capillaries might permit the use of animal islets for human implantation. However, such encapsulated islets often have been destroyed by tissue reactions in animal models with spontaneous diabetes.

E. **Genetically engineered pseudo β cells.** A potential approach to islet replacement therapy is the use of genetically engineered pseudo β cells, which have glucose-mediated insulin secretion. By gene transfer approaches, it is possible to program cells to synthesize and secrete insulin. Recent experiments, also genetically inserting other elements, have demonstrated the potential for programmed cells to sense glucose. The challenge is to develop a cell line that both responds to glucose and secretes insulin in a physiologic manner, and that is nonimmunogenic and will not be rejected.

F. **Development of insulin-producing β cells from stem cells.** A potential approach is the development of β cells with glucose-mediated insulin secretion from other cell types, including either adult or embryonic stem cells, cord blood cells, or transdifferentiation of non–β cells into β cells. These approaches have shown some promise in animal models of diabetes.

VIII. GLUCOSE CONTROL AND COMPLICATIONS

A. **Diabetes Control and Complications Trial (DCCT): study design.** In June 1993, the DCCT reported its findings to the American Diabetes Association. This decade-long study involved 1 441 patients with type 1 diabetes, who were randomly allocated to either conventional treatment or intensive treatment (similar to that described in Section VI.B). The intensive group received three to four insulin injections daily or used an insulin pump, performed SMBG at least four times daily, and used the data to make self-adjustments to achieve a treatment target of near-normoglycemia. The conventional group received no more than two insulin injections daily, did not use SMBG data to make self-adjustments, and had a treatment target of avoiding excessive hyperglycemia and ketosis.

B. **DCCT results**

1. The DCCT demonstrated the dramatic significant impact of intensive therapy in lessening complications of diabetes.

   a. **Eye disease.** Clinically important progression of retinopathy was reduced by 62% to 76% for those with no retinopathy at entry and by 54% for those with mild retinopathy at entry. Progression to severity requiring referral to an ophthalmologist for treatment was reduced by 46%. Treatment for sight-threatening retinopathy, using laser photocoagulation, was reduced by about 50%.

   b. **Renal disease.** Clinically important kidney damage (proteinuria >300 mg per 24 hours) was reduced by 56%. Incipient (subclinical) nephropathy, or microalbuminuria, was reduced by 46%.

   c. **Nerve disease.** Clinically important neuropathy was reduced by 61%.

   d. **Cardiovascular.** Although not statistically significant in the DCCT per se, there was a 44% reduction in cardiovascular events in the intensive-therapy group. Subsequently, in the long-term follow-up of the DCCT, called EDIC (Epidemiology of Diabetes Interventions and Complications), there was demonstrated a 50% decrement in cardiovascular events, which was statistically significant.

2. Some **side effects** were seen more frequently in the intensive-therapy group.

   a. **Hypoglycemia.** Severe hypoglycemia requiring the assistance of another person for treatment was increased 3.3 times in the intensive-therapy group. Hypoglycemia resulting in seizure or coma was also increased threefold. The preponderance of events occurred without warning, either while asleep or while awake without symptoms.

   b. **Weight gain.** There was greater weight gain in the intensive-therapy group, with a relative risk of 1.6 for reaching 120% of ideal body weight. Average weight gain was about 10 pounds.

C. **Conclusion.** The DCCT demonstrates that intensive therapy lessens the risk of complications, but not without extracting a price. Patients must be made aware of the study results, so that an informed choice can be made regarding treatment targets. In general, the benefits seem to far outweigh the side effects.

Selected References

American Diabetes Association. Standards of medical care in diabetes—2007. *Diabetes Care* 2007;30(suppl 1):S5–S41.

Atkinson MA, Eisenbarth GS. Type 1 diabetes: new perspectives on disease pathogenesis and treatment. *Lancet* 2001;358:221–229.

Barker JM. Clinical review: type 1 diabetes-associated autoimmunity: natural history, genetic associations, and screening. *J Clin Endocrinol Metab* 2006;91:1210–1217.

Bode B, ed. *Medical Management of Type 1 Diabetes Mellitus.* 4th ed. Alexandria, VA: American Diabetes Association; 2004.

Chatenoud L, Bluestone JA. CD3-specific antibodies: a portal to the treatment of autoimmunity. *Nat Rev Immunol* 2007;7:622–632.

Daneman D. Type 1 diabetes. *Lancet* 2006;367:847–858.

DeWitt DE, Hirsch IB. Outpatient insulin therapy in type 1 and type 2 diabetes mellitus: scientific review. *JAMA* 2003;289:2254–2264.

Diabetes Control and Complications Trial/Epidemiology of Diabetes Interventions and Complications (DCCT/EDIC) Study Research Group. Intensive diabetes treatment and cardiovascular disease in patients with type 1 diabetes. *N Engl J Med* 2005;353:2643–2653.

Diabetes Control and Complications Trial Research Group. The effect of intensive treatment of diabetes on the development and progression of long-term complications in insulin-dependent diabetes mellitus. *N Engl J Med* 1993;329:683–689.

Eisenbarth GS. Update in type 1 diabetes. *J Clin Endocrinol Metab* 2007;92:2403–2407.

Garg S, Zisser H, Schwartz S, et al. Improvement in glycemic excursions with a transcutaneous, real-time continuous glucose sensor: a randomized controlled trial. *Diabetes Care* 2006;29:44–50.

Gillespie KM, Dix RJ, Williams AJ. Type 1 diabetes: pathogenesis and prevention. *Can Med Assoc J* 2006;175:165–170.

Hirsch IB. Insulin analogues. *N Engl J Med* 2005;352:174–183.

Hirsch IB. Intensive treatment of type 1 diabetes. *Med Clin N Am* 1998;82:689–719.

Hirsch IB, Farkas-Hirsch R, Skyler JS. Intensive insulin therapy for treatment of type 1 diabetes. *Diabetes Care* 1990;13:1265–1283.

Kligensmith G, ed. *Intensive Diabetes Management.* 3rd ed. Alexandria, VA: American Diabetes Association; 2003.

Lebovitz H, ed. *Therapy for Diabetes Mellitus and Related Disorders.* 4th ed. Alexandria, VA: American Diabetes Association; 2004.

Liao YH, Verchere CB, Warnock GL. Adult stem or progenitor cells in treatment for type 1 diabetes: current progress. *Can J Surg* 2007;50:137–142.

Porat S, Dor Y. New sources of pancreatic beta cells. *Curr Diabetes Rep* 2007;7:304–308.

Pugliese A, Eisenbarth GS. Type 1 diabetes mellitus of man: genetic susceptibility and resistance. *Adv Exp Med Biol* 2004;552:170–203.

Schade DS, Santiago JV, Skyler JS, et al. *Intensive Insulin Therapy.* Princeton, NJ: Excerpta Medica; 1983.

Skyler JS. Prediction and prevention of type 1 diabetes: progress, problems, and prospects. *Clin Pharmacol Ther* 2007;81:768–771.

Staeva-Vieira T, Peakman M, von Herrath M. Translational mini-review series on type 1 diabetes: immune-based therapeutic approaches for type 1 diabetes. *Clin Exp Immunol* 2007;148:17–31.

Want LL, Ratner RE. Pramlintide: a new tool in diabetes management. *Curr Diabetes Rep* 2006;6:344–349.

Wood JR, Laffel LM. Technology and intensive management in youth with type 1 diabetes: state of the art. *Curr Diabetes Rep* 2007;7:104–113.

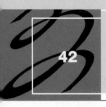

42 DIAGNOSIS AND MANAGEMENT OF TYPE 1 DIABETES MELLITUS
Stuart J. Brink

I. GOALS OF TREATMENT
A. The **primary goals** for the treatment of type 1 insulin-dependent diabetes mellitus (IDDM) are achievement of as near-normal blood sugar levels as possible, normal growth and development for children and adolescents, and avoidance of severe hypoglycemia. **Secondary goals** include avoidance of the long-term complications associated with type 1 diabetes: retinopathy, neuropathy, nephropathy, and atherosclerotic events such as heart attacks, stroke, and peripheral arteriosclerosis.

B. Overall goals of treatment must take into account:
1. The age of the patient, and how well he or she understands the management concepts
2. How much endogenous insulin remains available
3. Caloric needs for normal growth and avoidance of obesity
4. Activity patterns and their unique fuel requirements
5. Home glucose and ketone monitoring needs
6. Insulin choices, delivery, kinetics, absorption idiosyncracies, and adjustment guidelines
7. Psychosocial factors including financial and family issues

C. Diabetes treatment team. The goals of therapy usually are best achieved using a multidisciplinary approach to deal with all of these complex issues. A pediatric diabetologist should supervise the team for children and adolescents, and an internist diabetologist should do the same for adults. If specific complications exist, other subspecialists (i.e., opthalmologists, cardiologists, neurologists, nephrologists, gastroenterologists) will be extremely helpful.

II. INITIAL APPROACH TO THE PATIENT
A. Presentation and diagnosis
1. The classic manifestations of type 1 diabetes mellitus include:
   a. Hyperglycemia secondary to insulin insufficiency.
   b. Polyuria. As high glucose in the bloodstream is filtered through the kidneys, osmotic balance causes excess urination.
   c. Polydipsia. As more water is excreted, the body requires more water intake and, because thirst mechanisms are intact, thirst increases.
   d. Loss of weight. Loss of water as well as loss of muscle mass and fat mass all contribute to acute or subacute weight loss at the time of diagnosis of type 1 diabetes mellitus.
   e. Fatigue and weakness probably occur as a result of decreased glucose utilization and subtle electrolyte and/or mineral abnormalities as well as clinical and subclinical dehydration.
   f. Type 2 versus type 1 diabetes. With the obesity epidemic around the world, it is important to distinguish between type 1 and type 2 diabetes in children, adolescents, and young adults where type 2 diabetes is also epidemic. Classic type 2 diabetes in children and adolescents sometimes presents with ketoacidosis, but almost always with moderate to severe insulin resistance because of obesity. This is different than classic maturity onset of diabetes in youth (MODY), with a different pattern of family history and different pathogenesis. MODY are types of diabetes with monogenic inheritance patterns.

Several have been elucidated. Some have nonprogressive types of hyperglycemia, whereas others are more aggressive and more similar to classic type 2 diabetes, in which loss of insulin reserve over time is typical. Knowledge of the genetic types of diabetes may help to determine who needs more aggressive management, when to consider using insulin, who else in the family needs to be assessed, and whether certain types of oral agents should be considered.

Treatment of type 2 diabetes in younger patients focuses on weight loss, increasing caloric expenditure, and the same host of oral agents classically available for the older patient with type 2 diabetes. Sometimes, insulin is needed.

2. Laboratory findings in type 1 diabetes mellitus
   a. Fasting blood glucose. According to the latest diagnostic classification, if the fasting blood glucose value is >126 mg/dL on two or more separate days, the diagnosis of diabetes mellitus can be confirmed. **Random blood glucose** values >200 mg/dL are also diagnostic.
   b. Glucose tolerance test (2-hour). If the diagnosis is still in doubt, then perform a glucose tolerance test (usually not necessary):
   (1) Give at least 150 to 200 g carbohydrate daily for 3 days prior to test.
   (2) Overnight fast.
   (3) Have patient drink 75 g of glucose dissolved in 300 mL of water within a few minutes.
   (4) Measure serum glucose levels at 30-minute intervals for 2 hours. Usually it is not necessary to measure insulin levels quantitatively.
   c. Autoantibodies and genetic testing (islet cell antibodies, glutamic acid decarboxylase-65, and insulin antibodies). In combination, such autoantibodies are positive at least 60% to 80% of the time in children and adolescents with type 1 diabetes mellitus, which is thought to be an autoimmune disorder. Adults with positive antibodies will likely need insulin eventually, but early in the course of what is called latent autoimmune type 1 diabetes they may be treated only with typical type 2 diabetes treatment protocols.
   d. New genetic tests for **monogenic diabetes** can help identify rare cases of neonatal or early-childhood diabetes associated with potassium-channel or sulfonylurea-receptor abnormalities. These youngsters may present with severe diabetic ketoacidosis (DKA) at diagnosis but can be elegantly managed later (if diagnosis is confirmed genetically) without insulin but with sulfonylurea medications.
   e. C-Peptide is not affected by antibodies to exogenous insulin, so measurement may be helpful in classifying the diabetes in an already-diagnosed patient when drawn either fasting, postprandially (especially if concomitant with elevated blood glucose levels), or after glucagon or Sustacal stimulation testing.
B. Diabetic ketoacidosis. See Chapter 43.
C. Hyperglycemia without dehydration. If dehydration is not present and there is no vomiting, insulin can be started on an outpatient basis at the same time that preliminary meal planning and home blood glucose monitoring are taught.
D. Insulin treatment. Aggressive insulin therapy using basal-bolus concepts can be started as soon as possible in an attempt to "rest" the damaged islet cells and help to "induce" a remission ("honeymoon," see Section II.F.2). Evidence suggests that quick normalization and maintenance of blood sugars may allow for some recovery and prolong pancreatic function. Newer analogs such as glargine (Lantus) or detemir (Levemir) insulins can provide basal insulin coupled with bolus doses of fast-acting analogs (lispro [Humalog], aspart [Novolog] or glulisine [Apidra]) around meals and snacks. Prandial insulin provided by rapid-acting insulin before meals and snacks offers flexibility combined with carbohydrate counting and insulin-correction algorithms. Basal insulin can be provided as in the past with overlapping doses of NPH insulin (two, three, or four times a day). Detemir is almost always given twice a day, whereas glargine is sometimes needed only once

a day. Many youngsters nevertheless need glargine also on a twice-a-day regimen, but exact doses and proportions of daytime versus nighttime dosing are extremely varied and must be individualized based on frequent blood glucose test results. Other advantages include the following.

E. Other considerations regarding insulin therapy

1. <u>Insulin analogs</u> (lispro, aspart, and glulisine) are the most physiologic rapid-acting insulin preparations and can be given immediately before or after eating to mimic previous endogenous insulin delivery. Regular insulin takes longer to be absorbed, reaches a peak after injection later than such rapid-acting insulin analogs, and often has a more prolonged "tail effect," causing delayed hypoglycemia hours after use. Analogs also can be used in combination with intermediate-acting insulins in any patient with diabetes who demonstrates hyperglycemia after meals and/or snacks, with overlapping NPH or lente providing basal insulin function. Better still, they can be used with the longer-sustained analogs such as glargine and detemir, but must be given using different syringes or pens, because these longer-acting insulins have a different pH and do not readily mix.

2. In <u>a three-shot-per-day regimen</u>, prebreakfast, presupper, and bedtime insulin is given. This most commonly involves a combination of analog or regular insulins plus an intermediate-acting insulin prebreakfast, analog, or regular insulin alone presupper, and intermediate-acting insulin alone at bedtime. This has a major benefit of decreasing peak early nocturnal insulin effects between 2 A.M. and 4 A.M. Sometimes combinations of two types of insulin are used at two or three of these injection times, based on actual blood glucose readings.

3. Preprandial analog insulin doses with a prebedtime intermediate- or long-acting insulin work best for some patients with type 1 diabetes (<u>four- or five-shot regimen</u>). This regimen tends to provide greater flexibility with changing patterns of diet and activity. Overlapping doses of intermediate-acting insulins can be combined with any or all of these four injection times based on blood glucose data.

4. Glargine and detemir insulins help decrease hypoglycemia and are often now preferred basal insulins. Usually, glargine as a basal insulin can be started alone at bedtime. In very young children, glargine sometimes is given only at breakfast. Most youngsters, however, need glargine insulin twice a day to prevent a waning effect at the sixteenth to twenty-fourth hours. Detemir insulin as a basal insulin is almost always used via a twice-a-day regimen. All such basal insulin decisions should not be dogmatic but based on actual frequent blood glucose patterns and assessments.

5. In general, insulin doses with analog insulin should be given immediately before meals to best match food absorption and insulin absorption characteristics. If regular insulin is used, it should be given 30 to 60 minutes before food, but this is rarely sustained because of its inconvenience. For very young children in whom food intake is unpredictable, the newest fast-acting analogs (lispro, aspart, and glulisine) can be given immediately **after** food is consumed, so that less guessing and "food battling" occur.

6. Insulin absorption is variable in different parts of the body. Manufacturers use different buffers in their insulin preparations, and this may contribute to insulin–food mismatches if brands are changed frequently. Ideally, the same brand of insulin should be used unless a specific reason exists to change from one manufacturer to another or availability of insulin is problematic. Insulin absorption is most consistent in the abdominal and buttocks regions compared with the extremities. Exercise-related changes in extremity absorption of insulin can contribute to poor glucose control because of erratic absorption.

7. Insulin lipohypertrophy, though much less common and less intense than in years past, occurs when the same site is overused. Any insulin lipohypertrophy interferes with insulin absorption consistency and contributes to erratic hyperglycemia as well as hypoglycemia. Improved purity of insulin has likely helped decrease hypertrophy problems.

8. Lente and ultralente insulins have generally been discontinued, although they are still available in some parts of the world.

F. How much insulin is needed

1. Most youngsters at diagnosis need ~1.0 U/kg per day. With multidose insulin (MDI) regimens, ~50% of total dose is given as basal insulin. Usually this entails ~80% to 90% as bedtime glargine and ~10% to 20% as breakfast glargine but with varying amounts if detemir is used instead. About 10% of patients, particularly younger patients, need a "reverse" distribution, with more in the morning dose of glargine and less at bedtime (sometimes none at all at bedtime in toddlers). The prandial analogs constitute the other 50% distribution, with ~20% prebreakfast, ~10% prelunch, and ~10% predinner plus the remaining 5% to 10% presnacks.

   Because of overnight growth-hormone effects, the morning "dawn phenomenon" (explained in Section VII.G) may also be seen and require relatively larger boluses than would be needed at other times of the day. Reverse dawn phenomena, however, also occur not infrequently.

2. The remission stage (or **"honeymoon" phase**) results from a partial recovery of islet cell function (as measured by C-peptide). It occurs within 1 to 3 months after diagnosis and can last from weeks to a few months, during which time insulin requirements fall drastically, to < 0.3 U/kg per day and, in some, to no requirement for insulin at all. However, insulin administration usually is not discontinued during this time because of the potential development of insulin allergy (see Section II.G), as well as the need to reinforce the concept that type 1 IDDM is a life-long illness without potential for true remission with current treatment. Remission phases last longest in older teenagers and young adults compared with toddlers and young school-aged children.

3. Eventually, most prepubertal youngsters require between 0.6 and 0.8 U/kg per day. On a twice-a-day insulin regimen, two thirds of a total dose is given as a mixture of regular plus NPH (or lente) a half-hour before breakfast (in a ratio of about 1 U rapid-acting insulin for every 3 to 4 U of NPH [or lente]) plus one third of the total dose given as a mixture of rapid-acting insulin plus NPH (or lente) a half-hour before supper (in a ratio of 1:1–2). Using an intensified MDI regimen, small bursts of insulin analogs (i.e., lispro, aspart, or glulisine) are used immediately prior to big meals and snacks, with some type of basal insulin provided either at bedtime alone, bedtime plus breakfast, or in overlapping doses (if using NPH) throughout the day and night. This can be started at diagnosis or introduced when treatment goals are modified and intensified. Ratios are usually 50% basal plus 50% prandial boluses.

4. Teenagers may need as much as 1.0 to 1.5 U/kg per day during the rapid growth spurt at or around puberty; in subsequent years they return to lower insulin requirements.

5. The ratio of faster-acting insulins to NPH (or lente) insulin as well as basal analog insulins can vary according to the activity of the patient and the type of carbohydrate ingested. NPH, lente, and ultralente insulin are absorbed more irregularly and thus produce more peak effects in a much more variable fashion than faster-acting (regular and analog) insulin. The longer-acting insulins, glargine and detemir, produce more predictable insulin effects. Although they are supposed to be peakless, glargine and detemir sometimes have a small peak effect at 6 to 8 hours after being given; this can be determined by careful round-the-clock glucose monitoring. Under most circumstances, glargine and detemir insulin are associated with less hypoglycemia and better basal delivery characteristics.

6. Insulin doses at lunchtime and midafternoon, and the number of insulin injections, vary depending on activity intensity and consistency as well as food ingestion, glycemic effect, and which type of basal insulin is being utilized. Many youngsters do extremely well with overlapping doses of analog insulin and NPH prebreakfast, prelunch, predinner, and NPH at bedtime if the more expensive detemir or glargine basal insulin is unavailable or is not used. Some patients with

large afternoon snacks and relatively little afternoon activity also need presnack analog insulin to keep predinner blood glucose levels in target range.

G. Types of insulin. Human analog insulin is preferred at the time of diagnosis to reduce the likelihood of future allergic problems, such as itching, burning, redness, and hives. Because purity of insulin seems to be related to lipoatrophy at injection sites, such atrophic sites may be completely avoided with the use of either pure pork or human insulins.

H. Insulin allergy

1. Local allergy to insulin is now quite rare. It may occur minutes to hours after injection and may manifest with redness, pruritus, swelling, and heat. It usually occurs within the first few weeks of therapy and can be self-limiting. Subcutaneous insulin injections caused by poor technique sometimes can cause similar problems.

2. Rarely, systemic allergy to insulin occurs, with manifestations of urticaria, angioneurotic edema, and anaphylaxis, especially in an otherwise allergy-prone individual. This type of insulin allergy may be related to prior intermittent use of insulin. The immediate systemic reaction is more likely IgE-mediated (local allergy tends to be IgG-mediated). Insulin desensitization is the required preventive measure. Insulin allergy desensitization kits can be obtained from most insulin manufacturers on special request.

I. Administration of shots

1. In general, adults should retain the major responsibility for diabetes care of their young children and often even with teenagers. Gradual transfer of this responsibility is begun when the child with diabetes demonstrates age-appropriate readiness to accept the day-to-day burden of self-care.

2. Automatic injection or pen delivery systems may be preferred for children on MDI regimens.

3. Omitted insulin may occur up to 30% of the time in adults as well as in children and adolescents when prescribed insulin doses are compared with actual pharmacy vials distributed. Lack of comprehension of the importance of glucose control, eating disorders, depression and anger in patients, and patients feeling overwhelmed by the difficulties of modern diabetes treatment all contribute to insulin omission.

III. HOME MONITORING

A. Home blood glucose monitoring (HBGM) or self blood glucose monitoring (SBGM)

1. The best and most accurate home monitoring system involves the use of capillary blood glucose determinations. Automatic lancet injectors (e.g., Monojector Penlet, Autolance, and Autolet) are available for skin puncture to minimize trauma and discomfort using short and very fine disposable lancets. The drop of blood obtained is placed on a reagent strip on which colors are read with the naked eye, with the use of a colorimetric meter, or with a meter that reads blood glucose levels via electrical impedance.

2. Reflectance meters and electronic meters (LifeScan's Ultra and Profile; Abbott's Medisense Precision Xtra and Free Style series; Roche's Accucheck series meters; Free Style and Bayer's glucometer as well as Dex series meters; etc.) are widely used because of increased accuracy and ease of administration. Many diabetologists prefer memory meters, which can also be downloaded into home as well as office computers for data analysis and graphic displays to help analyze patterns of glucose control. The newest meters use minute amounts of capillary blood (1 to 5 μL) to decrease pain and discomfort, as well as semiautomatic capillary filling characteristics of their test strips. These features lead to more accurate testing. Some new meters also auto-calibrate when strips are inserted further, decreasing user errors.

3. Blood sugar monitoring should ideally be done every 2 to 3 hours around the clock, but such monitoring is impractical except with newer but expensive continuous monitoring systems. There is hope that such continuous

glucose monitoring systems will improve control, provide more feedback, and sustain such improvements, but this remains to be proven scientifically in longer-term usage. The more frequent the actual blood glucose monitoring, the more data áre available not only for pattern analysis but also for adjustments of food and/or insulin. Daily monitoring for type 1 diabetes is usually recommended before breakfast, before lunch, before dinner, and at bedtime, plus often before morning and/or afternoon snack times. Overnight monitoring can be extremely valuable but is usually done intermittently or on a monthly basis as well as for specific problem solving (see Table 42.1 for SBGM/HBGM protocol).

  4. There have been no problems with local cellulitis, abscess, or excess callus formation using this protocol in patients as young as neonates as long as reasonable common sense, site rotation, and hygienic technique are used. Routine alcohol swabbing is no longer recommended.

B. Urine testing
  1. Glucose testing
      a. Double-voided urine testing allows assessment of both sugar and acetone in a semiquantitative fashion. It should be realized that urine glucose testing is inaccurate because of changes in renal threshold, fluid intake, and output.
      b. Combination systems such as Chemstrip uGK and Keto-Diastix allow identification of glucose and ketone spillage. They are the standard urine testing systems for use on sick days and on days when blood sugars are either running high (>250 mg/dL) or are not being tested.
  2. Ketone testing
      a. Urine testing for ketones remains extremely valuable during sick days or whenever ketoacidosis may occur. If these are unavailable, older nitroprusside powder can also be used. All such systems test for acetone and acetoacetate, but not for β-hydroxybutyric acid, and provide guidance regarding the need for extra insulin under such circumstances.
      b. Newer **ketone capillary blood systems** (Precision Extra) are now available that will test specifically for blood β-hydroxybutyric acid and may eliminate the need for nonspecific urinary acetone and acetoacetate testing while also providing earlier data about ketonemia.

IV. HBGM (HOME BLOOD GLUCOSE MONITORING) WITH INSULIN AND CARBOHY-DRATE ALGORITHMS
Better decisions regarding insulin, food amounts, and food choices, as well as exercise, may result from using insulin algorithms (Table 42.2). These provide a basis for flexibility with insulin analogs as well as with regular insulin.

A. Tight blood sugar goals include the following:
  1. To achieve near-normal blood sugar levels ($\sim$100 mg/dL) **without frequent episodes of hypoglycemia** before breakfast and supper and throughout the night
  2. An overall target of 70 to 120 mg/dL preprandially and lower than 160 to 180 mg/dL postprandially
  3. A1c levels <7%

B. Considerations in achieving blood sugar goals
  1. Usually, 0.5 to 1.0 U of fast-acting regular insulin decreases blood sugar levels by 40 to 50 mg/dL for patients taking 20 to 40 U per day if blood sugar levels are <240 mg/dL; above 240 mg/dL, the patient may need proportionately more insulin to accomplish the same goal (1 to 2 U to decrease 40 to 50 mg/dL).
  2. In very young children and in those who are extremely sensitive to insulin, u100 preparations can be diluted (make u10 or u20 insulin with diluent supplied by manufacturer). Then algorithms can be created using 0.1-U to 0.2-U increments.
  3. HBGM/SBGM is used to double-check and adjust the algorithms being applied.
  4. Improvement (or lack of) is confirmed by hemoglobin A_{1c} (HbA$_{1c}$) measurements every 4 to 6 weeks as demonstrated in the DCCT (Diabetes Control and Complications Trial) (see Section VII.A).

TABLE 42.1 Home Blood Glucose Monitoring Protocol

Interval	Breakfast	Mid-morning	Lunch	Mid-afternoon	Dinner	Bedtime	11 P.M.–midnight	3:00–4:30 A.M.
				Check prior to				
"Profile" 3 days each month[a]	bG	bG	bG	bG	bG	bG	bG	bG
Daily	bG		bG	bG	bG			
Every 8 days (awake profile)	bG	bG	bG	bG	bG	bG		

bG, blood glucose.

Problem-solving profile should be obtained whenever there is a question of dose needing adjustment or change. Many patients can obtain 3–4 blood glucose measurements each day. Keeping written records is important so that patterns can be identified. 240mg/dL. than more is level glucose blood whenever

[a]On sick days, follow this profile for testing, sometimes more often, and remember to **check for acetone** whenever blood glucose level is >240 mg/dL.

TABLE 42.2 New England Diabetes and Endocrinology Center (NEDEC) Algorithms, Sick-Day Advice, and Hypoglycemia Information

INSULIN ALGORITHM - (how to adjust or **VARY INSULIN** for high and low blood glucose [BG])—this intensified insulin system only works if you know BG level and then allows adjustments for food, activity, stress....

FOR _____ DATE _____

BLOOD GLUCOSE	BREAKFAST HUMALOG OR NOVOLOG	LUNCH HUMALOG OR NOVOLOG	AFTERNOON SNACK HUMALOG OR NOVOLOG	DINNER HUMALOG OR NOVOLOG	BEDTIME SNACK HUMALOG OR NOVOLOG	
<69 (JUICE)	___	___	___	___	___	
70–100	___	___	___	___	___	
101–150	___	___	___	___	___	
151–200	___	___	___	___	___	
201–250	___	___	___	___	___	
251–300*	___	___	___	___	___	
301–350*	___	___	___	___	___	
351–400*	___	___	___	___	___	
401–450*	___	___	___	___	___	
451–500*	___	___	___	___	___	* = check ketones even if not sick
>501*	___	___	___	___	___	
BASAL INSULIN	___ +	___ +	___ +	___	___	

DAY-DAY GLYCEMIC INDEX ADJUSTMENTS: approximately 1:15 insulin:carbohydrate coverage ratio

DIFFERENT FOOD EFFECTS ON BG LEVELS: USE _____ MORE HUMALOG OR NOVOLOG INSULIN FOR HIGH GLYCEMIC INDEX FOODS SUCH AS: CORN PRODUCTS, POTATO PRODUCTS, ROLLS, CHINESE FOOD, PASTA, PIZZA AND MOST "FAST" FOOD. IF MERELY OVEREATING, DECIDE IF YOU NEED MORE HUMALOG OR NOVOLOG TO "COVER" BG EFFECTS.

BUT **DECREASE** HUMALOG OR NOVOLOG INSULIN BY _____ UNITS OR ADD EXTRA SNACK FOR PLANNED **ACTIVITY**

(continued)

TABLE 42.2 New England Diabetes and Endocrinology Center (NEDEC) Algorithms, Sick-Day Advice, and Hypoglycemia Information *(Continued)*

NEDEC SICK DAY ADJUSTMENTS: *CHECK BG EVERY 2–3 HOURS INCLUDING OVERNIGHT BGs*

1. GET WEIGHED AT LEAST THREE TIMES EACH DAY. WEIGHT LOSS MEANS POSSIBLE DEHYDRATION.
   DRINK MORE SALTY FLUIDS LIKE SOUPS.

2. CHECK KETONES AT LEAST EVERY 3–4 HOURS. IF +, MORE INSULIN NEEDED IF BG LEVELS ARE ALSO HIGH.

3. EXTRA INSULIN (**SICK DAY BOOSTER**) IS BASED ON 10–20% OF TOTAL DAY'S INSULIN DOSE (   ) IF YOUR BLOOD GLUCOSE WAS 100. THIS 10–20% SICK DAY BOOSTER IS GIVEN
   EVERY 3–4 HOURS DAY & NIGHT. THIS IS MUCH MORE THAN USUAL ALGORITHM CHANGES
   → 10% SICK DAY BOOSTER IF BG >240 & KETONES NEGATIVE: _____ **EXTRA HUMALOG OR NOVOLOG**
   → 20% SICK DAY BOOSTER IF BG >240 & KETONES POSITIVE: _____ **EXTRA HUMALOG OR NOVOLOG**

4. CALL IF NOT BETTER, SYMPTOMS DO NOT GO AWAY, SEVERE HEADACHE OR ACTING STRANGE, VOMITING DOES NOT STOP OR WEIGHT LOSS CONTINUES OR IF NOT SURE WHAT TO DO

5. RARELY, WITH ILLNESS, INSULIN NEEDS TO BE DECREASED - WHEN BG <100.

6. *USUALLY, EVEN IF NOT EATING WELL, ILLNESS BLOCKS INSULIN SO THAT EXTRA INSULIN IS NEEDED.*

HYPOGLYCEMIA RECOGNITION & TREATMENT: IF POSSIBLE, CHECK GLUCOSE

A. DECIDE IF EXTRA FOOD NEEDED AT BEDTIME SNACK FOLLOWING INCREASED AFTERNOON OR EVENING ACTIVITY
   TO PREVENT OVERNIGHT (NOCTURNAL) HYPOGLYCEMIA!!!

B. NEVER GO TO BED WITHOUT KNOWING YOUR BLOOD GLUCOSE LEVEL.

C. REMEMBER THAT MANY EPISODES OF HYPOGLYCEMIA DO NOT PRODUCE SYMPTOMS. CHECK YOUR BLOOD GLUCOSE LEVEL BEFORE A NAP.

D. IF ABLE TO TALK AND RESPOND, GIVE 4–6 OZ OF JUICE OR BFSERIES SUGAR-CONTAINING SODA OR 2–3 GLUCOSE TABLETS OR 7 LIFE SAVERS ® OR GLUCOSE GEL OR HONEY OR REGULAR
   TABLE SUGAR. RARELY THIS NEEDS REPEATING. (NOT CHOCOLATE **or other high fat foods**: TOO SLOW ACTING AND ALSO EXCESSIVE CALORIES)

E. DURING DAYTIME, USUALLY NO NEED FOR EXTRA SNACK AFTER TREATING REACTION. JUST JUICE OR OTHER SIMPLE CARBS.

F. IF MIDDLE OF THE NIGHT, BE SAFER AND GIVE AN EXTRA SNACK: 1 BREAD + 1 PROTEIN W/FAT.

G. IF LIMP, HAVING A CONVULSION OR SEIZURE, UNCONSCIOUS OR NOT ABLE TO TALK → THEN DO NOT PUT ANYTHING IN THE MOUTH, USE GLUCAGON SHOT $1/_4$–$1/_2$–1 CC IN MUSCLE.
   IF NOT BETTER BY 15 MINUTES, CALL US - ANY TIME DAY OR NIGHT - SO WE CAN DISCUSS AMBULANCE, EMERGENCY ROOM EVALUATION AND INTRAVENOUS GLUCOSE

5. One may establish and confirm carbohydrate algorithms in a similar fashion (i.e., how much fruit or bread must be changed to bring about an increase or decrease in blood sugar, which foods have what type of glycemic effect, effects of high fiber on food absorption, what types of adjustments with food are needed for different types, intensities, and timing of activities).

V. MEAL PLANNING

Dietary prescriptions must take into account individual and ethnic preferences as well as the family habits of the child, teenager, or adult with type 1 diabetes mellitus.

A. Carbohydrates

1. The total carbohydrate content of the diabetic meal plan is usually ~50% to 60% of total calories.
2. Concentrated sugars are avoided except for management of short activity bursts or actual hypoglycemia. Ten to fifteen grams of fast-acting sucrose or glucose (i.e., 4 to 6 oz of orange or apple juice or regular carbonated soda, seven small hard candies such as Lifesavers), or 10 to 15 g of a variety of prepackaged dextrose preparations (Monogel, BD Tablets, Instant Glucose, Glutose) is generally adequate treatment. Some diabetes specialists now recommend only concentrated carbohydrates during daytime hypoglycemic episodes, whereas others suggest that extra carbohydrate or protein also be given not just in the middle of the night but during the daytime hours as well. This author suggests that simple carbohydrates be used for most episodes of hypoglycemia except overnight, when more caution should be exercised. High-fat chocolate candies are not optimal because the fat tends to slow down the absorption of the simple sugars, thus delaying hypoglycemic correction.
3. Complex high-fiber carbohydrates (bran, whole-grain cereals and breads, legumes, vegetables, and whole fruit) are encouraged.
4. A small minority of diabetologists and nutritionists recommend a low-carbohydrate/high-protein approach to meal planning on the basis that less insulin may be needed and therefore it may be easier to counterbalance food and insulin needs under such circumstances. Such approaches are more often recommended for adults than for children and adolescents, and are more often associated with type 2 rather than type 1 diabetes.
5. Carbohydrate-counting concepts provide added flexibility and decrease the previous restriction on individual carbohydrates by allowing exchanges among all sources of carbohydrates.
6. Paying individual attention to variabilities in <u>glycemic index</u> allows for more appropriate adjustment of insulin according to different types of foods and snacks (i.e., prolonged pasta effects vs. rapid effects after eating potato, corn, or rice products).
7. In those with concomitant <u>celiac disease</u> (gluten sensitivity), occurring in the range of 5% to 10% of type 1 diabetes patients in many parts of the world, wheat and gluten restrictions demand changes to more rapid-acting types of carbohydrates with a concomitant need for higher doses of prandial insulin to cover these expected hyperglycemic surges.

B. Protein

1. The total protein content of the diabetic meal plan is usually ~15% to 20%. It may be prudent to limit animal-source protein rather than vegetable-source protein for general cardiovascular and/or renal benefits.
2. Protein and fat may be very helpful in the bedtime snack to help prevent overnight hypoglycemia, because they slow absorption of carbohydrates.
3. Sugar-containing high-fat <u>ice cream</u> may be an ideal bedtime snack because the protein and fat content in such ice cream preparations allows for slower glycemic availability throughout the nighttime hours and thus decreases the chances of overnight hypoglycemia. <u>Uncooked cornstarch</u> mixed with liquids or solid foods may also provide a source of long-acting carbohydrates to prevent overnight hypoglycemia.

C. Fats

1. Total fat content usually should be no more than 25% to 30% of total calories. Saturated animal fat intake should be reduced for improved cardiovascular effect, whereas intake of unsaturated fats—particularly those from vegetable sources—should not necessarily be restricted.

2. In many surveys of youngsters with type 1 diabetes, lipid values are increased, particularly in the subset of patients whose glucose remains out of control. This may occur in as many as 40% of such youngsters as well as in adults with type 1 diabetes.

3. The following guidelines should be used: skim or low-fat milk; no more than 2 or 3 eggs weekly (egg substitutes okay); margarine may not be any different than butter in terms of saturated fat content, so both should be decreased; decrease red and brown meats; increase poultry, tofu, fish, and vegetable-based oils; encourage skim milk–based cheeses.

4. With documented hypercholesterolemia and/or hypertriglyceridemia, more restrictions in dietary saturated fat and *trans*-fatty acids will be important—perhaps also supplemented by lipid-lowering medications.

D. General dietary considerations

1. Total calories are guided by body habitus and general appetite.

2. General rule of thumb: Start with 1 000 kcal per day for a 1-year-old and increase by ~100 kcal per year thereafter.

3. For boys, keep increasing calories to about 2 600 to 2 800 kcal for a base diet, but 3 000 to 3 500 kcal daily may be needed to cover prolonged and regular athletic activity or several weeks at camp.

4. Girls need to start calorie restriction at about age 10 to 12 years (early puberty), so meal plans are increased to about 1 800 to 2 000 kcal per day until this stage and then decreased to 1 100 to 1 700 kcal per day according to metabolic needs, activity patterns, and desired weight, with 1 200 to 1 400 kcal being the mean.

5. If the patient is overweight or frankly obese, caloric restriction plus increasing activity will be needed.

6. To counterbalance extra activity, extra food is provided or insulin doses should be adjusted downward in anticipation of such extra activity demands.

7. Attempts should be made to identify early signals of hypoglycemia with HBGM/SBGM, so that quick-acting carbohydrate may be used.

8. Holidays and special events often associated with extra food can be allowed, with appropriate extra insulin (or activity) counterbalanced.

9. For special religious fast days (e.g., Yom Kippur or Ramadan), education should be used to minimize hypoglycemia.

VI. EXERCISE

The goal of modern diabetes treatment includes consistent daily activity.

A. Burst activity

1. Short burst activity generally requires extra short-acting carbohydrate intake just before or just after such activity, whereas prolonged exercise requires a reduction in insulin as well as an increase in carbohydrates, proteins, and fats.

2. Blood glucose monitoring should be used to document such effects and learn what works as counterbalancing measures.

B. Prolonged, planned activity

1. The longer the activity (and the more aerobic), the more likely it is to cause a delayed hypoglycemic effect (accentuating insulin effect several hours afterward); recognizing this phenomenon allows for additional food to be provided several hours after the activity is completed. Ice cream, chocolate products, or uncooked cornstarch (available in some special "bars"), as well as foods that are high in protein and fat, may be used to counterbalance such prolonged activity effects on sugar levels, presumably through changes in liver and muscle insulin receptors.

2. If the activity is planned, one may decrease the amount of insulin taken, especially that peaking several hours after activity.

C. General considerations

1. In theory, it should not matter whether a patient reduces insulin in anticipation of activity or compensates with extra food in an attempt to balance energy expenditure. However, because as many as 20% to 30% of female teenagers with type 1 diabetes are >120% above ideal weight, it may be prudent to avoid additional calories under such circumstances.

2. Sports should be encouraged. Supervisory personnel at school or at a park or camp must be made aware of the presence of a person with diabetes and be provided with a source of quick-acting carbohydrate to manage hypoglycemia should it occur; guidelines must be given so that hypoglycemia can be recognized and avoided. Decisions about glucagon use and availability should be openly discussed and individual advice provided.

3. Medic-Alert tags must be worn in case of emergencies by all children and teenagers as well as by adults who take insulin.

VII. SPECIAL CONSIDERATIONS

A. Hemoglobin A1c (glycohemoglobin [GHb], HbA₁c).

A. Hemoglobin A1c (glycohemoglobin [GHb], HbA_{1c}). This test is an indicator of blood sugar control during the previous 4- to 12-week period. Blood is assayed after saline washing to detect the relative percentage of "stable" glycosylated hemoglobin present.

1. Glucose attaches to hemoglobin in a mostly irreversible fashion throughout the life span (120 days) of the red cell. At any given moment, a sample of blood will represent a collection of newly "born," middle-aged, and "dying" cells such that the glycohemoglobin level obtained represents an integrated glucose value that is reflective of the glucose environment confronting the red cell over the previous 1- to 3-month period. There does, however, seem to be an <u>overrepresentation</u> of <u>the most recent 2- to 4-week period</u> of glycemia in most A1c assays.

2. The most reliable methods use high-pressure liquid chromatography or gel electrophoresis, and separate out the subfraction called HbA_{1c}; alternatively, HbA_{1a+b+c} (total glycosylated hemoglobin, total HbA_1, or glycohemoglobin fractions) can be separated as an index of blood glucose control. Either HbA_{1c} or total GHb can be used to estimate the average blood sugar present for the past few months. Values <8% for HbA_{1c} are acceptable, whereas values <7% are ideal as long as excessive or severe episodes of hypoglycemia do not occur. According to the DCCT, the higher the HbA_{1c} value and the longer the HbA_{1c} stays out of ideal range, the more likely will be the long-term eye, kidney, and neurologic complications of diabetes as well as the more likely will be cardiovascular problems.

3. In patients with anemias or other hemoglobinopathies, alternatives such <u>as fructosamine assays</u> can serve similar purposes.

B. Limited joint mobility (LJM, joint contractures, diabetic hand syndrome).

B. Limited joint mobility (LJM, joint contractures, diabetic hand syndrome). LJM is present in as many as 15% to 30% of adolescents with type 1 diabetes and may be the harbinger of a subset of young people who are at 400% to 600% greater risk for developing the complications associated with hyperglycemia, such as retinopathy, nephropathy, hypertension, and neuropathy. LJM probably reflects <u>collagen glycosylation</u> based on long-standing ambient glucose concentrations in the body.

1. As originally described by Rosenbloom, the patient places the hands together in prayer position with the forearm parallel to the floor. Normal placement allows for juxtaposition of all fingers as well as the palm.

2. The Brink-Starkman classification is as follows: stage 0, no abnormality; stage I, skin thickening without contractures; stage II, bilateral fifth-finger contractures; stage III, other fingers involved bilaterally; stage IV, fingers plus wrist involvement bilaterally; stage V, fingers, wrist, and other joint involvement.

C. Sick-day guidelines and ketoacidosis.

C. Sick-day guidelines and ketoacidosis. Special attention because of potential acute insulin resistance and associated dehydration is required during illnesses, with more blood glucose monitoring, blood or urine ketone monitoring, as well as weight checks several times each day.

1. Unless there is a major vomiting component to the illness, more rapid-acting or regular insulin is given every 2 to 4 hours (calculated by adding up the total daily insulin requirement and using a sick-day booster dose of 10% to 20%) with each dose. This is either added to the usual insulin dose or given as a supplemental dose until the added stress of such infection subsides. With insulin pump treatment, basal doses can temporarily also be increased quite easily.

2. Antiemetic medications have been questioned because of reports associating these types of medicines with Reye syndrome, but prochlorperazine (Compazine) or trimethobenzamide (Tigan) suppositories, as well as bismuth-salicylic acid (Pepto-Bismol) liquid preparations, can be used to reduce nausea and vomiting. Recently, Zophran (Tabs or I.V.) is also uses.

3. The provision of large amounts of salty fluids (soups and broths, or electrolyte solutions such as Gatorade or Lytren) is perhaps more important than extra insulin in preventing hospitalization from dehydration caused by the osmotic effects of excessive glycosuria.

4. Obtaining frequent weights, several times each day, is a simple technique for assessing overall hydration status and gives family members an indication of how much additional fluid is required; acute weight loss over a 1- to 2-day period is attributable almost completely to fluid loss.

5. HBGM is a critical part of home monitoring during sick days but must be coupled with urinary ketone testing or blood β-hydroxybutyric acid levels; blood sugar levels >180 to 240 mg/dL associated with ketonuria or increasing levels of β-hydroxybutyric acid demand 10% to 20% more insulin given every few hours throughout the day as well as throughout the night to prevent hyperglycemia and dehydration from progressing to decompensated ketoacidosis, coma, and death.

6. Ketonuria can be present because of relative lack of food (starvation ketosis) as well as insulin deficiency. Blood sugar levels <180 mg/dL with ketonuria do not automatically call for additional insulin; instead, liquids containing carbohydrates should be added to the treatment program at home (i.e., Gatorade, sweetened juices, and sugar-containing carbonated soda) and alternated with salty fluids.

D. Uncontrolled diabetes mellitus and recurrent DKA. Children and teenagers who require frequent hospitalization and intravenous fluids generally are those who are not properly supervised by adults, those who are not routinely testing either blood or urine at home, and those who "forget" to take their insulin. Noncompliance and psychosocial problems are major causes of recurrent ketoacidosis.

E. Hypoglycemia

1. Most episodes of hypoglycemia are predictable and preventable.

2. Very young children may be at higher risk for severe hypoglycemic reactions (unconsciousness or seizures) because of their inability to recognize and/or communicate subtle symptoms of hypoglycemia.

3. The combination of alcoholic beverages and insulin (usually by teenagers or adults) can produce long-lasting and very severe hypoglycemia hours after alcoholic intake; such information must be made available to teenagers and adults with type 1 diabetes so that prevention is possible.

4. Purposeful insulin overdose is being recognized as a form of suicidal gesture by the adolescent or adult with severe but often unsuspected depression and/or severe family turmoil (i.e., physical, emotional, or sexual abuse).

5. Recent studies suggest an abnormality of counterregulatory response in many patients with diabetes, which may account for prolonged and unpredictable hypoglycemia.

6. Hypoglycemia unawareness is associated with recurrent and severe episodes of hypoglycemia. Frequent blood glucose monitoring is required. Efforts to minimize hypoglycemia under such circumstances focus on retraining (called hypoglycemia awareness training [HGAT] or blood glucose awareness training [BGAT]). HGAT and BGAT utilize frequent monitoring and focus on relearning early warning signals that presage additional, more severe episodes.

If severe episodes of hypoglycemia occur, evaluation for <u>celiac disease</u>, <u>adrenal insufficiency</u>, <u>thyroid disorders</u>, and <u>growth-hormone deficiency</u> should be considered (see also sections on CGMS and insulin pumps).

F. Somogyi phenomenon (rebound effect)

1. The Somogyi phenomenon is a series of events caused by overinsulinization. As the insulin dose is increased beyond the amount required for any given portion of the day, the effect of the excessive insulin is to cause either overeating or frank hypoglycemia, which is not always recognized or reported.

2. This excessive insulin effect elicits a <u>counterregulatory hormone response</u> followed by <u>"rebound" hyperglycemia</u>.

3. In its most common form, relatively minor hypoglycemia from any cause or combination of causes (inadequate meals or snacks, excess activity, unopposed insulin, alcohol) contributes directly to subsequent hyperglycemia, which lasts for 8 to 24 hours.

4. In rare instances, this counterregulatory response is so excessive as to produce not only ketonuria but also full-fledged DKA.

5. Recognition of the possibility that some episodes of high blood sugar levels might be caused by too much rather than too little insulin, especially in the middle of the night, leads to the correct conclusion that reduction of insulin can correct some causes of fasting hyperglycemia.

G. Dawn phenomenon

1. Many patients with type 1 diabetes mellitus demonstrate an early-morning (4 to 8 A.M.) rise in glucose levels that is aggravated by intake of food at breakfast (but not caused by it) and that tends to peak in midmorning. It often occurs because of <u>waning insulin</u> availability plus concomitant <u>increase in growth hormone</u> and <u>cortisol</u> overnight.

2. It appears to be unrelated to food intake or activity, and whether it represents an increase in hepatic glucose production or decreased peripheral utilization (or both) is not known. It does indicate a further requirement for basal insulin levels that may be ideally treated with continuous subcutaneous infusions such as those provided by insulin pumps.

3. It may be confused with the Somogyi phenomenon. Sampling of glucose levels throughout the night may help in differentiating the two conditions.

4. Some have recommended an earlier injection in the morning (5 to 6 A.M.), and most suggest a late-evening (before bedtime) injection of intermediate-acting insulin if an insulin pump is not being used. With an insulin pump, increasing the basal insulin in an effort to counterbalance the dawn phenomenon is usually successful, just as the new, long-lasting insulin analogs (glargine and detemir insulins) provide smoother insulinization, without overnight peaks.

H. Idiosyncratic insulin needs

1. <u>Reverse dawn phenomenon</u>, in which supper or evening insulin needs exceed those of the predawn breakfast hours, occurs in up to 10% to 20% of youngsters.

2. Other patients may have no dawn or reverse dawn phenomenon but relatively "flat" basal needs—some with a small dinnertime insulin need and others with an early-afternoon peak requirement.

I. Growth

1. Decreased growth velocity appears to be more common in boys than in girls with type 1 diabetes mellitus, and may be as common as 5% to 10% in large pediatric and adolescent cohorts.

2. Extreme growth failure can be associated with pubertal delay and hepatomegaly (<u>Mauriac syndrome</u>) caused by severe and chronic diabetes mellitus out of control as a result of long-standing lack of insulin or insulin underutilization. This is seen in parts of the world where insulin is not consistently available or when insulin is purposefully/surreptitiously omitted.

3. In the subset of children and adolescents who are prone to obesity (family history, bulimia and binge eating, inactivity, etc.), attention to body mass index (BMI) will help identify those in need of special dietary and/or psychosocial support.

J. Teenage and adult pregnancy

1. The teenager who has diabetes and becomes pregnant has many added burdens affecting both herself and the child. The first trimester is often associated with increasing episodes or severity of hypoglycemia, whereas the second and third trimesters are usually associated with rapidly increasing insulin resistance, and therefore insulin doses rise dramatically.

2. Discussions about contraception and birth-control options must become part of the repertoire of professionals responsible for diabetes care.

3. Patients ready to conceive must be made aware that improving blood sugar control at—or ideally *before* conception—reduces the risks of congenital anomalies, as well as prematurity and its associated complications.

4. Fetal monitoring and close collaboration with high-risk obstetric teams is extremely valuable.

K. Thyroid dysfunction and other autoimmune endocrinopathies

1. Thyroid problems often coexist with type 1 autoimmune diabetes mellitus (see Chapters 33, 41 and 42). In the type 1 diabetes population, 5% to 10% have a variety of thyroid dysfunctions including euthyroid goiters, hyperthyroidism, or hypothyroidism.

2. The vast majority of thyroid problems seen in association with type 1 diabetes are secondary to chronic Hashimoto thyroiditis, consistent with the concept that type 1 diabetes mellitus, to a large extent, is an autoimmune disorder. Thyroid antibodies should be checked yearly along with thyroid function tests, but euthyroid Hashimoto thyroiditis does not automatically require immediate hormone treatment.

3. Achlorhydria and mild iron deficiency related to possible iron malabsorption may occur (associated with positive gastroparietal antibodies).

4. Adrenal insufficiency (adrenalitis) and ovarian failure (oophoritis-gonadal antibodies) are also seen with type 1 diabetes.

5. Celiac disease with positive transglutaminase, endomysial, or other gluten-related antibodies (gliadin) is also significantly more common in many cohorts of patients with type 1 diabetes, particularly in those populations with ancestry in or around the Mediterranean Sea. Celiac disease associated with type 1 diabetes may coexist in as many as 6% to 10% and often is also associated with other vitamin and mineral deficiencies, such as iron deficiency and osteopenia from calcium and/or vitamin D malabsorption. Lactose intolerance also may coexist with celiac disease in otherwise asymptomatic patients.

L. Osteopenia

1. Prevalence and incidence in type 1 diabetes is unknown, but there are some research reports suggesting increases in this population.

2. There is increased prevalence and incidence of osteopenia if celiac disease coexists, even if the celiac disease is asymptomatic.

M. Hypertension

1. Hypertension should be treated aggressively in an effort to reduce morbidity and mortality associated with diabetic complications.

2. Essential hypertension can occur in any youngster or young adult with type 1 diabetes, and detailed family history of hypertension and cardiovascular disease should be reviewed. Most cases of hypertension are associated with diabetic nephropathy.

3. Thiazide diuretics can be safely used in most cases to control hypertension. Beta-blockade can also be used but with some caution because of the potential to mask symptoms of hypoglycemia. Angiotensin-converting enzyme (ACE) inhibitors now play a role not only in normalizing mild hypertension but also in reducing glomerular hyperfiltration and microalbuminuria. Therefore, ACE inhibitors may be the medication treatment of choice if hypertension exists.

4. Sequential evaluation of renal function with blood urea nitrogen (BUN), creatinine, overnight or 24-hour urine protein, and creatinine clearance are helpful in early detection of nephropathy. Microalbuminuria (>7 to 20 mg up to 200 to 300 mg per day obtained in overnight or 24-hour collections as well

as with random screening sampling) may identify subpopulations at risk for diabetic nephropathy. If values are abnormal, protein intake may need to be restricted (to as low as 12%), although this is a difficult meal-plan prescription for many to follow. ACE inhibitors also have been helpful under circumstances when microalbuminuria or proteinuria occurs even when hypertension is not present. Controlling hyperglycemia is most important to slow down kidney damage and possibly reverse such abnormalities. Smoking cessation is also helpful.

   5. Onset of proteinuria and hypertension during the first 10 years of type 1 diabetes mellitus should not be automatically considered as indicative of diabetic nephropathy (uncommon in the first 10 years of diabetes mellitus), and its etiology should be vigorously pursued despite the fact that all such hypertension may be effectively treated with ACE inhibitors.

N. Lipids. Fasting blood levels should be obtained for total cholesterol, triglyceride, and high-density lipoprotein (HDL) cholesterol, as well as direct or calculated low-density lipoprotein (LDL) cholesterol values at least every 6 to 12 months to identify which patients require further dietary lipid control as well as more intensified insulin therapy. Antilipid medications, including resins such as cholestyramine and colestipol, as well as gemfibrozil and statin medications (e.g., atorvastatin and simvastatin as well as others), can be used in conjunction with insulin treatment based on family risk analysis and individualized lipid data even in children. Plant sterols and stanols also can be safely prescribed.

O. Ophthalmologic evaluation. Baseline ophthalmology evaluation, including fundus photographs, is recommended within the first 2 to 3 years of developing diabetes and might be repeated at 1- to 2-year intervals after 5 years' duration of type 1 diabetes mellitus (or age 10 years) to pick up early vascular changes in the retina. Fluorescein angiograms may show the earliest abnormalities of diabetic retinopathy years before dilated-eye examinations or fundus photography and may be especially valuable in the cohort with the highest HbA$_{1c}$ values. Poor glycemic control is clearly associated with earlier and more severe types of retinopathy. Rapid improvement of long term poor control is also associated with retinopathy. Laser treatment of retinopathy can save vision.

VIII. CONTINUOUS GLUCOSE MONITORING SYSTEMS (CGMS)

A. CGMS (Glucowatch, Guardian, Dexcom, Navigator) is now available, although expensive, with results every 5 to 15 minutes.

B. Initial systems were useful for trend analysis but had error rates in the range of 20% to 30% for individual values, especially when registering hypoglycemia.

C. Newer models have a reduced the error rate to the range of 10% to 15% and offer alarms that identify decreasing as well as increasing glycemic trends.

IX. INSULIN PUMPS, INTENSIFIED MDI THERAPY, AND NEW RESEARCH

A. General considerations

   1. While totally implantable artificial endocrine pancreases and pancreas transplants (partial and β-cell) continue to be investigated, insulin pumps (continuous subcutaneous insulin infusion [CSII] systems) coupled with extensive SMBG are being used in adults and children more frequently than ever.

   2. CSII and MDI therapy has been applied successfully in research settings and in clinical practice in association with multidisciplinary health professional teams.

   3. Development of implantable and noninvasive glucose sensors is on the horizon and will revolutionize current diabetes care. Sensors are coupled to internally or externally situated programmable insulin delivery systems that potentially can feed appropriate amounts of insulin adjusted frequently according to glucose fluctuations in the blood or interstitium. Current CGMS units are available that communicate directly with CSII but are not yet fully automatic.

B. Continuous subcutaneous insulin infusion (CSII)

   1. Young children, teenagers, and adults can be treated successfully with insulin pumps. CSII may be the preferred treatment modality for infants and toddlers because of ability to immediately turn off delivery and for fine-tuning adjustments.

2. Hypoglycemia may be decreased with successful use of insulin pumps, particularly when insulin analogs are used.

3. A1c improvements using CSII are in the range of 0.5% to 2.0% in many large studies around the world.

C. Intensive MDI therapy

1. Whereas CSII uses analog or regular insulin delivered in small boluses over 24 hours with larger prefood boluses given as needed, MDI uses basal-bolus algorithms of subcutaneous insulin in a variety of programs. Some examples are the following:

   a. Glargine or detemir insulin before breakfast and again at bedtime, with additional analog or regular insulin before meals, and snacks as needed (b.i.d. long-acting insulin with premeal boluses)

   b. Analog or regular insulin given before breakfast, before lunch, and before supper, with glargine or detemir insulin at suppertime (bedtime long-acting insulin with premeal boluses)

   c. Glargine insulin prebreakfast with prandial analogs often used in preschoolers who do not need any bedtime insulin

   d. Analog or regular insulin plus NPH (or lente) before breakfast; analog or regular alone before supper; and NPH (or lente) alone at bedtime (b.i.d. NPH [or lente] with premeal boluses)

   e. Analog or regular insulin plus NPH (or lente) before all three meals, plus NPH (or lente) alone at bedtime (overlapping NPH [or lente] with premeal bolus mixtures)

   f. Same as example **e,** but also with analog insulin before afternoon snack (when there is no afternoon activity)

   g. Analog or regular insulin given before breakfast, before lunch, and before supper, with ultralente insulin at suppertime (ultralente at bedtime with premeal boluses)

2. The principles of insulin adjustment are similar to those for CSII and demand frequent SMBG each day to provide data to adjust insulin, food, and exercise accordingly.

D. Inhaled insulin may replace injected bolus insulin in MDI but still must be coupled with injected basal insulin analogs or overlapping intermediate-acting insulins. Short-term pulmonary safety has been established, but long-term pulmonary safety remains unknown.

X. ONGOING EDUCATION, PEER, AND PARENT SUPPORT GROUPS

A. Diabetes education

1. Education is a critical component of diabetes care. It should include survival skills shortly after diagnosis and evolve into a continuous and ongoing process with periodic updating and review by the health care team.

2. The patient's entire family should be included.

B. Peer and parent support groups

1. Groups provide an opportunity to complement office visits.

2. Groups can be informational, supportive, and therapeutic.

3. The Internet has many sites (e.g., www.childrenwithdiabetes.com) available for education and support internationally. Other excellent publications are produced privately (*Diabetes Health*) as well as via many other national and local diabetes organizations around the world.

XI. SUMMARY

Efforts to provide ongoing education and support for the patient with type 1 diabetes should be aimed at obtaining blood sugar levels as close to normal as possible without causing excessive hypoglycemia. With attention to the psychological needs of the child and family members, and with a positive, nonpunitive attitude on the part of the health care team, more patients should be able to live better, happier, and longer lives free of the complications of IDDM.

Selected References

Amin R, Ross K, Acerini CL, et al. Hypoglycemia prevalence in prepubertal children with type 1 diabetes on standard insulin regimen: use of continuous glucose monitoring system. *Diabetes Care* 2003:662–667.

Brink SJ. Complications of type 1 diabetes mellitus in children and teenagers. In: Cheta D, ed. *Vascular Involvement in Diabetes. Clinical, Experimental and Beyond*. Basel: Karger; 2005:375–388.

Brink SJ. Diabetes camping. In: Werther G, Court J, eds. *Diabetes and the Adolescent*. Melbourne, Australia: Miranova Publishers; 1998:281–294.

Brink SJ. Diabetic ketoacidosis. In: Chiarelli F, Dahl-Jorgensen K, Kiess W., eds. *Diabetes in Childhood and Adolescence*. Basel: Karger; 2005:94–121.

Brink SJ. Hypoglycaemia in children and adolescents with type 1 diabetes mellitus. *Diabetes Nutr Metab* 1999;12:108–121.

Brink SJ. Insulin treatment and home monitoring for type 1 diabetes mellitus. In: LeRoith D, Taylor SI, Olefsky JM, eds. *Diabetes Mellitus. A Fundamental and Clinical Text*. 3rd ed. Philadelphia: Lippincott Williams & Wilkins; 2004:683–700.

Brink SJ. Pediatric and adolescent IDDM meal planning 1992: our best advice to prevent, postpone and/or minimize angiopathy. In: Weber B, Burger W, Danne T, eds. *Structural and Functional Abnormalities in Subclinical Diabetic Angiopathy*. Basel: Karger; 1992:156–169.

Brink SJ. The very young child with diabetes. In: Brink SJ, Serban V, eds. *Pediatric and Adolescent Diabetes*. Timisoara, Romania: Brumar; 2004:189–232.

Brink SJ, Moltz K. The message of the DCCT for children and adolescents. *Diabetes Spectrum* 1997:248–267.

Brink SJ, Serban V, eds. *Pediatric and Adolescent Diabetes*. Timisoara, Romania: Brumar; 2004.

Brink S, Siminerio L, Hinnen-Hentzen D, et al. *Diabetes Education Goals*. Alexandria, VA: American Diabetes Association; 1995.

Danne T, Tamborlane WV, eds. Insulin pumps in childhood diabetes. In: *Pediatr Diabetes* 2006;7(S4):1–50.

DCCT/Epidemiology of Diabetes Interventions and Complications (EDIC) Research Group. Beneficial effects of intensive therapy of diabetes during adolescence: outcomes after the conclusion of diabetes control and complications trial (DCCT). *Pediatrics* 2001;139:804–812.

DCCT/Epidemiology of Diabetes Interventions and Complications Research Group. Retinopathy and nephropathy in patients with type 1 diabetes four years after a trial of intensive therapy. *N Engl J Med* 2000;342:381–389.

DCCT Research Group. The effect of intensive treatment of diabetes on the development and progression of long-term complications in insulin-dependent diabetes mellitus. *N Engl J Med* 1993;329:977–986.

Dorchy H. What glycemic control can be achieved in young diabetics without residual secretion of endogenous insulin? What is the frequency of severe hypoglycemia and subclinical complications? *Arch Pediatr* 1994;1:970–981.

Gonder-Frederick L, Cox D, Kovatchev B, et al. A biopsychobehavioral model of risk of severe hypoglycemia. *Diabetes Care* 1997;20:661–669.

Hassan K, Loar R, Anderson BJ, Heptulla RA. The role of socioeconomic status, depression, quality of life, and glycemic control in type 1 diabetes mellitus. *J Pediatr* 2006;149:526–531.

Hattersley AT, Ashcroft FM. Activating mutations in Kir6.2 and neonatal diab3ts: new clinical syndromes, new scientific insights and new therapy. *Diabetes* 2005;54:2503–2513.

Hirsch IB, Farkas-Hirsch R, Skyler JS. Intensive insulin therapy for treatment of type I diabetes. *Diabetes Care* 1990;13:1265–1283.

Holterhus P-M, Odendahl R, Oesingmann S, et al. The German/Austrian DPV Initiative and the German Pediatric CSII Working Group. Classification of distinct baseline insulin infusion patterns in children and adolescents with type 1 diabetes on continuous subcutaneous insulin infusion therapy. *Diabetes Care* 2007;30:568–573.

Iannotti RJ, Nansel TR, Schneider S, et al. Assessing regimen adherence of adolescents with type 1 diabetes. *Diabetes Care* 2006;29:2263–2267.

Ryan CM. Why is cognitive dysfunction associated with the development of diabetes early in life? The diathesis hypothesis. *Pediatr Diabetes* 2006;7:289–297.

Siminerio L, Brink SJ. Diabetes school issues. In: Brink SJ, Serban V, eds. *Pediatric and Adolescent Diabetes*. Timisoara, Romania: Brumar; 2004:27–44.

Siminerio LM, Charron-Prochownik D, Banion C, et al. Comparing outpatient and inpatient diabetes education for newly diagnosed pediatric patients. *Diabetes Educ* 1999;25:895–906.

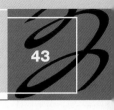

DIABETIC KETOACIDOSIS
Benjamin Fass

43

DIABETIC KETOACIDOSIS

I. GENERAL PRINCIPLES

Diabetic ketoacidosis (DKA) is the most common endocrine emergency seen by the primary care physician. Mortality rates from <1% to 10% have been reported, and in children it accounts for a major portion of diabetes-related deaths. DKA is much more common at presentation of type 1 diabetes, but it has also been reported at diagnosis of type 2 diabetes in children. The presence of DKA does not exclude a possible diagnosis of type 2 diabetes. All of the abnormalities associated with DKA can be traced to an absolute or relative lack of insulin that develops over several hours or days. In the newly diagnosed diabetic, insulin lack results from failure of endogenous insulin secretion, whereas in the known insulin-dependent diabetic, insulin deficiency can result from inadequate administration of exogenous insulin or from increased requirements for insulin caused by the presence of an underlying stressful condition, e.g., intercurrent infection (pneumonia, urinary tract infection, upper respiratory tract infection, meningitis, cholecystitis, pancreatitis), a vascular disorder (myocardial infarction, stroke), an endocrine disorder (hyperthyroidism, Cushing syndrome, acromegaly, pheochromocytoma), trauma, pregnancy, or emotional stress (especially in adolescence). The concomitant increased secretion of counterregulatory hormones or stress hormones (hormones antagonistic to the action of insulin—glucagon, epinephrine, cortisol, and growth hormone) explains the additional insulin requirements in such disorders. From 10% to 20% of patients presenting in DKA have no identifiable precipitating cause. A diagnosis of DKA is made when hyperglycemia (blood glucose >200 mg%) and metabolic acidosis (blood bicarbonate <15 mEq/L, arterial/capillary pH <7.3, or venous pH <7.25) exist in the presence of ketonemia.

II. PATHOPHYSIOLOGY OF DKA

A. Role of insulin

1. The sequence of events in DKA (Fig. 43.1) is one of insulin deficiency leading to hyperglycemia and a resulting osmotic diuresis that leads in turn to dehydration and electrolyte depletion.
2. The insulin deficiency activates glycogenolysis (glycogen breakdown to glucose) and gluconeogenesis (protein breakdown that leads to nitrogen loss and production of amino acids that serve as precursors in formation of new glucose). In addition, lipolysis results in production of free fatty acids (FFAs) as well as glycerol, which further helps fuel new glucose production.
3. Contributing further to the hyperglycemia are the decreased peripheral glucose utilization (secondary to both insulin lack and resistance) and the volume depletion (secondary to the osmotic diuresis), which reduce renal blood flow and consequently the amount of glucose filtered and excreted by the kidneys.
4. FFAs are delivered to the liver, where ketone bodies are produced (ketogenesis) with resultant ketonemia, which is intensified by decreased peripheral utilization. This leads to ketonuria, which further depletes electrolytes by an associated obligatory loss of cations.

617

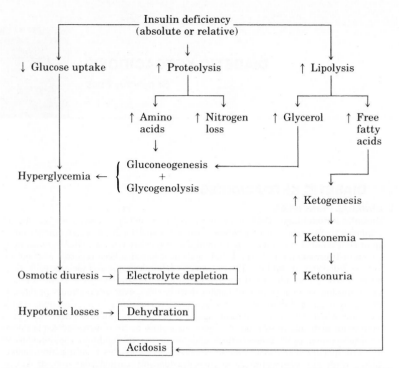

Figure 43.1. Pathophysiology of diabetic ketoacidosis. (From Davidson MD. Diabetes mellitus and hypoglycemia. In: Hershman JM, ed. *Endocrine Pathophysiology: A Patient-Oriented Approach.* Philadelphia: Lea & Febiger; 1982.)

5. Acidosis occurs as body bases are exhausted in the process of buffering the ketone anions that accumulate, accounting for the elevated plasma anion gap.

B. Role of counterregulatory hormones. The hypersecretion of epinephrine, glucagon, cortisol, and growth hormone contributes to ketoacidosis by:
   1. Inhibiting insulin-mediated glucose uptake by muscle, that is, peripheral utilization (epinephrine, cortisol, growth hormone)
   2. Activating glycogenolysis and gluconeogenesis (epinephrine, glucagon, cortisol)
   3. Activating lipolysis (epinephrine, growth hormone)
   4. Inhibiting residual insulin secretion (epinephrine, growth hormone)

III. CLINICAL PRESENTATION
A. Signs and symptoms
   1. **Polydipsia, polyuria,** and **weakness** are the most common presenting complaints; the severity depends on the degree of hyperglycemia as well as the duration of illness.
   2. **Anorexia, nausea, vomiting,** and **abdominal pain** (more common in children) may be present and may mimic an abdominal emergency. Ketonemia is thought to be responsible for most of these symptoms. Young children may present with dehydration, abdominal pain, or fatigue, and the presence of oral and perineal candidiasis.
   3. **Ileus** (secondary to potassium depletion from the ongoing osmotic diuresis) and **gastric dilatation** may occur and predispose to aspiration.
   4. **Kussmaul breathing** (deep, sighing respiration) is present as respiratory compensation for the metabolic acidosis and is usually apparent when the pH is <7.2.

    5. Neurologically, 20% of patients are without any sensorial changes at all, whereas 10% are actually comatose.

B. Physical examination

    1. Hypothermia is common in DKA. A fever should be taken as strong evidence of infection and vigorously pursued.

    2. Hyperpnea or Kussmaul respirations (depth and not rate of respirations is important) are present and are related to the degree of acidosis.

    3. Tachycardia is often present, but blood pressure is usually normal except in the presence of profound dehydration.

    4. Musty (fruity) breath odor can often be detected.

    5. Poor skin turgor may be prominent, depending on the degree of hydration.

    6. Hyporeflexia (associated with low serum potassium) can be elicited.

    7. Signs consistent with a "surgical abdomen" but that follow severe ketonemia can obscure the clinical picture.

    8. In extreme cases of DKA, one can see hypotonia, stupor, coma, incoordination of ocular movements, fixed dilated pupils, and, finally, death.

    9. Other signs from a precipitating illness can be present.

IV. LABORATORY DATA

A. Glucose

    1. Serum glucose is usually elevated above 300 mg/dL, although levels range from almost normal to very high levels characteristic of hyperosmolar coma.

    2. One important determinant of the glucose level is the degree of extracellular fluid depletion. Severe depletion results in decreased renal blood flow and decreased glucose excretion. The osmotic diuresis that results from the hyperglycemia causes severe fluid and electrolyte loss, dehydration, and hyperosmolality. At normal levels the contribution of blood glucose to osmolality is slight. In DKA the degree of hyperglycemia commonly seen can contribute significantly to the raised serum osmolality (generally up to 330 mOsm/kg), but not to the much higher levels seen in the hyperosmolar hyperglycemic state [HHS]).

B. Ketones. The three principal ketone bodies are **β-hydroxybutyric acid, acetoacetate,** and **acetone.** If measured, the total ketone concentration is usually >3 mM/L and can go as high as 30 mM/L (normal values are up to 0.15 mM/L).

    1. Serum acetone concentration (formed by nonenzymatic decarboxylation of acetoacetate) is high on admission. It is usually three or four times the concentration of acetoacetate. In contrast to other ketones, it does not contribute to the acidosis.

    2. β-Hydroxybutyric acid and acetoacetate (1:1 ratio in normal individuals) accumulate in the serum at a ratio of 3:1 (mild DKA) to as high as 15:1 (severe DKA).

    3. Standard nitroprusside reagents react with acetoacetate and not β-hydroxybutyric acid. They react only weakly with acetone. Therefore, a small ketone reading does not imply absence of ketoacidosis.

    4. As the DKA state is corrected, β-hydroxybutyric acid is converted to acetoacetate, giving a stronger or more positive reading when tested with nitroprusside. However, it does not indicate worsening of the DKA state.

C. Acidosis

    1. The metabolic acidosis is characterized by a serum bicarbonate of <15 mEq/L and an arterial pH of <7.3.

    2. It is due mainly to accumulation of β-hydroxybutyric acid and acetoacetate in the serum.

    3. The ketone bodies are strong acids that dissociate completely under physiologic conditions and thereby produce the acidemia.

    4. Some degree of lactic acidosis exists from hypoperfusion.

    5. Hyperchloremic acidosis can exist, especially after intravenous (IV) therapy and during the recovery phase of DKA. Patients who are less dehydrated and have better preservation of renal function have a greater tendency to develop this feature during treatment.

TABLE 43.1	Average Fluid and Electrolyte Losses in Diabetic Ketoacidosis	
	Maintenance requirements	**Losses**
Water	1 500–2 000 mL/m^2	100 mL/kg (range 60–100 mL/kg)
Sodium	45 mEq/m^2	6 mEq/kg (range 5–13 mEq/kg)
Potassium	35 mEq/m^2	5 mEq/kg (range 4–6 mEq/kg)
Chloride	30 mEq/m^2	4 mEq/kg (range 3–9 mEq/kg)
Phosphate^a	10 mEq/m^2	3 mEq/kg (range 2–5 mEq/kg)
Magnesium^b		0.5–1.5 mEq/kg

^{a}1 mM/L = 1.8 mEq/L = 3.1 mg/dL.
^{b}1 mM/L = 2 mEq/L = 2.4 mg/dL.
Adapted from Sperling MA. Diabetic ketoacidosis. *Pediatr Clin North Am* 1984;31:596.

D. Electrolytes

1. The serum sodium level may be low, normal, or high. The presence of the elevated serum glucose results in the obligatory movement of water from the intracellular to the extracellular space. This redistribution of body water can contribute to apparent hyponatremia despite dehydration and hyperosmolality. The presence of hypertriglyceridemia can also contribute to an artifactually lowered serum sodium.

2. Serum potassium levels can be low, normal, or high. Potassium levels reflect both egress of potassium from cells secondary to the existing acidosis and the degree of intravascular contraction. Because of this and other circumstances, a normal or high serum potassium level does not reflect the actual total-body deficits of potassium that uniformly exist secondary to the ongoing osmotic diuresis. An initial low potassium concentration attests to severe depletion and should be managed aggressively.

3. The serum phosphate level can be normal on admission but, like serum potassium, does not reflect the actual body deficits that uniformly exist while shifts of intracellular phosphate to the extracellular space occur as part of the catabolic state. This phosphate is subsequently lost in the urine as a result of osmotic diuresis (Table 43.1).

E. Other laboratory tests

1. **Blood urea nitrogen (BUN)** levels are usually in the range of 20 to 30 mg/dL, reflecting moderate volume depletion.

2. **Leukocytosis** in the range of 15,000 to 20,000/μL occurs frequently in DKA and therefore cannot be used as a sole indication of an infectious process.

3. **Serum amylase** levels can be elevated. The reason is unknown, but the elevation might be of pancreatic (but not indicating pancreatitis) or salivary gland origin.

4. **Transaminases** can be elevated, but their significance is unknown.

5. **Thyroid function studies** in the presence of DKA tend to be unreliable. This might be another example of the "euthyroid sick syndrome" (see Chapter 30).

V. TREATMENT

The goals of therapy include rehydration, reduction of hyperglycemia, correction of acid–base and electrolyte imbalances, and investigation of precipitating factors. Many correct approaches exist. The most important factor to emphasize is the frequent monitoring of the patient both clinically and chemically (as opposed to an "automatic pilot" approach) as the best way to minimize morbidity and mortality.

A. General management techniques

1. A flow sheet that includes data on glucose, serum ketones, electrolytes, BUN, creatinine, calcium, phosphorus, arterial gases, urine glucose, and ketones should be used. In addition, intake and output should be carefully recorded, as well as the type of hydrating solution used and the mode, timing, and amount of insulin

administered. Initially, laboratory data should be obtained every 1 to 3 hours and then less frequently once clinical improvement is noted. Patients with DKA should, in general, be admitted to an intensive care facility, where close monitoring is more easily assured.

2. If the patient is in shock, stupor, or coma, use of a nasogastric tube, especially if vomiting is present, and a urinary catheter is recommended.

3. Frequent assessment of potassium status is vital. A lead II electrocardiogram (EKG) can provide a rapid assessment of hyperkalemia (peaked T waves) and hypokalemia (flat T waves and presence of U waves). Hyporeflexia and ileus are clinical indications of potassium deficiency.

4. Careful observation of neurologic status is vital to detect the uncommon but devastating presence of cerebral edema.

5. Bedside glucose determinations can be obtained every 30 to 60 minutes at the onset of therapy to help determine the rate of serum glucose fall and to determine the point at which dextrose should be added to the IV solution.

6. A "two-bag" IV fluid method is an effective and rapid way of administering concentrations of glucose to children who have DKA. This system consists of two bags of IV fluids that contain identical electrolyte concentrations, but with one bag containing 10% dextrose and the other 0% dextrose. They are administered simultaneously in a piggyback fashion. The rates of administration of each bag are adjusted to give the desired concentration of dextrose while maintaining a constant overall rate of administration of fluid and electrolytes.

B. **Fluid and electrolyte therapy**

1. **General principles.** The underlying philosophy of therapy is for the metabolic disturbances characteristic of the DKA state to be corrected gradually, albeit tailored to each patient.

2. **Fluid replacement.** With hyperglycemia, water is drawn from the intracellular to the extracellular space, thus depleting the former. Simultaneous extracellular water depletion (specifically, the intravascular compartment) occurs as a result of the obligatory osmotic diuresis. Electrolytes (sodium, potassium, chloride, phosphate, magnesium) are considerably depleted as well, but the osmotic diuresis represents a hypotonic loss, as more water than electrolytes is excreted. This fluid loss can be aggravated further by other ongoing fluid loss, such as occurs with vomiting. The goal of fluid management is to replete both the extracellular and the intracellular compartments.

   a. **Volume-expansion phase**

      (1) **Severe hypovolemic shock.** The following is recommended.

         (a) **Adults.** Saline at about 20 mL/kg over 30 to 60 minutes, or colloid (albumin or plasma) is given to maintain the intravascular space and restore blood pressure and renal perfusion. Once restored, the fluid rate is re-evaluated.

         (b) **Children.** Shock is rare in children in DKA, but if it is present, saline at 10 to 20 mL/kg may be given over 30 to 60 minutes, though some prefer giving aliquots of 10 mL/kg of normal saline (NS) rapidly until blood pressure is normalized, capillary refill time improved (<3 seconds), and peripheral pulses are palpated. Usually, no more than two to three such infusions are needed to accomplish this.

      (2) **Volume expansion for other clinical presentations**

         (a) **Adults.** NS is infused at a rate of 15 to 20 mL/kg over an hour (usually 1 to 1.5 L in an average adult) until hypotension is corrected, blood volume and blood pressure are stabilized, and urine flow is normalized (50 to 100 mL per hour).

         (b) **Children.** If the patient is not in shock, the initial rate of NS infusion can be 5 to 10 mL over the first hour, while laboratory results are pending. Once electrolyte values are known, the addition of potassium to these solutions (See table 43.2 and Section B.3, p. 625) depends on the serum K^+ levels and the absence or presence of oliguria. A child admitted to the emergency department in a state of DKA may at times be overzealously hydrated. Therefore, it is recommended that during this transitional treatment phase while awaiting an inpatient bed (if the wait is not prolonged), the rate of IV infusion after the initial hour of re-expansion should be 1.5 times maintenance, not to exceed 125 mL per hour in most cases (Tables 43.2 and 43.3).

b. **Re-expansion solution.** The initial hydrating fluid should be NS, for the following reasons.

(1) As serum glucose levels decrease and tonicity falls, water shifts back into the intracellular space. This redistribution can unmask the degree of dehydration actually present in the intravascular space, which was previously "hidden" by the degree of water that shifted into this compartment in response to the elevated serum osmolality. This unmasking may further aggravate the circulatory losses and, in severe cases, may contribute to circulatory collapse. Therefore, use of NS rather than a hypotonic solution is recommended to minimize this effect.

(2) Because patients with DKA universally demonstrate hyperosmolality, even NS may be hypotonic in relation to serum osmolality (NS = 308 mOsm/L; $1/2$ NS = 154, 5% dextrose + NS = 560, 5% dextrose + $1/2$ NS = 406, and 5% dextrose in water = 250 mOsm/L). If a rapid fall in serum osmolality is an important contributor to cerebral edema, then a gradual lowering of tonicity is desirable; this is best obtained by avoiding the use of hypotonic IV solutions during the initial stages of therapy. (Some use lactated Ringer's solution, which has less chloride than NS and therefore can reduce the degree of hyperchloremic acidosis that may be associated with ongoing therapy. It has 4 mEq/L of potassium and 28 mEq/L of lactate, which is slowly metabolized to bicarbonate. It should be noted that it has 275 mOsm/L.)

c. **Rehydration phase**

(1) **Adults.** After re-expansion, the subsequent choice of fluid replacement depends on the state of hydration, urinary output, and serum electrolytes. In general, $1/2$ NS infused at 4 to 14 mL/kg per hour is appropriate if serum Na^+ is normal or elevated, and NS—at a similar rate—if corrected serum Na^+ is low. In general, fluid replacement in adults is estimated to correct deficits within the first 24 hours.

(2) **Children.** Because of the higher risk in children of cerebral edema that may occur during therapy for DKA, as well as a lack of an obvious cause, caution has been advocated as to the rate and type of IV solution to be used for rehydration after initial fluid re-expansion. If the occurrence of cerebral edema is influenced by excessive fluid administration and inadequate Na^+ replacement, then avoiding overzealous hydration and reduction of plasma osmolality are reasonable precautionary measures. Many have recommended fluid replacement rates of 3 000 mL/m² per day, not to exceed 4 000 mL/m² in the first 24 hours, regardless of initial deficit estimates and ongoing losses. Others distinguish deficit losses (which are necessarily proportional to weight) from maintenance requirements (which are proportional to energy expenditure, i.e., surface area). They calculate maintenance at 1 500 mL/m² per day and add to that estimated fluid deficits, and correct evenly over 48 hours. When fluid deficits are not reliably known (which is often the case), an estimated deficit of 10% can be assumed. If ongoing fluid losses are considered excessive, then some degree of replacement is advised. For those patients at greater risk for cerebral edema (e.g., young age at initial presentation of diabetes), some suggest that fluid replacement should not exceed 2 000 to 2 500 mL/m² per day. As to type of solution, it has been suggested that higher-tonicity fluids (greater than $1/2$ NS, e.g., $2/3$ NS, $3/4$ NS) should be used during the early replacement period (first 12 hours) to help prevent the rapid fall in osmolality that occurs when blood glucose concentrations drop with ongoing therapy.

TABLE 43.2	**Outline for Treatment of Diabetic Ketoacidosis (DKA) and Hyperglycemic Hyperosmolar State (HHS)**

Laboratory evaluation

After a brief history and physical examination, initial laboratory evaluation should include determination of complete blood count, blood glucose, serum electrolytes, SUN, creatinine, serum ketones, osmolality, arterial blood gases, and urinalysis. Admission electrocardiogram, chest radiograph, and cultures of blood, urine, and sputum may be ordered if indicated clinically. During therapy, capillary blood glucose should be determined every hour at the bedside using a glucose oxidase reagent strip, and blood should be drawn every 2 to 4 hours for determination of serum electrolytes, glucose, SUN, creatinine, phosphorus, and venous pH.

Fluids

Administer 1 000 mL normal saline (0.9% sodium chloride) first hour, then normal or 0.45% saline at 250 to 500 mL per hour, depending on serum sodium concentration. When plasma glucose is <200 mg/dL, change to 5% dextrose in .45% saline to allow continued insulin administration until ketonemia is controlled, while avoiding hypoglycemia.

Insulin

Administer 0.1 U/kg body weight as intravenous bolus, followed by 0.1 U/kg per hour as a continuous infusion. The goal is to achieve a rate of decline of glucose between 50 and 70 mg per hour. When plasma glucose is 200 mg/dL, change fluid to D5 $^1/_2$ NS and reduce insulin rate to 0.05 U/kg per hour. Thereafter, adjust insulin rate to maintain glucose levels to between 150 and 200 mg/dL until serum is $\geq$18 mEq/L and pH is >7.30. In patients who have mild to moderate DKA, subcutaneous rapid-acting analogs may be an alternative to intravenous insulin (see caveats discussed later).

Potassium

If serum K^+ is >5.0 mEq/L, no supplementation is required. If serum K+ is 4 to 5 mEq/L, add 20 mEq/L to each liter of replacement fluid after adequate renal function is established (urine flow at least 50 mL per hour). If serum K^+ is 3 to 4 mEq/L, add 40 mEq/L to each liter of replacement fluid. If serum K^+ is <3 mEq/L, hold insulin and give 10 to 20 mEq per hour until K^+ is >3.3, then add 40 mEq/L to each liter of replacement fluid.

Bicarbonate

If arterial pH is <7.0 or bicarbonate is <5 mEq, give 50 mEq in 200 mL of H_2O over 1 hour until pH increases to >7.0. Do not give bicarbonate if pH is >7.0. For pH <6.9, give 100 mEq of bicarbonate and 20 mEq of KCl in 400 mL of H_2O to run for 2 hours.

Phosphate

If indicated (serum levels <1 mg/dL), administer 20 to 30 mmol potassium phosphate over 24 hours. Monitor serum calcium level.

Transition to subcutaneous insulin

Insulin infusion should be continued until resolution of ketoacidosis (glucose <200 mg/dL, bicarbonate >18 mEq/L, and pH >7.30). When this occurs, start subcutaneous insulin regimen. To prevent recurrence of DKA during the transition period to subcutaneous insulin, intravenous insulin should be continued for 1 to 2 hours after subcutaneous insulin is given. A similar protocol should be used for HHS except that no bicarbonate is needed for HHS, and switching to glucose-containing fluid is done when blood glucose reaches 300 mg/dL. HHS is resolved when glucose is $\geq$300 mg/dL, osmolality is <320, and patient is alert.

Data from Kitabchi AE. Medical guidelines for clinical practice. Hyperglycemic crises in diabetes mellitus. Diabetic ketoacidosis and hyperglycemic hyperosmolar state. *Diabetes Care*, 2006 Dec; 24(12):2739–2748. Kitabchi AE, Murphy MB. Consequences of insulin deficiency. In: Skyler JS, ed. *Atlas of Diabetes*. 3rd ed. Philadelphia: Current Medicine; 2005, with permission.

TABLE 43.3 **Emergency Department Management of Pediatric Patients in Diabetic Ketoacidosis (DKA)**

The acute management of DKA in pediatric patients (<18 years old) is different from that of adults, because children are at risk for acute cerebral edema with accompanying high morbidity and mortality.

Initial approach
- Obtain and monitor vital signs, including blood pressure, on all patients.
- Assess the degree of hydration and mental status.
- Do a bedside glucose determination. Note: Many meters do not read above 600 mg% and will indicate only "HI."
- Obtain a urine sample for ketone determination. Note: Patients in ketoacidosis will have high ketones.
- Draw blood for serum glucose, ketones, electrolytes, BUN, creatinine (which may be artifactually elevated because of elevated ketones), and complete blood count. Obtain a venous pH.
- Start an IV and give **10 mL/kg** of normal saline (NS) or Ringer's lactate over 30 to 60 minutes. Note: *Shock rarely occurs in pediatric DKA.* However, if shock is present, give 20 mL/kg of NS, which may be repeated until the patient is hemodynamically stable.
- Order to bedside:
  (a) Insulin drip: Usually a concentration of regular insulin to NS of 100 U/100 mL (1 U/mL).
  (b) IV solutions:
  1. $^2/_3$ NS + 20 mEq Kphos/L + 20 mEq Kacetate/L (total: 40 mEq/L)
     as well as
  2. D10, $^2/_3$ NS + same electrolytes
     This is done now to avoid any delay in obtaining appropriate IV solutions later. One may vary the concentration of glucose infused by piggybacking these IVs and running each at different rates, but with both rates combined equaling the desired total hourly infusion rate.
- Consult with a pediatric endocrinologist as soon as possible.

Based on lab results and clinical assessment, patients can be stratified by the degree of acidosis:
1. Mild: pH >7.25, or CO_2 >12, and no alteration of mental status. Consider admission unless patient improves sufficiently.
2. Moderate: pH 7.10–7.25, or CO_2 7–12, and patient lethargic. Arrange for admission.
3. Severe: pH<7.10, or CO_2 <7, and patient c altered mental status. Arrange for admission.

Initial management for all three stratifications is essentially the same, with some caveats for each:
- After the initial hour of isotonic volume expansion, and if bedside blood glucose is >300 mg%, run $^2/_3$ NS plus above electrolyte solution (b) at a maximum rate of $1^1/_2$ times maintenance, not to exceed 200 mL per hour.[a] Note: Unless patient is hyperkalemic (>5.5 mEq/L), start K^+ within 2 hours of admission to the emergency department, or when insulin has been started. If patient is hypokalemic (<3.5 mEq/1L), increase IV K^+ replacement to 60–80 mEq/L added as KCL with close K^+ monitoring. If IV solution not ready, continue with NS. If bedside blood glucose <300 mg%, run the D10, $^2/_3$ NS + same electrolytes.
- Begin an insulin drip at 0.1 U/kg per hour of regular insulin. In *mild* DKA, may give 0.2 U/kg of Novolog SC if it is decided that IV insulin is unnecessary and continue with other monitoring guidelines.
- Follow electrolytes every 2 hours until bicarbonate trends upward and then every 4 hours. However, this schedule may be different (q1–2h) if hypokalemia (<3.5 mEq/L) or hyperkalemia (>5.5 mEq/L) is of concern.
- Do bedside glucose hourly. If blood glucose falls to <300 mg% and patient is being given IV insulin, change IV solution to D10, $^2/_3$ NS + electrolyte solution. Maintain blood glucose between 200 and 300 mg% while the acidosis is resolving.
- In moderate to severe DKA, monitor VS continuously with neuro checks. Arrange for a PICU bed ASAP.
- In severe DKA, if patient is in shock or obtunded, consider nasogastric tube, especially if vomiting, and urinary catheter.

(continued)

TABLE 43.3	Emergency Department Management of Pediatric Patients in Diabetic Ketoacidosis (DKA) (*Continued*)

Do nots (see text for further discussion):

■ Do not give more than 20 ml/kg as a single fluid bolus.

■ Do not give bolus insulin.

■ Do not give boluses of sodium bicarbonate.

■ Do not start insulin until a fluid bolus has been given and maintenance fluids begun. This may wait until admission to the hospital if this occurs within no more than 2 hours of admission to the emergency department.

[a]Calculation of maintenance fluids per 24 hours:

    100 mL/kg for first 10 kg of body weight
    50 mL/kg for the next 10 kg of body weight
    20 mL/kg for each additional 1 kg of body weight

Example: A 25-kg child would receive 1 000 mL + 500 mL + 100 mL = 1 600 mL per 24 hours, or 67 mL per hour of maintenance fluids.

If calculating maintenance as 1 500 mL/m^2 per 24 hours: 10 kg = 0.5 m^2, 30 kg = 1 m^2, 50 kg = 1.5 m^2, 70 kg = 1.7 m^2.

Note: Estimated osmolality: 2(Na + K) + blood glucose/18 + BUN/2.8; anion gap = Na − (Cl + HCO$_3$); normal: 8–16 mEq/L.

Calculated serum Na = Na measured + (blood glucose − 100)/100 × 1.6 mEq/L.

Source: The Southern California Kaiser Permanente Regional Pediatric Endocrinologists offer these guidelines, based on a document by the late Dr. James Seidel of Harbor–UCLA, for the acute management of pediatric DKA in the emergency department.

(3) In the later stages of therapy, $^1/_5$ to $^1/_2$ NS can be used as replacement fluid as free-water deficits are reversed after the extracellular fluid volume has been restored.

(4) If initial serum Na$^+$ exceeds 150 mEq/L, instead of NS, a solution of lesser tonicity can be used ($^1/_2$, $^2/_3$, $^3/_4$ NS). Although by no means a mathematical constant, it is helpful to consider that each 100 mg/dL elevation in blood glucose depresses serum Na$^+$ by 1.6 mEq/L. Thus, a "calculated" serum Na$^+$ is derived.

3. Potassium

a. As correction of acidosis proceeds (by hydration and use of insulin), potassium is shifted back to the cells and serum levels fall, with a possibility of hypokalemia resulting. Hypokalemia, rather than hyperkalemia, has been associated with more serious complications (e.g., life-threatening arrhythmias).

b. In adults, if K$^+$ levels are normal on admission, then adding 20 to 40 mEq of K$^+$ to each liter of IV fluid will keep serum K$^+$ at the 4- to 5-mEq/L range. In children, 3 mEq/kg per day of K$^+$ is recommended initially. Potassium levels may drop with initiation of therapy and correction of acidosis. Potassium infusion rates often have to be increased to maintain K$^+$ concentration >3.5 mEq/L. This is usually accomplished by adding 30 to 40 mEq of K$^+$ to each liter of hydrating solution. Potassium can be added as a combination of K$^+$ chloride, K$^+$ acetate, or K$^+$ phosphate ($^2/_3$ KCl and $^1/_3$ KPhos; $^1/_2$ KPhos and $^1/_2$ Kacetate). If potassium levels are elevated on admission (≥5.5 mEq/L), potassium supplementation is withheld and serum K$^+$ concentration is checked hourly. Adjustments of potassium supplementation should be based on electrocardiographic, clinical, and chemical parameters of K$^+$ deficiency, which should be frequently assessed.

c. If initial K$^+$ levels are low, then depletion is severe. In adults, if K$^+$ is ≤3.3 mEq/L, 40 mEq of K$^+$ per hour is given ($^2/_3$ KCl and $^1/_3$ KPhos), with the suggestion that insulin be held until K$^+$ ≥ 3.3 mEq/L. Higher amounts of K$^+$ may be needed if depletion is very severe (60 to 80 mEq K$^+$ per hour). In children, if serum K$^+$ concentration is ≤3.4, then 40 to 60 mEq/L of K$^+$ is added to the IV solution until K$^+$ is ≥3.5 mEq. K$^+$ should be monitored hourly.

d. If the patient is hypokalemic and anuric, K^+ supplementation is started at 10 to 30 mEq of KCl, given cautiously, per hour with close electrocardiographic monitoring. For children it is recommended that the maximal rate of K^+ administration should be 0.5 mEq/kg per hour, starting with 0.25 mEq. Almost hourly K^+ determinations are required along with electrocardiographic monitoring.

4. Bicarbonate

a. Continued controversy surrounds bicarbonate replacement. Although severe acidosis can impair myocardial contractility, predispose to arrhythmias, and decrease cardiac and peripheral vasculature response to catecholamine stimulation, several factors should be considered before utilizing alkali therapy.

(1) In diabetic ketoacidosis, 2,3-diphosphoglycerate (2,3-DPG) levels are decreased (mostly secondary to phosphorus depletion) with a resultant shift of the oxygen dissociation curve to the left (oxygen is held more tightly by hemoglobin). This effect is compensated for by the existing acidosis, such that the curve remains normal or essentially unchanged (Bohr effect) and oxygen is released to the tissues normally. If bicarbonate therapy is initiated, the curve again shifts to the left, with theoretically less oxygen being delivered to the tissues.

(2) With alkali therapy, potassium shifts back into the cell and may potentiate hypokalemia.

(3) Ketone bodies are themselves metabolized to bicarbonate once proper therapy is begun (fluids, electrolytes, insulin), and exogenous administration of bicarbonate can overcorrect, leading to alkalosis.

(4) Commercially available bicarbonate solutions are hyperosmolar and can aggravate the already-existing high serum osmolality.

(5) Alkali therapy can contribute to central nervous system (CNS) symptoms (from clouding of consciousness to frank coma). Bicarbonate combines with hydrogen ion and dissociates to water and carbon dioxide. This carbon dioxide easily crosses the blood–brain barrier, whereas bicarbonate does so with difficulty. Therefore, despite improved peripheral pH values, a paradoxical CNS acidosis may be created or aggravated and may affect cerebral consciousness.

(6) There is no evidence that bicarbonate therapy accelerates metabolic recovery.

b. At present there seems to be no evidence to support the routine use of bicarbonate. Situations where its use may be considered are as follows:

(1) In the presence of life-threatening hyperkalemia.

(2) When severe lactic acidosis complicates DKA.

(3) In adults, if arterial pH <7.0, especially when clinical condition is complicated by shock that is refractory to appropriate fluid resuscitation measures (NS, plasma, albumin, whole blood) in an attempt to improve cardiac output. In children, if pH remains below 7.0 after the initial few hours of hydration, it seems prudent to consider the use of bicarbonate.

c. In adults, if arterial pH <7.0 or bicarbonate <5 mEq/L, give 50 mEq of sodium bicarbonate in 200 mL of sterile water over 1 hour until pH increases to 7.0. Do not give bicarbonate if pH is >7.0.

d. In children, in those rare situations when pH <7.0 and clinical course dictates the use of bicarbonate, a dose of 1 to 2 mEq/kg of sodium bicarbonate is given over an hour, although some clinicians recommend 1 to 3 mEq/kg over 12 hours. The sodium bicarbonate can be added to NS, with any required K^+, and this solution can be used as the rehydration solution for that hour. No bicarbonate therapy is necessary if pH is ≥7.0. If one uses different hydrating solutions, the combination of the Na in sodium bicarbonate and the Na in the IV solution should not exceed the concentration of NS.

5. Phosphate

a. Phosphate therapy is also a somewhat controversial issue in the treatment of DKA. Total-body phosphate stores can be markedly depleted in DKA.

However, serum phosphate concentration is usually slightly elevated or in the high-normal range on admission because of the vascular contraction. In severe depletion (serum levels <0.5 mg/dL), serious organ dysfunction can ensue (rhabdomyolysis, altered consciousness, muscle weakness, impaired cardiac function, and respiratory failure). However, in reality, the deficiency is usually clinically silent and only detected chemically. It should also be remembered that vigorous phosphate replacement can precipitate both hypocalcemia and hypomagnesemia. It may be argued that to avoid cardiac and skeletal muscle weakness and respiratory depression as a result of hypophosphatemia, in patients with cardiac dysfunction, anemia, and respiratory depression, and in those with phosphate levels <1.0 mg/dL, replacement may be beneficial. Currently, some degree of phosphate replacement is routinely accepted.

b. If the phosphate is replaced, it is given as potassium phosphate, subtracting this amount of potassium from that given as potassium chloride. A minimum requirement of 90 mEq (50 mM) of phosphate in the first 24 hours can be anticipated in the adult. In children, phosphate replacement can be safely calculated at 1 mEq/kg per day. Generally, one may simply give one third of the total potassium requirement (Tables 43.1 and 43.2) as the phosphate salt. This can usually be done by adding 20 to 30 mEq/L potassium phosphate to replacement fluids. Phosphate therapy is not to be used in patients with renal insufficiency.

6. Magnesium. The normal magnesium concentration is 1.5 to 2.5 mEq/L. Although depleted (usually in prolonged ketoacidosis), it is usually not a problem in most cases of DKA. If the magnesium level is low (usually <1 mEq/L), replacement can be given as a magnesium sulfate solution.

C. Insulin therapy

1. Insulin can be administered by subcutaneous (SC), intramuscular (IM), or IV route, depending on the clinical situation. In mild DKA (pH >7.3, CO_2 >15), especially if IV hydration is deemed unnecessary, SC rapid-acting insulin analogs (lispro or aspart) have been used quite effectively. Patients receive 0.2 U/kg initially, followed by 0.1 U/kg every hour or an initial dose of 0.3 U/kg followed by 0.2 U/kg every 2 hours until blood glucose is <250 mg%, then the insulin dose is decreased by half to 0.05 U/kg or 0.1 U/kg, respectively, and administered every 1 or 2 hours until resolution of DKA. This form of therapy is not recommended for patients with severe DKA or HHS, and may not be effective in patients who have severe fluid depletion because these insulins are given SC.

2. In moderate to severe DKA, IV insulin is the preferred route. However, if IV access is difficult, and tissue perfusion is good, then one may give insulin SC or IM.

3. Low-dose insulin infusion is the mode of insulin administration that is now generally accepted for both children and adults. The benefits derived from continuous low-dose insulin infusion are as follows:

a. It avoids the potential hazards of rapid and erratic serum glucose and osmolar fluctuations.

b. It avoids, to a greater extent, episodes of late hypoglycemia and hypokalemia.

c. With a constant amount of insulin infused, a steady linear fall in glucose can be expected (usually 50 to 90 mg/dL per hour, although this varies from patient to patient) and appropriate changes in IV solution anticipated (i.e., addition of dextrose to initial hydration solution when serum glucose concentration falls to 250 mg/dL).

d. One has the advantage of instantaneously adjusting the insulin infused in response to sudden clinical and chemical changes.

4. Management of insulin infusion and IV glucose concentrations

a. Regular insulin is mixed with NS to give the desired concentration, usually 100 U in 100 mL, to give a 1:1 solution. In children, a more dilute concentration may be desired (125 U/250 mL, to give a 1:2 concentration) in order to give smaller doses of insulin, but the final volume of dilution should not be excessive.

b. A loading dose of 0.1 U/kg is recommended for adults but not for children, as this may increase the risk of cerebral edema. Flushing the IV tubing is recommended. A rate-control pump can be piggybacked onto the regular IV line.

c. The insulin solution is infused at the rate of 0.1 U regular insulin per kilogram per hour. This rate is calculated to decrease serum glucose by 50 to 90 mg/dL per hour.

d. The addition of glucose to the intravenous solution is necessary for correction of tissue lipolysis and acidosis. A solution of 5% to 10% dextrose is added to the IV line to avoid rapidly lowering the glucose level and to help maintain the blood glucose concentration at ~200 to 250 mg/dL in the first 12 to 24 hours of therapy. Please refer to the "two-bag" IV administration system described in Section V,A.6, p. 621.

e. Half-hourly to hourly bedside finger punctures for glucose determinations are recommended.

f. If the glucose level does not improve after an hour of infusion, the rate of insulin infusion is doubled until a response is noted. If after an additional hour there is still no response, the infusion of insulin is doubled again, with the proviso that the IV access should be checked for correct functioning.

g. If within 3 to 4 hours of onset of therapy, there is no metabolic improvement (no fall in serum glucose, and no change in or worsening of pH), then, after checking that the IV is functioning properly and has not infiltrated, underhydration, occult infection, or other coexisting medical problems might be complicating the medical response. If these last conditions are unlikely, then the increasing doses of insulin can indicate the more rare type of insulin resistance that requires very high doses.

h. The major goal of therapy is to stop ketogenesis and reverse acidosis in addition to lowering the glucose level. Over a period of hours, the glucose level responds to therapy more quickly than the ketoacidosis. A common mistake is to considerably decrease or shut off the insulin infusion when glucose levels approach the normal range (5% dextrose having already been added to the IV solution). Because the half-life of insulin is quite brief (4 to 5 minutes), this situation could lead to a worsening of the ketoacidosis. Therefore, when confronted with this situation, rather than decrease the insulin infusion, one can increase the rate of the IV hydrating solution if calculations of fluid requirements allow, or add more glucose substrate (7.5%, 10%, or 12.5%) to the IV solution.

i. As previously noted, measurement of serum ketone levels may not be reflective of the improving metabolic state. Improvement in serum bicarbonate and pH and a reduction of the anion gap are more reliable indicators. The normal anion gap $(Na - [CO_2 + Cl] = 12$ to $14)$ is increased in DKA.

j. Once started, the insulin infusion can be run until the acidosis is fully corrected and the serum bicarbonate is back to normal (usually 12 to 24 hours) before switching to SC insulin. However, if for any reason it is desired to discontinue the infusion and to start SC insulin, a serum bicarbonate of 18 mEq/L may be used as a suitable switching point. Another common error is to delay between the time the insulin infusion is discontinued and when the first SC regular or rapid-acting insulin dose is given. One should give the first SC regular dose about 30 minutes, rapid-acting dose 15 minutes before discontinuing the infusion (whether combined with NPH or not.)

k. After discontinuing the insulin infusion, it is not necessary to switch to the traditional sliding-scale regular insulin coverage q4h. Instead, the following methods of insulin coverage are recommended:

(1) A total daily insulin dose of about 0.7 U/kg should be administered, with a range of 0.5 to 1 U/kg per day.

(2) Give two thirds of this total amount before breakfast and one third before supper.

(3) Give one fourth to one half of the total doses as either short-acting insulin (regular) 30 minutes before the meals, or rapid-acting insulin (lispro, aspart), 15 minutes before the meals, and give the rest as NPH.

(4) Younger children may demonstrate a greater sensitivity to both rapid-acting and short-acting insulin. Therefore, it may be prudent to start with a lower dose of either.

(5) Glargine is a 24-hour peakless insulin, which may be well used in association with rapid-acting insulin in the management of children with diabetes and can be used after the DKA has resolved. Usually, 40% to 50% of the total daily NPH dose is given as glargine in the evening, around 9 to 10 P.M., in conjunction with rapid-acting insulin that is administered about 15 minutes before meals.

(6) Insulin is adjusted accordingly in subsequent days, based on fingerstick readings obtained at 8 and 10 A.M., noon, 4 P.M., midnight, and 4 A.M., as well as any dietary adjustment.

VI. COMPLICATIONS

A. Metabolic abnormalities must be watched for and quickly corrected (severe acidosis, hypokalemia, hypoglycemia, and hypocalcemia).

B. Nonmetabolic complications can also be devastating and therefore must be considered during patient evaluation.

1. Infection. Although infection occasionally accompanies ketoacidosis, it is rarely a cause of death. Elevated temperature should lead to a serious search for the focus of infection.

2. Shock. The severity of shock depends on the degree of volume depletion and acidosis. If the patient does not respond to the usual resuscitative techniques, then one should consider etiologic factors such as cardiogenic shock (secondary to myocardial infarction) and gram-negative sepsis.

3. Vascular thrombosis. This is usually secondary to severe dehydration, high serum viscosity, and low cardiac output. Cerebral vessels seem to be most susceptible. It occurs hours to days after onset of therapy.

4. Pulmonary edema can exist on a noncardiogenic basis. It is thought to be caused by aggressive crystalloid fluid therapy.

5. Cerebral edema

   a. Cerebral edema occurs in 1% to 2% of children with DKA, and its outcome is poor. The typical onset is 4 to 16 hours after initiation of therapy, despite indications of biochemical improvement. It should be noted that some patients present with cerebral edema prior to receiving any therapy at all.

   b. Typically, at the time of admission nothing separates these patients from those who do well with similar modes of therapy. Within hours of initiation of therapy, headache, lethargy, recurrence of vomiting, incontinence, hypertension, bradycardia, altered mental status, mental stupor, and unconsciousness supervene in the previously conscious patient.

   c. On examination, signs of increased intracranial pressure are noted, including papilledema, ophthalmoplegia, and fixed, dilated, or unequal pupils. Diabetes insipidus and hyperpyrexia have been described. Mortality rates from 25% to >70% have been reported, with a 25% rate of permanent neurologic morbidity. Only 7% to 14% of patients have been reported to recover without permanent neurologic deficits.

   d. Multiple causes have been suggested as etiologic factors, including a rapid fall in glucose levels with movement of water into the intracellular space resulting in swelling of brain cells; rapid decrease in plasma oncotic pressure (secondary to administration of protein-free solutions); CNS hypoxia; and altered cerebral pH with paradoxical cerebrospinal fluid acidosis aggravated by the use of exogenous bicarbonate. Newer data suggest that cerebral edema is the result of increased cerebral perfusion as shown on MRI; an activation of the cell membrane Na^+/H^+ exchanger: elevated H^+ allows more Na^+ into cells, thus activating more water into the brain cells, and a possible direct role of acetoacetate and β-hydroxybuyrate (ketone bodies) that affect vascular integrity and permeability, thus contributing to cerebral edema. It has been shown that those at greater risk of developing cerebral edema are those patients admitted with an unexpectedly elevated BUN, a marked decrease in partial pressure of CO_2, and, in general, those who present already neurologically compromised and with an altered mental status. During therapy, some suggest that a failure of the serum Na^+ concentration to rise as glucose concentrations decline is a marker of excessive administration of free water, and in these patients a risk of brain swelling may be present. However, it appears that at present no one factor can clearly be implicated as causative of cerebral edema, and it may be an interplay of all the above-indicated factors plus others that have not yet been identified. (The reader is advised to review the references for comprehensive viewpoints.)

e. It seems a reasonable precautionary measure to avoid rapid rehydration and rapid reduction of plasma osmolality in the initial hours of DKA therapy. This can be accomplished by using NS as the initial hydrating solution, followed by solutions of tonicity greater than $^1/_2$ NS in the first hours of therapy; allowing serum glucose levels to fall slowly over the first hours of therapy (delaying use of insulin for up to 2 hours while infusing NS has been recommended, but this obviously depends on the degree of hyperglycemia and acidosis and the clinical condition of the patient); using low-dose constant insulin infusion rather than large-bolus therapy; and extending therapy for 48 hours rather than 24 hours.

f. Cerebral edema may be abrupt and present without warning, or it may be heralded by lethargy, headaches, and incontinence. One should suspect impending cerebral edema with declining or fluctuating mental status; sudden development of hypertension not detected at presentation; an unexpected decline in urine output without clinical improvement or tapering of IV fluids; corrected Na^+ falling to hyponatremic levels; or a drop of effective osmolality (Eosm = $2 \times Na^+$ + glucose/18) to <275 mOsm/kg. More ominous signs include dilated, unresponsive, sluggish, or unequal pupils; hypotension and bradycardia; and coma. A noncontrast CT performed in the emergency department may be helpful, though changes of cerebral edema may be delayed.

g. If cerebral edema is diagnosed, <u>treatment</u> involves the immediate use of IV <u>mannitol</u> (0.25 to 0.5 or 1 g/kg over 20 minutes; this may be repeated hourly as necessary); use of a hypertonic saline solution; <u>furosemide</u> (1 mg/kg), and <u>dexamethasone</u> (0.25 to 0.5 mg/kg per dose) (anecdotal report by this author of successful use with one patient, though no evidence exists for its efficacy or that of furosemide). Other measures include raising the head of the bed, reducing the rate of IV infusion, and possible mechanical hyperventilation to help reduce brain swelling but clearly avoiding lowering the partial pressure of CO_2 to critical levels.

HYPEROSMOLAR HYPERGLYCEMIC STATE

Hyperosmolar hyperglycemic state (HHS) was previously termed hyperosmolar hyperglycemic nonketotic coma. The change in term reflects that altered mental status can occur without coma, and that HHS may exist with variable degrees of ketosis, albeit not severe. It occurs in middle-aged and elderly patients, though it has been described in children. Most patients have type 2 diabetes or no prior history of diabetes, but it has been described in type 1 diabetes associated with DKA. When seen in the pediatric population, case series have suggested that obese African American children with type 2 diabetes are at greater risk for HHS. As in DKA, it is characterized by an absolute or relative lack of insulin. When there is lack of ketosis in this syndrome, it has been traditionally explained by the presence of insulin in sufficient levels to prevent lipolysis and ketogenesis but not sufficiently high to prevent hyperglycemia. However, other mechanisms must be at play, because it has been noted that in some cases of HHS, insulin levels are not markedly different from those observed in DKA. The extreme hyperglycemia might be explained by the coexistence of decreased renal function in a great majority of these patients, limited access to fluids, and, in general, an osmotic diuresis that may exist for a prolonged period before presentation to the emergency department. Thus, DKA and HHS may represent points along a continuum of clinical presentations of poorly controlled diabetes, differing only in the severity of dehydration, ketosis, and metabolic acidosis.

See Chapter 45 for a full discussion of hyperosmolar hyperglycemic state.

Selected References

American Diabetes Association. Hyperglycemic crises in patients with diabetes mellitus. *Clin Diabetes* 2001;19:2.

Bell DSH, Alele J. Diabetic ketoacidosis. *Postgrad Med* 1997;101:4.

Boschert S. Cerebral edema in diabetic ketoacidosis. *Pediatr News* 2000 Nov.

Bull SV, et al. Mandatory protocol for treating adult patients with diabetic ketoacidosis decreases intensive care unit and hospital lengths of stay: results of a nonrandomized trial. *Crit Care Med* 2007;35:41.

Butkiewicz EK, et al. Insulin therapy for diabetic ketoacidosis. *Diabetes Care* 1995;18:8.

Cardella F. Insulin therapy during diabetic ketoacidosis in children. *Acta Biomed* 2005; 76(3):49.

Cefalu W. Diabetic ketoacidosis. *Crit Care Clin* 1991;7:89.

Davidson M. *Diabetes Mellitus: Diagnosis and Treatment.* 3rd ed. New York: Churchill Livingstone; 1991.

Delaney MF, Zisman A, Kettyle WM. Diabetic ketoacidosis and hyperglycemic, hyperosmolar nonketotic syndrome. *Endocrinol Metab Clin North Am* 2000;29:4.

Duck SC, et al. Factors associated with brain herniation in the treatment of diabetic ketoacidosis. *J Pediatr* 1988;113:10–13.

Dunger DB, Edge JA. Predicting cerebral edema during diabetic ketoacidosis. *N Engl J Med* 2001;344:4.

Dunger DB, Sperling MA, Acerini CL, et al. ESPE/LWPES consensus statement on diabetic ketoacidosis in children and adolescents. *Arch Dis Child* 2004 Feb;89(2):188–194.

Editorial. Choosing the right fluid and electrolyte prescription in diabetic ketoacidosis. *J Pediatr* 2007 May:455.

Editorial. Strategies to diminish the danger of cerebral edema in a pediatric patient presenting with diabetic ketoacidosis. *Pediatr Diabetes* 2006;7:191.

Eledrisi MS, et al. Overview of the diagnosis and management of diabetic ketoacidosis. *Am J Med Sci* 2006;331:243.

Ersoz HO, et al. Subcutaneous lispro and intravenous regular insulin treatments are equally effective and safe for the treatment of mild and moderate diabetic ketoacidosis in adult patients. *Int J Clin Pract* 2006;60:429.

Finberg L. Why do patients with diabetic ketoacidosis have cerebral swelling, and why does treatment sometimes make it worse?. *Arch Pediatr Adolesc Med* 1996;150.

Fleckman AM. Diabetic ketoacidosis. *Endocrinol Metab Clin North Am* 1993;22:2.

Flordalisi I, Harris GD. Diabetic ketoacidosis. In: *Saunders Manual of Pediatric Practice.* 2nd ed. In press.

Foster DW, McGarry JD. The metabolic derangements and treatment of diabetic ketoacidosis. *N Engl J Med* 1983 Jul 21;309(3):159–169.

Ginde AA, Pelletier AJ. National study of US emergency department visits with diabetic ketoacidosis, 1993–2003. *Diabetes Care* 2006;29:2117.

Glaser N. New perspectives on the pathogenesis of cerebral edema complicating diabetic ketoacidosis in children. *Pediatr Endocrinol Rev* 2006;3:379.

Glaser N, et al. Frequency of sub-clinical cerebral edema in children with diabetid ketoacidosis. *Pediatr Diabetes* 2006;7:75.

Glaser N, et al. Risk factors for cerebral edema in children with diabetic ketoacidosis. *N Engl J Med* 2001;344:4.

Glaser NS, Kupperman N, Yee CKJ, et al. Variation in the management of pediatric diabetic ketoacidosis by specialty training. *Arch Pediatr Adolesc Med* 1997;151.

Gonzalez-Campy JM, Robertson BP. Diabetic ketoacidosis and hyperosmolar nonketotic state. *Postgrad Med* 1996;99:6.

Hafeez W, Vuguin P. Managing diabetic ketoacidosis: a delicate balance. *Contemp Pediatr* 2000;17:6.

Harris G, et al. Minimizing the risk of brain herniation during treatment of diabetic ketoacidemia: a retrospective and prospective study. *J Pediatr* 1990;117:22.

Harris G, et al. Safe management of diabetic ketoacidemia. *J Pediatr* 1988;113:567.

Harris GD, Fiordalisi I. Physiologic management of diabetic ketoacidosis. *Arch Pediatr Adolesc Med* 1994;148.

Hekkala A, et al. Ketoacidosis at diagnosis of type 1 diabetes in children in Northern Finland. *Diabetes Care* 2007;30:861.

Hoorn EJ, et al. Preventing a drop in effective plasma osmolality to minimize the likelihood of cerebral edema during treatment of children with diabetic ketoacidosis. *J Pediatr* 2007 May:467.

Israel R. Diabetic ketoacidosis. *Emerg Med Clin North Am* 1989;7:859.

Kaufman FR, Halvorson M. The treatment and prevention of diabetic ketoacidosis in children and adolescents with type 1 diabetes. *Pediatr Ann* 1999;28:9.

Kitabchi AE, Nyenwe EA. Hyperglycemic crisis in diabetes mellitus: diabetic ketoacidosis and hyperglycemic hyperosmolar state. *Endcrinol Metab Clin North Am* 2006;35:725.

Lebovitz HE. Diabetic ketoacidosis. *Lancet* 1995;345.

Leonard RCF, et al. Acute respiratory distress in diabetic ketoacidosis: possible contribution of low colloid osmotic pressure. *Br Med J* 1983;286:760.

Lipsky MS. Management of diabetic ketoacidosis. *Am Fam Physician* 1994;49:7.

Munk MD. Pediatric DKA. *JEMS* 2006 Jun;31:70.

Pediatric diabetic ketoacidosis and hyperglycemic hyperosmolar state. *Pediatr Clin North Am* 2005;52:1611.

Quinn M, et al. Characteristics at diagnosis of type 1 diabetes in children younger than 6 years. *J Pediatr* 2006 Mar:366.

Rewers A, et al. Bedside monitoring of blood b-hydroxybutyrate levels in the management of diabetic ketoacidosis in children. *Diabetes Technol Ther* 2006;8:671.

Rosenbloom AL. Intracerebral crisis during treatment of diabetic ketoacidosis. *Diabetes Care* 1990;13(1):22–33.

Rosenbloom AL. Letter to the editor. *J Pediatr* 1990;117:1009.

Seidel J. *New Protocols for DKA in the ED*. Los Angeles: Los Angeles Pediatric Society; 2000 Sep:10.

Siperstein MD. Diabetic ketoacidosis and hyperosmolar coma. *Endocrinol Metab Clin North Am* 1992;21:45.

Sperling MA. Diabetic ketoacidosis. *Pediatr Clin North Am* 1984;31:591.

Sulli N, Shashaj B. Long-term benefits of continuous subcutaneous insulin in children with type 1 diabetes: a 4-year follow-up. *Diabetic Med* 2006;23:900.

Type 1 diabetes mellitus: etiology, presentation, and management. *Pediatr Clin North Am* 2005;1553.

Umpierrez GE, Khajavi M, Kitabchi AE. Review: diabetic ketoacidosis and hyperglycemic hyperosmolar nonketotic syndrome. *Am J Med Sci* 1996;311:8.

Wachtel TJ. The diabetic hyperosmolar state. *Clin Geriatr Med* 1990;6:797.

White NH. Diabetic ketoacidosis in children. *Endocrinol Metabol Clin North Am* 2000; 29:4.

Wittlesey CD. Case study: diabetic ketoacidosis complications in type 2 diabetes. *Clin Diabetes* 2000;18.

Wolfsdorf J, et al. Diabetic ketoacidosis in infants, children, and adolescents. *Diabetes Care* 2006;5:1150.

Wolfsdorf JC, et al. ISPAD clinical practice consensus guidelines 2006–2007. Diabetic ketoacidosis. *Pediatr Diabetes* 2007;8:28–43.

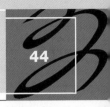

DIABETES MELLITUS TYPE 2, OBESITY, DYSLIPIDEMIA, AND THE METABOLIC SYNDROME IN CHILDREN

44

Norman Lavin

DIABETES MELLITUS TYPE 2

I. INTRODUCTION

A. Type 2 diabetes mellitus (DM) is no longer exclusively a disease of adults, as evidenced by an emerging epidemic of type 2 DM in children throughout the world. Twenty years ago, type 2 DM accounted for <3% of all cases of new-onset diabetes in children and adolescents, but now 45% of cases are attributed to it. Because of the close link between obesity and type 2 DM, there are comorbidities including hypertension, dyslipidemia, nonalcoholic fatty liver disease, and the metabolic syndrome, all of which are associated with increased cardiovascular risk. This disorder is polygenic, resulting from an interaction of genetics and environmental factors, such as obesity, inactivity, and a high-fat and/or high-calorie diet leading to insulin resistance. Among Pima Indian children, both low and high birth weight, maternal diabetes during pregnancy and bottle-feeding from birth are associated with type 2 diabetes.

B. There is an increased risk of type 2 DM in patients with polycystic ovary syndrome because of insulin resistance that is independent of obesity. Thirty-one percent of these patients have impaired glucose tolerance, and 7% to 16% have or will develop overt type 2 diabetes.

C. MODY/ADM

1. In addition to type I and type 2 DM, there is another specific type of diabetes: **mature-onset diabetes of the young (MODY).** MODY is characterized by early-onset diabetes inherited in an autosomal dominant pattern, and it is believed to be a subtype of non–insulin-dependent diabetes mellitus. Classic MODY occurs predominantly in Caucasians and presents before age 25 years, is nonketotic, and is generally not insulin-requiring. Fewer than 5% of cases of childhood diabetes in Caucasians are caused by MODY. Mutations in five genes can cause this entity. These genes include hepatocyte nuclear factor-4α (HNF-4α, MODY 1), glucokinase (MODY 2), hepatocyte and nuclear factor-1α (HNF-1α, MODY 3), insulin-promoter factor-1 (IPF-1, MODY 4), and hepatocyte and nuclear factor-1β (HNF-1β, MODY 5). Patients with MODY do not usually require long-term insulin for survival. Genetic studies to search for the various MODY mutations are usually limited to research investigations.

2. Atypical diabetes mellitus (ADM) is a subtype of diabetes that occurs in ~10% of African Americans with youth-onset diabetes. In contrast to MODY in Caucasians, ADM presents clinically as acute-onset diabetes, often associated with weight loss, ketosis, and even diabetic ketoacidosis. Approximately 50% of patients with ADM are obese. Initially, it is sometimes difficult to distinguish ADM from type 1 diabetes. Many months or years later, a non–insulin-dependent clinical course develops in patients with ADM that is clearly different from type 1 diabetes.

II. INCIDENCE

The highest incidence of type 2 DM is evident in Native Americans, Hispanics, and African Americans. There are also many family members with type 2 DM in children with this disorder. The peak incidence is age 13 to 14 years, probably secondary to physiologic insulin resistance during pubertal maturation. In lean African American children ages 7 to 11 years, insulin levels are significantly higher than in age-matched white children, which may predispose this group to obesity and type 2 diabetes. There is as much as a 30% decline in insulin action in comparison with preadolescent children or adults. Therefore, minority children may have a genetic predisposition to insulin resistance.

III. INSULIN RESISTANCE SYNDROME/METABOLIC SYNDROME

A. Definition

Risk factors for the development of the insulin resistance/metabolic syndrome are more prevalent during childhood than was previously thought. This syndrome reflects a wide array of factors, including adiposity, dyslipidemia, hypertension, hyperinsulinemia, impaired glucose metabolism, microalbuminuria, and abnormalities in fibrinolysis and inflammation. Many health organizations define the metabolic syndrome differently, but most agree that a low high-density lipoprotein (HDL) level and a high triglyceride level are two characteristics. Even though there is no general agreement regarding clinical assessment or potential treatment for the pediatric metabolic syndrome, the American Diabetes Association and the American Heart Association agree that obesity prevention and treatment in childhood should be the first-line approach to this problem. In addition to the body mass index (BMI) percentile, the inclusion of waist circumference is a fairly good surrogate marker for insulin resistance. That is, the greater the circumference, the greater is the likelihood of insulin resistance. Waist circumference percentiles have been developed for children and adolescents.

B. Obesity

Elevated fasting serum insulin concentration correlates significantly with serum lipids and blood pressure, which, in turn, are linked to obesity and diabetes. There is a strong relationship in childhood between obesity and subsequent dyslipidemia and hypertension. Obesity in teens is associated with an increased risk of premature death from coronary heart disease, especially among males. High birth weight is also a marker for subsequent cardiovascular risk. Larger infants born to diabetic mothers have an increased incidence of hypertension and hyperinsulinemia at ages 10 to 16 years in comparison with controls.

C. The fetus

Fetal life is a critical time for the ultimate development of cardiovascular risk factors in later life. Many studies have shown that insulin resistance in adults is related to birth weight—either small for gestational age or large for gestational age (a U-shaped curve). The long-term effects of fetal nutritional abnormalities may result in later insulin resistance, or certain genes may cause both low birth weight and insulin resistance. Low birth weight is associated with increased risk for the insulin resistance syndrome, probably evolving from undernutrition in utero. The risk is independent of that associated with adult obesity. The poor fetal nutrition emanates from chronic maternal malnutrition. When these infants become adults, they may ultimately have high blood pressure, hyperglycemia, hyperinsulinemia, and elevated triglyceride levels.

D. Measure of insulin resistance

1. A biochemical measure of insulin resistance is the Homeostasis Model of Insulin Resistance (HOMA-IR) index.
2. In the adolescent population, the HOMA-IR index is an excellent noninvasive technique with sensitivity of 76% and specificity of 66%, with a cutoff value of 3.16. In adults, it is >2.50. Therefore, >3.16 is high HOMA-IR, which is calculated as fasting insulin (μU/mL) × fasting glucose (mg/dL) divided by 22.5.
3. A HOMA-IR of 3 or lower is considered normal. Anything above 7 to 10 is considered insulin resistance. There is great lab-to-lab variation in insulin assay

results. Consequently, insulin values or HOMA indices cannot be compared between labs. A rising HOMA within the same lab, however, indicates a rising risk of diabetes.

IV. DIABETES PATHOPHYSIOLOGY

Type 2 DM emanates from a combination of insulin resistance, increased hepatic glucose output, and progressive decline of insulin sensitivity in response to glycemic stimulation. Chronic hyperglycemia gradually impairs β-cell function and leads to more insulin resistance and more hyperglycemia. The β cell loses its ability to compensate, leading to lower insulin concentration despite the presence of hyperglycemia. The failure of the β cell to continue to hypersecrete insulin underlies the transition from insulin resistance to clinical type 2 DM.

V. SCREENING FOR DIABETES OR PREDIABETES (adapted from Yale University)

The first step in evaluating an obese child is to measure fasting glucose and insulin levels as well as hemoglobin A_{1c}. The hemoglobin A_{1c} may be in the normal range despite abnormal glucose metabolism, but if it is >6, this should be considered a "red flag" that warrants further evaluation. Insulin levels may be elevated during puberty. Fasting insulin levels that are >20 μU/mL indicate insulin resistance, and prepubertal fasting insulin levels of 10 to 15 are a cause for concern. But actual glucose values are more important than insulin levels. A fasting glucose of 100 to 125 mg/dL indicates impaired fasting glucose. A level of 126 mg/dL or higher is consistent with a diagnosis of diabetes. A 2-hour postchallenge blood sugar of 140 to 199 mg/dL indicates impaired glucose tolerance. A blood sugar of 200 mg/dL or higher indicates diabetes. A recent pediatric study found that half of the cases of impaired glucose tolerance were missed using fasting assessments of glucose alone. They recommend that any adolescent who is obese, who has acanthosis nigricans, and who has a family history of diabetes, should undergo a 2-hour oral glucose tolerance test even when the fasting blood glucose is <100 mg/dL.

VI. DIFFERENTIAL DIAGNOSIS (Table 44.1)

Type 1 and type 2 DM may have clinical presentations that are indistinguishable from each other, so distinguishing between them may be difficult at the onset. Nevertheless, whether a patient is type 1 or type 2 may be established by the clinical presentation. Children with type 1 DM present with weight loss rather than obesity, as in type 2. Polyuria and polydipsia and a high incidence of diabetic ketoacidosis (DKA) are more typical of type 1. Insulin administration is required for survival in type 1, and 5% of these children have a first- or second-degree relative with the same disorder. Some children with type 2 DM present with DKA, and they initially require insulin as well. Acanthosis nigricans, found in 90% of children with type 2 DM, is a skin lesion that is prominent around the neck and in the intertriginous areas. There is a high correlation with insulin resistance. Polycystic ovary syndrome is also associated with insulin resistance and may be more common in children with type 2 DM as well. Lipid disorders and hypertension are also found in such children.

In children with type 2 DM, 17% to 32% have hypertension and 4% to 32% manifest elevated triglyceride levels. In the Pima Indian population, 22% of the children have abnormal urine albumin excretion at diagnosis.

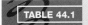

TABLE 44.1   **Diagnosis of Diabetes Mellitus**

1. Signs and symptoms (polyuria, polydipsia) plus random glucose >200 mg/dL
   or
2. Fasting blood glucose ≥126 mg/dL
   or
3. Two-hour oral glucose tolerance test ≥200 mg/dL

TABLE 44.2	Classification of Diabetes Mellitus by Etiology

A. Type 1 diabetes mellitus (immune-mediated)
B. Atypical diabetes mellitus (ADM)
C. Maturity-onset diabetes of youth (MODY)
D. Type 2 diabetes mellitus
   1. Insulin resistance; insulin deficiency; secretory defect
   2. Maturity-onset diabetes of youth; genetic defects of β-cell function
   3. Lipotropic diabetes
   4. Cystic fibrosis
   5. Cushing syndrome
   6. Drug-induced (glucocorticoids)
   7. Infections (congenital rubella)
   8. Gestational
   9. Other genetic defects

Atypical DM (which has been known as type 1.5 [or "Flatbush" DM]) is usually found in African American children with a positive family history of early-onset DM. Insulin is required at onset but may not be needed at later stages (Table 44.2).

VII. CLINICAL PRESENTATION OF TYPE 2 DM IN CHILDREN

Unrecognized hypoglycemia 42%
Polyuria 58%
Hispanic 47%
Black 37%
Caucasian 11%
Mean age 14.3 years
Acanthosis nigricans 90%
Type 2 family history 80%
Hypertension 15% to 25%
Mean glucose 397 mg/dL

Hemoglobin A_{1c} equal 9.3%
Average insulin level 76.8 mIU/L
C-peptide 5.5 ng/dL
Elevated total cholesterol
Elevated low-density lipoprotein (LDL)
Centripetal obesity
Weight >120% of ideal body weight or
BMI >85th percentile for age and sex
No recent weight loss
DKA 30%

VIII. DIABETES DIAGNOSIS AND EVALUATION

For high-risk populations, such as obese members of minority groups, I order a fasting glucose, insulin level, and C-peptide level, and, if needed, a 2-hour glucose tolerance test. If I have a strong index of suspicion, I order the glucose tolerance test even with a normal fasting blood glucose (Fig. 44.1).

At presentation, the child with type 2 DM has hyperglycemia, which is usually not as high as in type 1. There are also high insulin and C-peptide levels, as well as absence of autoimmune markers, such as the islet-cell and GAD antibody and the tyrosine phosphatase insulin antibody (1A-2 and 1A-2β), which argues strongly against type 1.

IX. ACUTE COMPLICATIONS OF TYPE 2 DM

A. Diabetic ketoacidosis. In a study in Cincinnati, 42% of African American adolescents presented with ketonuria and 25% met criteria for DKA at presentation. DKA in patients with type 1 diabetes is associated with substantial morbidity and a small incidence of mortality. Currently, no reports have been published on morbidity or mortality associated specifically with the DKA in type 2 DM.

B. Hyperglycemic hyperosmolar state. This is a life-threatening emergency. Standard diagnostic criteria are blood glucose concentrations >600 mg/dL and serum osmolality >330 mOsm/L with mild acidosis (serum bicarbonate >15 mmol/L and

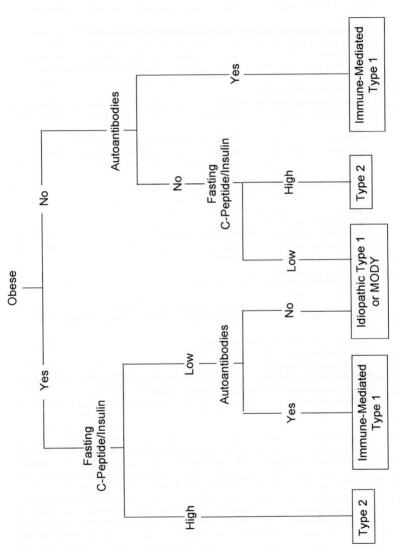

Figure 44.1. Classification of diabetes mellitus in children.

mild ketonuria ≤ 15 mg/dL). Precipitating causes include infections, medications, nonadherence to diabetes treatment, undiagnosed diabetes, substance abuse, and coexisting chronic illness. In the literature, 29 cases have been reported of adolescents with a hyperglycemic hyperosmolar state, of whom 26 were African American and 22 were male. As in adults, this complication is associated with substantial mortality.

   C. Malignant hyperthermialike syndrome with rhabdomyolysis. This is a rare syndrome that includes the hyperglycemic hyperosmolar state complicated by a malignant hyperthermialike event with fever, rhabdomyolysis, and severe cardiovascular instability after administration of insulin. Mortality is a common outcome.

X. DIABETES MANAGEMENT

   A. Weight reduction and exercise. Reducing weight and increasing physical exercise can reduce the incidence of type 2 DM as well as improve control in children who already have type 2 DM.

   1. Goal. The goal is to normalize blood sugar values and hemoglobin A_{1c} as well as to control hypertension and dyslipidemia. If weight loss and normalizing glucose are not achieved by diet and physical exercise, then pharmacologic therapy should be considered.

   2. Lifestyle changes. Many factors will increase insulin sensitivity and most can be accomplished through lifestyle changes. These include:

   a. Institute aerobic and resistance exercise.

   b. Increase muscle mass.

   c. Reduce body fat, particularly visceral fat.

   d. Reduce levels of circulating fats, including triglycerides and free fatty acids.

   e. Eat foods rich in antioxidants.

   f. Increase physical activity.

   g. Reduce mental and physical stressors.

   h. Increase intake of dietary fiber.

   i. Decrease consumption of saturated fats and *trans*-fats.

   j. Decrease consumption of highly refined foods with high glycemic index values.

   k. Eat a healthy breakfast every day.

   l. Get adequate sleep.

   m. Treat sleep apnea.

   B. Oral drugs. Most pediatric diabetologists now use oral agents for type 2 DM after insulin is administered on admission to the hospital.

   1. Metformin (biguanide) decreases hepatic glucose production and enhances hepatic and muscle insulin sensitivity. The first oral agent I generally recommend is metformin, because it can contribute to weight loss and not cause hypoglycemia. Compared with placebo, metformin was associated with a loss of 4.8% of total body weight and statistically significant reductions in BMI, waist circumference, fasting glucose, and fasting insulin. LDL and triglyceride concentrations decrease as well. It may also normalize ovulatory abnormalities in girls with polycystic ovary syndrome (PCOS). Metformin should be discontinued during administration of radioactive material if a patient has impaired renal function, hepatic disease, serious infection, alcohol abuse, or pregnancy. Side effects are usually gastrointestinal disturbances, but these usually diminish with time. The correct dosing in children has not been fully evaluated. I start at low levels, such as 250 mg at dinner for 1 week, and then titrate upward to 2 000 mg per day maximum.

   If monotherapy with metformin is unsuccessful, then consider adding a sulfonylurea or insulin. Also consider a meglitinide or glucosidase inhibitor. In teens with irregular eating habits, consider giving meglitinide.

   For patients with high levels of glucose who are very symptomatic or ketonuric, I begin with insulin administration as for a type 1 patient. Then, when glucose control is established, I add metformin while reducing the insulin dose.

   2. Sulfonylureas promote insulin secretion and are used in both adults and children with MODY. These agents can cause hypoglycemia and weight gain.

3. **Meglitinide** (repaglinide) causes short-term promotion of glucose-stimulated insulin secretion.
4. **Glucosidase inhibitors** (acarbose; miglitol) slow carbohydrate absorption and slow the hydrolysis of complex carbohydrates, which decreases postprandial rise in glucose. Because of flatulence, children may not want to use these medications.
5. **Thiazolidinediones (TZDs)** improve peripheral insulin sensitivity and reduce triglyceride concentration. Triglitazone has been associated with hepatic failure and is no longer recommended. Rosiglitazone (Avandia) and pioglitazone (Actos) are now available but, as of 2007, there were reports of cardiac side effects with Avandia and many endocrinologists are questioning whether they should continue using this class of medication.
6. **Exenatide** belongs to a class of drugs called **incretin mimetics,** so-called because they imitate natural hormones known as incretin. It was noticed that the pancreas releases more insulin when a person eats more carbohydrate-containing foods than when a comparable amount of glucose is infused intravenously. This led to finding a hormone in the gastrointestinal (GI) tract that plays a role in blood glucose control. The incretins are released from cells in response to food. One of these is glucagonlike peptide-1 or GLP-1. GLP (or exenatide) lowers blood glucose in the following ways: **(a)** it improves the normal release of insulin from the pancreas; **(b)** it decreases glucagon release; and **(c)** it slows the speed with which food leaves the stomach and promotes a feeling of fullness.

    Exenatide can be used in type 2 patients along with a sulfonylurea or metformin and is given by injection. Side effects include moderate nausea, which is most common when first starting. It rarely causes hypoglycemia and it tends to cause gradual weight loss.
7. **Liraglutide** is another incretin mimetic, which is currently being investigated in clinical trials.
8. **Sitagliptin (Januvia)** and **vildagliptin (Galvus).** GLP-1is rapidly broken down by enzymes called DPP-4. These two drugs act by inhibiting DPP-4, which increases the level of GLP-1 in the body. This improves insulin production and suppresses glucagon secretion, as does exenatide. These drugs reduce blood glucose levels after meals and affect the signal to the liver to stop producing glucose. They are once-a-day medications and are given orally. The most commonly reported side effects include stuffy or runny nose, sore throat, headache, diarrhea, and joint pain. Neither medication has been associated with weight gain.
9. **Pramlintide (Symlin).** A healthy pancreas releases both insulin and amylin in response to food intake. Without enough amylin, as seen in diabetes, glucose from food enters the bloodstream more quickly than normal, causing blood glucose levels to rise. Pramlintide, a synthetic analog of human amylin, prevents the rise in blood glucose after meals in the following ways: **(a)** it slows the speed with which food leaves the stomach; **(b)** it suppresses the secretion of glucagon after meals, which decreases the amount of glucose released from the liver; and **(c)** it decreases appetite. Pramlintide is approved for use in type 1 and type 2 diabetics who have not achieved adequate blood glucose control using intensive insulin therapy. As of this writing, it is approved only for adults. It is also an injectable medication. The most common side effect is mild to moderate nausea.

C. **Insulin.** Insulin may aggravate an existing hyperinsulinemic state with problems of hypoglycemia and weight gain. Some endocrinologists recommend the use of oral agents in the morning and insulin at bedtime, which decreases nocturnal hepatic glucose (reducing fasting glucose) and enhances the effects of the sulfonylureas.

    Rapid-acting or a combination of rapid/NPH, e.g., Humalog 75/25, helps to lower postprandial elevated glucose levels.

D. **Chronic complications**
1. **Hypertension.** There is a prevalence of hypertension at presentation of type 2 DM, varying between 10% and 32%. Hypertension at diagnosis is eight times as frequent in adolescents with type 2 DM compared to those with type 1.
2. **Nephropathy.** Microalbuminuria can also occur at presentation, particularly in Pima Indians, of whom 22% demonstrated this finding. The rate of progression of microalbuminuria and nephropathy seems to be rapid in adolescents with

type 2, whereas the rate of progression in microalbuminuria in adolescents with type 1 diabetes for the same duration was significantly less.

3. **Retinopathy.** Similar to nephropathy, retinopathy can be present at diagnosis of diabetes type 2. Retinopathy is significantly more frequent in individuals with type 1 diabetes than in those with type 2 (20% vs. 4%). However, median duration of diabetes was strikingly shorter in patients with type 2 diabetes, making conclusions difficult to draw.

4. **Dyslipidemia.** Many adolescents had substantial dyslipidemia at time of diagnosis of type 2 diabetes.

5. **Nonalcoholic fatty liver disease.** This is the most frequent cause of chronic liver disorder in obese and diabetic individuals. In a study of young people with type 2 diabetes in Canada, 22% had high liver enzymes compared to normals.

6. **Cardiovascular and atherosclerotic complications.** As many as 71% of patients with type 2 diabetes had diminished nocturnal decline in blood pressure, which is a known predictor of cardiovascular risk. Ultrasonographic variables indicating posterior and septal wall thickness were above the reference range in 47% of the children in one study. Another study reported left ventricular hypertrophy in 22% of adolescents with type 2 DM.

7. **Neuropathy.** There are no systemic reports on the incidence of neuropathy in children and adolescents with type 2 DM.

8. **Psychiatric disorders.** A significant number of patients had neuropsychiatric disease at presentation of DM type 2, including depression, schizophrenia, bipolar disorder, autism, mental retardation, attention-deficit disorder (ADD), obsessive-compulsive disorders, and behavior disorders.

9. **Conclusion.** Because of the epidemic of type 2 diabetes in children, early-age screening should be encouraged and early-age DM prevention programs should be explored further. Unfortunately, early onset of type 2 DM is associated with risk for complications qualitatively similar to that seen in adult patients. Because of hesitation and inexperience on the part of some pediatricians, many medications are not initiated early, such as drugs for hypertension, dyslipidemia, and type 2 DM.

OBESITY

I. INTRODUCTION

The International Obesity Task Force estimates that >300 million individuals worldwide are obese, and a billion are overweight. Childhood obesity may shorten life expectancy. If current trends in obesity among children continue, life expectancy will begin to decline for the U.S. population. This generation of children could become the first in modern history to live shorter and less healthy lives than their parents' generation. Statistics show that the problems of overweight in U.S. children ages 6 to 11 rose from 4% to 15.3% between 1963 and 2000, and during the past 10 years the prevalence of overweight also increased among children ages 2 to 5 years, to as much as 10%. About 66% of adult Americans are either obese or overweight, but the most significant increases over the past 20 years have been among children and among minority populations.

Our current Western food environment has become highly "insulinogenic," as demonstrated by food with increased energy density, high fat content, high glycemic index, increased fructose composition, decreased fiber, and decreased dairy content. As a result, insulin increases and acts on the brain to encourage eating through two separate mechanisms: **(a)** it blocks the signals that travel from the body's fat stores to the brain by suppressing the effectiveness of the hormone leptin, resulting in increased food intake and decreased activity; and **(b)** it promotes the signal that seeks the reward of eating, carried by the chemical dopamine, which makes a person want to eat to get the pleasurable "rush."

Calorie intake and expenditure are regulated by leptin. When leptin is functioning properly, it increases physical activity, decreases appetite, and increases feelings of well-being. Conversely, when leptin is suppressed, feelings of well-being and activity decrease and appetite increases, a state called "leptin resistance."

Metabolic consequences of obesity often begin in childhood. According to adult studies, obesity is one of the most important risk factors in the development of type 2 DM and is often associated with elevated insulin levels. Childhood obesity may lead to adult cardiovascular diseases that are independent of adult weight. Early onset of obesity is found in many groups, such as Native Americans (Pima, Cherokee, Mescalaro, Apache, Onandago, and Navajo), African Americans, and Hispanics.

As in adults, it is visceral fat rather than total body fat that correlates with basal and stimulated insulin levels and inversely correlates with insulin sensitivity. The Bogaloosa Heart Study showed that African American teens were more obese and had higher insulin levels to oral glucose challenge and higher insulin-to-glucose ratios compared to their Caucasian counterparts.

There are also current reports correlating childhood weight with an adult abnormal atherogenic lipid profile. The Bogaloosa Heart Study, the Muscutane Study, and the Minneapolis Children's Blood Pressure Study showed evidence of these abnormalities in children developing into cardiovascular disease in adults.

II. INCIDENCE

Thirty-three percent of U.S. adults are above the 80th percentile for BMI. According to the National Health and Nutritional Examination Surveys (NHNES) 1, 2, and 3, 23% of U.S. children aged 6 to 17 are above the 85th percentile for BMI and 11% are above the 95th percentile. African American girls aged 6 to 11 years are more likely than Caucasians to be overweight. Obesity is more prevalent among African Americans and Native Americans and among poor or less educated families. The prevalence of pediatric obesity is increasing at the rate of ~30% per decade. This significant change over a single decade must reflect major changes in nongenetic factors. Therefore, obesity results from the interactions of genetic susceptibility to store excess calories as fat, as well as heritable predilections toward insulin resistance, impaired β-cell function, dyslipidemia, and hypertension, with an environment that favors the expression of these susceptibilities.

III. DEFINITION

A child is **overweight** if his or her BMI is above the 80th percentile and **obese** if the BMI is above the 95th percentile. BMI is calculated by dividing the child's weight (kg) by the square of the height (m), or kg/m². Standard graphs are also used by most pediatricians to plot weight for height and age to determine whether a child is obese.

BMI	Weight status
Below 18	Underweight
18.5–24	Normal
25.0–29	Overweight
30.0 and above	Obese

Body fat distribution is usually defined on the basis of waist circumference. Central distribution of body fat is an independent predictor of insulin resistance and dyslipidemia in prepubertal and pubertal children and of type 2 diabetes, cardiovascular disease, stroke, and death in adults. Free fatty acids from omental fat drain directly into the portal circulation, exposing the liver to circulating free fatty acids, which results in increased hepatic glucose production and decreased insulin clearance and which, in turn, leads to insulin resistance and dyslipidemia.

IV. COMPLICATIONS

In children, as in adults, there are many complications associated with obesity (Table 44.3).
A. Insulin resistance.
B. Non–insulin-dependent diabetes mellitus or type 2 DM.
C. Dyslipidemia.

TABLE 44.3 Complications Associated with Obesity

Signs and symptoms	Disorder	Additional findings
Snoring	Sleep apnea	Hypertrophy of tonsils or adenoids
Daytime somnolence	Pickwickian syndrome or sleep apnea	
Abdominal pain	Gallbladder disease	
Hip pain or limp	Slipped capital femoral epiphysis	
Irregular menses or amenorrhea	Polycystic ovary disease	Hirsutism, visceral adiposity, insulin resistance
	Prader-Willi syndrome	Short stature, hypogonadism, small hands and feet, infantile hypotonia
Short stature or growth arrest	Hypothyroidism, Cushing syndrome	
Developmental delay	Prader-Willi syndrome, other genetic syndromes	
Fatigue/tiredness	Depression	
Elevated blood pressure	Cardiovascular disease	Consider Cushing syndrome
Postaxial polydactyly	Bardet-Biedl syndrome	Retinitis pigmentosa, hypogonadism, mental retardation
Eyes		
Papilledema	Pseudotumor cerebri	
Retinitis pigmentosa	Bardet-Biedl syndrome	
Skin		
Acanthosis nigricans	Obesity, glucose intolerance, metabolic syndrome	
Violaceous striae	Cushing syndrome	
Hirsutism	Polycystic ovary disease, Cushing syndrome	
Hepatomegaly	Nonalcoholic fatty liver disease	Elevated serum aminotransferases
Genitalia		
Undescended testicles	Prader-Willi syndrome	
Delayed puberty	Cushing syndrome	
	Prader-Willi syndrome in girls	
	Bardet-Biedl syndrome	
Bowed legs	Blount disease, bowed femurs	Bowed tibias

D. Premature atherosclerosis. The Bogaloosa Heart Study showed that atherosclerosis can be found in early childhood and that a high BMI is associated with early plaque formation—hence the necessity of early intervention to prevent cardiovascular disease in the adult. C-reactive protein (CRP) and lipoprotein (a) [Lp(a)] show promise as markers in children of future atherosclerosis.

E. Hypertension (Even as young as 2 to 5 years in overweight children). In one study, 10.6% of overweight and obese children had elevated blood pressure values in comparison with normal subjects.

F. The insulin resistance/metabolic syndrome is a clustering of factors including hypertension, dyslipidemia, and insulin resistance. This newly described entity is the most common cause of early cardiovascular disease (see Chapter 45).

G. Low self-esteem.

H. Pseudotumor cerebri.

I. Sleep apnea.

J. Slipped capital femoral epiphysis.

K. NASH or NAFLD. Nonalcoholic steatohepatitis (NASH) or nonalcoholic fatty liver disease (NAFLD) is a common cause of chronic liver disease in adults. In adolescents, the most common cause of elevated liver enzymes is obesity. Up to 10% of obese children may have abnormal alanine aminotransferase levels. Abnormal liver enzymes in overweight children may emanate from a combination of hyperinsulinemia, hyperlipidemia, and a decrease in antioxidant levels.

The diagnosis of NAFLD is first suspected because of an elevation of liver enzymes, or in the setting of an echogenic liver detected by ultrasound. Diagnosis requires exclusion of other causes of chronic hepatitis. Pediatric NAFLD is increasing in prevalence, at least in the United States, in parallel with the prevalence of obesity. The liver pathology encompasses a range from isolated fatty liver to steatohepatitis, advanced fibrosis, and cirrhosis. NASH may progress to cirrhosis even in children. NAFLD occurs most commonly in conditions associated with insulin resistance, including obesity, diabetes mellitus, and the insulin resistance syndrome.

There are some data by Levine suggesting that vitamin E may normalize aminotransferase levels in these patients. Additionally, modest alcohol ingestion may exacerbate obesity-associated liver disease. Therefore, in a child with elevated liver enzymes, I recommend immediate weight loss and exercise, vitamin E supplements, and, obviously, no ingestion of alcohol.

V. EVALUATION AND WORKUP

A. Rule out various conditions of which obesity is a sign, including hypothyroidism, Cushing syndrome, and certain genetic syndromes (e.g., Prader-Willi, Lawrence-Moon-Bidel, Alstrom, and Cohen syndromes (Table 44.3).

Also, rule out certain medications as a cause, such as anticonvulsants, corticosteroids, antipsychotics, and tricyclics. Albeit rare, ischemic injuries that affect the appetite center in the lateral hypothalamus can cause obesity.

B. Laboratory tests

1. Lipid profile
2. Serum chemistries
3. Fasting glucose
4. Glucose tolerance test
5. Fasting insulin
6. C-peptide
7. T4 and TSH
8. Cortisol levels (serum; 24-hour urine)
9. Repeat electrolytes and the lipid profile 6 to 12 weeks after the first test and after initiating the dietary program.

VI. MANAGEMENT

Management of obesity in children includes increase in physical exercise, reduction in television or computer time, and decrease in caloric intake. Drug therapy to reduce weight has not been well studied in children.

For a child 2 to 6 years of age who has a BMI at or above the 95th percentile, the goal of treatment is to achieve weight maintenance. Weight loss is indicated for this age group if there are weight-related complications. For older children, weight reduction is the goal if the BMI is at or above the 95th percentile, whether or not there is a weight-related complication, including pseudotumor cerebri, sleep apnea, orthopedic abnormalities, type 2 DM, hypertension, as well as major psychological or social issues.

A. Recommendations

1. Discourage ingestion of high-fat snacks and beverages that are high in calories and sugar. There is evidence that economics plays a large part in the obesity epidemic, as food has become cheaper during the past several decades, especially foods that are high in fat and sugar. Obesity rates among the poor, who are more

likely to depend on high-fat, high-sugar foods for their meals, are substantially higher than the rates seen in higher-income groups. The Cardia study showed that frequent <u>fast-food</u> consumption is associated with weight gain and risk of insulin resistance. The study also demonstrated that the bigger the portion size provided, the more people consume.

2. Very-low-calorie or high-protein diets are not recommended.

3. Drinking of skim milk is not associated with any negative effect on growth in early childhood.

4. Replace sedentary activity with exercise. Sixty minutes of physical activity every day is recommended for children, and 30 minutes for adults.

5. Do not recommend a semistarvation diet. Such diets usually lead to failure because the body defends itself against starvation by metabolic, hormonal, and behavioral processes establishing a set point of weight that the body attempts to maintain. Because of a lowered metabolic rate, the patient may gain weight back rapidly—even more than was lost ("Yo-Yo" dieting).

6. Set reasonable goals for weight loss to avoid frustration; slowing of weight gain rather than loss should be considered.

7. Consider the "stoplight" diet, in which foods are grouped as red, yellow, or green lights according to their lipogenic potential.
   a. Green-light food (unlimited quantities) includes fruits, nonstarchy vegetables, fat-free dairy products, and baked or broiled skinless poultry and fish.
   b. Yellow-light foods (moderate quantities) are the starchy vegetables (potatoes, corn, peas), rice, pasta, and breads.
   c. Red-light foods (infrequent ingestion) are high in fat and sugar; these include cakes, fatty meats, pizza, fruit juices, and other fast foods.

8. Behavior modification may be helpful.

9. The child should be seen by a physician and/or nutritionist at regular and frequent intervals.

10. Limit meals at fast-food restaurants. Individuals who ate meals from fast-food restaurants more than twice a week gained 4.5 kg more weight and had a greater increase in insulin resistance than those who ate at such restaurants less frequently.

B. Questionable treatment

1. Weight-loss programs that supply food that are usually not individualized for a child's taste and often do not teach children how to make healthy food choices.

2. Weight-loss summer camps are not always successful because the child is out of the family environment, which may be part of the problem. Therefore, the child often regains the lost weight upon returning home.

3. Herbal diet products containing ma-huang or ephedrine should be avoided because they may result in hypertension, agitation, insomnia, arrhythmia, and sudden death.

C. Pharmacotherapy

Most pediatric obesity centers do not use medications for obesity, at least initially, because long-term safety and efficacy have not been shown. A few drugs have proven to be harmful, such as fenfluramine (Pondimin) and dexphenfluramine (Redux) and have been discontinued.

1. Currently, some centers are exploring the use of **sibutramine (Meridia),** a psychostimulant, and **orlistat (Xenical),** a lipase inhibitor that prevents fat absorption.

2. The side effects of orlistat are steatorrhea and anal leakage, whereas the side effects of sibutramine are nervousness, irritability, headache, dry mouth, nausea, and constipation. The safety and efficacy of sibutramine have not been established for patients <16 years of age, and orlistat has not been evaluated in patients <12 years of age.

3. The adverse effects of orlistat include fatty and oily stool, fecal urgency, and oily spotting in up to 30% of patients. Fecal incontinence was observed in 7%, and to prevent deficiencies in fat-soluble vitamins, a co-prescription of a daily multivitamin was recommended. Sibutramine does not increase release of serotonin and

has not been associated with valvular heart disease or pulmonary hypertension, in contrast to fenfluramine and dexfenfluramine. It has, however, been associated with small increases in blood pressure and pulse rate, therefore it is not recommended for patients with uncontrolled hypertension, pre-existing cardiovascular disease, or tachycardia.

4. **Metformin** reduces food intake, inhibits lipogenesis, and reduces fasting glucose and insulin concentrations, all of which may lead to some weight loss.

5. **Rimonabant.** The ability of recreational marijuana to stimulate appetite generated interest in the use of endogenous cannabinoid agonists and antagonists for weight-related disorders. The endocannabinoid system includes two major receptors, the CB-1 and CB-2 receptors. Endocannibinoids increase motivation to eat and stimulate food intake. Ribonabant, the first CB-1 receptor blocker, enhances thermogenesis, diminishes hepatic and adipocyte lipogenesis and augments adiponectin concentrations, and inhibits preadipocyte proliferation and increases adipocyte maturation without lipid accumulation. It significantly reduced weight (in one study by 4.6 kg), reduced waist circumference, and improved triglyceride and HDL cholesterol profiles. Adverse effects include nausea, dizziness, diarrhea, and insomnia in a small percentage of patients.

6. **Benefits.** There are no definitive data showing benefit of one antiobesity drug over another. No matter which drug is used, if there is no effectiveness within the first 3 to 6 months, then these drugs should be discontinued. Combination treatment has not been well researched at this time, and the optimum duration of treatment is unclear. Drugs that improve surrogate endpoints, such as weight loss, might not necessarily improve endpoints judged to be more clinically relevant.

7. **Future therapy.** New drugs are being tested, including some that act on the central melanocortin pathway, a group of neurons centered in the arcuate nucleus and hypothalamus that controls appetite and energy expenditure. Examples include ciliary, neurotrophic factor, and other melanocortin-4 receptor agonists, ghrelin, neuropeptide-Y antagonists, melanin-concentrating hormonal antagonists, and peptide YY. It is possible that multiple drugs with different mechanisms may be needed to produce significant and persistent weight loss.

D. **Treatment for morbidly obese adolescents**
   1. Ketogenic (carbohydrate-restricted diet).
      a. Improved lipid profile
      b. Decreased insulin resistance
   2. Other than bariatric surgery, which is not an encompassing population-based treatment for obesity, no intervention has produced consistent, effective, long-term weight loss. It is essential for society to address all aspects of the environment that are thought to be obesogenic. There have been limited published reports of experience with bariatric surgery in the pediatric age group. Recommendations suggest limiting its use to adolescents with a body mass index of at least 40 or more who also have obesity-related coexisting illnesses.

E. **Risks of treatment.** Lowering of dietary fat in infancy does not alter growth patterns during the first 3 years of life according to the STRIP Study in Finland. Likewise, the Dietary Intervention Study in Children (DISC) shows no negative effect of lowering dietary fat on growth in preteens.

VII. SUMMARY

To prevent cardiovascular disease in adults, prevent or manage obesity aggressively in childhood.

LIPID DISORDERS

I. INTRODUCTION

Cardiovascular disease in adults has its roots in childhood. I believe that by correcting lipid disorders at an early age, we can help prevent coronary heart disease. The American

Heart Association (March 21, 2007) panel statement reflects research showing that the pathogenesis of cardiovascular disease begins many years before it is manifested in adulthood. It has become clear, the panel said, that atherosclerotic cardiovascular disease begins in childhood and is progressive. There is still not total agreement regarding when to measure lipids in children, how to interpret them, and what medications to use, if any, in pediatric dyslipidemias.

Fatty streak formation can begin in the fetus and is greatly increased by maternal hypercholesterolemia leading to subsequent atherosclerosis, according to the FELIC (Fate of Early Lesions in Children) study. Cholesterol-lowering intervention of hypercholesterolemia in pregnancy may reduce the incidence of atherogenesis in children. (Of course, the use of statins is contraindicated during pregnancy.) During fetal life, the placenta may be permeable to certain fatty acids or native lipoproteins. Maternal hypercholesterolemia may also increase oxygen radical production and peroxidative compounds that may permeate the placenta. As a result, signaling processes as well as gene expression and transcription in the arterial wall may be altered.

Hyperlipidemia or dyslipidemia means that high levels of fats or lipids are found in the blood when the diet contains too much cholesterol and fat, when the body produces too much cholesterol and fat, or both. Fats do not dissolve in water. In order for them to be carried in the blood, which is mostly water, they combine with a protein to create a lipoprotein. There are three kinds of lipoproteins in the body: LDL, HDL, and triglycerides. Hyperlipidemia can run in families as a genetic disorder:

- Familial hypercholesterolemia—LDL levels are high.
- Familial hypertriglyceridemia—triglyceride levels are high.
- Familial combined hyperlipidemia—levels of cholesterol, triglycerides, or both are high, and HDL is low.

There are medications that can lower LDL cholesterol and triglycerides or raise HDL. *Statins* are the most common medications for lowering LDL cholesterol. *Fibrates* and *niacin* are used to lower triglycerides and to raise HDL cholesterol (see Tables 44.7, 44.9, and 44.11, later).

II. LIPOPROTEIN PHYSIOLOGY

Triglyceride and cholesterol are combined with apolipoproteins and phospholipids and then are transported through the body as lipoproteins.

Lipoproteins are classified according to their density and their ratio of cholesterol and triglycerides to protein. The five main classifications of lipoprotein are chylomicrons, very-low-density lipoprotein (VLDL), LDL, intermediate-density lipoprotein (IDL), and HDL (Table 44.4).

Chylomicrons are the largest, most buoyant lipoproteins, with relatively more triglyceride within their core and less cholesterol than LDL and HDL particles. They are comprised of ~90% triglyceride, which is less dense than cholesterol and gives them

TABLE 44.4 Classification of Lipoproteins

Phenotype (old classification)	Particles with elevated levels	Major lipid abnormality	Frequency
I	Chylomicron	TG	Very rare
IIA	LDL	LDL-C	Common
IIB	LDL and VLDL	LDL-C, TG	Common
III	IDL	TC, TG	Rare
IV	VLDL	TG	Common
V	Chylomicron	TG	Uncommon

IDL, intermediate-density lipoprotein; LDL, low-density lipoprotein; LDL-C, low-density lipoprotein cholesterol; TG, triglycerides; VLDL, very-low-density lipoprotein.

their buoyancy. They are made in the intestines following the absorption of digestive fat. From there, they are transported to the bloodstream to such tissues as skeletal muscle, body fat, and the liver. In these tissues, an enzyme called **lipoprotein lipase** breaks down the triglycerides within the chylomicrons into free fatty acids. These free fatty acids are then either used by muscle cells to create energy, stored in muscle or fat tissues, or broken down and transported into other substances by the liver. The lipoproteins enter two major pathways.

A. Exogenous pathway. Triglycerides hook onto chylomicrons and circulate systemically, where they are acted on by lipoprotein lipase. The triglycerides are then released as free fatty acids and monoglycerides, which are resynthesized in fat tissue where they are stored, subsequently resulting in production of chylomicron remnants.

B. Endogenous pathway. VLDL produced in the liver also interacts with lipoprotein lipase to release IDL particles, which are either removed by the liver or metabolized to LDL. Some of the LDL is brought to the subintimal space, where atheromas develop, causing atherosclerosis. Elevated LDL cholesterol (LDL-C), decreased HDL cholesterol (HDL-C), and an elevated ratio of total cholesterol to HDL predict increased risk for atherosclerosis in adults.

III. EVALUATION

A. Studies to exclude secondary dyslipidemia should be instituted, including thyroid function tests as well as liver and renal function tests.

B. Lipids in all first and secondary relatives of the affected child should be measured.

C. I recommend ordering a lipid panel that includes total cholesterol, HDL, LDL, and triglycerides, as well as measurement of the size of the LDL particles.

D. Measurement of total cholesterol and HDL does not require fasting. Triglyceride and LDL levels should be measured following an overnight fast, but new methods to measure LDL directly do not require fasting specimens (these methods can be used to measure LDL when the triglyceride level is >400 mg/dL) (Table 44.5).

IV. INTERPRETING AND MANAGING ABNORMAL LIPID LEVELS (Table 44.6)

A. Evaluation of elevated cholesterol

1. If the total cholesterol is between 170 and 199 mg/dL, repeat the test in 2 to 4 weeks and average the two levels.

2. If the average is >170 mg/dL, or if the initial total cholesterol is >200 mg/dL, I recommend ordering a complete lipid profile (Table 44.6).

a. If the LDL is between 110 and 129 mg/dL, I recommend the Step 1 diet developed by the National Cholesterol Education Program (NCEP), which provides for <30% total fat (of which <10% is saturated fat, and <300 mg cholesterol per day is permitted), 55% carbohydrate, and 15% to 20% protein. This diet is safe and does not interfere with growth. The goal is to achieve an LDL level <110 mg/dL by beginning the Step 1 diet and changing to the Step 2 diet if significant improvement has not been achieved in 3 months. This latter diet reduces saturated fat to <7% of total calories and dietary cholesterol to <200 mg per day. If dietary and exercise interventions have not reduced LDL to <160 mg/dL in 6 to 12 months, then pharmacotherapy should be considered (see Table 44.11).

TABLE 44.5   Goals for Lipid Levels in Children

Lipid	Goal (mg/dL)
Cholesterol	<170
Low-density lipoprotein	<110
High-density lipoprotein	>45
Triglycerides	<125

TABLE 44.6   Dyslipidemia and Atherosclerosis

Dyslipidemia that increases the risk of atherosclerosis	Dyslipidemia that decreases the risk of atherosclerosis
Elevated levels of the following:	Decreased levels of the following:
TC	TC
LDL	LDL
ApoB	ApoB
TC/HDL-C ratio	TC/HDL-C ratio
ApoB/HDL-C ratio	ApoB/HDL-C ratio
ApoB/apoA-I ratio	ApoB/apoA-I ratio
Lipoprotein(a), or Lp(a)	Lipoprotein(a), or Lp(a)
Decreased levels of the following:	Elevated levels of the following:
HDL	HDL
HDL-C	HDL-C
ApoA-I	ApoA-I
LDL-C/apoB ratio	LDL-C/apoB ratio

apoA-I, apolipoprotein A-I; apoB, apolipoprotein B; HDL, high-density lipoprotein; HDL-C, high-density lipoprotein cholesterol; LDL-C, low-density lipoprotein cholesterol; TC, total cholesterol.

  b. Because adding fiber to the diet is benign and can lower total cholesterol and LDL in adults, also consider this product for children.
  c. If the LDL is >130 mg/dL, consider familial dyslipidemias and secondary causes of dyslipidemia (see Table 44.7).
  d. Restriction of dietary cholesterol, saturated and *trans*-fat, along with liberal intake of dietary fiber and plant sterols, can lower LDL. High intake of omega-3 fatty acids can reduce serum triglyceride. Jenkins et al., reported a 28%

TABLE 44.7   Clinical Characteristics and Treatment Options for High-Risk Adolescents with Hyperlipidemia

	Familial combined hyperlipidemia	Metabolic syndrome	FH hetero-zygote	FH homo-zygote
Total cholesterol (mg/dL)	200–250	200–250	250–350	600–700
Triglycerides (mg/dL)	175–350	>150	100–150	100–150
LDL cholesterol (mg/dL)	150–200	130–200	160–250	600–650
HDL cholesterol (mg/dL)	25–35	<35	45–55	45–55
Xanthomata	Rare	None	10% of teens	Common
Adolescent's 10-y risk of myocardial infarction	<1%	<1%	15–20%	Very high, 90%
Treatment used if TLC fails	Extended-release niacin, omega-3 fatty acids, fibrates, statins	Extended-release niacin, omega-3 fatty acids fibrates, statins	Statins with or without ezetimibe, extended-release niacin, or bile acid seques-trant	Biweekly apheresis

HDL, high-density lipoprotein; LDL, low-density lipoprotein; TLC, therapeutic life change.

TABLE 44.8   Dosing of HMG-CoA-Reductase Inhibitors

Statin	Adult dose	Pediatric dose
Lovastatin (Mevacor)	Initial: 20 mg/d PO qhs Followed by 10–80 mg/d PO qhs or divided b.i.d.	10–17 y: 10 mg/d PO; not to exceed 40 mg/d
Simvastatin (Zocor)	Initial: 5–10 mg/d PO qhs Followed by 5–80 mg/d PO qhs or divided b.i.d.	10–17 y: 10 mg/d PO; not to exceed 40 mg/d
Pravastatin (Pravachol)	Initial: 10–20 mg/d PO qhs Followed by 5–40 mg/d PO qhs	8–13 y: 10 mg/d PO initially; not to exceed 20 mg/d 14–17 y: 10 mg/d PO initially; not to exceed 40 mg/d
Fluvastatin (Lescol)	Initial: 20–30 mg/d PO qhs Followed by 20–80 mg/d PO qhs; divide 80 mg into b.i.d.	<18 y: Not established
Atorvastatin (Lipitor)	Initial: 10 mg/d PO qhs Followed by 10–80 mg/d PO qhs	10–17 y: 10 mg/d PO initially; not to exceed 20 mg/d

TABLE 44.9   Medications for Dyslipidemia

Drug class	Examples	Action	Contraindications and side effects
Statins	Atorvastatin Fluvastatin Lovastatin Pravastatin Rosuvastatin Simvastatin	Inhibits hepatic cholesterol synthesis	Myalgia, myositis, raised aspartate, aminotransferase (AST [SGOT]) and alanine aminotransferase (ALT [SGPT])
Niacin	Extended-release niacin	Impairs VLDL (high TG)	Flushing, elevated AST and ALT
Fibrate	Gemfibrozil Fenofibrate	Impairs VLDL (high TG)	Dyspepsia, constipation, myositis, anemia
Bile acid sequestrant	Cholestyramine Colesevelam	Binds intestinal bile acids, interrupts entero-hepatic recirculation	Gas, bloating, constipation, cramps
Cholesterol absorption inhibitor	Ezetimibe	Inhibits cholesterol absorption from small intestine	Gas, bloating, constipation

VLDL, very-low-density lipoprotein; TG, triglyceride.

TABLE 44.10 Dyslipidemias—Frederickson Classification

Phenotype	Elevated particle	Lipid disorder	Frequency	Etiology
I	Chylomicron	Triglycerides > 1000 mg/dL	Rare	Lipoprotein lipase deficiency
IIA	LDL	LDL > 130 mg/dL	Common	Familial hypercholesterolemia, familial combined hyperlipidemia (also DM, hypothyroidism, and nephrosis)
IIB	LDL VLDL	LDL > 130 mg/dL triglycerides > 125 mg/dL	Common	
III	IDL	Total cholesterol > 200 mg/dL triglycerides > 125 mg/dL	Rare	Apolipoprotein E2 homozygosity (also diabetes and kidney disease)
IV	VLDL	Triglycerides > 125 mg/dL	Common	Familial combined hyperlipidemia, familial hypertriglyceridemia (also diabetes, hypothyroidism, Cushing, nephrosis, drugs, e.g., glucocorticoids, GH, androgens)
V	VLDL chylomicron	Triglycerides > 1000 mg/dL	Uncommon	

LDL, low-density lipoprotein; VLDL, very-low-density lipoprotein; IDL, intermediate-density lipoprotein; DM, diabetes mellitus; GH, growth hormone.
Modified from *Contemp Pediatr* May 1999.

reduction in LDL cholesterol levels with a diet that was low in saturated fat and cholesterol and rich in soluble fiber, plant sterols, soy proteins, and nuts.
e. The original ATP-3 guidelines were updated in 2004 and introduced an optimal LDL goal of <70 mg/dL for patients at very high risk of heart disease and also recommended drug therapy for these patients even at baseline LDL

TABLE 44.11 American Heart Association (AHA) 2007 Statement for the Treatment of Children with High-Risk Lipid Disorders

Lipid	Frederickson class	Medication First choice	Second choice
LDL	IIA	Statins (lovastatin, simvastatin, provastatin, atarvastatin)	Bile acid-binding resin or niacin
LDL + triglycerides	IIB	Statins	Niacin or fibric acid derivatives
Triglycerides	IV	Statins	Fibric acid derivatives

LDL, low-density lipoprotein; HMG-Co, 3-hydroxy-3-methylglutanyl.
Note: Types I, III, and V are uncommon.

TABLE 44.12	Pharmacotherapy for Dyslipidemia

I. Children with type IIA or IIB hyperlipoproteinemia
  A. LDL >160–190 + family history of early CV disease
  B. LDL >160–190 + risk factors for CV disease (e.g., hypertension), HDL <35 mg/dL, obesity, diabetes mellitus
  C. LDL >190
II. Children with fasting hypertriglyceridemia

Triglyceride level (mg/dL)	Management (see Tables 44.10 and 44.11)
125–300	Weight reduction, exercise
300–500	If HDL <35 mg/dL, consider medication
500–1 000	Medication
>1 000	Medication

CV, cardiovascular; HDL, high-density lipoprotein; LDL, low-density lipoprotein.

cholesterol levels <100. A recent meta-analysis of the four recent trials suggested a 16% reduction in the incidence of coronary death or any cardiovascular event with LDL cholesterol reduction to 75 mg/dL with high-dose statin therapy.

B. Management of elevated triglycerides (see Tables 44.9, 44.11, 44.12). If the triglyceride level is >300 mg/dL, especially with an HDL level <35 mg/dL, pharmacotherapy should be instituted. It is well known that severe hypertriglyceridemia (>1 000 mg per day) can predispose to acute pancreatitis and needs immediate therapy. Triglycerides are most responsive to lifestyle interventions, such as diet, and particularly low-fat diets. If there is no resolution, then pharmacologic intervention should be instituted with fibrates, niacin, and/or omega-3 polyunsaturated fatty acids. Although elevated serum triglycerides are considered to be an independent risk factor for heart disease, the benefit of treating mild to moderate hypertriglyceridemia on mortality is still not entirely clear. Key points to remember for lipoproteins and the significance of hypertriglyceridemia are the following:

1. Triglyceride levels >1 000 to 2 000 mg/dL are associated with an increased risk for pancreatitis.

2. Consider familial or inherited forms of hypertriglyceridemia (e.g., familial combined hyperlipidemia, familial hypertriglyceridemia, and LPL deficiency).

3. Consider underlying diseases that could cause hypertriglyceridemia (such as diabetes mellitus, renal insufficiency, obesity, and alcoholism).

4. Be aware of associated decreases in HDL levels.

5. Increased risk for cardiovascular disease independent of a low HDL level is possible.

C. Dyslipidemias
Concurrent with instituting a diet and exercise program, eliminate <u>secondary causes</u> of lipid disorders. These include obesity, poor diet, lack of exercise, smoking, alcohol, DM, hypothyroidism, liver and renal diseases, as well as drugs such as diuretics, beta-blockers, glucocorticoids, retinoid acid derivatives, and interferons ($-\alpha$, $-\beta$, $-\gamma$). These are all well known to increase serum triglycerides. Cyclosporine can increase LDL cholesterol levels, and sirolimus and HIV-1 proteus inhibitors can cause severe hypertriglyceridemia. Tamoxifen can cause hypertriglyceridemia in certain individuals but reduces LDL cholesterol levels. Aromatase inhibitors can modestly raise LDL cholesterol levels.

Hyperlipoproteinemia types 1, 3, and 5 are uncommon. Elevated levels of LDL suggest a Frederickson 2A phenotype. A Frederickson type 2B phenotype includes elevations in both LDL and triglyceride levels. These two types are often associated with familial hypercholesterolemia and familial hyperlipidemia.

1. Familial hypercholesterolemia is an autosominal dominant lipid disorder marked by an elevated LDL with or without a concurrent hypertriglyceridemia (1 in 500 people). Cord-blood LDL and total cholesterol are elevated in babies with familial hypercholesterolemia. Coronary heart disease can begin in the third decade in this disorder.

   Homozygous familial hypercholesterolemia is caused by loss-of-function mutations in both alleles of the LDL receptor gene. Patients have a poor response to conventional drug therapy, which generally lowers LDL levels through upregulation of the hepatic LDL receptor.

   A potentially effective therapy for homozygous familial hypercholesterolemia is to reduce LDL production. The microsomal triglyceride transfer protein is responsible for transferring triglyceride onto apolipoprotein B within the liver in the assembly of VLDL, the precursor to LDL. In certain patients, there is a rare disorder of an absence of this protein; it is called **abetalipoproteinemia** and leads to the absence of all lipoproteins containing apolipoprotein B in the plasma. Therefore, an inhibitor was developed.

   The **microsomal triglyceride transfer protein inhibitor** was effective in reducing cholesterol levels. There were, however, major side effects on liver enzymes. Therefore, this type of medication will need to be carefully studied to determine its safety.

2. Familial combined hyperlipidemia (1 in 200 to 300 people) is autosomal dominant, with elevated total cholesterol or triglyceride in some, and increased LDL and triglyceride in others. Premature coronary heart disease occurs in this group as well.

3. Lipid disorders in type 1 and type 2 diabetes. One of five children in a study called SEARCH and one of three children with type 2 diabetes had elevated total cholesterol levels, and 50% of either type 1 or type 2 diabetics had elevated LDL levels. The optimal levels are the same as in nondiabetic children, which include an LDL <100, HDL >35, and triglycerides <125. The American Diabetes Association recommends initiation of pharmacologic treatment in children 10 years or older with type 1 or type 2 DM if the LDL is >160 mg/dL after glycemic control is established and other nonpharmacologic interventions fail. It should also be considered if the LDL is >130 to 159.

V. PHARMACOTHERAPY FOR PEDIATRIC DYSLIPIDEMIAS (see Tables 44.7, 44.8, 44.9, 44.11, 44.12)

A. **Bile acid–binding resins** were for many years considered first-line drugs for management of type 2A hyperlipoproteinemia (increased LDL), but resins are poorly tolerated in children. The use of statins, therefore, is an obvious therapeutic choice. The American Heart Association says that *statins* should be the first-line therapy in these children. Statins have similar safety and efficacy in lipid disorders in children as in adults.

   Cholestyramine and **cholestipol** are taken with meals, when bile acids are secreted. Begin with one or two packets or scoops per day, given in orange juice or water with meals (breakfast and dinner). The dose is increased monthly until LDL is <130 mg/dL or the maximal dose has been reached. Because bile acid–binding resins can elevate triglycerides, they are not indicated in the condition of hypertriglyceridemia found in type 2B hyperlipoproteinemia. Remember that these resins can bind other drugs and vitamins in addition to bile salts. Therefore, the child should not take other medications for at least 1 hour before or 3 hours after consuming resins.

B. **Niacin** (nicotinic acid) has been effective in adults for types 2A, 2B, 4, and 5 hyperlipoproteinemia and is also effective in children. Beginning at a dose of 50 mg per day, increase the dose gradually at monthly intervals until the LDL is <160 mg/dL (types 2A, 2B), or the triglycerides are <300 mg/dL (type 4), or until a maximal dose of 1 500 to 3 000 mg/m² is reached without liver toxicity. Split the dose as soon as you reach 100 mg per day. Once the LDL falls to <130 mg/dl, or the triglycerides fall to <125 mg/dL, either reduce the niacin dose or attempt a trial off medication.

Side effects of niacin include liver disease, nausea, gastrointestinal upset, and facial flushing. The flushing may be reduced by ingestion of aspirin, but this is not generally recommended for children, especially if a viral illness is present or suspected.

Slow-release preparations of niacin include Slo-niacin, Niacor, Nicolar, and Niaspan, but these may be associated with a higher incidence of liver toxicity because higher niacin levels are sustained for longer periods. Liver function tests should be measured every 3 months in all children treated with niacin products.

C. "Statins" (3-hydroxy-3-methylglutaryl, coenzyme A [HMG-CoA] reductase inhibitors) (Table 44.8). These "statins" inhibit production of HMG-CoA reductase, which controls the rate-limiting step in cholesterol biosynthesis. We begin treatment in children at the lowest dose available, with increases every 6 to 12 weeks until the LDL is <160 mg/dL or the maximal adult dose is reached without toxicity. Remember to scale back the dose in proportion to the child's weight compared with that of an adult. Using lovastatin as an example, I would not exceed 40 mg per day in a young child, compared to the maximal adult dose of 80 mg per day. If the LDL drops to <130 mg/dL, consider reducing the statin dose or discontinuing the medication. This group of drugs has been shown to be effective and safe in children. Included in the group are lovastatin (Mevacor), pravastatin (Pravachol), simvastatin (Zocor), fluvastatin (Lescol), and atorvastatin (Lipitor) (Table 44.9). Weigman et al. reported findings of a 2-year trial of pravastatin for the treatment of familial hypercholesterolemia in children aged 8 to 18 years. The primary efficacy variable was change from baseline of carotid intima-medial thickness (IMT) as measured by ultrasound. The mean carotid IMT was attenuated after 2 years of treatment, while there was a trend toward an increase in the placebo group. LDL levels were reduced in the treatment group, while HDL, triglyceride, and lipoprotein (a) levels remained unchanged. This statin was both effective and well tolerated, with minimal observable side effects. There were no negative effects on growth or sexual development. Weigman et al. stated further that resins were poorly tolerated in this age group, therefore, the use of statins is an obvious therapeutic choice. Lovastatin in teenage boys with familial hypercholesterolemia showed no adverse effects on growth or sexual development over the 48-week course of the study. Side effects include hepatocellular toxicity and, rarely, rhabdomyolysis. Liver functions should be monitored every 3 months.

D. Fibric acid derivatives. These drugs are useful in adults for treating types 2A, 2B, 4, and 5 hyperlipoproteinemias, but there are few data on their use in children. They include chlofibrate (Atromid-S), gemfibrozil (Lopid), and fenofibrate (Tricor). Tricor is indicated as adjunctive therapy in patients with primary hypercholesterolemia or mixed dyslipidemia (Frederickson types 2A and 2B). It increases HDL, reduces triglycerides, reduces LDL, reduces total cholesterol, and reduces apolipoprotein (apoB). The combined use of Tricor and statins should be avoided unless the benefit of further alterations in lipid levels is likely to outweigh the increased risk. This combination has been associated with rhabdomyolysis, marked elevated creatinine kinase levels, and mild globulinuria leading to acute renal failure.

Before using fibric acid derivatives in children to treat a type 2 lipid disorder, I recommend using statins, bile acid–binding resins, or niacin. With elevated triglyceride, niacin, gemfibrozil, and atorvastatin should be considered.

Side effects include myalgias, myositis, myopathy, rhabdomyolysis, liver toxicity, gallstones, and glucose intolerance. Gemfibrozil is less likely to cause gallstones than gemfibrate. I recommend monitoring liver functions every 3 months in children treated with this group of drugs.

VI. SUMMARY

Occasionally, combination medications are indicated. For those with high LDL levels, various combinations of statins, bile acid-binding sequestrants, ezetimibe, and niacin, can be used. For severe hypertriglyceridemia, a combination of statins, fibrates, and fish oils may be used. The combination of statins and fibrates, however, may be associated with increased risk of serious myopathy and rhabdomyolysis and therefore should be used with great caution.

Evaluate children with dyslipidemias every 3 months to re-establish diet and exercise programs, explore symptoms of drug toxicity, and review vital signs as well as growth, height, and weight.

Because premature cardiovascular disease is increasing, studies of the safety and efficacy of lipid-lowering drugs in children should be expanded. If the pediatrician or generalist is unaccustomed to interpreting lipid results or prescribing and monitoring hypolipidemic drugs, the patient should be referred to a pediatric lipid specialist.

Selected References

Alberti KG, Zimmet P, Shaw J, et al. The metabolic syndrome—a new worldwide definition. *Lancet* 2005;366:1059–1062.

American Diabetes Association. Type 2 diabetes in children and adolescents. *Pediatrics* 2000;105:671–680.

Arslanian SA. Type 2 DM in children: pathophysiology and risk factors. *J Pediatr Endocrinol Metab* 2000;13:1385–1394.

Barter P, Gotto AM, LaRosa JC, et al. HDL cholesterol, very low levels of LDL cholesterol, and cardiovascular events. *N Engl J Med* 2007;357:1301–1310.

Bell LM, Watts K, Siafarakis A, et al. Exercise alone reduces insulin resistance in obese children independently of changes in body composition. *J Clin Endorcinol Metab* 2007; 92:4230–4235.

Brunkhorst FM, Engel C, Bloos F, et al. Intensive insulin therapy and pentastarch resuscitation in severe sepsis. *N Engl J Med* 2008;358:125–139.

Ganderson EP, Lewis CE, Tsai AL, et al. A 20-year prospective study of childbearing and incidence of diabetes in young women, controlling for glycemia before conception. *The Cardia study. Diabetes.* 2007 Dec;56(12)2990–2996.

Circulation 2007, April 10

Dietz WH, Robinson TH. Overweight children and adolescents. *N Engl J Med* 2005;352: 2100–2109.

Eckel RH, Grundy SM, Zimmet PZ. The metabolic syndrome. *Lancet* 2005;365:1415–1428.

Fagot-Campagna A, et al. Type 2 diabetes among North American children and adolescents. *J Pediatr* 2000;136:664–672.

Falkner B, et al. Hypertension in children *Pediatr Ann* 2006;35:795–801.

Fernández JR, Redden DT, Pietrobelli A, et al. Waist circumference percentiles in nationally representative samples of African-American, European-American, and Mexican-American children and adolescents. *J Pediatr* 2004;145:439–444.

Holman RR, Thorne KI, Farmer AJ, et al. Addition of biphasic, prandial, or basal insulin to oral therapy in type 2 diabetes. *N Engl J Med* 2007;357:1716–1730.

Kastelein JJP, Akdim F, Stroes ESG, et al. Simvastatin with or without ezetimibe in familial hypercholesterolemia. *N Engl J Med* 2008;358:1431–1443.

Kershner AK, Daniels SR, Imperatore G, et al. Lipid abnormalities are prevalent in youth with type 1 and type 2 diabetes: The SEARCH for Diabetes in youth study. *J Pediatr.* 2006 Sep;149(3)314–319.

Kotronen A, Westerbacka J, Bergholm R, et al. Liver fat in the metabolic syndrome. *J Clin Endocrinol Metab* 2007;92:3490–3497.

Lee S, Bacha F, Arslanian SA. Waist circumference, blood pressure, and lipid components of the metabolic syndrome. *J Pediatr* 2006;149:809–816.

Ngyen TT, Keil MF, Russell DL, et al. Relation of acanthosis nigricans to hyperinsulinemia in overweight children. *J Pediatr* 2001;138:474–480.

Rodden AM, Diaz VA, Mainous AG 3rd, et al. Insulin resistance in adolescents. *J Pediatr* 2007;157:275–279.

Sondike SB, et al. Obesity. *Contemp Pediatr* 2000;17:133–138.

Srinivasan S, Ambler GR, Baur LA, et al. Randomized, controlled trial of metformin for obesity and insulin resistance in children and adolescents: improvement in body composition and fasting insulin. *J Clin Endocrinol Metab.* 2006 Jan;91(6)2074–2080.

Srinivasan SR, Myers L, Berenson GS. Predictability of childhood adiposity and insulin for developing insulin resistance syndrome (syndrome X) in young adulthood. *The Bogalusa Heart Study. Diabetes.* 2002 Jan;51(1)204–209

Steinberger J, Moran A, Hong CP, et al. Adiposity in childhood predicts obesity and insulin resistance in young adulthood. *J Pediatr* 2001;138:469–473.

Utriainen P, Jääskeläinen J, Romppanen J, Voutilainen R. Childhood metabolic syndrome and its components in premature adrenarche. *J Clin Endocrinol Metab* 2007;92:4282–4285.

Winter WE, et al. Hyperlipidemia. *Contemp Pediatr* 1999;16(5).

Zappalla FR. Evaluation of dyslipidemia in children. *Pediatr Ann* 2006;35:808–813.

Zhu H, Yan W, Ge D, et al. Relationships of cardiovascular phenotypes with healthy weight, at risk overweight, and overweight in US youths. *Pediatrics* 2008;121:115–122.

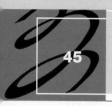

45 TYPE 2 DIABETES MELLITUS
Stephanie Smooke Praw and Andrew J. Drexler

I. INTRODUCTION

Type 2 diabetes mellitus (T2DM) accounts for >90% of all cases of diabetes in the United States. The prevalence of diabetes is increasing, with the disease affecting 20.8 million Americans or 7% of the U.S. population. More than 200,000 people die each year because of complications of diabetes, making it the sixth leading cause of death. Diabetes is also a leading cause of renal failure, new blindness in adults, and nontraumatic limb amputations. Heart disease and stroke are the leading causes of death in individuals with diabetes. All evidence suggests that the prevalence of type 2 diabetes will continue to increase both in the United States and in the rest of the world.

II. ETIOLOGY

The origin of type 2 diabetes mellitus is multifactorial, including genetic and environmental factors. Studies of identical twins document the genetics of type 2 diabetes mellitus, in whom concordance rates are nearly 100%. The strong environmental and genetic contribution to diabetes may be best seen in the Pima Indians of the Gila River Valley in Arizona. As they turned to a more Western European lifestyle, not only did the tribe members become more obese, the incidence of diabetes increased from a negligible number to nearly 50%. Another portion of the tribe returned to a more physically active lifestyle, in Mexico. They performed >40 hours of physical labor per week, compared to <3 hours among those living a Western European lifestyle. In the Mexican Pimas, the prevalence of diabetes in males decreased to 6.3%, compared to 54% in the Arizona Pimas. This example demonstrates that even though the genetics of the tribe did not change, their environment did, and this in turn had a significant impact on the development of diabetes. Researchers believe that populations inherit genes that help them survive in times of drought and famine. Though these genes are helpful for peoples living a traditional lifestyle, those same genes put us at risk for diabetes, obesity, and their associated complications when living a Western European lifestyle.

III. PATHOPHYSIOLOGY

T2DM is a complex, progressive disease. Current understanding suggests that type 2 diabetes results from the combination of pancreatic β-cell deficiency, insulin resistance in the adipose tissues and skeletal muscles, and excessive hepatic glucose production.

A. Insulin resistance. The earliest defect in patients with type 2 diabetes is insulin resistance. This concept has now been broadened as the **metabolic syndrome,** although other names are also used. Although the role of insulin resistance in the pathogenesis of diabetes has been recognized since the first radioimmunoassays for insulin, Gerald Reaven showed that the combination of hyperinsulinemia, hypertension, high triglycerides, and low high-density lipoprotein (HDL) cholesterol predicted the development of atherosclerosis even in people who were not yet diabetic and not obese. These individuals also had a high incidence of developing diabetes and eventually becoming obese. Reaven called this **syndrome X.** Current thinking has attributed some etiologic component of the metabolic syndrome to visceral adiposity. Since the original description, the concept of metabolic syndrome has also come to include patients who are diabetic or who have impaired fasting

TABLE 45.1	Metabolic Syndrome	
Risk factor	**Defining level**	
Abdominal obesity (waist, in)	Men >40	Women >35
Triglycerides (mg/dL)	≥150	
HDL-C (mg/dL)	Men <40	Women <50
Blood pressure (mmHg)	≥130/85	
Fasting glucose (mg/dL)	(ADA ≥100)	

ADA, American Diabetes Association; HDL-C, high-density lipoprotein cholesterol.

glucose. For this reason, waist circumference has become a key element in the signs used to make the diagnosis.

Current U.S. criteria as outlined in the NCEP ATP III guidelines are given in Table 45.1.

B. Controversy and the metabolic syndrome. Regardless of the controversy surrounding the metabolic syndrome, the importance of insulin resistance in the etiology of type 2 diabetes is not in dispute. The body initially compensates by increasing insulin production to maintain normal glucose levels. However, a subset of patients with decreased β-cell secretory capacity, is unable to sustain the necessary level of insulin production and develops diabetes. Early on in the course of the disease, these patients may have higher-than-normal circulating insulin levels, but these levels remain below those needed to maintain euglycemia, and hence, these patients are still insulin-deficient.

C. Progression to diabetes mellitus. As the disease progresses, fasting blood glucose levels or the 2-hour post–oral glucose challenge test levels increase further. Again, insulin secretion continues to increase in response, but it continues to be less than is needed, and by an increasing margin. This is the result of decreased pancreatic β-cell function. The results from the United Kingdom Prospective Diabetes Study (UKPDS) demonstrated that affected individuals may have lost 50% of their β-cell function by the time of diagnosis, and that this level decreases in a linear fashion over time. More specifically, the initial defects in insulin secretion are usually the loss of the first-phase insulin release and the loss of the pulsatory insulin secretion pattern. The clinical correlate is elevated postprandial blood glucose values. As a result, patients may have normal or near-normal fasting blood sugars, but their blood sugars are not controlled after eating.

Further decline in insulin release leads to inadequate suppression of hepatic gluconeogenesis, resulting in further fasting and postprandial hyperglycemia. Thus, the combination of insulin resistance and diminished insulin secretion creates the setting for profound hyperglycemia. So, although the circulating levels of insulin rise and subsequently fall early in the disease process, at all times these circulating insulin levels are diminished for the glucose levels present, when compared with normal subjects.

Despite extensive investigation, the molecular mechanisms of diminished insulin secretion and insulin resistance have not been fully clarified. Chronic elevation of free fatty acids, a characteristic of T2DM, as well as structural changes in the islets of Langerhans as a result of amyloid accumulation may contribute to reduced insulin secretion and apoptosis. Histopathologic findings have not been elucidated in insulin resistance, but weight loss has been demonstrated to improve insulin sensitivity. Many therapies are now targeted at the reduction of insulin resistance in hopes of improving insulin secretion and reducing hyperglycemia.

D. Other hormones and pathogenesis. Other hormones have also been demonstrated to have a role in the pathogenesis of diabetes. These include amylin and incretin hormones (glucagonlike peptide 1 [GLP-1], glucose-dependent insulinotropic polypeptide, etc.). New therapies for T2DM are now targeting these hormonal pathways as well.

IV. DIAGNOSIS

A. Hyperglycemia. Individuals at risk of developing diabetes may be identified before the clinical onset of disease. It is important to remember that mild to moderate hyperglycemia while asymptomatic contributes to the development of the complications of diabetes. In the UKPDS, a significant proportion of the patients presented at diagnosis with both macrovascular disease and, more surprisingly, microvascular disease, including retinopathy. Although we often think of polyuria and polydipsia as presenting symptoms of diabetes, these symptoms do not develop until the renal threshold for glucose has been exceeded. Depending on the patient's age, this may occur with blood glucose values in excess of 180 mg/dL.

Given the significant number of Americans with undiagnosed diabetes and prediabetes, early detection and treatment is essential to prevent complications of T2DM. The American Association of Clinical Endocrinologists (AACE), in a 2007 position paper, recommends annual screening of all individuals 30 years or older who are at risk for having or developing T2DM.

B. Risk factors are defined as follows:

1. Family history of diabetes
2. Cardiovascular disease
3. Overweight or obese status
4. Sedentary lifestyle
5. Latino/Hispanic, non-Hispanic black, Asian American, Native American, or Pacific Islander ethnicity
6. Previously identified impaired glucose tolerance (IGT) or impaired fasting glucose (IFG)
7. Hypertension
8. Increased triglycerides, low concentrations of high-density lipoprotein cholesterol, or both
9. History of gestational diabetes
10. History of delivery of an infant with a birth weight >9 lb
11. Polycystic ovary syndrome
12. Psychiatric illness

C. Definitions. According to the American Diabetes Association (ADA), subjects may be classified as normal, impaired fasting glucose, or diabetic, based on their blood glucose values. Based on the 2003 ADA guidelines, **normal** is defined as fasting glucose concentration <100 mg/dL; IFG or **prediabetes** as 100 to 125 mg/dL; and **overt diabetes mellitus** as ≥126 mg/dL.

The World Health Organization (WHO) criteria permit a diagnosis of two- to threefold more individuals with IGT than the ADA's IFG criteria through the use of an additional diagnostic measure, the **oral glucose tolerance test** (OGTT). The OGTT is the centerpiece of the WHO guidelines. The WHO criteria reflect a fasting glucose of <115 mg/dL as potentially normal and that between 115 and 140 mg/dL as tentative for IGT or diabetes; thus, a 2-hour OGTT is required. A 2-hour OGTT value of <140 mg/dL is normal, whereas one between 140 and 200 mg/dL is diagnostic for IGT, and >200 mg/dL is diagnostic for diabetes.

IGT patients have an increase in cardiovascular risk of up to 60%. Therefore, recognition of these patients is imperative in the prevention of disease-associated risk. As a result, patients who have repeated fasting plasma glucose levels >90 mg/dL may benefit from further diagnostic testing using the OGTT.

Of note, patients with IFG and IGT are considered to have "prediabetes." These diagnoses are associated with the metabolic syndrome, described earlier.

Finally, it should be noted that the glycated hemoglobin test or home blood glucose monitoring equipment cannot be used for diagnostic purposes, based on current standards.

D. Interpretation of plasma glucose values. See Table 45.2.

E. Diagnostic criteria for diabetes mellitus. See Table 45.3.

TABLE 45.2	Diagnosis of DM type 2

Glucose concentration (mg/dL)	Interpretation
Fasting	
<100	Within normal reference range
100–125	Impaired fasting glucose/prediabetes
≥126	Diabetes mellitus
2-hour OGTT (75 g)	
<140	Within normal reference range
140–199	Impaired fasting glucose/prediabetes
≥200	Diabetes mellitus

OGTT, oral glucose tolerance test.

F. Diagnosis of gestational diabetes mellitus (GDM). The criteria used for the diagnosis of GDM are those of Carpenter and Coustan and are endorsed by the ADA in their 1997 position paper from the Fourth International Workshop Conference on Gestational Diabetes Mellitus. Patients at increased risk for GDM include age >25 years, overweight or obese state, family history of diabetes mellitus, history of abnormal glucose metabolism, history of poor obstetric outcome, history of delivery of an infant weighing >9 lb, history of polycystic ovary syndrome, ethnicities including Latino/Hispanic, non-Hispanic black, Asian Americans, Native American, or Pacific Islander, <u>fasting plasma glucose >85 mg/dL</u>, or 2-<u>hour postprandial glucose concentration >140 mg/dL</u>. Patients with these risk factors should be screened at their initial obstetric visit with glucose testing. If they are not found to have diabetes mellitus at that time, they should be retested between 24 and 28 weeks of gestation. Women with a history of gestational diabetes should also be tested at initial presentation to exclude the possibility of previously undiagnosed type 2 diabetes, which is associated with the possible consequence of congenital anomalies in the fetus. These congenital anomalies occur during embryogenesis (early in the first trimester), so waiting until 24 to 28 weeks of pregnancy to discover hyperglycemia may be too late to prevent complications in the fetus.

Patients with average risk require screening only between 24 and 28 weeks of gestation. Practitioners should perform an initial screening by measuring plasma or serum <u>glucose 1 hour after a 50-g oral glucose load</u> (glucose challenge test or GCT). OGTT should be performed on women who exceed the glucose threshold on the GCT (1-hour postchallenge glucose concentration ≥140 mg/dL). OGTT can be performed using either a 75-g or a 100-g glucose load. The 100-g OGTT is better validated in the literature. The two step diagnostic approach, using a glucose

TABLE 45.3	Diagnostic Criteria

Two or more of the following criteria should be met for diagnosis:
- Symptoms of diabetes (polyuria, polydipsia, unexplained weight loss) and random plasma glucose concentration ≥200 mg/dL

or
- Fasting plasma glucose concentration ≥126 mg/dL (fasting is defined as no caloric intake for at least 8 h)

or
- Two-hour postchallenge glucose concentration ≥200 mg/dL during a 75-g oral glucose tolerance test

TABLE 45.4	**Diagnosis of Gestational Diabetes**

Time	Plasma glucose concentration (mg/dL)
75-g challenge	
Fasting	>95
1 h post–glucose administration	>180
2-h post–glucose administration	>155
100-g challenge	
Fasting	>95
1 h post–glucose administration	>180
2 h post–glucose administration	>155
3 h post–glucose administration	>140

threshold value of >140 mg/dL, identifies ~80% of women with GDM. This yield may be increased to 90% by using a glucose threshold value >130 mg/dL. It is important to note that patients should be instructed to carbohydrate-load prior to the OGTT.

G. Diagnostic criteria for gestational diabetes mellitus using OGTT. See Table 45.4.

V. PREVALENCE

In 2005 epidemiologic studies of individuals in the United States 20 years of age or older, it was reported that 20.6 million people or 9.6% of people have diabetes. This includes ~6.2 million people who are not aware of their disease. Diabetes affects 20.9% of people over the age of 60. Even more alarming is that another 35 million people (33.8%) in the United States between 40 and 74 years of age have IFG; 16 million (15.4%) have IGT. 1.5 million new cases of diabetes were diagnosed in 2005 alone.

For individuals born in the year 2000, the estimated lifetime risk for developing diabetes (type 1 diabetes mellitus [T1DM] or T2DM) is 33% for males and 39% for females. The latest data from the Centers for Disease Control and Prevention also show an increased prevalence of diabetes in Mexican Americans and non-Hispanic black individuals. The estimated direct and indirect cost associated with diabetes was $132 billion in 2002.

VI. CLINICAL EVALUATION

The clinical evaluation of a patient with diabetes should include documentation of the onset and progression of diabetes, the need for hospitalization for either hyper- or hypoglycemia, medication history, and history of glycemic control. Notation should also be made of cardiovascular risk factors, history of retinopathy, date of most recent retinal examination, presence of microalbuminuria, and any history of neuropathy or lower-extremity ulcers. Given the correlation between diabetes and obesity, patients should also be evaluated for nonalcoholic steatohepatitis (NASH) with measurement of liver function tests.

Patients should also be questioned for symptoms of polyuria, polydipsia, blurry vision, and weight loss. Patients with these complaints are likely to have significant blood glucose elevation. Additionally, history of extremity pain, numbness or tingling, sexual dysfunction, or visual changes because of retinopathy should be documented.

If patients do not fit the typical presentation of type 2 diabetes, it is important to consider the possibility of late-onset type 1 diabetes. While we are seeing more adolescents with type 2 diabetes or **mature-onset diabetes of youth (MODY),** we are also encountering more adults with **latent autoimmune diabetes in adults (LADA).** This is an important distinction to make, as these patients require a very different treatment strategy.

VII. POTENTIAL COMPLICATIONS ASSOCIATED WITH T2DM

The management of diabetes should be directed at the control of hyperglycemia as well as the prevention of the long-term complications of diabetes. The long-term complications of diabetes may be classified as microvascular diseases (affecting the eyes, kidneys, and nerves) or macrovascular diseases (affecting the heart, brain, and peripheral vascular system).

A. Prevention. The Diabetes Control and Complications Trial (DCCT), completed in 1993, was a long-term, randomized, prospective study involving 1 441 patients with T1DM, which demonstrated that near-normalization of blood glucose with intensive therapy was able to prevent or delay the development of diabetic retinopathy, nephropathy, and neuropathy.

B. Pathophysiology of complications. Several molecular mechanisms of glucose-induced damage have been proposed. These include: **(1)** increased polyol pathway flux; **(2)** increased intracellular advanced glycation end-product (AGE) formation; **(3)** activation of protein kinase C; and **(4)** increased hexosamine pathway flux. We will explore one of these mechanisms in more detail.

   1. Glycation end-product mechanism. One of the central pathogenic processes of chronic diabetic complications is mediated by advanced glycation end products. These glycation end products are a direct result of glucose attaching to protein through nonenzymatic reactions. Damage of target tissues occurs through modification of intra- and extracellular proteins and matrix components. The glycation of proteins results in protein dysfunction because of structural changes occurring at sites that are important for protein action, or by an alteration of protein half-lives brought about by a decrease in the enzymatic cleavage and disposal of proteins. When proteins are glycated, the glucose moiety that glycates the protein becomes unusually chemically reactive, forming free radicals. These activated glucose derivatives, as free radicals, polymerize and induce the "browning reaction," which is why diabetic patients' scars are dark brown when their glucose levels are poorly controlled. The free radicals can also induce cross-linking, thereby decreasing the effectiveness of normal degradative enzymes. Glycation reactions also occur with smaller molecules, leading to the formation of soluble AGEs that are cleared by a number of mechanisms including specific receptors that bind to them. The relative importance of soluble versus insoluble AGEs is not currently known. Of note, it is the glycation of hemoglobin that permits us to assess hyperglycemia management.

   2. Smoking. Smoking can drive advanced glycation end products because it results in the inhalation of particulate matter composed of glycated proteins from the tobacco plant. During smoking, AGEs are elevated in the plasma. Therefore, encouraging smoking cessation is a vital part of diabetes care.

   3. Hypertension. Glycated end products can also affect arteriolar muscle cells, resulting in hypertension. Normally, the synthesis of nitric oxide induces relaxation of smooth muscles of arterioles, preventing hypertension. However, in the setting of glycation, nitric oxide levels are diminished because of impaired synthesis, and there is a higher likelihood of vasoconstriction and associated hypertension. From a systemic point of view, the vasoconstriction causes microvascular damage in the eye, kidney, and nerve.

   4. Kidneys. Finally, AGEs can affect renal glomerular function, through disturbances of the structural integrity of the glomerular filter. Such filtration abnormalities result in increased hydrostatic pressure in the glomerulus and the excretion of albumin into the urine, which, if >20 mg/dL, is known as microalbuminuria.

VIII. HYPEROSMOLAR NONKETOTIC COMA (HONC) OR HYPEROSMOLAR HYPERGLYCEMIC STATE (HHS)

Hyperosmolar nonketotic coma is one of the more devastating complications of T2DM. Recognition of this condition and prompt action to correct it is vital to caring for patients. Mortality may be as high as 20% and increases with increasing age.

A. Definition. The physiologic response to hyperglycemia is primarily regulated by insulin and glucagon. Insulin acts to restore euglycemia by decreasing hepatic glucose production, via reduction in glycogenolysis and gluconeogenesis, and by increasing glucose uptake by skeletal muscle and adipose tissue. Insulin-induced inhibition of glucagon secretion then further inhibits hepatic glucose production. Therefore, in uncontrolled hyperglycemia, several major abnormalities are largely responsible for the decompensation of euglycemia, including insulin deficiency and/or resistance, glucagon excess, and increased secretion of catecholamines and cortisol. The development of ketoacidosis then occurs when ketones are needed to provide an alternate source of energy because of impaired glucose utilization.

B. Clinical manipulations. These disorders in glucose metabolism and catabolism may be manifested as either diabetic ketoacidosis (DKA) (see Chapter 42) or hyperosmolar nonketotic coma. These are related disorders that differ according to the presence of ketoacidosis and the degree of hyperglycemia. In HONC, circulating insulin levels are likely adequate to control ketogenesis but are insufficient to maintain euglycemia. Therefore, in HONC, there is little to no ketoacid accumulation and plasma glucose concentrations may exceed 600 to 1 000 mg/dL. To accumulate this degree of hyperglycemia it is necessary for the patient to have limited access to water. A typical patient will exhibit polydipsia to a sufficient degree to prevent blood sugar from being sustained at these levels. For that reason, HONC usually occurs in elderly or neurologically impaired individuals, partially explaining the high mortality. Other differences between DKA and HONC include the degree of hyperosmolality, which may reach as high as 380 mosmol/kg in HONC. In addition, neurologic abnormalities are frequently present in HONC, with coma occurring in 25% to 50% of affected patients. Finally, HONC may develop over the course of a week or longer, whereas DKA develops over 1 to 2 days.

C. Underlying causes. Similar to DKA, HONC may be triggered by infections (including pneumonia, which is present in 40% to 60% of cases, and urinary tract infections), alcohol and drug abuse, myocardial infarction, stroke, pancreatitis, trauma, medications that impair insulin secretion or action (for example, corticosteroids, phenytoin, diuretics, immunosuppressants), hot weather or dehydration, and nonadherence to insulin therapy.

D. Signs and symptoms. The presenting signs and symptoms include polyuria, polydipsia, fatigue, weakness, lethargy, drowsiness, anorexia, mental status changes, seizures, aphasia, or even hemiplegia. Diagnosis of this condition is based on serum glucose >600 to 800 mg/dL, serum osmolality >320 mosmol/kg, mental status changes, absent to low ketones, and absence of acidosis. Of note, neurologic symptoms usually develop when the serum osmolality exceeds 350 mosmol/kg.

This condition should be suspected in patients who exhibit evidence of volume contraction, altered mental status/coma, sensory deficits, and an absence of Kussmaul respirations. The initial evaluation should include a complete blood count, chemistry panel, glucose, serum and urine ketones, urinalysis, arterial blood gas, chest radiograph, electrocardiogram, and blood cultures.

E. Treatment. Once a diagnosis of HONC is made, treatment should be as follows:

1. **Intravenous fluid:** Rapid repletion of 2 to 3 L of normal saline (NS); replete one half of estimated fluid deficit within the first 6 hours (the usual deficit is 10 L), then change to NS. Continue to monitor fluid status carefully to avoid volume overload, especially in patients with underlying cardiac disease.
2. **Insulin:** Start an insulin infusion with the goal of decreasing blood glucose by 100 mg/dL per hour, but only after fluid repletion has been initiated.
3. Treat the underlying issue, including considering antibiotics if infection is suspected (Table 45.5).

IX. GOALS OF TREATMENT

Long-term prospective trials, such as the Diabetes Control and Complications Trial (DCCT) in the United States, the United Kingdom Prospective Diabetes Study (UKPDS), and the Japanese Kumomoto study, clearly indicate that chronic complication rates

TABLE 45.5 Differentiating between Diabetic Ketoacidosis (DKA) and Hyperosmolar Nonketotic Coma (HONC)

	DKA			HONC
	Mild	**Moderate**	**Severe**	
Plasma glucose (mg/dL)	>250	>250	>250	>600
Arterial pH	7.25–7.30	7.00–7.24	<7.0	>7.30
Serum bicarbonate (mEq/L)	15–18	10–15	<10	>15
Urine ketones	Positive	Positive	Positive	Small
Serum ketones	Positive	Positive	Positive	Small
Effective serum osmolality (mOsm/kg)[a]	Variable	Variable	Variable	>320
Anion gap	>10	>12	>12	Variable
Alteration in sensorium	Alert	Alert/drowsy	Stupor/coma	Stupor/coma

[a]Effective osmolality = $2Na + (glucose/18)$.

are directly proportional to the prolongation of hyperglycemia (as defined by elevated levels of glycated hemoglobin).

A. Prevention of complications. Thus, the evidence exists for aggressive and intensive glucose control for prevention of microvascular disease in type 1 diabetes, and both macro- and microvascular diseases in type 2 diabetes. Furthermore, these studies suggest that macrovascular events require lower glycated hemoglobin levels when compared with microvascular complications. Despite concerns about study design, findings from the UKPDS and other studies clearly indicate that decreased epidemiologic risk for macrovascular disease is associated with blood glucose levels in or near the normal range (UKPDS, hemoglobin A_{1c} <6.2%) when compared with higher blood glucose levels. The UKPDS data further indicate that in patients with type 2 diabetes, intensive or aggressive glucose control reduces mortality and cardiovascular event rates. Thus, for every 1% reduction in A_{1c}, there is about a 10% to 15% cardiovascular event rate reduction. In addition, studies such as the DECODE study have demonstrated that postprandial hyperglycemia, independent of HgA_{1c} values, has been linked to the development of macrovascular disease.

B. HgA_{1c} goals. Recent recommendations from the ADA propose a goal HgA_{1c} of <7.0%, while the AACE recommends tighter control, with goal HgA_{1c} of <6.5%. Additionally, the AACE, in its 2007 practice guidelines, recommends fasting plasma glucose concentration <110 mg/dL and 2-hour postprandial glucose concentration <140 mg/dL.

Several recent studies have investigated the contribution of fasting versus postprandial blood glucose values to overall glycemia. In a study by Monnier et al., investigators concluded that, in patients with HgA_{1c} >10.2%, fasting blood glucose levels contribute 70% to overall glycemia. In patients with HgA_{1c} <7.3%, the overall contribution of fasting glucose is only 30%. The contribution of fasting and postprandial blood glucose values to overall glycemia is approximately equal in patients with HgA_{1c} levels between 7.3% and 8.4%. Based on these findings, therapies for diabetes may be targeted at different types of blood glucose impairment depending on HgA_{1c}.

X. BLOOD GLUCOSE MONITORING

Home blood glucose monitoring permits adjustments of drugs and dosages; glycated hemoglobin levels indicate whether the adjustments did or did not result in achieving the goal.

A. Home blood glucose monitoring. It is important that *all* diabetic patients have access to home blood glucose monitoring. Although there is some question regarding the need for blood glucose monitoring in patients who are not on insulin, several recent trials demonstrated that self-monitoring of blood glucose values results in greater reductions in HgA$_{1c}$ values in non–insulin-treated patients.

Of course, it is also recommended that insulin-treated patients check their glucose level before administering insulin. Checking fasting and postprandial glucose values is also very helpful in this patient population for fine-tuning insulin regimens.

Patients whose blood glucose levels continue to be above target range on oral agents and/or once-daily insulin should be encouraged to check their blood glucose more frequently. Again, we recommend that patients vary the time of day at which they check their blood glucose, sometimes checking fasting and sometimes checking postprandial values. The AACE recommends that patients periodically obtain preprandial and 2-hour-postprandial values and during the week prior to a physician visit, so that a comprehensive set of data may be reviewed. It is also recommended that patients bring their glucometers to physician visits for review. Patients should also be encouraged to check their blood glucose if they suspect hypo- or hyperglycemia based on physical symptoms.

Blood glucose goals are as follows: morning fasting blood glucose 85 to 110 mg/dL; preprandial blood glucose <110 mg/dL; 1-hour postprandial <180 mg/dL; 2-hour postprandial <140 mg/dL. It is important to recognize that goals may be individualized.

Home blood glucose monitoring at various times should assist the provider to determine **(1)** which medications should be used, **(2)** when patients should be taking their medicines, and **(3)** what the doses should be, regardless of whether treatment is an oral agent or insulin.

B. Glycated hemoglobin testing

1. **Gestational diabetes.** Data from the early 1980s from East Germany indicated that glycated hemoglobin levels were strongly linked with the prevalence of congenital malformations observed among offspring of diabetic mothers. Thus, the higher the glycated hemoglobin level, the higher was the congenital malformation rate. With >12% glycated hemoglobin levels, offspring from diabetic mothers had a 15% malformation rate, and with a glycated hemoglobin level <8% or normal for the assay used, the malformation rate was the same as for offspring from nondiabetic mothers, at 1.5%. For complications such as retinopathy and microalbuminuria, Scandinavian data by the mid-1980s indicated that the glycated hemoglobin level was a good measure of the potential for chronic diabetic complications.

2. **Complications.** It has now been determined from a variety of studies, including several Scandinavian trials, the DCCT, and the UKPDS, that chronic diabetes complications are a manifestation of increased blood glucose levels, measured most effectively as elevated glycated hemoglobin levels. Furthermore, it has been shown that complication rates increase very sharply after the glycated hemoglobin exceeds 8% for eye disease and 9% for microalbuminuria. Importantly, the first statistical differences in microvascular complication rates (e.g., for the eye) occur at a glycated hemoglobin of 6%, and for macrovascular disease the threshold is 6% to 7%. Thus, the only recommended monitoring test for the prevention or slowing of chronic microvascular or macrovascular diabetic complications is the glycated hemoglobin test.

3. **Frequency of testing.** HgA$_{1c}$ should be checked every 3 months as a measure of the patient's longer-term blood glucose control. As mentioned earlier, if a discrepancy is noted between the patient's fasting blood glucose and A$_{1c}$ values, postprandial blood glucoses should be measured. For example, if the HgA$_{1c}$ is 6.4%, the average blood glucose is ~110 mg/dL; an HgA$_{1c}$ of 7.2% correlates with a blood glucose of 150 mg/dL; an HgA$_{1c}$ of 9.2% correlates with a blood glucose of 230 mg/dL, and so on.

4. **Errors.** The glycated hemoglobin test can be altered by significant anemia, hemoglobinopathies (including hemoglobins C, D, and S), and in any condition that reduces the lifespan of erythrocytes. Other substances may cause falsely high HgA$_{1c}$ values. These include prehemoglobin A$_{1c}$ (reversible aldimine intermediate), carbamylated hemoglobin (uremia), or hemoglobin F.

Another major caveat regarding the HgA$_{1c}$ is that there are ~60 to 70 different assays available for the glycated hemoglobin test, but only 30 of these assays were used in the two major chronic complication studies, the DCCT and UKPDS. The various assays can differ by as much as 3 glycated hemoglobin percent. As a result, efforts should be made to use the same assay when following an individual patient's HgA$_{1c}$ values.

5. **Fructosamine test.** If a measure of blood glucose values over a shorter period of time is desired or abnormal hemoglobin or hemoglobinopathies exist, a serum fructosamine may be measured. Fructosamine is formed by nonenzymatic glycosylation of serum proteins (predominantly albumin), which have a much shorter half-life than erythrocytes, ~14 to 21 days. This test may be affected by low albumin states. It is important to note that fructosamine has not been standardized to the degree that HgA$_{1c}$ has and is not accepted as useful by all investigators.

XI. THERAPY

As mentioned previously, the management of diabetes should be directed at control of hyperglycemia as well as prevention of associated complications. This chapter is limited to the management of hyperglycemia. The management of hyperglycemic patients should include medical nutrition therapy, exercise recommendations, weight management, pharmacologic therapy, and diabetes self-management education. In order to maximize the likelihood of attaining glycemic goals, therapy should be tailored to each individual patient.

Multiple algorithms have been proposed for the stepped-care treatment of patients with type 2 diabetes. Specific protocols can be found through the ADA or AACE.

A. **Diet and exercise.** Lifestyle modifications are the initial therapy for the prevention and treatment of newly diagnosed T2DM. Weight loss and reduction in adipose tissue, especially abdominal obesity, decreases insulin resistance. The UKPDS demonstrated that only 3% of patients treated with dietary therapy alone were able to maintain glycemic control over a 6-year period. Despite these discouraging statistics, weight loss has been proven to reduce the amount and dosage of medications needed to control hyperglycemia and potential complication of T2DM.

B. **Medications.** The next step in care of the type 2 diabetes mellitus patient is pharmacologic therapy. These agents may be used individually or in combination to achieve glycemic control.

Although the initial treatment for diabetes is often monotherapy, through our understanding of the pathophysiology of the disease, most patients eventually require combination therapy. Based on mechanism of action, medications may be split into two categories: medications to help overcome insulin resistance or insulin sensitizers (e.g., biguanides, thiazolidinediones) and medications to help with the β-cell defect (e.g., sulfonylureas, meglitinides/amylin analogs, incretin mimetics, dipeptidyl-peptidase 4 [DPP-4] inhibitors). Here, we will discuss the mechanism of action of the various medications and their potential for benefit.

1. **Biguanides (metformin).** Metformin is often the initial choice of medication for patients with newly diagnosed diabetes characterized by insulin resistance. However, it is important to remember that this may not be the right choice for all patients, especially if the patient appears to have more β-cell dysfunction than insulin resistance.

a. **Mechanism of action.** Metformin acts primarily by reducing hepatic gluconeogenesis in the presence of insulin. It takes ~1 to 2 weeks for the effects of the medication to begin. Therefore, biguanides will not immediately decrease blood glucose values. Because this medication functions independently of β-cell activity, it does not produce hypoglycemia. An additional benefit of metformin is that monotherapy is associated with weight loss. Studies have also shown that use of metformin may decrease HgA$_{1c}$ by 1 to 1.5%.

b. **Adverse reactions.** The potential adverse reactions to metformin include gastrointestinal upset, including nausea, diarrhea, and abdominal pain. For most patients, these side effects abate with long-term use of the medication.

Side effects can also be minimized by slow titration of the medication. Metformin should be avoided in patients with impaired renal function, as it may lead to an increased risk of medication-associated lactic acidosis. This medication should also be avoided in patients of advanced age (>80 years old) and in those with hepatic dysfunction, congestive heart failure, metabolic acidosis, dehydration, or alcoholism. It is also advised that metformin be withheld prior to contrast studies or surgery, when the patient is at a higher risk of developing renal insufficiency. The medication should be held for 48 hours following the procedure, or longer if renal insufficiency develops.

    c. Indications. Metformin may be used as monotherapy or in combination with sulfonylureas, thiazolidinediones, insulins, or incretin mimetics.

2. Thiazolidinediones

    a. Controversies. Thiazolidinediones (TZDs) have recently become controversial medications secondary to a meta-analysis by Nissen et al. published in the *New England Journal of Medicine* in 2007, which described an increased risk of myocardial infarction in patients using rosiglitazone compared with a control group (OR, 1.43; 95% CI 1.03 to 1.98; p <0.03). Further studies are needed to formally investigate this risk. These data are controversial, and it is currently uncertain whether these findings can be extended to the entire class of medications. The reports from the recently stopped ACCORD trial seem to exonerate rosiglitazone, but no data are yet available.

        It is important not to ignore these medications, as their potential benefit in the appropriate patient population may be significant.

    b. Mechanisms of action. TZDs appear to function by increasing insulin sensitivity in the liver and peripheral tissues. Currently, two thiazolidinedione medications are commercially available, rosiglitazone and pioglitazone. The TZDs are pharmacologic ligands that bind to and activate peroxisome proliferator–activated receptors (PPARs), which in turn regulate gene expression in response to ligand binding. Specifically, these drugs interact with PPAR-γ nuclear receptors, which are responsible for the transcription of various genes that regulate carbohydrate and lipid metabolism. It is presumably through this process that TZDs increase insulin-stimulated glucose uptake into skeletal muscles.

        Of note, PPAR-γ is found predominantly in adipose tissue, pancreatic β-cells, vascular endothelium, and macrophages. This may explain why, in addition to lowering blood glucose, TZDs have also demonstrated modest reductions in blood pressure, enhanced fibrinolysis, and improved endothelial function. TZDs may also help preserve pancreatic β-cell function.

    c. Indications. TZDs lower HgA$_{1c}$ comparably to the biguanides and sulfonylureas. They are approved for monotherapy or in combination with metformin, sulfonylureas, or insulin.

    d. Adverse effects. Though TZDs are widely considered to be very effective medications, when choosing therapy with these drugs, a myriad of potential adverse effects must be considered. These include weight gain (time- and dose-dependent), fluid retention, heart failure, decreased bone density, and increased fracture risk.

3. Secretagogues (sulfonylureas and glinides)

    a. Sulfonylureas. This class of medications includes glipizide, glyburide, and glimepiride, among others.

        (1) Mechanisms of action. Sulfonylureas act by increasing insulin secretion from the pancreatic β cells. More specifically, these drugs bind to the sulfonylurea receptors on the β cells, leading to the closure of voltage-dependent potassium adenosine triphosphate (ATP) channels. This facilitates cell-membrane depolarization, calcium entry into the cell, and subsequent insulin release. Sulfonylurea therapy may reduce HgA$_{1c}$ by 1% to 2%.

        (2) Adverse effects. Because of the increase in insulin release, sulfonylurea medications may induce hypoglycemia. In addition, because these medications are cleared by the liver and kidneys, they should be used with caution in patients with hepatic or renal insufficiency.

The various medications in this class have different side-effect profiles. For example, glyburide is known to cause more weight gain compared to other sulfonylureas. Glyburide is also thought to cause more hypoglycemia, making glimepiride or glipizide a better choice in patients such as the elderly, in whom hypoglycemia can be more dangerous. Some of the other classes of secretagogues may be even safer and hence more desirable for the elderly.

(3) Indications. These medications are approved for monotherapy and for combination treatment with most other oral medications and insulin.

b. Glinides

(1) Mechanisms of action. Similar to the sulfonylureas, the glinides increase insulin secretion from the pancreatic β cells. These medications differ in that glinides have a much shorter duration of action. When taken at meal times, these medications improve prandial insulin release, decreasing postprandial hyperglycemia. Given their short duration of action, they also decrease the risk of hypoglycemia during the late postprandial phase, which may occur with sulfonylureas, because their effect on insulin release has largely diminished by that time. This said, hypoglycemia can certainly occur with these medications.

Of the two available glinides, repaglinide and nateglinide, the latter seems to be somewhat less potent.

(2) Adverse effects. Both repaglinide and nateglinide are metabolized by the liver and excreted by the kidneys and should be used with caution in patients with hepatic insufficiency and dose-adjusted in patients with severe renal insufficiency. Of note, repaglinide is only minimally cleared by the kidneys and may be safe for use in patients with renal impairment.

(3) Indications. Glinides are often beneficial early on in the care of diabetes, or in patients with $HgA_{1c} <7.2\%$ when control of postprandial hyperglycemia is of greater concern. Coupled with an insulin-sensitizer, they can be helpful in curtailing glucose fluctuations associated with eating.

4. α-Glucosidase inhibitors

a. Mechanisms of action. α-Glucosidase inhibitors, including acarbose and miglitol, lower blood glucose by decreasing the absorption of carbohydrates from the gastrointestinal tract. Specifically, they competitively inhibit the enzyme in the small intestine that is responsible for breaking down disaccharides and more complex carbohydrates, delaying their absorption and attenuating postprandial blood glucose elevations. α-Glucosidase inhibitors have been shown to decrease HgA_{1c} by 0.55 to 1%.

b. Adverse effects. Adverse effects include abdominal discomfort, flatulence, and diarrhea. Slow titration of the medication may help lessen side effects.

c. Indications. These agents are approved for use as monotherapy or in combination with sulfonylureas.

These medications are not tremendously effective in controlling blood glucose values and should really be considered only as adjunctive therapy.

5. Amylin analog (pramlintide)

a. Mechanisms of action. Amylin is a hormone that is cosecreted with insulin by the pancreatic β cells. It regulates glucose levels by suppressing glucagon release, delaying gastric emptying, and possibly reducing appetite. Pramlintide is a synthetic analog of amylin. In studies, when used as an adjunctive therapy for patients using prandial insulin, it has been shown to reduce postprandial blood glucose excursions, improve weight control, and reduce HgA_{1c} more than in patients taking insulin alone. When starting pramlintide, patients should reduce their prandial insulin doses by 50% to prevent hypoglycemia.

b. Adverse effects. Pramlintide should not be used in patients with gastroparesis or in those who are unable to sense hypoglycemia.

6. Incretin mimetics (exenatide)

a. Mechanisms of action. This new class of medications, including exenatide, mimics the effects of human incretin hormone glucagonlike peptide 1 (GLP-1). GLP-1 or incretins are secreted in response to food intake and work via multiple mechanisms, including enhancing glucose-stimulated insulin release, inhibiting the release of glucagon after meals, delaying absorption of nutrients, and causing the sensation of satiety.

Exenatide is the first incretin mimetic to become commercially available. It has been approved for use in patients who have not achieved glycemic goals on metformin and/or sulfonylureas.

b. Indications. Exenatide is indicated for combination therapy with a sulfonylurea, metformin, combination of sulfonylurea and metformin, or thiazolidinedione with or without metformin. Exenatide is administered via twice-daily subcutaneous injections. The small gauge of needles used today, as small as 31 gauge, has made injections less objectionable for many patients than in the past. This medication has also been shown to produce modest weight loss and decreased appetite. Therefore, in patients who would benefit from additional weight loss, this may be a good choice.

c. Adverse effects. Adverse effects include gastrointestinal upset, nausea, vomiting, diarrhea, dizziness, headache, and feeling jittery. Slow titration of the medication dose may help mitigate these side effects. New studies have suggested a possible increased incidence of pancreatitis in patients using exenatide. This risk has not yet been validated in trials, but pancreatitis should be considered in the differential diagnosis when patients on exenatide complain of abdominal pain.

7. Dipeptidyl-peptidase 4 inhibitors. Dipeptidyl-peptidase 4 inhibitors (DPP4-I) slow the inactivation of incretin hormones. GLP-1 has a half-life of 1 minute in the circulation. DPP4-I inhibit dipeptidyl-peptidase 4, which is responsible for degrading this hormone and hence allows higher levels to accumulate. The mechanism of the incretin hormones has been described previously. As a result of the aforementioned actions, DPP4-I help target postprandial glucose elevations but have also been demonstrated to reduce fasting blood glucose values.

Sitagliptin, a daily pill, is the commercially available form. It has been approved for monotherapy as well as in combination with metformin, thiazolidinediones, and sulfonylureas. There are few side effects associated with this medication, and reported adverse effects were similar to those of placebo. Sitagliptin was comparable to glipizide in one study in terms of HgA_{1c} reduction over 52 weeks of follow-up, making it a reasonable alternative to sulfonylurea therapy, although not all studies have found the same degree of efficacy.

Sitagliptin should be considered for patients who need some additional help in reaching blood glucose goals. Its affects are less dramatic than those of exenatide, but it is a good choice in patients who are averse to injections but would benefit from the multiple ways in which this medication addresses the pathophysiology of diabetes (Table 45.6).

8. Insulin therapy for type 2 diabetes. Our current understanding of type 2 diabetes, emanating from the UKPDS and other studies suggests that most diabetics will eventually require insulin therapy as a consequence of progressive β-cell loss. This can be seen in patients treated with secretagogues, such as glyburide and chlorpropamide, and with the insulin-sparing agents such as metformin, who eventually go on to require insulin therapy. Some of the newer agents are suggested to reverse or slow this trend, but the data are still very preliminary and often derived from studies of rodent islets, which may not be a good model for human islets. Unlike the situation with type 1 diabetes, about which there is general agreement that basal bolus insulin therapy is the standard, there are still questions as to how to initiate and use insulin in type 2 diabetes. Five different approaches are currently most common:

- Bedtime NPH insulin
- Bedtime long-acting basal insulin, either glargine or detemir

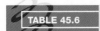 **TABLE 45.6**   Medications for Type 2 DM

Class/name	Mechanism of action	Hypoglycemia?	Caution
Sulfonylureas (tolbutamide, chlorpropamide, tolazamide, acetohexamide, glipizide [Glucotrol], glyburide, glimepiride)	Insulin secretagogue, improves β-cell function	Yes	Weight gain, hypoglycemia, caution if hepatic or renal dysfunction (may prolong duration)
Meglitinides (repaglinide [Prandin], nateglinide [Starlix])	Also insulin secretagogue, but fast onset and short duration of action	Yes	As above, must take before meal
Biguanides (metformin [Glucophage])	Insulin sensitizer, decrease hepatic glucose output and increase peripheral glucose uptake and usage	No	Lactic acidosis (esp. if renal, hepatic, or cardiac dysfunction); hold doses prior to IV contrast, GI disturbances common
α-Glucosidase inhibitors (acarbose, miglitol [Glyset])	Inhibit GI tract enzymes that digest oligosaccharides, thus delaying glucose absorption	No	Flatulence, diarrhea; warn patients they cannot treat hypoglycemia via usual mechanisms
Thiazolidinediones (rosiglitazone [Avandia], pioglitazone [Actos])	Bind to nuclear receptors (peroxisome proliferator–activated receptors), enhance expression of proteins that enhance cellular insulin action	No	Idiosyncratic hepatic failure; ↑LDL levels; weight gain; fluid retention (caution in CHF)
GLP-1 Mimetics (exenatide [Byetta])	Main mechanism of action is the stimulation of glucose-dependent insulin release from the pancreatic islet cells; also reduces the secretion of glucagons	No*	May slow gastric emptying and cause nausea; *Mild to moderate hypoglycemia may occur when given with sulfonylureas
DPP4 inhibitors (vildagliptin [Galvus], sitagliptin [Januvia])	Function as "incretin enhancers," inhibiting DPP4, an enzyme that breaks down GLP-1.	No*	*Hypoglycemia may occur when used with other agents

CHF, congestive heart failure; DPP4, dipeptidyl-peptidase 4; GI, gastrointestinal; GLP-1, glucagonlike peptide 1; IV, intravenous; LDL, low-density lipoprotein.

- Premixed insulin analog, either Novolog 70/30 or Humalog 75/25 or 50/50.
- Preprandial rapid-acting insulin without basal insulin
- Full basal bolus therapy

    In addition, oral agents are often used in conjunction with many of these approaches. And the same patient may require different approaches at different stages of β-cell loss.

    Each of these approaches has advantages and disadvantages.

a. **Bedtime NPH therapy.** Human NPH has a peak action of 5 hours and a duration of action of ~12 hours. These time intervals or durations of action, as with all insulins with the exception of the rapidly acting analogs, increase with increasing dosage. The usual starting dose is 10 U, which is then titrated up as needed to produce a normal fasting blood sugar while avoiding nocturnal hypoglycemia. When given at bedtime, NPH is primarily designed to produce a normal fasting glucose. Following the administration of a nighttime dose of NPH, there is little benefit on the subsequent daytime prandial glucose levels. For this reason, treatment with an oral secretagogue is also necessary. This approach is only successful if the patient still has endogenous insulin production. The disadvantages of this approach are twofold: First, the peak effect of NPH occurs at 5 hours with many dosages, increasing the risk of nocturnal hypoglycemia. Second, because NPH is a suspension rather than a solution, NPH insulin has greater variability than the basal analogs. This effect may be exaggerated if there is inadequate mixing prior to the insulin being drawn up. An advantage of NPH insulin is lower cost than for the newer basal analogs.

b. **Bedtime basal insulin analogs** . The two currently available basal insulin analogs, <u>glargine</u> and <u>detemir</u>, can also be given at bedtime to control fasting blood sugar. They differ from NPH in that they produce less of a peak and have a longer duration of action. Again, the duration of action is dependent on the dosage. Studies have clearly shown that patient-reported symptomatic hypoglycemia is less with these insulins than with NPH, although few studies have evaluated absolute rates of hypoglycemia. This effect may be explained by the absence of a peak of action, causing less dramatic drops in blood glucose. Therefore, the rates of glucose fall will be less severe and thus less likely to produce a catecholamine surge and subsequent adrenergic symptoms even at the same ultimate glucose level.

    What can be either an advantage or a disadvantage is the greater increase in daytime basal rates consequent to the longer duration of action of the basal insulin analogs compared to NPH insulin. In patients with significant β-cell loss, this longer duration of action is an advantage when there is daytime basal insulin deficiency. In the type 2 diabetic who is continuing to gain weight, increased daytime basal insulin may be a disadvantage. Again, when providing basal insulin levels, these analogs should not provide prandial coverage and hence a secretagogue and adequate residual insulin-secretory capacity is necessary to maintain euglycemia. At very high doses, some prandial insulin coverage may be present, but only at the risk of excessive basal insulin coverage with the probability of either weight gain, intermeal hypoglycemia, or both.

c. **Premixed insulin analogs, including 70/30 (Novo), 75/25 (Lilly), and 50/50 (Lilly).** Premixed insulin analogs are mixtures of a rapid-acting analog and protamine formulated to produce a ratio of 70% protomated analog plus 30% free analog, 75% protamine analog plus 25% free analog, or 50% protamine analog plus 50% free analog. Insulin mixed analogs provide mealtime free analog insulin along with protomated analog for longer duration of action to cover the postpraudial period.

    These protomated analogs behave similarly to protomated regular insulin, i.e., NPH insulin, with some important differences. They are usually given before breakfast and dinner; in some studies, a third dose was also given before lunch. No data have been released on the action of the protomated rapid-acting analog alone. The advantage is premeal insulin coverage at breakfast and dinner with some basal coverage because of the protomated analog. The use of these analogs helps to avoid the problem of requiring an insulin secretagogue to cover the expected prandial rise in blood sugar as well as limiting the number of injections a patient must administer on a daily basis.

The major disadvantages are similar but more severe compared to those described for bedtime NPH. The protomated analog taken even earlier, i.e., at dinner, is even less likely to provide sufficient insulin to control fasting blood sugar overnight. Nocturnal hypoglycemia is also a risk based on the kinetics of the protomated analog. A further risk is hypoglycemia before lunch, because use of the protomated analog at breakfast requires a carbohydrate meal 5 hours after administration. For patients in whom regular PO intake cannot be guaranteed, premixes should be used with caution.

d. **Preprandial rapid-acting analog only.** Most studies of insulin secretion in type 2 diabetes have shown the loss of prandial insulin occurring before the loss of basal insulin. It therefore seems logical that insulin replacement should start with prandial insulin, with basal insulin added later on, as needed. The risk of hypoglycemia is less with these regimens because the use of insulin is always accompanied by food. However, the success of these regimens is dependent on adequate endogenous basal insulin. Therefore, this regimen may be most suitable for patients who eat at widely varying times of the day or who frequently skip meals. To the degree that one believes glucose fluctuations are important factors in the development of complications, these regimens should have the benefit of avoiding postprandial hyperglycemia. Of note, most of these insulin regimens also involve the use of metformin to control fasting blood sugar.

e. **Full basal bolus therapy.** This regimen has the advantage of coming closest to replacing the body's physiologic insulin secretory pattern. It requires the use of two types of insulin, a basal insulin as described in option **b** and preprandial insulin as described in option **d**. If the basal dose is chosen correctly (which is often not the case), the risk of hypoglycemia should be minimal and approximately equivalent to that of using preprandial rapid-acting insulin analogs only. Finally, insulin pump therapy is not commonly used for type 2 diabetes but may become more so in the future. The effect on blood glucose control should be similar to that described in combination basal bolus therapy.

f. **How to choose.** Which of the five options is chosen depends on the patient's and the physician's priorities. If minimizing the number of injections is the major concern, then bedtime NPH, glargine, detemir, or premixed analogs will be preferred. If avoidance of hypoglycemia is most important or if control of postprandial sugars is the priority, then preprandial or combination basal bolus therapy may be the appropriate method of management. The amount of residual insulin secretory capacity will also be important in the success of any of the described regimens except for combination basal bolus therapy.

The success of any regimen depends on choosing the correct dose of insulin. The recommendations described are only starting points and must be individualized for each patient. The average type 2 diabetic will require between 0.4 and 1.0 U of insulin per kilogram of body weight. Of this, half of the dose should be administered as basal and half as bolus. The latter should be divided into three doses and given at mealtimes. The correct basal dose is one that maintains the blood sugar and does not cause it to either rise or fall, in the absence of food. This requires titrating the dose overnight as well as during the day. Only titrating the dose to achieve a normal fasting blood sugar without monitoring the bedtime blood sugar will often result in higher-than-desired basal rates, which are associated with weight gain and hypoglycemia. The rapid-acting analog dose should be titrated by observing the rise in blood sugar from fasting until 1 to 2 hours after the meal.

XII. CONCLUSION

Type 2 diabetes mellitus is rapidly increasing in prevalence. The financial burden of this disease exceeds $130 billion per year. More important, early diagnosis and effective management of this condition can greatly improve the associated complication rates and quality of life of patients.

Selected References

American Association of Clinical Endocrinologists medical guidelines for clinical practice for the management of diabetes mellitus. *Endocr Pract* 2007;13:S4–S68.

American Diabetes Association. Diagnosis and classification of diabetes mellitus. *Diabetes Care* 2004;27:S1–S10.

American Diabetes Association position statement on gestational diabetes mellitus. *Diabetes Care* 2003;26:S103–S105.

Carpenter MW, et al. Criteria for screening tests for gestational diabetes. *Am J Obstet Gynecol* 1982;144:768.

DECODE Study Group, European Diabetes Epidemiology Group. *Diabetes Care* 2003;26: 2626–2632.

Diabetes Control and Complications Trial Research Group. The effect of intensive treatment diabetes on the development and progression of long-term complications in insulin-dependent diabetes mellitus. *N Engl J Med* 1993;329:977–986.

Kitabchi AE, et al. Hyperglycemic crises in patients with diabetes mellitus, position statement. *Diabetes Care* 2003;26:S109–S117.

Monnier L, Colette C, Dunseath GJ, Owens DR. The loss of postprandial glycemic control precedes stepwise deterioration of fasting with worsening diabetes. *Diabetes Care* 2007; 30:263–269.

Monnier L, Lapinski H, Colette C. Contributions of fasting and postprandial plasma glucose increments to the overall diurnal hyperglycemia of type 2 diabetic patients: variations with increasing levels of HbA(1c). *Diabetes Care* 2003;26:881–885.

Monnier L, Mas E, Ginet C, et al. Activation of oxidative stress by acute glucose fluctuations compared with sustained chronic hyperglycemia in patients with type 2 diabetes. *JAMA* 2006;295:1681–1687.

Nathan DM, et al. Management of hyperglycemia in type 2 diabetes: a consensus algorithm for the initiation and adjustment of therapy. A consensus statement from the American Diabetes Association and the European Association for the Study of Diabetes. *Diabetes Care* 2006 Aug;29:1963–1972.

Nauck MA, Meininger C, Sheng D, et al. Efficacy and safety of the dipeptidyl peptidase-4 inhibitor, sitagliptin, compared with the sulfonylurea, glipizide, in patients with type 2 diabetes inadequately controlled on metformin alone: a randomized, double-blind, non-inferiority trial. *Diabetes Obesity Metab* 2007;9:194–205.

Proceedings of the 4th International Workshop-Conference on Gestational Diabetes Mellitus. *Diabetes Care* 1998;21(suppl 2).

Stratton IM, et al. Association of glycaemia with macrovascular and microvascular complications of type 2 diabetes (UKPDS 35): prospective observational study. *Br Med J* 2000;321:405–412.

46

TYPE 1.5 OR TYPE 3 DIABETES MELLITUS
Anna Pawlikowska-Haddal and Emily Swant

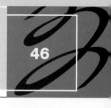

I. INTRODUCTION
Diabetes mellitus (DM) is a disorder characterized by fasting and postprandial hyperglycemia resulting from a deficiency of insulin secretion and/or resistance to its action.

II. ETIOLOGY
Etiologic classification of DM in children and adolescents recognizes two major forms of this illness: type 1 diabetes, insulin-dependent or ketosis-prone; and type 2, non–insulin-dependent or ketosis-resistant.

A. Type 1 diabetes mellitus (T1DM). T1DM is caused by autoimmune destruction of β cells of the pancreas. It generally affects genetically predisposed patients who, after being exposed to environmental triggers, develop autoimmune destruction of β cells. This process leads to the release of antigens and production of antibodies to these antigens. These antibodies include islet-cell antibodies (ICA), glutamic acid decarboxylase (GAD), insulin autoantibodies (IAA), and antibodies to tyrosine phosphatase (IA-2 pr ICA512). As the autoimmune process continues, a gradual loss of β cells occurs, leading ultimately to loss of insulin secretion.

B. Type 2 diabetes mellitus (T2DM). The diagnosis of T2DM relies on the clinical criteria of hyperglycemia and the presence of one or more of the following: belonging to a high-risk minority population; T2DM in at least one parent; obesity; and acanthosis nigricans as a sign of insulin resistance. Presence of any of the β-cell autoimmune markers, IAS, GAD, and IAA, is used classically to negate the diagnosis of T2DM.

C. Type 2 DM with Antibodies. This classification was straightforward until the late 1970s, when the presence of pancreatic islet-cell antibodies in adult patients with T2DM treated with oral hypoglycemia agents was reported. Moreover, the presence of antibodies in T2DM predicted future insulin requirement.

It was also noted that obese children with acanthosis nigricans and T2DM can present with pancreatic antibodies, a hallmark of T1DM. Over the last 30 years, DM has emerged as a syndrome of hyperglycemia, obesity, and autoimmunity in young patients. It is the fastest-growing chronic disorder in the pediatric population, and distinguishing between T1DM and T2DM has become more difficult. The unifying concept of T1DM and T2DM is still controversial; however, ethnic, genetic, autoimmune, and clinical overlays between these two types of DM have become more distinct.

III. ETHNIC OVERLAY
T2DM can present with ketosis in African American patients who are antibody-negative. Ketosis is an outcome of glucotoxicosis that eventually resolves, and these patients do not require insulin therapy. Hispanic adolescents and adults with T2DM and negative antibodies may present with ketoacidosis similar to African American patients. It is not clear why African American and Hispanic patients with hyperglycemia, obesity, and acanthosis nigricans are more prone to diabetic ketoacidosis. It has been theorized that it may be due to a more severe relative insulin deficiency.

673

IV. AUTOIMMUNE OVERLAY

The absence of autoimmune markers in T2DM has given rise to the notion of latent autoimmune diabetes of adults (LADA). LADA was introduced by Zimmet to describe an important minority of patients with diabetes. Typical patients are positive for GAD antibodies, and they present without ketoacidosis and weight loss. Their C-peptide concentrations are lower than in antibody-negative patients. Age criteria for LADA vary in different studies. Zimmet described LADA patients who were at least 35 years old. In Sweden, LADA is defined in a patient clinically classified not as T1DM, but as T2DM, or unclassifiable, and positive for either ICA, GADA, or IA-2; onset has been as early as 15 years of age. LADA patients maintain good glycemic control for several years with oral therapy; however, they become insulin-dependent more rapidly than antibody-negative type 2 diabetic patients.

Studies in children and adolescents with T2DM found that some children may also have autoimmune markers. The incidence of diabetes antibody markers is significantly lower in T2DM versus T1DM; however, up to 30% of T2DM patients can be GAD-positive, 35% can be IAA-positive, and 8% can be ICA-positive. It is currently recognized that the absence of autoimmune markers is not a prerequisite for the diagnosis of T2DM in children and adolescents, that positive antibodies in adolescents with non–insulin-requiring diabetes may represent a form of early-onset LADA, and that some type 2 patients, particularly those who require insulin, are actually obese patients with T1DM.

Libman studied 130 African American children and adolescents diagnosed with diabetes and treated with insulin at time of diagnosis matched with an equal number of white children by age of onset, sex, and year of diagnosis. It was found that one of four of the black children with ICA was obese and/or had acanthosis nigricans. Among white children, the absence of ICA was not associated with any differences in obesity or acanthosis nigricans compared with those with ICA. The authors concluded that their pediatric subjects, regardless of autoimmunity state, often showed characteristics of T2DM. They suggested that childhood diabetes may constitute a spectrum of pathogenic mechanisms associated with T1DM and T2DM that may overlap.

V. GENETIC OVERLAY

A genetic link between type 1 and type 2 diabetes through HLA Class II risk haplotypes has been reported. In 695 Finnish families in which more than one member had T2DM, 14% also had members with T1DM, and there was a marked overlap of risk haplotypes independent of the presence of GADA. The data were suggestive of genetic interaction between T1DM and T2DM, mediated by the HLA locus. Studies in adult patients with LADA and with adult-onset T1DM did not find any difference in obesity, lipid profile, or hypertension frequency between those two groups, and HLA high-risk haplotype frequencies did not differ between the LADA and adult-onset type 1 patients. The authors concluded that LADA is a slowly progressive form of T1DM.

The classical model for type 1 diabetes research has been the nonobese diabetic (NOD) mouse. The numerous genes differentially regulated in the NOD mouse are more commonly associated with T2DM rather than T1DM. Changes in gene expression were related to insulin resistance, vascular pathology, and endoplasmic reticulum stress.

Interesting reports have shown familial clustering of T1 and T2DM genes, and recent studies suggest that selected susceptibility gene variants may be involved in the pathogenesis of T1DM and T2DM.

VI. CLINICAL OVERLAY

Misclassification of some children and adolescents with diabetes has been reported. These patients demonstrate at the onset the classical features of T1DM, including the presence of antibodies and ketoacidosis. However, they also have cardinal features of T2DM, such as acanthosis nigricans, obesity, and positive family history of T2DM. Recognizing these patients is very important for accurate estimation of the magnitude of the problem of T2DM and for appropriate therapy. These patients require full replacement insulin doses to stabilize their glycemic control at the onset of DM but ultimately are not entirely insulin-dependent.

VII. THERAPEUTIC LINK

Patients with clinical T2DM but who are antibody-positive may inevitably require insulin therapy. There is an increased likelihood of decompensation to insulin therapy in individuals who are antibody-positive. The UK Prospective Diabetes Study Group (UKPDS) study showed that the presence of GAD antibodies predicted insulin therapy at 6 years in 84% of patients, and the presence of ICA predicted insulin therapy in 94% of patients. If neither antibody was present, only 14% of patients required insulin therapy at 6 years. This study also showed that the positive predictive values of GADA alone, or both GADA and ICA, for insulin therapy were 52% and 68%, respectively.

Management strategy for patients who present clinically with T2DM but who have positive autoimmune markers relies usually on oral therapy and long-acting insulin such as glargine or detemir. Insulin therapy might possibly arrest the destructive β-cell process and protect endogenous insulin secretion.

However, insulin treatment of patients who are not insulin-dependent should be avoided, because it has been implicated in additional weight gain and an increase in diabetic complications such as atherosclerosis, ischemic heart disease, and hypertension.

VIII. IMPLICATIONS OF THE OVERLAY, OR THE ACCELERATOR HYPOTHESIS

Welkin proposed the accelerator hypothesis, which envisages overlay between T1DM and T2DM. Because the distinctions between T1DM and T2DM are becoming increasingly blurred both clinically and etiologically, where β-cell insufficiency is the shared characteristic, Welkin identifies three processes that accelerate the loss of β cells through apoptosis: constitution, insulin resistance, and autoimmunity. These accelerators will not lead to diabetes without a central trend, which is excess weight gain. The first accelerator is a constitutionally high rate of β-cell apoptosis, the second accelerator is determined by insulin resistance resulting from weight gain and physical inactivity, and the third accelerator is β-cell autoimmunity, which develops in a small and genetically defined subset of patients with both intrinsic lesions and insulin resistance. The first accelerator is necessary for diabetes to develop but not sufficient to cause it alone. The second accelerator triggers the effect of the first accelerator and overall is responsible for the rising incidence of T1DM and T2DM in developed societies.

Thus, the hypothesis postulates that body mass is a primary risk factor in the etiology of T1DM and T2DM, and views T1DM and T2DM as the same disorder, distinguishable only by their rate of β-cell loss and the accelerators responsible. Only tempo distinguishes the types. Both T1DM and T2DM have been simultaneously rising in frequency as the result of changes in body fat and fitness. Welkin further postulates that if the rising incidence and earlier presentation of diabetes were to be explained by a heavier population at all ages, weight gain would have as much a role in the demography changes of T1DM and T2DM.

The hypothesis was tested, and it was proven that increasing body weight was also associated with the earlier presentation of T1DM. The relationship between obesity and age at diagnosis was examined in context of birth weight, weight change since birth, weight at diagnosis, body mass index (BMI) at diagnosis, and BMI 12 months later in 49 boys and 45 girls aged 1 to 16 years presenting for management of acute-onset type T1DM. It was found that BMI standard deviation score (SDS) at diagnosis, weight SDS change since birth, and BMI SDS 12 months later were all inversely related to age at presentation.

IX. CLINICAL IMPLICATIONS

The etiologic and clinical distinctions between T1DM and T2DM have become increasingly blurred. At the same time, the prevalence of childhood obesity has created an epidemic, and the prevalence of being overweight at the onset of T1DM tripled from the 1980s to the 1990s, following a parallel rise in obesity among the general population. These factors alone should urge everyone to undertake all preventive measures against childhood obesity and sedentary lifestyle. In the meantime, doctors have to be able to diagnose DM and initiate appropriate therapy not under influence of classification but rather under the influence of a constellation of clinical and biochemical characteristics of their young patients.

Selected References

Donath MY, Ehses JA. Type 1, type 1.5, and type 2 diabetes: NOD the diabetes we thought it was. *Proc Natl Acad Sci U S A* 2006;103:12217–12218.

Fagot-Campagna A. Type 2 diabetes among North American children and adolescents: an epidemiologic review and a public health perspective. *J Pediatr* 2000;136:664–672.

Gale EAM. Declassifying diabetes. *Diabetologia* 2006;49:1989–1995.

Gale EAM. The rise of childhood diabetes in the twentieth century. *Diabetes* 2002;12:3353–3361.

Hathout EH, Thomas W, El-Shahawy M. Diabetic autoimmune markers in children and adolescents with type 2 diabetes mellitus. *Pediatrics* 2001;107(6):E102.

Hermann R, Knip M, Veijola R. Temporal changes in the frequencies of HLA genotypes in patients with type 1 diabetes-indication of an increased environmental pressure? *Diabetologia* 2003;46:420–425.

Juneja R, Hirsch IB, Naik RG, et al. Islet cell antibodies and glutamic acid decarboxylase antibodies, but not clinical phenotype, help to identify type 1½ diabetes in patients presenting with type 2 diabetes mellitus. *Metabolism* 2001;50:1008–10013.

Juneja R, Palmer JP. Type 1½ diabetes: myth or reality? *Autoimmunity* 1999;29:65–83.

Karvonen M, Pitkaniemi J, Tuomilehto J. The onset age of type 1 diabetes in Finnish children has become younger. (The Finnish Childhood Diabetes Registry Group). *Diabetes Care* 1999;22:1066–1070.

Kibrige M, Metcalf B, Renuka R, Welkin TJ. Testing the accelerator hypothesis. The relationship between body mass and age at diagnosis of type 1 diabetes mellitus. *Diabetes Care* 2003;26:2865–2870.

Kordonouri O, Hartmann R. Higher body weight is associated with earlier onset of type 1 diabetes mellitus in children: confirming the "accelerator hypothesis." *Diabet Med* 2005;22:1783–1784.

Libman IM, Pietropaolo M, Arslanian SA, et al. Islet cell autoimmunity in white and black children and adolescents with IDDM. *Diabetes Care* 2003;10:2876–2882.

Torn C, Landin-Olsson J, et al. Glutamic acid decarboxylase autoantibodies (GADA) is the most important factor for prediction of insulin therapy within 3 years in young adult diabetic patients not classified as Type 1 diabetes on clinical grounds. *Diabetes Metab Res Rev* 2000;16:442–447.

Turner R, Stratton I, Horton V, et al. Autoantibodies to islet-cell cytoplasm and glutamic acid decarboxylase for prediction of insulin requirement in type 2 diabetes: UK Prospective Diabetes Study Group. *Lancet* 1997;350:1288–1293.

Welkin TJ. The accelerator hypothesis: weight gain as the missing link between type I and type II diabetes. *Diabetologia* 2001;44:914–922.

Welkin TJ. Changing perspectives in diabetes: their impact on its classification. *Diabetologia* 2007;50:1587–1592.

Zimmet PZ, Tuomi T, Mackay IR, et al. Latent autoimmune diabetes mellitus in adults (LADA): the role of autoantibodies to glutamic acid decarboxylase in diagnosis and prediction of insulin dependency. *Diabetes Med* 1994;11:299–303.

47

PRE-EXISTING DIABETES AND PREGNANCY
Siri L. Kjos, Marie U. Beall, and John Kitzmiller

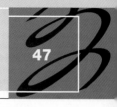

I. GENERAL PRINCIPLES
A. Intensive management of diabetes is required during pregnancy for optimal perinatal outcome. The hormonal and metabolic effects of pregnancy increase the risk of ketoacidosis from the physiologic accelerated starvation and the risk of hypoglycemic reactions from aggressive insulin therapy. The amount of insulin required to control hyperglycemia usually increases by two- to threefold throughout gestation. In addition, a woman with severe obesity or diabetes-associated vascular disease faces serious health challenges as a result of the physiologic alterations of pregnancy.

B. The fetus of a diabetic woman is also at increased risk for a poor perinatal outcome. Aggressive maternal glucose control can reduce these risks, which include major congenital abnormalities, neonatal hypoxia and stillbirth, preterm delivery, and both extremes of fetal growth abnormalities, i.e., restricted and accelerated growth. Fetal monitoring for these risks includes screening for birth defects using biochemical markers and ultrasound examination of fetal anatomy, serial evaluation of fetal growth, and, in the third trimester, weekly antepartum monitoring for well-being using either fetal heart rate testing and/or biophysical profiles.

C. The mother's medical condition may be further complicated by the pregnancy. During pregnancy, the combination of pregnancy-related metabolic changes (preprandial accelerated starvation and postprandial facilitated anabolism) and the desire to achieve tight glycemic control, increases the incidence of hyper- and hypoglycemic episodes. In addition, physiologic changes of pregnancy may negatively affect women with pre-existing cardiac, renal, or vascular disease, or obesity. Preconception care of the diabetic woman should establish and/or assess any pre-existing diabetic sequelae or disease and evaluate the superimposed risk of pregnancy to optimize her health and reduce any identified risks.

II. PHYSIOLOGIC CHANGES OF PREGNANCY
A. Glucose utilization. Pregnancy produces major changes in the homeostasis of all metabolic fuels, which in turn affect the management of diabetes.

1. Postabsorptive or fasting state. Plasma concentrations of glucose decline in normal women as pregnancy advances, as a result of increasing placental uptake of glucose. Although fat deposition is accentuated in early pregnancy, lipolysis is enhanced by human placental lactogen later in gestation, with higher plasma levels of glycerol and free fatty acids. Ketogenesis is thus accentuated during pregnancy, probably secondary to increased substrate free fatty acids and because of hormonal effects on the maternal liver cells. In sum, the occurrence of postabsorptive hypoglycemia is more frequent and may more easily lead to ketogenesis. Both tendencies are clinically important in the management of type 1 and type 2 diabetes during pregnancy.

2. Fed state. In normal pregnancies, the disposal of glucose is impaired because of postreceptor changes in muscle and liver, resulting in higher rates of maternal insulin secretion being required to normalize maternal glucose levels. Despite this relative hyperinsulinism in normal pregnancy, postprandial maternal blood glucose (BG) levels are somewhat higher. This contrainsulin effect seen during pregnancy is caused by the placental production of lactogen and progesterone. Glucagon secretion continues to be suppressed by glucose, and the secretory

677

response of glucagon to amino acids is not increased above nonpregnant levels. After meals, more glucose is converted to triglyceride in pregnancy, leading to conservation of calories and enhanced fat deposition. Both of these normal changes in glucose utilization may significantly affect diabetes management in pregnancy.

B. Cardiovascular and renal changes.
   1. Pregnancy is accompanied by an increase in blood volume of 40% to 60% and an increase in cardiac output of 30% to 50%; with an increased maternal heart rate and stroke volume. The majority of these increases occur prior to the end of the first trimester. Labor and delivery are associated with further increases in cardiac output; these increases are both constant and episodic (associated with uterine contractions) and may total almost 60% above prelabor values by the time of delivery. Systemic vascular resistance falls during normal pregnancy, producing a concurrent fall in blood pressure. In pregnancy, renal blood flow increases by ~20%, and glomerular filtration rate (GFR) by 40% to 60%. Urinary excretion of albumin increases only slightly during pregnancy, remaining within the normal range. However, protein excretion does increase, with rates of up to 300 mg per day considered normal during pregnancy. Diabetic women with pre-existing renal or cardiovascular disease may not tolerate these changes well. Pre-eclampsia, defined as development of blood pressure >140/90 mm Hg, and proteinuria can develop *de novo* or more commonly in diabetic women superimposed on pre-existing hypertension. It can affect up to 20% of diabetic gravidas. In diabetic women with underlying renal dysfunction or hypertension, superimposed pre-eclampsia can produce dangerous increases in blood pressure, serum creatinine, and proteinuria, often requiring preterm delivery.

C. Obesity. Obesity is a common accompaniment of type 2 diabetes and is an independent risk factor for pregnancy. Obese women, even in the absence of diabetes, have an increased risk of poor perinatal outcome, including stillbirth and need for cesarean delivery. After surgery, obese diabetic women are at substantial risk for infection, poor wound healing, and thromboembolic events.

III. PRECONCEPTION MANAGEMENT OF THE DIABETIC WOMAN

Optimally, every woman should enter pregnancy informed of her risk and what the best condition is to withstand the rigors of pregnancy. Preconception care has been shown to improve pregnancy outcome (Table 47.1). A woman presenting for care prior to conception should be:

A. Counseled regarding her health risk from a pregnancy. This includes an assessment of possible complications resulting from pre-existing medical conditions, notably hypertension, nephropathy, and retinopathy, including the possible deterioration of these complications with pregnancy. Medications that are possibly teratogenic should be discontinued. In particular, angiotensin-converting enzyme (ACE) inhibitors are generally contraindicated in pregnancy, but may be advisable to prevent or limit renal damage.

B. Counseled regarding the risk of an abnormal pregnancy outcome, including the risk of a fetal congenital malformation, fetal death, or premature delivery.

C. Optimized glycemic control. Team management should be utilized to institute appropriate medical nutritional therapy, daily exercise, and appropriate medical treatment. The preconception treatment goal is glucose levels within the normal range and glycosylated hemoglobin levels of <7%.

D. Optimized medically. Assessment of possible or pre-existing diabetic sequelae should be undertaken. Medical therapeutic goals include steps to normalize blood pressure, stabilize renal function, and treat any significant retinopathy.

IV. MANAGEMENT DURING PREGNANCY: ACHIEVING GLYCEMIC CONTROL

A. Medical nutritional therapy. Caloric intake should be adjusted to achieve the desired pregnancy weight gain based on prepregnancy body mass index (BMI) following the recommendations of the Institute of Medicine (Table 47.2). The majority of expected weight gain occurs during the second half of pregnancy. Weight loss is

TABLE 47.1 Stages of Care in Diabetes of Pregnancy

Preconception
  Normalize glucose levels (HbA$_{1c}$ <7%), monitor glycemic control
  Evaluate for presence and severity of diabetic sequelae, institute appropriate medical therapy
  Optimize general health, minimize risks
  Institute beneficial lifestyle changes (diet, exercise, stop smoking, daily folate supplement)
First trimester (glycemic target: PPBG <120 mg/dL; <160 if frequent hypoglycemic episodes)
  Reduce abortion risk and anomalies
  Monitor for ketonemia
  First-trimester fetal screening for anomalies (biochemical markers and ultrasound)
Second trimester (glycemic target: PPBG <130 mg/dL)
  Reduce risk of macrosomia
  Second-trimester fetal screening for anomalies (biochemical markers and ultrasound)
Third trimester (glycemic target: PPBG <130 mg/dL)
  Reduce risk of macrosomia
  Reduce risk of respiratory distress syndrome
  Reduce risk of stillbirth
  Monitor for ketonemia
  Initiate discussion regarding breast feeding, contraception, future pregnancies
Postpartum (glycemic target: PPBG <180 mg/dL)
  Counseling and education regarding breastfeeding, contraception, future pregnancies and
    child development

PPBG, postprandial blood glucose.

not recommended, however, there is evidence to support modest energy (30% reduction of estimated energy needs) and carbohydrate restriction in overweight and
obese women with glucose intolerance. It has generally been considered inappropriate to recommend a weight-loss diet in pregnancy, although there is evidence that
in very obese women (BMI >40), perinatal outcome may be optimized with a small
weight loss during pregnancy. Currently there are no evidence-based recommendations for dietary guidelines for obese women during pregnancy. Ketonemia, either
from starvation or ketogenesis, should be avoided. The amount and distribution of
carbohydrate should be adjusted based on clinical outcomes including hunger, glucose levels, weight gain, and ketone levels, with a minimum of 175 g per day of
carbohydrate intake, distributed in 3 meals and 2 to 4 snacks throughout the day

TABLE 47.2 Institute of Medicine Recommendations for Weight Gain in Pregnancy

Prepregnancy BMI	Recommended weight gain in pregnancy (kg)
<19.8	12.7–18.2
19.8–26	11.4–15.9
26.1–29	6.8–11.4
>29	6.0–?

BMI, body mass index (kg/m^2).
Targets are chosen to optimize perinatal outcome, not normalize maternal weight. African American women
and adolescents are recommended to target the upper limit of weight gain.

to avoid nocturnal and preprandial hypoglycemia. For normal-weight women, the Institute of Medicine calculations estimate no additional energy requirements (EER) in the first trimester, with progressive increases in caloric requirement in the second and third trimesters—an additional 300 to 450 kcal per day, based on activity and increased metabolic needs. Sedentary individuals may not need additional caloric intake.

Controlled studies demonstrate better glycemic balance with a diet containing ~40% carbohydrates. The meal plan should include ~70 g per day of protein in the first half of pregnancy, increasing to about 100g per day after 20 weeks of gestation. Individuals with diabetic microalbuminuria are counseled to lower protein intake slightly, to 0.8 g/kg body weight, and increase natural fiber intake.

B. Self-monitoring of blood glucose. Patients should self-monitor their blood glucose levels throughout the day; in pregnancy, sugars should be checked fasting and 2 hours postprandial (four times daily) at a minimum. Women with pre-existing diabetes generally require more frequent monitoring schedules that include preprandial glucose levels to modify premeal insulin doses optimally, and postprandial/bedtime glucose levels to avoid hyperglycemia and reduce the risk of macrosomic fetal growth.

Fasting plasma glucose levels between 60 and 95 mg/dL and postprandial levels between 100 and 129 mg/dL appear to be most appropriate to sustain normal fetal growth. This degree of euglycemia may not be attainable during the first trimester because of increased insulin sensitivity and symptomatic nausea and hyperemesis. Thus, more lax glucose targets (fasting ≤120 mg/dL and postprandial ≤160 mg/dL) may be safer.

Women should be cautioned not to overtreat hypoglycemic reactions so as to minimize rebound hyperglycemia. For moderate symptoms, 8 oz of nonfat milk is generally sufficient; for glucose levels <60 mg/dL, 10 g of fast-acting carbohydrate (dextrosols, or 4 oz orange juice followed by crackers or 6 oz milk) is recommended. To avoid the possibility of developing severe hypoglycemia or unconsciousness, patients and their family members must keep glucagon on hand, and know how to inject glucagon subcutaneously.

C. Medical treatment. Insulin preparations and many oral hypoglycemic agents have been used successfully in pregnancy without known fetal harm. A patient with type 2 diabetes on oral antidiabetic therapy should be counseled not to stop her medication upon discovering that she is pregnant until a pregnancy-appropriate therapy can be initiated. All women with type 1 and most with type 2 diabetes require insulin therapy to achieve adequate blood glucose control.

In pregnancy, most diabetic women require at least two injections of a mixture of rapid-acting DNA analog (lispro or aspart) or short-acting (regular) insulin and intermediate (NPH) insulin. Insulin therapy may be initiated by calculating the total anticipated insulin requirement as a proportion of actual body weight (Table 47.3). Two thirds of the total dose is given before breakfast (two thirds as intermediate/one third as short- or rapid-acting insulin). Of the remaining insulin, one half is given as short- or rapid-acting insulin before dinner and one half as intermediate-acting insulin. In many patients, better control of fasting glucose levels is achieved by delaying the evening dose of intermediate-acting insulin until bedtime, which prevents nocturnal hypoglycemia and may help deal with the dawn phenomenon of increased insulin requirement between 4 and 8 A.M. Other patients need to use more stringent regimens, administering rapid-acting insulin 3 to 5 times each day or by continuous subcutaneous insulin infusion with a portable pump to achieve euglycemia. Alternatively a long-acting insulin DNA analog (e.g., glargine), which provides 24-hour basal insulin coverage, can be taken at night. Rapid-acting insulin is taken prior to each meal and dosed according to carbohydrate ingestion and premeal glucose levels (Table 47.3).

V. FETAL DEVELOPMENT

The incidence of **major congenital anomalies** in infants of type 1 and type 2 diabetic mothers has been reported to be 6% to 13%, compared with 2% to 4% in the nondiabetic population. (Table 47.4) In women with poorly controlled diabetes, identified

TABLE 47.3 Total Anticipated Insulin Requirement by Stage of Pregnancy— Guidelines for Daily Insulin Dose in 60-kg Woman with Type 1 Diabetes

Calculate daily insulin needs

Type 1: Before conception, 0.5 U/kg DBW; during pregnancy (second and third trimester), 0.7 U/kg DBW

Type 2: Optimize glycemic control with diet, exercise, weight loss, and combination of oral antidiabetic medications, including insulin as needed

First trimester

A. Standard dose allocation: 0.7 U/kg DBW × 60 kg = 42 U

Prebreakfast: Two thirds of total daily dose	Predinner: One third of total daily dose
(NPH:rapid-acting = 2:1)	(NPH:rapid-acting or regular = 1:1)
18 U NPH:9 U rapid-acting or regular	7 U NPH:7 U rapid-acting or regular

B. Intensive insulin regimen (4 doses daily using carbohydrate counting (carbohydrate: insulin ratio plus premeal adjustments) based on prandial glucose levels)

1. Basic dosing scheme

Breakfast	Lunch	Dinner	Before bedtime
9 U	8 U	8 U	17 U NPH or
rapid-acting	rapid-acting or	rapid-acting or	long-acting
or regular	regular	regular	

2. Carbohydrate intake in relation to meals
(patient's weight: 60 kg; daily calories @ 35 kcal/kg = 2 100; 45% carbohydrates = 237 g/d)

Breakfast	(Snack)	Lunch	(Snack)	Dinner	(HS)
45 g	(22 g)	55 g	(30 g)	55 g	(30 g)

3. Carbohydrate (g):insulin (U) ratio
(may decrease with advancing gestation and with individual patient)

Breakfast	Lunch	Dinner
5:1	7:1	7:1

4. Basic dose insulin adjustment (based on premeal blood glucose algorithm)

Premeal blood glucose (mg/dL)	Rapid-acting or regular insulin (U)
<60	(−) 3
60–80	(−) 2
81–100	Use basic dose
101–130	(+) 1
131–160	(+) 2
161–190	(+) 3
191–220	(+) 4
>220	(+) 5

DBW, desirable body weight.

by elevated glycosylated hemoglobin and/or glucose levels during embryonic development, anomaly rates up to 22% to 30% have been reported. Although many anomalies are found, cardiac, neural tube, and urogenital malformations are especially common in infants of diabetic mothers (Table 47.5). Thus the initial glycosylated hemoglobin percent obtained during early pregnancy is useful for counseling women regarding their risk of having a fetus with a major congenital anomaly. As perinatal deaths, because of unexplained stillbirth and respiratory distress syndrome have declined, congenital anomalies are now associated with the majority of fetal–neonatal deaths in infants of diabetic mothers.

Interventions to reduce the incidence of major congenital anomalies must be initiated very early in pregnancy, as the formation of all major organ systems is complete by 8 weeks after the last menstrual period (6 weeks embryologic age). For practical reasons, this means that good control (postprandial glucose <160 mg/dL, HbA$_{1c}$ <7%)

TABLE 47.4 Prevention of Major Congenital Malformations in Infants of Diabetic Women in Preconception Clinical Trials

| | Preconception group | | Registered already pregnant | |
Author	Infants	Anomalies[a] (%)	Infants	Anomalies[a] (%)
Fuhrmann (1983, 1984)	185	2 (1.1)	473	31 (6.6)
Goldman (1986)	44	0	31	2 (6.5)
Damm (1989)	197	2 (1.0)	61	5 (8.2)
Steel (1990)	143	2 (1.4)	96	10 (10.4)
Kitzmiller (1991)	84	1 (1.2)	110	12 (10.4)
Total	653	7 (1.1)	771	60 (7.8)

[a]Estimated costs of neonatal care for infants with anomalies: $400 260 for preconception group; $3 430 900 for registered group.

must be instituted **before conception** in diabetic women planning pregnancy. It also means that effective contraceptive counseling must be offered to all diabetic women of reproductive age.

A. Screening for congenital abnormalities. Screening for congenital abnormalities can begin with first-trimester serum screening using biochemical markers, followed by ultrasound examination between 10 and 13 completed weeks of gestation. This first-trimester sonogram is also used to establish the accuracy of the estimated length of gestation, and to serve as a baseline for future evaluation of fetal growth.

B. Although the fetal anatomy survey is traditionally performed at 18 to 20 weeks of gestation, acceptable fetal anatomy surveys using transvaginal ultrasound imaging are often possible at 13 or 14 weeks. In a very obese woman, this may represent the

TABLE 47.5 Congenital Malformations in Infants of Diabetic Women

Malformation	Ratio of incidences (diabetic vs. control group)	Latest gestational age for occurrence (week after menstruation)
Caudal regression	252	5
Anencephaly	3	6
Spina bifida, hydrocephalus, or other central nervous system defect	2	6
Cardiac anomalies	4	
Transposition of great vessels		7
Ventricular septal defects		8
Atrial septal defects		8
Anorectal atresia	3	8
Renal anomalies	5	
Agenesis	6	7
Cystic kidney	4	7
Ureter duplex	23	7
Situs inversus	84	6

Modified from Kucera J. Rate and type of congenital anomalies among offspring of diabetic women. *J Reprod Med* 1971;7:61; and from Mills JL, Baker L, Goldman MS. Malformations in infants of diabetic mothers occur before the seventh gestational week: implications for treatment. *Diabetes* 1979;28:292.

best opportunity to visualize the fetus. Maternal serum screening may be performed at 15 to 20 weeks in place of, or in addition to, first-trimester screening. In any case, **maternal serum α-fetoprotein** should be measured in the second trimester to screen for fetal neural tube defects, as this test is not effective in the first trimester. Fetal anatomy survey, if not previously completed, and fetal echocardiography, are generally performed at 20 to 22 weeks.

VI. OBSTETRIC MANAGEMENT

A. **Fetal growth.** Maternal hyperglycemia is related to excessive birth weight in **infants of diabetic mothers,** and has been explained by the causal chain of fetal hyperglycemia → fetal hyperinsulinemia → excess growth and fat deposition. Strict glucose control in pregnancy has been associated with a reduction in fetal macrosomia, but in exchange there may be an increase in the number of fetuses born small for gestational age. Both extremes of growth disturbance are associated with higher rates of obesity, metabolic syndrome, and type 2 diabetes in the later life of these offspring. The fetus of a woman with diabetes and vascular disease may suffer **intrauterine growth retardation** related to inadequate uteroplacental perfusion. In addition to total fetal growth, the growth of the abdominal circumference is a key feature. Failure of the abdomen to grow appropriately signifies fetal undernutrition and poor fat deposition. Conversely, accelerated abdominal circumference growth has been used as a proxy for fetal hyperinsulinemia, i.e., elevated fetal amniotic insulin levels, which has been associated with an increased risk for biochemical and somatic fetopathy. Accelerated abdominal growth (and amniotic fluid insulin levels) have been used as an indication for increased stringency of glucose control in diabetic patients, both pregestational and gestational. Thus periodic assessment of the fetal growth pattern can be useful to identify fetopathy in utero to modify management strategies and initiate close fetal surveillance if needed.

B. **Fetal well-being.** In addition to the ultrasound studies of fetal growth, **antepartum fetal surveillance** is utilized to reduce the chance of stillbirth. The gestational age to initiate surveillance depends on maternal–fetal risk factors. For most patients, testing will begin at 32 to 34 weeks of gestation and most commonly consists of a modified biophysical profile (nonstress test that monitors the fetal heart rate pattern and the ultrasound measurement of amniotic fluid volume). Testing is typically performed twice weekly. Earlier or more frequent testing, or testing by other methods, such as the biophysical profile, may be appropriate for some patients, e.g., those with renal disease, vascular disease, or fetal growth disturbances.

C. **Delivery planning.** A well-controlled diabetic patient can be managed expectantly until 40 weeks of gestation. Generally, continuation of pregnancy after 40 weeks is not recommended. A patient whose control is more problematic may be delivered whenever fetal pulmonary maturity is attained; this may be assessed by the fetus reaching 39 weeks of gestation, or by measurement of pulmonary lecithin obtained through amniocentesis. With current obstetric and diabetic management, well-dated term pregnancies complicated by diabetes have low rates of neonatal respiratory distress ($\leq 0.5\%$) whether or not fetal lung maturation was assessed. The route of delivery should be determined by the usual obstetric indications. Estimated fetal weight $>4\,250$ g or a head circumference-to-abdominal circumference ratio ≤ 0.8 has been associated with a higher risk of fetal birth injury during vaginal delivery, and cesarean section is recommended. If estimated fetal weight is $3\,800$ to $4\,200$ g by 38 weeks of gestation, induction of labor is recommended.

D. **Labor management.** Maternal blood glucose is usually easily kept within 80 to 100 mg/dL during labor by alternating intravenous infusions of 5% dextrose with normal saline solution. In type 1 diabetic patients, insulin infusion (0.5 to 2.0 U per hour of regular or rapid-acting insulin) is administered to prevent ketonemia. The need for insulin in patients with type 2 diabetes generally is more variable. During active labor and in the postpartum period there is a marked increase in insulin sensitivity, often producing low or normal glucose levels. This period requires continued close monitoring and a reduction in or temporary withholding of insulin if low glucose levels are present. Postpartum, the insulin requirement typically drops rapidly and often remains low for several days.

E. Diabetic women should be encouraged to breast-feed their infants. The quality of milk is not affected by diabetes, and breast feeding appears to reduce the risk of childhood allergies, obesity, and later diabetes.

F. Diabetic women have several safe options for contraception. Data indicate that intrauterine devices are effective and safe in diabetic women, and that oral contraceptives, either low-dose combination or progestin-only pills, are safe and do not significantly alter glycemic control or lipid levels, at least in nonsmoking diabetic women without vascular disease.

Selected References

ACOG Practice Bulletin. Clinical management guidelines for obstetrician-gynecologists. *Pregestational diabetes* 2005;105:675–685.

American Diabetes Association. Nutrition recommendations and interventions for diabetes. A position statement of the American Diabetes Association. *Diabetes Care* 2008; 31(suppl 1):S61–S78.

American Diabetes Association. Preconception care of women with diabetes. *Diabetes Care* 2004;27(suppl 1):S76–S78.

American Diabetes Association. Standards of medical care in diabetes—2008. *Diabetes Care* 2008;31(Suppl 1):S12–S54.

Chew EY, Mills JL, Metzger BE, et al. The Diabetes in Early Pregnancy Study. Metabolic control and progression of retinopathy. *Diabetes Care* 1995;18:631–637.

Clausen TD, Mathiesen E, Ekbom P, et al. Poor pregnancy outcome in women with type 2 diabetes. *Diabetes Care* 2005;28:323–328.

De Veciana M, Major CA, Morgan M, et al. Postprandial versus preprandial blood glucose monitoring in women with gestational diabetes mellitus requiring insulin therapy. *N Engl J Med* 1995;333:1237–1241.

Gold AE, Reilly R, Little J, et al. The effect of glycemic control in the pre-conception period and early pregnancy on birth weight in women with IDDM. *Diabetes Care* 1998;21:535–538.

Kaiser LL, Allen L; American Dietetic Association. Position of the American Dietetic Association: nutrition and lifestyle for a healthy pregnancy outcome. *J Am Diet Assoc* 2002;102:1479–1490.

Kimmerle R, Heinemann L, Delecki A, et al. Severe hypoglycemia incidence and predisposing factors in 85 pregnancies of type 1 diabetic women. *Diabetes Care* 1992;15:1034–1037.

Kitzmiller JL. Clinical diabetic nephropathy before and during pregnancy. In: Reese EA, Coustan DR, Gabbe SG, eds. *Diabetes in Women, Adolescence, Pregnancy and Menopause*. 3rd ed. Philadelphia: Lippincott Williams & Wilkins; 2004:383–424.

Kjos SL, Buchanan TA. Postpartum management, lactation and contraception. In: Reece AE, Coustan DR, Gabbe SG, eds. *Diabetes in Women: Adolescence, Pregnancy and Menopause*. Philadelphia: Lippincott Williams & Wilkins; 2004.

Kjos SL, Schaefer-Graf UM. Modified therapy for gestational diabetes using high-risk and low-risk fetal abdominal circumference growth to select strict versus relaxed maternal glycemic targets. *Diabetes Care* 2007;(suppl 2):S200–S205.

Major CA, Henry MJ, de Veciana M, et al. The effects of carbohydrate restriction in patients with diet-controlled gestational diabetes. *Obstet Gynecol* 1998;91:600–604.

Reece EA, Homko C, Wiznitzer A. Metabolic changes in diabetic and non-diabetic subjects during pregnancy. *Obstet Gynecol Surv* 1994;49:64–71.

Schaefer-Graf UM, Buchanan TA, Xiang A, et al. Patterns of congenital anomalies and relationship to initial maternal fasting glucose levels in pregnancies complicated by type 2 and gestational diabetes. *Am J Obstet Gynecol* 2000;182:313–320.

Towner D, Kjos SL, Leung B, et al. Congenital malformations in pregnancies complicated by NIDDM. *Diabetes Care* 1995;18:1446–1451.

Visser J, Snel M, Van Vliet HAAM. Hormonal vs non-hormonal contraceptives in women with diabetes type 1 and 2 (review). *Cochran Collab* 2008;1:1–19.

DIABETES MELLITUS: RECENT DEVELOPMENTS AND CLINICAL IMPLICATIONS

48

Charles Choe and Steven V. Edelman

I. INTRODUCTION

This chapter focuses on devices and therapies that have recently been approved, or are nearing the review process, by the U.S. Food and Drug Administration (FDA). We briefly overview and highlight the important advances that have significant clinical implications for the management of diabetes.

II. ADVANCES IN GLUCOSE MONITORING

A. Home glucose monitoring (HGM). HGM devices are continually being improved to facilitate their use for patients and to provide more helpful information for both patients and practitioners. Each HGM has its own unique combination of features that a patient should consider when selecting an HGM device best suited for him or her.

There have been several advances in the functionality of HGM devices. Their development has progressed to smaller and lighter versions, and they come in a variety of shapes to suit each patient's preference. The speed at which they are able to measure blood glucose has improved, with some providing results in as fast as 5 seconds. The volume of blood required has decreased, with some requiring only 0.3 μL of blood. Some devices are approved for testing at alternative sites (e.g., the forearm). Some use test-strip cartridges, so individual test strips do not need to be loaded for each glucose measurement. Others no longer need to be coded or calibrated each time a new supply of test strips is used. Finally, some HGM devices can be combined or integrated into other commonly carried devices, such as cell phones, personal digital assistants (PDAs), or insulin pumps.

Most HGM devices have data analysis capabilities. Data stored on HGM devices and downloaded with computer software programs can create charts and graphs that help reveal patterns in blood glucose values.

B. Continuous glucose monitoring (CGM). The development of CGM devices represents a quantum leap forward in the management of diabetes and holds tremendous promise for allowing near-normalization of glucose levels while avoiding the most serious complication of intensive glucose management, hypoglycemia. CGM devices measure glucose levels from the subcutaneous interstitial fluid or through the skin at frequent intervals. These values are then sent to a display device that shows real-time glucose values and trends.

There are many benefits of CGMs. Unlike traditional fingersticks, which provide a glucose value at one point in time, continuous readings create a trend line that displays whether glucose levels are rising or falling, and how fast these changes are occurring. Monitoring these trends allows for better interpretation of a given glucose reading at a specific time. The significance of the same glucose value varies significantly if one's glucose is rapidly rising, falling, or stable, and this knowledge allows for very different yet appropriate interventions for the same glucose reading. CGMs also inform patients how insulin, food, exercise, and other variables affect their glucose values. Finally, CGM devices have alerts that will alarm for both low and high glucose levels, thus helping to prevent and manage hypo- and hyperglycemia.

The advent of these devices does not mean that traditional blood glucose monitoring by fingersticks can be abandoned. Currently, CGM devices are approved as

685

an adjunct to traditional glucometers, not as replacements for them. In fact, it is recommended that patients confirm continuous glucose readings with a fingerstick blood glucose reading before taking any action such as eating or injecting insulin. In addition, blood glucose meters are needed to calibrate CGM devices.

Even with frequent traditional blood glucose monitoring, the amount of time patients with diabetes are hyperglycemic and hypoglycemic during a 24-hour period is vastly underappreciated. Recent trials have demonstrated that when patients have access to real-time, continuous glucose readings, the time spent hypo- and hyperglycemic can be significantly decreased. In a recent controlled trial, 91 insulin-requiring subjects given CGM devices were randomized either to a control group that was blinded to the real-time CGM readings or to a group that was able to see their continuous glucose readings. Availability of CGM data reduced the time subjects spent <55 mg/dL and >240 mg/dL by 9% and 15% from baseline, respectively, and increased the time spent between 80 and 140 mg/dL by 16%. Compared to the control group, the group with real-time access to CGM data spent 21% less time <55 mg/dL, 23% less time >240 mg/dL, and 26% more time in the 81- to 140-mg/dL range.

The first CGM device to be FDA-approved was the **GlucoWatch** automatic glucose biographer (Animas). The GlucoWatch obtains noninvasive glucose measurements through the skin by reverse iontophoresis, taking measurements as frequently as every 10 minutes for up to 13 hours. It displays glucose values as an average of the last two 10-minute measurements. Concerns regarding its accuracy and correlation with blood glucose tests (especially at low glucose values), skin irritation, and problems during sweating have prevented its widespread use.

More recently, two minimally invasive CGM devices have been approved for commercial use—the **DexCom STS** (Dexcom; Fig. 48.1A) and the **Guardian RT** (Medtronic). These devices measure interstitial fluid glucose from a sensor the size of a fine wire that is self-inserted by the patient into the subcutaneous tissue. The sensor wirelessly transmits data to a pager-sized device that receives and displays averaged measurements every 5 minutes. Medtronic has also combined the CGM receiver and display with an insulin pump into a single device, the **Paradigm RT** (Fig. 48.1B). A third CGM device, the **Freestyle Navigator** (Abbott), is being reviewed by the FDA for approval.

One of the key features of CGM devices is that glycemic control can be improved, with associated decreases in hypoglycemia. This is in stark contrast to the fact that most therapies that improve glycemic control also typically increase rates of hypoglycemia. CGM is not indicated for all patients with diabetes, and for many patients with diabetes, the additional information provided by CGM may not have a significant effect on HbA$_{1c}$ or diabetic complications. However, for patients who

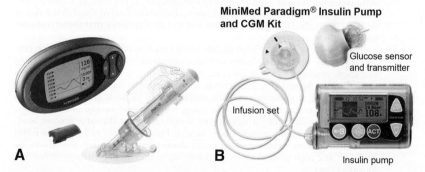

Figure 48.1. **A.** DexCom STS continuous glucose monitor device. **B.** Paradigm RT combined continuous glucose monitor and insulin pump device.

are on insulin, have labile blood sugars, have hypoglycemic unawareness, or require extremely tight control, the potential benefit that CGM provides may be enormous. Although many issues, including clear indications for CGMs and insurance coverage, have yet to be resolved, there is no doubt that current CGM devices and future CGM technology will be an integral part of diabetes management.

C. Home glycosylated hemoglobin. Because treatment strategies are in part determined by HbA_{1c} levels, the ability for patients to determine HbA_{1c} at home represents another potentially useful tool. With currently available test kits, patients send a sample of blood from a fingerstick to a lab, which then sends the HbA_{1c} result back to the patient. An important factor to be aware of is that the methodology for determining HbA_{1c} in these kits differs and may not be certified by the National Glycohemoglobin Standardization Program (NGSP). The NGSP serves as a reference laboratory for manufacturers to standardize HbA_{1c} results so that results from their assays are comparable to those of other labs that are NGSP-certified and to data from the large Diabetes Control and Complications Trial (DCCT).

D. 1,5-Anhydroglucitol (1,5-AG). The GlycoMark assay, recently approved by the FDA, measures blood levels of 1,5-AG, a unique monosaccharide that, like HbA_{1c} and fructosamine, serves as a measure of glycemic control in a patient. However, unlike other measures, 1,5-AG levels fall when glucose levels are elevated. It reflects glycemic control for the preceding 1 to 2 weeks. In addition, 1,5-AG levels have been demonstrated to be a more robust reflection of postprandial hyperglycemia than HbA_{1c} or fructosamine. At this point, the outcomes or complications data using this measure of glycemic control are limited. How best to use this test has yet to be determined.

III. NEW TYPES OF INSULINS

A. Rapid-acting analog insulins. The development of rapid-acting analog insulins has been an extremely important advance in the management of diabetes, but it is not new—the insulins lispro (Humalog, Lilly) and aspart (NovoLog, NovoNordisk) were FDA-approved in 1996 and 2000, respectively. Nevertheless, a third rapid-acting analog insulin approved by the FDA in 2004, **glulisine** (Apidra, Sanofi-Aventis), has expanded the available options. Glulisine, like the other rapid-acting analogs, has an approximate onset of action of <15 minutes, peak action at 30 to 90 minutes, and a duration of action of 3 to 4 hours. Glulisine is approved for dosing from 15 minutes before to 20 minutes after starting a meal, and it is approved for use with insulin pumps.

B. Long-acting analog insulins. The development of long-acting analog insulins followed on the heels of the rapid-acting analogs. Glargine (Lantus, Sanofi-Aventis) was the first of these, FDA-approved in 2000. The second and latest long-acting insulin analog, approved by the FDA in 2005, is **detemir** (Levemir, NovoNordisk). It is indicated for patients with type 1 diabetes and for adults with type 2 diabetes who require long-acting insulin. Detemir is relatively peakless, its approximate onset of action is 45 to 120 minutes, and its duration of action is 6 to 23 hours, depending on dose. Its prolonged duration of action occurs because of slow absorption from the injection site and slow distribution to target tissues from strong self-association and albumin binding. Clinical trials comparing basal-bolus regimens using detemir versus NPH insulin in type 1 diabetes and comparing add-on basal insulin using detemir versus NPH insulin in type 2 diabetes demonstrate detemir to have equivalent reductions in $HbA1c$ and glucoses with less within-subject variability in fasting glucoses and somewhat less weight gain than with NPH.

C. Inhaled insulin. The search for a noninjectable alternative means of delivering insulin has been ongoing for over a decade. Investigators have pursued oral, buccal, and intranasal routes of delivery. However, with the FDA approval of Pfizer's **inhaled insulin** (**Exubera**, Pfizer; Fig. 48.2) in 2006, it was the inhaled route that was the first noninjectable insulin to be successful. At the time of this publication, despite its FDA approval, Pfizer has decided to no longer market Exubera for commercial use. However, other pharmaceutical companies are also developing inhaled insulin products that are currently in Phase II and Phase III clinical trials.

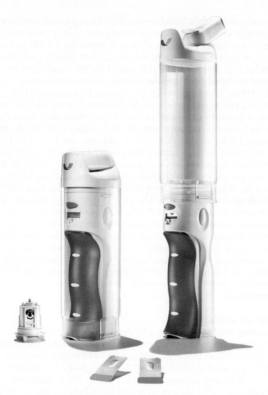

Figure 48.2. The Exubera inhaled insulin device.

The insulin in Exubera is recombinant human insulin in dry-powder form. The dry insulin powder is aerosolized within a chamber and then inhaled from a mouthpiece. The insulin is delivered into the pulmonary tree, where it is rapidly absorbed into the blood via the large alveolar vascular bed.

Inhaled insulin has an onset of action that is similar to that of subcutaneous rapid-acting insulin analogs and has a duration of action that is comparable to that of subcutaneous regular insulin. As such, it does not replace long-acting or basal insulins. In the major Exubera clinical trials of type 1 diabetes, inhaled insulin was demonstrated to have efficacy comparable to that of subcutaneous regular insulin administered premeal three times a day. In clinical trials of patients with type 2 diabetes, Exubera was shown to be effective as monotherapy, as add-on therapy to oral antidiabetic medications, or as prandial insulin in patients using longer-acting insulin.

Exubera was contraindicated in patients who have smoked within 6 months of starting, or who have unstable or poorly controlled pulmonary disease. Although some patients with mild-moderate asthma or chronic obstructive pulmonary disease (COPD) participated in the Phase III trials of Exubera, its safety and efficacy in these patients were not systematically assessed. Declines in pulmonary function tests (PFTs) were seen with Exubera.

IV. INSULIN PUMPS

Although insulin pumps have been around for many years, they have also had significant advances in the last few years. Each pump has its own specific combination of features that must be considered when deciding which is best suited for a particular patient.

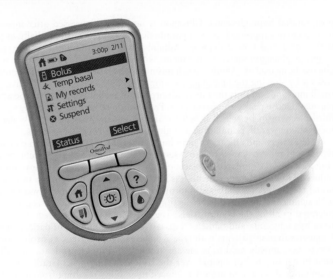

Figure 48.3. OmniPod Insulin System. The OmniPod *(right)* attaches to the skin. It holds the insulin and self-contained catheter. The personal device manager *(left)* is used to program and control insulin delivery by the OmniPod.

Pumps have been improved so that the amount of insulin being delivered can be adjusted in extremely small increments for insulin-sensitive patients—some can be adjusted by as small as 0.025 U per hour for basal rates and 0.05 U per hour for bolus doses. Manufacturers have made pumps smaller and lighter, and some are waterproof. Similar to blood glucometers, software programs have also been improved so that data are downloadable from pumps to provide user-friendly reports.

One of the unique advances in insulin pump technology has come with the **Omni-Pod System** (Insulet Corporation; Fig. 48.3), which was approved by the FDA in 2005. It is the first insulin pump system that does not use an infusion line. The OmniPod, which holds the insulin and a self-contained canula, which automatically inserts under the skin, is attached to the skin with an adhesive. A wireless hand-held device is then used to control the OmniPod, programming basal rates and bolus doses. After 3 days, the empty OmniPod is replaced with a new one.

V. ANTIDIABETIC MEDICATIONS
Until the mid-1990s, insulin and sulfonylureas (SFUs) were the only classes of medications available to treat type 1 and/or type 2 diabetes. The next 10 years saw the introduction of insulin analogs, α-glucosidase inhibitors, nonsulfonylurea insulin secretagogs, biguanides, and thiazolidinediones (TZDs). Now, in the last few years, three new drugs in completely different classes of antidiabetic medications have been FDA-approved, and a fourth is in the process of FDA review.

A. Amylin analog. Amylin is a 37-amino-acid hormone that is collocated and cosecreted with insulin from the β cell in response to nutrient intake. Amylin acts to regulate the glucose homeostasis during the postprandial period, but in people with diabetes, amylin secretion is abnormal; an absolute <u>deficiency in amylin is seen in type 1 diabetes</u>, and insufficient amylin secretion is seen in type 2 diabetes.

Pramlintide (Symlin, Amylin) is a synthetic analog of amylin that has all the effects of amylin, namely, it suppresses inappropriate postprandial glucagon secretion, slows gastric emptying, and enhances satiety to help maintain glucose homeostasis in patients with diabetes. Glucagon secretion is an important contributor to postprandial hyperglycemia. Glucagon is normally suppressed after meals but is inadequately suppressed or even paradoxically elevated postprandially in patients with type 1 and type 2 diabetes. Administration of pramlintide suppresses inappropriate glucagon secretion in patients with diabetes, thereby helping to maintain glucose homeostasis. Another mechanism by which pramlintide helps control glucoses is by slowing the rate of gastric emptying. By slowing nutrient delivery to the small intestine and thus the rate of absorption of carbohydrates, early postprandial plasma glucose peaks are diminished. Pramlintide's effect of enhancing satiety is a third mechanism by which it helps maintain glucose homeostasis. By decreasing food intake overall, pramlintide acts globally to control glucose levels.

The safety and efficacy of pramlintide as an adjunct to insulin in patients with type 1 and type 2 diabetes were assessed in several long-term, placebo-controlled clinical studies. Compared to placebo, adjunctive pramlintide therapy consistently reduced HbA$_{1c}$, and did so with less total daily insulin. In contrast to most traditional treatments for diabetes, improvements in glycemic control were associated with significant and sustained reductions in weight. Pramlintide was generally well tolerated in all of the clinical trials. The most commonly reported adverse effects were hypoglycemia and nausea. Nausea was more common in patients with type 1 diabetes than in patients with type 2 diabetes. Nevertheless, gastrointestinal side effects were mostly mild to moderate in intensity, dose-dependent, generally transient in nature, and dissipated over the course of treatment. Gradual titration of pramlintide dosing minimizes the reduced tolerability resulting from nausea.

Pramlintide is FDA-approved as an adjunct to mealtime insulin in patients with type 1 or type 2 diabetes who are unable to achieve glycemic goals despite optimized insulin therapy. In patients with type 2 diabetes who are using insulin, pramlintide can be used concurrently with metformin and/or sulfonylureas. It is important to note that although pramlintide itself does not cause hypoglycemia, the addition of pramlintide to an insulin-based regimen can increase the risk of insulin-induced hypoglycemia. Therefore, patients should pre-emptively reduce mealtime insulin doses to prevent insulin-induced hypoglycemia upon initiation of pramlintide.

B. Incretin mimetics. It had been observed that insulin secretion was more robust following an oral glucose load than an intravenous glucose load despite producing the same glucose excursion. Hormones released from the gastrointestinal tract in response to oral intake, called incretins, are responsible for this phenomenon of enhanced insulin secretion, termed the incretin effect (Fig. 48.4). The incretin effect is diminished or even absent in patients with type 2 diabetes.

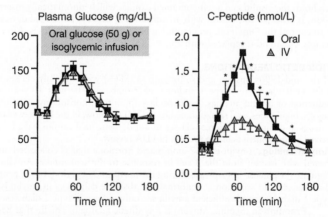

Figure 48.4. The incretin effect. Endogenous insulin secretion is greater for the same glucose excursion if glucose is given orally versus intravenously. (Adapted from Nauck MA, et al. *J Clin Endocrinol Metab.* 1986;63:492–498.)

GLP-1 is a naturally occurring incretin in humans that is rapidly degraded within minutes of release. Infusions of GLP-1 in patients with type 2 diabetes increase insulin secretion and improve fasting and postprandial glucose levels. Furthermore, the enhanced insulin secretion is glucose-dependent, which means that when glucose levels are elevated, insulin secretion is increased; but when glucose levels are normal or low, insulin secretion is no longer stimulated. GLP-1 has additional biologic effects that make it a particularly attractive therapeutic agent for type 2 diabetes. GLP-1 infusions have been shown to inhibit inappropriate glucagon secretion that occurs in type 2 diabetes. It slows the absorption of carbohydrates by slowing gastric emptying and serves to blunt peak postprandial glucose excursions. GLP-1 also has direct effects on appetite and enhances satiety, resulting in weight loss in most treated patients. Finally, from in vitro and in vivo studies, GLP-1 may improve β-cell function and preserve or increase islet cell mass.

Exenatide (Byetta, Amylin Pharmaceuticals, San Diego, CA, and Eli Lilly Co., Indianapolis, IN) is the first GLP-1 mimetic to be approved by the FDA. It is an injectable medication that is a synthetic version of exendin-4, a 39-amino-acid peptide originally purified from the saliva of the Gila monster (*Heloderma suspectum*). Exenatide has all the same effects of native GLP-1 but has greater potency and longer duration of action. Twice-daily exenatide is FDA-indicated as an adjunct for patients with type 2 diabetes who are inadequately controlled on a sulfonylurea, metformin, a TZD, a combination of metformin and a sulfonylurea, or a combination of metformin and a TZD.

In large randomized, placebo-controlled trials, the safety and efficacy of exenatide were examined as add-on therapy to sulfonylureas, metformin with and without sulfonylureas, and TZDs with or without metformin. Exenatide significantly reduced fasting and postprandial glucoses. In these trials, exenatide, 10 μg twice a day, reduced HbA$_{1c}$ by 0.9% to 1.0% compared to placebo. In addition, compared to placebo, there was weight loss of 1.3 to 2.8 kg by the studies' end. In 82-week open-label extensions of three of these studies, progressive weight loss (4 to 5 kg total weight loss) has been seen while maintaining glycemic control over that period. The adverse effects of exenatide were generally gastrointestinal in nature but were mild in severity, tended to occur at the initiation of therapy, and improved over time. Hypoglycemia rates with exenatide were slightly increased when added to sulfonylureas, either alone or in combination, but were not greater than placebo when added to metformin or TZDs. Other studies showed that in type 2 diabetes patients who were inadequately controlled on metformin and a sulfonylurea, the addition of exenatide versus insulin glargine or 70/30 biphasic aspart achieved comparable improvements in HbA$_{1c}$. However, significant weight gain was seen with the addition of insulin and weight loss seen with the addition of exenatide, producing a difference of 4.1 to 5.4 kg between the treatment groups by the end of the studies.

Liraglutide (NovoNordisk) is a GLP-1 analog that has recently entered the Phase III stage of development. Liraglutide binds noncovalently to albumin, resulting in a half-life of ~10 to 14 hours, so it can be given as a once-daily and possibly a once-weekly injection. Early data show that liraglutide significantly reduces fasting and postprandial glucose, improves levels of HbA$_{1c}$ by as much as 1.75%, and prevents weight gain or induces modest weight loss.

C. Dipeptidyl peptidase-4 (DPP-4) inhibitors. The incretins, GLP-1 and glucose-dependent insulinotropic polypeptide (GIP), are rapidly inactivated by the ubiquitous DPP-4 enzyme within minutes of release. Therefore, an alternative approach to harness the benefits of incretins is to increase endogenous levels of GLP-1 and GIP by inhibiting their metabolism. DPP-4 inhibitors reduce serum DPP-4 enzyme activity by >80% and increase active GIP and GLP-1 levels. In contrast to GLP-1 mimetics, which are injected subcutaneously, DPP-4 inhibitors are oral medications. DPP-4 inhibitors are generally not associated with slowing of gastric emptying and do not induce weight loss, though they do not cause weight gain.

Sitagliptin (Januvia, Merck) is the first DPP-4 inhibitor to be approved by the FDA. The efficacy and safety of add-on sitagliptin therapy have been demonstrated in several randomized, placebo-controlled trials of patients with type 2 diabetes treated with diet and exercise alone, metformin, or TZDs. Sitagliptin, 100 mg daily, significantly lowers fasting and postprandial glucose. Placebo-subtracted reductions in HbA_{1c} ranged from $\sim$0.65% to 0.79% in these studies. Overall, sitagliptin was well tolerated, hypoglycemia and gastrointestinal adverse events were no different than with placebo, and there were no significant changes in weight.

Sitagliptin was compared against glipizide monotherapy in patients with type 2 diabetes who were previously uncontrolled by metformin alone. Comparable reductions in HbA_{1c} were seen with sitagliptin, 100 mg daily, and glipizide, up to 20 mg daily. In this study, sitagliptin-treated patients had mean weight loss of 1.5 kg, compared to mean weight gain of 1.1 kg in glipizide-treated patients. Sitagliptin-treated patients also had less hypoglycemia.

Sitagliptin is currently FDA-indicated to improve glycemic control in patients with type 2 diabetes as monotherapy or as combination therapy with metformin or TZDs.

Vildagliptin (Galvus, Novartis) is a second DPP-4 inhibitor that is currently in the FDA approval process. In placebo-controlled studies, vildagliptin induced placebo-subtracted reductions in HbA_{1c} of 0.5% to 1.1% when added to diet and exercise, metformin, or pioglitazone. Vildagliptin has also been demonstrated to lower fasting and postprandial glucose and to enhance insulin secretion. There was no significant weight loss, nor were there differences in adverse events compared to placebo. In a noninferiority study, vildagliptin monotherapy had comparable HbA_{1c} reductions to rosiglitazone monotherapy, and it did not produce the weight gain seen with rosiglitazone. The FDA's decision on approval is expected in the near future.

D. **Endocannabinoid (CB) receptor antagonists.** Investigation of the endocannabinoid system has revealed that it plays a complex role in the regulation of metabolic, cardiovascular, and inflammatory response. CB1 receptors are found extensively throughout the central nervous system (CNS), and it is believed that activity in the CNS plays an important role in food intake. In addition, CB1 receptors are found in peripheral tissues such as the gut, liver, pancreas, muscle, and adipose tissue. In many in vitro, in vivo, and animal studies, the metabolic effects of these peripheral CB1 receptors have been elucidated. CB1 antagonism has been demonstrated to enhance glucose uptake, decrease hepatic enzymes involved in fatty acid synthesis, decrease adipose cell size, induce adipose cell differentiation, decrease adipose tissue lipoprotein lipase, increase adiponectin levels, and decrease ghrelin, leptin, and resist secretion. Meanwhile, activation of the CB1 receptor has been demonstrated to have opposite effects. CB1 receptor–knockout mice and CB1 receptor antagonist–treated mice are lean and resistant to diet-induced obesity.

Rimonabant (Accomplia, Sanofi-Aventis) is the first CB receptor antagonist to be used in clinical practice, approved in 2006 for use in Europe. It is a potent antagonist of the CB1 receptor. A series of studies called the RIO (Rimonabant in Obesity) trials has been conducted in different specific populations to examine its effects on weight as well as other cardiometabolic parameters. In the RIO-Diabetes study, overweight or obese patients with type 2 diabetes treated with metformin or a sulfonylurea were randomized to receive placebo or rimonabant. After 1 year, patients treated with 20 mg of rimonabant daily had a mean weight change of -5.3 kg from baseline, which was significantly greater than with placebo (-1.4 kg). In fact, $\sim$50% of rimonabant-treated subjects achieved >5% weight loss from baseline. HbA_{1c} improved significantly, by 0.7% compared to placebo (placebo +0.1%), which could not be accounted for by weight loss alone. The incidence of adverse events that led to discontinuation was slightly greater in the 20-mg/day rimonabant group, mainly because of depressed mood disorders, nausea, and dizziness.

What impact emerging therapies that target this system will have in type 2 diabetes is yet to be determined. The endocannabinoid system plays an important role in food intake, weight, lipogenesis, and glucose homeostasis.

VI. ISLET CELL TRANSPLANTATION

Following successful islet cell transplantation in rodent models of diabetes in 1972, there was a great deal of excitement about this modality as a feasible option for humans with type 1 diabetes. In the following decades, success rates in humans were far from impressive, but recently, 7 consecutive patients with type 1 diabetes were successfully treated with islet cell transplantation and were able to remain off insulin for 1 year; therefore, excitement in islet cell transplantation as a viable treatment option was renewed.

The success from this study using the "Edmonton protocol" has been partially attributed to stringent patient selection, preparation of islet cells using a xenoprotein-free medium, increased number of transplanted islets, and use of a glucocorticoid-free immunosuppressive regimen. The results of an international multicenter trial organized by the Immune Tolerance Network and designed to test the reproducibility of the Edmonton protocol were published in 2006. Of 36 patients with type 1 diabetes who underwent islet cell transplantation, 16 (44%) were insulin-independent with adequate glycemic control, 10 (28%) had partial graft function, and 10 (28%) had complete graft loss 1-year posttransplant. Five of the 16 who had achieved insulin independence at 1 year remained insulin-independent at 2 years. Even with only partial graft function, there was still benefit to glycemic control compared to baseline.

However, long-term success has yet to be determined. Furthermore, although glycemic control is improved and reduced rates of diabetic complications may be extrapolated from other outcomes studies (e.g., DCCT), there are no outcomes data to demonstrate that islet cell transplantation affects micro- or macrovascular complications. Another limiting factor in the widespread use of this treatment modality is the availability of sufficient islet cells. Given these issues, widespread implementation of islet cell transplantation will be slow to come, and selection of recipients for current transplantation must be strict.

With renewed interest in islet cell transplantation during the last handful of years, refinements in all aspects of the process are being made. There have been improvements in the collection of islets, from pancreas harvesting to pancreas transportation to islet isolation. New techniques and novel pharmacotherapies are being discovered and tested to enhance islet survival, prevent islet cell apoptosis, and even promote islet growth.

VII. CONCLUDING COMMENTS

There have been many exciting new developments in the management of diabetes. Developments in blood glucose meters and insulin pumps have improved the devices already available. The release of new insulin analogs has increased the options available to caregivers. Although islet cell transplantation remains largely an experimental procedure, the many advances in islet cell transplantation have brought it closer to being a viable treatment for some patients with type 1 diabetes.

In addition, the last few years have seen the development and release of several novel first-in-class devices and medications. The advent of continuous glucose monitors holds great promise to allow more intensive glucose management without increasing hypoglycemia rates. The approval of the first noninjectable insulin has made insulin more palatable for many patients. Therapies are now available that take advantage of multiple pancreatic and gut hormones not previously targeted. Moreover, these medications do not cause weight gain, which has been a major disadvantage of older therapies. How these new advances will ultimately be used is yet to be determined, but they will no doubt play central roles in how we will manage diabetes.

Selected References

Apidra [package insert]. Kansas City, MO: Aventis Pharmaceuticals; 2005.

Aschner P, Kipnes MS, Lunceford JK, et al. Sitagliptin Study 021 Group. Effect of the dipeptidyl peptidase-4 inhibitor sitagliptin as monotherapy on glycemic control in patients with type 2 diabetes. *Diabetes Care* 2006;29:2632–2637.

Blonde L, Klein EJ, Han J, et al. Interim analysis of the effects of exenatide treatment on A1C, weight and cardiovascular risk factors over 82 weeks in 314 overweight patients with type 2 diabetes. *Diabetes Obes Metab* 2006;8:436–447.

Bosi E, Camisasca RP, Collober C, et al. Effects of vildagliptin on glucose control over 24 weeks in patients with type 2 diabetes inadequately controlled with metformin. *Diabetes Care* 2007;30:890–895.

Charbonnel B, Karasik A, Liu J, et al. Sitagliptin Study 022 Group. Efficacy and safety of the dipeptidyl peptidase-4 inhibitor sitagliptin added to ongoing metformin therapy in patients with type 2 diabetes inadequately controlled with metformin alone. *Diabetes Care* 2006;29:2638–2643.

Dreyer M; for the Exubera Phase 3 Study Group. Efficacy and 2-year pulmonary safety data of inhaled insulin as adjunctive therapy with metformin or glibenclamide in type 2 diabetes patients poorly controlled with oral monotherapy. *Diabetologia* 2004;47(suppl 1):A44.

Dungan KM, Buse JB, Largay J, et al. 1,5-Anhydroglucitol and postprandial hyperglycemia as measured by continuous glucose monitoring system in moderately controlled patients with diabetes. *Diabetes Care* 2006;29:1214–1219.

Garg S, Schwartz S, Edelman S. Improved glucose excursions using an implantable real-time continuous glucose sensor in adults with type 1 diabetes. *Diabetes Care* 2004;27:734–738.

Garg S, Zisser H, Schwartz S, et al. Improvement in glycemic excursions with a transcutaneous, real-time continuous glucose sensor. *Diabetes Care* 2006;29:44–50.

Haak T, Tiengo A, Draeger E, et al. Lower within-subject variability of fasting blood glucose and reduced weight gain with insulin detemir compared to NPH insulin in patients with type 2 diabetes. *Diabetes Obes Metab* 2005;7:56–64.

Hermansen K, Davies M, Derezinski T, et al. A 26-week, randomized, parallel, treat-to-target trial comparing insulin detemir with NPH insulin as add-on therapy to oral glucose-lowering drugs in insulin naive people with type 2 diabetes. *Diabetes Care* 2006;29:1269–1274.

Hollander PA, Blonde L, Rowe R, et al. Efficacy and safety of inhaled insulin (Exubera) compared with subcutaneous insulin therapy in patients with type 2 diabetes: results of a 6-month, randomized, comparative trial. *Diabetes Care* 2004;27:2356–2362.

Hollander PA, Levy P, Fineman MS, et al. Pramlintide as an adjunct to insulin therapy improves long-term glycemic and weight control in patients with type 2 diabetes: a 1-year randomized controlled trial. *Diabetes Care* 2003;26:784–790.

Kolendorf K, Ross GP, Pavliv-Renar I, et al. Insulin detemir lowers the risk of hypoglycemia and provides more consistent plasma glucose levels compared with NPH insulin in type 1 diabetes. *Diabet Med* 2006;23:729–735.

McGill JB, Cole TG, Nowatzke W, et al. Circulating 1,5-anhydroglucitol levels in adult patients with diabetes reflect longitudinal changes of glycemia: a U.S. trial of the Glyco-Mark assay. *Diabetes Care* 2004;27:1859–1865.

Nauck MA, Homberger E, Siegel EG, et al. Incretin effects of increasing glucose loads in man calculated from venous insulin and C-peptide responses. *J Clin Endocrinol Metab* 1986;63:492–498.

Quattrin T, Belanger A, Bohannon N, et al. Efficacy and safety of inhaled insulin (Exubera) compared with subcutaneous insulin therapy in patients with type 1 diabetes: results of a 6-month, randomized, comparative trial. *Diabetes Care* 2004;27:2622–2627.

Rosenstock J, Baron MA, Dejager S, et al. Comparison of vildagliptin and rosiglitazone monotherapy in patients with type 2 diabetes: a 24-week, double-blind, randomized trial. *Diabetes Care* 2007;30:217–223.

Scheen AJ, Finer N, Hollander P, et al.; RIO-Diabetes Study Group. Efficacy and tolerability of rimonabant in overweight or obese patients with type 2 diabetes: a randomised controlled study. *Lancet* 2006;368:1660–1672.

Shapiro AM, Ricordi C, Hering BJ, et al. International trial of the Edmonton protocol for islet transplantation. *N Engl J Med* 2006;355:1318–1330.

Whitehouse F, Kruger DF, Fineman M, et al. A randomized study and open-label extension evaluating the long-term efficacy of pramlintide as an adjunct to insulin therapy in type 1 diabetes. *Diabetes Care* 2003;26:3074–3079.

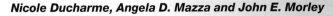
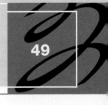

DIABETES MELLITUS AND THE GERIATRIC PATIENT

49

Nicole Ducharme, Angela D. Mazza and John E. Morley

$\mathcal{D}$iabetes mellitus is a common disease in the elderly population. The prevalence of diabetes increases dramatically with age. By the age of 75 years, ~20% of the U.S. population is afflicted with this illness. It is estimated that by 2025, the incidence of diabetes will increase by 42%, affecting 300 million people. The interaction of many factors, including increased body mass, decreased exercise, medications, coexisting illness, and insulin secretory defects associated with the aging process, all play a role in the development of alteration in glucose tolerance in older people. Elderly people with diabetes have experienced not only an increase in its associated morbidity and mortality but also a decline in function and quality of life. Diabetes in this population is associated with an increase in falls that can result in severely debilitating injury. Diabetes is also associated with vascular dementia, which ultimately leads to decline in cognitive function. Diabetes puts patients at risk for pressure ulcers and congestive heart failure secondary to diastolic dysfunction. Diabetes is a common cause of urinary incontinence and increases the propensity to develop life-threatening infections, such as tuberculosis. Elderly diabetics are more likely to develop hyperosmolar nonketotic coma and have worse outcomes (higher mortality) than middle-aged diabetics. Despite the high prevalence of diabetes and its associated morbidity and death in the aged, most studies on diabetes have focused on middle-aged subjects. Although there are many similarities between diabetes in middle-aged and elderly subjects, there are unique aspects of diabetes in the elderly.

I. PATHOPHYSIOLOGY OF HYPERGLYCEMIA OF AGING

Spence first described aging in association with increase in fasting and postprandial blood glucose levels. Some potential aspects of pathophysiology involved in the development of this "hyperglycemia of aging" are briefly discussed in the following.

A. Metabolic changes and autoimmune abnormalities.
Recent studies found that all elderly diabetic patients had absent first-phase insulin release. Second-phase insulin release was impaired profoundly in lean elderly type 2 diabetics. Also, compared with younger subjects, the elderly type 2 diabetics had normal fasting hepatic glucose production, and fasting hepatic glucose production was suppressed normally in response to insulin infusion. Unlike middle-aged subjects, lean elderly type 2 diabetic patients seldom had minimal resistance to insulin-mediated glucose disposal. However, consistent with the evidence in middle-aged subjects, marked resistance to insulin-mediated glucose disposal was observed in obese elderly type 2 diabetic patients. These data suggest that an impairment in glucose-induced insulin release is the primary metabolic defect in lean elderly type 2 diabetics, whereas in obese elderly subjects, the primary abnormality is resistance to insulin-mediated glucose disposal, which often occurs in middle-aged persons with type 2 diabetes.

It is well known that autoimmune phenomena play an important role in the pancreatic β-cell failure in type 1 diabetics. Studies have shown that autoimmune abnormalities also may be an important contributing factor to the marked impairment in insulin release that occurs in a significant proportion of lean elderly type 2 diabetics. Human leukocyte antigen haplotypes with associated type 1 diabetes are found with increased frequency in lean elderly type 2 diabetics. Increased frequency of islet-cell antibodies and antibodies to glutamic acid decarboxylase was also found in these subjects.

695

B. In the Health, Aging and Body Composition Study, it was found that diabetes is associated with <u>increased levels of inflammatory markers</u> (C-reactive protein [CRP], interleukin 6 [IL-6], tumor necrosis factor α [TNF-α]). The study also found that among diabetics, those with poor glycemic control had higher levels of CRP. Whether the elevation of inflammatory markers could predict the development of diabetes still needs to be determined by future studies.

C. Additional defect in non–insulin-mediated glucose uptake. Insulin-mediated and non–insulin-mediated-glucose uptake (NIMGU) are the two mechanisms by which the human body uses glucose. Under basal conditions, non–insulin-mediated glucose uptake occurs primarily in the central nervous system. During hyperglycemia, NIMGU is enhanced to a greater extent in skeletal muscle. It is increasingly recognized that alterations in NIMGU play an important role in the pathogenesis of carbohydrate metabolism. The effect of glucose on glucose uptake is impaired in elderly patients with type 2 diabetes; hence, interventions that have been proven to enhance NIMGU in younger diabetics (decrease in free fatty acid levels, exercise, certain oral antihyperglycemic agents, and glucagonlike peptide-1), may have important therapeutic implications in the management of the elderly population afflicted with diabetes.

D. Effects of leptin and amylin

1. Leptin. Leptin is a hormone secreted by fat cells and is a major <u>regulator of adiposity</u>. In rodents, leptin has been demonstrated to decrease food intake and cure the obesity of the congenitally obese mouse, which fail to produce leptin. In humans, the level of leptin in the blood correlates strongly with body weight, percentage of body fat, and body mass index. Abdominal fat cells appear to produce more leptin per cell than do fat cells in the thigh. An analysis of 15-year longitudinal data from the New Mexico Process Study found that leptin levels were highly correlated with the development of insulin resistance in older persons. In addition to the relationship between leptin and waist-to-hip ratio, leptin levels are also influenced strongly by sex hormones. Males have lower leptin levels than females, and testosterone replacement in aging men with androgen deficiency reduces leptin levels. Current data suggest that <u>high leptin levels are at least a marker for insulin resistance</u> and the hyperglycemia of aging and may actually play a role in the pathogenesis of metabolic syndrome.

2. Amylin. Amylin is a peptide hormone secreted along with insulin from pancreatic β cells. Amylin inhibits the second phase of insulin secretion and inhibits effects of insulin on the liver and the muscle. Amylin also decreases food intake, slows gastric emptying, and modulates memory processing. Edwards et al. demonstrated that amylin levels are reduced in middle age at the time of an increase in adiposity. However, as persons grow older, this appropriate decrease in amylin is no longer maintained, so that older people have higher levels of amylin than do middle-aged people. Amylin levels have been found to be highly correlated with elevated postprandial glucose levels.

II. METABOLIC SYNDROME

Metabolic syndrome, popularized by Reaven as syndrome X after the original description by Camus, is a cluster of cardiovascular risk factors, including components of hyperinsulinemia, hypertriglyceridemia, hypertension, hyperglycemia, hyperuricemia, and altered clotting factors. Metabolic syndrome is more prevalent with increasing age, <u>affecting half of adults aged 60 years and over</u>. Emerging evidence has suggested new insight into the pathogenesis of this syndrome. The production of TNF-α from adipocytes has been correlated with the development of diabetes and insulin resistance. TNF-α and other cytokines activate inducible nitric oxide synthase. There is evidence that nitric oxide synthase has a role in the production of insulin resistance. Insulin sensitizers, such as metformin and the thiazolidinediones, have been shown to inhibit nitric oxide synthase activity. The increasing available data strongly suggest that nitric oxide has an important role in the pathogenesis of insulin resistance and the metabolic syndrome. By definition, metabolic syndrome incorporates some established risk factors (e.g., hypertension and diabetes) that contribute to its association with cardiovascular disease. However, there is conflicting evidence about whether metabolic syndrome itself may predict cardiovascular risk more strongly than its individual components. Data showing that metabolic syndrome is associated with increased coronary risk independent of Framingham risk score category suggests that metabolic syndrome is associated with risk that is not entirely accounted for by traditional vascular risk factors. This highlights the important association between metabolic syndrome and other nontraditional atherogenic risk factors linked to insulin resistance (e.g., elevated triglyceride-rich lipoproteins, small dense low-density lipoprotein [LDL] particles, postprandial lipemia, endothelial dysfunction, low-grade inflammation, and prothrombotic state, which are not routinely measured in clinical practice. Prospective studies have established that metabolic syndrome is associated with a doubling of the risk of cardiovascular disease. This risk also extends to people with metabolic syndrome who do not have diabetes. **The presence of metabolic syndrome in individuals without diabetes markedly increases the likelihood of developing type 2 diabetes (approximately sevenfold).** The treatment for metabolic syndrome is aimed primarily at reducing long-term risk of cardiovascular disease and diabetes. Current guidelines recommend focusing on intensive therapeutic lifestyle interventions (such as increased physical activity, dietary modification, and modest weight reduction) that address many of the metabolic risk factors in metabolic syndrome, including insulin resistance. When necessary, pharmacologic agents should be used to achieve recommended therapeutic target goals set forth by guidelines. Among nursing home residents, 50% have either diabetes mellitus or metabolic syndrome.

III. MONITORING OF LONG-TERM DIABETIC CONTROL

A. Glycated hemoglobin. Hemoglobin is a protein that transports oxygen throughout the body and is located inside red blood cells (RBCs). The lifespan of a RBC is 120 days, and in turn the lifespan of hemoglobin is related to the lifespan of the RBC in which it resides. During the 120 days, hemoglobin is exposed to glucose in the circulation. Glycation of the glucose to the hemoglobin is what we are measuring when we order a HbA_{1c}, the most widely used measure for monitoring diabetic control. However, any condition that interferes with the RBC lifespan will affect the HbA_{1c}, and this should be taken into consideration when interpreting the value. Conditions such as hereditary spherocytosis, hemolysis, sickle cell anemia, thalassemias, and acute/chronic blood loss all decrease the time of exposure of hemoglobin protein to circulating glucose, therefore decreasing the glycosylation process, which results in a falsely low HbA_{1c} being reported. On the other hand, any condition that lengthens the lifespan of the RBC, such as vitamin B_{12} deficiency, folate-deficiency anemia, or iron-deficiency anemia, increases the glycation process and results in a falsely elevated HbA_{1c}.

B. Fructosamine. Fructosamine is a glycosylated albumin that provides information on shorter periods (2 to 3 weeks) of diabetic control than does HbA_{1c} (3 to 4 months). Results differ between the two measurements mainly because of the difference in turnover times of the underlying glycation targets, hemoglobin versus serum proteins. Fructosamine is inexpensive and performs well in elderly diabetic subjects when corrected for albumin, which is why **we believe that fructosamine is preferable to HbA_{1c} for monitoring glucose control in elderly diabetics.** However, one must take into consideration certain conditions, such as paraproteinemias and nephropathies, which may interfere with the result.

C. Hyperglycemic coma. There are three typical types of hyperglycemic coma: ketoacidotic, hyperosmolar nonketotic, and lactic acidotic. Approximately 10% of elderly persons with new-onset diabetes manifest the type 1 form of the disease and therefore may present with ketoacidotic coma, which usually occurs in young subjects. Moreover, older persons with long-standing type 2 diabetes can develop pancreatic β-cell "exhaustion" and convert to type 1 diabetes. Therefore, mixed hyperosmolar ketotic comas may be seen in these older persons with diabetes. The diagnosis of ketoacidotic coma is confirmed by detection of ketones in the blood.

Urine ketones often are a nonspecific marker of starvation if an elderly diabetic subject person has negative ketones in the blood.

D. Ketoacidosis. Malone et al. analyzed the unique characteristics of ketoacidosis in the elderly and found that elderly diabetics were more likely to be on insulin or to have had a prior episode of ketoacidosis than younger subjects. In contrast to younger persons, more insulin was needed in older persons to stabilize their glucose levels. The mortality rate was much higher in older patients than in younger subjects. Older patients were hospitalized 6 days longer than younger persons following an episode of ketoacidosis.

E. Nonketotic hyperosmolar coma. Nonketotic hyperosmolar coma was first described and characterized in 1957 by Sament, DeGraef, and Lips. It only occurs predominantly in elderly type 2 diabetics, with the mean age of patients being between 57 and 69 years, in whom dehydration and severe hyperglycemia may occur without development of ketoacidosis. The diagnosis is made by a serum osmolality >320 mOsm/L and a glucose >600 mg/dL. Associated findings may include severe azotemia, lactic acidosis (giving a mixed presentation), and hypernatremia or hyponatremia (secondary to hyperglycemia inhibiting arginine vasopressin). Nursing home residents are particularly more likely to develop hyperosmolar coma. Acute infection is the most common precipitating factor. Mortality rates are relatively high, with most recently reported rates ranging between 14% and 17%. Severe hyperosmolarity, residence in a nursing home, and advanced age are the major prognostic factors associated with death.

F. Hypoglycemia. In general, hypoglycemia occurs when the capillary blood glucose level is <40 mg/dL. Hypoglycemia is a serious complication of therapy in elderly patients with diabetes. The frequency of these episodes increases with increasing quality of glycemic control assessed with HbA_{1c}. In the elderly, hypoglycemia can have serious consequences in terms of heart and brain function, and thus can be life-threatening, in addition to increasing morbidity and causing a decline in quality of life. The major reason that clinicians undertreat diabetes in the elderly population is the fear of hypoglycemia, although in reality severe hypoglycemia is relatively rare. Therefore, the risk of hypoglycemia must be evaluated and balanced against the potential benefit of tight glycemic control in each individual. Elderly diabetics are at risk for hypoglycemic events because they tend to experience fewer symptoms. Hypoglycemic unawareness can be related to intensification of the insulin therapy and to repeated, sometimes nonperceived, episodes of hypoglycemia, leading to defective counterregulation that is reversible by strict avoidance of hypoglycemic events. This can be worsened by the duration of diabetes and the presence of autonomic neuropathy. Regarding the frequency of severe hypoglycemic episodes, this is an easier factor to analyze: Such events are recorded because of the resulting emergency hospitalization. The rate could be considered low for patients with type 2 diabetes (0.4 episode per 100 patient-years) or treated with insulin (1.5 episodes per 100 patient-years), according to results observed in a recent study from Germany. These results are in agreement with those observed in a Chinese population of diabetics, for whom it was reported that the annual incidence was 1.4% for all diabetic patients, but higher in men (3.5%) and women (6.8%) >60 years of age, with 24% of the population aged 70 to 74 years having experienced severe hypoglycemia. In general, the consequences of hypoglycemia can be more serious in the elderly subject: increased risk of myocardial infarction, ventricular rhythm disorders, and stroke (in a population with an already high cardiovascular risk), as well as the risk of injury and fractures in a predisposed population. The highest risk factor for the development of hypoglycemia in older persons was in the 30 days following hospitalization, with a relative risk of 4.5 (3.5 to 5.7). Other predisposing factors include advanced age, black race, polypharmacy (more than five medications), lack of self-monitoring, unawareness of symptoms, decreased counterregulatory hormones, missed meals, comorbidities such as renal insufficiency, insulin use with or without antihyperglycemic agents, increased number of injections, and the use of rapid-acting insulin. Prevention requires reinforced education, knowledge of signs of hypoglycemia, and appropriate management treatment.

IV. PREVENTION OF LONG-TERM COMPLICATIONS

A. Microvascular. Microvascular complications include <u>retinopathy</u>, which can lead to various degrees of visual impairment; <u>neuropathy</u>, leading to pain and numbness, which is a risk for infected skin ulcers that can lead to amputations; and <u>nephropathy</u>, which can ultimately lead to renal failure. In one study, nearly 10% of subjects had experienced a microvascular complication by 9 years after diagnosis. Nearly half of the cost of treating type 2 diabetes complications has been attributed to microvascular complications. Although tight glycemic control has been clearly demonstrated to significantly decrease long-term complications of diabetes by the Diabetes Control and Complications trial (DCCT) and the UK Prospective Diabetes Study (UKPDS), the question of whether similar outcomes would occur in elderly type 2 diabetics was left unanswered. The Veterans Affairs Cooperative Trial demonstrated the feasibility of tight glucose control in middle-aged and elderly diabetics. Recent evidence showed that progression of retinopathy is markedly decreased with good diabetic control in persons over the age of 60 years. **Almost no retinopathy progression was found in patients with HbA$_{1c}$ levels <7%.** In a retrospective cohort study of 250 patients with at least one microvascular complication, tight glycemic control was associated with <u>reduced risk of additional complications in other organ systems</u>. The Wisconsin Eye Study demonstrated that for each 1% decrease in HbA$_{1c}$ levels in type 2 diabetes, there is an exponential decrease in long-term diabetic complications. These data strongly support the concept that tight glycemic control is also important in elderly diabetic patients even if the resulting effort results in only minor changes.

B. Macrovascular. Whether tight glycemic control reduces macrovascular complications of diabetes is still uncertain. Laakso demonstrated that the lower the HbA$_{1c}$ level, the less likely diabetics are to develop coronary artery disease end points, such as myocardial infarction or death.

V. GLUCOTOXICITY

Hyperglycemia causes numerous signs and symptoms in elderly diabetic patients.

A. Osmotic diuresis. Elevated glucose levels lead to a hyperosmolar diuresis, which has three major consequences: nocturia, incontinence, and dehydration. Older persons are <u>impaired in their ability to recognize thirst</u>. Both animal and human studies have demonstrated that this is secondary to a failure in the u-opioid drinking drive. With diabetes-induced polyuria, the failure to have a normal thirst response leads to mild dehydration, which in turn leads to a generalized feeling of malaise and orthostatic hypotension, increasing the risk of falls and syncope. Incontinence in many older diabetics is not caused by autonomic neuropathy, but rather by polyuria. This incontinence is similar to diuretic-induced incontinence.

Osmotic diuresis leads to:

- Nocturia, dehydration, and orthostasis
- Incontinence
- Hyperosmolar state
- Trace mineral loss; decreased zinc and magnesium

Hyperglycemia leads to a loss of trace elements in the urine. Older diabetics tend to be zinc-deficient. <u>Zinc deficiency</u> becomes important when the diabetic patient develops peripheral vascular disease or pressure ulcers. In this situation, <u>zinc replacement</u> is important for healing the ulcer.

B. Cognitive defects. Studies have shown that hyperglycemia is associated with cognitive difficulties. There is a high prevalence of cognitive dysfunction, depression, and functional impairment among elderly diabetic patients, which causes challenges in their management. Elderly diabetics need to be screened for barriers to safe and effective diabetes control. Goals for diabetes control need to adjusted and simplified based on the patients' cognitive abilities. In diabetic mice, hyperglycemia interferes with memory retention, and a single insulin injection that normalizes glucose levels reverses the retention deficit. Evidence indicates that <u>treatment of diabetes in older persons enhanced cognitive function</u>. Thus, hyperglycemia plays an important role in decreasing compliance in older persons with diabetes.

C. Increased infections. Diabetes has been associated with increased infections, which may be partially explained by a <u>decreased T-cell–mediated immune response</u>. There is conflicting evidence regarding whether common and rare infections are more prevalent among patients with diabetes in comparison to the general population. Patients with diabetes appear to have an increased risk of asymptomatic bacteriuria urinary tract infections, and skin and mucous membrane infections, including *Candida* infections and infections of the foot. Epidemiologic studies support the fact that patients with diabetes are at high risk for complications, hospitalization, and death from influenza and pneumococcal disease. Studies have shown that influenza and pneumococcal vaccines in patients with diabetes have the potential to significantly reduce morbidity and mortality related to influenza and pneumococcal disease. The current recommendation regarding immunizations is that patients should receive the <u>influenza vaccine yearly and the pneumonia vaccine every 5 years</u>. Despite national goals, immunization rates for at-risk patient groups remain low, so we must continue to implement effective strategies to identify at-risk patients and closely monitor their immunization record.

D. Increased pain perception. Hyperglycemia is associated with an increased perception of painful stimuli because elevated glucose levels interfere with the ability of β-endorphin to bind to the opioid receptor and downregulate pain impulses. A classic population based study found some degree of <u>neuropathy in 66%</u> of patients with diabetes. Among those with type 1 and type 2 diabetes, 54% and 45%, respectively, had diabetic peripheral neuropathy, and 15% and 13%, respectively, had subjective complaints. Several studies have demonstrated that the duration of diabetes correlates strongly with the risk of developing peripheral neuropathy. In addition, intensive glycemic control (maintaining HbA_{1c} <7%), particularly when initiated early in the disease process, has also been shown to reduce the prevalence of diabetic peripheral neuropathy. Among patients with type 1 diabetes, intensive glucose control also delays or prevents the development of clinical manifestations of peripheral neuropathy. Comorbidities associated with diabetic peripheral neuropathy include sleep disturbance, depression, and interference with activities of daily living, which has a huge impact on quality of life. The treatment of diabetic peripheral neuropathy includes <u>tricyclic antidepressants,</u> <u>anticonvulsants,</u> and <u>analgesics,</u> but there are no strict guidelines for treatment. Hence, treatment should be geared to each individual patient, and the benefits versus the adverse effects of medications should be assessed and discussed in detail with the patient before prescribing any medication for treatment. This is extremely important in the elderly, in whom polypharmacy, declining renal function, and decline in cognitive skills are issues that can cause adverse events when prescribing any of the above medications.

E. Decreased responsiveness to sulfonylureas. Finally, glucotoxicity can lead to sluggish islet-cell response to sulfonylureas. Lowering the circulating glucose level with insulin can result in improved responsiveness to sulfonylureas.

VI. DIABETES AND FUNCTION

Diabetes mellitus has been identified as a major <u>cause of functional impairment</u> and activities-of-daily-living dependence. Our studies have shown that this impaired function is multifactorial. Diabetes, arthritis, and age of 80 years or older were the three best indicators of inability to complete tests of lower-extremity functioning in a population of 2 873 Mexican Americans aged 6 years and older. Diabetes also is associated with an <u>increase in falls</u> and in particular injurious falls. There is a strong association between diabetes and hip fractures. Type 1 diabetes is associated with a decrease in bone mineral density (BMD); however, type 2 diabetics have normal BMD, likely because of increased body mass index (BMI), but studies have found associations between type 2 diabetes and fractures. A population-based study, assessing the risk of hip fractures in older individuals with diabetes revealed that diabetes was associated with <u>a 20% increase in the risk of hip fractures in both women and men</u>. The risk was 11% for women and 18% for men after adjusting for risk factors for fracture, such as age, medications, comorbidities, and health care utilization.

It is hypothesized that uncontrolled glucose may lead to increased accumulation of advanced glycation end products in bone collagen, which may increase bone stiffness and fracture susceptibility. Hyperglycemia may impair calcium deposition and subsequent mineralization, which impairs bone quality and increases fracture risk. Some studies have also reported an increased risk of fractures with insulin treatment, which might be explained by the fact that insulin treatment may suggest a longer duration of disease or insulin use increases the risk of hypoglycemic events, leading to increased fall risk.

VII. CONGESTIVE HEART FAILURE

The incidence of congestive heart failure (CHF) has doubled in diabetics compared to nondiabetics, and age is one of the major risk factors. The occurrence of CHF in diabetics is probably related to the degree of glycemic control. In some studies, every 1% increase in HbA_{1c} corresponds to a 15% increase in the risk of developing CHF. Of 31 600 U.S. subjects 65 years and older hospitalized for CHF, 27% of whom were 85 years or older, 40% were diabetics. Through advanced glycation end products, chronic hyperglycemia has a specific role in the pathophysiology of myocardial fibrosis leading to diastolic dysfunction. Theoretically, at least at an early stage, strict blood sugar control should be able to slow down left ventricular remodeling. However, at this time there is no evidence of this benefit. The use of antihyperglycemic agents on cardiac function is unknown. However, the use of metformin can be complicated by lactic acidosis in the setting of acute CHF. The insulin-sensitizing effects of thiazolidinediones may have a positive effect on the prevention or treatment of myocyte hypertrophy related to hyperinsulinemia. However, a major side effect of these drugs is water and salt retention, leading to edema and weight gain, which increases the risk of CHF by 1.6 to 1.8 times. Therefore, current recommendations advise against prescribing glitazones to subjects with known left ventricular dysfunction, despite the stage, or to discontinue them if symptoms of CHF develop.

In conclusion, age, diabetes, and arterial hypertension are risk factors for CHF. Myocardial changes that are seen with normal aging are similar to those seen in patients with diabetes, with diabetes considered an accelerator of aging. At this time there is no evidence on how to treat diastolic dysfunction, and prevention should be optimized utilizing tight blood pressure and glucose control.

VIII. DEPRESSION IN ELDERLY DIABETICS

Several cross-sectional studies have found an increased risk in the prevalence of depression among those with diabetes, usually secondary to either poor glycemic control or diabetes-related complications. Prospective studies have also suggested that the course of depression in diabetics is often unfavorable and that persistent depression is common. A recent cohort study of 2 522 subjects aged 70 to 79 years, without baseline depression, showed that diabetes was associated with a 30% increased incidence of depressed mood. A strong relationship was also noted in this study between those with depression and poor glycemic control.

IX. SEXUAL DYSFUNCTION

It is estimated that 40% to 60% of men with diabetes have erectile dysfunction (ED). ED in diabetics is often multifactorial and can result from impaired blood flow, nerve damage, or psychological factors. It is very important to inquire about ED and to take a comprehensive history. A physical exam and a thorough laboratory investigation should be conducted, including a complete blood count, basal metabolic panel, lipid profile, HbA_{1c}, total testosterone, prolactin, luteinizing hormone (LH), and thyroid-stimulating hormone (TSH). An endocrinologist should be consulted if hyperprolactinemia, abnormal thyroid function tests, or a low to normal LH in the setting where a morning total testosterone of <200 is detected. There are no studies to confirm that intensive glycemic control prevents the progression of other complications of diabetes mellitus. Improvement in erectile dysfunction can usually be achieved with a phosphodiesterase-5 inhibitor, e.g., sildenafil, intracavernosal administration of PGE1, or a vacuum device. If none of these treatments is effective, a surgical prosthesis should be considered as an alternative. Diabetes produces a decrease in testosterone levels in men, which accelerates the onset of the androgen deficiency in aging men (ADAM) syndrome. The ADAM syndrome is associated with erectile dysfunction, retrograde ejaculation, and decreased libido, as well as decreased strength and cognitive abnormalities. In women, diabetes may result in vaginal dryness and vaginal infections, particularly *Candida* infections.

X. THERAPEUTIC MANAGEMENT

Diabetes management is a multifaceted task with objectives of decreasing microvascular and macrovascular complications while increasing quality of life. However, in contrast to the general medicine patient, management of the geriatric patient is complicated by different degrees of disease, comorbidities, and polypharmacy, not to mention other considerations, such as living environment (nursing home or home alone).

A. Medical nutrition therapy (MNT). Therapeutic management of diabetes, both type 1 and type 2, in the general population aims initially towards lifestyle modification by way of MNT. The goal of MNT is glucose homeostasis by means of weight management, if not weight loss, usually by way of decreased intake and increased energy expenditure while maintaining sufficient macronutrient as well as micronutrient intake. Although these principles may be appropriately applied to young and middle-aged patients, MNT in the elderly population is less clear because of insufficient data.

1. Diet. Dietary restriction and subsequent weight loss in the geriatric patient results in inadequate micronutrient intake and increased frailty. Moreover, studies in long-term-care facilities have not shown any utility of dietary intervention to control diabetes. Another single study demonstrated increased mortality in older persons with diabetes who lose weight. To date, the American Diabetes Association guidelines do not recommend a therapeutic diet for diabetics in nursing homes.

2. Exercise. Exercise is a key component of all diabetes management. Exercise physiology is based on the shift of fuel usage by the muscle from a fatty acid source to an energy source progression/combination that includes muscle glycogen, circulating glucose, and fatty acids. Glucose uptake continues long after the activity is ceased. Furthermore, exercise, independent of body weight, is effective in reducing HbA_{1c}. For the older diabetic patient, aerobic exercise may be challenging, if not dangerous, considering individual issues, such as vision impairment or peripheral neuropathy. Resistance exercise in older persons, on the other hand, is highly recommended. Resistance exercise training increases muscle mass and endurance while improving body composition and functional status. Increasing evidence shows beneficial effects of resistance training and results in improved overall glucose management.

3. Teamwork approach. The best results are seen with an interdisciplinary approach that involves, most importantly, the patient and/or the patient's family, as well as the physician, nutritionist, and ancillary nursing staff. The patient should be educated about the complications, both short-term and long-term, of poor glucose control, not only to enable the patient to feel a certain amount of personal control over his or her own condition, when feasible, but also to prevent hospitalization and incurrence of substantial medical cost.

B. Medical therapeutics. Therapeutic focus in the long-term-care population shifts toward medical management, ranging from insulin to alternate interventions, such as metformin, sulfonylureas, thiazolidine diones (TZDs), α-glucosidase inhibitors, and, more recently, modulators of the incretin system, listed in Table 49.1. These treatment options have different profiles with regard to risk versus benefit in the geriatric patient. Most of these drugs are well studied in general populations but not in elderly populations, so it is vital to be careful in choosing the specific agent to be implemented and the specific patient who will be taking the agent.

1. Insulin. Insulin is often used when oral hypoglycemic agents fail after a long period of time, and its institution is often too long delayed to produce optimal results. Insulin therapy tends to carry some unnecessary stigmata in the

| TABLE 49.1 | Comorbidities and Barriers in the Management of Diabetic Older Individuals |

Hypertension	Dementia
Depression	Foot problems
Congestive heart failure	Increased frailty
Stroke	Immobility
Decreased vision	Impaired communication
Food and medication allergies	Incontinence

general population, as well as among medical professionals; however, insulin can produce predictable glucose control in the geriatric population if it is implemented correctly. Insulin preparations vary according to structure and resulting half-life. The most common insulin and insulin analog preparations are listed in Table 49.2. Insulin initiation should be tailored to the patient (i.e., renal function, hypoglycemic unawareness) and requires regular blood glucose monitoring. There are a number of different approaches to insulin use in long-term facilities. A common one is to start with a long-acting insulin and use short- or rapid-acting insulin before meals. For those working in long-term-care facilities, bear in mind that meals are not always served punctually and can lead to

| TABLE 49.2 | Currently Available Diabetes Treatment Options for the Geriatric Patient |

Medical nutrition therapy (MNT)	Includes education, exercise, and multidisciplinary team approach

Insulin and insulin analogs	Rapid-acting:
	     Insulin lispo (Humalog)
	     Insulin aspart (Novolog)
	     Insulin glulisine (Apidra)
	 Short-acting:
	     Regular (Humulin R, Novolin R)
	 U-500
	 Intermediate-acting:
	     NPH (Humulin N, Novolin N)
	 Long-acting:
	     Insulin glargine (Lantus)
	     Insulin detemir (Levemir)

Oral agents: Sulfonylureas	Inhaled insulin (Exubera) Glipizide Glyburide Glimepiride Chlorpropamide
Meglitinides	Nateglinide Repaglinide
Biguanides	Metformin
Thiazolidinediones (TZDs)	Rosiglitazone Pioglitazone
α-Glucosidase inhibitors	Acarbose Miglitol
Incretin mimetics and dipeptidyl-peptidase IV (DPP IV) inhibitors	Exenatide (Byetta) Sitagliptan (Januvia)

hypoglycemia, Multiple insulin mixtures (not listed), either intermediate/rapid or intermediate/short, exist. Insulin mixtures, although they may seem in theory to be easy to use, do not allow "fine tuning" of therapy and often lead to extreme peaks and valleys. It is also important to reassess any previous oral hypoglycemic agents once insulin therapy is initiated, to prevent augmenting hypoglycemia.

2. **Sulfonylureas.** Sulfonylureas are a class of drugs that target hyperglycemia through enhancing insulin secretion from the β cells of the pancreas. Their principal target is the adenosine triphosphate (ATP)-sensitive potassium (K-ATP) channel of the β-cell membrane. Inhibition of this channel, by either glucose or sulfonylureas, results in the triggering and opening to voltage-gated calcium channels, leading to calcium influx into the cell and insulin exocytosis. Members of this class are mostly similar, varying mainly in half-time and potency, depending largely on level of K-ATP channel activity and its subunits. Sulfonylureas should be used cautiously in elderly patients, as well as in anyone with hepatic and renal failure, for fear of hypoglycemia.

3. **Meglitinides.** A class of insulin secretagogs with rapid onset and short half-life are the meglitinides. Available members are **repaglinide** and **nateglinide**. Side effects of meglitinides are quite similar to those of sulfonylureas, and the meglitinides should be used cautiously, if at all, in geriatric patients.

4. **Biguanides. Metformin** is the sole available member of the biguanide class. It works to decrease hepatic glucose production while increasing hepatic glucose uptake, without having any effect on insulin secretion. Metformin is widely used in the general obese type 2 diabetic population for these hepatic effects. Anorexia and weight loss are also seen commonly, most probably through inhibition of nitric oxide synthase. Although weight loss is desirable in the obese younger patient, it is not desirable in the geriatric patient and leads to frailty. Metformin is not recommended for use in persons over the age of 80 years or in persons with renal failure. Older persons frequently have muscle breakdown, or sarcopenia, that can mask renal insufficiency, further limiting its use in this population.

5. **Thiazolinediones (TZDs).** TZDs are a class of drugs that can also improve insulin sensitivity. **Rosiglitazone** and **pioglitazone** are members of this class. These drugs have recently been found to be important in our understanding of diabetes as well as the subject of recent controversy. TZDs work via the peroxisome proliferator-activated receptor-γ (PPARγ) to promote insulin sensitivity at the level of the liver as well as muscle. Recent research has focused on TZDs and adipokines, most importantly adiponectin. Adiponectin is produced by adipocytes and appears to enhance insulin effects on hepatic gluconeogenesis. Activators of PPAR-γ have also been shown to increase adiponectin levels, a concept that may be important to current research in diabetes prevention. On a more clinical level, the DREAM trial showed substantial reductions in the incidence of diabetes in high-risk individuals with TZD treatment for 3 years. In the long-term-care setting, insulin resistance is associated with a proinflammatory state, while TZD treatment has been observed, through ubiquitin-proteasome activity analysis, to decrease inflammation. Improvement in homocystinemia in diabetic patients was also recognized with the addition of this pharmacologic agent. Alternately, the benefits of TZDs have been questioned, especially in the older population, by research that shows that activation of PPAR-γ may promote differentiation of bone marrow–derived progenitor cells toward adipocytes. A later clinical observational study supports the hypothesis that TZDs may cause bone loss in older women, thereby putting patients, already at risk for falls, at a superimposed increased risk of fracture. In addition, recent research has emerged with regard to the long-term cardiovascular safety of TZDs, and data are currently being re-evaluated. It appears that TZDs may increase the rates of heart failure and possibly myocardial infarction and therefore should be avoided in susceptible individuals.

6. **α-Glucosidase inhibitors.** α-Glucosidase inhibitors are a class of drugs that target postprandial hyperglycemia by decreasing carbohydrate absorption at the intestinal brush border. The net result is more of an increase insulin sensitivity

as opposed to release in elderly patients. Currently available class members are **acarbose** and **miglitol.** Recent studies suggest that that these drugs may also increase glucagonlike peptide I (GLP-1), an incretin hormone, which will be discussed in more detail later. However, the mechanism is unclear at this time. These drugs have a good overall safety profile for older populations, with the most common side effects being gastrointestinal, such as bloating and loose stools, which, unfortunately, limit their use in some patients. Postprandial hypotension is a significant clinical condition that predisposes elderly patients to events such as syncope and falls. Also, this postprandial hypotension severity tends to be augmented with greater carbohydrate content. The addition of α-glucosidase inhibitors appears to attenuate postprandial hypotension and its resulting effects, possibly by slowing gastric emptying.

7. **Incretin mimetics and dipeptidyl peptidase IV (DPP IV) inhibitors.** A recent group of diabetes medications has centered on incretin hormones. The gut hormones, GLP-1 and gastric inhibitory polypeptide (GIP), are incretin hormones that are released postprandially and appear to augment insulin secretion by way of β-cell glucose sensitization as well as decreasing hepatic glucose production. In healthy persons, GLP-1 dose-dependently inhibits gastric emptying. It is this effect that may decrease food intake through either neuronal or endocrine signaling. With increased aging and glucose impairment, insulin release patterns are altered and become more chaotic, which can be improved with GLP-1 infusion. The enzyme dipeptidyl peptidase IV (DPP IV) rapidly degrades GLP-1, giving it a half-life of <1 minute.

   a. The first clinically available incretin mimetic was **exenatide.** Exenatide has a significantly longer half-life as well as greater glucose-lowering potential compared with GLP-1. Statistically significant reductions in HbA_{1c} and both fasting and postprandial glucose levels, as well as body weight, have been recognized in placebo-controlled studies performed by adding exenatide to regimens of inadequately controlled patients on metformin, a sulfonylurea, or both, to show significant reductions in HbA_{1c}, overall glucose control, and body weight. Despite improved glucose management, this drug should most probably not be used in older populations considering this decrease in body weight (at least until more studies are available), bearing in mind that weight loss can result in worsening frailty.

   b. Another class of drugs that increase GLP works through inhibition of DPP IV activity. In human studies, DPP IV inhibition appears to improve glucose homeostasis through stimulation of insulin secretion and inhibition of glucagon release without altering gastric emptying. **Sitagliptin** is a highly selective oral DPP IV inhibitor. Sitagliptin treatment up to 600 mg was generally well tolerated without side effects, such as increased hypoglycemia or gastrointestinal complaints, compared with placebo in healthy euglycemic men. Sitagliptin has been found to have similar HbA_{1c} reductions and side-effect profile compared to sulfonylurea without significant hypoglycemia. No specific studies on DPP IV inhibitor therapy in the geriatric population exist, but considering the favorable gastrointestinal profile and effects on weight, this medication may be a reasonable alternative.

XI. SUMMARY

Diabetes is a chronic progressive condition that becomes more common as well as more complicated in the older population. The management of diabetes should be approached from a number of different angles, and its management needs to be tailored to the individual patient to achieve the best results.

Selected References

Ahren B, Simonsson E, Larsson H, et al. Inhibition of dipeptidyl peptidase IV improves metabolic control over a 4-week study period in type 2 diabetes. *Diabetes Care* 2002;25: 869–875.

American Diabetes Association. Evidence-based nutrition principles and recommendation for the treatment and prevention of diabetes and related complication. *Diabetes Care* 2002;25:202–212.

American Diabetes Association. Immunization and the prevention of influenza and pneumococcal disease in people with diabetes. *Diabetes Care* 2003;26:S126–S128.

American Diabetes Association. Nutrition recommendations and interventions for diabetes—2006. *Diabetes Care* 2006;29:2140–2157.

American Diabetes Association. Nutrition recommendations and interventions for diabetes: a position statement of the American Diabetes Association. *Diabetes Care* 2007; 30(suppl 1):S48–S65.

Argoff C, Cole E, Fishbain D, Irving G. Diabetic peripheral neuropathic pain: clinical and quality-of-life issues. *Mayo Clin Proc* 2006;81:S3–S9.

Arnold J, Mcgowan H. Delay in diagnosis of diabetes mellitus due to inaccurate use of hemoglobin A1c levels. *J Am Board Family Med* 2007;20:93–96.

Banks WA, Willoughby LM, Thomas DR, Morley JE. Insulin resistance syndrome in the elderly: assessment of functional, biochemical, metabolic, and inflammatory status. *Diabetes Care* 2007;30:2369–2373.

Berg AH, Combs TP, Du X, et al. The adipocyte-secreted protein Acrp30 enhances hepatic insulin action. *Nat Med* 2001;7:947–953.

Boule NJ, Hadda E, Kenny GP, et al. Effects of exercise on glycemic control and body mass in type 2 diabetes mellitus: a meta-analysis of controlled clinical trials. *JAMA* 2001;286:1218–1227.

Buse JB, Henry RR, Han J, et al. Exenatide-113 Clinical Study Group: Effects of exenatide (exendin-4) on glycemic control over 30 weeks in sulfonylurea-treated patients with type 2 diabetes. *Diabetes Care* 2004;27:2628–2635.

Castaneda C, Layne JE, Munoz-Orians L, et al. A randomized controlled trial of resistance exercise training to improve glycemic control in older adults with type 2 diabetes. *Diabetes Care* 2002;25:2335–2341.

Chew G, Gan SK, Watts G. Revisiting the metabolic syndrome. *Med J Austr* 2006;185:445–449.

Cicero DG, D'Angelo A, Gaddi A, et al. Effects of 1 year of treatment with pioglitazone or rosiglitazone added to glimepiride on lipoprotein (a) and homocysteine concentrations in patients with type 2 diabetes mellitus and metabolic syndrome: a multicenter, randomized, double-blind, controlled clinical trial. *Clin Ther* 2006;28:679–688.

Cohen R, Holmes Y, Chenier T, Joiner C. Discordance between HbA1c and fructosamine. *Diabetes Care* 2003;26:163–167.

Combs TP, Wagner JA, Berger J, et al. Induction of adipocyte complement-related protein of 30 kilodaltons by PPAR-γ agonists: a potential mechanism of insulin sensitization. *Endocrinology* 2002;143:998–1007.

Coulston AM, Mandelbaum D, Reaven GM. Dietary management of nursing home residents with non-insulin-dependent diabetes mellitus. *Am J Clin Nutr* 1990;51:67–71.

Crosson JT, Majika SM, Grazia T, et al. Rosiglitazone promotes development of a novel adipocyte population from bone marrow-derived circulating progenitor cells. *J Clin Invest* 2006;116:3220–3228.

DeFronzo RA, Ratner RE, Han J, et al. Effects of exenatide (exendin-4) on glycemic control and weight over 30 weeks in metformin-treated patients with type 2 diabetes. *Diabetes Care* 2005;28:1092–1100.

DeLeon MJ, Chandurkar V, Albert SG, et al. Glucagon-like peptide-1 response to acarbose in elderly type 2 diabetic subjects. *Diabetes Res Clin Pract* 2002;56:101–106.

De Rekeneire N, Peila R, Ding J, et al. Diabetes, hyperglycemia, and inflammation in older individuals. *Diabetes Care* 2006;29:1902–1907.

Dunstan DW, Daly RM, Owen N, et al. High-intensity resistance training improves glycemic control in older patients with type 2 diabetes. *Diabetes Care* 2002;25:1729–1736.

Egan JM, Clocquet AR, Elahi D. The insulinotropic effect of acute exendin-4 administered to humans: comparison of nondiabetic state to type 2 diabetes. *J Clin Endocrinol Metab* 2002;87:1282–1290.

Gentilcore D, Bryant B, Wishart JM, et al. Acarbose attenuates the hypotensive response to sucrose and slows gastric emptying in the elderly. *Am J Med* 2005;118:1289.

Gerstein HC, Yusuf S, Bosch J, et al. Effect of rosiglitazone on the frequency of diabetes in patients with impaired glucose tolerance or impaired fasting glucose: a randomized controlled trial. *Lancet* 2006;368:1096–1105.

Herman GA, Stevens C, Van Dyck K, et al. Pharmacokinetics and pharmacodynamics of single doses of sitagliptin, an inhibitor of dipeptidyl peptidase-IV, in healthy subjects. *Clin Pharm Ther* 2005;78:675–688.

Hijazi R, Betancourt-Albrecht M, Cunninghan G. Gonadal and erectile dysfunction in diabetics. *Med Clin North Am* 2004;88:933–945.

Home PD, Pocock ST, Beck-Nielsen H, et al. Rosiglitazone evaluated for cardiovascular outcomes—an interim analysis. *N Engl J Med* 2007:28–38.

Hvidberg A, Nielsen MT, Hilsted J, et al. Effect of glucagon-like peptide 1 (proglucagon 78–107 amide) on hepatic glucose production in healthy men. *Metabolism* 1994;43:104–110.

Josse RG, Chiasson JL, Ryan EA, et al. Acarbose in the treatment of elderly patients with type 2 diabetes. *Diabetes Res Clin Pract* 2003;59:37–42.

Kendall DM, Riddle MC, Rosenstock J, et al. Effects of exenatide (exendin-4) on glycemic control over 30 weeks in patients with type 2 diabetes treated with metformin and a sulfonylurea. *Diabetes Care* 2005;28:1083–1091.

Kim MJ, Rolland Y, Cepeda O, et al. Diabetes mellitus in older men. *Aging Male* 2006;9:139–147.

Kumar VB, Bernardo AE, Vyas K, et al. Effect of metformin on nitric oxide synthase in genetically obese (ob/ob) mice. *Life Sci* 2001;69:2789–2799.

Lassmann-Vague V. Hypoglycemia in elderly diabetic patients. *Diabetes Metab* 2005;31:5S53–5S57.

Lee A, Morley JE. Metformin decreases food consumption and induces weight loss in subjects with obesity with type II non-insulin-dependent diabetes. *Obes Res* 1998;6:47–53.

Lee A, Patrick P, Wishart J, et al. The effects of miglitol on glucagon-like peptide-1 secretion and appetite sensations in obese type 2 diabetics. *Diabetes Obes Metab* 2002;4:329–335.

Lipscombe LL, Jamal SA, Booth GL, Hawker GA. The risk of hip fractures in older individuals with diabetes. *Diabetes Care* 2007;30:835–841.

MacIntosh C, Morley JE, Chapman IM. The anorexia of aging. *Nutrition* 2000;16:983–995.

Maraldi C, Volpato S, Penninx B, et al. Diabetes mellitus, glycemic control, and incident depressive symptoms among 70- to 79-year-old persons: the health, aging, and body composition study. *Arch Intern Med* 2007;11:1137–1144.

Marfella R, D'Amico M, Di Filippo C, et al. Increased activity of the ubiquitin-proteasome system in patients with symptomatic carotid disease is associated with enhanced inflammation and may destabilize the atherosclerotic plaque: effects of rosiglitazone treatment. *J Am Coll Cardiol* 2006;47:2444–2455.

Mazza AD, Morley JE. Metabolic syndrome in the older male population. *Aging Male* 2007;10:3–8.

Meneilly GS, Ryan EA, Radziuk J, et al. Effect of acarbose on insulin sensitivity in elderly patients with diabetes. *Diabetes Care* 2000;23:1162–1167.

Meneilly GS, Veldhuis JD, Elahi D. Deconvolution analysis of rapid insulin pulses before and after six weeks of continuous subcutaneous administration of glucagon-like peptide-1 in elderly patients with type 2 diabetes. *J Clin Endocrinol Metab* 2004;90:6251–6256.

Morley JE. Editorial: Postprandial hypotension—the ultimate Big Mac Attack. *J Gerontol A Biol Sci Med Sci* 2001;56:M741–M743.

Morley JE. Weight loss in the nursing home. *J Am Med Dir Assoc* 2007;8:201–204.

Morley JE, Flood JF. Effect of competitive antagonism of NO synthetase on weight and food intake in obese and diabetic mice. *Am J Physiol* 1994;266(1 pt 2):R164–R168.

Morley JE, Kim MJ, Haren MT, et al. Frailty and the aging male. *Aging Male* 2005;8:135–140.

Muller LMAJ, Gorter KJ, Hak E, et al. Increased risk of common infections in patients with type 1 and type 2 diabetes. *Clin Infect Dis* 2005;41:281–288.

Munshi M, Capelson R, Grande L, et al. Cognitive dysfunction is associated with poor diabetes mellitus control in older adults. *Diabetes Care* 2006;8:1794–1799.

Nauck MA, Meininger G, Sheng D, et al. Efficacy and safety of the dipeptidyl peptidase-4 inhibitor, sitagliptin, compared with the sulfonylurea, glipizide, in patients with type

2 diabetes inadequately controlled on metformin alone: a randomized, double-blind, non-inferiority trial. *Diabetes, Obes Metab* 2007;9:194–205.

Nauck MA, Niedereichholz U, Ettler R, et al. Glucagon-like peptide 1 inhibition of gastric emptying outweighs its insulinotropic effects in healthy humans. *Am J Physiol* 1997; 273:981–988.

Nielsen LL, Young AA, Parkes DG. Pharmacology of exenatide (synthetic exendin-4): a potential therapeutic for improved glycemic control of type 2 diabetes. *Regul Pept* 2004; 117:77–88.

Nissen NE, Wolski K. Effect of rosiglitazone on the risk of myocardial infarction and death from cardiovascular causes. *N Engl J Med* 2007;356:2457–2471.

Proks P, Reimann F, Green N, et al. Sulfonylurea stimulation of insulin secretion. *Diabetes* 2002;51:S368–S376.

Schellhase K, Keopsell TD, Weiss N. Glycemic control and the risk of multiple microvascular diabetic complications. *Family Med* 2005;37:125–130.

Schwartz AV, Sellmeyer DE, Vittinghoff E, et al. Thiazolidinedione use and bone loss in older diabetic adults. *J Clin Endocrinol Metab* 2006;91:3349–3354.

Schwartz RS. Exercise training in treatment of diabetes mellitus in elderly patient. *Diabetes Care* 1990;13(suppl 2):77–85.

Shibao C, Gamboa A, Diedrich A, et al. Acarbose, an α-glucosidase inhibitor, attenuates posprandial hypotension in autonomic failure. *Hypertension* 2007;50:54–61.

Sigal RJ, Kenny GP, Wasserman DH, et al. Physical activity/exercise and type 2 diabetes. *Diabetes Care* 2004;27:2518–2537.

Tariq SH, Karcic E, Thomas DR, et al. The use of no-concentrated-sweets diet in the management of type 2 diabetes in nursing homes. *J Am Diet Assoc* 2001;101:1463–1466.

Vella A, Bock G, Giesler PD, et al. Effects of dipeptidyl peptidase-4 inhibition on gastrointestinal function, meal appearance, and glucose metabolism in type 2 diabetes. *Diabetes* 2007;56:1475–1480.

Verny C. Congestive heart failure in the elderly diabetic. *Diabetes Metab* 2007;33:S32–S39.

Wedick NM, Barrett-Connor E, Knoke JD, Wingard DL. The relationship between weight loss and all-cause mortality in older men and women with and without diabetes mellitus: the Rancho Bernardo Study. *J Am Geriatr Soc* 2002;50:1810–1815.

Winer N, Sowers JR. Epidemiology of diabetes. *J Clin Pharm* 2004;44:397–405.

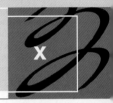

Special Topics in Clinical Endocrinology

X

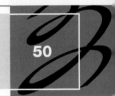

ENDOCRINE DISEASES IN PREGNANCY
Jorge H. Mestman

50

$\mathcal{E}$ ndocrine diseases in pregnancy present a challenge to the physician, not only because they may complicate the maternal course of gestation, but also because they may affect the growth and development of the fetus. It is imperative that a team approach be used in the management of these conditions; the close cooperation of the obstetrician, endocrinologist, and anesthesiologist will offer the patient the best maternal and neonatal outcomes.

I. PITUITARY DISEASES

The pituitary gland enlarges during gestation as a result of hyperplasia of the lactotroph cells, producers of prolactin (PRL); however, the growth does not have clinical repercussions unless a pathologic process is present.

A. Anterior pituitary insufficiency. Anterior pituitary insufficiency is a result of a pituitary tumor in almost 80% of patients, a result of extrapituitary disease in 13%, of sarcoidosis in 1%, and of Sheehan syndrome in 0.5%.

Sheehan syndrome or **postpartum pituitary necrosis** is a result of severe <u>blood loss</u> during or a few hours after delivery. In some patients, acute adrenal insufficiency with hypotension, hypoglycemia, and shock is the presenting picture; in most cases, however, a more insidious onset occurs, with anorexia and nausea, lethargy, weakness, weight loss, lack of lactation following delivery, amenorrhea, loss of pubic and axillary hair, or failure of pubic hair to grow back following cesarean section.

Partial pituitary insufficiency is not uncommon. In a review of anterior pituitary function in patients with a history of pituitary apoplexy due to different causes, growth hormone deficiency occurred in almost 90% of patients, ACTH deficiency in ~66% of patients, hypothyroidism because of thyroid-stimulating hormone (TSH) deficiency in ~42% of patients, hypogonadism in 65% of patients, and the incidence of diabetes insipidus was <5%.

Anterior pituitary insufficiency may also develop for the first time during pregnancy, unrelated to delivery. Clinical manifestations are related to the etiology, local signs and symptoms resulting from acute expansion of the pituitary gland, or to specific hormone deficiencies. Severe, deep, mid-line headaches and nausea, vomiting, and visual disturbances characterize the symptoms of an acute expansion of a pituitary tumor. Acute endocrine deficiency symptoms are related mainly to <u>cortisol deficiency</u>: protracted hypoglycemia that responds to glucocorticoid therapy. <u>Lymphocytic hypophysitis</u> is being recognized with increasing frequency as a cause of partial or total hypopituitarism during pregnancy. It is considered to have an autoimmune pathogenesis and occurring mainly in women during pregnancy or in the postpartum period. The clinical presentation is characterized by headaches and visual disturbances, related to pressure from the expanding lesion mimicking a pituitary tumor, or symptoms and signs of hypopituitarism such as hypoglycemia, hypotension, nausea, and vomiting. It may also present in the postpartum period as pituitary insufficiency, similar to Sheehan syndrome without the history of profound bleeding. Hyperprolactinemia with partial pituitary insufficiency and diabetes insipidus, with or without a pituitary mass, have been reported. When available, the pathologic specimen showed significant lymphocytic infiltration. The <u>differential diagnosis between pituitary tumor and lymphocytic hypophysitis</u> is made only by histologic examination; in fact, in some cases, surgery was performed during pregnancy with the preoperative diagnosis of pituitary tumor. Spontaneous regression of the pituitary mass with recovery of endocrine function has been reported. Based on the above information, in the presence of a clinical diagnosis of lymphocytic hypophysitis and absence of visual field defects, surgical therapy may be safely withheld, with periodic reassessment of endocrine function and size of the lesion. In the majority of cases reported, gonadotropin function has been spared, suggesting a possibility of future spontaneous pregnancies.

Patients with partial or total hypopituitarism, who become pregnant spontaneously or after treatment with gonadotropin, may have a normal pregnancy with successful neonatal outcome. In women on glucorticoid replacement therapy, no increase in the dose is needed; the usual amount of hydrocortisone in patients with pituitary insufficiency is between 20 and 30 mg per day, two thirds of the total amount in the morning and one third in the evening. The equivalent amount of prednisone is 5.0 to 7.5 mg daily and of dexamethasone is 0.5 to 0.75-mg daily. Aldosterone secretion is preserved, because adrenal secretion is independent of ACTH; therefore, compared to primary adrenal insufficiency, there is <u>no need for mineralocorticoid replacement therapy</u>. In the presence of thyroid deficiency, the usual amount of l-thyroxine may need to be increased from early pregnancy. The usual replacement dose is between 0.075 and 0.15 mg daily, and the amount should be adjusted to keep the FT4 in the upper third of normal. In patients with secondary hypothyroidism (such as in women with hypopituitarism), serum TSH levels are not a good marker of proper thyroxine replacement as is the case in primary hypothyroidism.

B. Prolactinomas. Prolactinoma is the most common pituitary tumor diagnosed in women of child-bearing age. Serum prolactin increases early in normal pregnancy, reaching values close to 140 ng/mL by the end of pregnancy.

Medical therapy with bromocriptine, a dopamine-receptor agonist, is effective in producing ovulation in 80% to 90% of hyperprolactinemic women. In women who wish to become pregnant, it is advisable to use mechanical contraception in the first few months of bromocriptine therapy, until the menstrual period rhythm is established.

<u>Once conception takes</u> place, <u>bromocriptine should be discontinued</u> and the patient followed closely. The determination of serum prolactin during gestation is not very helpful in evaluating tumor growth; with a few exceptions, serum prolactin levels in women with prepregnancy hyperprolactinemia remained unchanged during pregnancy. For those women whose <u>initial prolactin levels are >200 pg/mL</u>, or who <u>have an abnormal magnetic resonance imaging (MRI) with suprasellar extension, bromocriptine therapy during pregnancy should be continued</u>. Potential <u>perinatal complications</u> resulting from the use of bromocriptine have been reported; abortion rates (11.1%), multiple pregnancy rates (1.2%), and prematurity rates (10.1%) are similar to those seen in the infertile population. The congenital malformation rate

of 3.5% (major and minor lesions) is comparable to the rate of 2.7% reported in a control group.

Cabergoline, a dopamine agonist with a long duration of action, has been used in a few patients with prolactinoma. Bromocriptine is preferred over cabergoline because of its extensive safety record. More than 6 000 bromocriptine-treated pregnant women have been reported in the literature, compared with ~350 treated with cabergoline.

Breastfeeding is not contraindicated in mothers with prolactinoma.

Complications during pregnancy are related directly to tumor size. In patients with microadenomas, headaches and visual field disturbances occurred in between 1% and 4% of the patients. Determination of visual fields during pregnancy is indicated only if there are signs and symptoms of tumor enlargement. For patients with macroadenomas, enlargement of the tumor is close to 35%; however, in patients treated by surgery or radiation therapy before conception, potential enlargement of the residual tumor during pregnancy was reduced to 4%. Women with macroadenomas should have their visual fields examined each trimester of gestation. In the presence of worsening of visual fields, an MRI of the pituitary gland should be obtained. If there is objective evidence of tumor enlargement, bromocriptine should be resumed and continued throughout pregnancy (up to 20 mg per day). If there is no improvement after a few days, dexamethasone, 4 mg every 6 hours, is indicated. Surgery is performed when there is no response to these therapies. Following delivery, women should be followed carefully for assessment of tumor growth. In patients with microadenomas, prolactin levels are measured a few months after delivery; drug therapy is reinstituted in the presence of persistent hyperprolactinemia. An MRI should be repeated in cases of hyperprolactinemia soon after delivery, to detect any change in the size of the tumor. The choice of treatment for patients who wish to conceive is summarized in Table 50.1.

Postdelivery, prolactin levels lower than before conception and complete remission of hyperprolactinemia have been reported in 17% to 37% of women after pregnancy.

C. Acromegaly. Women with acromegaly rarely ovulate spontaneously; however, with the advent of new medical therapies, successful pregnancies have been reported with increased frequency. Herman-Bonert et al. reported 24 cases of pregnancies in acromegalic women.

Pregnancy complications include gestational diabetes, worsening of impaired glucose metabolism, and enlargement of the pituitary tumor. It is estimated that overt diabetes mellitus will develop in 10% to 20% of patients and impaired glucose tolerance in 30% of them; hypertension develops in 25% to 35% of cases. Carpal tunnel syndrome symptoms may worsen during gestation.

Several cases have been reported of successful pregnancy in acromegalic women treated with a long-acting analog of somatostatin (Octreotide). Octreotide was usually discontinued at the time of pregnancy diagnosis; in two cases, however, the drug

TABLE 50.1 **Management of Women with Hyperprolactinemia before Conception**

Tumor	Management	Pregnancy follow-up
No tumor	Bromocriptine	Visual field (?)
Microadenoma	Bromocriptine[a] or surgery	Visual field if clinically indicated
Macroadenoma	(a) Surgery + bromocriptine	Visual field each trimester
	(b) Radiotherapy + bromocriptine	Visual field each trimester

[a]Therapy for 1 year before conception.
Reprinted with permission from Mestman JH. Endocrine diseases in pregnancy. In: Sciarra JJ, ed. *Gynecology and Obstetrics*. Philadelphia: Lippincott-Raven; 1997:chap 23:6.

TABLE 50.2	Clinical Presentations of Diabetes Insipidus in Pregnancy

1. Pregestational diabetes insipidus
2. Presenting for the first time in pregnancy and persisting thereafter
3. Transient, occurring during gestation or in the immediate postpartum period, associated with pre-eclampsia, liver disease, or HELLP syndrome
4. Transient, recurrent in pregnancy, patients with latent diabetes insipidus, manifesting only in pregnancy because of the increase in the placenta enzyme vasopressinase
5. Postpartum diabetes insipidus in patients with acute pituitary insufficiency, such as Sheehan syndrome or hypophysitis
6. An unusual transient form of diabetes insipidus that is resistant both to vasopressin and dDAVP administration

dDAVP, desmopressin; HELLP, hemolysis, elevated liver enzyme levels, and low platelet count.

was continued throughout pregnancy. The dose of octreotide is 300 to 1 500 μg in three divided doses by subcutaneous injection.

It is generally recommended to discontinue drug therapy after conception, although to our knowledge there is no information on potential side effects based on evaluation of pregnancy outcomes. As in cases of prolactinoma, it is advisable to perform visual fields examination each trimester or as clinically indicated, such as in the event of severe headache or visual disturbances; MRI is reserved for those patients who develop abnormal visual fields. If an enlargement of the pituitary tumor is detected, reinstitution of medical therapy and close follow-up is recommended.

Pegvisomant, a growth hormone antagonist, was reported in one case of a woman with persistent active disease after surgery, not responding to other medical therapies (cabergoline and octreotide). She had a successful response to pegvisomant, with normal fetal growth and term delivery.

D. Diabetes insipidus (DI). Women with isolated DI antedating pregnancy, and with normal anterior pituitary function, carry their pregnancies uneventfully, and infant outcome is normal. Worsening of symptoms during pregnancy occurred in >50% of cases, spontaneous improvement of symptoms in 20%, and no changes were reported in the rest.

Diabetes insipidus during pregnancy may occur in different clinical settings (Table 50.2).

Desmopressin (dDAVP) is the drug of choice in the treatment of diabetes insipidus. The prepregnancy dose does not need to be modified in most cases. There are no side effects on the fetus, and it is safe to use in lactating mothers.

II. PARATHYROID DISEASES
Parathyroid diseases, uncommon in pregnancy, may produce significant perinatal and maternal morbidity and mortality if not diagnosed and properly managed.

A. Calcium homeostasis during pregnancy. Total serum calcium during gestation is 8% below the postpartum level; the upper limit of normal is 9.5 mg/dL. This decrease in total serum calcium is a result of the physiologic hypoalbuminemia secondary to the normal expansion of the intravascular volume seen from early pregnancy. The ionized calcium levels, however, remain unchanged throughout gestation.

Maternal serum parathyroid hormone (PTH) levels, when measured by a sensitive two-sided immunoradiometric (IRMA) assay that accurately measured the levels of intact PTH, are slightly decreased in the second half of pregnancy.

B. Hyperparathyroidism. The most common cause of primary hyperparathyroidism in pregnancy is a single parathyroid adenoma, present in ~80% of all cases. Primary hyperplasia of the four parathyroid glands occurs in ~15% of the cases reported; 3% are the result of multiple adenomas; and a few cases due to parathyroid carcinoma have been reported in the English-language literature.

During pregnancy, because routine calcium determinations are not performed, manifestations of the disease are present in almost 70% of diagnosed patients; gastrointestinal symptoms such as nausea, vomiting, and anorexia; weakness and fatigue; mental symptoms including headaches, lethargy, agitation, emotional liability, confusion, and inappropriate behavior have been reported. Nephrolithiasis occurred in 36%, bone disease in 19%, acute pancreatitis in 13%, hypertension in 10% of cases.

Acute pancreatitis is a complication of hyperparathyroidism; it has been reported in 13% of women with primary hyperparathyroidism (PHP). The incidence in nonpregnant hyperparathyroid women is ~1.5% and it is <1% in normal pregnancies.

Hyperparathyroid crisis, a serious complication of PHP, has been reported during gestation and in the postpartum period. Severe nausea and vomiting, generalized weakness, changes in mental status, and severe dehydration characterize it. Hypertension may be present and should be differentiated from pregnancy-induced hypertension (PIH). The serum calcium is frequently >14 mg/dL; hypokalemia and elevation in serum creatinine are routinely seen. If not recognized and treated promptly, it may progress to uremia, coma, and death. Of the 12 cases reported in the literature, 4 occurred in the postpartum period. Maternal and perinatal mortality is high.

The two most common causes of neonatal morbidity are prematurity and neonatal hypocalcemia, the latter related to levels of maternal hypercalcemia, and in the early reports, it was frequently the only clue of maternal hyperparathyroidism. It develops between the 2nd and 14th days of life and lasts for a few days.

Surgery is the only effective treatment for primary hyperparathyroidism. The proper management of PH in pregnancy has not been uniformly agreed on. For asymptomatic pregnant women in whom serum calcium is <11 mg/dL, close follow-up with proper hydration and avoidance of medications that could elevate calcium (thiazides diuretics) are reasonable, although there are not studies in the literature supporting this or any other approach. Because most of the neonatal complications have been reported in patients with symptomatic disease, a surgical approach is indicated in symptomatic patients, those with complications (nephrolithiasis, bone disease), and those with persistent hypercalcemia >11 mg/dL. It is preferable to perform the surgery in the second trimester of pregnancy. However, a recent report of a good outcome was reported when surgery was performed in the third trimester of gestation.

Medical therapy is reserved for those patients with significant hypercalcemia who are not surgical candidates. Oral phosphate therapy, 1.5 to 2.5 g per day, has been shown to be effective in controlling hypercalcemia.

C. **Hypoparathyroidism.** Treatment of hypoparathyroidism in pregnancy does not differ from treatment during the nonpregnant state. Treatment includes a normal high-calcium diet and vitamin D supplementation. The normal calcium supplementation of pregnancy is about 1.2 g per day. Vitamin D requirement may decrease in some patients by the second half of gestation. Calcitriol (1,25[OH]D$_2$), 0.5 to 3 μg per day, is used almost routinely in most patients affected with hypoparathyroidism.

Following delivery, the dose of vitamin D needs to be reduced, because severe hypercalcemia has been reported during lactation.

D. **Osteoporosis.** Osteoporosis is suspected in pregnancy or in the postpartum period when the patient presents with severe, persistent back or hip pain; because radiography cannot be performed during pregnancy, symptomatic treatment is indicated. In the few studies available, there was an improvement in bone density following delivery.

In patients receiving heparin, attention needs to be given to symptoms such as back pain or hip pain. Heparin-associated osteoporosis has been reported in several cases during pregnancy.

III. ADRENAL DISEASES

A. **Cushing syndrome.** The most common cause of Cushing syndrome in women of child-bearing age is bilateral adrenal hyperplasia, which accounts for 75% of all cases; 20% are due to adrenal tumor, most commonly a single adenoma; a few cases are due to bilateral nodular adrenal hyperplasia; and the rest are due to ectopic ACTH production. In pregnancy, however, adrenal adenomas account for >50% of Cushing syndrome. Adrenal carcinoma is rare, although it appears to be more common than in nonpregnancy.

The clinical diagnosis may present some difficulty during pregnancy because characteristically similar abdominal striae, weight gain, and hypertension are seen in both conditions. Comparisons of close-up photographs from earlier years are helpful in detecting subtle changes. Some clinical features, such as severe hypertension in the second trimester, significant hyperglycemia, mental changes, and proximal muscle weakness, may alert the physician to the possibility of this rare disorder.

A persistent elevation in urinary free cortisol in a 24-hour urine collection is the best indicator of its overproduction by the adrenal gland(s). It should be kept in mind, however, that an elevation does occur in normal pregnancy during the second and third trimesters. Mean urinary free cortisol levels of 127 μg per day (range, 68 to 252 μg per day), compared to nonpregnant levels of 37 μg per day (range, 11 to 83 μg per day), have been reported.

The dexamethasone suppression test is blunted in pregnancy, giving false positive results. Lack of diurnal cortisol variation may be used as a complementary test.

A few more than 100 cases have been reported in the English-language literature, most of them isolated reports with spontaneous exacerbation or amelioration of symptoms throughout the course of pregnancy. Maternal and perinatal morbidity and mortality are significant. Arterial hypertension occurs in >70% of cases, overt diabetes in 30%, pre-eclampsia in 7%, and congestive heart failure in 7%. Maternal death occurs in 4% of cases as a result of congestive heart failure in the postpartum period. Fetal wastage, including abortions, stillbirth, and neonatal death, is close to 30%. Prematurity has been reported in 52% of infants, and intrauterine growth retardation in 25%.

The modality of treatment depends on the severity of the disease, the etiology, and gestational age at the time of diagnosis. A frank discussion of potential benefits and risks of therapy with the patient and her family is of outmost importance; there is some evidence, in the sparse literature, that treatment during pregnancy improved fetal outcome. A group of 32 patients treated during pregnancy were compared to 73 untreated women; the perinatal mortality was 6.3% in the former and 15.1% in the untreated group. The outcome of pregnancy was significantly better in patients in whom surgery was performed during pregnancy (bilateral adrenalectomy for hyperplasia or unilateral adrenalectomy for adenoma), with fewer fetal losses (1 of 11 vs. 9 of 30 pregnancies) and less prematurity.

Transsphenoidal pituitary surgery was performed in several cases.

Ketoconazole has shown beneficial effects in some patients during pregnancy.

In summary, etiology and gestational age determine management of Cushing syndrome in pregnancy. In the first two trimesters, adrenal surgery is indicated in the presence of an adrenal tumor; if MRI localizes the lesion in the pituitary gland, transsphenoidal surgery may be attempted in specialized centers. For patients in the third trimester, or for in whom the source of hypercorticalism cannot be localized, drug therapy with ketoconazole should be considered. Drug therapy during embryogenesis, however, should be used with great caution, in view of the possible teratogenicity of the drug.

B. Addison disease. Primary adrenal insufficiency is rarely diagnosed during pregnancy, and in most reported cases, the diagnosis antedated gestation.

The ACTH stimulation test is the standard test for the diagnosis of adrenal insufficiency.

Women with Addison disease have very few complications during pregnancy. If the patient is on hydrocortisone therapy, the dose of glucocorticoid does not need to be increased, because there is a potentiation of hydrocortisone action during normal pregnancy. However, when prednisone is used, the daily amount may be increased by a few milligrams a day, according to patient symptomatology. The requirement for glucocorticoid increases during the stress of labor or during intercurrent illnesses; mineralocorticoid requirements remain the same throughout pregnancy.

Neonatal adrenal insufficiency is rare in infants of mothers receiving corticosteroid therapy. In a review of 260 pregnancies during which steroids were given to the mother for variable periods, only one infant was believed to have adrenal corticosteroid insufficiency.

C. Congenital adrenal hyperplasia. Reproductive function may be impaired, particularly in women with the salt-wasting form. The causes of low rate of conception are multiple, including anovulation, reconstructive surgery, and sexuality. If a female fetus is exposed to high levels of androgen during early development, clitoromegaly, labioscrotal fusion, urethral abnormalities, and virilization are common findings at birth. Maternal evaluation and treatment with glucocorticoids at the onset of pregnancy may reduce complications. A total of 258 cases from 235 families with a sibling, parent, or close relative with 21-hydroxylase deficiency were studied, with 229 pregnancies/live births. Prenatal diagnosis was made by amniocentesis, measuring 17-hydroxyprogesterone (17-OHP) in amniotic fluid or by direct molecular analysis of the 21-hydroxylase (CYP21) gene performed after chorionic villus sampling (CVS). The latter method can be carried out at 10 weeks' gestation. Treatment with dexamethasone, 20 μg/kg body weight per day, in two or three divided doses, was started before 10 weeks' gestation in those mothers whose babies would potentially be affected. Treatment was discontinued if the fetus was found to be male or an unaffected female. The authors concluded that <u>dexamethasone administered at or before 10 weeks' gestation</u> was effective in reducing and in some cases preventing virilization. Follow-up of the 84 newborns treated prenatally showed normal birth weight, birth length, and head circumference compared to untreated fetuses.

D. Primary aldosteronism. Primary hyperaldosteronism is diagnosed in the presence of arterial <u>hypertension and persistent hypokalemia</u>. Serum bicarbonate is in most patients in the upper limit of normal, in contrast to the below-normal levels seen in normal pregnancy.

Treatment is based on the cause of aldosteronism. An MRI of the abdomen is effective in localizing the adrenal lesion. In most cases reported in pregnancy, a single adrenal tumor was the etiology, in which case adrenalectomy is the treatment of choice.

E. Pheochromocytoma. As with many other endocrine diseases, pheochromocytoma associated with pregnancy is <u>uncommon</u>; however, when it is present, it poses a life-threatening situation for mother and fetus. Clues to the diagnosis are paroxysmal hypertension, diaphoresis, palpitations, gestational age <20 weeks, significant blood pressure changes from supine to recumbent position, postural hypotension, and aggravation of the blood pressure in patients given beta-blocker agents. The differential diagnosis from pregnancy-induced hypertension can be difficult, particularly in the presence of proteinuria.

As soon as the diagnosis is confirmed, administration of an <u>α-adrenergic blocking agent</u> should be started; both maternal and fetal morbidity and mortality have greatly improved in the last three decades, since the introduction of α-adrenergic receptor–blocking agents. The drug most frequently used is <u>phenoxybenzamine (Dibenzyline)</u>, with a starting dose of 10 mg a day; the dose is increased by 10 mg every 2 to 3 days until blood pressure and symptoms are controlled. The blocking dose is about 1.0 mg/kg per day. It may need to be adjusted because it has a half-life of ~24 hours and hence it is cumulative. The usual dose of phenoxybenzamine is 40 to 80 mg per day; a 2-week course of an α-adrenergic–receptor blocker is the cornerstone of preoperative management. <u>Beta-blockers</u> are added to the regimen when tachycardia develops following administration of α-adrenergic–blocking agents. <u>Propranolol</u>, 10 mg 3 to 4 times a day, is useful in maintaining the pulse rate between 80 and 100 beats per minute. <u>Labetalol should not be used</u>, because it has α- and β-blocking properties in a ratio of 1:5. Hypertensive crises are treated with <u>intravenous phentolamine</u> in doses of 1 to 5 mg. Intravenous therapy also may be used in cases of unstable hypertension in preparation for surgery. A course of 10 and 14 days of α- and β-adrenergic blockers is used in preparation for surgery. Indicators of

TABLE 50.3	**Causes of Fetal and Maternal Virilization in Pregnancy**

Drugs
Dilantin
Danazol[a]
Progesterone
Stilbestrol[a] (large doses)

Ovarian lesions
Arrhenoblastomas[a]
Luteoma of pregnancy[a]
Krukenberg tumor[a]
Mucinous cystadenomas
Leydig cell tumor
Lipoid cell tumor
Granulosa—theca cell tumor
Dermoid cysts
Hyperreactio luteinalis
Polycystic ovarian syndrome

Adrenal lesions
Virilizing adenoma[a]
Virilizing carcinoma[a]
Aldosterone-producing tumor

[a]Lesions and drugs that produce fetal virilization.
Reprinted with permission from Mestman JH. Endocrine diseases in pregnancy. In: Sciarra JJ, ed. *Gynecology and Obstetrics*. Chapter 23 p 25, Philadelphia: Lippincott-Raven; 1997:chap 23:25.

acceptable control include a blood pressure <165/90 mm Hg, orthostatic hypotension, but with standing blood pressure >90/45 mm Hg; no changes on electrocardiogram for the last 2 weeks (no ST-segment or T-wave abnormalities); and less than one premature ventricular contraction every 5 minutes.

Surgical intervention is the treatment of choice. Localization of the tumor is imperative; magnetic resonance imaging is the method of choice.

When the diagnosis is made during the first trimester of pregnancy, some authorities recommend elective termination of the pregnancy followed by tumor excision, whereas others recommend selective tumor resection without interruption of pregnancy. However, the incidence of spontaneous abortion is high.

During the last two trimesters of pregnancy, medical treatment is preferable, with removal of the tumor at the time of delivery during a cesarean section. Laparoscopic adrenal surgery has been performed. An anesthesiologist should be consulted and become closely involved in the management of patients with pheochromocytoma.

F. Virilization. When signs of hyperandrogenism appear for the first time in pregnancy, a complete investigation is warranted because of the possibility, albeit small, of a malignant lesion as the cause of the excess androgen production (Table 50.3). A medical history will reveal potential drugs responsible for hirsutism, the time of onset of the symptoms and signs, similar history in previous pregnancies, degree of virilization, and the presence of systemic symptoms. Virilization of the newborn is not always dependent on the concentration of maternal androgens.

The most common cause of hirsutism and virilization in pregnancy is luteoma of pregnancy, which is defined as a benign human chorionic gonadotropin-dependent ovarian tumor that develops during pregnancy.

IV. THYROID DISEASES

Thyroid disorders in pregnancy present a unique opportunity for health care professionals to use a similar "team approach" as has successfully improved the care of diabetic women. Autoimmune thyroid diseases occur five to eight times more often in women than in men, and its course may be affected by the immunologic changes that occur during pregnancy and in the postpartum period.

From early pregnancy on, the maternal thyroid gland is challenged with an increased demand for thyroid hormone secretion, mainly as a result of three different factors: the increase in thyroxine-binding globulin (TBG), the stimulatory effect of human chorionic gonadotropin hormone (hCG) on the TSH thyroid receptor, and the available supply of iodine to the thyroid gland. This last factor is of importance in terms of iodine deficiency. The normal thyroid gland is able to compensate for these demands by increasing the secretion of thyroid hormones and maintaining the serum levels of free hormones within normal limits. However, if there is a subtle pathologic abnormality of the thyroid gland, such as chronic autoimmune thyroiditis, the normal increases in the production of thyroid hormones do not occur; as a consequence, the pregnant women may develop biochemical markers of hypothyroidism (elevation in serum TSH) and even an increase in the size of the thyroid gland. Studies in the last decade have suggested that mild maternal thyroid deficiency in the first trimester of pregnancy may result in long-term neuropsychologic damage to the offspring.

Human chorionic gonadotropin is a weak thyroid stimulator, acting on the thyroid TSH receptor. If there is high production of hCG or more potent molecular variations, such as in multiple pregnancies, hydatidiform mole, and hyperemesis gravidarum (HG), serum free thyroxine (T_4) concentrations may rise to levels seen in thyrotoxicosis, with a transient suppression in serum TSH values (gestational thyrotoxicosis). Therefore, in addition to Graves disease, there are other situations in the first half of pregnancy in which abnormal tests may present a diagnostic challenge to the physician (Table 50.4).

A. Thyroid function tests (TFTs). Thyroid autoimmune disease, mainly chronic or Hashimoto thyroiditis, is diagnosed in 5% to 15% of women of child-bearing age. In many of these women, the diagnosis is made for the first time during pregnancy; they are at risk of perinatal complications such as miscarriages and preterm delivery. Furthermore, untreated hypothyroidism, even mild, may affect fetal and childhood neurologic development. Controversy still exists about whether routine thyroid screening in pregnant women is necessary. A recent consensus statement of experts representing the major endocrine societies recommended aggressive screening before or very early in pregnancy in women at high risk for thyroid disease (Table 50.5). However, selective screening may miss 30% of women at risk for thyroid disease.

Serum TSH determination is the most practical, simple, and economic screening test for thyroid dysfunction. The normal range of values for serum TSH varies according to the trimester of pregnancy. Serum TSH values decrease in early pregnancy;

TABLE 50.4   Hyperthyroidism in Pregnancy—Etiology

Intrinsic thyroid disease
Graves disease
Iatrogenic hyperthyroidism
Excessive levothyroxine intake
Gestational thyrotoxicosis
Normal pregnancy (up to 15% of them)
Multiple gestations
Mild nausea and vomiting
Hyperemesis gravidarum (transient hyperthyroidism of hyperemesis gravidarum)
Trophoblastic disease
Mutation in the TSH receptor (one case)
TSH, thyroid-stimulating hormone.

TABLE 50.5 Screening for Thyroid Disease in Pregnancy

1. Women on thyroid therapy
2. Previous history of thyroid disease
3. Symptoms and signs of thyroid disease (i.e., presence of goiter)
4. Family history of thyroid disease
5. Type 1 diabetes mellitus
6. Autoimmune disorders (lupus erythematosus, rheumatoid arthritis, Addison disease)
7. History of postpartum depression
8. History of miscarriage(s) and/or preterm delivery
9. Previous history of high-dose neck radiation
10. Previous birth of a child with intellectual impairment
11. Infertility

a range of 0.1 to 2.5 mU/L is considered normal in the first trimester. Values between 0.3 and 3.0 mU/L are considered normal in the second and third trimesters. A high TSH value is consistent with a diagnosis of primary hypothyroidism, whereas a suppressed one, with few exceptions, suggests hyperthyroidism (Fig. 50.1). A determination of serum free T4 or an equivalent FT4 index is helpful in distinguishing clinical from subclinical thyroid dysfunction. Serum anti–thyroid peroxidase antibodies (anti-TPO) determination is indicated in addition to the TSH determination, because this value is a marker of autoimmunity, the most common etiology of thyroid pathology in women of child-bearing age. Furthermore, it was reported that L-thyroxine therapy in the first trimester of pregnancy, in euthyroid women with chronic thyroiditis, prevents miscarriages and premature deliveries.

The determination of TSH receptor antibodies (TSHRAb) is indicated in patients with a history of Graves hyperthyroidism treated with ablation therapy in the past or in women with active Graves hyperthyroidism during gestation. These antibodies (immunoglobulins of the IgG subclass), with TSH-stimulating activity, cross the placenta and act on the TSH receptor of the thyroid fetal gland, and if present in high titers may produce fetal or neonatal hyperthyroidism. These antibodies may be present in patients with Graves disease even after thyroid ablation.

SCREENING FOR THYROID
DISEASE IN PREGNANCY

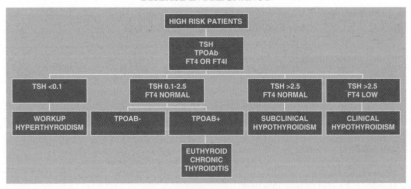

Figure 50.1. Algorithm for the diagnosis of thyroid disease. FT4, free thyroxine; TPOAb, thyroid peroxidase antibodies; TSH, thyroid-stimulating hormone.

B. Prepregnancy counseling. The physician may be faced with various clinical situations in the presence of a woman with thyroid disease who is contemplating pregnancy. With the advent of available information in the electronic media, it is important for the health care professional to offer the patient and her family objective and scientific data, supported by medical literature published in recognized peer-reviewed medical journals. The clinical situations may be summarized as follows.

1. **Hyperthyroidism under drug treatment.** Potential side effects of antithyroid drugs on the fetus should be discussed. If the patient chooses ^{131}I ablation therapy, it is customary to wait 6 months after the therapeutic dose is administered before pregnancy is contemplated. If she decides to conceive while on antithyroid drugs, propylthiouracil (PTU) is the drug of choice, in view of sporadic reports of specific congenital malformations in infants from mothers taking methimazole in the first trimester of pregnancy.

2. **Previous ablation treatment for Graves disease.** Two points are important to consider: **(a)** as in all women on thyroid therapy, the dose of thyroid replacement therapy needs to be increased in most cases soon after conception; and **(b)** in spite of euthyroidism, high maternal titers for TSHRAb may be present, with the fetus being at risk of developing hyperthyroidism despite the mother being euthyroid. Close follow-up during pregnancy and communication between obstetricians and endocrinologists are essential.

3. **Previous treatment with ^{131}I for thyroid carcinoma.** Pregnancy does not affect the natural history of women previously treated for thyroid cancer. It appears reasonable for patients with thyroid carcinoma to wait for 1 year after completion of radioactive treatment before conception.

4. **Treated hypothyroidism.** Women under treatment with thyroid hormone replacement usually require higher doses soon after conception. Following delivery, the dose should be reduced to the prepregnancy amount. Common medications may affect the absorption of l-thyroxine, including ferrous sulfate and calcium, among others. Patients should take l-thyroxine at least 2 hours apart from other medications.

5. **Euthyroid chronic thyroiditis.** Patients with Hashimoto thyroiditis are at greater risk of spontaneous abortions, preterm delivery, and the development of postpartum thyroiditis. As mentioned earlier, L-thyroxine treatment early in pregnancy decreased obstetrical complications.

C. Hyperthyroidism. Hyperthyroidism is diagnosed in pregnancy in ~0.1% to 0.4% of patients. Classically, it has been stated that Graves disease is the most common cause of hyperthyroxinemia in pregnancy, with other etiologies being uncommon (Table 50.4). However, transient hyperthyroidism (gestational thyrotoxicosis) is becoming recognized now as the most common cause of hyperthyroidism in pregnancy.

Single toxic adenoma and multinodular toxic goiter are seen in <10% of cases; subacute thyroiditis is rarely seen during gestation.

1. **Transient hyperthyroidism of hyperemesis gravidarum (THHG).** THHG is characterized by severe nausea and vomiting, with onset between 4 and 8 weeks of gestation, weight loss of at least 5 kg, ketonuria, and, depending on the severity of vomiting and dehydration, abnormal liver function tests and hypokalemia. Free thyroxine levels are elevated, sometimes up to four to six times the normal values, while free tri-iodothronine (FT_3) is elevated in up to 40% of affected women. The T_3/T_4 ratio is <20, in comparison to Graves hyperthyroidism, in which the ratio is usually >20. Serum TSH is consistently low or suppressed. In spite of the significant biochemical hyperthyroidism, signs and symptoms of hypermetabolism are mild or absent. Patients may complain of mild palpitations and heat intolerance, but perspiration, proximal muscle weakness, and frequent bowel movements are rare. Spontaneous normalization of hyperthyroxinemia parallels the improvement in vomiting and weight gain, with most cases resolving spontaneously between 14 and 20 weeks of gestation. Suppressed serum TSH may lag for a few more weeks after normalization of free thyroid hormones (Fig. 50.2). No antithyroid medication is needed; furthermore, because of the severity of the vomiting, drug therapy is poorly tolerated.

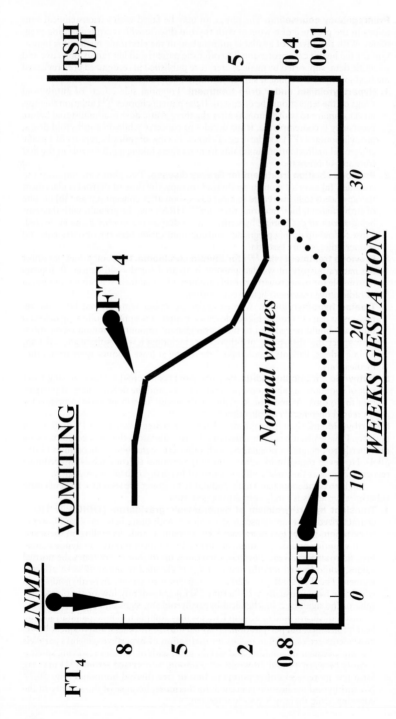

Figure 50.2. Clinical course of transient hyperthyroidism of hyperemesis gravidarum (THHG). FT4, free thyroxine; LNMP, last normal menstrual period; TSH, thyroid-stimulating hormone.

TABLE 50.6	**Maternal and Fetal Complications of Hyperthyroidism**

Maternal	Fetal
Miscarriage	Low birth weight
Pregnancy-induced hypertension	Prematurity
Preterm delivery	Small for gestational age (SGA)
Congestive heart failure	Intrauterine growth restriction or SGA
Thyroid storm	Stillbirth
Placenta abruptio	Hyperthyroidism (fetal and neonatal)
	Hypothyroidism (inappropriate antithyroid drug therapy)

2. **Graves disease.** The natural course of hyperthyroidism as a result of Graves disease in pregnancy is characterized by an exacerbation of symptoms in the first trimester and during the postpartum period, and amelioration in the second half of pregnancy.

When hyperthyroidism is properly managed throughout pregnancy, the outcome for mother and fetus is good; however, maternal and neonatal complications in untreated or poorly controlled mothers are significantly increased (Table 50.6).

In the vast majority of patients in whom the diagnosis is made for the first time during pregnancy, hyperthyroid symptoms antedate conception. The clinical diagnosis of thyrotoxicosis may present difficulties during gestation, because many symptoms and signs are commonly seen in normal pregnancy, such as mild palpitations, heart rate between 90 and 100 beats per minute, mild heat intolerance, shortness of breath on exercise, and warm skin. There are some clinical clues to incline the physician toward the diagnosis of hyperthyroidism: presence of goiter, ophthalmopathy, proximal muscle weakness, tachycardia with a pulse rate >100 beats per minute, and weight loss or inability to gain weight in spite of a good appetite.

The goal of treatment is normalization of thyroid tests as soon as possible and to maintain euthyroidism with the minimum amount of antithyroid medication. Thyroid tests should be performed every 2 weeks at the beginning of treatment, and every 2 to 4 weeks when euthyroidism is achieved. The two antithyroid drugs available are PTU and methimazole (Tapazole). Both drugs are effective in controlling symptoms. When the efficacy of these two drugs was compared in gestation, euthyroidism was achieved with equivalent amounts of drugs and in the same period of time. Several rare birth defects have been reported in women taking methimazole in the first trimester; none of these congenital malformations has been reported in women on PTU therapy. Therefore, it is advisable to avoid Tapazole therapy during the period of organogenies.

The initial recommended dose of PTU is 100 to 450 mg a day, and methimazole 10 to 20 mg a day in two divided daily doses. Rarely, doses of PTU up to 600 mg or methimazole up to 40 mg a day are needed. In patients with minimum symptoms, an initial dose of 10 mg of Tapazole daily or 50 mg of PTU two or three times a day may be initiated. In most patients, clinical improvement is seen in 2 to 6 weeks. Improvements in thyroid tests occur within the first 2 weeks of therapy, with normalization into chemical euthyroidism in 3 to 7 weeks. Resistance to drug therapy is very unusual, most often a result of poor patient compliance. Once clinical improvement occurs, mainly weight gain and reduction in tachycardia, the dose of antithyroid medication may be reduced by half of the initial dose. The daily dose of antithyroid drug is adjusted every few weeks according to the clinical response and the results of thyroid tests. The goal of therapy is to keep the FT_4 in the one third of the upper limit of normal with the minimum amount of medication; if there is an exacerbation of symptoms or worsening of the thyroid tests, the dose of antithyroid medication is doubled. Serum TSH may remain suppressed throughout pregnancy in spite of normal FT_4 concentrations. Excessive amounts of antithyroid drug have induced fetal hypothyroidism and goiter. The diagnosis of goiter is made by ultrasonography.

β-Adrenergic-blocking agents (propranolol, 20 to 40 mg every 6 hours, or atenelol, 25 to 50 mg daily) are very effective in controlling hyperdynamic symptoms and are indicated for the first few weeks in symptomatic patients. One situation in which β-adrenergic–blocking agents may be very effective is in the treatment of severe hyperthyroidism during labor. In a case reported in which both mother and fetus were affected, labetalol was infused at a rate of 2 mg/min, controlling maternal and fetal tachycardia within 45 minutes.

Subtotal thyroidectomy in pregnancy may be performed preferably in the second trimester of pregnancies. Indications for surgical treatment are few: allergy to antithyroid drugs, very large goiters, and patient and physician preference.

^{131}I therapy is contraindicated in pregnancy, because when it is given after 10 weeks' gestation it may produce fetal hypothyroidism. A pregnancy test is mandatory in any woman of child-bearing age before a therapeutic dose of ^{131}I is administered.

Breastfeeding is permitted if the daily dose of PTU is <150 to 200 mg per day or of methimazole is <10 mg per day.

Fetal well-being assessment with the use of ultrasonography, nonstress test, and biophysical profile is indicated for cases in poor metabolic control, in the presence of fetal tachycardia and/or intrauterine growth retardation, in pregnancies complicated by pregnancy-induced hypertension, or with any other obstetric or medical complications. Fetal goiter is one of the complications seen during antithyroid drug therapy.

D. Neonatal hyperthyroidism. Neonatal hyperthyroidism may affect from 1% to 5% of infants born to mothers with Graves disease. In the vast majority of cases, the disease is cause by the maternal transfer of high titers of thyroid-stimulating immunoglobulins (TSIs) to the fetus producing fetal or neonatal hyperthyroidism. When the mother is treated with antithyroid medication, the fetus can benefit from maternal therapy, remaining euthyroid during pregnancy. However, the protective effect of antithyroid drug is lost after delivery, and neonatal clinical hyperthyroidism may develop within a few days after birth if neonatal hyperthyroidism is not recognized and treated properly. Mortality may be as high as 30%. Because the half-life of the receptor is only a few weeks, complete resolution of neonatal hyperthyroidism is the rule.

E. Fetal hyperthyroidism. In mothers with a history of Graves disease, previously treated with ablation therapy, either surgery or ^{131}I, concentrations of TSIs may remain elevated in spite of maternal euthyroidism. Symptoms of fetal hyperthyroidism are not evident until the 22nd to 24th week of gestation; they consist of fetal tachycardia, intrauterine growth retardation, oligohydramnios, and occasionally a goiter, which is seen on ultrasonography. The diagnosis may be confirmed by measuring thyroid hormone levels in cord blood obtained by cordocentesis (performed only in specialized obstetric centers, because of a high rate of complications). Treatment consists of antithyroid medication given to the mother, 100 to 400 mg PTU daily or 10 to 20 mg methimazole a day; the dose is guided by the improvement of fetal tachycardia, resolution and normalization of fetal growth, and resolution of fetal goiter, which are indicators of good therapeutic response. The diagnosis of fetal hyperthyroidism should be suspected in the presence of fetal tachycardia with or without fetal goiter, in mothers with a history of Graves disease treated by ablation therapy, and with high titers of serum TSI antibodies.

F. Neonatal central hypothyroidism. Infants of untreated hyperthyroid mothers may be born with transient central hypothyroidism (pituitary or hypothalamic origin). High levels of thyroxine crossing the placenta barrier feed back to the fetus pituitary with suppression of fetal pituitary TSH. The diagnosis is made in the presence of low FT4 and normal or low TSH in cord blood. This is another complication that is easily avoided with proper management of maternal hyperthyroidism.

| TABLE 50.7 | Maternal and Fetal Complications of Hypothyroidism |

Maternal	Fetal
Miscarriage	Low birth weight
Pregnancy-induced hypertension	Small for gestational age
Preterm delivery	Prematurity
Postpartum hemorrhage	Intrauterine growth restriction
	Rare transient congenital hypothyroidism
	Intellectual deficiency

G. Hypothyroidism. The incidence of hypothyroidism in pregnancy, defined as any elevation in serum TSH above normal values, is between 0.19% and 2.5%. The spectrum of women with hypothyroidism in pregnancy includes **(1)** women with subclinical and overt hypothyroidism diagnosed for the first time during pregnancy; **(2)** hypothyroid women who discontinue thyroid therapy at the time of conception because of poor medical advice or because of the misconception that thyroid medication can affect the fetus; **(3)** women on thyroid therapy who require larger doses during pregnancy; **(4)** those previously diagnosed but noncompliant with their medication; **(5)** hyperthyroid patients on excessive amounts of antithyroid drug therapy; and **(6)** some patients on lithium or amiodarone therapy—both drugs may affect thyroid production, particularly in women with chronic thyroiditis.

As in the case of hyperthyroidism, the most common complication in poorly treated hypothyroid pregnant women is PIH, with an incidence of 21% in a study of 60 patients with overt hypothyroidism (Table 50.7); complications were significantly decreased when women achieved euthyroidism before 24 weeks' gestation.

The impact of maternal hypothyroidism (both clinical and subclinical) on the intellectual development of the offspring has been the subject of recent studies. Therefore, it is imperative to screen mothers who are at risk early in pregnancy and adjust the amount of thyroid medication. Levothyroxine is the drug of choice in the treatment of hypothyroidism. In view of the complications mentioned previously, it is important to normalize thyroid tests as soon as possible. An initial dose of 0.150 mg of L-thyroxine is well tolerated by the majority of young hypothyroid patients. In those with severe hypothyroidism, there is a delay in the normalization of serum TSH, but normal serum FT4 values are achieved in the first 2 weeks of therapy. The maintenance dose required for most patients is between 0.125 and 0.250 mg of L-thyroxine per day. Higher doses may be required for patients after total thyroidectomy for thyroid carcinoma, because the goal in these cases is suppression of serum TSH.

Patients on thyroid therapy before conception should have their TSH checked on their first visit and the amount of L-thyroxine adjusted accordingly. In most cases, an increase in the dose of L-thyroxine from 50 to 100 μg a day is required, according to the initial TSH level. Serum TSH tests should be repeated every 4 weeks for the first 20 weeks of gestation and then between 28 and 32 weeks. Immediately after delivery, dosage should be returned to the prepregnancy amount. Interference in the absorption of thyroxine was discussed previously.

H. Single nodule of the thyroid gland. It is estimated that nodular thyroid disease (NTD) is clinically detectable in 10% of pregnant women; in most cases, it is discovered during the first routine clinical examination or is detected by the patient herself.

In a retrospective study, a conservative approach in the management of a single thyroid nodule was recommended. In a group of 61 pregnant women with thyroid carcinoma, 14 of them were operated on during pregnancy, whereas the other 47 women underwent surgical treatment 1 to 84 months after delivery. The median follow-up was 22.4 years. The treatment and outcomes were similar in both groups,

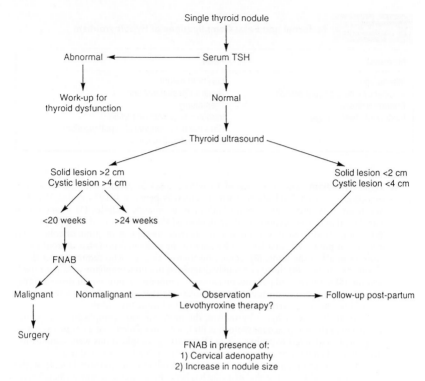

Figure 50.3. Evaluation of single thyroid nodules in pregnancy.

i.e., those operated on during pregnancy as in those in whom thyroidectomy was performed postpartum. The authors concluded that both diagnostic studies and initial therapy may be delayed until after delivery in most patients. In the presence of a single thyroid nodule detected on physical examination, the approach shown in Figure 50.3 is recommended in our institution.

I. Chronic autoimmune thyroiditis (Hashimoto thyroiditis). The importance of diagnosing chronic thyroiditis in women of childbearing age relates to the potential repercussions in pregnancy and in the postpartum period. Women with chronic thyroiditis are at higher risk of spontaneous abortion, premature delivery, hypothyroidism in the first trimester, and postpartum thyroiditis.

Women with a history of euthyroid chronic thyroiditis should be evaluated early in pregnancy. Even if they are euthyroid, one study reported that treatment with L-thyroxine prevented miscarriages and premature delivery.

J. Postpartum thyroid dysfunction. Postpartum thyroiditis (PPT), a variant of Hashimoto or chronic thyroiditis, is the most common cause of thyroid dysfunction in the postpartum period. The prevalence is between 5% and 10% of all women, with the exception of women with type 1 diabetes, in whom the incidence is close to 30%. The clinical diagnosis is not always obvious, and the clinician should be concerned about nonspecific symptoms such as tiredness, fatigue, depression, palpitations, and irritability following birth, or a miscarriage or abortion. These symptoms are not specific, fatigue being the most common complaint. In some cases, the clinical symptoms resemble the syndrome of "postpartum depression."

PPT is characterized by symptoms of thyroid dysfunction that present in different forms: **(1)** an episode of hyperthyroidism (2 to 4 months), followed by

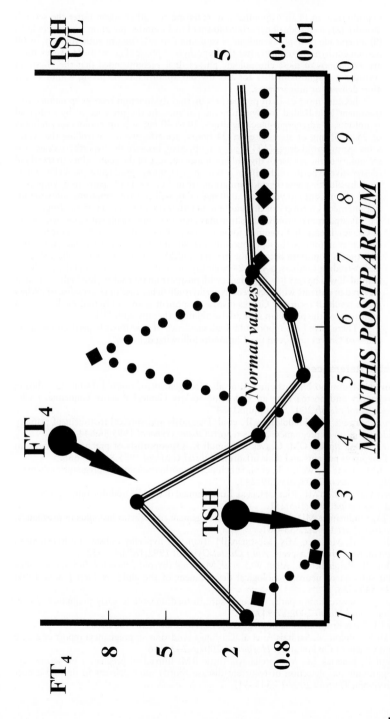

Figure 50.4. Clinical course of postpartum thyroiditis.

hypothyroidism (4 to 6 months) and reverting to euthyroidism (after the seventh month); **(2)** an episode of hyperthyroidism (3 to 4 months) reverting to euthyroidism; **(3)** an episode of hypothyroidism (4 to 6 months) reverting to euthyroidism; or **(4)** permanent hypothyroidism after the hypothyroid phase (Fig. 50.4). However, there are exceptions to these chronologic phases. It is recommended that the physician consider a diagnosis of PPT for any thyroid abnormality occurring within 1 year after delivery or miscarriages.

Because most cases of postpartum thyroid dysfunction recover spontaneously, treatment is indicated for symptomatic patients. In the presence of hyperthyroid symptoms, β-adrenergic–blocking drugs, 20 to 40 mg of propranolol every 6 hours or 25 to 50 mg of atenolol every 24 hours, are effective in controlling the symptoms. Antithyroid drugs (ATDs) are not effective, because the hyperthyroxinemia is secondary to the release of thyroid hormones because of the acute injury to the gland (destructive hyperthyroidism); there is no new hormone production, so ATDs, which work by blocking new thyroid formation, are ineffective. For hypothyroid symptoms, small amounts of L-thyroxine, 0.050 mg a day, will control symptoms, allowing for a spontaneous recovery of thyroid function after discontinuation of the drug.

Postpartum thyroid dysfunction may also occur in patients with a known history of Graves disease. It is common for women with Graves disease to have exacerbation of their symptoms in the first 2 months postpartum. The differential diagnosis in this situation is important because the treatment is different. If not contraindicated, as in breast-feeding mothers, a 4- or 24-hour thyroid radioactive iodine uptake (RAIU) is helpful. It will be very low in patients with postpartum thyroiditis, but high-normal or elevated in patients with recurrent hyperthyroidism because of Graves disease. When it is a result of recurrent Graves disease, treatment with antithyroid medications is indicated, or the physician may advise ablation therapy with [131]I.

There have been reports of a high incidence of new-onset hyperthyroidism because of Graves disease in the 12 months following delivery.

Selected References

Abalovich M, Amino N, Barbour LA, et al. Management of thyroid dysfunction during pregnancy and postpartum: an Endocrine Society Clinical Practice Guideline. *J Clin Endocrinol Metab* 2007;92(suppl):S1–S47.

Baron F, Sprauve ME, Huddleston JF, et al. Diagnosis and surgical treatment of primary aldosteronism in pregnancy: a case report. *Obstet Gynecol* 1995;86:644–645.

Carbone LD, Palmieri GM, Graves SC, Smull K. Osteoporosis of pregnancy: long term follow up of patients and their offspring. *Obstet Gynecol* 1995;86:664–666.

Casey BM, Dashe JS, Wells CE, et al. Subclinical hypothyroidism and pregnancy outcome. *Obstet Gynecol* 2005;105:239–245.

Doherty CM, Shindo ML, Rice DH, et al. Management of thyroid nodules during pregnancy. *Laryngoscope* 1995;105:251.

Durr JA, Lindheimer MD. Diagnosis and management of diabetes insipidus in pregnancy. *Endocr Pract* 1996;2:353–361.

Goodwin TM, Montoro MN, Mestman JH. Transient hyperthyroidism and hyperemesis gravidarum: clinical aspects. *Am J Obstet Gynecol* 1992;167:648–652.

Haddow JE, Palomaki GE, Allan WC, et al. Maternal thyroid deficiency during pregnancy and subsequent neuropsychological development of the child. *N Engl J Med* 1999; 341:549–555.

Karlsson F. Severe embriopathy and exposure to methimazole in early pregnancy. *J Clin Endocrinol Metab* 2002;87:947.

Keely EJ. Pheochromocytoma in pregnancy. *Curr Obstet Med* 1995;3:73.

Kita M, Sakalidou M, Saratzis A, et al. Cushings syndrome in pregnancy: report of a case and review of the literature. *Hormones* 2007;6:242–246.

Leboeuf R, Emerick LE, Martorella AJ, Tuttle RM. Impact of pregnancy on serum thyroglobulin and detection of recurrent disease shortly after delivery in thyroid cancer survivors. *Thyroid* 2007;17:543–547.

Leung AS, Millar LK, Koonings PP, et al. Perinatal outcome in hypothyroid pregnancies. *Obstet Gynecol* 1993;81:349.

Lindsay JR, Nieman LK. The hypothalamic-pituitary-adrenal axis in pregnancy: challenges in disease detection and treatment. *Endocr Rev* 2005;26:775–799.

Mercado AB, Wilson RC, Cheng KC, et al. Prenatal treatment and diagnosis of congenial adrenal hyperplasia owing to steroid 21-hydroxylase deficiency. *J Clin Endocrinol Metab* 1995;80:2014–2020.

Mestman JH. Hyperthyroidism in pregnancy. *Best Pract Res Clin Endocrinol Metab* 004;18:267.

Mestman JH. Parathyroid disorders in pregnancy. *Semin Perinatol* 1998;22:485–496.

Millar LK, Wing DA, Leung AS, et al. Low birth weight and preeclampsia in pregnancies complicated by hyperthyroidism. *Obstet Gynecol* 1994;84:946–949.

Montoro MN, Mestman JH. Pituitary diseases during pregnancy. *Infertil Reprod Med Clin North Am* 1994;24:41–71.

Montoro MN, Paler RJ, Goodwin TM, Mestman JH. Parathyroid carcinoma during pregnancy. *Obstet Gynecol* 2000;96:841.

Negro R, Formoso G, Mangieri T, et al. Levothyroxine treatment in euthyroid pregnant women with autoimmune thyroid disease: effect on obstetrical complications. *J Clin Endcrinol Metab* 2006;91:2587–2591.

Nelson DH, Tanney H, Mestman JH, et al. Potentiation of the biologic effect of administered cortisol by estrogen treatment. *J Clin Endocrinol* 1963;23:261–265.

Polak M, Le Gac I, Vuillard E, et al. Fetal and neonatal thyroid function in relation to maternal Graves' disease. *Best Pract Res Clin Endocrinol Metab* 2004;18:289.

Pressman EK, Zeidman SM, Reddy UM, et al. Differentiating lymphocytic adenohypophysitis from pituitary adenoma in the peripartum patient. *J Reprod Med* 1995;40:251–259.

Stagnaro-Green A. Recognizing, understanding and treating postpartum thyroiditis. *Endocrinol Metab Clin North Am* 2000;29:414–417.

Thomas E, Mestman JH, Henneman C, et al. Bilateral luteomas of pregnancy with virilization. *Obstet Gynecol* 1972;39:577–584.

Wing DA, Miller LK, Koonings PP. A comparision of propylthiouracil versus methimazole in the treatment of hyperthyroidism in pregnancy. *Am J Obstet Gynecol* 1994;170:90–95.

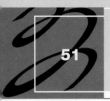

51 HORMONES AND AGING
Rani Nair, Srivalli Vegi, Asif Bhutto, and John E. Morley

By the middle of the 21st century, 16% of the global population will be elderly. This contrasts with only 5% of the world population being older than 65 years in 1950.

Aging is any change in an organism over time. The aging process is a continuous and linear one, beginning in the early thirties and continuing throughout life. In women, the first clear aging event is the onset of menopause around the mean age of 52 years. Menopause has been demonstrated to be a marker for longevity; the later the onset, the longer the woman's life. In most, but not all countries, women live longer than men but also live more years with some degree of disability. The longest documented lifespan is that of a woman, Jeanne Calment of France, who died at age 122 years.

The onset of the **hormonal signs of aging in men** begins in the early thirties, but decreased testosterone in the hypogonadal range is not commonly seen until most men are in their sixties or seventies. Erectile dysfunction was found in 5% of 40-year-old men and 15% of 70 year-old-men among the 3 607 men included in the Men's Health Survey. However, erectile dysfunction appears to be more related to the development of vascular diseases than to aging effects per se.

One of the greatest conundrums to be solved in the 21st century is the role of hormones and nutritional factors in the pathogenesis of sarcopenia (muscle wasting of aging). Baumgartner et al. found that the testosterone levels, Insulinlike growth factor I (IGF-I) levels, physical activity, nutritional factors, and age were related to the development of sarcopenia. Hormones have also been suggested to be factors in age-related cognitive decline and in the pathogenesis of atherosclerosis. Age-related decline of IGF-I and gonadal hormones have been postulated to play an important role in the pathogenesis of age-related bone loss in men. Figure 51.1 provides a conceptual framework of the factors involved in the pathogenesis of frailty.

This chapter first briefly reviews the hormonal changes associated with aging. It then focuses on the potential role of some hormones on the aging process. Finally, it reviews hip fractures in the old and the anorexia of aging.

I. HORMONAL CHANGES ASSOCIATED WITH AGING

A. Factors affecting hormone levels. Numerous hormone levels decline with aging. Some increase and others remain unchanged (Table 51.1). With aging, it is particularly important to distinguish the changes that are due directly to aging and those that are associated with disease or with protein-energy malnutrition, such as euthyroid sick syndrome. In addition, it is important to recognize that polypharmacy is common in older persons, and that drugs can have direct effects on circulating hormone levels (e.g., high doses of β-adrenergic blockers may increase thyroxine levels by blocking entry into cells). Psychiatric disease may also result in hormonal changes. For example, psychosis leads to stress-induced hyperthyroxinemia, and Alzheimer's disease is associated with multiple changes in hormonal levels.

B. Target-organ functioning. With aging there are changes in receptors and postreceptor function. The classical changes are the decline in postreceptor adrenergic β function. Mooradian et al. have demonstrated that there are marked decreases in the tissue responsiveness to thyroid hormones with aging. There are abnormalities in the urinary cyclic adenosine monophosphate and cyclic guanosine monophosphate production to arginine vasopressin (AVP) and atrial natriuretic factor with aging. The decline in AVP-2 receptor activation leads to a decrease in aquaporin-2 receptors.

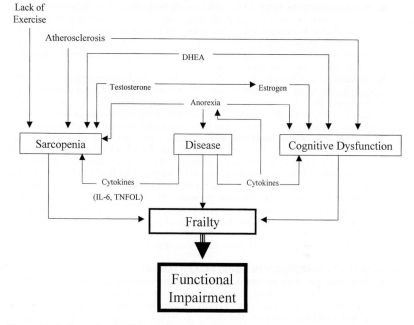

Figure 51.1. Factors involved in the pathogenesis of frailty. IL-6, interleukin-6; TNFOL, tumor necrosis factor-ol.

These hormone/receptor mismatches are certainly a component of the cause of the high incidence of hyponatremia in older persons.

C. Circadian rhythms. Alterations in circadian rhythms are common with aging. Thus, while circulating AVP levels increase during the day with aging, the nocturnal peak is attenuated. This attenuation of AVP is the reason for the physiologic nocturia that develops with aging. In rodents, the age-related decline in AVP is related to the decline in testosterone and can be restored with testosterone replacement.

TABLE 51.1	Alterations in Hormones with Aging

Increase	No change	Decrease
Luteinizing hormone (women)	Luteinizing hormone (men)	Growth hormone
Follicle-stimulating hormone	Prolactin	IGF-I
Parathyroid hormones	Thyroid-stimulating hormone	Testosterone
Atrial natriuretic factor	Amylin	Estradiol (women)
Vasopressin (basal)	Thyroxine	DHEA
Insulin	Tri-iodothyronine	Vasopressin (noctural)
Norepinephrine	Epinephrine	
Vasoactive intestinal polypeptide	Glucagonlike peptide type 1	Vitamin D
Cortisol (mild)	Gastric inhibitory peptide	DHEA sulfate
Cholecystokinin	Calcitonin gene-related peptide	Melatonin

DHEA, dehydroepiandrosterone; IGF-I, insulinlike growth factor type I.

D. Plasma clearance rates. In the case of some hormones, when the production rate declines, there is also a <u>decline in plasma clearance rates</u>, resulting in maintenance of circulating hormone levels. Thus, when the thyroxine production rate declines with aging, so does the plasma clearance rates, resulting in no decline in plasma thyroxine levels. Circulating cortisol levels are slightly increased with aging as a result of a decline in clearance rate.

E. Vitamin D. 25(OH)$_2$-D levels have been shown to <u>decrease even in very healthy elderly men</u> living in a sunny climate. This results in an increase in parathormone, leading to loss of calcium from bone and osteopenia. Recent studies have indicated that low levels of 25(OH)$_2$-D are associated with increased falls, sarcopenia, and a decline in functional status that can be reversed with vitamin D replacement.

F. Thyroid-stimulating hormone (TSH). There is a tendency for TSH to increase with aging, but not out of the normal range. If the TSH level is borderline elevated, an increase in thyroid peroxidase autoantibodies is associated with progression to hypothyroidism. <u>In the old-old, a mildly elevated TSH level has been associated with a decrease in mortality</u>, suggesting that mild hypothyroidism in persons >80 years of age may not benefit from treatment. In older persons, low supersensitive TSH levels are not diagnostic of hyperthyroidism. The supersensitive TSH assay has poor sensitivity and specificity in older persons and cannot be relied on to diagnose hyperthyroidism in these persons. Low TSH is associated with development of atrial fibrillation, but neither with other cardiovascular disease nor mortality.

II. ANDROGEN DEFICIENCY IN AGING MALES (ADAM)

A. Testosterone measurement. It has now been clearly demonstrated in cross-sectional and longitudinal studies that serum testosterone concentrations in men <u>decrease by 1% per year as they age</u>. As testosterone declines, sex hormone–binding globulin (SHBG) increases. The change in SHBG with aging makes the change in total testosterone a poor measurement of tissue-available testosterone. It is now accepted that bioavailable testosterone (free and albumin-bound) testosterone is the most appropriate measurement to diagnose hypogonadism in older persons.

B. Pathogenesis . The cause of the decline in testosterone in aging males is multifactorial. There is a deficit in the production of testosterone by the Leydig cells of the testis. More important, however, there is a failure of the hypothalamic–pituitary unit. Thus the majority of older men present with secondary hypogonadism. With aging, gonadotropin-releasing hormone (GnRH) is secreted chaotically, resulting in a lesser stimulus to the gonadotropes. In addition, the GnRH is less capable of stimulating the pituitary to produce luteinizing hormone (LH). Thus, despite the low circulating testosterone level with aging, the LH level remains in the normal range. In very old men (>80 years old), primary hypogonadism with elevated LH levels is more common.

C. Sperm cells. Although spermatozoa levels decline with aging, most men usually have sufficient sperm to procreate. With aging there is a <u>decline in sertoli cell production of inhibin</u>, leading to an increase in follicle-stimulating hormone.

D. Clinical presentations. Cross-sectional data have suggested that the testosterone decline in older men is associated with decreased libido, decreased strength of erection, decreased muscle mass and strength, increased visceral fat and leptin levels, dysphoria, decreased cognition, osteopenia, and a decline in functional status. Subsequently, interventional studies confirmed the capacity of testosterone to restore these age-related changes to normal. Whether testosterone replacement can improve the insulin resistance associated with low testosterone is controversial.

E. Treatment. The effects of testosterone in older men are summarized in Table 51.2. Testosterone increases upper-arm strength and possibly lower-limb strength. Low testosterone levels have been associated with minimal hip trauma fracture, and testosterone replacement increased bone mineral density. Testosterone has improved some cognitive elements. Recently, orally active selective androgen-receptor molecules (SARMs) have become available. In a pilot study the SARM ostarine increased lean mass and power in healthy persons >60 years of age when they received it for 3 months.

TABLE 51.2	Effects of Testosterone in Older Men

Increased libido
Increased strength of erection
Increased lean body mass
Increased upper-limb strength
Increased bone mineral density
Decreased adiposity
Decreased leptin
Increased hematocrit
Improved cognition
Coronary artery vasodilation
Decreased angina

F. Side effects of treatment. The major side effect of testosterone therapy in older men is <u>erythrocytosis</u>. <u>Sleep apnea</u> occasionally develops or worsens during androgen-replacement therapy. The accumulation of lean body mass and fluid retention generally cause <u>weight gain</u>. Mild <u>gynecomastia</u> may result occasionally, as testosterone can be aromatized to estradiol in peripheral tissues. Recent studies have suggested that low testosterone levels are associated with coronary artery disease prevalence and that testosterone replacement causes coronary artery vasodilatation and either positive or no effects on lipids. Testosterone replacement does not appear to be particularly deleterious in men with benign prostatic hypertrophy, but it should <u>not be given to men with prostatic cancer</u>.

G. ADAM questionnaire. In order to identify older males with hypogonadism, we have developed the ADAM questionnaire (Table 51.3). This questionnaire has been demonstrated to have high sensitivity and adequate specificity. The major false positives are to the result of depression. The questionnaire is easily used in the primary care physician's office. The ADAM is shorter and performs at a similar level to the Aging Male Survey.

III. GROWTH HORMONE (GH)

A. Physiology. Human aging leads to a decline in circulating concentration of both GH and IGF-I. Much of the decline in GH begins at 40 years of age, and by 70 years of age mean GH concentration are approximately one quarter of the values seen in adults in their twenties. GH secretion <u>decreases by ~1.6% per year</u> over the life span. GH continues to demonstrate a nocturnal peak in older persons. With aging, there is a reduction in the GH response to growth hormone–releasing hormone (GHRH), insulin-induced hypoglycemia, and exercise. Overall, animal and human

TABLE 51.3	The Saint Louis University Androgen Deficiency in Aging Males (ADAM) Questionnaire

Yes	No	**1.** Do you have a decrease in libido (sex drive)?
Yes	No	**2.** Do you have a lack of energy?
Yes	No	**3.** Do you have a decrease in strength and/or endurance?
Yes	No	**4.** Have you lost height?
Yes	No	**5.** Have you noticed a decreased enjoyment of life?
Yes	No	**6.** Are you sad and/or grumpy?
Yes	No	**7.** Are your erections less strong?
Yes	No	**8.** During sexual intercourse, has it been more difficult to maintain your erection to completion of intercourse?
Yes	No	**9.** Are you falling asleep after dinner?
Yes	No	**10.** Has there been a recent deterioration in your work performance?

studies suggest that with aging there is both an increase in somatostatin tone and a reduction in GHRH input to the pituitary that result in the decline in GH production. Ghrelin is a peptide hormone that is produced from the fundus of the stomach and that increases growth hormone and improves appetite and memory.

B. GH treatment. Rudman noticed the similarity between the effects of GH deficiency and physiologic aging and suggested that older persons go through a "growth hormone menopause." This spawned a panoply of GH replacement studies in older persons. GH increases lean body mass and decreases fat mass in older persons. However, these changes do not appear to be associated with an increase in strength, and GH fails to produce any additional benefit in older persons who are exercising. GH has not been shown to produce any clear-cut positive effects on bone mineral density. GH increases skin thickness. GH therapy in the elderly has been associated with numerous side effects, including carpel tunnel syndrome, fluid retention, fatigue, arthralgias, gynecomastia, joint swelling, and headache. These side effects are dose-related. When given short term, growth hormone has been shown to improve function in malnourished older persons.

C. Alternative treatments. Because of the problems with side effects, numerous studies have attempted to produce physiologic increases in GH by stimulating the hypothalamic–pituitary axis. Nightly subcutaneous injections of GHRH for 16 weeks in healthy older persons increased GH and IGF-I secretion. The GH-related peptide hexarelin, which can be given orally, increased secretion of both GH and IGF-I in older persons. The nonpeptide GH-related peptide analog MK-677 has been shown to produce nearly a doubling of GH and IGF-I after chronic oral administration in older persons. Studies with ghrelin agonists have been shown to increase food intake in cachetic individuals.

D. Side effects. Of greater concern are the facts that high-normal physiologic GH levels in the Paris policeman study were associated with increased mortality, and the Snell dwarf (GH-deficient) mouse lives longer than control mice. These findings suggest that the long-term administration of GH may increase mortality in older persons. At present the antiaging effects of GH are clearly not proven, and a number of troublesome side effects suggest that GH should not be used for this purpose.

IV. DEHYDROEPIANDROSTERONE (DHEA) AND PREGNENOLONE

A. Physiology. Both pregnenolone and DHEA and their sulfated moieties decline dramatically with aging. By age 80 years, both DHEA and its sulfate (DHEAS) are 20% of the values seen in young persons. These low serum levels of DHEAS have been associated with increased cardiovascular mortality (in some but not all studies), premenopausal breast cancer, functional decline, gastric cancer, and osteoporosis.

B. DHEA treatment. At least 25 studies have examined the effect of DHEA replacement in older persons, with mixed results. DHEA administration results in an increase of other circulating androgenic hormones, namely, testosterone, androstenedione, and dihydrotestosterone. At a high dose of DHEA (100 mg), Yen et al. demonstrated an increase in lean body mass in men but not in women. IGF-I levels increased in both groups. A year-long study with 50 mg DHEA daily failed to increase muscle mass and strength. Some studies have found positive effects of DHEA on the immune system, whereas others have not. Some have suggested a positive effect of DHEA on carbohydrate metabolism, but, again, there are insufficient data from which to draw firm conclusions.

DHEA has been reported to improve perceived physical and psychological well-being in middle-aged men and women. Again, other studies have failed to reproduce this finding. An open-label study suggested that DHEA decreased dysphoric symptoms and improved memory in six subjects with major depression. DHEA has been clearly demonstrated to have positive effects on mood in younger women with adrenal insufficiency. The dramatic effects of DHEA on memory in mice have yet to be demonstrated in humans.

C. Pregnenolone treatment. Pregnenolone is the true "mother hormone," being the precursor of all known steroid hormones. Studies in the 1940s suggested that pregnenolone was a safe and effective therapy for many symptomatic persons with arthritis. Pregnenolone improves sleep, decreases fatigue, and improves production efficiency. In mice, pregnenolone is the most potent memory-enhancing substance to have been discovered. However, the effect of pregnenolone on memory in humans is yet to be established. In a pilot study, we found no effect on strength, balance, or memory of a daily 50-mg dose of pregnenolone given for 12 weeks.

D. Summary. Like GH, pregnenolone and DHEA have occasioned much excitement among antiaging enthusiasts. However, the experimental evidence lags far behind the excitement. A further concern is that many of the DHEA products on the market contain minimal amounts of absorbable DHEA. Overall, there is a need for carefully controlled long-term studies to establish the role of DHEA and pregnenolone in aging. At present, the positive effects of these hormones in humans have yet to be convincingly established.

V. MELATONIN

Melatonin is produced by the pineal gland, "the seat of the soul." Melatonin levels increase in the evening and peak in the middle of the night. Melatonin in animals has been demonstrated to extend the life span. Free radicals have been considered to be a major factor in support of the aging process. Melatonin is a potent scavenger of the highly toxic hydroxyl radical and other oxygen-centered radicals. Melatonin seemed to be more effective than other known antioxidants, e.g., mannitol, glutathione, and vitamin E, in protecting against oxidative damage. Serum melatonin concentrations vary considerably according to age. Most studies suggest that melatonin levels decline in middle and old age. In humans, higher melatonin levels have been correlated with better cognitive function. Patients with Alzheimer's disease have lower melatonin levels than healthy older persons. Unfortunately, we lack controlled trials in humans to allow any prognostications on the effect of melatonin on aging.

VI. HIP FRACTURES

"We come into the world through the brim of the pelvis and go out through the neck of the femur."

Hip fracture is one of the most seriously debilitating but preventable injuries among individuals aged 65 years and older. Among this group, approximately one half of white women and one quarter of white men will sustain at least one osteoporotic fracture in their remaining lifetime. The burden of hip fracture among older adults requires continued vigilance in primary and secondary prevention. Osteoporosis causes 1.5 million fractures each year. In the United States, the cost of fall injuries is expected to reach $32.4 billion by 2020.

A. Causes. Hip fracture rates increase with aging. The causes of hip fracture are multifactorial and include osteoporosis, falls, prostate cancer, orchiectomy, androgen-deprivation therapy, and malnutrition (Fig. 51.2). Persons who have had a hip fracture are often not treated for osteoporosis despite the fact that they are two and a half times as likely to have another fracture within the next 2 years.

B. Risk factors. The risk factors for osteoporosis, according to the World Health Organization (WHO) and the International Osteoporosis Foundation, are advanced age, prior fragility fracture, parental history of proximal femur fracture, low body mass index, low bone mass, glucocorticosteroid treatment, rheumatoid arthritis, smoking, and the overuse of alcohol. A major risk factor for the loss of bone with aging is the decline in vitamin D levels. $24(OH)_2$-D levels have been found to decline longitudinally in a highly healthy, elderly population living in a sunny climate. The decline in vitamin D levels with aging has many causes, including decreased synthesis of cholecalciferol in aging skin, decreased conversion of $25(OH)_2$-D to $1,25(OH)$-D in the kidney, and decreased vitamin D receptor function.

C. Treatment. Mortality is increased after a hip fracture, and strategies that improve outcomes are needed. Treatment combines a limitation of fracture risk-factor effects, including fall prevention and improvement of bone quality, by applying pharmacotherapy. Newly admitted nursing facility residents only infrequently received an indicated osteoporosis treatment despite the expected high prevalence of osteoporosis in this setting.

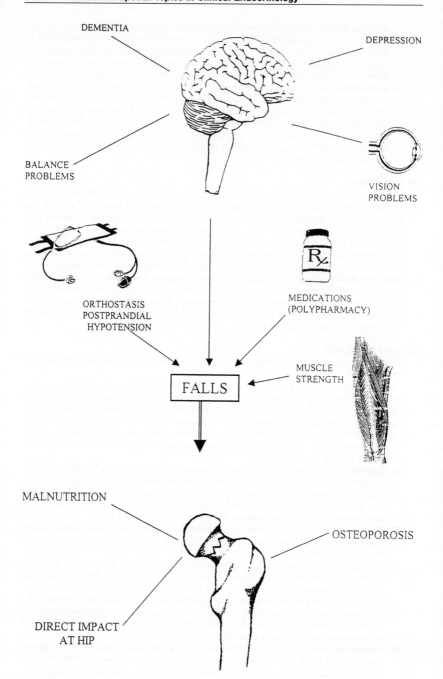

Figure 51.2. Causes of falls and hip fractures.

Prevention of hip fracture in older persons requires administration of calcium and vitamin D. When osteoporosis is established, bisphosphonates should be added. The three approved bisphosphonates are alendronate, risedronate, and ibandronate. Alendronate and risedronate are dosed daily or weekly, and ibandronate has been approved for monthly oral dosing or as an intravenous formulation to be given intermittently (every 3 months). In addition, zoledronic acid is the only once-yearly treatment for women with postmenopausal osteoporosis.

Risk factors for falls are either intrinsic factors, extrinsic factors, or situational factors. New-onset falls in older persons are often due to delirium. Intrinsic causes of falls include muscle weakness, balance problems, gait problems, orthostasis, postprandial hypotension, depression, visual problems, arthritis, activities-of-daily-living impairment, cognitive impairment, and polypharmacy (hypnotics, antidepressants, and antipsychotics). Selective serotonin receptor–inhibitor antidepressants are more likely to be associated with hip fractures than are tricyclics.

The Cochrane Collaboration found in their meta-analytic review that interventions aimed at a single cause are unlikely to protect against falls. Falls interventions need to identify and manage multiple patient-specific factors and involve an interdisciplinary approach if they are to succeed. In nursing home residents, the use of hip protectors, when worn regularly, may reduce hip fracture rate, though this is controversial. Restraints are not fall-prevention devices.

The 30-day mortality after hip fracture was 7.2%. Patients who were operated on within 2 days of admission had a 30-day postoperative mortality rate of 5.8%, versus 9.4% in those patients who experienced a delay of more than 2 calendar days. Recent studies on the benefit of multidisciplinary rehabilitation for people who have sustained hip fracture showed that there is a 16% reduction in the pooled outcome, combining death or admission to a nursing home.

VII. ANOREXIA OF AGING

A. Diet and exercise. Food intake declines throughout the life span. Thus, at middle age, in which obesity is endemic in the United States, persons are actually eating less than when they were younger. This suggests that the major cause of middle-aged obesity is a decrease in physical activity coupled with a decrease in resting metabolic rate. Over age 50, weight loss without an exercise program results in loss of muscle as well as fat. With aging, replacement of muscle mass becomes harder. Thus, in older persons, dieting can lead to a vicious cycle of fat and muscle loss followed by regaining of fat mass only. This can eventually lead to the development of "the fat frail syndrome." Persons who develop "fat frail syndrome" have worse outcomes than underweight frail older persons. Thus, from middle age on, exercise is the key to weight loss. The exercise regimen should include muscle strengthening as well as endurance exercises.

B. Anorexia. People tend to experience less hunger and become rapidly satiated as they age. With aging, the energy expenditure decreases and results in overall less food consumption. This age-related physiologic decline in food intake over the life span has been termed anorexia of aging. The etiology of anorexia of aging is multifactorial, including both central and peripheral causes. Alterations in taste and smell sensitivity with aging appear to play a minor role in the decreased food intake. The cause of this change is mainly age-related decline in taste-bud receptors with decreased food palatability, as well as potential side effects of multiple medications the elderly population is prescribed because of their multiple comorbidities. However, alterations in satiating signals from the stomach appear to play a major role in the early satiation that occurs with aging. Hormonal factors contributing to development of anorexia of aging include decreased levels of testosterone, higher circulating levels of cholecystokinin, possible reduced activity of ghrelin, alterations in leptin release and sensitivity, and decreased endorphin concentrations in brain cerebrospinal fluid. The role of increased activity of certain cytokines such as interleukins (IL) IL-1, IL-2, IL-6, and tumor necrosis factor-α (TNF-α) with aging has also been studied in different studies. The nonendocrine factors linked to anorexia of aging include social isolation, psychological factors, and coexisting medical illnesses.

C. Anatomic characteristics. With aging, the ability of the fundus of the stomach to demonstrate adaptive relaxation to the presence of food particles declines, which results in less food being eaten at each meal. Aging has also been shown to be associated with delayed gastric emptying for both liquids and solids, which is probably caused by increased phasic pyloric pressures or autonomic neuropathy seen in elderly populations. Another important factor is decreased production of nitric oxide locally in the stomach in response to food, which is considered the major reason for the age-related decline in adaptive relaxation. With the decrease in adaptive relaxation, food fills the antrum more quickly, resulting in earlier antral stretch and early satiety.

D. Cholecystokinin (CCK). In addition, circulating levels of the satiating hormone CCK increase with aging. Studies have shown that older subjects have more CCK levels in their small intestine compared to younger age groups. CCK also has a greater satiating effect when administered to older persons. CCK is released in response to fat in the meals, and these findings explain the decline in the fat calories ingested as a person ages.

E. Leptin. Leptin is a peptide hormone produced by the adipose cell. It decreases food intake and increases metabolic rate. With aging, leptin levels increase in men and decline in women. This decrease in leptin level in men is associated with the age-related decline in testosterone, and testosterone administration to older men caused a decrease in leptin levels. Men have a more dramatic decrease in food intake with aging than women, and the testosterone–leptin interaction appears to explain this difference.

F. Neuropeptides. Animal studies have suggested that aging results in the alterations in the levels or responsiveness of a number of neuropeptides involved in food intake, including the endogenous kappa opioid and neuropeptide Y. Neuropeptide Y is one of the mediators of leptin's effects in the central nervous system.

G. Cytokines. Not only do cytokines produce anorexia, they also lead to muscle wasting (cachexia) and a reduction in circulating albumin levels. The cytokines most active in this regard are TNF-α, IL-2, IL-6, and ciliary neurotrophic factor. Older persons suffer multiple inflammatory conditions that result in cytokine elaboration. Certainly, cytokines appear to play a major role in the anorexia seen in frail sick older persons. Studies have shown that aging is associated with increased levels of cortisol and catecholamines, which in turn also lead to increased cytokine activity in this population.

H. Ghrelin. Ghrelin is a ligand for the growth-hormone receptor, which is produced mainly in the gastric mucosa. It exerts its effects by stimulating the release of neuropeptide Y from the arcuate nucleus, which in turn leads to increased appetite. Ghrelin stimulates the release of growth hormone, and it regulates energy balance and adipose tissue metabolism. Studies have shown that ghrelin also inhibits the production of inflammatory cytokines. Data exist that older individuals have impaired secretion of ghrelin in response to nutritional deficiencies, which could possibly contribute to decreased food intake. The role of ghrelin in improving anorexia of aging is still under investigation.

I. Glucagonlike peptide-1 (GLP-1). GLP-1 is secreted from gut endocrine cells, mediates its effects by vagal afferent signals from the liver, and slows gastric emptying. Some studies have shown a possible role of glucagon in satiation associated with older age, particularly in postmenopausal women. Peripheral administration of GLP-1 has been shown to suppress food intake and increase satiety. In diabetics, glucagon administration has been shown to decrease appetite and increase satiety. However, further research is needed to confirm these findings.

J. Treatable causes of weight loss. Besides cancer, numerous treatable conditions result in anorexia and subsequent weight loss. Depression is considered the most common condition leading to weight loss in the elderly, with this cause representing 30% to 36% in community and nursing home settings. The other significant causes include medications, for example, digoxin, theophylline, and excessive levothyroxine

TABLE 51.4	MEALS-ON-WHEELS Mnemonic as an Easy Method to Screen for Causes of Weight Loss in Older Persons

Medications (e.g., digoxin, theophylline, cimetidine)
Emotional (e.g., depression)
Alcoholism, elder abuse, anorexia tardive
Late-life paranoia
Swallowing problems

Oral factors
Nosocomial infections (e.g., tuberculosis)

Wandering and other dementia-related factors
Hyperthyroidism, hypercalcemia, hypoadrenalism
Enteral problems (e.g., gluten enteropathy)
Eating problems
Low-salt, low-cholesterol, and other therapeutic diets
Stones (cholecystitis)

replacement. Metabolic causes include hyperthyroidism, Addison disease, pheochromocytoma, and hypercalcemia. Chronic medical conditions include rheumatoid arthritis, AIDS-related cachexia, temporal arteritis, malabsorption syndromes, *Helicobacter pylori* infection, chronic obstructive pulmonary disease (COPD), congestive heart failure (CHF), alcoholism, and infections. Therapeutic diets may result in excessive weight loss and malnutrition if their effects are not carefully monitored. Other conditions such as bad oral hygiene and poor dentition play an important role in malnutrition in elderly. Table 51.4 provides a simple mnemonic as a reminder of the treatable causes of weight loss in older persons.

K. Anorexia treatment. The key components of treatment include identification and management of the underlying cause, followed by administration of oral liquid calorie supplements with corrections of vitamin and mineral deficiencies, especially vitamin D, folate, and calcium. A meta-analysis has demonstrated their efficacy at increasing food intake and producing weight gain. Supplements should be administered between meals. More aggressive measures such as tube feeding are considered in cases of severe malnutrition and disorders that cause difficulty in swallowing and digestion. A number of orexigenic agents have also been used to increase food intake, including megace, dronabinol, and anabolic steroids. Megestrol acetate was found to decrease cytokine levels and increase food intake in older individuals, especially those with cancer-related cachexia. Nandrolone has been shown to lead to improvement of nutrition in patients with renal failure. Although originally it was thought that growth hormone might improve outcomes in persons with malnutrition, Takata et al. suggested that in critically ill, severely malnourished patients, use of GH increased mortality. In cachexia related to chronic medical conditions such as COPD, CHF, and end-stage renal disease, ghrelin injections have been shown to be effective in improving weight. Some studies have shown the benefit of mirtazapine, an antidepressant, in improving appetite and causing weight gain in patients with underlying depression and weight loss.

Selected References

Abrahamsen B, Nielsen MF, Eskildsen P, et al. Fracture risk in Danish men with prostate cancer: a nationwide register study. *Br J Urol* 2007;100:749–754.

Barrett-Connor E, Khaw KT, Yen SS. A prospective study of dehydroepiandrosterone sulfate, mortality, and cardiovascular disease. *N Engl J Med* 1986;315:1519–1524.

Baumgartner RN, Waters DL, Gallagher D, et al. Predictors of skeletal muscle mass in elderly men and women. *Mech Ageing Dev* 1999;107:123–136.

Canalis E, Giustina A, Bilezikian JP. Mechanisms of anabolic therapies for osteoporosis. *N Engl J Med* 2007;357:905–916.

Cappola AR, Fried LP, Arnold AM, et al. Thyroid status, cardiovascular risk, and mortality in older adults. *JAMA* 2006;295:1033–1041.

Chapman IM. Hypothalamic growth hormone-IGF-I axis. *Endocrinol Aging* 2000;20:23–40.

Chapuy MC, Arlot ME, Delmas PD, et al. Effect of calcium and cholecalciferol treatment for three years on hip fractures in elderly women. *Br Med J* 1994;308:1081–1082.

Evers MM, Marin DB. Mood disorders. Effective management of major depressive disorder in the geriatric patient. *Geriatrics* 2002;57:36–40.

Flint A, Raben A, Astrup A, et al. Glucagon-like peptide 1 promotes satiety and suppresses energy intake in humans. *J Clin Invest* 1998;101:515–520.

Gussekloo J, van Exel E, deCraen AJ, et al. Thyroid status, disability and cognitive function, and survival in old age. *JAMA* 2004;292:2591–2599.

Haren MT, Malmstrom TK, Banks WA, et al. Lower serum DHEAS levels are associated with a higher degree of physical disability and depressive symptoms in middle-aged to older African American women. *Maturitas* 2007;57:347–360.

Johansen KL, Mulligan K, Schambelan M. Anabolic effects of nandrolone decanoate in patients receiving dialysis: a randomized controlled trial. *JAMA* 1999;281:1275–1281.

Johnell, O, Kanis J. Epidemiology of osteoporotic fractures. *Osteoporosis Int* 2005;16:S3–S7.

Kim MJ, Morley JE. The hormonal fountains of youth: myth or reality? *J Endocrinol Invest* 2005;28:5–14.

Kumanov P, Tomova A, Robeva R, et al. Influence of ageing and some lifestyle factors on male gonadal function: a study in Bulgaria. *Andrologia* 2007;30:136–140.

Lainscak M, Andreas S, Scanlon PD, et al. Ghrelin and neurohumoral antagonists in the treatment of cachexia associated with cardiopulmonary disease. *Intern Med* 2006; 45:837.

Melanson KJ, Saltzman E, Vinken AG, et al. The effects of age on postprandial thermogenesis at four graded energetic challenges: findings in young and older women. *J Gerontol A Biol Sci Med Sci* 1998;53:B409–B414.

Mooradian AD, Morley JE, Korenman SG. Endocrinology in aging. *Disease-A-Month* 1988; 34:393–461.

Mooradian AD, Wong NC. Age-related changes in thyroid hormone action. *Eur J Endocrinol* 1994;131:451–461.

Morley JE. Anorexia of aging: physiologic and pathologic. *Am J Clin Nutr* 1997;66:760–773.

Morley JE. Growth hormone: fountain of youth or death hormone? *J Am Geriatr Soc* 1999; 47:1475–1476.

Morley JE. Should all long-term care residents receive vitamin D? *J Am Med Dir Assoc* 2007;8:69–70.

Morley JE, Kaiser F, Raum WJ, et al. Potentially predictive and manipulable blood serum correlates of aging in the healthy human male: progressive decreases in bioavailable testosterone, dehydroepiandrosterone sulfate, and the ratio of insulin-like growth factor 1 to growth hormone. *Proc Natl Acad Sci U S A* 2000;94:7537–7542.

Morley JE, Kraenzle D. Causes of weight loss in a community nursing home. *J Am Geriatr Soc* 1994;42:583–585.

Morley JE, Perry HM III. Androgen deficiency in aging men: role of testosterone replacement therapy. *J Lab Clin Med* 2000;135:370–378.

Morley JE, Thomas DR, Wilson MM. Cachexia: pathophysiology and clinical relevance. *Am J Clin Nutr* 2006;83:735–743.

Nagaya N, Itoh T, Murakami S, et al. Treatment of cachexia with ghrelin in patients with COPD. *Chest* 2005;128:1187–1193.

Nagaya N, Noritoshi M, Junji Y, et al. Effects of ghrelin administration on left ventricular function, exercise capacity, and muscle wasting in patients with chronic heart failure. *Circulation* 2004;110:3674–3679.

Nair KS, Rizza RA, O'Brien RA, et al. DHEA in elderly women and DHEA or testosterone in elderly men. *N Engl J Med* 2006;355:1647–1659.

Neary NM, Small CJ, Wren AM, et al. Ghrelin increases energy intake in cancer patients with impaired appetite: acute, randomized, placebo-controlled trial. *J Clin Endocrinol Metab* 2004;89:2832–2836.

Perry HM III, Horowitz M, Morley JE, et al. Longitudinal changes in serum 25-hydroxyvitamin D in older people. *Metabolism* 1999;48:1028–1032.

Rae HC, Harris IA, McEvoy L, et al. Delay to surgery and mortality after hip fracture. *ANZ J Surg* 2007;77:889–891.

Rhoden EL, Morgentaler A. Risks of testosterone-replacement therapy and recommendations for monitoring. *N Engl J Med* 2004;350:482–492.

Rucker D, Ezzat S, Diamandi A, et al. IGF-I and testosterone levels as predictors of bone mineral density in healthy, community-dwelling men. *Clin Endocrinol* 2004;60:491–499.

Rudman D. Growth hormone, body composition and aging. *J Am Geriatr Soc* 1985;33:800–807.

Sih R, Morley JE, Kaiser FE, et al. Effects of pregnenolone on aging. *J Invest Med* 1997;45:348A.

Sih R, Morley JE, Kaiser FE, et al. Testosterone replacement in older hypogonadal men. A 12-month randomized controlled trial. *J Clin Endocrinol Metab* 1997;82:1661–1667.

Snowdon D. Early natural menopause and duration of post-menopausal life. *J Am Geriatr Soc* 1990;38:402.

Sturm K, MacIntosh CG, Parker BA, et al. Appetite, food intake, and plasma concentrations of cholecystokinin, ghrelin, and other gastrointestinal hormones in undernourished older women and well-nourished young and older women. *J Clin Endocrinol Metab* 2003;88:3747–3755.

Takala J, Ruokonen E, Webster NR, et al. Increased mortality associated with growth hormone treatment in critically ill adults. *N Engl J Med* 1999;341:785–792.

Tariq SH, Haren MT, Kim MJ, et al. Andropause: is the emperor wearing any clothes? *Rev Endocr Metab Disord* 2005;6:77–84.

Truica T, Sweeney M. Prevalence of erectile dysfunction with respect to age, culture and socioeconomic status as assessed by the Men's Health Survey. *Aging Male* 1998;suppl 1:11.

Uchida K, Okamoto N, Ohara K, et al. Daily rhythm of serum melatonin in patients with dementia of the degenerate type. *Brain Res* 1996;717:154–159.

Wurtman JJ, Lieberman H, Tsay R, et al. Calorie and nutrient intakes of elderly and young subjects measured under identical conditions. *J. Gerontol* 1988;43:B174–B180.

Wynne K, Giannitsopoulou K, Small CJ, et al. Subcutaneous ghrelin enhances acute food intake in malnourished patient who receive maintenance peritoneal dialysis: a randomized, placebo-controlled trial. *J Am Soc Nephrol* 2005;16:2111–2118.

Xu X, Pang J, Yin H, et al. Hexarelin suppresses cardiac fibroblast proliferation and collagen synthesis in rat. *Am J Physiol Heart Circ Physiol* 2007;293:H2952–H2958.

Yen SS, Morales AJ, Khorram O. Replacement of DHEA in aging men and women. Potential remedial effects. *Ann N Y Acad Sci* 1995;774:128–142.

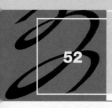

52 APUD SYNDROMES
Adrian Langleben*

I. GENERAL PRINCIPLES
The APUD cell, a term coined by Pearse in 1968, constitutes a family of neurosecretory cells that are widely distributed throughout the body. These cells display electron-dense granules on ultrastructural microscopy and contain neuron-specific enolase, characteristics that persist as malignant degeneration occurs. These cells share a common synthetic pathway for hormone production, from which the acronym APUD has been derived. This includes the capacity for **a**mine **p**recursor **u**ptake and subsequent **d**ecarboxylation, resulting in the synthesis of bioactive amines or polypeptide hormones. This classification remains valid even though subsequent experimental evidence has challenged the notion of a common embryologic origin, i.e., the neural crest for the APUD cells, as originally proposed by Pearse.

A. **Location.** APUD cells are found in:
1. The central and peripheral neuroendocrine system (from the hypothalamus and pituitary to the peripheral autonomic ganglia and adrenal medulla)
2. The gastrointestinal tract (from the pharynx to the anus)
3. The pulmonary mucosa

B. The **function** of the APUD cells is the neuroendocrine regulation of normal homeostatic mechanisms, including vasomotor tone, as well as carbohydrate, calcium, and electrolyte metabolism. Each APUD cell normally synthesizes, stores, and secretes its single amine or polypeptide and is responsive to its environment for stimulation or suppression.

C. **Classification.** Three classes of hormones are produced or regulated by APUD cells: **(1)** the amines (produced by APUD cells), **(2)** the polypeptides (produced by APUD cells), and **(3)** the steroids (produced by the mesodermal adrenal cortex and the gonads). Steroids are not APUD cell products but are involved in the APUD syndromes because they are responsive to the trophic actions of the APUD polypeptides. The specific hormones in the first two categories are listed in Table 52.1.

Hyperplasia or neoplasms of cells that produce these hormones are called **APUDomas,** a term first used by Szijj in 1969 to describe a medullary carcinoma of the thyroid that was secreting adrenocorticotropic hormone (ACTH).

Depending on the location of the tumor and the specific hormone produced, an APUDoma may be characterized as either:
1. **Entopic (orthoendocrine).** The APUD cell in its normal location produces excessive amounts of its native hormone. For example, a β-cell adenoma of the pancreas oversecretes insulin.
2. **Ectopic (paraendocrine).** Polypeptides and occasionally amines are produced by tumors, usually malignant, that are located in areas that do not normally produce that humoral substance. The term **ectopic** is sometimes used to describe embryologically misplaced adenomas such as mediastinal parathyroid adenomas or pheochromocytomas of a sympathetic ganglion. In these instances, the secretion is entopic, but the tumor tissue is embryologically misplaced. The true ectopic syndromes arise from tumors of either endocrine glands or organs not considered endocrine that, when malignant, hypersecrete polypeptide hormones that are not native to that gland or tissue. For example:

*The author wishes to acknowledge Avrum Bluming, author of this chapter in the previous edition.

TABLE 52.1	APUD Cell Hormones

I. Amines
  1. Catecholamines
     a. Epinephrine
     b. Norepinephrine
     c. Dopamine
  2. Serotonin
  3. Histamine
  4. Thyroxine
  5. Acetylcholine
II. Polypeptides
  1. Hypothalamic and pituitary tropic hormones
     a. Adrenocorticotropic hormone
     b. Prolactin
     c. Growth hormone
     d. Melanocyte-stimulating hormone
     e. Thyroid-stimulating hormone
     f. Somatostatin
  2. Thyrocalcitonin
  3. Parathyroid hormone
  4. Gastropancreatic hormones
     a. Gastrin
     b. Secretin
     c. Cholecystokinin-pancreozymin
     d. Gastric inhibitory peptide
     e. Substance P
     f. Insulin
     g. Glucagon
     h. Somatostatin
     i. Human pancreatic polypeptide
     j. Vasoactive intestinal polypeptide

APUD, amine precursor uptake and decarboxylation.

    a. An islet cell malignancy producing the **Zollinger-Ellison syndrome** by elaboration of a high-molecular-weight prohormone of gastrin, not native to the pancreas

    b. An oat cell carcinoma of the lung hypersecreting the prohormone of ACTH, resulting in **Cushing syndrome**

II. APUDOMA SYNDROMES

APUDoma syndromes (Table 52.2) may be categorized as follows.

A. Entopic

  1. Gastrointestinal tract

    a. Carcinoid. First described by Obendorfer in 1907, this tumor is the most frequently encountered tumor of the APUD system. The incidence of carcinoid tumors is estimated to be ~1.5 cases per 100 000 of the general population (about 2 500 cases per year in the United States). Carcinoid tumors have been identified throughout the gastrointestinal tract, including the esophagus, stomach, duodenum, jejunum, ileum, Meckel diverticulum, appendix, colon, rectum, bile ducts, pancreas, and liver. They have also been found in the larynx, thymus, lung, breast, ovary, urethra, and testis.

      (1) The secretory product of the tumor is primarily 5-hydroxytryptamine (serotonin), although there are other hormones reportedly elaborated by

TABLE 52.2 APUDoma Syndromes

Tumor type	Clinical syndrome	Site	Hormone(s)
Entopic			
Carcinoid	Flushing/diarrhea/wheezing	Midforegut Pancreas/foregut Adrenal medulla	Serotonin
Insulinoma	Hypoglycemia	Pancreas/uterus Retroperitoneal liver	Insulin, IGF
Pancreatic glucagonoma	Dermatitis/dementia Diabetes/DVT	Pancreas	Glucagon
Gastrinoma	Ulcer disease	Stomach Duodenum	Gastrin
Somatostatinoma	Diabetes/steatorrhea, cholelithiasis	Pancreas	Somatostatin
Anterior pituitary adenoma	Cushing syndrome Hyperpigmentation Acromegaly, gigantism Galactorrhea	Anterior pituitary gland	ACTH MSH GH Prolactin
Medullary carcinoma	Diarrhea	Thyroid gland	Calcitonin Prostaglandin
Pheochromocytoma	Hypertension	Adrenal medulla	Epinephrine
Ganglioneuroma Neuroblastoma	Abdominal mass	Sympathetic ganglia	Norepinephrine
Bronchogenic carcinoma	Cushing syndrome	Lung	ACTH
Carcinoid of bronchus or gut		Bronchus or gut	
Epithelial cancer of thymus		Thymus	
Islet cell tumor of pancreas		Pancreas	
Medullary cancer of thyroid		Thyroid	
Pheochromocytoma		Adrenal medulla	
Gastrinoma	Zollinger-Ellison syndrome	Pancreas	Gastrin
VIPoma	Watery diarrhea Hypokalemia Alkalosis	Pancreas	VIP

ACTH, adrenocorticotropic hormone, corticotropin; APUD, amine precursor uptake and decarboxylation; DVT, deep venous thrombosis; GH, growth hormone, somatotropin; IGF, insulinlike growth factor; MSH, melanocyte-stimulating hormone; VIP, vasoactive intestinal polypeptide.

this tumor, including bradykinin, hydroxytryptophan, prostaglandins, substance P, neurokinin A (NKA), thyrocalcitonin, pancreatic polypeptide, calcitonin gene–related peptide (CGRP), vasoactive intestinal polypeptide (VIP), and histamine.

(2) Symptoms associated with the classic carcinoid syndrome (which occur in <10% of patients with carcinoid tumors) include the following.

(a) Flushing (found in 49% of symptomatic patients; a pellagralike eruption in severe cases). This symptom is usually attributed to the effects of secreted bradykinin, hydroxytryptophan, and prostaglandins. It is occasionally responsive to a combination of the H_1 blocker diphenhydramine and the H_2 blocker cimetidine. Niacin may partially alleviate the pellagralike eruption.

(b) Diarrhea (found in 83% of symptomatic patients) is attributed to the effects of serotonin, prostaglandin, and bradykinin. It may respond to the serotonin antagonists cyproheptadine or methysergide.

(c) Bronchospasm (found in 6% of symptomatic patients) is attributed to bradykinin, histamine, and prostaglandins, and may also be responsive to methysergide.

The following are all attributed to the effects of serotonin:

(d) Coronary artery spasm leading to angina pectoris

(e) Endocardial fibrosis

(f) Arthropathy

(g) Glucose intolerance

(h) Hypotension

Only 7% to 10% of patients with carcinoid tumors, but up to 45% of those with liver metastases, have been reported to exhibit any of the above symptoms of the carcinoid syndrome. This observation has been attributed to the short half-life of serotonin (<1 minute) and the very high hepatic extraction of this chemical from the circulation.

(3) Diagnosis of a nonfunctioning carcinoid tumor is by biopsy and histologic section. Patients with functioning carcinoid tumors may be diagnosed by measuring the 24-hour urine excretion of 5-hydroxyindoleacetic acid (5-HIAA). A value >9 mg per 24 hours in a patient without malabsorption, or >30 mg per 24 hours in a patient with malabsorption, is reported as diagnostic.

(4) Treatment of choice is surgical excision of the primary tumor and, when possible, of the hepatic or nodal metastases, because this tumor generally grows at an indolent pace. When symptomatic metastases cannot be removed, palliative therapy with the long-acting analog of somatostatin (octreotide acetate, Sandostatin) has been of reported benefit for both symptom control and occasionally for actual reduction of tumor burden.

A review of 300 patients with carcinoid tumors treated with interferon-α for a median of 2.5 years concluded that this agent has significant antitumor effects in 70% to 80% of patients, as manifested by biochemical control and inhibition of tumor growth. Tumor progression generally occurred within 3 to 9 months after cessation of the drug. However other studies have questioned the efficacy of interferon-α. Traditional single-agent and combination chemotherapy have only modest activity. However, targeted therapies with recombinant human endostatin and with sunitinib have shown very high rates of "clinical benefit" and prolonged stable disease. Furthermore, imatinib, an inhibitor of the platelet-derived growth-factor receptor (PDGFR-B), has recently been shown to produce a high rate of disease stabilization.

Until recently, the median 5-year survival rate for all cases of carcinoid tumors was 82%, increasing to 94% if the tumor was localized and falling to 64% with regional lymph node involvement, and to 18% with the presence of distant metastases. It remains to be seen if the new targeted therapies will improve these statistics.

b. Insulinoma. This tumor usually arises from the β cells of the islets of Langerhans. This tumor, which accounts for >75% of functional islet-cell tumors, is usually benign and may be a solitary lesion, but in 10% of cases it is part of a multiple endocrine neoplasia (MEN) syndrome.

(1) Symptoms are the result of hypoglycemia from excessive or inappropriate insulin secretion.

(2) Diagnosis is by radioimmunoassay (RIA) of plasma insulin level, which is generally high or high-normal.

(3) Treatment, ideally, consists of surgical removal of the tumor, if possible. Resection or radiofrequency ablation of metastatic lesions should be considered when necessary. If the tumor is malignant and cannot be completely excised, hypoglycemic symptoms may be controlled with diazoxide, corticosteroids, or the long-acting analog of somatostatin (Sandostatin). Conventional chemotherapy has only modest activity, but sunitanib has been specifically associated with a high clinical benefit in this histology.

c. Pancreatic glucagonoma is usually the result of a malignant tumor of the α cells of the islets of Langerhans. From 60% to 85% of patients have metastatic disease at the time of diagnosis, even though the growth rate tends to be slow.

(1) The **clinical picture** is a characteristic rash in a diabetic patient. The rash, called **necrolytic erythema migrans,** consists of superficial epidermal blistering, central healing, and peripheral spreading with a defined edge. The erythema may occur anywhere but has a predilection for the lower abdomen and areas of chafing, such as the groin or thighs. Glossitis, anemia, thromboembolic phenomena, and weight loss have been reported as well.

(2) **Diagnosis** is by RIA of elevated plasma glucagon. Plasma insulin is also often elevated as a compensatory reaction. The tumor may be localized by pancreatic angiography.

(3) **Treatment** of this catabolic syndrome is surgical excision when possible. Selective intra-arterial streptozotocin infusion for symptomatic liver metastases may be of benefit. Symptom control and reduction of glucagon levels has been reported using the long-acting analog of somatostatin (Sandostatin). Specific data evaluating the efficacy of the targeted tyrosine kinase and mTOR inhibitors in this histology is not yet available. However, in a preliminary study, everolimus, an effective inhibitor of the mammalian target of rapamycin (mTOR), achieved clinical benefit in 86% of patients with low-grade islet-cell tumors.

d. Gastrinoma is a result of G- (gastrin-secreting) cell hyperplasia or carcinoma in the stomach or duodenum. The inappropriate hypergastrinism is stimulated by an ingested meal and is not affected by secretin stimulation. The possibility of gastrinoma syndrome should be entertained in all patients with ulcer disease and in those with unexplained secretory diarrhea.

(1) The **clinical picture** varies from an almost asymptomatic duodenal ulceration to acute perforation of a jejunal ulcer. This clinical picture may be indistinguishable from that due to a pancreatic gastrinoma and is therefore termed **pseudo-Zollinger-Ellison syndrome.**

(2) **Treatment.** The ulcerative symptoms usually respond completely to surgical antrectomy. Alternative therapies include omeprazole, a benzimidazole that suppresses gastric acid secretion by inhibiting the sodium-potassium ATPase of the parietal cell, and the long-acting analog of somatostatin (octreotide acetate, Sandostatin).

e. Somatostatinoma. Somatostatin, first identified as a polypeptide of the hypothalamus, is an inhibitor of release of somatotropin (growth hormone) from the anterior pituitary. It is also present entopically in the D cells of the pancreas, from where it inhibits the release of insulin and glucagon. The tumor responsible for this syndrome is usually a malignant pancreatic neoplasm, with 83% of patients reported to have metastatic disease at the time of diagnosis.

(1) **Signs and symptoms** of this syndrome include:
  (a) Mild diabetes mellitus
  (b) Steatorrhea (usually with dyspepsia and diarrhea)
  (c) Gallstones
  (d) Anemia
  (e) Weight loss

(2) **Diagnosis** is confirmed when plasma levels of somatostatin are elevated while those of insulin and glucagon are depressed, distinguishing this APUDoma from a glucagonoma.

(3) **Treatment** is surgical removal of the tumor, if possible.
  Streptozotocin may help shrink symptomatic metastases.

2. Anterior pituitary gland
  a. Clinical features
  (1) ACTH overproduction leads to Cushing syndrome.
  (2) Melanocyte-stimulating hormone overproduction leads to hyperpigmentation.
  (3) Growth-hormone overproduction leads to acromegaly or gigantism.
  (4) Prolactin overproduction leads to galactorrhea.
  b. Treatment for all the above is ablation of the pituitary gland by irradiation or surgery, followed by appropriate replacement therapy.
3. Thyroid gland. Medullary carcinoma of the thyroid produces calcitonin, which causes no symptoms, and prostaglandin, which often is responsible for diarrhea.
  a. Treatment is total thyroidectomy and removal of all involved lymph nodes.
  b. This tumor may be a solitary lesion or part of MEN type 2.
4. Adrenal medulla and other sympathetic ganglia. These tumors range from the relatively well-differentiated and benign pheochromocytoma (which may be a solitary lesion or part of MEN), ganglioneuroma, and paraganglioma, to the highly malignant neuroblastoma.

B. Ectopic
1. Cushing syndrome
  a. This is the **most frequently encountered ectopic APUD syndrome**, and it is usually a result of one of the following:
  (1) Bronchogenic carcinoma (most often of the small-cell type)
  (2) Carcinoid tumors of the bronchus or the gut
  (3) Epithelial carcinoma of the thymus
  (4) Islet-cell tumors of the pancreas
  (5) Medullary carcinoma of the thyroid
  (6) Pheochromocytoma.
  (7) Cushing syndrome has been reported as well in primary malignancies of the ovary, liver, and breast. Interestingly, in 1928, Brown reported clinical stigmata of adrenal cortical overactivity in a patient with cancer of the lung, 4 years before Cushing described this symptom complex to which his name has been appended.
  b. Symptoms include:
  (1) Hypokalemia, often with associated alkalosis
  (2) Hyperglycemia
  (3) Hypertension
  (4) Hirsutism
  (5) Edema
  (6) Profound muscle weakness and atrophy.
     The other features seen in pituitary Cushing syndrome or exogenous corticosteroid excess, such as centripetal obesity, cutaneous striae, moon facies, buffalo hump, and increased pigmentation, are less common, and are reported to be more common in the relatively indolent carcinoids, thymomas, and pheochromocytomas.
  c. Diagnosis begins by thinking about the possibility in the appropriate clinical setting. When the previously described features are present, a plasma ACTH >200 pg/mL is highly suggestive of ectopic ACTH production. The simplest biochemical approach is to obtain an 8 A.M. and a 6 P.M. cortisol level (in ectopic ACTH syndromes, these are usually >40 μg/mL, showing loss of the diurnal variation), followed by an 8 A.M. cortisol and ACTH level after 2 mg of dexamethasone given every 6 hours for 8 doses (48 hours). In 95% of cases of ectopic hormone production, the ACTH and cortisol levels will not suppress (i.e., will not fall to at most 60% of the prior values). If results of these studies are consistent with ectopic ACTH production, a careful evaluation for a tumor should be undertaken and continued until the source of ACTH overproduction has been identified.

   d. Treatment should be directed at eradicating the primary tumor when possible, using surgery, radiotherapy, and/or chemotherapy as determined by the histologic characteristics and location of the primary tumor. If treatment directed at the primary tumor fails, drugs that inhibit adrenal corticoid production may be tried, including aminoglutethimide, metyrapone, or mitotane. In rare cases of chronic ectopic ACTH excess and indolent tumors, bilateral adrenalectomy may be considered.

2. Zollinger-Ellison syndrome (pancreatic gastrinoma). In 1955, Zollinger and Ellison described two patients with fulminant peptic ulcer disease and non-β islet-cell tumors of the pancreas. The gastrin produced by these pancreatic tumors is believed to arise from the pancreatic D cell. Most of the tumors are multifocal within the pancreas, and though ~25% are benign adenomas, 60% to 75% are malignant and have metastasized by the time of diagnosis. Thirty percent to 50% of patients belong to kindreds with a history of MEN syndromes.

   a. Symptoms include:

   (1) Severe peptic ulcer disease manifested usually by pain. The ulcers are commonly multiple, often recurrent, and frequently located in atypical sites.

   (2) Diarrhea, which may precede the ulcer symptoms or which may be the dominant feature of presentation in 15% to 20% of cases.

   b. Diagnosis is by RIA for circulating <u>gastrin levels</u> that are 10 times greater than normal. In 60% to 70% of patients the tumor cannot be localized radiographically in the absence of metastases. The use of selective venous catheterization in association with a provocative stimulus, such as secretin, may provide accurate localization of the tumor. In 30% to 50% of patients, associated MEN syndromes coexist.

   c. Treatment entails parietal cell receptor blockade with cimetidine, ranitidine, or omeprazole and complete extirpation of the tumor if possible. If surgical removal of the gastrinoma is not possible, antrectomy or total gastrectomy may be required.

3. VIPoma (WDHA syndrome, also called pancreatic cholera). The responsible hormonal agent is a <u>vasoactive intestinal polypeptide</u> that is normally secreted by both the small and large intestinal mucosa cells, and, in this case, ectopically secreted by δ cells, usually located in the body and tail of the pancreas. This syndrome has also been seen in patients with bronchogenic carcinoma and neuroblastoma.

   a. Symptoms typically include the following (and make up the acronym for WDHA syndrome):

   (1) Watery **d**iarrhea, with a volume of 6 to 8 L per day

   (2) Hypokalemia

   (3) Alkalosis

   b. Treatment is surgical excision, if possible, of both the primary and metastases. Some reports have implicated <u>prostaglandins</u> in the pathogenesis of this syndrome, and <u>indomethacin</u>, an inhibitor of prostaglandin synthesis, has sometimes been of benefit. Symptoms may also be controlled with the long-acting analog of somatostatin (octreotide acetate, Sandostatin).

C. MEN syndromes. The endocrinopathies, whether entopic or ectopic, may occur in combinations sufficiently often to be designated MEN syndromes. These associations are usually genetic and transmitted as an autosomal dominant trait. The pathologic changes of dysplasia range from hyperplasia to malignant neoplasia. The endocrinopathies may present in a synchronous fashion with simultaneous aberrant endocrine manifestations or, more commonly, in a metachronous fashion in which one component of MEN precedes the others by several years. There are now three well-established genetic associations of MEN.

1. MEN1. Initially described by Wermer, this syndrome is composed of three component endocrinopathy sites: parathyroid, anterior pituitary, and pancreatic islet cells. A genetic defect, allelic loss in the 11q12-11q13 region, has been linked to this disorder.

   a. Parathyroid. Usually hyperplasia leading to elevated parathyroid hormone levels.

b. Anterior pituitary
  (1) Increased prolactin leading to lactation and amenorrhea in the female
  (2) Increased human growth hormone leading to acromegaly
  (3) Increased ACTH–melanocyte-stimulating hormone leading to Cushing syndrome and/or hyperpigmentation
  (4) Increased thyroid-stimulating hormone leading to hyperthyroidism
  (5) Increased gonadotropins leading to feminizing or masculinizing syndromes
c. Pancreatic islet cells
  (1) Ectopic hypergastrinemia with Zollinger-Ellison syndrome.
  (2) Ectopic release of VIP with WDHA syndrome.
  (3) Ectopic ACTH leading to Cushing syndrome.
  (4) Ectopic parathyroid hormone leading to hyperparathyroidism.
  (5) Entopic hyperinsulinism.
  (6) Entopic hyperglucagonism.
  (7) Entopic release of human pancreatic polypeptide. This peptide, which by itself is identified with no clinical syndrome, has pharmacologic and, presumably, physiologic actions that appear to be antagonistic to cholecystokinin-pancreozymin (i.e., it relaxes gallbladder contractions and inhibits exocrine pancreatic enzyme release). It is deficient in patients with obesity and with cystic fibrosis of the pancreas, and is excessively elaborated in response to a meal in MEN1 patients. Most important, it has been found to be an excellent marker in the fasting state of MEN1 patients with islet-cell tumors.

2. **MEN2A.** Initially described by Sipple, this syndrome is also composed of three endocrinopathy components: medullary carcinoma of the thyroid, adrenal pheochromocytoma, and secondary parathyroid hyperplasia.
  a. Medullary carcinoma of the thyroid is usually present in both lobes of the thyroid gland and consists of microscopic, nonpalpable tumors. A diagnostic histologic feature is the presence of amyloid in the thyroid carcinoma, which is reported to contain the prohormone of thyrocalcitonin. This tumor may also elaborate ectopic ACTH and prostaglandins.
  b. Adrenal pheochromocytoma is bilateral in 70% of cases and is seldom malignant. Satellite lesions may be present in the sympathetic ganglia ranging from the mediastinum to the urinary bladder. It is important to **exclude pheochromocytoma before operating on medullary thyroid carcinoma,** because general anesthesia administered to patients with untreated pheochromocytomas may lead to hypertensive crisis and death.
  c. Secondary parathyroid hyperplasia with elevated circulating parathormone levels usually disappears when the medullary carcinoma of the thyroid (with associated increase in circulating thyrocalcitonin) is resected.
3. **MEN2B**
  a. This syndrome, originally described by Schimke et al., is similar to MEN2A. In addition to the medullary carcinoma of the thyroid and pheochromocytomas seen in the latter syndrome, these patients are often found to have:
    (1) Multiple mucosal neuromas of lips, mouth, and tongue
    (2) Marfanoid habitus
    (3) Prominent jaw
    (4) Pectus excavatum
      In contrast to MEN2A, hyperparathyroidism is rare in MEN2B. As well, medullary thyroid carcinoma tends to develop in younger MEN2B patients, and often pursues a more aggressive course.
  b. Management of the thyroid and adrenal components of this syndrome is surgical, as it is for type 2A. Bilateral adrenal resection and total thyroidectomy with central node dissection are recommended. Activating mutations of the RET proto-oncogene have been found in sporadic as well as MEN2-related medullary thyrohyoid cancer. Recently, targeted therapy with small-molecule tyrosine kinase inhibitors that inhibit RET signaling has been shown to be active in medullary thyroid cancer.

Selected References

Averbuch SD, Baylin SB, Chahinian AP, et al. Neoplasms of the neuroendocrine system. In: Holland JR, Frei D III, Bast RC Jr, et al., eds. *Cancer Medicine*. 3rd ed. Philadelphia: Lea & Febiger; 1993.

Bajetta E, Ferrari L, Procopio G, et al. Efficacy of a chemotherapy combination for the treatment of metastatic neuroendocrine tumours. *Ann Oncol* 2002;13:614–621.

Baylin SB. APUD cell fact and fiction. *Trends Endocrinol Metab* 1990;1:1981.

Bluming AZ, Berez RR. Successful treatment of unstable angina in malignant carcinoid syndrome using the long acting somatostatin analogue SMS 201-995 (Sandostatin). *Am J Med* 1988;85:872–874.

Brown WH. A case of pluriglandular syndrome. Diabetes of bearded women. *Lancet* 1928; 2:1022.

Edney JA, Hoffmann S, Thompson JS, et al. Glucagonoma syndrome is an underdiagnosed entity. *Am J Surg* 1990;160:625.

Faiss S, Pape UF, Böhmig M, et al. Prospective, randomized, multicenter trial on the antiproliferative effect of lanreotide, interferon alfa, and their combination for therapy of metastatic neuroendocrine gastroenteropancreatic tumors—the International Lanreotide and Interferon Alfa Study Group. *J Clin Oncol* 2003;21:2689–2696.

Friesen SR. The APUD syndromes. *Prog Clin Cancer* 1982;8:75.

Gordon P, Comis RJ, Maton PN, et al. Somatostatin and somatostatin analogue (SMS 201-995) in treatment of hormone secreting tumors of the pituitary and gastrointestinal tract and non-neoplastic disease of the gut. *Ann Intern Med* 1989;110:35.

Journal of Clinical Oncology, vol 23, #16S, part 1 of 2, page 310s, Proceedings of ASCO 2005, abstract 4008c.

Kulke M, Bergsland E, Ryan DP, et al. A phase II, open-label safety, pharmacokinetic, and efficacy study of recombinant human endostatin in patients with advanced neuroendocrine tumors. *Proc Am Soc Clin Oncol* 2003;22:A958.

Kulke M, Lenz HJ, Meropol J, et al. A phase 2 study to evaluate the efficacy and safety of SU11248 in patients (pts) with unresectable neuroendocrine tumors (Nets) *Proc Am Soc Clin Oncol* 2005;23:A4008.

Kvols LK, Perry RR, Vinik AI, et al. Neoplasms of the neuroendocrine system and neoplasms of the gastroenteropancreatic endocrine system. In: Holland JF, Frei E III, eds. *Cancer Medicine*. 5th ed. Hamilton, Ontario: BC Decker; 2000:1121.

Larsson C, Skogseid B, Oberg K, et al. Multiple endocrine neoplasia type 1 gene maps to chromosome 11 and is lost in insulinoma. *Nature* 1988;332:85.

Oberg K. The action of interferon alpha on human carcinoid tumors. *Semin Cancer Biol* 1992;3:35.

Pearse HGE. Common cytochemical and ultrastructural characteristics of cells producing polypeptide hormones (the APUD series) and their relevance to thyroid and ultimobranchial C cells and calcitonin. *Proc R Soc Lond* 1968;170:171.

Ram MD. Apudomas. *Curr Surg* 1981;38:230.

Sipple JH. The association of pheochromocytoma with carcinoma of the thyroid gland. *Am J Med* 1961;31:163.

Szijj I, et al. Medullary cancer of the thyroid gland associated with hypercorticism. *Cancer* 1969;24:16.

Temple WJ, Sugarbaker EV, Ketcham AS. The APUD system and its apudomas. *Int Adv Surg Oncol* 1981;4:255.

Välimäki M, Järvinen H, Salmela P, et al. Is the treatment of metastatic carcinoid tumor with interferon not as successful as suggested? *Cancer* 1991;67:547–549.

Vidal M, Wells S, Ryan A, Cagan R. ZD6474 suppresses oncogenic RET isoforms in a *Drosophila* model for type 2 multiple endocrine neoplasia syndromes and papillary thyroid carcinoma. *Cancer Res* 2005;65:3538–3541.

Vinik AI, Thompson NW, Averbuch SD. Neoplasms of the gastroenteropancreatic endocrine system. In: Holland JF, Frei D III, Bast RC Jr, et al., eds. *Cancer Medicine*. 3rd ed. Philadelphia: Lea & Febiger; 1993.

Phan AT, Wang L, Xie J, et al. Association of VEGF Expression with peer prognosis among patients with low-grade neuroendocrine carcinoma. *J Clin Oncol* {Asco proceedings. June 20 supplement} 2006;24[18S]:A4091.

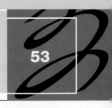

I. INTRODUCTION

The term **multiple endocrine neoplasia (MEN),** which succeeds the earlier designation "multiple endocrine adenomatosis," refers to a group of syndromes of familial disorders manifested by multiple endocrine abnormalities, neoplasms (frequently malignant), and often other associated tissue dysplasias. They are "ectopic hormone" syndromes, are usually marked by multiple hormonal abnormalities, and are considered genetic disorders. In recent years there have been no major changes in the basic principles of MEN syndromes, but current research is at the molecular and cellular level. There still are the three basic "syndromes": MEN1, MEN2 (also known as MEN2A), and MEN3 (also known as MEN2B). MEN3 familial medullary thyroid carcinoma (FMTC) is now thought by some to be a separate form of this disease without the other manifestations.

A. History. Modern recognition is credited to Wermer, who first proposed the term multiple endocrine adenomatosis, describing a syndrome of tumors involving the pituitary gland, pancreatic islet cells, and parathyroid gland. Sipple described a syndrome of thyroid carcinoma and pheochromocytoma. Schimke noted a subgroup of the Sipple syndrome manifested by neurofibromatoses and other genetic abnormalities in association with the Sipple features. Zollinger-Ellison (ZE) syndrome, thought at first to be separate, is now considered a variant of MEN without other manifestations (it is rarely seen in MEN1 and more often in MEN2).

B. Genetics. These disorders are autosomal dominant and highly penetrant, although frequently asynchronous and periodic in expression. Even though half of newly diagnosed cases are sporadic (i.e., mutant), 50% of the offspring of such individuals will develop the same MEN syndrome as their parents. The genetic disorders are complex and have not yet been completely identified. Family and linkage studies have mapped MEN1 to long-arm deletions in chromosome 11 and MEN2A to the pericentromeric region of chromosome 10. For example, it has been suggested that MEN1 is caused by a mutation in a tumor-suppressor gene or genes when two gene copies in a tumor precursor cell have been segmentally inactivated ("two-hit" oncogenesis). Currently, testing for such mutations is only possible in research facilities. In medullary carcinoma (MEN2A and 2B, familial type), the *RET* oncogene has been identified and is probably 100% predictive for development of this tumor. Genetic probe studies of markers will be helpful in the future for identification and risk evaluation of patients and families. New variations are being described and reported, each containing some of the mutant conditions, but it is clear that rigid classification of these syndromes is not possible. An international consensus recommends that MEN1 be defined as the presence of two of the three MEN tumor types and "familial" MEN is an index case that has one of the three main tumor types (parathyroid, enteropancreatic adenomas, and pituitary adenomas). The primary purpose of familial screening is to prevent morbidity and mortality, with little evidence of efficacy of prevention of morbidity or mortality, but with much concern about insurance eligibility in a healthy person.

C. Pathogenesis. In 1966, Pearse proposed the APUD theory (amine precursor uptake and decarboxylation; see Chapter 52). This concept embodies the assumption that the involved tissues are of embryonic neural crest origin and are potential producers of peptide hormones. They share the common ability to take up amine precursors and

749

convert them to neurotransmitter hormones. This theory is controversial and does not seem to fit all the embryologic data and the clinical observations of involvement of nonectodermal tissues. It is believed that there probably is a genetic tissue with a propensity to overstimulation, hyperplastic, and neoplastic activity mediated by an as-yet-unknown growth-stimulating factor(s).

II. MEN CLASSIFICATION

MEN syndromes are grouped by cluster of manifestations and are recognized by consensus of most authorities. As mentioned earlier, variations and exceptions to the rule are common. However, most authorities feel that there is no reason for such syndromes as Von Hippel-Lindau, peripheral neurofibromatoses, and McCune-Albright to be reclassified as new MEN syndromes, although awareness of endocrine manifestations of these disorders is necessary. Genetic testing for MEN2A, FMTC, and MEN2B is now commercially available, but not for MEN1.

A. MEN1

  1. Manifestations

   a. Hyperparathyroidism occurs in >75% of patients and is the most common disorder associated with MEN1 as a consequence of hyperplasia of more than one gland. Renal and bone disorders are not frequently associated.

   b. Pituitary lesions occur in >50% of these patients. Generally, they are nonfunctional tumors associated with pituitary hypofunction resulting from mechanical destruction of the gland, although it is possible that many of those thought to be nonfunctional in the past were prolactinomas that were not detected because of the unavailability of appropriate assays. Less commonly seen are functioning prolactinomas and tumors producing acromegaly and Cushing syndrome. Silent lesions are frequently detected only by imaging techniques (computed tomography [CT] and magnetic resonance imaging [MRI]) performed in patients suspected of having MEN1. Secondary acromegaly with pituitary adenoma can be caused by ectopic growth hormone–releasing factor (GHRF) production from pancreatic, adrenal, and carcinoid tumors and may be entirely reversible by removal of such sources.

   c. Pancreatic tumors. More than 75% of patients have pancreatic tumors. These are usually multiple and may be of β- or other islet-cell origin. They can be associated with hypergastrinemia (ZE syndrome). The most common complaint of patients with these tumors is peptic disease. Hyperinsulinemia and secreting vasoactive intestinal polypeptide tumor, or VIPoma (pancreatic cholera), can be a manifestation of these pancreatic tumors or a VIPoma ("pancreatic cholera").

   d. Adrenal cortex. About 40% of patients have adrenal adenomas or hyperplasia. Such lesions are generally nonfunctional but are detected as incidental findings.

   e. Thyroid disease. About 20% of patients have thyroid disorders. These include tumors, benign or malignant (nonmedullary), occasional thyrotoxicosis, colloid goiter, and Hashimoto thyroiditis.

   f. Uncommon lesions. These include carcinoids, particularly of the bronchus, as well as lipomata, gastric polyps, testicular tumors, and nerve sheath tumors.

  2. Diagnostic evaluation and screening. MEN1 is rare before the age of 10 years but can develop at any age, peaking between the second and fourth decades. Hyperparathyroidism is the usual presenting feature. Screening of the family should be done after the diagnosis is established in an individual, and the patient should be tested periodically for the other manifestations. This is especially important in patients with ZE syndrome (50% of these have MEN1). Hypergastrinemia may be associated with hyperparathyroidism and relieved by parathyroidectomy.
  Testing should include:

   a. Serum calcium

   b. Serum prolactin

   c. Serum gastrin and pancreatic polypeptides

    d. Assessment for hypoglycemia (e.g., fasting blood sugar)

    e. CT or MRI of the pituitary to detect early or silent lesions

        Pancreatic imaging is inefficient for early detection of pancreatic tumors. Early diagnoses of endocrine lesions are biochemical (e.g., screening test, stimulation meals after basal levels of serum pancreatic peptides, and gastrin response).

B. MEN2 or MEN2A

  1. Manifestations

    a. Medullary thyroid carcinoma. Medullary thyroid carcinomas occur in >90% of cases. They are usually multicentric and are preceded by C-cell hyperplasia. These tumors produce calcitonin and occasionally other hormones, including adrenocorticotropic hormone (ACTH) (with Cushing manifestations) or serotonin. Hypercalcitoninemia has no known physiologic significance (e.g., does not lead to hypocalcemia) but is invaluable for diagnosis.

    b. Pheochromocytoma

      (1) Pheochromocytomas develop in >70% of cases. They are usually bilateral and are either intra-adrenal or extra-adrenal, and they are frequently multiple with sustained or intermittent hypertension. They usually appear in the third or fourth decade of life.

      (2) Zeller and colleagues noted 11 patients who had pheochromocytoma and islet-cell tumors. This overlap syndrome had no other manifestation of the MEN syndrome. Therefore, all pheochromocytoma patients should be screened for pancreatic tumors by imaging or chemical studies, or both. [131]MIBG (*meta*-iodobenzylguanidine) imaging is particularly useful for detecting adrenal medullary tumors and pheochromocytomas.

    c. Hyperparathyroidism, secondary to hyperplasia, occurs in ~50% of patients. This is probably not a response to hypercalcitoninemia, because it can occur in the absence of medullary carcinoma.

    d. Rare familial cutaneous lichen amyloidosis, a localized (scapular) pruritic eruption with MEN2A, is clearly associated and is defined as an autosomal dominant syndrome.

  2. Diagnostic evaluation and screening. Suspected individuals should probably be evaluated every 1 to 2 years. Studies should include serum calcium and plasma calcitonin determinations, especially after pentagastrin- or calcium-infusion provocative testing. Catecholamines, vanillylmandelic acid, and metanephrine studies may be performed. ACTH assays also may be warranted. Carcinoembryonic antigen may be a good prognostic marker for medullary carcinoma of the thyroid, but *RET* gene determination is the most valuable test. The high predictive value of the finding of the *RET* oncogene mutation makes testing of patients with a familial history (MEN2A and MEN2B) of medullary carcinoma of the thyroid extremely important. Such a finding warrants prophylactic total thyroidectomy, even in asymptomatic patients, at early ages.

C. MEN3 or MEN2B

  1. Clinical manifestations

    a. Multiple gangliomas. These occur in >95% of patients. They are especially seen on the lips, eyelids, and tongue, producing the characteristic "lumpy lips" appearance. Also frequently noticed are marfanoid habitus, hyperplastic corneal nerves, and gastrointestinal ganglioneuromatosis and megacolon. Hypertrophy or prominence of corneal nerves can be found in MEN2A as well. Gastrointestinal symptoms include diarrhea and motility disorders such as megacolon and severe constipation (Hirschsprung disease). These may be manifested in infancy and might be the first sign of MEN3.

    b. Medullary carcinoma of the thyroid appears nearly universally, and early thyroidectomy may be the only hope of cure. *RET* gene determination is confirmatory.

    c. Pheochromocytoma has an incidence of ~33% in MEN3.

    d. Unlike in MEN2A, hyperparathyroidism is uncommon, occurring in <5% of patients.

2. Diagnostic evaluation and screening. In this form of MEN, which may have an indolent course, the most important diagnostic evaluation is clinical. Assessment for hypertension, ganglioneuromas, corneal nerve hypertrophy, and gastrointestinal lesions is the key to diagnosis. The lumpy lips and tongue abnormality are pathognomonic, but biopsy studies of apparently normal skin can reveal nerve sheath abnormalities microscopically. The endocrine assessment of MEN3 is the same otherwise as for MEN2.

III. TREATMENT

A. Treatment is directed to the individual conditions with the added conditions and complications brought about by multicentricity of the lesions. For example, a thyroid carcinoma is almost always multicentric, whether or not there are palpable lesions. Therefore, treatment must be total thyroidectomy.

B. Pancreatic lesions are also multicentric; however, total excision is impossible or impractical in most situations. For example, surgical management of MEN1 may include parathyroidectomy with implantation of one gland or a fragment in the forearm plus resection of an endocrine tumor of the tail and enucleation of tumors in the head and body of the pancreas. Total pancreatectomy should be avoided.

C. Many authorities recommend bilateral adrenalectomy for pheochromocytoma because of the frequent bilateral occurrence and high degree of recurrence.

D. Screening for all possible components of the syndrome should be done before treatment is begun. For example, if a pheochromocytoma and medullary carcinoma exist simultaneously, adrenal surgery should be performed first to prevent hypertensive crises during thyroid surgery. Early detection of the MEN syndrome is important because prognosis and cure rates are far better with prompt recognition and vigorous, aggressive treatment.

E. Hypergastrinemia may be associated with hyperparathyroidism and relieved by parathyroidectomy.

F. It appears that with the incredible advances in medical genomics that are being made, any hormonal secreting tumor should require further investigation for additional tumors.

Selected References

Decker RA, Wells SA Jr. Multiple endocrine neoplasia. *Jpn J Surg* 1989;19:645–657.

Hilden JM, Watterson J, Carr CL. Genetic testing for familial cancer. A clinician's perspective. *Minn Med* 1996;79:29–32.

Lallier M, St-Vil D, Giroux M, et al. Prophylactic thyroidectomy for medullary carcinoma in gene carriers of MEN2 syndrome. *J Pediatr Surg* 1998;33:846–848.

Lips CJ, Hoppener JW, Van Nesselrooij BP, et al. Counselling in multiple endocrine neoplasia syndromes: from individual experience to general guidelines. *J Intern Med* 2005;257:69–77.

Marx S, Spiegel AM, Skarulis MC, et al. Multiple endocrine neoplasia type I: clinical and genetic topics. *Ann Intern Med* 1998;129:484–494.

Pearse AGE. The APUD concept and hormone production. *Clin Endocrinol Metab* 1980;9:211–222.

Schimke RN. Multiple endocrine adenomatosis syndromes. *Adv Intern Med* 1976;21:249–265.

Schimke RN. Multiple endocrine neoplasia. How many syndromes? *Am J Med Genet* 1990;37:375–383.

Schimke RN, Hartmann WH, Prout TE, et al. Syndrome of bilateral pheochromocytoma, medullary thyroid carcinoma and multiple neuromas. A possible regulatory defect in the differentiation of chromaffin tissue. *N Engl J Med* 1968;279:1–7.

Second International Workshop on Multiple Endocrine Neoplasia Type II Syndromes. Cambridge, UK, Sept. 17–20, 1986. *Henry Ford Hosp Med J* 1987;35:93–175.

Sipple JH. The association of pheochromocytoma with carcinoma of the thyroid gland. *Am J Med* 1961;31:163–166.

Skinner MA, Moley JA, Dilley WG, et al. Prophylactic thyroidectomy in multiple endocrine neoplasia type 2A. *N Engl J Med* 2005;353:1105–1113.

Third International Workshop on MEN Type II syndromes. Heidelberg, West Germany, Sept. 28–30, 1989. *Henry Ford Hosp Med J* 1989;37:98–203.

Yip L, Cote GJ, Shapiro SE, et al. Multiple endocrine neoplasia type 2: evaluation of the genotype-phenotype relationship. *Arch Surg* 2003;138:409–416.

Wermer P. Genetic aspects of adenomatosis of endocrine glands. *Am J Med* 1954;16:363–371.

Zeller JR, Kauffman HM, Komorowski RA, et al. Bilateral pheochromocytoma and islet cell adenoma of the pancreas. *Arch Surg* 1982;117:827–830.

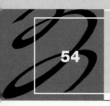

RADIOLOGY, NUCLEAR MEDICINE, AND ENDOCRINOLOGY*

54

Sing-Yung Wu

I. IMAGING MODALITIES RELATED TO ENDOCRINE DISEASE

A. Isotopic

1. Radioactive iodine. Radioactive iodine uptake (RAIU) and imaging reveals the functional status of thyroid tissue, including nodules, ectopic tissue, and metastatic foci. The sodium/iodide symporter (NIS) mediates iodide uptakes.

a. Iodine 131 (^{131}I) is reserved for thyroid cancer imaging and therapy, and for management of a hyperfunctioning thyroid gland or nodule.

b. Iodine 123 (^{123}I) replaces other iodine isotopes for routine thyroid RAIU and scan because of its short half-life (13.3 hours) and low radiation dose to the patient.

c. Patient preparation

(1) For a patient on **no** thyroid medication (either thyroid hormone or antithyroid) who has not received iodine-containing agents recently, no patient preparation is necessary.

(2) For a thyroid cancer patient on suppressive dose of **thyroxine (T$_4$),** stop the T$_4$, which has a half-life (T$_{1/2}$) of 6 to 8 days, for 3 weeks, or stop the T$_4$ and switch to **tri-iodothyronine (T$_3$)** (25 μg two or three times a day; T$_3$ has a shorter T$_{1/2}$ of about 1 day) for 2 to 4 weeks, then stop the T$_3$ for 2 weeks. Both methods of preparation can achieve serum thyroid-stimulating hormone (TSH) levels >30 mU/L in >90% of patients. It is also good practice to get a blood sample for thyroglobulin (Tg) measurement before giving the ^{131}I dose.

To avoid the morbidity of hypothyroidism that is often associated with thyroid hormone withdrawal, recombinant human TSH (rhTSH) (Thyrogen) has been developed for clinical use. Patients are given 10 U (0.9 mg) of rhTSH, two doses 24 hours apart. Twenty-four hours after the second dose, 1 to 3 mCi of ^{131}I ("stunning" may occur with doses of 5 to 10 mCi) is administered orally, and a total-body scan is obtained 48 hours later.

(3) For a hyperthyroid patient on **antithyroid medication,** such as propylthiouracil (PTU) or methimazole (MMI), stop the PTU or MMI for 3 days, then do the uptake and scan; give a treatment dose of ^{131}I if indicated. After administration of ^{131}I (for Graves disease or toxic nodular goiter), PTU or MMI can be resumed in 48 hours.

(4) For a patient who has received a large dose of iodine (e.g., water-soluble computed tomography [CT] radiocontrast agent), one should usually should wait 2 to 4 weeks for an accurate RAIU study, ^{131}I total-body scan, or ablative treatment for thyroid cancer.

2. ^{99m}Tc-MIBI (methoxy-isobutyl-isonitrile). Preoperative localization of an abnormal parathyroid gland (2 to 3 hours delay and/or ^{123}I substrate imaging) can reduce operative time, postoperative morbidity, and the need for repeat surgery. A total-body scan may be helpful for ^{131}I-negative metastatic thyroid cancer lesions. No patient preparation is needed.

*This work has been supported by the U.S. Department of Veterans' Affairs.

3. **Iodocholesterol (^{131}I-labeled 6-iodomethyl-19-norcholesterol, NP-59)** for adrenocortical imaging in Cushing disease, cortisol-producing adenoma, and primary aldosteronism.

 Patient preparation: One drop saturated solution of potassium iodide (SSKI) or Lugol solution PO t.i.d. started 1 day before imaging and continued throughout the study. For a suppression scan, patients receive 2 mg of dexamethasone PO q6h beginning 2 to 3 days before injection of NP-59. The medication is continued until imaging is completed.

4. **MIBG (^{131}I- or ^{123}I-metaiodobenzylguanidine)** for adrenomedullary imaging in pheochromocytoma, neural crest tumors (paragangliomas), carcinoid, and medullary thyroid carcinoma. ^{131}I-MIBG may be used for palliative therapy.

 Patient preparation: Same as with iodocholesterol.

5. **Indium 111(^{111}In) octreotide scan.** Somatostatin (SS) analog is used to show neural crest tumors, including pheochromocytoma, carcinoid, paraganglioma, medullary thyroid carcinoma, islet-cell tumor, gastrinoma. If available, one should also consider receptor imaging other than SS.

 Patient preparation: Discontinue somatostatin analog therapy 1 week before study. Administration of a laxative may be considered.

6. **^{18}FDG PET/CT or SPECT/CT (fluorodeoxyglucose positron emission tomography [PET]/computed tomography or single photon emission computed tomography [SPECT]/CT).** FDG PET or SPECT imaging in combining with multislice CT provides anatomic and metabolic information; it may be helpful in detecting ^{131}I-negative/thyroglobulin-positive thyroid carcinoma and evaluating its prognosis, as well as in characterizing a variety of endocrine tumors.

 Patient preparation: Fasting for 4 to 6 hours.

7. **Thallium 201 (^{201}Tl).** Imaging techniques using ^{201}Tl facilitate the detection of ^{131}I-negative metastatic thyroid cancer lesions in total-body scan.

 Patient preparation: None.

8. **Other isotopic scans.** Isotope bone scan is extremely useful in Paget bone disease to determine disease location and activity.

 Patient preparation: None.

B. **Nonisotopic.** Adrenal, thyroid (<1.5 cm in diameter and nonpalpable), and pituitary "incidentaloma" found by CT/ultrasonography (US)/magnetic resonance imaging (MRI) for unrelated problems are often benign, nonfunctioning lesions, such as adenomas or cysts.

1. **MRI** is the first choice for imaging of pituitary and parasellar lesions. Gadolinium diethylenediaminepenta-acetic acid has been used as an MRI contrast agent. Dynamic scan may be obtained at 20- to 30-second intervals.

 Patient preparation: None.

 MRI is contraindicated in patients with an indwelling metal prosthesis or pacemaker or claustrophobia. **Caution:** The use of gadolinium-containing contrast agents in patients with renal or liver dysfunction has been associated with nephrogenic systemic fibrosis (NSF) or nephrogenic fibrosing dermopathy (NFD).

2. **Multislice CT** is the first choice for imaging adrenal and abdominal endocrine lesions. Patients are often given both oral and intravenous iodine-containing contrast. Quantitative CT is the first choice for evaluating osteoporosis, particularly in early postmenopausal bone loss.

 Patient preparation: NPO after midnight.

 Caution: CT with contrast is contraindicated in patients who are allergic to iodine-containing agents and those whose serum creatinine is >1.5 mg/dL.

3. **PET-CT** combines complementary modalities, thereby allowing precise structural and functional characterization of a variety of endocrine conditions.

4. **US** provides excellent and reproducible anatomic images for thyroid, parathyroid, and neighboring structures. It can be used to guide fine-needle aspiration for cytologic diagnosis of an endocrine/thyroid/adrenal nodule. **Endoscopic or intraoperative US** may be useful in making an early diagnosis of pancreatic/abdominal endocrine tumors.

5. **Venography (phlebography)** is usually accompanied by venous sampling to determine hormonal output from a gland (e.g., adrenal, parathyroid) or a suspected area of functional metastatic lesion. Venous samples usually are obtained before injection of contrast agent.
6. **Intra-arterial angiography (arteriography)** has been largely replaced by multislice CT angiography (CTA) or MRA.
7. **Planar x-ray radiography** is useful in screening for bone age, bone disease, sellar size, and tumor metastases (lytic lesions).

II. ENDOCRINE DISORDERS
Table 54.1 lists recommended multitechnique imaging approaches for various endocrine disorders.

A. **Pituitary abnormalities**
1. **Functional adenoma** is usually a microadenoma (<10 mm), a growth hormone–secreting adenoma (acromegaly), an adrenocorticotropic hormone (ACTH)–secreting adenoma (Cushing disease), or a prolactinoma. Imaging modalities are MRI (may use dynamic to increase the detection rate) and CT (thin-section). Localization of microadenomas within the pituitary gland demands highest standards of imaging technique and interpretation. The diagnosis is made on clinical and laboratory grounds.
2. **Nonfunctional adenoma** is often a macroadenoma. Imaging modalities are MRI and CT. MRI has distinct advantages over CT in the delineation of the extent of macroadenoma. Cavernous sinus involvement and basilar skull invasion are shown best on coronal and sagittal images.
3. **Hypopituitarism.** MRI is used for delineation of common anatomic abnormalities in patients with hypopituitarism that may be the result of developmental, toxic, hypoxic, or traumatic etiologic factors.
B. **Adrenal abnormalities.** Thin-section CT is the imaging technique of choice for the initial evaluation in adults; US is used in children.
1. **Cushing syndrome.** Clinical and biochemical studies usually first establish the diagnosis of ACTH-dependent Cushing syndrome (MRI of the pituitary is the first choice) or adrenal tumor. Imaging techniques are used to determine on which side an adrenal tumor is located. Imaging modalities include:
   a. **CT** to determine the location and size of the lesions
   b. **MRI** to assess the size and extent of a pituitary lesion
   c. **Radioiodinated iodocholesterol scan (NP-59)**
      (1) **ACTH-dependent cortical hyperplasia** (70% of cases involve excess secretion of glucocorticoids). Bilateral symmetric (NP-59) visualization, with nonvisualization after suppression with dexamethasone.
      (2) **ACTH-independent adenoma.** Unilateral visualization (adenoma) versus hyperplasia seen with bilateral heterogeneous uptakes.
   d. **PET-CT** ACTH-independent adenoma, hyperplasia, and carcinoma (and metastasis) are visualized concordantly.
2. **Primary aldosteronism (Conn syndrome).** After biochemical documentation of primary aldosteronism, the next step is to localize the lesion and determine whether one or both adrenals are affected. Imaging modalities include the following.
   a. **CT,** thin-section, to differentiate a unilateral adenoma (80% of cases) from bilateral hyperplasia. One difficulty is that there is a 2% to 8% incidence of a small nonfunctioning adrenal adenoma in the general population. MRI is an alternative imaging modality.
   b. **Venous sampling.** Technical difficulties and complications, such as rupture of the adrenal veins, should also be considered.
   c. **Iodocholesterol scanning** is most useful if the patient is on a dexamethasone suppression protocol.
3. **Pheochromocytoma.** The diagnosis must be first made clinically and biochemically. About 85% of pheochromocytomas arise in the adrenal medulla, and 15% are found in extramedullary sites. Imaging modalities include the following:

TABLE 54.1 **Optimal Imaging Modalities in the Management of Endocrine Disorders**[a]

Disorder	131I	123I	PET/CT	MIBI	Octre	MIBG	Tl	Chol	US	CT	MRI	Venogram
Pituitary												
Functional adenoma (acromegaly, Cushing, prolactinoma)										2	1	
Nonfunctional adenoma										2	1	
Cushing disease			4					3	1	2		
Conn syndrome								3	1			2
Pheochromocytoma			3		2	2				1		
Adrenogenital syndrome			3						2	1		
Addison disease										1	2	
Adrenocortical carcinoma			3							1	2	
Carcinoid					2	3				1		
Paraganglioma					2	3				1		
Thyroid												
Graves disease	2[b]	1										
Nodules		2							1[c]			
Thyroiditis												
Subacute		1										
Painless		1										
Congenital hypothyroidism	1[d]											
Carcinoma	1		2	3			4					
Parathyroid												
Adenoma				2					1			3
Pancreas												
Insulinoma					1[e]	4			3[f]	1[e]	2	
Glucagonoma					1[e]	4			3[f]	1[e]	2	
Gastrinoma					1[e]	4			3[f]	1[e]	2	
Islet-cell tumor					1[e]				3[f]	1[e]	2	
Struma ovarii	1										2	

[a]Numbers indicate order of preference for administration of tests.
[b]Treatment with 131I.
[c]Fine-needle aspiration can be done concurrently.
[d]Radioactive iodine uptake and perchlorate discharge test.
[e]PET may be combined with CT as PET/CT fusion imaging.
[f]Endoscopic ultrasound may be extremely helpful for insulinoma in pancreatic head.
CT, computed tomography (may be combined with an angiography, CTA); FDG, fluorodeoxyglucose; MIBG, metaiodobenzylguanidine; MIBI, methoxy methylpropyl isonitrile; MRI, magnetic resonance imaging; PET, positron emission tomography.

a. **CT** has been the imaging modality of choice; MRI is an alternative to CT. Both have high sensitivity in detecting sporadic tumors but not as sensitive in NEM2.

b. **¹¹¹In-Octeotide or ¹³¹I-MIBG** is useful if CT findings are equivocal or if recurrent or metastatic disease is suspected. ¹³¹I-MIBG is much more sensitive than CT or MRI for diagnosing adrenal medullary hyperplasia (a precursor) and also has been used to treat patients with unresectable or metastatic pheochromocytomas. Overall, octreotide and MIBG scanning score similarly with respect to the diagnosis of pheochromocytoma, both having a specificity of 88%.

c. **PET-CT** may be helpful in detecting occult pheochromocytomas.

4. Adrenogenital syndrome. The differential diagnosis includes congenital adrenal hyperplasia, ovarian neoplasia, polycystic ovarian disease, and autonomous adrenal tumors. Imaging modalities include the following.

   a. CT. Hyperplasia or tumor can be detected.

   b. US may be used to delineate adrenal masses in children and thin adults.

5. Addison disease. A biochemical distinction between pituitary and adrenal causes must be established first. Imaging modalities include CT, which is valuable in distinguishing certain specific adrenal causes (e.g., dense calcification from previous granulomatous disease, hemorrhage, metastasis) from idiopathic adrenal atrophy.

6. Adrenocortical carcinoma. This is a rare malignant neoplasm that accounts for <0.2% of all cancer deaths. The CT findings are not specific. The differential diagnosis includes metastasis, lymphoma, adenoma, and granulomatous infection. MRI may be useful to differentiate benign adenoma from malignancy. In this respect, ^{18}FDG PET/CT may also be helpful as well as to identify additional unsuspected lesions.

C. Neural crest tumors (other than pheochromocytoma). These include paragangliomas, neuroblastoma, and carcinoid tumors. CT or MRI is sensitive in the initial diagnosis and follow-up. ^{111}In-octreotide, ^{131}I-MIBG or PET/CT may be used in demonstrating metastatic lesions.

D. Thyroid

1. Graves disease. Diffuse enlargement of the thyroid gland, characteristic eye signs, suppressed TSH, increased serum free thyroxine, and elevated RAIU usually confirm the diagnosis.

   a. ^{123}I. An elevated uptake in the face of elevated serum T_3/T_4 is important evidence to differentiate Graves disease from other entities such as thyroiditis (subacute, painless, or postpartum) and iodine-induced (amiodarone-induced, type 1) or factitious thyrotoxicosis. Imaging is important in Graves disease only when toxic nodular goiter is in the differential diagnosis.

   b. ^{131}I is used for therapy.

2. Thyroid nodule

   a. US is used to determine whether a palpated nodule is part of a focal, multifocal, or diffuse disease process; whether that nodule is solid, cystic, or calcified; as well as to document and follow up the size. Fine-needle aspiration (US-guided, if necessary) often is used to make a cytologic diagnosis in cases involving a solitary hypofunctioning nodule.

   b. Radioactive iodine (^{123}I) provides a true physiologic picture of the thyroid tissue because it determines the functional status of the nodule (cold, warm, or hot). ^{131}I is used for the management of toxic nodular goiter.

   c. CT is not generally used as a first-line imaging modality in this field, but it can provide valuable data detailing extrathyroid tumor extension and invasion of malignant thyroid nodules; it is particularly effective in the areas of the superior mediastinum and the cervical lymph nodes.

3. Thyroiditis. RAIU with ^{123}I is useful in determining different phases of subacute, painless, and postpartum thyroiditis. In the acute phase, when the patient has elevated T_3 and T_4, the RAIU is characteristically suppressed. In the recovery phase, the RAIU can rise transiently to even above normal. Occasionally, patients with Hashimoto thyroiditis and a relatively high RAIU need a perchlorate discharge test to document a defect in organification, if antithyroid antibodies are negative.

4. Dyshormonogenesis. RAIU and perchlorate discharge tests are used to detect dyshormonogenesis, including an organification defect.

5. Carcinoma. Treatment of differentiated thyroid carcinoma involves a postablative ^{131}I total-body scan and therapy with 30 to 200 mCi of oral ^{131}I. **FDG PET** is used in posttherapy ^{131}I scan–negative patients and may have prognostic value.

E. Parathyroid. Once the diagnosis of primary hyperparathyroidism is established, localization of a parathyroid adenoma may be helpful to the surgeon.

1. US provides correct preoperative localization of 60% to 70% in new cases where the parathyroid glands are close to the thyroid gland, but it is less reliable in identifying ectopic glands in the mediastinum.

2. **⁹⁹ᵐTc-MIBI scans** have 83% sensitivity and specificity and compare favorably with ultrasound and MRI.
3. **Venography with selected venous sampling** technique is used after other non-invasive procedures have failed to locate an adenoma.

F. **Insulinoma and glucagonoma.** Insulinomas are uncommon in patients <20 years of age. After the diagnosis is confirmed biochemically, radiographic localization includes pancreatic US and CT (with CTA) as well as venography with sampling in the case of glucagonoma. Endoscopic US may be extremely helpful in the early diagnosis of insulinoma in the pancreatic head. Somatostatin receptor scintigraphy and PET/CT are also noninvasive methods.

G. **Ovarian teratoma.** Modalities to detect struma ovarii, or a thyroxine-producing teratoma, include RAIU and CT scanning.

III. SUMMARY

The advancement in structural and functional characterization (multislice CT, CTA, MRI, and PET/CT) discussed in this chapter has altered the way we manage endocrine disease to a large extent. In addition, use of these techniques has either eliminated unnecessary endocrine surgery or resulted in greater postoperative success.

Selected References

Cooper DS, Doberty GM, Haugen BR, et al. Management guidelines for patients with thyroid nodules and differentiated thyroid cancer, the American Thyroid Association Guidelines Taskforce. *Thyroid* 2006;16:109–142.

Elaini AB, Shetty SK, Chapman VM, et al. Improved detection and characterization of adrenal disease with PET-CT. *Radiographics* 2007;27:755–767.

Hoang JK, Lee WK, Lee FM, et al. US features of thyroid malignancy: pearls and pitfalls, *Radiographics* 2007;27:847–865.

Lau JH, Drake W, Matson M. The current role of venous sampling in the localization of endocrine disease. *Cardiovasc Intervent Radiol* 2007;30:555–570.

Rennert J, Doerfler A. Imaging of sellar and parasellar lesions. *Clin Neurol Neurosurg* 2007;109:111–124.

Robbins RJ, Wan Q, Grewal RK, et al. Real-time prognosis for metabolic thyroid carcinoma based on 2-[18F]fluoro-2-deoxy-D-glucose-positron emission tomographic scanning. *J Clin Endocrinol Metab* 2006;91:498–505.

Rufini V, Calcagni ML, Baum RP. Imaging of neuroendocrine tumors. *Semin Nuclear Med* 2006;36:228–247.

Scarsbrook AF, Thakker RV, Wass JAH, et al. Multiple endocrine neoplasia: spectrum of radiologic appearances and discussion of a multitechnique imaging approach. *Radiographics* 2006;26:433–452.

Schima W. MRI of the pancreas: tumours and tumour-stimulating processes. *Cancer Imaging* 2006;6:199–203.

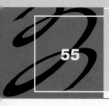

SURGERY FOR ENDOCRINE DISORDERS
Orlo H. Clark

THYROID NODULES AND THYROID CANCER

I. GENERAL PRINCIPLES

About 4% of people in the United States have thyroid nodules, yet only 40 persons per million per year develop clinical thyroid cancer and 6 persons per million per year die from this tumor. A selective approach must therefore be used in determining whether a patient will benefit from observation or thyroidectomy. Well-differentiated thyroid cancers generally have an indolent and favorable course, especially in patients <45 years of age. However, some thyroid cancers are lethal. Thyroid cancer is the most rapidly increasing cancer in women.

A. Factors suggesting that a thyroid nodule is benign are
   1. Multinodular goiter
   2. Diffuse goiter
   3. Family history of benign goiter
   4. High antithyroid antibody titers (Hashimoto thyroiditis)
   5. Increased thyroid-stimulating hormone (TSH)
   6. Cystic lesion
   7. Decrease in size in response to TSH-suppression treatment
   8. Benign cytology by aspiration biopsy

B. Factors suggesting that a thyroid nodule might be malignant are
   1. History of low-dose therapeutic irradiation
   2. Family history of thyroid cancer, multiple endocrine neoplasia type 2 (MEN2; also termed Sipple syndrome, comprising medullary carcinoma of the thyroid, hyperparathyroidism, and pheochromocytoma), or Cowden syndrome
   3. History of thyroid cancer in other lobe
   4. Solitary
   5. Young male
   6. Growing nodule
   7. Hard nodule
   8. Solid or mixed solid–cystic lesion
   9. Palpable ipsilateral lymph nodes
   10. Vocal cord palsy
   11. Suspicious appearance on ultrasonography
   12. Suspicious or diagnostic cytology for cancer by aspiration biopsy

C. About 13% of persons exposed to low-dose, therapeutic irradiation (6.5 to 3 000 rad calculated dose to thyroid gland) develop thyroid cancer. Parathyroid tumors, salivary gland tumors, and breast tumors are also more common in irradiated persons.

D. About 40% of persons exposed to low-dose therapeutic radiation who also have a discrete thyroid nodule have thyroid cancer in the thyroid gland. In 60%, the index nodule is the cancer, and in 40% the cancer is found elsewhere in the thyroid gland.

E. Most persons with thyroid nodules are euthyroid with a normal serum TSH level. TSH levels are increased in hypothyroidism and decreased in hyperthyroidism.

F. Benign thyroid nodules include colloid and involutional nodules, adenomas, cysts, and focal thyroiditis.

G. Malignant thyroid tumors include papillary, mixed papillary–follicular, follicular variant of papillary thyroid cancer, and follicular thyroid cancer, Hürthle cell cancer, medullary cancer, undifferentiated or anaplastic thyroid cancer, lymphosarcoma, teratoma, squamous cell cancer, and secondary or metastatic tumors.

II. EVALUATION OF THE NODULE

Patients with clinically solitary thyroid nodules or a discrete or growing nodule in a multinodular goiter should be evaluated by a sensitive TSH test, ultrasound examination of the thyroid and cervical nodes, and percutaneous aspiration cytology. If a lesion is malignant by cytologic examination, the thyroid gland and tumor should be removed; if a lesion is benign, it can be safely followed; and if it is a follicular neoplasm, and the TSH level is suppressed, a radioactive iodine scan is recommended. If the follicular neoplasm is "hot" by scanning, it can be followed; if it is "cold" and >2 cm, it should usually be removed. This approach is safe and cost-effective. Fine-needle aspiration (FNA) is less effective in patients with a history of irradiation or a family history of thyroid cancer because both benign and malignant thyroid neoplasms exist, so that thyroidectomy is usually recommended.

III. MANAGEMENT

Thyroid nodules that are growing, that occur in patients with a family history of thyroid cancer or who have been irradiated, that are unusually hard on palpation, or that are suspicious on ultrasound examination or diagnostic of cancer by aspiration biopsy cytology should be surgically removed by thyroid lobectomy or thyroidectomy.

A. Multinodular goiters should be evaluated by ultrasound, and any suspicious area or nodule in a nodular goiter should be biopsied by a fine needle (23 gauge) for cytology. Ultrasonography using the 10-MHz real-time scanner is a good method for quantitating nodule size, suspicious nodules for cancer, and adjacent lymphadenopathy. Blood thyroglobulin levels usually correlate with goiter size.

B. Solitary nodule. If the lesion is benign by aspiration biopsy cytology, some clinicians recommend treatment with enough thyroxine (T_4) to suppress TSH but keep tri-iodothyronine (T_3) and T_4 levels in the normal range. Lesions suspected of malignancy should be removed with the entire lobe of the thyroid gland. If they are malignant, a total or near-total thyroidectomy should usually be done.

C. Irradiated patients. All palpable nodules in these patients should be removed because of the increased risk of cancer ($\sim$40%). Treatment should be total thyroidectomy or near-total thyroidectomy.

D. Familial thyroid cancer. All family members of patients with familial medullary thyroid cancer should have a *RET* oncogene test. *RET* oncogene–positive patients warrant a prophylactic total thyroidectomy prior to age 6 years. They also need to be screened for pheochromocytoma and hyperparathyroidism. Patients with a family history of familial nonmedullary thyroid cancer also are at increased risk of thyroid cancer and should have a careful physical and ultrasound examination.

E. Surgical treatment. There is considerable controversy concerning the extent of surgery necessary for patients with suspicious thyroid nodules. The minimal operation for any lesion that may be cancer, except for small lesions in the isthmus, is a total thyroid lobectomy on the side of the nodule. Excisional biopsy is acceptable treatment for lesions in the isthmus, but excisional biopsy, partial lobectomy, or subtotal thyroidectomy for all but the smallest of lesions should be discouraged. Near-total or total thyroidectomy has advantages over lobectomy for differentiated thyroid cancers >1.0 cm, but they have higher complication rates than lobectomy. Total thyroidectomy should be performed only on patients with medullary thyroid cancer and those with differentiated thyroid cancer when it can be performed with minimal morbidity (<2% rate of hypoparathyroidism or recurrent laryngeal nerve injury). The advantages of total thyroidectomy are that it **(1)** results in removal of all thyroid cancer within the thyroid gland, **(2)** allows use of radioactive iodine to identify and ablate micrometastases, **(3)** allows use of blood thyroglobulin levels as a sensitive indicator of persistent disease, **(4)** decreases local recurrence and improves survival rate, and **(5)** decreases the risk of change from a differentiated tumor to an undifferentiated tumor.

Patients with clinically palpable, cervical or ultrasound-positive lymphadenopathy should be treated by a modified neck dissection (preserving the sternocleidomastoid muscle, spinal accessory nerve, and internal jugular vein) on the side of lymphatic metastases. An ipsilateral prophylactic central neck dissection is recommended by some thyroid cancer guidelines.

F. Postsurgical treatment. All persons with differentiated thyroid cancer should be treated with enough **thyroid hormone** to suppress TSH. **Radioactive iodine** is used for scanning the patient to determine the extent of the disease and for ablation of micrometastases. Ablative treatment with radioactive iodine is recommended for differentiated thyroid cancers >2 cm, for multifocal tumors, for tumors extending to the margin of the resected specimen, and for all locally invasive tumors or for local (lymphatic) or distant metastases. **External radiation** is used in patients >45 years old for invasive or metastatic thyroid cancer that fails to take up radioactive iodine, for distant metastases, and for undifferentiated thyroid carcinomas or unresectable medullary thyroid carcinomas. Chemotherapy is palliative in some patients with recurrent unresectable thyroid cancer or with undifferentiated thyroid cancer and is usually used in conjunction with external radiation. Some clinical trials are now in progress using "target therapy" against certain oncogenes or tumor-suppressor genes.

G. Follow-up evaluation

1. Question the patient about bone pain, cough, and headache at intervals of 6 months to 1 year. Perform thorough cervical examination by ultrasonography for lymph node metastases and recurrent thyroid masses.

2. A serum thyroglobulin level should be monitored after withdrawl of thyroid hormone or after recombinant TSH. If the level is increased after total thyroidectomy, a thyroid ultrasound examination is recommended because recurrent cancer is likely. For patients with medullary thyroid cancer, basal and serum calcitonin levels should be obtained, as should a carcinoembryonic antigen level, and *RET* oncogene. Patients with medullary thyroid cancer should also be screened for a pheochromocytoma and hyperparathyroidism.

3. A sensitive TSH should be obtained to ascertain whether the patient is receiving enough thyroid hormone.

4. A radioactive iodine scan is recommended 3 months after thyroidectomy for patients with thyroid cancers >2 cm and for invasive tumors or for patients with distant metastases who have been treated by total thyroidectomy. The patient should discontinue T_3 (Cytomel, 50 to 75 μg per day) for 2 weeks or T_4 (125 to 200 μg per day) for 6 weeks prior to scanning so that serum TSH levels will be elevated. Patients should receive a low-iodine diet for 2 weeks and can also be scanned after receiving recombinant TSH. Once the scan reveals no uptake, additional scans are unnecessary unless other tests, such as an elevated blood thyroglobulin level, suggest recurrent tumor.

5. A chest radiograph should be obtained yearly in patients with thyroid carcinoma. About 60% of pulmonary metastases take up radioactive iodine. A positron emission tomography (PET) scan or PET/computed tomography (CT) scan is recommended for patients who are thyroglobulin- or calcitonin-positive and ultrasound- or scan-negative.

H. Factors predicting prognosis. Differentiated thyroid cancers (papillary, mixed papillary–follicular, follicular, and Hürthle cell) generally have a favorable prognosis. These tumors should be classified into stages (DeGroot classification).

Stage 1. Localized to thyroid

Stage 2. Thyroid and adjacent cervical lymph nodes

Stage 3. Invasion into adjacent structures

Stage 4. Distant metastases

The prognosis for thyroid cancer is worse in older patients (men over 40 years and women over 50 years) and gets worse as the stage progresses. Medullary thyroid cancer has a poorer prognosis (~50% dead in 10 years) than papillary, follicular, or Hürthle cell thyroid cancer (20% dead in 15 years); poorly differentiated have ~40% mortality at 10 years, and undifferentiated thyroid cancer has an extremely poor prognosis.

HYPERTHYROIDISM (SEE CHAPTER 30)

I. GENERAL PRINCIPLES
See Chapter 30.

II. DIFFERENTIAL DIAGNOSIS
See Chapter 30.

III. MANAGEMENT
Graves and Plummer diseases may be treated by antithyroid drugs, radioactive iodine, or subtotal thyroidectomy. Patients with small goiters and minimal hyperthyroidism respond well to antithyroid drugs, whereas patients with larger goiters require treatment with radioactive iodine or surgery. All patients should be prepared with antithyroid medications prior to definitive treatment.

A. Drug therapy with antithyroid drugs. See Chapter 30.

B. Radioactive iodine (^{131}I). See Chapter 30.

C. Subtotal or near-total thyroidectomy

    1. This is the treatment of choice for young patients (children and pregnant women) who are not readily controlled by antithyroid medications, for patients with large diffuse or nodular goiters with low radioactive iodine uptake (RAIU), for patients with coexisting suspicious or malignant thyroid nodules, for patients with exophthalmos, and for psychologically or mentally incompetent patients who probably will not take thyroid hormone. It is also excellent treatment for all patients with Graves disease if an experienced thyroid surgeon is available. The incidence of hypothyroidism the first year after subtotal thyroidectomy depends on remnant size. After the first year the incidence increases at a rate of <1% per year. This is lower than the 3% per year after treatment with radioiodine.

    2. Preparation for surgery includes maintaining the patient euthyroid by continuing antithyroid medications and then adding potassium iodide solution or Lugol solution (3 drops twice a day) for 10 days prior to thyroidectomy.

    3. Complications of thyroidectomy include a low (1%) incidence of hypoparathyroidism or injury to the recurrent laryngeal nerve with permanent hoarseness. Hypothyroidism develops in ~15%, depending on the size of the thyroid remnant, and recurrent hyperthyroidism in ~5%.

    4. The thyroid remnant should range from 4 to 8 g. For children, smaller remnants are required to avoid recurrence. Many surgeons today prefer total or near-total thyroidectomy because it avoids recurrence and may help patients with Graves ophthalmopathy.

D. Special situations

    1. Thyroid storm (hyperthyroid crisis). See Chapter 30.

    2. Severe exophthalmos. See Chapter 30.

    3. Hyperthyroidism in pregnancy. See Chapter 30.

OTHER THYROID DISORDERS

I. THYROIDITIS
See Chapter 29.

II. ECTOPIC THYROID
Aberrant placement of thyroid tissue occurs because of the failure of normal migration of the thyroid during embryologic development. It results in development of a sublingual

thyroid or thyroglossal duct cyst (midline cyst) anywhere from the foramen cecum at the base of the tongue to the normal position of the thyroid. Thyroglossal duct cysts occasionally must be removed for cosmetic or diagnostic reasons or because of infection. <u>About 1% of these cysts contain papillary or squamous cell carcinoma.</u> Occasionally, it is difficult to differentiate histologically between a thyroid rest and metastatic thyroid cancer. Thyroid rests are situated in the midline, whereas laterally located thyroid tissue in lymph nodes (lateral aberrant thyroid) almost always is metastatic thyroid cancer.

 HYPERCALCEMIA AND HYPERPARATHYROIDISM

I. GENERAL PRINCIPLES (Table 55.1)
See Chapters 25 and 26.

II. CLINICAL MANIFESTATIONS AND ASSOCIATED CONDITIONS
See Chapters 25 and 26.

III. DIAGNOSIS (Table 55.2)
See Chapters 25 and 26.

TABLE 55.1	Differential Diagnosis of Hypercalcemia

Malignancy
Solid
Metastatic to bone
Secretion of PTH-like protein
Hematogenous
Myeloma, leukemia, lymphoma
Endocrine
Hyperparathyroidism (plus malignancy account for 90% of all hypercalcemic cases)
Other endocrine
Hyperthyroidism, hypothyroidism, hypoadrenalism, acromegaly, and VIPoma
Increased intake
Calcium and alkali (milk–alkali syndrome)
Vitamin D or A
Thiazides
Lithium
Estrogen
Granulomatous disorders
Sarcoidosis
Tuberculosis
Berylliosis
Other disorders
Benign familial hypocalciuric hypercalcemia
Immobilization
Error or artifact
Idiopathic hypercalcemia of infancy
Acute renal failure with rhabdomyolysis
PTH, parathyroid hormone.

TABLE 55.2	Laboratory Tests for Hypercalcemia or Possible Hyperparathyroidism

General tests (serum)
Calcium
Phosphorus
Parathyroid hormone
Chloride
pH
Alkaline phosphatase
Protein electrophoresis
Uric acid
Creatinine
Hematocrit

Other tests
Urinalysis
24-hour urinary calcium
Chest radiography
Intravenous pyelography

Specialized tests
Hydrocortisone suppression test
1,25-Dihydroxyvitamin D
Nephrogenous cyclic AMP
Tubular resorption of phosphorus
Industrial-grade hand films
Bone biopsy

AMP, adenosine monophosphate.

IV. MANAGEMENT

A. **Surgical management—selection of patients for parathyroidectomy.** There is general agreement that patients with symptomatic hyperparathyroidism (HPT), those <50 years old, and those with a serum calcium level 1 mg/dL above the upper limit of normal should be treated with parathyroidectomy. Because "asymptomatic patients" with primary HPT receive the same metabolic benefits of parathyroidectomy as symptomatic patients, many people believe that these patients should also be treated by parathyroidectomy. However, operative treatment is not urgent, and in all patients the diagnoses must be certain. Patients who are pregnant and have primary HPT should be treated surgically during the second trimester. Patients with hypercalcemic crisis should be treated surgically as soon as the diagnosis is confirmed and they are appropriately hydrated.

B. **Medical management of hypercalcemia.** See Chapters 25 and 26.

C. **Localization.** Preoperative localization of parathyroid tumors can now be accomplished by experienced individuals in ~75% of patients using 10-MHz real-time ultrasonography or sestamibi imaging. These tests are especially helpful in patients who have previously had an unsuccessful parathyroid operation or extensive thyroid surgery. All localization procedures have problems in identifying the smaller abnormal parathyroid glands in patients with hyperplasia. Only the largest gland is seen in many of these cases. Because an experienced surgeon can cure 95% of patients with primary HPT without using localization tests, such tests are not required but are helpful for surgeons who perform unilateral or focal explorations with or without intraoperative parathyroid hormone (PTH) testing and to identify ectopically situated parathyroid glands.

Magnetic resonance imaging (MRI) and invasive localization procedures, including digital subtraction arteriography, plain arteriography, and selective venous catheterization for PTH, are recommended only for patients who have previously undergone parathyroid or thyroid surgery. Fine-needle aspiration (FNA) biopsy cytology and PTH sampling via ultrasound or CT guidance have been used successfully to confirm that an observed mass is a parathyroid gland. Preoperative FNA evaluation of suspicious coexisting thyroid nodules is indicated when a focal parathyroidectomy is planned.

D. Operative approach and pathology

1. Many surgeons recommend bilateral neck exploration and identification of the abnormal and normal parathyroid glands, but most endocrine surgeons today recommend a focused approach directed by sestamibi and ultrasound localization in patients with sporadic HPT.

a. A solitary adenoma occurs in 85% of patients with sporadic primary HPT. Today, surgeons usually perform a unilateral or focal exploration and determine whether the PTH level falls by 50% within 10 minutes following removal of the parathyroid tumor. This suggests a successful operation.

b. When all glands are hyperplastic (12%), a subtotal parathyroidectomy is done, leaving about 50 mg (the size of a normal parathyroid gland) of the smallest and most accessible parathyroid gland. In such patients there may be considerable variation in size of the parathyroid gland.

c. When there is more than one abnormal parathyroid gland and several normal-appearing parathyroid glands (4%), all abnormal glands should be removed and normal glands biopsied and marked with a clip in case reoperation is required.

d. Total parathyroidectomy and parathyroid autotransplantation has been recommended by some experts for patients with familial HPT, multiple endocrine neoplasia type 1 (MEN1), or primary or secondary hyperplasia. I prefer a subtotal parathyroid resection in such patients, leaving approximately a 50-mg remnant of the most normal parathyroid gland. I reserve total parathyroidectomy and autotransplantation for patients with recurrent or persistent HPT or for children with neonatal HPT.

e. Pregnant patients, except those with very mild disease, should be operated on during the second trimester of pregnancy.

f. When a parathyroid tumor invades its surrounding structures, parathyroid carcinoma must be suspected. This parathyroid gland should be removed along with contiguous structures, including the thyroid lobe. Parathyroid cancer should be considered in any patient with profound hypercalcemia and a palpable parathyroid gland.

2. The possible **complications** of parathyroidectomy include hemorrhage, vocal cord injury, hypocalcemia, infection, and, very rarely, hypomagnesemia. These complications should occur in <2% of patients. Patients with more severe HPT and with extensive bone disease are more likely to develop hypocalcemia following parathyroidectomy because of "bone hunger" (influx of calcium and phosphorus into the metabolically active bone).

3. The **benefits** of parathyroidectomy include metabolic cure and/or improvement of symptoms such as fatigue, arthralgias, bone pain, renal colic, weakness, and peptic ulcer in ~75% of patients. Serum calcium, phosphorus, alkaline phosphatase, and PTH return to normal; subperiosteal resorption disappears; osteoporosis decreases; left ventricular hypertrophy and cardiac calcification as well as urinary calcium decrease. Life expectancy is also reported to improve.

SECONDARY HYPERPARATHYROIDISM

I. GENERAL PRINCIPLES

Secondary HPT occurs most often in patients with chronic renal failure but may develop from any condition that causes hypocalcemia, such as malabsorption.

A. Secondary HPT in patients with chronic renal failure can usually be prevented by good **medical treatment,** including **(1)** a low-phosphorus diet and binding phosphorus with calcium carbonate or aluminum hydroxide (Alucaps with meals); **(2)** maintaining a positive calcium balance with supplemental calcium intake and high calcium concentration (3.5 mEq/L) in dialysate; **(3)** treating with 1,25-dihydroxyvitamin D (Rocaltrol, 0.25 to 1.0 μg PO b.i.d.); **(4)** treating with cinacalcet HCI (Senispar, 60 mg PO b.i.d.), which reduces PTH and the product of calcium × phosphate (CaXP).

B. Indications for surgical treatment include **(1)** a calcium × phosphorus product of 70 or greater, **(2)** progressing renal osteodystrophy with bone pain, **(3)** severe pruritus, **(4)** soft-tissue calcification, **(5)** a calcium level >11.0 mg/dL with markedly increased PTH level, and **(6)** calciphylaxis.

II. SURGICAL MANAGEMENT

A. Surgical treatment includes the following:

   1. Dialysis 1 day before operation to correct electrolyte abnormalities and to lower potassium level.

   2. Subtotal parathyroidectomy, leaving 50 to 60 mg of an accessible, histologically confirmed hyperplastic parathyroid gland (preferred); or total parathyroidectomy and autotransplantation of fifteen 1-mm pieces to individual muscle pockets in the forearm. The <u>upper thymus</u> situated cephalad to the innominate should be removed in these patients, because as many as 15% of persons will have a fifth hyperplastic parathyroid gland.

B. Postoperatively, these patients are prone to develop tetany because of "hungry bones" and a small parathyroid remnant. They should be treated with 1,25-dihydroxyvitamin D (0.25 to 1.0 μg PO b.i.d.) and calcium supplementation.

C. Complications include hemorrhage, hypoparathyroidism, recurrent laryngeal nerve injury, infection, and hyperkalemia with respiratory arrest. All these complications are rare except for hypocalcemia.

D. The **prognosis** after successful parathyroidectomy is good. Bone pain and pruritus usually disappear, and patients develop an improved state of well-being. However, patients' calcium balance must be corrected by vitamin D supplementation or else the secondary HPT will recur. Some patients with secondary HPT also develop bone pain and have a low-turnover type of osteomalacia, which may be caused or aggravated by aluminum toxicity. The PTH values in these patients, though increased because of renal failure, are generally much lower than in patients with osteitis fibrosa cystica.

 ADRENALS

I. GENERAL PRINCIPLES

Clinically important functioning and nonfunctioning adrenal tumors are rare and arise from the cortex, causing <u>hyperaldosteronism</u> or <u>Cushing syndrome</u>, or from the adrenal medulla or other chromaffin cells in the sympathetic nervous system, <u>causing pheochromocytomas</u>. Adrenal tumors may secrete one or more hormones. Many nonfunctioning adrenal tumors are frequently identified today because of the use of CT, MRI, or ultrasonography. If these adrenal tumors are asymptomatic, nonfunctional, homogeneous with a smooth capsule, and <4 cm in diameter, they can be followed. CT should be repeated in 6 months.

<u>Adrenalectomy is recommended for functioning adrenal tumors, whether benign or malignant,</u> for growing or enlarging tumors, for complex tumors, and for nonfunctioning adrenal tumors 4 cm and larger and for those with adjacent lymphadenopathy.

II. PRIMARY HYPERALDOSTERONISM

A. Diagnosis

   1. Clinical manifestations. See Chapter 12.

   2. Laboratory tests. See Chapter 12.

B. Differentiating between adenoma and hyperplasia. See Chapter 12.

C. Treatment
  1. Medical. Spironolactone, a competitive aldosterone antagonist, or **amiloride,** a potassium-sparing diuretic, will normalize blood pressure and correct the hypokalemia. Either of these medications is the treatment of choice for patients with adrenocortical hyperplasia and for preparing patients with adrenocortical adenomas or carcinomas for operation. In patients with mild biochemical abnormalities and symptoms, potassium supplementation (8 g potassium chloride daily) and sodium restriction can correct the electrolyte abnormalities.
  2. Surgical
    a. Once the patient has been prepared medically for the operative procedure, laparoscopic adrenalectomy is the treatment of choice. The posterior twelfth-rib approach is used when an experienced laparoscopic surgeon is not available.
    b. Total or subtotal adrenalectomy (leaving 30% of the left adrenal gland) for patients with hyperplasia is controversial, because few patients become normotensive. Therefore, most of these patients are treated medically.
  3. Postoperative care
    a. Most patients require only the usual postoperative care.
    b. A few patients will require supplemental saline because of transient (1-day to 1-month) aldosterone deficiency. Fludrocortisone (50 to 100 μg per day PO) may be needed.
    c. Glucocorticoids are rarely required if only one gland is removed, but a high unexplained fever or profound weakness warrants obtaining a plasma cortisol level to rule out Addisonian crisis and the need for immediate glucocorticoid treatment.
D. Prognosis. The response rate to adrenalectomy can usually be predicted by the preoperative response to spironolactone. Young, slim female patients with a relatively short period of hypertension have the best response. Blood pressure decreases in $\sim$80% of patients, although this may take several months, and virtually all patients become normokalemic. In patients with hyperplasia, some degree of hypertension normally remains, but the hypokalemia is usually corrected.

III. HYPERADRENOCORTICISM (Fig. 55.1)
  See Chapter 12.
  A. Diagnosis and differential diagnosis. See Chapter 12.
    1. Clinical manifestations. See Chapter 12.
      a. Symptoms. See Chapter 12.
      b. Physical findings. See Chapter 12.
    2. Laboratory tests. See Chapter 12.
  B. Complications. See Chapter 12.
  C. Treatment
    1. Medical treatment. Temporary control of Cushing syndrome can be accomplished with ketoconazole, metyrapone, and aminoglutethimide, which inhibit steroid production, and with 1,1-dichloro-2-(*o*-chlorophenyl)-2-(*p*-chlorophenyl)ethane (mitotane), which is toxic to the adrenal cortex. Mitotane with steroid replacement and documentation of mitotane levels have been used for patients with adrenocortical carcinomas.
    2. Surgical treatment
      a. Cushing syndrome is managed by transsphenoidal hypophysectomy with microsurgical excision of the pituitary adenoma or with pituitary irradiation. Excision of the pituitary adenoma results in rapid relief of symptoms, although ACTH deficiency is common. The clinical response to irradiation takes longer (up to 18 months) and frequently results in panhypopituitarism.
      b. Laparoscopic adrenalectomy is the treatment of choice for patients with benign-appearing adrenal tumors <6 cm in size and for some patients with pituitary Cushing syndrome who fail to respond to pituitary irradiation or microsurgery. Before operation, hypokalemia and other electrolyte abnormalities should be corrected and diabetes mellitus controlled. Exogenous corticosteroid must be provided.

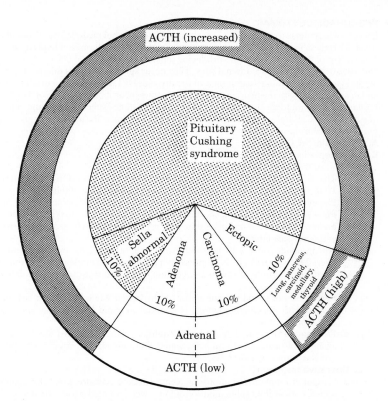

Figure 55.1. Approximate distribution and adrenocorticotropic hormone levels in patients with Cushing syndrome. (Modified from Welbourn RB. Some aspects of adrenal surgery. *Br J Surg* 1980;67:723.)

(1) Postoperative care. Cortisol hemisuccinate (100 mg IV q8h) is given to all patients. After total adrenalectomy, permanent replacement is necessary (hydrocortisone, 20 mg in the morning and 10 mg in the evening). After unilateral adrenalectomy, the dose of cortisol is tapered over several weeks to physiologic levels (30 mg per day). The dosage is then gradually reduced to alternate-day treatment for several months before all steroids are discontinued. Alternate-day treatment minimizes inhibition of endogenous ACTH and leads to earlier resumption of the normal pituitary–adrenal axis. A few patients may require fludrocortisone (0.1 mg PO daily). Postoperative complications include wound infection, wound dehiscence, peptic ulceration with bleeding, and pulmonary problems.

(2) The **prognosis** in patients after removal of an adrenal adenoma and after treatment of pituitary Cushing syndrome is generally excellent. Hypoadrenocorticism and panhypopituitarism occur after total adrenalectomy and pituitary ablation, respectively, and these patients require life-long corticosteroid replacement, which must be increased in times of stress. **Nelson syndrome,** which causes hyperpigmentation, headaches, exophthalmos, and blindness because of growth of the pituitary tumor, develops in 20% of patients after total bilateral adrenalectomy. When Cushing syndrome is the result of adrenocortical carcinoma, the prognosis is grave. Palliation with mitotane, started soon after adrenalectomy, is helpful in ~20% of patients.

IV. PHEOCHROMOCYTOMAS

Pheochromocytomas (see Chapter 13) are tumors of the adrenal medulla and chromaffin tissues elsewhere in the body and account for 0.1% to 0.2% of all cases of hypertension. Ten percent of these catecholamine-producing tumors are malignant, 10% are bilateral, and 10% are found in extra-adrenal sites. They occur sporadically, in association with Sipple syndrome (medullary carcinoma of the thyroid, HPT, and ganglioneuromatosis) and in association with the neurocutaneous syndromes (neurofibromatosis, von Hippel-Lindau disease—multiple endocrine neoplasia type 2, Sturge-Weber disease, and tuberous sclerosis). Children and patients with familial syndromes are more likely to have multiple pheochromocytomas.

A. Diagnosis. See Chapter 13.

B. Treatment. See Chapter 13.

  1. Medical treatment includes:

  a. The α-adrenergic–blocking agent phenoxybenzamine, 1 to 3 mg/kg per day; 10 to 40 mg q.i.d. starting with a low dose; maximal dose 300 mg per day.

  b. Phentolamine (Regitine, (1.0 to 2.5 mg IV followed by 1 mg/min, or 50 mg PO 4 to 6 times daily) is a shorter-acting α blocker, but phenoxybenzamine is preferred because of its longer duration of action, better hypertension control, and fewer side effects.

  c. Nitroprusside (0.01% IV infusion) is the drug of choice for managing intra-operative hypertension. Nitroprusside has replaced phentolamine because of its shorter duration of action and because it has no direct cardiac-stimulating effects.

  d. Restoration of blood volume by forced hydration while the patient is being treated with phenoxybenzamine is essential to avoid hypotension upon removal of the tumor.

  e. Propranolol (Inderal, 5 to 40 mg PO q6h), a β blocker, is used for the management of tachycardia and arrhythmias, but only after treatment with phenoxybenzamine has been started.

  2. Operative treatment

  a. Careful intraoperative monitoring (central venous pressure, arterial pressure, and electrocardiographic monitoring) in a well-hydrated patient treated with phenoxybenzamine for at least 10 days is the initial step.

  b. A laparoscopic approach is recommended when tumors are <6 cm. These tumors sometimes may be multiple and in ectopic sites, so preoperative localization tests are indicated.

  c. Avoid hypotension after removal of the tumor by ensuring that the patient is well hydrated prior to operation and is adequately blocked with phenoxybenzamine.

  d. Complications include sequelae of hypertension (stroke, renal failure, myocardial infarction), arrhythmias, hypotension, bleeding, and hypoglycemia.

C. Prognosis. The results of surgery are excellent for benign lesions, with an operative mortality rate of <5%. About 95% of patients with paroxysmal hypertension and 65% of those with sustained preoperative hypertension become normotensive. Malignant pheochromocytoma has a poor prognosis. Treatment with phenoxybenzamine and metyrosine (Demser) as well as with external irradiation or with ^{131}I-MIBG sometimes gives effective palliation.

VIRILIZATION AND FEMINIZATION

I. GENERAL PRINCIPLES

A. Diagnosis and differential diagnosis. See Chapters 21, 22, 23.

B. Treatment. See Chapters 21, 22, 23.

  1. Congenital adrenal hyperplasia

  2. Tumor

C. Course. See Chapters 21, 22, 23.

Selected References

Clark OH, Duh QY, Kebebew E. *Textbook of Endocrine Surgery.* 2nd ed. Philadelphia: Elsevier Saunders; 2005.

Clark OH, Duh QY, Perrier ND, Jahan TM, eds. *Endocrine Tumors.* 3rd ed. Hamilton, Ontario: BC Decker; 2003.

Jossart GH, Clark OH. Thyroid and parathyroid procedures. In: Souba W, Fink M, Jurkovich G, et al, eds. *ACS Surgery: Principles and Practice.* Web MD; 2005:185–194.

Lal G, Clark OH. Endocrine surgery. In: Gardner DG, Shoback D, eds. *Greenspan's Basic and Clinical Endocrinology.* New York: McGraw-Hill Medical; 2006:911–932.

Lee J, Clark OH. Diagnosis and management of thyroid cancer. In: Silberman H, Silberman AW, eds. *Principles and Practice of Surgical Oncology: Multidisciplinary Approach to Difficult Problems.* 2nd ed. Philadelphia: Lippincott Williams & Wilkins; 2007.

Ogilvie J, Piatigorsky E, Clark OH. Advances in surgery: current status of fine needle aspiration for thyroid nodule. *Adv Surg* 2006;40:223–238.

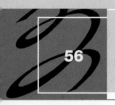

56 DERMATOLOGIC MANIFESTATIONS OF ENDOCRINE DISORDERS
Anne W. Lucky

*S*kin lesions may be specific to a variety of endocrine disorders as well as manifestations of secondary conditions. Classic conditions as well as newly described genetic syndromes with cutaneous and endocrine features are outlined in this chapter.

I. THYROID
A. Hyperthyroidism
1. **General features** of hyperthyroidism include warmth, increased sweating, flushing, and a smooth velvety texture of the skin. In severe cases, there may be generalized hyperpigmentation as a result of skin deposition of both melanin and hemosiderin.
2. **Hair and nails.** Hair may become thin, fine, limp, and oily. There is distal onycholysis (separation of the nail plate from the nail bed), characteristically starting on the fourth finger (Plummer nail).
3. **Pretibial myxedema (PTM, Graves dermopathy).** Localized accumulations of acid mucopolysaccharides (glycosaminoglycans such as hyaluronic acid) appear as red to brown to yellow plaques, usually on the shins. There is a "peau d'orange" pebbly surface with dilated hair follicles and coarse hairs. Lesions are nonpitting, cool, nontender, and may be pruritic. PTM is seen with active Graves disease as well as in hypo- or euthyroid "burned-out" or treated patients. High thyroid-stimulating immunoglobulin levels have been associated with PTM.
4. **Thyroid acropachy.** Diffuse thickening of the distal extremities, clubbing, and periosteal new-bone formation with characteristic perpendicular bone spicules are associated with Graves disease, often with ophthalmopathy and pretibial myxedema.

B. Hypothyroidism
1. **Congenital** hypothyroid signs are subtle and should be vanishing with the advent of newborn screening programs for hypothyroidism. **General features** include cool, pale, translucent "alabaster" skin with a yellow hue. This color and texture are a result of decreased blood flow, anemia, infiltration with mucopolysaccharides, prolonged jaundice, and/or carotenemia. Sweating is reduced. Thermal instability and frank hypothermia are accompanied by persistent cutis marmorata, a violaceous mottling in a vascular pattern. Umbilical hernia, short proximal limbs, depressed nasal bridge, and large tongue complete the picture of congenital hypothyroidism.
2. **Acquired** hypothyroidism has many of the same general features seen in the congenital disease. In addition, children and adults have more prominent dry and scaling skin resembling ichthyosis. Sweating is minimal as eccrine ducts become atrophic. Generalized myxedema makes the skin puffy, pale, and doughy with a nonpitting edema, especially noticeable around the face and eyelids, resulting from the accumulation of acid mucopolysaccharides.
3. **Hair.** Scalp hair is lost in a generalized pattern. The remaining scalp hair is coarse and dry. Loss of the lateral one third of the eyebrows (St. Ann sign) is characteristic. Pubic and axillary hair is sparse. Children may get a paradoxical **hypertrichosis** of the arms, back, and legs, which is reversible with treatment.

II. ADRENAL

A. Hypoadrenalism (adrenocortical insufficiency, Addison disease)

1. Patients gradually develop generalized **hyperpigmentation,** often noted as failure to lose a summer suntan. There is darkening of the areolae, genital skin, pre-existing nevi, palmar and plantar creases, and recent scars. Blue-black pigment deposits are seen on the gums at the tooth margin and on the hard palate. The etiology of hyperpigmentation is debatable, but it is probably a result of excessive secretion of melanocyte-stimulating hormone (MSH).

2. **Hair** in pubic and axillary areas becomes sparse. **Nails** may develop hyperpigmented, linear streaks.

3. **Vitiligo** has occurred in patients with Addison disease.

B. Hyperadrenalism. Pituitary Cushing syndrome, adrenal tumors, and autonomous nodular adrenal hyperplasia may have features of androgen excess as well as glucocorticoid excess. Iatrogenic Cushing syndrome, resulting from systemic or topical glucocorticosteroids, does not have the androgenic features. Some forms of congenital adrenal hyperplasia are associated with elevated androgens and normal glucocorticosteroids.

1. **Glucocorticoid excess**

a. **Primary features**

(1) **General features** include plethora, telangiectasias, and increased growth of fine, downy vellus hairs, especially on the sides of the face. With prolonged exposure, there is generalized atrophy of the skin and easy bruisability.

(2) **Striae** represent both dermal and epidermal atrophy and occur in areas of skin tension. A medusalike pattern over the abdomen is typical. In adrenocorticoid excess, they are pigmented red to blue because the dermal and subcutaneous blood vessels show through the translucent, atrophic skin. In some cases, they may become hyperpigmented with melanin.

(3) **Steroid acne** appears on the upper arms, chest, and back as well as on the face. The follicular lesions are erythematous, hyperkeratotic papules, although in late stages they may become pustular and comedonal. They all erupt at the same stage of development.

(4) Redistribution of subcutaneous **fat** to the cheeks ("moon facies"), upper back ("buffalo hump"), buttocks, and abdomen causes the characteristic body habitus.

(5) In pituitary disease or in syndromes of ectopic adrenocorticotropic hormone (ACTH) production, there may be **hyperpigmentation,** such as seen in Addison disease.

(6) The androgenic effects from weak adrenal androgens, such as dehydroepiandrosterone sulfate, which may be converted peripherally to more potent androgens such as testosterone and dihydrotestosterone, produce classic **acne vulgaris** as well as **hirsutism** and male-pattern **hair loss** in women.

b. **Secondary features**

(1) **Tinea versicolor** appears as scaly, oval macules and patches on the upper trunk, back, and arms with variable hyper- and hypopigmentation. It is caused by a superficial colonization with the fungus *Malassezia furfur (Pityrosporum ovale).*

(2) **Candida (Monilia)** infections of the skin and mucous membranes include buccal mucosa (thrush), vaginal mucosa, nails and surrounding tissues (onychomycosis and paronychia), interdigital webs (blastomycetes interdigitalis erosion), corners of the mouth (perleche), and intertriginous folds (intertrigo).

(3) There is an increased occurrence of cutaneous bacterial infections with pustules, furuncles, and abscesses, especially caused by *Staphylococcus aureus.*

(4) Cushing syndrome can accompany McCune-Albright syndrome (polyostotic fibrous dysplasia) with large **café-au-lait macules** as well as bony abnormalities and precocious puberty.

c. Premature adrenarche (pubarche). Early development of pubic hair with elevation of serum dehydroepiandrosterone sulfate before other signs of puberty has been termed premature adrenarche. It occurs primarily in girls. In children who also have **acanthosis nigricans,** premature adrenarche may represent an early sign of insulin resistance and eventuate in polycystic ovarian disease (PCOS) and/or non-insulin–dependent diabetes mellitus (NIDDM). It is hypothesized that high levels of insulin may stimulate epidermal growth factor–like substances that promote acanthosis (i.e., hypertrophy) of the epidermis.

2. Congenital adrenal hyperplasia (CAH)

a. In **infancy,** severe forms of CAH caused by enzyme defects in the biosynthetic pathway to the synthesis of cortisol may have only mild cutaneous signs, primarily hyperpigmentation of genital skin from excessive pituitary production of ACTH or MSH, or both.

b. In **later childhood,** early onset of pubic and axillary hair **(premature adrenarche)** and acne are signs of androgen excess.

c. In postpubertal **adult** women and perhaps in some men, "mild" (or "partial" or "late-onset") forms of CAH are now being recognized primarily from their skin manifestations of severe late-onset or persistent **acne,** female-pattern **hair loss,** and **hirsutism** in women. Hirsutism is defined as excessive hair growth in androgen-dependent areas, such as the upper lip, chin, areolae, linea alba, and upper inner thighs. Female-pattern hair loss (androgenic alopecia) is thinning of the hair over the crown of the scalp with relative sparing of the sides and back. Affected hairs are of smaller diameter and grow to shorter length before entering the resting phase and falling out. The diagnosis of CAH is made by finding elevations of the hormone that is the immediate substrate for the deficient enzyme, usually as abnormal responses to ACTH stimulation.

III. OVARY

A. Androgen excess from the **ovary** causes the same skin manifestations of **acne, hair loss, hirsutism, and androgenic alopecia** as in androgen excess from the adrenal. Rarely, ovarian tumors are the cause. The most common cause of androgen excess from the ovary is **polycystic ovarian syndrome (PCOS).** In addition to acne, hirsutism and androgenetic alopecia as well as acanthosis nigricans are common, especially in obese patients, reflecting insulin resistance. Some patients with PCOS also have metabolic syndrome and are at risk for non-insulin–dependent diabetes mellitus, hyperlipidemia, and cardiovascular disease.

B. Acanthosis nigricans has also been associated with a wide variety of other endocrine disorders, including pituitary Cushing syndrome, pituitary tumors, acromegaly, and Addison disease. Most patients with acanthosis nigricans have underlying insulin resistance.

IV. DIABETES MELLITUS

A. Primary skin diseases associated with diabetes mellitus

1. Diabetic dermopathy (pigmented pretibial patches, shin spots). Lesions of diabetic dermopathy are <1 cm and are red-brown, atrophic macules on the shins, which may begin as papules. Capillary basement membranes appear to be thickened.

2. Necrobiosis lipoidica diabeticorum. These lesions also characteristically appear on the shins and are oval, atrophic plaques that can reach several centimeters in size. They have a raised, erythematous border and a yellow-brown, waxy central atrophic area through which telangiectatic subcutaneous vessels are easily visible. These lesions may ulcerate. Histologically, there is necrobiosis of collagen and inflammation around blood vessels. The histologic picture is similar to that seen in granuloma annulare and rheumatoid nodules.

3. **Disseminated granuloma annulare.** Development of multiple small, grouped, erythematous to flesh-colored papules, which coalesce into small plaques covering the entire body surface, has been associated with diabetes mellitus. However, most patients with granuloma annulare do not have diabetes mellitus.

4. **Acanthosis nigricans** and insulin resistance may be associated with polycystic ovarian syndrome in young women (type A) or with the presence of antibodies to insulin receptors and other autoimmune phenomena (type B). These patients typically have type 2 (non-insulin–dependent) diabetes mellitus and are at risk for cardiovascular disease.

5. **Bullous diabeticorum.** Development of tense blisters that appear suddenly on apparently normal skin, usually on the extremities, occurs in diabetics. Histologically, the blisters may be intraepidermal or subepidermal. Lesions may tend to ulcerate.

6. **Eruptive xanthomas** are accumulations of lipid in macrophages to form widespread yellow to red papules, which may occur in a linear array in response to trauma (the Koebner phenomenon). These lesions appear in patients with poorly controlled <u>diabetes mellitus</u> who have <u>massive hypertriglyceridemia</u>.

7. **Scleredema** (adultorum of Buschke) is a rare condition seen in severe insulin-dependent diabetes in which there is thickening of the collagen of the dermis and deposition of acid mucopolysaccharides between collagen bundles. The clinical lesions are broad areas of nonpitting edema and hardening of the skin, especially on the face, neck, and upper trunk. It is <u>not related to scleroderma</u>.

8. **Idiopathic hemochromatosis,** a disorder of excessive iron storage, consists of a triad of hepatic cirrhosis, cardiac insufficiency, and diabetes. There is striking hyperpigmentation as a result of increased melanin deposition in the basal layer of the epidermis.

9. **Thickened skin and "finger pebbles."** Thickened, waxy skin, especially over the backs of the hands, and tiny papules ("pebbles") on the tops of the fingers are characteristic of both types 1 and 2 diabetes. Joint stiffness and contractures often prevent the flat opposition of both palms. The mechanism of these findings has not been elucidated but is presumed to be a result of changes in collagen and/or dermal mucopolysaccharides.

B. **Secondary skin disorders**
1. **Candida** infections of the skin and mucous membranes occur in similar locations as those described for glucocorticoid excess.
2. Cutaneous bacterial infections, especially **staphylococcal** infections, such as folliculitis, furunculosis, and frank abscess formation, occur in people with poorly controlled diabetes.
3. Opportunistic infections by fungal organisms, such as *Mucor* and *Rhizopus* (phycomycosis), are rarely seen in diabetics. Such lesions may be fatal.
4. **Tinea pedis** is a dermatophytic infection affecting the interdigital web spaces of the feet. It is common in diabetes, and the ensuing fissures between the toes serve as portals of entry for bacteria, especially streptococci, producing cellulitis of the foot and lower leg.
5. **Diabetic ulcers.** Poorly healing ulcerations, especially on the lower legs and feet, are common. On the sole, these can be deep and penetrating and can result in osteomyelitis because of diabetic neuropathy and loss of sensation (mal penetrons). Eventually, severe ischemic changes (gangrene) resulting from angiopathy may necessitate amputations.

V. LIPODYSTROPHIES
A. **Congenital** generalized lipodystrophies (Beradinelli-Seip, CGL types 1 and 2) are autosomal recessive disorders caused by mutations in AGPAT@ and GNG3L1, respectively. The cutaneous features include acanthosis nigricans, thick hair, hypertrichosis, hyperhidrosis, hyperpigmentation, and parchmentlike skin with prominent blood vessels because of the absence of fat. Noncutaneous hallmarks are severe lipoatrophy (sparing abdominal fat), insulin resistance with progression to diabetes, high anabolic rate, precocious puberty, large muscle mass, high triglycerides, liver

cirrhosis, cardiomyopathy, and early death. The **acquired** (Lawrence-Seip) form has similar but milder features.

B. Familial partial lipodystrophies may also be congenital or acquired and may involve the face and upper body or lower extremities (Dunnigan-Kobberling, FPLD 1, 2, and 3). Acanthosis nigricans is common.

C. Rare inherited disorders of the insulin receptor include **leprechaunism** (Donohue syndrome) with acanthosis nigricans, generalized lipoatrophy, failure to thrive, elfin facies, and severe insulin resistance; and **Rabson-Mendenhall** syndrome with acanthosis nigricans, hypertrichosis, coarse facies, precocious puberty, insulin resistance, and, eventually, diabetes.

D. Localized lipoatrophy and lipohypertrophy may appear at sites of insulin injection. The mechanism for this is unclear. Local injections of glucocorticoids may also cause lipoatrophy at the injection site.

VI. GLUCAGONOMA SYNDROME

The **glucagonoma syndrome** consists of a diffuse, scaly, brightly erythematous rash made up of gyrate, serpiginous plaques with clear centers and superficial scale. The lesions tend to expand—thus the name **necrolytic migratory erythema.** Such lesions are seen in association with malignant neoplasms of the α cells of the pancreas and have regressed when the tumor has been surgically removed.

VII. OTHER GENETIC SYNDROMES WITH CUTANEOUS AND ENDOCRINE MANIFESTATIONS

The genetic, cutaneous and endocrine manifestations of these syndromes are summarized in Table 56.1. Some pertinent features are described below.

A. Gonadal dysgenesis (Turner syndrome, XO). Turner syndrome exhibits a few special cutaneous features such as lymphatic malformations (puffy feet and pterygium colli or webbed neck), hemangiomas, short fourth and fifth metatarsals, hyperconvex nails, wide-spaced nipples, multiple nevi, high-arched palate), W-shaped hairline, distichiasis (accessory row of eyelashes), and keloids. The hemangiomas tend to resolve in childhood, but lymphatic malformations often enlarge when puberty is induced. Girls with mosaic forms of Turner syndrome may have more subtle features. The differential diagnosis includes Noonan syndrome.

B. Pseudohypoparathyroidism (PHP, Albright hereditary osteodystrophy) and pseudopseudohypoparathyroidism (PPHP). PHP is a hormone resistance disorder due in most cases to loss-of-function mutations in the GNαS gene. The classic phenotype includes short stature, delayed development, brachydactyly with a short fourth metacarpal, hyperphosphatemia, and hypocalcemia because of end-organ resistance to parathyroid and often thyroid hormones. **Osteoma cutis,** the ectopic deposition of bone, in the dermis, is the cutaneous hallmark of this disease and may precede the biochemical changes. The phenotype without calcium abnormalities is called PPHP. When carried on the maternal allele, PHP occurs; the same mutation on the paternal allele results in progressive osseous heteroplasia (POH) with heterotopic ossification including osteoma cutis.

C. McCune Albright syndrome (MAS, polyostotic fibrous dysplasia with multiple endocrine abnormalities and café-au-lait spots). McCune-Albright syndrome results from mosaic, postzygotic gain-of-function mutations in the GNAS gene. The hallmark is overstimulation of tissue growth that causes a variety of endocrinopathies. The characteristic **café-au-lait macules** are large and segmental, reflecting their mosaic origin.

D. Autoimmune polyglandular syndrome

1. APS-1. APS-1 is a result of mutations in the AIRE gene. Mucocutaneous candidiasis is the hallmark, along with alopecia, vitiligo and nail pitting, and hypoplasia.

2. APS-2 (Schmidt's syndrome) does not have a known single-gene mutation. Autoimmune vitiligo and alopecia may occur.

E. Multiple endocrine neoplasia (MEN) syndromes

1. MEN1 is the result of mutations in the MEN1 gene and is characterized by multiple cutaneous overgrowths such as angiofibromas, collagenomas, leiomyomas,

TABLE 56.1 Genetic Syndromes with Cutaneous and Endocrine Manifestations

Eponym	Descriptive name	Gene	Chromosome	Cutaneous manifestations	Endocrine manifestations
Turner	Gonadal dysgenesis	Absent X	X	Lymphatic malformations (puffy feet) Hemangiomas Short fourth and fifth metatarsals Hyperconvex nails Wide-spaced nipples Multiple nevi High-arched palate Pterygium colli (webbed neck) W-shaped hairline Distichiasis (accessory row of eyelashes) Keloids	Ovarian dysgenesis
Albright hereditary osteodystrophy	Pseudohypoparathyroidism (PHP and PPHP)	GNAS1 (LOF)	20q13.3	Osteoma cutis	Resistance to PTH, TSH $\downarrow Ca^{2+}$ $\uparrow PO_4$ $\uparrow PTH$ Hypothyroidism
McCune Albright	Polyostotic fibrous dysplasia with multiple endocrine abnormalities and café-au-lait spots	GNAS1 (mosaic GOF)	20q13.3	Café au lait macules	Precocious puberty $\uparrow GH$ $\uparrow Prolactin$ $\uparrow T_4$ Nodular adrenal hyperplasia with glucocorticoid excess

(continued)

TABLE 56.1 Genetic Syndromes with Cutaneous and Endocrine Manifestations (*Continued*)

Eponym	Descriptive name	Gene	Chromosome	Cutaneous manifestations	Endocrine manifestations
APS 1	Autoimmune polyglandular syndrome 1 (APECED)	AIRE	21q22.3	APS 1 Mucocutaneous candidiasis (MCC) Alopecia Vitiligo Nail pitting Enamel hypoplasia	APS1 Hypoparathyroidism Adrenal failure Gonadal failure Parietal cell atrophy IDDM Autoimmune thyroid
Schmidt (APS 2)	Autoimmune polyglandular syndrome 2	Unknown		APS 2 Vitiligo (rare) Alopecia (rare)	APS2 Adrenal failure Autoimmune thyroid IDDM Gonadal failure Myasthenia gravis Celiac disease Pernicious anemia
MEN 1	Multiple endocrine neoplasia 1	MEN-1	11q13	MEN 1 Angiofibromas Collagenomas Leiomyomas Lipomas Collagenomas Confettilike ↓ pigmentation Café au lait macules Gingival papules Melanoma	

Disease	Name	Gene	Locus	Skin Features	Associated Features
Sipple (MEN2A)	Multiple endocrine neoplasia 2A	RET	10q11.2	MEN 2A Lichen amyloidosis	MEN 2A Medullary carcinoma of the thyroid Pheochromocytoma Parathyroid hyperplasia
MEN 2B	Multiple endocrine neoplasia 2B	RET	10q11.2	MEN 2B Marfanoid habitus Elongated facies Mucosal neuromas Café au lait macules	MEN 2B Pheochromocytoma Medullary carcinoma of the thyroid (MCT)
Carney complex	Primary pigmented nodular adrenocortical disease (PPNAD)	PRKARIA	2p16 17q22-24	Lentigines Cutaneous and mucosal myxomas Multiple epithelioid blue nevi Conjunctival pigmentation Combined nevi Small café au lait macules Depigmented macules Skin tags Lipomas Pigmented schwannomas Pilonidal sinus	Adrenal tumors (PPNAD) Cushing syndrome Pituitary tumors Gigantism & acromegaly Precocious puberty Sertoli cell tumors (LCCST) Thyroid nodules and carcinomas

APECED, autoimmune polyendocrinopathy-candidiasis-ectodermal dystrophy; GOF, gain-of-function mutation; IDDM, insulin-dependent diabetes mellitus; LCCST, large-cell calcifying Sertoli cell tumors; LOF, loss-of-function mutation; PHP, pseudohypoparathyroidism; PPHP, pseudopseudohypoparathyroidism.

lipomas, confettilike hypopigmentation, café au lait macules, gingival papules, and melanoma. The "3 P" tumors—parathyroid, pituitary and pancreatic islet cells—are the most common.

2. **MEN2A and MEN2B** have fewer skin findings such as lichen amyloidosis, mucosal neuromas, and café-au-lait macules with Marfanoid habitus and elongated facies, but are most important because recognition of mutations in the RET proto-oncogene can be predictive of medullary carcinoma of the thyroid and an indication for prophylactic thyroidectomy.

F. Carney complex. Also known as primary pigmented nodular adrenocortical disease (PPNAD), these patients have mutations in the protein kinase gene PKAR1A on two different chromosomes. The striking clinical feature is the multiple pigmented lesions, especially lentigines and cutaneous and mucosal myxomas. Other cutaneous findings include multiple epithelioid blue nevi, conjunctival pigmentation, combined nevi, small café au lait macules, depigmented macules, skin tags, lipomas, pigmented schwannomas, and pilonidal sinuses. There are multiple endocrine tumors in this syndrome.

Selected References

Ahmed I, Goldstein, B. Diabetes mellitus. *Clin Dermatol* 2006;24:237–246.

Bauer AJ, Stratakis CA. The lentiginoses: cutaneous markers of systemic disease and a window to new aspects of tumourigenesis. *J Med Genet* 2005;42:801–810.

Eisenbarth GS, Gottlieb PA. Autoimmune polyendocrine syndromes. *N Engl J Med* 2004;350:2068–2079.

Fuleihan Gel-H, Rubeiz N. Dermatologic manifestations of parathyroid-related disorders. *Clin Dermatol* 2006;24:281–288.

Hengge UR, Ruzicka T, Schwartz RA, Cork MJ. Adverse effects of topical glucocorticosteroids. *J Am Acad Dermatol* 2006;54:1–15.

Heymann WR. Advances in the cutaneous manifestations of thyroid disease. *Int J Dermatol* 1997;36:641–645.

Jabbour SA. Cutaneous manifestations of endocrine disorders: a guide for dermatologists. *Am J Clin Dermatol* 2003;4:315–331.

Jabbour SA, Davidovici BB, Wolf R. Rare syndromes. *Clin Dermatol* 2006;24:299–316.

Lee AT, Zane LT. Dermatologic manifestations of polycystic ovary syndrome. *Am J Clin Dermatol* 2007;8:201–219.

Lucky AW. Cutaneous manifestations of endocrine, metabolic and nutritional disorders. In: Schachner LA, Hansen RC, eds. *Pediatric Dermatology*. 3rd ed. New York: Churchill Livingstone; 2003.

Monajemi H, Stroes E, Hegele RA, Fliers E. Inherited lipodystrophies and the metabolic syndrome. *Clin Endocrinol (Oxf)* 2007;67:479–484.

Nieman LK, Chanco Turner ML. Addison's disease. *Clin Dermatol* 2006;24:276–280.

Perheentupa J. Autoimmune polyendocrinopathy-candidiasis-ectodermal dystrophy. *J Clin Endocrinol Metab* 2006;91:2843–2850.

Prendiville JS, Lucky AW, Mallory SB, et al. Osteoma cutis as a presenting sign of pseudohypoparathyroidism. *Pediatr Dermatol* 1992;9:1–18.

Rosenfield RL, Lucky AW. Acne, hirsutism and alopecia in adolescent girls. *Endocrinol Metab Clin North Am* 1993;22:507–532.

Schwartz RA. Acanthosis nigricans. *J Am Acad Dermatol* 1994;31:1–19.

Seip M, Trygstad O. Generalized lipodystrophy, congenital and acquired (lipoatrophy). *Acta Paediatr Suppl* 1996;413:2–28.

Shibli-Rahhal A, Van Beek M, Schlechte JA. Cushing's syndrome. *Clin Dermatol* 2006; 24:260–265.

Völkl TM, Dörr HG. McCune-Albright syndrome: clinical picture and natural history in children and adolescents. *J Pediatr Endocrinol Metab* 2006;19(suppl 2):551–559.

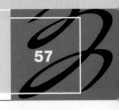

AUTOIMMUNE ENDOCRINE SYNDROMES

George S. Eisenbarth

57

I. GENERAL PRINCIPLES

Immunoendocrinopathy syndromes include (in approximate order of prevalence) autoimmune polyendocrine syndrome type II (APS2; depending on specific diseases, some authors subdivide type II into types II, III, and IV [see later]), autoimmune polyendocrine syndrome type I (APS1), immunodysregulation, polyendocrinopathy, and enteropathy, X-linked(IPEX), anti-insulin receptor antibody syndrome, plasma cell dyscrasia with polyneuropathy, organomegaly, endocrinopathy, M-protein gammopathy, and skin changes (POEMS), and thymic tumors with associated endocrinopathy. These syndromes are characterized by the presence of multiple overt autoimmune disorders, the presence of autoantibodies to multiple organs, often without overt disease, and high probability for patients and their relatives to develop new autoimmune diseases. APS1, APS2, and IPEX have major identifiable genetic determinants and established disease associations that allow physicians to suspect and screen for additional unrecognized illnesses in patients or their family members. Table 57.1 is a simple handout that can be given to APS2 patients with instructions to distribute it to their relatives.

A. Type II autoimmune polyendocrine syndrome. Also known as Schmidt syndrome, APS2 is characterized by the classic triad of Addison disease, autoimmune thyroid disease (Graves disease or primary hypothyroidism), and type 1A (immune-mediated) diabetes. Other illnesses seen in these patients include primary hypogonadism, pernicious anemia, alopecia, serositis, myasthenia gravis, celiac disease, and stiff-man syndrome. Disease onset is usually in adulthood, and as in many autoimmune diseases, there is a female predominance. Inheritance is polygenic and there is a strong human leukocyte antigen (HLA) DQ and DR allele association, specifically DR3, DQB1*0201, and DR4, DQB1*0302 (with DR4 most often DRB1*0404 for familial Addison disease). Other DR3-associated illnesses such as Sjögren syndrome, selective IgA deficiency, juvenile dermatomyositis, chronic active hepatitis, and dermatitis herpetiformis, also indicate that a patient is susceptible to the type II syndrome illnesses (most commonly autoimmune thyroid disease). Some authors subdivide the type II syndrome (type II, Addison with type 1A diabetes or autoimmune thyroid; type III, thyroid plus other autoimmune (not Addison or diabetes); and type IV, two or more organ-specific autoimmune.

B. Type I autoimmune polyendocrine syndrome. Also known as APECED (autoimmune polyendocrinopathy-candidiasis-ectodermal dystrophy), this syndrome is characterized by the classic triad of hypoparathyroidism (80% of patients), Addison disease (70% of patients), and mucocutaneous candidiasis (90% of patients). Other autoimmune illnesses seen in these patients include primary hypothyroidism, type 1A diabetes, primary hypogonadism, chronic active hepatitis, pernicious anemia, malabsorption syndromes, keratopathy, vitiligo, and alopecia. In contrast to the type II syndrome, APS1 onset is usually in infancy and early childhood. Inheritance is autosomal recessive with a single gene defect, mutation of the *AIRE* (autoimmune regulator) gene on chromosome 21q22.3. There is evidence that the *AIRE* gene controls negative selection of T lymphocytes within the thymus, and in particular expression of a series of "peripheral" antigens such as insulin, which are organ-specific molecules of which very small amounts are expressed in the thymus. Thus, a leading hypothesis is that mutations of the *AIRE* gene contribute to many autoimmune disorders by allowing self-reactive T cells to more often escape from the thymus and

781

TABLE 57.1	Associated Illnesses Found in Relatives
Illness	**Signs and symptoms**
Hypothyroidism	Weight gain, high blood pressure, feeling cold
Hyperthyroidism	Weight loss, bulging eyes, feeling warm and anxious
Pernicious anemia	Low blood count, nerve disability with imbalance and fine-movement problems
Adrenal insufficiency	Skin darkening, weight loss, dizziness, nausea, and weakness
Testicular failure	Decreased sexual interest, infertility
Ovarian failure	Decreased sexual interest, infertility, hot flashes, and decreased/absent menstrual periods
Diabetes mellitus	Increased urination, increased thirst and appetite

cause disease. Many patients have autoantibodies that precede autoimmune disorders, and, of note, it is reported that 100% of these patients have autoantibodies that react with interferon-α. Firm diagnosis is usually made with direct sequencing of the *AIRE* gene, with several populations having an increased frequency of specific mutations, including Iranian, Jewish, and Finnish populations. Chronic candidiasis may develop into oral squamous cell carcinoma, and evidence of ectodermal changes includes hypoplastic dental enamel and pitted dystrophic nails.

C. **Immunodysregulation, polyendocrinopathy, and enteropathy, X-linked (IPEX).** This syndrome is also known as XPID syndrome and occurs in neonates with overwhelming autoimmunity, frequently leading to death associated with severe enteropathy. Mutations of the *FOXP3* gene inherited in an X-linked manner are causative. The *FOXP3* gene encodes a transcription factor that is essential for the development of a major subset of regulatory T lymphocytes. In the absence of these regulatory T lymphocytes, multiple autoimmune disorders develop, including neonatal diabetes with β-cell destruction and presence of anti-islet autoantibodies (e.g. GAD65 autoantibodies). Of note, bone marrow transplantation can replace missing regulatory T lymphocytes and is an important consideration for this fatal disorder.

D. **Anti-insulin receptor antibody syndrome.** Also known as type B insulin resistance, this syndrome is characterized by marked insulin resistance, hyperglycemia, and acanthosis nigricans. Approximately one third of patients also have other autoimmune diseases, usually disorders such as lupus erythematosus. Paradoxically, the anti-insulin receptor antibodies can also lead to episodes of hypoglycemia via a partial agonist effect.

E. **Polyneuropathy, organomegaly, endocrinopathy, M protein, and skin changes (POEMS syndrome).** This syndrome is characterized by severe sensorimotor polyneuropathy, organomegaly (liver, spleen, and lymph nodes), endocrinopathy, monoclonal antibody production with bony lesions secondary to a plasma cell dyscrasia, and skin changes (hyperpigmentation, hypertrichosis, sclerosis, and Raynaud phenomenon). The endocrinopathies include hyperestrogenism leading to impotence and gynecomastia in men (79% of patients), amenorrhea (70% to 100% of patients), primary hypothyroidism (16% of patients), and diabetes mellitus (16% of patients, and 32% with impaired glucose tolerance). Disease onset is in adulthood (fourth or fifth decade). It has a male predominance and is more common in the Japanese population. There is evidence of increased VEGF levels associated with the syndrome as well as response to therapy of the plasmacytoma and reports of response to auto–peripheral blood stem cell transplantation following chemotherapy.

F. **Thymic tumors.** Thymomas are associated with autoimmune disease in ∼40% of patients. The most common autoimmune diseases include myasthenia gravis, red blood cell aplasia, and hypogammaglobulinemia. Occasionally, type 1A diabetes, Addison disease, autoimmune thyroid disease, and stiff-man syndrome have been reported.

II. EVALUATION

A. As a general rule, given a patient with one or more diseases of APS type II, the likelihood of developing an additional type II syndrome disease in the patient or the patient's family members reflects the prevalence of the disease in the general population increased 10- to 100-fold. Approximately one in six relatives of patients with APS type II has an unsuspected illness, most commonly hypothyroidism. Therefore, a screening thyroid-stimulating hormone is recommended every 5 years for otherwise asymptomatic patients and their family members. Assays for 21-hydroxylase autoantibodies can have a high positive predictive value for Addison disease with high sensitivity (>90%). Although autoantibodies can be disease-specific (e.g., antithyroglobulin antibody), they can also be involved in multiple diseases. Both **stiff-man syndrome** (a rare neurologic disorder involving painful muscle contractions of the neck, trunk, and limbs) and type 1A diabetes have in common the glutamic acid decarboxylase autoantibody (GADAA). Approximately 30% of patients with stiff-man syndrome will develop type 1A diabetes, and they are also at increased risk for other APS type II diseases. Therefore, patients with any APS type II disease should undergo regular focused history and physical examinations for associated diseases. In addition, evaluation for organ-specific autoantibodies or even HLA typing of families can be useful in the detection of individuals at highest risk. For example, one could predict the risk of developing type 1 diabetes among first-degree relatives of diabetics using a combination of three autoantibodies: insulin autoantibody (IAA), GADAA, and insulinoma-associated autoantibody (IA-2AA, also termed ICA512) (Fig. 57.1). For relatives, who are positive for two or more autoantibodies, the 3- and 5-year risks of developing diabetes were 39% and 68%, respectively. A fourth major islet autoantigen has recently been discovered, zinc transporter 8 (ZnT8), and research assays for this autoantibody are now available at a number of centers. Given the ability to measure four major "biochemical" autoantibodies, I usually do not measure cytoplasmic islet cell autoantibodies (ICAs), though rarely a patient may be ICA-positive and lack the other four antibodies. Difficulty in standardizing the ICA assay, which utilizes sections of human pancreas, limits the utility of this assay.

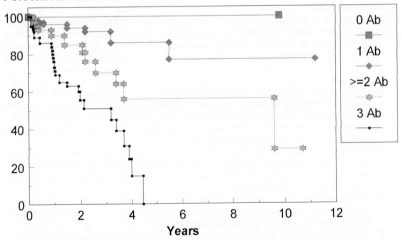

Figure 57.1. The diabetes-free survival of first-degree relatives, according to the number of autoantibodies (Ab) present at baseline, considering insulin autoantibody, glutamic acid decarboxylase autoantibody, and islet-cell autoantibody. (From Verge CF, et al. Prediction of type I diabetes in first-degree relatives using a combination of insulin, GAD, and ICA512bdc/IA-2 autoantibodies. *Diabetes* 1996;45:930.)

Patients with type 1 diabetes or who have first-degree relatives with type 1 diabetes are also at higher risk for developing celiac disease, which is often asymptomatic in this "at-risk" patient population. Furthermore, the celiac patients are at increased risk for gastrointestinal lymphoma. In celiac disease, tissue transglutaminase has been identified as the major antigen for endomysial autoantibody. A positive transglutaminase autoantibody among at-risk asymptomatic children has a positive predictive value of 70% to 80% for small-bowel biopsy evidence of celiac disease if the level of transglutaminase antibodies is high (e.g., 10 times the 99th percentile of normal controls, dependent on the assay), and the antibody level is related directly to the likelihood of biopsy positivity. Therefore, screening of high-risk patients may lead to the discovery of otherwise asymptomatic disease, and initiation of intervention (e.g., a gluten-free diet) may decrease the risk of subsequently developing a life-threatening condition, such as lymphoma.

B. The most common first presentation in APECED is persistent mucocutaneous candidiasis, with endocrine involvement developing in the subsequent several months to several years. The syndrome almost universally presents before age 20 years. This is in contrast to candidiasis presenting in adults, which is frequently associated with thymoma or immunodeficiency (e.g., acquired immunodeficiency syndrome). Siblings' are at high risk for the component illnesses, and periodic evaluation for hypocalcemia, cortisol deficiency, and hepatic enzyme abnormalities are indicated. With identification of mutations of the AIRE gene, sequencing and identification of siblings with the mutation are now possible. There are extremely rare autosomal dominant AIRE mutations, however.

C. Anti-insulin receptor antibodies should be suspected in a patient with marked hyperinsulinemia (before insulin therapy), resistance to intravenous insulin on an intravenous tolerance test, and (rarely) fasting hypoglycemia. Specialized laboratories can directly quantitate the antireceptor antibodies to aid in the differential diagnosis.

D. Radiographic demonstration of a localized sclerotic bone lesion in a patient with other associated symptoms is strongly suggestive of POEMS syndrome.

E. Patients with aplastic anemia or myasthenia gravis with concurrent autoimmune endocrine disease should have computed tomography (CT) of the thorax to search for a thymoma. Transient remission of the syndrome often allows thymectomy.

III. MANAGEMENT

A. In patients with untreated Addison disease and hypothyroidism, steroids should be given prior to thyroxine (T$_4$) replacement to avoid precipitating an adrenal crisis. Thyroxine replacement increases the metabolism of the residual cortisol remaining in adrenal-insufficient patients, thereby worsening the insufficiency. In APS type I and APS type II patients and their relatives, early detection of hypothyroidism, adrenal sufficiency, and pernicious anemia prior to morbidity is a major goal.

B. In addition to appropriate hormonal replacement therapy, patients with APECED-associated hepatitis should also be placed on immunosuppressive therapy. Given the adverse growth effects in children with chronic glucocorticoids, azathioprine may be preferred, but careful monitoring and specialized care is essential, as cirrhosis is often preventable with appropriate therapy.

C. The clinical course of patients with anti-insulin receptor antibodies has been extremely varied, with some patients remitting, others developing severe hypoglycemia, and others having no benefit from massive doses of intravenous insulin. No immunologic therapy is of proven efficacy.

D. Therapy of POEMS syndrome is initially directed at the plasmacytoma, which is quite responsive to radiotherapy or radiotherapy plus surgery. Choice of chemotherapy should avoid neurotoxic agents such as vincristine.

E. Surgical resection of thymic tumors can result in at least temporary remission of life-threatening associated autoimmune diseases.

IV. FRONTIERS

Over the past several years, there have been major advances in defining the genetics of a series of autoimmune disorders, development of highly specific and sensitive autoantibody assays that can predict disease, and development of potent novel immunotherapeutics. Identifying risk or subclinical autoimmune disorders in those at risk allows early intervention to prevent morbidity (or the rare mortality at diagnosis of disorders such as type 1A diabetes or Addison disease) at onset, or treat "asymptomatic" disorders such as chronic active hepatitis or celiac disease. A major goal is the immunologic prevention of diseases such as type 1A diabetes, and multiple trials prior to disease onset among individuals expressing multiple anti-islet autoantibodies or at the onset of diabetes (to preserve remaining islet β cells) are under way. For instance, relatives of patients with type 1A diabetes can be screened for anti-islet autoantibodies through Trialnet (1-800-HALT-DM1) for potential entry into prevention studies.

Selected References

Bao S, et al. Type B insulin resistance syndrome associated with systemic lupus erythematosus. *Endocr Pract* 2007;13:51–55.

Barker JM. Type 1 diabetes associated autoimmunity: natural history, genetic associations and screening. *J Clin Endocrinol Metab* 2006;91:1210–1217.

Barker JM, Eisenbarth GS. "Autoimmune Polyendocrine Syndromes." Type I Diabetes: Molecular, Cellular and Clinical Immunology 2007. www.barbaradaviscenter.org.

Eisenbarth GS, Gottlieb P. Immunoendocrinopathy syndromes. In: Larsen PR, Kronenberg H, Melmed S, Polonsky KS, eds. *Williams Textbook of Endocrinology*. 10th ed. Philadelphia: WB Saunders; 2003:1763–1776.

Gandhi GY, et al. Endocrinopathy in POEMS syndrome: the Mayo Clinic experience. *Mayo Clin Proc* 2007;82:836–842.

Hoffenberg EJ, et al. Clinical features of children with screening-identified evidence of celiac disease. *Pediatrics* 2004;113:1254–1259.

Kondo K, Monden Y. Thymoma and myasthenia gravis: a clinical study of 1,089 patients from Japan. *Ann Thorac Surg* 2005;79:219–224.

Meager A, et al. Anti-interferon autoantibodies in autoimmune polyendocrinopathy syndrome type 1. *PLoS Med* 2006;3:e289.

Neufeld M, et al. Two types of autoimmune Addison's disease associated with different polyglandular autoimmune (PGA) syndromes. *Medicine (Balt)* 1981;60:355–362.

Perheentupa J. Autoimmune polyendocrinopathy-candidiasis-ectodermal dystrophy. *J Clin Endocrinol Metab* 2006;91:2843–2850.

Villasenor J, et al. AIRE and APECED: molecular insights into an autoimmune disease. *Immunol Rev* 2005;204:156–164.

Wildin RS, et al. IPEX and FOXP3: clinical and research perspectives. *J Autoimmun* 2005; 25(suppl):56–62.

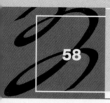

MANAGEMENT OF SOME HORMONE-DEPENDENT CANCERS WITH ANALOGS OF HYPOTHALAMIC HORMONES

Andrew V. Schally and Norman L. Block

PROSTATE CANCER

I. GENERAL PRINCIPLES

A. Carcinoma of the prostate is the most common noncutaneous malignancy and the second leading cause of cancer-related deaths among adult American men. In 2006 an estimated 32 000 men in the United States died from prostate cancer and about 230 000 new cases were diagnosed. Adenocarcinoma of the prostate is rare before the age of 40 years, but the incidence increases with advancing age. Men who have first-degree relatives with prostate cancer and African American men have a higher lifetime risk for developing the disease. Carcinoma of the prostate is androgen-dependent in ~70% of cases. Twenty percent to 30% of patients with prostate cancer already have metastatic disease when they are first diagnosed.

II. EVALUATION

A. Screening tests for prostate cancer offer the best chance for early diagnosis of organ-confined, potentially curable disease. The American Cancer Society currently recommends that both the prostate-specific antigen (PSA) blood test and digital rectal examination (DRE) be offered annually, beginning at age 50 years, to men with a life expectancy of at least 10 years. In addition, the American Urologic Association currently recommends that African American men and all men with a family history of prostate cancer have the screening tests initiated at age 40 years.

B. Digital rectal examination. DRE is routinely used for diagnosis and for evaluating the local extent of prostate cancer. The positive predictive value of DRE for prostate cancer is ~50% and varies relatively little with age. The predictive value of the DRE is enhanced by combination with the results of the PSA test.

C. Prostate-specific antigen. The PSA and DRE are complementary in the detection of prostate cancer. It has been shown that PSA and DRE combined increase the rate of detection by 81% over DRE alone and 22% over PSA alone. PSA levels >4.0 ng/mL are often considered suspicious of prostate cancer. PSA is a glycoprotein produced by prostate cells and is specific to the prostate, but not to prostate cancer. Thus, PSA is not detected in the serum of 30% of patients with prostate cancer and is found in increased concentrations in the serum of 20% of men who do not have prostate cancer. PSA levels can also be elevated in benign prostatic hyperplasia and for several weeks after acute prostatitis, transrectal needle biopsy, prostatic manipulation, prostate surgery, acute urine retention, catheters, bicycle riding, etc. PSA is more sensitive than prostatic acid phosphatase (PAP) for the detection of prostatic cancer and is more useful in monitoring responses and recurrence after therapy.

D. Transrectal ultrasound (TRUS) examination of the prostate. TRUS is useful for detecting small lesions and for guiding biopsy procedures, but it is not recommended for screening. TRUS rarely detects cancer in the presence of both a normal DRE and PSA and should be reserved for further evaluation in patients who have abnormal results of DRE and/or PSA-level testing.

E. Computed tomography (CT) and/or magnetic resonance imagining (MRI). CT and MRI of the pelvis and/or the abdomen have been used extensively for staging prostate cancer; however, they cannot easily detect microscopic extension of cancer and are useful only in patients with signs of advanced cancer.

F. Radioisotope bone scan. A bone scan is the most sensitive method for detection of osseous metastases. However, it is relatively nonspecific and should be used in conjunction with roentgenography, such as thin-slice CT scanning with bone windows.

G. Pelvic lymphadenectomy. Pelvic lymph node metastases are often asymptomatic and are uncommonly visualized even with the most sophisticated radiologic imaging modalities. Guidelines have been developed for assessing the probabilities of a patient having nodal metastases based on a combination of clinical tumor stage, PSA, and biopsy Gleason grade. Such information allows a further staging of pelvic lymphadenectomy to be selectively performed in those patients in whom this procedure is likely to influence management decisions.

III. MANAGEMENT OF PROSTATE CANCER

The treatment of prostate cancer is based on the patient's clinical stage of disease. Clinical stage is usually assigned to the patient with prostate cancer in accordance with the TNM classification system (primary tumor, regional nodes, and metastasis).

A. Clinically localized prostate cancer. The best therapy for patients with clinically localized prostate cancer remains to be determined. The options for management of patients with clinically localized prostate cancer (stage T1–T2N0M0) include watchful waiting, radical prostatectomy, external-beam irradiation, brachytherapy, and hormonal therapy. Watchful waiting is offered to patients with a life expectancy of <10 years presenting with small and well-differentiated cancers. Radical prostatectomy, external-beam irradiation, and brachytherapy are recommended for those patients who have a life expectancy of >10 years. These modalities of treatment may be associated with urinary and sexual dysfunction.

1. Clinical course. Recurrence of prostate cancer after local therapy is becoming a significant medical problem. Tumor grade, pathologic stage, and rate of PSA change are important factors for predicting recurrence. PSA recurrence usually precedes clinical recurrence by several years.

2. Follow-up. Patients should have their PSA levels monitored periodically following local therapy for prostate cancer. Various studies show that after radical prostatectomy, a rising PSA predicts an eventual failure. Tumor eradication following radiation is associated with a PSA of <0.5 ng/mL.

3. Use of analogs of luteinizing hormone–releasing hormone (LHRH) after relapse following local therapy. Treatment with agonists of LHRH, also known as GnRH, for gonadotropin-releasing hormone, is now recommended in men with a rising PSA level after surgery or radiotherapy. However, long-term follow-up is needed to determine the benefits of adjuvant hormonal treatment in terms of local control, disease progression, and improvement in patient survival.

B. Locally advanced prostate cancer. There are various opinions as to the best mode of therapy for men with locally advanced (T3) nonmetastatic disease. Subjects with stage T3 disease, especially those with poorly differentiated tumors, are usually treated with adjuvant hormonal therapy combined with radiotherapy. LHRH agonists can be used in combination with an antiandrogen prior to radical prostatectomy in those patients having surgery for T3 prostate cancer. In addition, neoadjuvant therapy with LHRH agonists started at the beginning of external-beam radiotherapy, and continued for 3 years, can improve the 5-year overall survival of patients with locally advanced prostate cancer.

C. Advanced prostate cancer. The treatment of men with advanced prostate cancer is palliative and based on the accomplishment of androgen deprivation. Endocrine therapy improves quality of life and prolongs survival. Standard therapies for advanced prostate cancer consist of bilateral orchiectomy or long-term administration of LHRH agonists, each with and without an antiandrogen. Approximately 70% to 80% of patients with prostate cancer show symptomatic and objective responses to androgen ablation. Androgen deprivation leads to a decrease in libido, impotence, "hot flashes," weight gain, muscle loss, cognitive change, and osteopenia. In addition, surgical castration has a psychological impact. Acceptance of LHRH analogs is excellent, and in surveys of patients who are offered a choice between orchiectomy and LHRH agonists, the analogs are selected as primary treatment >70% of the time. However, because superactive agonists of LHRH initially stimulate the release of gonadotropins and sex steroids, an occasional temporary flare of the disease during the first week of administration has been observed. This can be of concern in patients with vertebral metastases and/or impending urinary obstruction, and may lead to neurologic problems (i.e., spinal cord compression) or increase in urinary obstruction. Administration of antiandrogens before and during early therapy with agonists can prevent such disease flare.

D. Use of LHRH antagonists in men with advanced prostate cancer. Clinical trials in patients with advanced prostate cancer have also been carried out with the LHRH antagonists cetrorelix (acetyl-D-2-naphthylalanyl-D-4-chlorophenylalanyl-D-3-pyridylalanyl-seryl-tyrosyl-D-citrullyl-leucyl-arginylprolyl-D-alanylamide), (available commercially as Cetrotide; Zentaris) and Abarelix (Praecis Pharm). Cetrorelix and other LHRH antagonists could be beneficial as a monotherapy for patients with prostate cancer and metastases in the brain, spine, liver, and bone marrow in whom the LHRH agonists cannot be used as single drugs because of the possibility of flare. These antagonists act on the same receptor sites as LHRH and cause an immediate inhibition of the release of gonadotropins and sex steroids. Because the inhibition of LH and sex steroids can be induced with a single injection of a potent LHRH antagonist such as cetrorelix, the time of the onset of therapeutic effects is greatly reduced. It was also demonstrated that cetrorelix can produce long-term improvement in patients with benign prostatic hyperplasia (BPH). Orally active nonpeptide LHRH antagonists are also being developed.

E. Hormone-refractory prostate cancer. Most patients with metastatic prostatic carcinoma eventually relapse because all hormonal therapies aimed at androgen deprivation, including bilateral orchiectomy, antiandrogens, LHRH analogs, and their combinations, can only provide a remission of limited duration. The relapse is manifested clinically, radiologically, and biochemically by a rise in serum PSA levels. These patients eventually die of androgen-independent prostatic cancer. This androgen-independent growth of prostate cancer cells is apparently stimulated by various growth factors. The prognosis for patients with hormone-refractory prostate cancer is very poor, and no effective treatment exists at present. Chemotherapy produces poor response rates, although Docetaxel-based therapy confers an improvement in survival. Palliative responses to mitoxantrone plus prednisone were recently demonstrated. Ketoconazole, Estramustin, and Suramin have also been used to improve the clinical outcome in these patients.

F. New approaches. Epidermal growth factor (EGF), insulinlike growth factor I (IGF-I), and their receptors may be involved in neoplastic transformation. Interference with endogenous growth factors and their receptors by somatostatin analogs, bombesin/GRP (gastrin releasing peptide) antagonists, and GHRH antagonists or the use of targeted cytotoxic peptide analogs could inhibit the growth of androgen-independent prostate cancers and improve the tumor treatment outcome.

G. Preparations of LHRH agonists used clinically in tumor therapy
  1. Decapeptyl (Triptorelin): (pyro)Glu-His-Trp-Ser-Tyr-D-Trp-Leu-Arg-Pro-Gly-NH$_2$ (D-Trp-6-LHRH), Ipsen-Biotech, Ferring, Akzo-Organon, Ache.
  2. Buserelin (Suprefact): (pyro)Glu-His-Trp-Ser-Tyr-D-Ser(Bu^t)-Leu-Arg-Pro-ethylamide, Hoechst-Marion-Roussel, Aventis (Canada).
  3. Leuprolide (Lupron): (pyro)Glu-His-Trp-Ser-Tyr-D-Leu-Leu-Arg-Pro-ethylamide (D-Leu-6-Des-Gly-10-LHRH ethylamide), Abbott-Takeda, TAP Pharmaceuticals.
  4. Zoladex (Goserelin): (pyro)Glu-His-Trp-Ser-Tyr-Ser-(Bu^t)-Leu-Arg-Pro-Azgly-NH$_2$ (ICI 118630), Zeneca Pharmaceuticals, Astra Zeneca.
  5. The therapeutic regimens are based on long-acting depot formulations consisting of analogs dispersed in microcapsules or implants of biodegradable polymers. Lupron depot and decapeptyl LP are available in the form of slow-release formulations containing 3.75 mg analog in microcapsules of poly(D,L-lactide-co-glycolide) and administered intramuscularly at monthly intervals through an

18- to 22-gauge needle. Depot formulations of leuprolide acetate 22.5 mg and 30 mg Triptorelin (Trelstar LA) containing 11.25 mg of the active drug have been developed. These formulations release the drugs for 3 to 4 months at the same daily dose as the monthly preparations. There are also implantable devices (Viadur, containing 65 mg Leuprolide) for year-long release.

Zoladex implant containing 3.6 mg goserelin is designed for subcutaneous injection with continuous release over a 28-day period. The analog is dispersed in a matrix of D,L-lactic and glycolic acids copolymer and supplied as a 1-mm-diameter cylinder preloaded in a single-use syringe with a 16-gauge needle. Zoladex 3-month goserelin implant contains 10.8 mg of goserelin and is designed for subcutaneous implantation with continuous release over a 12-week period. It is supplied as a 1.5-mm-diameter cylinder, preloaded in a single-use syringe with a 14-gauge needle. Suprefact depot (buserelin 2-month depot) is supplied in an applicator containing two implant rods, equivalent to a total of 6.3 mg buserelin, and is injected subcutaneously into the lateral abdominal wall every 8 weeks. About 7 days before the first injection of depot preparations of LHRH agonists, an antiandrogen such as bicalutamide (Casodex) should be administered in accordance with the manufacturer's directions. This comedication is to be continued at least for 2 to 4 weeks after the first agonist injection, until the testosterone levels have been lowered to the surgical castration range, or indefinitely.

BREAST CANCER

I. GENERAL PRINCIPLES

A. Breast cancer is the most common malignancy among American women. The American Cancer Society estimates that ~185 000 new cases of breast cancer are diagnosed in the United States annually and ~41 000 patients die of the disease. Although <10% of patients with breast cancer are diagnosed as having advanced disease at the time of presentation, cancer statistics indicate that 40% to 70% will eventually develop metastases in the course of their disease. Endocrine treatment alone or in combination with chemotherapy has been utilized for the palliation of advanced breast cancer, as well as for adjuvant therapy to surgery and irradiation in patients with primary breast cancer.

II. PRIMARY BREAST CANCER AND RISK FACTORS FOR RELAPSE

Special clinical problems exist concerning the initial evaluation of patients with early-stage breast cancer. A significant number of these patients are at risk of relapse following local treatment. Thus, it is important to assess the risk factors for relapse at the time of diagnosis. For patients at risk of relapse, adjuvant treatment based on hormonal therapy, chemotherapy, or combinations should be given immediately after local treatment. The panel of the 6th International Conference on Adjuvant Therapy of Primary Breast Cancer has identified the following factors as defining the patients at increased risk at the time of diagnosis:

A. Nodal status (node-positive breast cancer) and the number of regional lymph nodes involved are considered the most important factors for the estimation of risk.

B. For patients without histologic evidence of lymph node involvement (node-negative disease), the following factors are relevant: tumor size, histologic and nuclear grade, steroid hormone receptor status, presence of lymphatic and/or vascular invasion, and age of the patient at diagnosis.

C. Hormone receptors. The expression of estrogen receptors (ER) and progesterone receptors (PR) in tumor cells is the decisive factor predicting treatment response to endocrine therapy. Patients with ER-positive tumors appear to have longer survival rates compared to those with ER-negative tumors who are at high risk of relapse.

III. ENDOCRINE THERAPY

Endocrine therapy is used as adjuvant therapy to surgery and irradiation in patients with primary breast cancer as well as in the palliation of advanced breast cancer.

Approximately 30% to 40% of unselected premenopausal patients with breast cancer have estrogen-dependent tumors and can be treated with hormonal approaches, such as surgical oophorectomy, the antiestrogen tamoxifen, and agonists of LHRH.

A. Early-stage breast cancer. Adjuvant <u>tamoxifen</u> has been used extensively in premenopausal and postmenopausal patients with early breast cancer who present with detectable ER in the tumors. Prolonged treatment with LHRH analogs or surgical oophorectomy is being investigated in randomized trials. The use of tamoxifen following chemotherapy might be also considered for patients with minimal/trace levels of ER or PR.

B. Advanced breast cancer. Tamoxifen is the therapy of choice for the initial management of premenopausal and postmenopausal women with advanced breast cancer, particularly those with ER-positive tumors. However, for premenopausal women, some clinicians prefer the use of LHRH agonists or oophorectomy. Tumor remissions after therapy with LHRH agonists occur primarily in women with well-differentiated, slow-growing, and ER-positive tumors. A large trial in premenopausal women with breast cancer, using depot implants of Zoladex, demonstrated 53% objective tumor responses. In premenopausal women with estrogen receptor–positive breast cancer, adjuvant treatment with LHRH agonists for 2 to 3 years is as effective as chemotherapy and is burdened with fewer side effects. Combinations of agonists in long-acting depot preparations and tamoxifen produced a superior response rate in premenopausal women with breast cancer than either modality alone. Aromatase inhibitors such as letrozole, which block the conversion of adrenal androgens to estrogens, are primarily effective in postmenopausal women with breast cancer but can also be used in premenopausal women if they are combined with an agonist of LHRH, which produces ovarian estrogen deprivation. LHRH antagonists, such as cetrorelix, have been shown to be very effective in the management of experimental breast cancers but have not been evaluated clinically. Because receptors for LHRH are found in >50% of human breast cancer specimens, cytotoxic analogs of LHRH that contain doxorubicin have been developed. These cytotoxic analogs, such as AN-152, target breast cancers expressing LHRH receptors and are in Phase II clinical trials.

IV. CHEMOPREVENTION

The incidence of breast cancer in the United States declined after millions of women stopped taking hormone replacement therapy (HRT) following the release of the Womens Health Initiative Study in July 2002, which indicated that HRT led to more risks than benefits. The U.S. Food and Drug Administration (FDA) approved the use of tamoxifen citrate (<u>Nolvadex</u>) for prevention of breast cancer in women considered at high risk. However, tamoxifen does not completely antagonize the effect of ovarian estrogens and <u>may contribute to an increase in endometrial carcinomas</u>. A large clinical trial with tamoxifen and raloxifene, which includes 22 000 postmenopausal women with a high risk of breast cancer, is assessing breast cancer efficacy and endometrial safety of these agents. <u>Raloxifene (Evista)</u> is a selective estrogen receptor modulator (SERM). <u>Fulvestrant (Faslodex)</u> is also a novel antiestrogen without any agonistic activity and is approved for treatment of postmenopausal women with breast cancer.

A. Use of radiolabeled somatostatin analogs for localization and treatment of tumors. Radioiodinated analogs of somatostatin, such as [^{111}In-DTPA-D-Phe^1]-octreotide (OctreoScan), can be used clinically for the imaging of tumors that express receptors for somatostatin. Thus, the presence of somatostatin receptors, particularly subtypes 2 and 5, on tumors may permit their localization using such scanning techniques. Somatostatin receptor scintigraphy has now been carried out in thousands of patients and it is well established that various primary tumors, either neuroendocrine or non-neuroendocrine, containing high numbers of somatostatin receptors, can be localized in vivo. In addition, the sites of metastatic spread can also be visualized by scintigraphy with radiolabeled somatostatin analogs. Neuroendocrine tumors that can be localized with OctreoScan include growth hormone–secreting pituitary tumors, gastrinomas, insulinomas, glucagonomas, medullary thyroid carcinomas, neuroblastomas, pheochromocytomas, carcinoids, and small-cell lung cancers.

Among non-neuroendocrine tumors that could be imaged by scintigraphy are non-small-cell lung cancers, meningiomas, breast cancers, and astrocytomas. Information from scintigraphy improves therapeutic planning.

B. **Use of radiolabeled somatostatin analogs for tumor therapy.** Attempts are being made to use somatostatin analogs labeled with radionuclides, such as [111]Indium or [90]Yttrium, for cancer therapy. Radiolabeled somatostatin analogs to deliver therapeutic doses of a radioactive isotope to the cancer cell may improve the treatment of somatostatin receptor–positive tumors.

Selected References

American College of Physicians. Clinical guideline: part III. Screening for prostate cancer. *Ann Intern Med* 1997;126:480–484.

Catalona WJ, Ramos CG, Carvalhal GF. Contemporary results of anatomic radical prostatectomy. *CA Cancer J Clin* 1999;49:282–296.

Crown J. Evolution in the treatment of advanced breast cancer. *Semin Oncol* 1998;25:12–17.

Dawson NA. Response criteria in prostatic carcinoma. *Semin Oncol* 1999;26:174–184.

Early Breast Cancer Trialists' Collaborative Group. Tamoxifen for early breast cancer: an overview of the randomised trials. *Lancet* 1998;351:1451–1467.

Goldhirsch A, Glick JH, Gelber RD, et al. Commentary: meeting highlights—International Consensus Panel on the Treatment of Primary Breast Cancer. *J Natl Cancer Inst* 1998;90:1601–1608.

Gonzalez-Barcena B, Vadillo-Buenfil M, Cortez-Morales A, et al. LH-RH antagonist SB-75 (cetrorelix) as primary single therapy in patients with advanced prostatic cancer and paraplegia due to metastatic invasion of spinal cord. *Urology* 1995;45:275–281.

Gonzalez-Barcena D, Vadillo-Buenfil M, Gomez Orta F, et al. Responses to the antagonistic analogue of LH-RH (SB-75) (cetrorelix) in patients with benign prostatic hyperplasia and prostatic cancer. *Prostate* 1994;24:84–92.

Hegarty NJ, Fitzpatrick JM, Richie JP, et al. Future prospects in prostate cancer. *Prostate* 1999;40:261–268.

Jemal A, Murray T, Ward E, et al. Cancer statistics, 2005. *CA Cancer J Clin* 2005;55:10–30.

Kaufmann M, Jonat W, Blamey R, et al. Zoladex Early Breast Cancer Research Association (ZEBRA) Trialists' Group. Survival analyses from the ZEBRA study. Goserelin (Zoladex) versus CMF in premenopausal women with node-positive breast cancer. *Eur J Cancer* 2003;39:1711–1717.

Kaufmann M, Jonat W, Kleeburg U, et al. The German Zoladex Trial Group: goserelin, a depot gonadotropin releasing hormone agonist in the treatment of premenopausal patients with metastatic breast cancer. *J Clin Oncol* 1989;7:1113–1119.

Klijn JG, Beex LV, Mauriac L, et al. Combined treatment with buserelin and tamoxifen in premenopausal metastatic breast cancer: a randomized study. *J Natl Cancer Inst* 2000;92:903–911.

Krenning EP, Kwekkeboom DJ, Bakker WH, et al. Somatostatin receptor scintigraphy with [111In-DTPA-D-Phe[1]]- and [123I-Tyr[3]]-octreotide: the Rotterdam experience with more than 1000 patients. *Eur J Nucl Med* 1993;20:716–731.

McCarthy KE, Woltering EA, Espenan GD, et al. In situ radiotherapy with ^{111}In pentetreotide: initial observations and future directions. *Cancer J* 1998;4:94–102.

Oh WK, Kantoff PW. Management of hormone refractory prostate cancer: current standards and future prospects. *J Urol* 1998;160:1220–1229.

Ornstein DK, Oh J, Herschman JD, et al. Evaluation and management of the man who has failed primary curative therapy for prostate cancer. *Urol Clin North Am* 1998;25:591–601.

Perrotti M, Fair WR. Patient evaluation. In: Resnick MI, Thompson IM, eds. *Surgery of the Prostate*. New York: Churchill Livingstone; 1998:1–19.

Schally AV, Comaru-Schally AM. Hypothalamic and other peptide hormones: analogues of peptide hormones. In: Holland JF, Frei III E, Bast Jr RC, et al., eds. *Cancer Medicine*. 7th ed. Hamilton, Ontario, Canada: BC Decker; 2006:802–816.

Smith RA, Mettlin CJ, Davis KJ, et al. American Cancer Society guidelines for the early detection of cancer. *CA Cancer J Clin* 2000;50:34–49.

Stanford JL, Feng Z, Hamilton AS, et al. Urinary and sexual function after radical prostatectomy for clinically localized prostate cancer: the prostate cancer outcomes study. *JAMA* 2000;283:354–360.

Trump DL, Shipley WU, Dillioglugil O, et al. Neoplasms of the prostate. In: Holland JF, Bast RC Jr, Morton DL, et al., eds. *Cancer Medicine*. 4th ed. Baltimore: Williams & Wilkins; 1997:2125–2164.

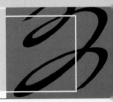

Appendices

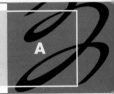

PROTOCOLS FOR STIMULATION AND SUPPRESSION TESTS COMMONLY USED IN CLINICAL ENDOCRINOLOGY

A

Etty Osher and Naftali Stern

ANTERIOR PITUITARY

I. DIAGNOSIS OF GROWTH HORMONE (GH) DEFICIENCY

In adults, the diagnosis of GH deficiency should be considered in subjects with known hypothalamic-pituitary disorders, particularly in the presence of significant or likely organic disease, such as the presence of a large pituitary tumor, pituitary trauma or significant head trauma, previous radiation treatment to the brain or the hypothalamic-pituitary region, and a childhood diagnosis of GH deficiency.

In subjects with significant organic pituitary disorders, the likelihood of GH deficiency in subjects with hypopituitarism increases in relation to the number of coexisting hormonal deficiencies in the anterior pituitary, rising from ~40% in the absence of coexisting deficiency to ~60% with a single impairment, ~80% with impaired secretion of two pituitary hormones, and ~100% when the secretion of three or more additional anterior pituitary hormones is deficient.

A. Measurement of serum IGF-1. In subjects with organic pituitary disease, serum IGF-1 concentration less than the age-defined lower limit of the normal range confirms the diagnosis of GH deficiency. Care must be taken, however, to exclude the presence of conditions known to lower serum IGF-I levels independent of pituitary disease, such as malnutrition, hepatic disease, poorly controlled diabetes mellitus, and hypothyroidism. Additionally, the presence of two or more pituitary hormone deficiencies in association with low serum IGF-I level is highly suggestive of GH deficiency. Still, if the pursuit of the diagnosis of GH deficiency is driven by intent to prescribe GH replacement therapy, confirmation of the diagnosis by a provocative test of GH release is advisable. In patients with subnormal IGF-I, a single GH stimulation test is apparently sufficient to confirm the diagnosis. When GH deficiency is considered in the absence of organic pituitary disease or in a subject with

793

known pituitary disease but normal IGF-1, performing two stimulatory tests appears preferable.

B. Growth hormone stimulation tests

1. Insulin-induced hypoglycemia test

a. Purpose. This is the most robustly validated test available to assess growth hormone secretion and also the "gold standard" test to diagnose hypofunction of the hypothalamic–pituitary–adrenal axis.

b. Procedure

(1) Perform the test in the morning, after an overnight fast.

(2) An indwelling intravenous (IV) line should be placed and maintained patent so that 50% glucose solution can be administered promptly if necessary.

(3) Blood samples for glucose and growth hormone should be obtained immediately before and at 15, 30, 45, 60, 90, and 120 minutes after insulin injection. (If evaluation of adrenocorticotropic hormone [ACTH] reserve is also desired, samples for cortisol should be obtained immediately before and at 30, 60, 90, and 120 minutes after insulin injection.)

(4) Inject regular insulin, 0.1 U/kg IV. Higher doses (0.15 U/kg or 0.2 U/kg) may be needed in states of insulin resistance such as obesity, pituitary Cushing syndrome, or acromegaly. A lower dose is advisable (i.e., 0.05 U/kg) in patients suspected of having hypopituitarism.

(5) This test may be performed in sequence with an arginine tolerance test. Also, it can be performed simultaneously with the thyrotropin-releasing hormones (TRH) and luteinizing hormone–releasing hormone (LHRH) tests if indicated.

c. Interpretation

(1) Growth hormone levels generally peak at 40 to 90 minutes after insulin administration. Attention should be paid to the type of growth hormone assay used. Newer immunoradiometric (IRMA) or immunofluorometric (IFMA) assays are more sensitive and specific and yield results that are 30% to 50% lower than the traditional radioimmunoassay (RIA) tests. For appropriate stimulation of growth hormone secretion, a fall in serum glucose levels of at least 50% from baseline levels (i.e., <40 mg/dL) is usually necessary. Thus mild hypoglycemic symptoms (e.g., nervousness, sweating, or tachycardia) are to be expected and do not require termination of the test. In children evaluated for short stature, most pediatric endocrinologists use a cutoff serum concentration of 10 ng/mL as evidence of normal response. In adults, peak growth hormone levels of <3 ng/mL are considered unequivocal evidence for growth hormone deficiency, whereas levels 5 mg/mL are seen in normal individuals. Recently, a diagnosis of partial GH deficiency, "GH insufficiency," has been proposed for subjects with pituitary disease whose insulin-stimulated GH ranges between 3 and 7 ng/mL. Obesity and insulin resistance complicate the interpretation of this test in that lower insulin-stimulated GH levels are seen in normal obese individuals.

(2) In assessing the **pituitary–adrenal axis,** a glucose level of <40 mg/dL provides an appropriate stimulus for sufficient ACTH/cortisol release. A peak cortisol exceeding 18 to 20 μg/dL implies an intact pituitary/adrenal response. Subnormal response suggests primary or secondary adrenal insufficiency. This test has been particularly reliable in patients with previous glucocorticoid therapy.

(3) In patients with **severe depression** who have elevated plasma and urinary corticosteroid levels that are relatively resistant to suppression by dexamethasone, the plasma cortisol response to insulin-induced hypoglycemia is preserved. Lack of cortisol response is characteristic in patients with Cushing syndrome.

d. Precautions. Severe hypoglycemia may occur, particularly if the pituitary–adrenal axis is also impaired. Therefore, close monitoring is indicated, and a meal should be given upon termination of this test. This test is contraindicated in patients with epilepsy or coronary artery disease, and we usually resort to alternative tests in patients >55 years old, to avoid the risk of occult ischemic disease.

2. Arginine infusion test

a. **Purpose:** Assessment of growth hormone secretion

b. **Procedure**

   (1) Perform the test in the morning, after an overnight fast.

   (2) Draw a baseline blood sample for growth hormone.

   (3) Infuse a sterile solution of arginine hydrochloride (0.5 g/kg IV, not to exceed 30 g) over 30 minutes.

   (4) Obtain blood samples for growth hormone at 30, 60, 90, and 120 minutes.

   (5) In men and postmenopausal women, the response to arginine infusion is improved by <u>pretreatment with Premarin, 5 mg (2.5 mg in patients <30 kg) twice daily for 2 or 3 days.</u>

   (6) This test may be performed in sequence with an insulin-induced hypoglycemia test (see Section I.B.1). One method is to infuse arginine as described, and after drawing the 60-minute sample, follow with the insulin-induced hypoglycemia test.

   A recent variation of the arginine infusion test is the combination of arginine administered as outlined previously with growth hormone–releasing hormone (GHRH), given intravenously together with arginine as a bolus (1 μg/kg)—see Section I.B.3.

c. **Interpretation.** In adults, peak growth hormone levels <3 ng/mL indicate severe GH deficiency, and those between 3 and 5 ng/mL are equivocal. Only 65% to 75% of healthy subjects display normal responses, although premenopausal women generally have a more consistent response to arginine than men. The response is better in men and postmenopausal women given estrogen pretreatment. As with the other growth hormone stimulation tests, hypothyroidism and obesity inhibit growth hormone stimulation by arginine. In children, peak level should be 10 ng/mL or higher. Because normal children may fail any single growth hormone stimulation test, an additional provocative test should be performed before the diagnosis of growth hormone deficiency is established. Whenever the possibility of constitutional delay in growth and puberty (CDGP) is considered in a prepubertal child with short stature, sex hormone priming with estrogen or androgen will often separate severe growth hormone deficiency from CDGP: In CDPG the growth hormone response is normalized after priming, whereas it is unaffected by this maneuver in severe growth hormone deficiency.

d. **Precautions.** Late hypoglycemia resulting from insulin stimulation can occur. Arginine should be given with caution to patients with severe hepatic or renal disease.

3. Combined arginine and GHRH test

a. **Purpose.** This test is now considered, along with the insulin stimulation test, as one of the two tests of choice to assess growth hormone secretion.

b. **Procedure**

   (1) Perform the test in the morning, after an overnight fast.

   (2) Draw a baseline blood sample for growth hormone (time −30 and 0).

   (3) Infuse **(a)** 1 μg/kg of GHRH intravenously as a bolus dose; **(b)** a sterile solution of arginine hydrochloride (0.5 g/kg IV, not to exceed 30 g) over 30 minutes.

   (4) Collect samples for the measurement of GH at, 30, 60, 90, and 120 minutes following the initiation of the test.

c. **Interpretation.** As is the case for other methods GH stimulation, attained peak levels are highly dependent on fat mass, and this has been particularly well studied with this test. Suggested minimal values for normalcy in lean (body mass index [BMI] <25), overweight (BMI ≥25 to <30), and obese (BMI ≥30) subjects are 11.5, 8.0, and 4.2 ng/mL. Others regard GH ≤4.1 ng/mL in a subject with organic pituitary disease as indicative of GH deficiency.

    d. Precautions. See Section I.B.2d. Additionally, transient facial flushing may be encountered in response to GHRH administration.

4. Glucagon test

    a. Purpose: Assessment of growth hormone secretion

    b. Procedure

        (1) Perform the test in the morning. after an overnight fast.

        (2) Draw a baseline blood sample for growth hormone (time -30 and 0).

        (3) Inject 1 mg glucagon intramuscularly.

        (4) Collect samples for the measurement of GH at 30, 60, 90, 120, 150, 180, 210, and 240 minutes following the injection of glucagon.

    c. Interpretation. As is the case for other methods of GH stimulation, attained peak levels are highly dependent on fat mass, and results in obese subjects are often difficult to interpret. Peak levels of 3 ng/mL or higher have high sensitivity and specificity in the exclusion of GH deficiency in adults. Because glucagon also stimulates cortisol and insulin release, this test should not be combined with any of the tests for assessing ACTH release.

    d. Precautions. Glucagon may cause vomiting and abdominal cramping.

II. DIAGNOSIS OF ACROMEGALY

A. IGF-1. Serum IGF-I concentrations are elevated in virtually all acromegaly patients, thereby providing, in principle, a powerful and highly reliable tool for the diagnosis of acromegaly. Although IGF-1 can be viewed as an integrated measure of GH secretion, free of such transient effects as stress, glucose levels, or circadian rhythm (which affect GH levels), it is strongly modified by age, peaking at puberty and declining steadily thereafter, which leaves room for some error in the interpretation.

B. Glucose tolerance test for acromegaly

    1. Purpose: To help establish the diagnosis of acromegaly

    2. Procedure

        a. The patient should fast overnight. Ambulation should be minimal prior to and during the test.

        b. Draw baseline blood samples for glucose and growth hormone.

        c. Give patients 75 to 100 g of glucose (or 1.75 g/kg to a maximum of 100 g) PO.

        d. Draw blood samples for glucose and growth hormone at 30 minutes and at 1, 2, and 3 hours.

    3. Interpretation. Interpretation is highly dependent on the type of assay used to measure GH. Using IRMA, growth hormone falls to <1-ng/mL levels within 30 minutes to 2 hours in normal subjects. Using various chemiluminescence assays, nadir posttest levels vary between 0.14 and 0.7 ng/mL, depending on the particular assay used. Patients with <u>acromegaly may demonstrate no suppression, incomplete suppression, or a paradoxical rise in GH levels.</u> In addition, blood glucose levels commonly show glucose intolerance. Exercise, ambulation, surgery, and hypoglycemia can elevate fasting GH levels. Stress can result in a false positive test. Mild acromegaly, concomitant pituitary infarction, or prior therapy for acromegaly may lead to false negative results. Incomplete <u>or lack of GH suppression can be also seen in Laron dwarfism,</u> pubertal or pregnant patients or subjects with malnutrition, diabetes mellitus, renal failure, or hepatic disease.

III. TRH TESTS AND ANTERIOR PITUITARY DISORDERS

A. TRH test

    1. Purpose

        a. Assessment of pituitary thyroid-stimulating hormone (TSH) secretion as a means to detect pituitary insufficiency or equivocal hyperthyroidism or hypothyroidism

        b. Ancillary test in the diagnosis of acromegaly

        c. Assessment of apparently nonfunctioning pituitary tumors

d. Differential diagnosis between TSH-secreting pituitary adenoma and the syndrome of resistance to thyroid hormones

2. **Procedure**
   a. Draw a blood sample for baseline TSH, growth hormone, or luteinizing hormone (LH)/follicle-stimulating hormone (FSH) and their β subunits.
   b. Give 400 mg of synthetic thyroid-releasing hormone (TRH) by IV injection.
   c. Draw blood samples for TSH at 30 and 60 minutes following TRH administration; for growth hormone or LH, FSH, β-LH, and β-FSH at 15, 30, 60, 90, and 120 minutes after TRH injection.

3. **Interpretation**
   a. Assessing TSH response. Following TRH administration, TSH normally rises by 5 mU or more, the adult average peak response being 15 to 16 mU (20 to 40 minutes after TRH injection). In men over the age of 40 years, the response is smaller and increments of 2mU or greater above baseline are considered normal.

   As TSH assays are now highly sensitive and specific, TRH-induced TSH levels provide little information beyond basal TSH. The only remaining indication for testing TRH-stimulated TSH secretion in the context of hypothyroidism is the consideration of subtle central hypothyroidism reflected by low-normal free thyroxine (FT_4) and/or free tri-iodothyronine (FT_3) and suspiciously "normal" to low-normal TSH, such as is seen in survivors of childhood irradiation or head trauma. Pharmacologic doses of glucocorticoids, L-dopa, bromocriptine, oral contraceptives, acetylsalicylic acid, and cyproheptadine can all decrease the TSH response to TRH. Decreased responses may also be seen in patients with renal failure, depression, and hypogonadotropic hypogonadism. TSH may typically remain low and unresponsive to TRH for several weeks following withdrawal of thyroid hormone replacement or after treatment of thyrotoxicosis.

   b. Assessing growth hormone response. In normal individuals, growth hormone levels are unaffected by TRH, although "false positive" responses have been reported in normal adolescent girls. In contrast, growth hormone levels will rise above baseline levels in most cases of acromegaly. The test may be helpful when basal growth hormone and/or IGF-1 levels are borderline, but is usually unnecessary and is less well standardized than the oral glucose tolerance test in this disease.

   c. Assessing gonadotroph and other clinically nonfunctioning pituitary adenomas. In normal subjects, TRH has no effect on gonadotropin secretion. Increased LH or FSH accompanied by normal to high testosterone concentration in a man with a pituitary mass suggests the diagnosis of an adenoma of a gonadotroph origin. This diagnosis is further strengthened if LH and or FSH rise in response to TRH by 30% to 50% or more. In postmenopausal women with pituitary masses, high LH or FSH per se are of limited diagnostic value, but increase in gonadotropin secretion in response to TRH is again indicative of gonadotroph adenoma. Finally, upon stimulation with TRH, most nonfunctioning pituitary adenomas release β-LH, β-FSH, or both. Thus, a 50% or more increase in these gonadotropin subunits in subjects harboring a pituitary mass is consistent with the diagnosis of nonfunctioning pituitary adenoma. The usefulness of this testing is limited, however, because of the lack of commercial assays for β-LH and or β-FSH, and because the measurement of these peptides is currently restricted to very few laboratories.

   d. TSH-secreting adenoma versus the syndrome of resistance to thyroid hormones. In the differential diagnosis between these conditions, particularly in the presence of a pituitary lesion of uncertain significance, TRH testing is often helpful in that serum TSH concentration increases in response to TRH in patients with the syndrome of resistance to thyroid hormone, but not in most patients with TSH-secreting adenomas.

4. Precautions. Transient nausea, warmth or flushing sensations, mild headache, or the urge to void may occur. Occasionally, subjects may display large increases in both systolic and diastolic blood pressure. In subjects with hypertension, we perform this test only after reasonable control of blood pressure has been achieved.

IV. GONADOTROPIN-RELEASING HORMONE (GnRH)

A. Purpose: Assessment of pituitary gonadotropin secretion

B. Procedure

1. Studies in women should preferably be done in the early follicular phase of the menstrual cycle (days 1 to 7).
2. Because of the known pulsatile release of gonadotropins, at least two blood samples should be obtained 15 minutes prior to and immediately before GnRH administration. The average of the two samples serves as the baseline LH and FSH values.
3. GnRH, 100 μg, is given as a subcutaneous bolus or by rapid IV injection.
4. Draw blood samples for LH and FSH at 30, 60, 90, and 120 minutes after GnRH injection. Because the time of peak response is quite variable, additional samples at 15 and 45 minutes may enhance the reliability of this test.

C. Interpretation

1. The LH response to GnRH is usually more pronounced and is seen earlier than the FSH response. **In normal adults,** LH peaks are generally found at 15 to 45 minutes, whereas FSH peaks may occur later in some patients. In adults, LH levels will at least double following GnRH administration, and even greater increments are common. In women, the LH response to GnRH (but normally not the FSH response) is affected significantly by menstrual-cycle variability, with greater stimulation of LH observed during the luteal phase. In adults, the rise in FSH levels is usually of the magnitude of a 1.5- to 2-fold increase, but it is not unusual to see little change in FSH levels even in normal subjects.
2. The GnRH test is helpful for evaluating the functional capacity and response of the pituitary gonadotropins in adults, but not in prepubertal children, in whom both basal and GnRH-stimulated gonadotropins levels are typically low. The test does not differentiate pituitary from hypothalamic disorders, as decreased response of plasma gonadotropins may indicate either pituitary disease or prolonged endogenous deficiency of GnRH. Furthermore, absent, impaired, or normal responses to the test can be seen in patients with known hypothalamic or pituitary disorders. When responses are normal, however, the test does imply that the pituitary is capable of gonadotropin release when stimulated. Exaggerated LH response to GnRH is observed in **men with primary hypogonadism,** and in women **with polycystic ovarian disease.**

D. Precautions. Transient thirst during the test has been reported.

V. COMBINED TESTING OF THE ANTERIOR PITUITARY GLAND

Although specific tests for the secretory capacity of the anterior pituitary hormones have been traditionally performed separately, sufficient evidence has now accumulated to warrant **simultaneous dynamic testing** of several hypophyseal hormones. These tests have now been shown to be safe, reproducible, and, most significantly, to yield results identical to those obtained by testing the same pituitary–hypothalamic functions on separate days. Although the cost-effectiveness benefits are obvious, published experience with the combined testing in disease is limited.

A. Procedure

1. Place an indwelling catheter in the antecubital fossa. Keep the line open by means of a very slow saline drip or a heparin lock.
2. Obtain baseline samples for GH, TSH, prolactin, LH, FSH, and cortisol (or ACTH).
3. Inject IV insulin (0.15 U/kg), TRH (400 μg), and LHRH (100 μg) consecutively as close together as possible, by means of three separate syringes.
4. Obtain repeat blood samples at 30, 60, 90, and 120 minutes.

B. Interpretation. Criteria for the interpretation of results obtained from the combined test should be the same as indicated for the corresponding tests when carried out separately.

 POSTERIOR PITUITARY

I. WATER-DEPRIVATION TEST

A. Purpose: Diagnosis and differential diagnosis of diabetes insipidus. The test is particularly useful when the diagnosis is considered in the context of polyuria ($\geq$40 mL/kg bodyweight per day), urine osmolality <300 mOsmol/kg, in the absence of hypernatremia (suspected "compensated diabetes insipidus").

B. Procedure

1. This test requires close observation of the patient, to ascertain complete withholding of fluids and carefully monitor the patient's status.
2. Withhold fluids from 6 A.M. Record body weight.
3. Obtain baseline sodium, plasma and urinary osmolality, and, whenever feasible, plasma antidiuretic hormone (ADH).
4. As water deprivation continues, collect hourly urine samples for osmolality until the increment in urine osmolality observed from two consecutive determinations is <30 mOsmol/kg; or until urine osmolality has reached 600 to 700 mOsmol/kg; or until plasma osmolality has reached 295 to 300 mOsmol/kg. This normally occurs by early afternoon. Record body weight hourly.
5. At that time, obtain a blood sample for osmolality and, whenever possible, plasma ADH. Record body weight and then administer aqueous vasopressin (Pitressin; 5 U SC) or 10 μg of dDAVP by nasal insufflation or 4 μg of dDAVP subcutaneously. Avoid the use of vasopressin in pregnancy, as it is subject to increased degradation by high circulating vasopressinase present in pregnancy.
6. Obtain repeat urine and blood samples for osmolality 30 and 60 minutes later.

C. Interpretation

1. **A normal response** consists of maximal urinary osmolality ranging between 800 and 1 400 mOsmol/kg by the end of the dehydration test and only a small rise, if any (<9%), in urine osmolality after vasopressin. Maximal urine osmolality is greater than plasma osmolality both prior to and following the administration of vasopressin. Subjects with **primary polydipsia** have an essentially normal response, but a more prolonged dehydration period may be needed. Still, the maximal urine osmolality in primary polydipsia (500 to 600 mOsmol/kg) often falls short of the normal response (800 mOsmol/kg because of partial washout of the real medullary interstitial gradient and downregulation of ADH secretion. In patients with chronic debilitating diseases, the maximal urinary osmolality may be as low as 450 to 800 mOsmol/kg, but the response to vasopressin is normal. Patients with **partial antidiuretic hormone (ADH) deficiency** display some endogenous capacity for urine concentration (i.e., maximal urine osmolality is more than plasma osmolality before the injection of vasopressin), but in response to vasopressin, urine osmolality increases significantly (i.e., >9%). These patients occasionally fail to respond to exogenous ADH because, once high plasma osmolality has been reached during the test, endogenous ADH released has increased already, eliciting maximal stimulation during the dehydration period.
2. With both severe ADH deficiency and nephrogenic diabetes insipidus, maximal urine osmolality is lower than plasma osmolality. However, in response to vasopressin, urinary osmolality increases by >50% in severe ADH deficiency, but only by <45% in nephrogenic diabetes insipidus. A more striking difference between partial central diabetes insipidus and nephrogenic diabetes insipidus in this setting is that urine remains very dilute in the latter condition, whereas patients with ADH deficiency usually attain urine osmolality of 300 mOsmol/kg or higher.

D. Precautions. Unless polyuria is mild or questionable, overnight fluid restriction should be avoided, because potentially severe volume depletion and hypernatremia can be induced in patients with marked polyuria. Severe weight loss and dehydration may occur in patients with true diabetes insipidus. Weight loss should not be allowed to exceed 5% of initial body weight. However, symptoms may occur even after 3% to 5% dehydration, and prompt measures to restore hydration should be taken.

 # DIABETES MELLITUS

I. ORAL GLUCOSE TOLERANCE TEST (OGTT)

The 2003 recommendations of the American Diabetes Association (ADA), now in agreement with World Health Organization (WHO) guidelines, indicate that both fasting glucose and OGTT are useful to diagnose diabetes mellitus. An elevated casual blood glucose ≥ 200 mg% in association with classic symptoms of diabetes including polyuria, polydipsia, and unexplained weight loss is also diagnostic and obviates the need for OGTT.

A. Purpose: Diagnosis of diabetes mellitus

B. Procedure

1. This test should be reserved for ambulatory subjects without fever or infection. Carbohydrate content in the diet should be at least 150 g per day for the last 3 days before the test.
2. The test should be done in the morning, following a fast of at least 8 hours but not exceeding 16 hours. Water is allowed during the fast. Coffee should be avoided.
3. Subjects should remain seated throughout the test and should refrain from smoking.
4. Glucose, 75g (anhydrous glucose dissolved in water; 1.75 g/kg ideal body weight, not to exceed 75 g), is given PO to nonpregnant adults. Pregnant women receive 50 or 100 g PO, as specified in the following paragraph.
5. Blood samples for glucose determination are obtained before glucose ingestion as well as 120 minutes later (2 h PG). For pregnant women, obtain samples at 0, 60, 120, and 180 minutes.

C. Interpretation (glucose levels in venous plasma). Subjects are classified as normoglycemic, having impaired fasting glucose (IFG), impaired glucose tolerance (IGT), or diabetes mellitus based on the following parameters, predominantly fasting and 2h post-glucose loading (PG) serum levels.

1. Nonpregnant adults

Normoglycemia	IFG and IGT	Diabetes mellitus
Fasting plasma glucose <100 mg/dL	Fasting plasma glucose ≥100 mg/dL and <126 mg/dL (IFG)	Fasting plasma glucose ≥126 mg/dL
2 h PG <140 mg/dL	2h PG ≥140 mg/dL and <200 mg/dL (IGT)	2 h PG ≥200 mg/dL
—	—	Symptoms of diabetes mellitus and casual plasma glucose concentration 200 mg/dL

In the absence of unequivocal hyperglycemia, a diagnosis of diabetes must be confirmed on a subsequent day by any one of the three methods indicated in the chart, but in the ADA guidelines, reliance on fasting plasma glucose is preferred because of ease of administration, convenience, acceptability to patients, and lower cost.

2. Pregnant women. The estimated risk for diabetes dictates the need for OGTT, the timing of OGTT, and the type of recommended OGTT. Early screening and diagnosis of gestational diabetes mellitus (GDM), as soon as feasible, is indicated for women at high risk (positive family history, history of GDM, marked obesity, high-risk ethnic group). Even if the initial screening is negative, women at high risk should undergo retesting at 24–48 weeks. Women of average risk should have the initial screen performed at 24 to 48 weeks of gestation.

For high risk women, the "one-step approach," consisting of a diagnostic OGTT (100 g) without prior plasma or serum glucose screening, appears suitable. In women with average risk, the "two step approach" may be more cost-effective. In this approach the first step consists of a 50-g oral glucose challenge, administered without regard to the time elapsed since the last meal. Plasma or serum glucose is measured 1 hour later; a value ≥130 to 140 mg/dL is considered abnormal. The full 100-g OGTT is administered as the second step to women showing such abnormal results. In this test, plasma glucose levels are determined at baseline, 1 hour, 2 hours, and 3 hours postchallenge. The diagnosis of GDM is made if two or more of the plasma glucose values in the following table are met or exceeded:

Diagnosis of GDM with a 100-g Glucose Load

Time	Plasma glucose
Fasting	≥95 mg/dL (5.3 mmol/L)
1 h	≥180 mg/dL (10.0 mmol/L)
2 h	≥155 mg/dL (8.6 mmol/L)
3 h	≥140 mg/dL (7.8 mmol/L)

Two or more values must be met or exceeded for a diagnosis of diabetes to be made. The test should be done in the morning, after an 8- to 14-hour fast.

II. INSULINOMA
A. Prolonged fasting test
   1. Purpose: Evaluation of hypoglycemia resulting from suspected insulinoma
   2. Procedure
   a. The patient should be hospitalized for this test and placed on a 72-hour fast. Only water and noncaloric, caffeine-free soft drinks are allowed during the test. Activity is not restricted. Some investigators even prefer to exercise the patient mildly at the end of the fast.
   b. Blood samples for glucose, insulin, C-peptide, and proinsulin (if available) should be obtained every 6 hours. In addition, blood samples should be drawn when hypoglycemic symptoms occur. Thus, the patient should be kept under close observation throughout the entire test. Glucometers can be used to allow better orientation as to current glucose range, but termination of the fast must always be decided on using lab glucose levels. Once glucose levels decline to <60 mg%, sampling frequency should be increased to every 1 to 2 hours.
   c. If any serious neuroglycopenic or other hypoglycemic symptoms occur, blood samples for insulin and glucose should be drawn and the test immediately terminated. Also, the test should be ended when plasma glucose concentration falls to <45 mg/dL.
   d. At the end of the fast (72 hours or earlier as specified above), a sample for plasma β-hydroxybutyrate and sulfonylurea is also collected (in addition to glucose, insulin, and C-peptide). Ancillary measurements may also include <u>chromogranin A, a general marker for neuroendocrine tumors</u>. Insulin antibodies, anti-insulin receptor antibodies, IGF-1, and plasma cortisol or growth hormone can be measured if a non-islet–cell tumor, autoimmune etiology, or hormone deficiency is suspected.
   e. At this time, 1 mg of glucagon is administered intravenously, and samples for plasma glucose are collected 10, 20, and 30 minutes later.
   f. The patient must be fed prior to his or her discharge from the hospital.
   3. Interpretation. In the normal patient, insulin levels will be appropriate for the serum glucose level. Normal serum glucose levels during a 72-hour fast may fall to the range of 30 mg/dL in women and to 50 mg/dL or lower in men. However, patients with serum glucose in these range will generally have low (<4 μU/mL)

or undetectable serum insulin levels. In contrast, patients with insulinoma will not only often develop symptoms (sometimes severe) of hypoglycemia, they will present with inappropriately high levels (>10 μU/mL) of serum insulin. A plasma insulin of ≥6 μU by RIA or ≥3 μU by radioimmunometric assay in connection with plasma glucose <45 mg/dL provides sufficient evidence for insulin excess. C-peptide levels (>0.2 nm/dL) will differentiate between endogenous and exogenous hyperinsulinemia. Additionally, if hypoglycemia(<45 mg%) is recorded during the 72-hour fast, proinsulin levels >5 pmol/L are indicative of insulinoma, with nearly 100% specificity and sensitivity. Because of the antiketogenic effects of insulin, patients with insulinoma have low plasma β-hydroxybutyric acid levels (<2.7 mmol/L) despite the prolonged fast. High sulfonylurea levels suggest factitious hyperinsulinemia. Finally, because hepatic glycogen stores are entirely depleted in normal individuals subjected to prolonged fasting, no significant increase in glucose (<25 mg/dL) is normally expected following the injection of glucagon at the end of the fast. In contrast, patients with chronic hyperinsulinemia have larger hepatic glycogen stores owing to the antiglycogenolytic effect of insulin. Thus, in patients harboring an insulinoma, glucose will rise by 25 mg/dL or more following glucagon administration.

4. **Precautions.** Glucose for rapid IV injection should be readily available. Severe hypoglycemic symptoms can occur and are an indication to terminate the test and institute immediate corrective measures.

THE ADRENAL GLAND

I. SCREENING TESTS FOR THE CONFIRMATION OF CUSHING SYNDROME

Unless exceptionally high cortisol values are seen, no single positive test should be taken as sufficient proof for the diagnosis of Cushing syndrome. At least three of the following tests should be considered: the overnight 1-mg dexamethasone suppression test; 24-hour urinary corticosteroid excretion, usually urinary free cortisol; the standard 2-day, 2-mg dexamethasone test; assessment of diurnal variation of circulating cortisol, usually through midnight salivary cortisol. Sufficient time should be allowed for follow-up and retesting. We consider two positive tests as requiring further workup, i.e., performing tests intended to differentiate among the various forms of true hypercortisolism. A single positive test requires careful clinical consideration and, when appropriate, further follow-up and laboratory reassessment. Though cyclic Cushing syndrome is rare, the potential for variation in cortisol secretion should be considered and requires repeat testing.

A. **Overnight dexamethasone suppression test.** This test is done in an outpatient setting and is a practical screening test for hypercortisolism.

1. **Procedure**
   a. Dexamethasone, 1 mg PO, given at 11 to 12 P.M. A nonbarbiturate sedative may also be given to help the patient sleep.
   b. Obtain plasma cortisol at 8 A.M. the following morning.

2. **Interpretation.** Most laboratories do not presently use the same assays for the measurement of cortisol that served to establish the normal serum cortisol response to dexamethasone suppression as reported in published studies. In general, though, normal subjects should suppress plasma cortisol levels to <1.8 to 2 μg/dL following 1 mg of dexamethasone administered the previous night. Cortisol levels at this range may be around the lower detection limit for some assays and should be viewed with caution. Acquaintance with the laboratory's performance and methods, repeated testing, or referral to another, preferably a reference laboratory, are some of the options available to the clinician at this point. Levels between 2 and 7 μg/dL may be difficult to interpret, as they are commonly seen in subjects with mental depression and alcohol- and stress-induced adrenocortical activation, referred to, collectively, as pseudo-Cushing disorders. Additional forms of testing are therefore recommended under these circumstances. On the other hand,

some patients with pituitary Cushing can be quite sensitive to dexamethasone and may sometimes show rather low cortisol levels following dexamethasone. Constitutive variation in the metabolic clearance of dexamethasone and acceleration in dexamethasone metabolism by alcohol and drugs such as nifedipine, rifampin, hydantoin, carbamazepine, phenobarbital, tamoxifen, and topiramate because of the induction of CYP3A4 enzymes, which also metabolize dexamethasone, can lead to false negative results. Suppression of cortisol can be incomplete in chronic renal failure because of decreased cortisol clearance, or high-estrogen states, resulting from increased cortisol-binding globulin level (CBG). Hence, the measurement of plasma dexamethasone, to verify that proper levels of dexamethasone have indeed been attained, can add much to the interpretation of any of the dexamethasone suppression tests.

B. Urinary steroid excretion. Absolute elevations of urinary steroid levels can be used to diagnose Cushing syndrome. The measurements are made on baseline 24-hour collections of urine, using creatinine and total volume as estimates of the adequacy of the collection.

   1. Urinary free cortisol excretion (UFC) is the measurement of choice for the initial diagnosis of hypercortisolism. It represents a direct measurement of cortisol not bound to plasma protein and is the most reliable and useful test for assessing cortisol secretion rate as long as the assay methods and normal ranges are well defined. Because it is a specific measurement of cortisol rather than its metabolites, it circumvents problems of variable metabolite excretion. Proper measurement of UFC requires extraction of cortisol from the urinary sample, followed by radioimmunoassay. The upper range is 90 to 100 μg per 24 hours. High-performance liquid chromatography (HPLC)-based methods provide a more specific way to assess UFC, with an upper range of $\sim$50 μg per 24 hours. Urinary free cortisol is elevated in $\sim$95% of Cushing syndrome patients, but only if several samples are assayed. High water intake will elevate the urine free cortisol, as will the drug carbamazepine. Incomplete urine collection, low urine output, and renal failure may cause false negative results. Some authorities advocate reliance on UFC levels exceeding three times the upper limit of the normal range as proof of true hypercortisolism, but as specificity of detection increases by raising cutoff values, sensitivity is much diminished. We recommend repeat testing over time and consideration of at least two additional screening tests.

   2. Urinary 17-hydroxycorticosteroids (17-OHCS), a traditional measure of the metabolites of cortisol, is occasionally of supplementary value. A limitation of the urinary 17-OHCS measurement is the dependence of metabolite excretion on body weight. One advantage of urinary 17-OHCS over UFC is that, unlike UFC, the excretion rate of 17-OHCS is not increased in subjects who drink very large volumes of liquid. The urinary 17-OHCS measurements are elevated in 76% to 89% of cases.

C. Standard 2-day, 2-mg test. This test provides essentially the same type of information derived from the shorter overnight 1-mg dexamethasone suppression test, but it offers the opportunity to examine more parameters, including urinary excretion of cortisol and its metabolites (17 hydroxycorticosteroids), as well as serum cortisol. It may also have higher specificity than the shorter overnight test.

   1. Procedure
   a. Baseline: Collect 24-hour urine samples for UFC and 17-OHCS.
   b. Day 1: Administer dexamethasone, 0.5 mg PO q6h, as of 9 A.M. Collect 24-hour urine sample for UFC and 17-OHCS.
   c. Day 2: Administer dexamethasone, 0.5 mg PO q6h, with the last dose administered at 3 A.M. on the morning of day 3. Collect 24-hour urine sample for UFC and 17-OHCS.
   d. Day 3: Collect blood sample for serum cortisol at 8 A.M.

   2. Interpretation. Normal subjects show suppression of 24-hour urinary cortisol excretion to <10 μg (27 nmol) per day and in urinary 17-OHCS excretion to <2.5 mg (6.9 μmol) per day. Proper suppression of serum cortisol is considered by most to be a better tool in this setting, but it suffers from the same practical limitations outlined for the 1-mg dexamethasone overnight test. The performance of this test is significantly enhanced if dexamethasone is also measured. In normal subjects, serum cortisol should decline to 1.8 to 3.6 μg/dL 6 hours following the last dexamethasone dose (last dose at 3 A.M.; sample collected at 9 A.M.). The cutoff level of 1.8 μg/dL enhances sensitivity, but few commercial assays have been tested for performance in this context.

D. Diurnal variation of circulating cortisol. Plasma cortisol values are highest from 6 to 8 A.M., declining during the day to less than 50% to 80% of morning values from 10 P.M. to midnight. This rhythm is typically lost very early in the course of Cushing syndrome.

1. **Salivary cortisol** concentration in the saliva is correlated with free or biologically active cortisol levels in serum or plasma. A sampling device is available with which saliva can be collected by chewing on a cotton tube for 2 to 3 minutes. This commercially available device is best used at the patient's home, followed by delivery to a reference laboratory the next morning. Cortisol in the saliva is quite stable and can be sent for determination over several days. Testing is done at bedtime to 11 or 12 P.M., but timing may actually affect the result, as the true nadir of circulating cortisol typically takes place at midnight or even later. A salivary cortisol >5.6 nmol/L is suggestive of true hypercortisolism, but variation in reference values among laboratories and methods (e.g., radioimmunoassay vs. tandem mass spectrometry) requires attention. False positive cases have been noted in older obese hypertensive and /or type 2 diabetic men.

2. **Midnight serum cortisol** seems intuitively to be a direct measure of circulating cortisol, but sample drawing requires hospitalization or some other special setting with obligatory disruption of normal late-night activities. This in itself may weaken the specificity of the measurement of serum cortisol.

   a. **Procedure.** Sampling is best performed with an indwelling needle and basal conditions maintained for 30 minutes prior to sampling. Because cortisol is secreted in pulsatile bursts, multiple samples are taken: Sampling for cortisol is done at 30-minute intervals between 10 P.M. and midnight. Patients should be in the supine position before and during the study.

   b. **Interpretation. A midnight plasma cortisol of 7.5 μg/dL or greater** strongly suggests a diagnosis of Cushing syndrome. Values of 5.0 μg/dL or less are unlikely to be Cushing syndrome, and values of 2.0 μg/dL nearly exclude Cushing. This test has value in moderate cases of hypercortisolism (in which urine free cortisol is normal), especially in distinguishing pseudo-Cushing, in which a normal diurnal pattern may be retained. A timed or spot urinary free cortisol-to-creatinine ratio at midnight can also be used to establish the presence of hypercortisolism. Also, a midnight "sleeping" plasma cortisol of 1.8 μg/dL or greater is shown to have a 100% diagnostic sensitivity for Cushing syndrome, but specificity at this level is apparently low. In general, it has been difficult to obtain a nonstressed late-night cortisol value.

II. RULING OUT PSEUDO-CUSHING SYNDROME

A. Corticotropin-Releasing Hormone (CRH) after low-dose dexamethasone suppression test. This test was developed to distinguish between patients with pseudo-Cushing and those with Cushing syndrome. The test is based on the premise that suppression of ACTH by dexamethasone is more profound in normal subjects and depressed patients than in patients with Cushing disease, such that following proper suppression with dexamethasone, serum cortisol cannot be stimulated by CRH in these patients, but only in subjects with Cushing disease.

1. **Choice of patients.** This test should be considered only for subjects who show normal suppression following dexamethasone administration but in whom Cushing syndrome continues to be seriously suspected because of clinical considerations or other anomalous (positive) screening test(s) for Cushing states.

2. **Procedure.** Give 0.5 mg dexamethasone at 6-hour intervals for 2 days, as of 12 A.M. on day 1. The CRH stimulation test is initiated at 8 A.M., 2 hours after completion of the last dexamethasone dose (at 6 A.M.). Both human and ovine

CRH are available and can be administered as an intravenous bolus of 1 μg/kg body weight or as a fixed dose of 100 μg intravenously.

3. **Interpretation.** A measurable serum cortisol response to CRH (e.g., cortisol level >1.4 to 2.5 μg/dL measured 15 minutes after CRH administration) identifies patients with Cushing syndrome compared to those with pseudo-Cushing conditions, with a sensitivity of ~90% but with much lower specificity, ranging overall around 70% in reports published thus far. Although abnormal results, consistent with increased hypothalamic-pituitary arousal, have been reported in anorexia nervosa, patients with this condition are unlikely to be worked up for Cushing syndrome.

III. DIFFERENTIAL DIAGNOSIS OF CUSHING SYNDROME: IS HYPERCORTISOLISM ACTH-DEPENDENT?

A. **Plasma ACTH.** Plasma ACTH is now a powerful tool to address this question, but dynamic testing is still required for many patients. Immunoradiometric measurement (IRMA) of ACTH offers good sensitivity and specificity in the differential diagnosis of Cushing syndrome. Samples should be taken at 8 A.M. under basal condition. As ACTH is rapidly degraded by circulating peptidases, the sample must be chilled and plasma-separated, aliquoted, and frozen immediately. The concomitant measurement of ACTH and cortisol provides a straightforward means to assess whether hypercortisolemia, once established and if present at the time of testing, is ACTH-dependent. Whenever basal levels of ACTH are measurable (ACTH values >10 pg/mL) in a patient with high levels of plasma cortisol, ectopic or pituitary (ACTH-dependent) forms of Cushing syndrome should be suspected. Plasma ACTH is sometimes extremely high in **ectopic Cushing syndrome,** most often because of lung carcinoma, but it may be only mildly elevated or normal in patients with bronchial carcinoid tumor. Patients with **pituitary Cushing syndrome** have elevated baseline plasma ACTH values in about half of cases, often ranging between 50 and 250 pg/mL, with the remainder of patients having levels within the normal range. However, even very high levels of a slightly modified ACTH molecule formed by the ectopic tissue can be missed by the current highly specific assays for ACTH. Nevertheless, undetectable levels of ACTH (ACTH values <5 pg/mL) in the presence of increased plasma cortisol levels suggest the diagnosis of adrenal Cushing syndrome (ACTH-independent forms of Cushing syndrome).

B. **High-dose 8-mg dexamethasone suppression test.** Administration of large doses (8 mg per day for 2 days) of the potent synthetic glucocorticoid dexamethasone will suppress urinary or plasma cortisol by >50% of baseline in pituitary but not in adrenal or ectopic Cushing syndrome. The test <u>distinguishes pituitary Cushing syndrome from other causes in ~85% of cases.</u> Some maintain that the high-dose dexamethasone suppression test has been made obsolete by the availability of reliable methods for the measurement of plasma ACTH, pituitary imaging, and inferior petrosal sinus sampling. The inconvenience of the latter procedure, pitfalls in plasma ACTH, and the high rate of pituitary and adrenal incidentalomas (up to 10% of the general population) comprise sufficient grounds for continued performance of this test.

1. **Procedure**
   a. **Baseline.** Collect 24-hour urine samples for UFC and 17-OHCS.
   b. **Day 1.** Administer dexamethasone, 2 mg PO q6h (usually at 8 A.M., 2 P.M., 8 P.M., and 2 A.M.). Collect 24-hour urine sample for UFC and for 17-OHCS.
   c. **Day 2.** Administer dexamethasone, 2 mg PO q6h. Collect 24-hour urine sample for UFC and 17-OHCS.

2. **Interpretation.** Suppression to >50% of baseline of urinary UFC or 17-OHCS on day 2 indicates lack of complete autonomy of ACTH secretion and is therefore compatible with pituitary Cushing disease or, occasionally, bronchial carcinoid tumor; failure to suppress on 8 mg per day implies adrenal or ectopic Cushing syndrome. **Anomalous responses** to high-dose dexamethasone suppression include:
   a. Suppression in ectopic Cushing because of bronchial tumors of low-grade malignancy

  b. Paradoxical increases in 17-OHCS in an occasional case of pituitary Cushing syndrome

  c. Lack of suppression of cortisol and or its metabolites in subjects harboring a large pituitary macroadenoma

   This test has a diagnostic sensitivity and specificity of 80% to 85%, so as many as 15% of pituitary Cushing patients will not be detected by this test. More recent criteria have been established that improve diagnostic accuracy. A decrease from baseline levels in urinary free cortisol of >90% and in 17-OHC excretion of >64% will detect 100% of patients with pituitary Cushing and exclude most ectopic cases.

C. The 8-mg overnight dexamethasone suppression test. This test can be used in place of the 2-day dexamethasone suppression test, because it has roughly similar accuracy and specificity.

 1. Procedure. Obtain a plasma cortisol at 8 A.M. as baseline, then give 8 mg dexamethasone at 11 P.M. and draw another blood sample for plasma cortisol the next morning at 8 A.M.

 2. Interpretation. More than a 50% reduction in plasma cortisol from the baseline level strongly indicates pituitary Cushing syndrome.

D. CRH stimulation test. Corticotropin releasing hormone, upon its release from the hypothalamus, selectively stimulates the pituitary corticotrope cells to increase ACTH; this is followed by a rise in cortisol. Both human and ovine CRH are available and are administered as an intravenous bolus of 1 μg/kg body weight or as a fixed dose of 100 μg intravenously. This dose increases ACTH and cortisol levels in up to 90% of patients with pituitary Cushing syndrome, because most pituitary ACTH-secreting tumors have CRH receptors. Patients with ectopic and adrenal Cushing syndrome have no ACTH or cortisol response to CRH. This test differentiates ACTH-dependent from ACTH-independent Cushing syndrome but might not always distinguish pituitary (eutopic) from ectopic causes, mostly because some pituitary patients do not respond to CRH. In this situation, a more precise method to localize the source of ACTH, such as inferior petrosal sinus sampling, is required.

E. CRH stimulation test during inferior petrosal sinus sampling

 1. Purpose: To distinguish between pituitary Cushing disease and Cushing syndrome secondary to ectopic ACTH secretion. The most common setting in which this test is helpful is suspected pituitary Cushing with a negative magnetic resonance imaging (MRI) scan of the pituitary (can be up to 50%) and equivocal levels of plasma ACTH versus an ectopic ACTH-secreting tumor, usually a bronchial carcinoid, that might be roentgenographically occult and have equivocal ACTH levels.

 2. Procedure

  a. Baseline samples for ACTH and prolactin are obtained from a peripheral vein as well as from catheters preinserted into the veins draining both the left and right inferior petrosal sinuses (IPS). Correction for prolactin level in the obtained samples may assist in identifying problems related to localization of the draining catheter and dilution.

  b. CRH (100 μg) is administered intravenously. Samples for ACTH are obtained simultaneously from each inferior petrosal sinus before as well as 2 to 3 and 5 to 6 minutes after CRH administration.

 3. Interpretation. Basal IPS-to-peripheral (P) ACTH ratio $\geq$2.0 to or post-CRH ratio $\geq$3.0 confirms the presence of a pituitary ACTH-secreting tumor. Other values are assumed to have an ectopic source. CRH testing is needed because up to 15% of pituitary tumors will not show an abnormal basal gradient. Correct preoperative lateralization of an ACTH-secreting microadenoma to the right or left hemisphere of the pituitary gland can be accomplished much less frequently than was initially believed, probably because of asymmetric venous drainage in many pituitary glands. The procedure carries some risk, including false positive and false negative results. Direct procedure-related risks are not common but include, besides inguinal and jugular hematomas or transient arrhythmias, rare serious consequences such as perforation of the right atrium, cavernous sinus thrombosis, and cerebrovascular events (0.2%), sometimes with permanent brainstem damage. Hence, IPS should be reserved for clearly equivocal cases such as normal pituitary MRI or the presence of very small pituitary lesions and/or atypical response to dexamethasone and/or CRH. Sources of error include some cases of Cushing disease that show no response to CRH, incorrect identification of the petrosal sinus or anomalous draining of the petrosal sinus, and rare cases of ectopic CRH-producing tumors.

IV. WORKUP OF ACTH-INDEPENDENT MACRONODULAR ADRENAL (AIMAH) HYPER-PLASIA: DYNAMIC TESTS TO DETECT EXCESSIVE CORTISOL SECRETION IN-DUCED THROUGH ANOMALOUS ROUTES

Ectopically expressed G-protein–coupled hormone receptors can be abnormally activated by hormones that do not normally affect adrenal cortical function, resulting in anomalous stimulation of cortisol secretion. This mechanism not infrequently underlies excess cortisol secretion in AIMAH as well as in some unilateral adrenal adenomas. Aberrant receptors thus far reported to be functionally coupled to steroidogenesis include receptors for gastric inhibitory peptide (GIP), vasopressin, β-adrenergic, LH/human chorionic gonadotropin (hCG), serotonin angiotensin II, leptin, glucagon, interleukin-1 (IL-1), and TSH. Some of these conditions can be treated medically. Lacroix's group has developed clinical protocols to screen for such dysfunctional activation of the adrenal cortex, which have been subsequently widely adopted, particularly for the workup of AIMAH. A 3-day protocol offers opportunity to capture the most common forms of anomalous cortisol secretion under these conditions.

A. Day 1

  1. Purpose: To detect potential modulation of cortisol by posture-induced signals such as increase in angiotensin II, vasopressin, or catecholamines, or a decline in atrial natriuretic peptide.

  2. Procedure

    a. Baseline samples are collected after 2 hours in the supine position.

    b. Subjects are then ambulated for 2 hours and samples are collected at 30- to 60-minute intervals.

    c. A standard mixed meal follows, to identify activation of cortisol release through GIP or other gastrointestinal hormones whose receptors might be abnormally and functionally expressed in cortisol-producing cells. Again, samples are collected at 30- to 60-minute intervals.

    d. Finally, the short 250-μg ACTH test is carried out, to serve as a reference test.

B. Day 2

  1. Purpose: To detect anomalous activation of cortisol through GnRH, LH, FSH, TRH, TSH, or prolactin receptors.

  2. Procedure

    a. Administer 100 μg GnRH intravenously, as described earlier (detects increases related to GnRH, LH, FSH).

    b. After 2 hours, administer 200 μg TRH intravenously (detects increases in cortisol induced by TSH, PRL, TRH).

C. Day 3

  1. Purpose: To assess the possibility that cortisol secretion is modulated by glucagon, AVP, or serotoninergic receptors.

  2. Procedure

    a. Inject 1 mg glucagon IV and collect samples at times 0, 30, and 60 minutes.

    b. Inject 10 IU AVP IM, and collect samples at times 0, 30, and 60 minutes.

    c. Inject metoclopramide IV and collect samples at times 0, 30, and 60 minutes.

D. Interpretation. Arbitrarily defined, increase in cortisol <25% is considered as lack of response, whereas increments $\geq$25% are seen as significant responses (25% to 49%, "partial response"; $\geq$50%, "positive response." Any positive change warrants further investigation to identify the precise pathway involved. Detailed description of these further lines of testing is available elsewhere (see Lacroix et al., *Endocr Rev* 2001;22:75–110).

V. ASSESSING ADRENAL CORTICAL SECRETORY FUNCTION

A. Rapid ACTH stimulation test (cosyntropin [Cortrosyn] test)

1. **Purpose**
   a. Evaluation of adrenocortical function cases of suspected <u>primary or secondary adrenal insufficiency</u>
   b. Diagnosis of late-onset or mild congenital adrenal hyperplasia (<u>CAH</u>) secondary to 21 hydroxylase deficiency.

   Cosyntropin is a potent and rapid stimulator of cortisol and aldosterone secretion. The cosyntropin test can be used on an inpatient or outpatient basis, and is apparently unaffected by time of day and food intake. In a previously undiagnosed patient it can, and indeed should, be performed even in the emergency room, while glucocorticoid replacement with dexamethasone is concomitantly initiated.

2. **Procedure**
   a. Draw blood for baseline serum cortisol, aldosterone, and ACTH. Aldosterone and ACTH will help differentiate primary from secondary adrenal hypofunction.
   b. Inject 250 μg of cosyntropin by IV or IM route. For IV use, dilute cosyntropin in 2 to 5 mL sodium chloride 0.9% and inject over 2 minutes.
   c. Obtain repeat samples for serum cortisol (and aldosterone) 30 and 60 minutes following ACTH administration.

3. **Interpretation**
   a. **Hypoadrenalism.** A normal adrenal response to ACTH consists of a rise in serum cortisol to 18 μg/dL or greater. A higher cutoff of 20 μg/dL is also used to increase the sensitivity of the test. A normal response effectively rules out primary adrenal insufficiency. Patients with secondary adrenal insufficiency usually show a blunted response to cosyntropin but occasionally have a normal response. Baseline ACTH levels in primary adrenal insufficiency are high, generally >50 to 100 pg/mL, whereas levels in secondary adrenal insufficiency are low or normal (10 pg/mL or less).

   Evaluation of ACTH-induced aldosterone responses also help to distinguish primary from secondary adrenal insufficiency. In primary adrenal insufficiency, baseline aldosterone levels are low and there is no response to cosyntropin. In secondary adrenal insufficiency, baseline aldosterone levels may be low or normal, but at 30 minutes, there is an increase in plasma aldosterone of at least 4 ng/dL over baseline.

   b. **CAH.** <u>21-Hydroxylase deficiency</u> is the most common form of late-onset/mild CAH detected by the ACTH test. Exaggerated response of 17-OH progesterone, the compound proximal to the enzymatic block, to levels >10 ng/mL (at 60 minutes) is the hallmark of this condition. In normal subjects, levels are <10 ng/mL. Heterozygotes for the various forms of 21-hydroxylase deficiency may have 60-minute post-ACTH levels as low as 5 ng/mL, which overlaps with values in the general population. Patients with more severe forms may present with high basal levels of 17-OH progesterone that are not further stimulated by exogenous ACTH. Less commonly, the diagnosis of relatively rare forms of CAH can be established using the ACTH test. In patients with <u>11β-hydroxylase deficiency</u>, ACTH-stimulated values of 11-deoxycortisol, the steroid most proximal to the 11β-hydroxylasion step, are very high (>1 μg/dL) compared to the normal population. In the rare condition of <u>3β-hydroxysteroid dehydrogenase deficiency</u>, 17-OH pregnenolone rises more steeply than in normal subjects following the injection of ACTH, resulting in a ratio of 17-OH pregnenolone to 17-OH progesterone >10 (and usually >20). Recently, modified age-related criteria have been proposed for genetically proven 3β-hydroxysteroid dehydrogenase deficiency based on ACTH-stimulated 17-OH pregnenolone values: infants, $\geq$12 600 ng/dL; Tanner stage I children, $\geq$5 490 ng/dL; children with premature pubarche, $\geq$9 790 ng/dL; adults, $\geq$9 620 ng/dL. In all, the number of adults studied for ACTH responses in this condition is limited.

B. Low-dose (1-μg) ACTH test
   1. Purpose: A screening test for impaired hypothalamic–pituitary–adrenal (HPA) axis
   2. Procedure
      a. The test can be performed at any time during the day.
      b. Draw a blood sample for cortisol. A sample for ACTH is optional
      c. Inject 1 μg of ACTH intravenously. As no standard packaging for this dose is currently available, the 250-μg Cortrosyn vial must be serially diluted in saline to a final volume of 2 mL containing 1 μg of ACTH.
      d. Draw blood for serum cortisol 20, 30, and 40 minutes after the injection of ACTH.
   3. Interpretation. This test is more sensitive and accurate than the 250-μg dose of ACTH in detecting partial adrenal gland insufficiency, especially in patients with secondary adrenal deficiency. The 250-μg dose of ACTH produces massive pharmacologic concentrations of ACTH, exceeding blood concentrations of 10 000 pg/mL, which is way above the ACTH level seen even under extreme conditions in real life. Therefore, the 250-μg dose tends to test only for maximum adrenocortical capacity and overrides any more partial loss of cortisol function. The 1-μg cosyntropin test should replace the 250-μg dose, because it is more likely to detect partial or more subtle forms of adrenal insufficiency, in particular secondary adrenal insufficiency resulting from pituitary tumors or chronic glucocorticoid treatment. Two important limitations, however, should be considered with this test: **(a)** Standard 1-μg cosyntropin packaging is not commercially available at the present time and care must be taken to produce the 1-μg dose accurately by serial dilutions; **(b)** the test may be unreliable in the first few weeks after acutely induced secondary hypoadrenalism (e.g., after pituitary surgery), because the evolution of impaired adrenal reserve (cortisol response to ACTH) under these conditions requires some time, yet the HPA axis may already be severely damaged as a result of ACTH deficiency.
C. Metyrapone tests
   1. Single-dose metyrapone test
      a. Purpose. Metyrapone activates the HPA axis by blocking cortisol production at the 11-hydroylase step, which leads to lowering of cortisol levels. This test is used to establish or confirm the diagnosis of adrenal insufficiency and is particularly useful when secondary adrenal insufficiency is suspected. Metyrapone is an inhibitor of 11β-hydroxylase, the adrenal enzyme responsible for catalyzing the conversion of 11-deoxycortisol (compound S) to cortisol—the last step in cortisol synthesis. Following metyrapone administration, cortisol synthesis is blocked and the low levels of cortisol lead to increased ACTH release, which accelerates the production of adrenal steroids proximal to the enzymatic block, particularly the immediate preblock precursor 11-deoxycortisol. 11-Deoxycortisol can be measured in serum or urine (as tetrahydrol 11-deoxycortisol [THS]).
      b. Procedure
         (1) Metyrapone, 2 to 3 g as a single dose, depending on body weight (<70 kg, 2 g; 70 to 90 kg, 2.5 g; >90 kg, 3 g), is given at midnight with a snack, to minimize the nausea accompanying metyrapone.
         (2) Serum cortisol and 11-deoxycortisol are collected at 8 A.M. the following morning.
      c. Interpretation. A normal response is an increase in serum 11-deoxycortisol >7 μg/dL; patients with primary or secondary adrenal insufficiency exhibit <5 μg/dL. Cortisol levels should fall below 5 μg/dL to confirm adequate metyrapone-induced blockade of cortisol synthesis. An abnormal metyrapone test in a subject with a near-normal response to the rapid ACTH stimulation test suggests **secondary adrenal insufficiency.** The dose of metyrapone dose needs to be increased in patients receiving phenytoin (Dilantin), rifampin, mitotane, or phenobarbital, which enhance the clearance of both metyrapone and steroids. Alternatively, short-term discontinuation of these agents or

reliance on tests other than metyrapone should be considered. Adverse effects of metyrapone include gastric irritation, nausea, and vomiting. The overnight (single-dose) metyrapone test is generally safer than the standard multiple-dose metyrapone test; however, caution must be applied, especially in patients in whom primary adrenal disease is likely, because <u>adrenal crisis can be precipitated</u>. Hospitalization with proper monitoring of the patient's condition is therefore suggested for this test. It is advisable to demonstrate some responsiveness of the adrenal cortex to ACTH before initiating a metyrapone test. If the ACTH stimulation test is already markedly blunted, then the metyrapone test may not be required.

2. **Standard (multiple-dose) metyrapone tests**
   a. **Purpose:** Assessment of the functional capacity of the pituitary-adrenal axis. This test can be used to establish or confirm the diagnosis of primary or secondary adrenal insufficiency and, for this purpose, should be carried out as an <u>inpatient procedure</u> only. It may also be helpful in the differential diagnosis of established Cushing syndrome.
   b. **Procedure: serum**
      (1) Administer metyrapone, 750 mg PO q4h, for 6 doses from 8 A.M. on the first morning to 4 A.M. on the following morning.
      (2) Four hours following the last metyrapone dose (at 8 A.M.), draw blood for serum cortisol and 11-deoxycortisol levels.
   c. **Procedure: urine**
      (1) Day 1. Beginning at 8 A.M., collect a 24-hour urine sample for baseline creatinine and 17-OHCS levels.
      (2) Day 2. Repeat day 1. (Some investigators skip day 2 and use only one 24-hour urine collection, on day 1, for baseline determinations.)
      (3) Day 3. Repeat day 1. In addition, starting at 8 A.M., 750 mg metyrapone is given PO q4h for 6 doses.
      (4) Day 4. Repeat day 1.
   d. **Interpretation**
      (1) The normal response is a serum 11-deoxycortisol level of 10 μg/dL or greater at 8 A.M., 4 hours following the last dose of metyrapone. The plasma cortisol levels should be <5 μg/dL, indicating effective blockade by metyrapone. If a normal 11-deoxycortisol response is not seen and the cortisol levels are >5 μg/dL, the test should be repeated.
      (2) The normal response using the urine test is a two- to fourfold rise in 17-OHCS on the day of metyrapone treatment or on the day after. Generally, 17-OHCS will increase by at least 6 mg over baseline levels. In patients with primary or secondary adrenal insufficiency, little or no increase in 17-OHCS excretion is seen.
      (3) Because of enhanced metabolism of metyrapone, <u>patients on phenytoin (Dilantin)</u> generally have subnormal increases in serum 11-deoxycortisol levels after standard metyrapone administration. This can be corrected by administering a <u>double dose of metyrapone</u>, 750 mg q2h (12 doses), instead of 750 mg q4h (6 doses). Patients receiving estrogens (or who are pregnant) as well as those with hypothyroidism, renal failure, cirrhosis of the liver, or malnutrition may all have subnormal urine 17-OHCS responses to metyrapone. Exaggerated peak plasma 11-deoxycortisol has been encountered in women taking oral contraceptives and patients with hypothyroidism, diabetes mellitus, chronic renal failure, or congestive heart failure.
      (4) In the differential diagnosis of Cushing syndrome, stimulation of 17-OHS excretion by >70% or of a plasma 11-deoxycortisol level by >400-fold is indicative of pituitary (ACTH-dependent, cortisol feedback–sensitive) disease. The latter criterion, however, is difficult to implement, because most assays do not measure low basal (unstimulated) levels of plasma 11-deoxycortisol reliably.
   e. **Precautions.** Metyrapone-induced gastric irritation leading to nausea and vomiting can be reduced by administering the drug with food or milk.

Headaches and dizziness may be seen with the multiple-dose test and can be alleviated by bed rest. Caution should be observed when administering metyrapone to patients suspected of having primary adrenal insufficiency, because there is a risk of adrenal crisis. They should be closely observed during the test so that supportive measures can be given if needed.

D. Insulin-induced hypoglycemia test. Although this test remains the "gold standard" to diagnose hypofunction of the hypothalamic–pituitary–adrenal axis, the need for careful surveillance of hypoglycemic symptoms and potential complications, especially in individuals >55 years old, and the convenience and reliability of the rapid ACTH test, especially the 1-μg ACTH test, it is now performed less often than previously. Insulin-induced hypoglycemia is now reserved for the workup of equivocal or special cases as a second-line test. For details, see Anterior Pituitary, Section I.B.1.

 DYNAMIC ASSESSMENT OF HYPER- AND HYPOALDOSTERONISM

I. DYNAMIC TESTING FOR THE DIAGNOSIS OF PRIMARY HYPERALDOSTERONISM

A. Salt-volume loading tests

1. Purpose: Confirmation of the diagnosis of primary hyperaldosteronism (primary aldosteronism; PA), following initial screening based on the aldosterone/plasma renin activity (PRA) ratio (ARR). These tests should be deferred until hypokalemia is corrected and are not recommended in individuals with severe hypertension, renal or congestive heart failure, or cardiac arrhythmia. Given the variability of basal aldosterone levels in this disorder, the effect of blood pressure–lowering drugs on both PRA and aldosterone levels and the age-related decline in PRA, nonsuppressibility of aldosterone in response to volume-expansion maneuvers has proved to be an excellent indicator of primary hyperaldosteronism. Volume expansion via saline infusion, high salt intake, or mineralocorticoid administration in any condition other than primary hyperaldosteronism suppresses aldosterone levels by >50%. In primary hyperaldosteronism, an additional volume load has only a minimal effect on aldosterone concentration. Spuriously increased ARR may be corrected by the use of one or more of the following tests.

2. Saline infusion test

a. Procedure

(1) Patients should be on a regular diet. Obtain serum K^+ and proceed only if concentration is $\geq$4 mmol/L.

(2) Obtain baseline aldosterone levels.

(3) Infuse 0.9% sodium chloride solution for 4 hours (500 mL per hour, a total of 2 L).

(4) Obtain repeat samples for aldosterone and potassium.

b. Interpretation. Following the infusion, plasma aldosterone will normally suppress by at least **50%** or to <5 ng/dL, whereas patients with primary hyperaldosteronism will display postinfusion levels >10 ng/dL.

3. Oral salt loading test

a. Procedure

(1) Increase sodium intake to >200 mmol/L and add slow-release potassium chloride tablets to keep serum potassium in the normal range.

(2) Obtain 24-hour urine collection to verify that the intended intake has been attained.

(3) Obtain 24-hour urine collection starting on the morning of day 3 for the measurement of urinary aldosterone.

b. Interpretation. Urinary aldosterone excretion >12 to 14 μg per 24 hours is highly suggestive of PA, whereas excretion <10 μg per 24 hours practically excludes this diagnosis. HPLC/tandem mass spectrometry is the preferred method of measurement, because radioimmunoassays for urinary aldosterone perform poorly in this setting.

B. Captopril challenge test

1. **Purpose:** To confirm or exclude the diagnosis of primary hyperaldosteronism. Under normal conditions, inhibition of angiotensin-converting enzyme leads to an acute increase in PRA because of acute disinhibition of renin release, whereas plasma aldosterone declines because of the reduction in angiotensin II generation. In PA, PRA remains suppressed because of hypervolemia, and plasma aldosterone does not change appreciably because it is secreted autonomously.

2. **Procedure**
   a. After 1 hour in the sitting position, obtain blood for PRA, aldosterone, and cortisol.
   b. Administer 25 to 50 mg of captopril as a single oral dose and keep the patient in the sitting position for 1 to 2 hours.
   c. Draw a second blood sample for PRA, aldosterone, and cortisol

3. **Interpretation.** In normal subjects, plasma aldosterone declines by at least 30%, but it is hardly affected in primary aldosteronism. The test is not suitable for patients receiving angiotensin-converting enzyme inhibitors or angiotensin receptor blockers. Plasma aldosterone may be decreased in this test in some patients with idiopathic hyperaldosteronism. Equivocal or false negative results are not uncommon.

II. ALDOSTERONE POSTURE TEST: AN ANCILLARY TEST FOR EQUIVOCAL CASES OF PRIMARY HYPERALDOSTERONISM

A. Background. Aldosterone-producing adenoma appears to be quite responsive to ACTH, but not to angiotensin II. The opposite pertains to bilateral adrenal hyperplasia, in which angiotensin II is the major regulator.

B. Procedure for posture test

1. Samples for PRA and plasma aldosterone are obtained between 8 and 9 A.M., after the patient has been in the supine position for 30 minutes.

2. The patient assumes upright posture and ambulates moderately for 4 hours, at which time samples are collected again.

C. Interpretation. Normal subjects assuming upright posture always increase plasma renin activity and, therefore, plasma aldosterone levels, and this is further enhanced with ambulation. Because PRA is suppressed in aldosterone-producing adenoma (APA), plasma aldosterone does not respond to posture and declines in association with the diurnal reduction in ACTH (8 A.M. to noon). Patients with bilateral adrenal hyperplasia (BAH) show a normal increase (>25% of the baseline value) in aldosterone levels with upright posture, accounted for by a partially intact renin response and enhanced adrenal gland sensitivity to angiotensin II. However, up to 50% of patients with APA demonstrate posture increases in plasma aldosterone. In fact, the reliability of the test in distinguishing APA and BAH has been questioned in light of recent information that the magnitude of posture response depends on baseline levels of aldosterone, independent of adrenal pathology. This should therefore be seen as an ancillary procedure and interpreted only in the context of additional functional and imaging procedures.

III. RENIN STIMULATION TEST: CONFIRMING A "LOW RENIN STATUS"

A. Purpose. This test is suitable to confirm the presence of a low renin status. The test is useful to detect low-renin forms of hypertension, including mineralocorticoid excess syndromes, and to confirm the diagnosis of hyporeninemic hypoaldosteronism.

B. Procedure

1. This test should be performed between 8 A.M. and noon. Patients may be on a regular diet. If possible, all antihypertensive medications should be discontinued for 2 weeks prior to testing.

2. The patient should rest supine for at least 30 minutes, and a blood sample for plasma renin should then be drawn.

3. Furosemide, 60 to 80 mg PO, is given. The patient should then ambulate for 3 to 4 hours, after which a sample for plasma renin analysis is taken with the patient in the sitting or upright position.

C. Interpretation. Basal levels <1 ng/mL per hour and stimulated levels <2 ng/mL per hour are considered suppressed. Suppressed levels are typically seen in patients with primary aldosteronism, low-renin essential hypertension, Cushing syndrome, mineralocorticoid ingestion, 11-hydroxylase– and 17-hydroxylase–deficient forms of congenital adrenal hyperplasia, and Liddle syndrome. Lack of an increase in renin can also be seen in hyporeninemic hypoaldosteronism.

 THE ADRENAL MEDULLA

I. DYNAMIC TESTING FOR PHEOCHROMOCYTOMA
A. Clonidine suppression test
   1. Purpose: Evaluation of suspected pheochromocytoma
   2. Procedure
   a. If possible, all medications should be discontinued 1 week prior to the test.
   b. The patient should be fasted overnight prior to the test and prohibited from drinking coffee or smoking on the day of the test.
   c. An indwelling IV line kept open with normal saline should be inserted for blood drawing at least 30 minutes prior to the test.
   d. The patient should be kept supine in quiet surroundings for at least 30 minutes prior to and during the entire test.
   e. Draw baseline blood samples for epinephrine and norepinephrine, twice, at 5-minute intervals. A baseline blood pressure and heart rate should also be obtained.
   f. Give 0.3 mg clonidine PO with water.
   g. Draw blood samples for epinephrine and norepinephrine levels at hourly intervals for 3 hours. Blood pressure and heart rate measurements should be obtained every 30 minutes.
   3. Interpretation. Very high basal catecholamine levels (>2 000 pg/mL for norepinephrine) are indicative of pheochromocytoma. However, the vast majority of subjects evaluated for this condition will have much lower values. Patients usually have significant decreases in both blood pressure and heart rates, which are maximal 3 to 4 hours after clonidine administration. In patients with pheochromocytoma, the baseline high levels of norepinephrine are typically not affected by clonidine. In contrast, patients without pheochromocytoma may or may not have elevated baseline norepinephrine values, but levels of norepinephrine + epinephrine fall significantly after clonidine administration, to <500 pg/mL, or by more than 50% for norepinephrine.
   4. Precautions. Hypotension, sometimes marked, has been described during this test and may be a particular problem in patients who have received antihypertensive medications within a few days prior to the test. Patients should be observed during the entire test and frequent blood pressure readings obtained. **Clonidine is not recommended for use during pregnancy.**
B. Glucagon stimulation test
   1. Purpose: Evaluation of suspected pheochromocytoma, especially in subjects in whom the diagnosis is highly suspected on clinical grounds, but biochemical evidence cannot be recorded despite adequate attempts. With the current availability of assays for free plasma metanephrine and normetanephrine, which are present at increased levels independent of episodic secretion by the tumor, this as well as other types of stimulation tests should be reserved for truly unusual cases.
   2. Procedure
   a. An indwelling intravenous line should be in place to allow glucagon injection and, if necessary, intravenous Regitine therapy. Regitine ampoules should be prepared to counteract any extreme rises in blood pressure.

b. Blood sample for catecholamine measurements is collected at time 0.

c. Glucagon, 1 μg, is given IV as a bolus dose.

d. Two minutes after the injection, a second sample for catecholamine is collected.

e. Blood pressure should be monitored continuously at 1-minute intervals from 10 minutes to 20 minutes after the injection.

f. Patients may be pretreated with prazosin or nifedipine in preparation for this test if the diagnosis of pheochromocytoma appears likely. The test can be performed before the clonidine suppression test (in one session), but 1 hour should be allowed before the baseline levels for the clonidine test are drawn.

3. **Interpretation.** A peak level of norepinephrine >2 000 pg/mL or an increase of threefold or more over the baseline norepinephrine establishes the diagnosis of pheochromocytoma.

THE THYROID GLAND

I. HUMAN RECOMBINANT TSH ("THYROGEN") TEST

A. Purpose: Detection, through TSH-stimulated thyroglobulin (Tg) secretion, of residual/recurrent local or metastatic thyroid cancer in subjects who have already undergone total thyroidectomy for differentiated thyroid cancer.

B. Procedure. Although this test can be performed either in conjunction with or in independent of total-body radioiodine scan, it is presently most often performed with the total-body scan (TBS). The test is intended to assess Tg secretion in subjects receiving TSH-suppressive doses of T_4 on a regular basis. **Patients with increased circulating anti-Tg antibodies are not candidates for this test because of interference of the antibodies with the Tg assay, but they can still undergo Thyrogen-stimulated TBS.**

1. If the test is combined with TBS, patients are placed on a low-iodine diet for 2 to 4 weeks and urine iodine is determined to verify that a low iodine state has been attained.

2. While the patient continues to receive the usual dose of L-thyroxine required to attain TSH suppression, administer Thyrogen (0.9 mg) IM, on day 1 and again on day 2.

3. If TBS is to be performed, administer the diagnostic dose of radioiodine on day 3 and proceed with scanning on day 5 (72 hours after the last Thyrogen injection).

4. On day 5, 72 hours after the last Thyrogen injection, collect blood for the measurement of Tg, anti-Tg antibodies, and TSH.

C. Interpretation. It is presently recommended that in patients with initial T1–2 N0–1 M0 disease, who have already undergone total thyroidectomy + adjuvant radioiodine treatment and show no clinical evidence of residual disease, a stimulated Tg >2 ng/mL warrants immediate evaluation. On the other hand, under the same clinical circumstances, stimulated Tg of <0.6 ng/mL could be followed with annual measurement of TSH-suppressed Tg. Finally, an intermediate value requires repeat periodic stimulation testing.

II. TRH TEST

See Anterior Pituitary, Section III.A.

III. DYNAMIC TESTING IN MEDULLARY THYROID CARCINOMA (MTC)

The widely available genetic testing for *RET* mutations has made dynamic calcitonin stimulation tests largely obsolete. Calcitonin stimulation tests are optional under the following circumstances: **(a)** thyroid nodule of uncertain nature by fine-needle aspiration, with borderline or mildly elevated circulating calcitonin levels; **(b)** follow-up of patients with established MTC; **(c)** diagnosis of MTC in a patient with multiple endocrine neoplasia type 2 (MEN2) who did not undergo prophylactic thyroidectomy and who has no other evidence of MTC; **(d)** diagnosis of MTC in seemingly unaffected members of the rare families with MEN2 without identifiable *RET* mutations; **(e)** young children with MEN2 in whom the parents wish to delay thyroidectomy; **(f)** occasional patients with MEN2 who have already had thyroidectomy but who are being evaluated for the appearance of a new lesion in the neck or elsewhere.

A. Pentagastrin stimulation test

1. Purpose: Screening and diagnostic test for medullary thyroid carcinoma

2. Procedure

  a. The patient is fasted overnight.

  b. The next morning, draw baseline blood sample for calcitonin.

  c. Give pentagastrin (Peptavlon), 0.5 μg/kg as an IV bolus in <5 seconds.

  d. Collect samples for calcitonin levels at 2, 5, and 15 minutes after pentagastrin injection.

3. Interpretation

  a. Normal basal levels for calcitonin are assay-dependent but generally <70 pg/mL. Maximal responses to pentagastrin stimulation generally occur within 2 minutes after injection, and levels return to normal or undetectable within 10 to 30 minutes. Stimulated levels in normal subjects seldom exceed the normal range. Those patients with MTC whose baseline levels are elevated usually show a marked response (up to 20-fold increase above baseline levels) to pentagastrin and have clearly abnormal stimulated values. Many patients with MTC may have normal or borderline basal values but will show a similarly marked response. Furthermore, some subjects with low basal calcitonin but a pronounced response to pentagastrin with a peak value still within the normal range may indeed harbor early MTC or C-cell hyperplasia.

  b. An occasional patient with MTC may not respond to either pentagastrin or calcium (see later), and therefore both procedures should be used before ruling out the diagnosis. Sequential testing over a period of months or years may be required to confirm or rule out the diagnosis. Like the calcium infusion test, pentagastrin is not specific for MTC, and a variety of conditions can be associated with elevated calcitonin levels (see Section B.4 following).

4. Precautions. Pentagastrin commonly produces side effects, including vaguely defined, unpleasant sensations, nausea, epigastric tightness, vomiting and diarrhea, chest discomfort, headache, light-headedness, weakness, flushing, and hyperventilation. All side effects are brief, generally lasting no longer than a few minutes. It is advisable to avoid this test in hypocalcemic patients.

B. Calcium infusion tests

1. Purpose: Screening and diagnostic test for medullary thyroid carcinoma

2. Procedure: short calcium infusion

  a. The patient is fasted overnight.

  b. The following morning, draw a blood sample for baseline calcitonin.

  c. Infuse 150 mg calcium chloride (in 50 mL of 0.9% NaCl solution) over 10 minutes.

  d. Draw blood samples at 10, 20, 30, and 60 minutes after beginning the infusion.

3. Procedure: standard 4-hour infusion

  a. The patient is fasted overnight.

  b. The following morning, draw a blood sample for baseline calcitonin level.

  c. Infuse a total of 15 mg calcium/kg as calcium gluconate in 500 mL of 0.45% NaCl solution over a 4-hour period (i.e., 125 mL per hour).

  d. Blood samples are drawn at 60, 120, 180, and 240 minutes after beginning the infusion.

4. Interpretation. In normal subjects, baseline calcitonin levels are <70 pg/mL and seldom stimulate beyond the normal range. Those patients with MTC whose baseline levels are elevated usually show a marked response (up to a 20-fold increase above baseline levels) to calcium and have clearly supernormal stimulated values. A similar response is also seen in many patients with MTC who have normal or borderline basal values. A pronounced response to calcium stimulation even if stimulated levels are still within the normal range may indicate that early MTC or C-cell hyperplasia exists. Sequential testing over a period of months or years may be required to confirm or rule out the diagnosis.

Increased levels of calcitonin may be seen in pregnancy, hypercalcemic states, renal failure, subacute thyroiditis, pernicious anemia, various bone diseases, and a variety of tumors, particularly oat-cell carcinoma of the lung and carcinoma of the breast.

5. **Precautions.** The calcium load infused in the 4-hour test is large, and the serum calcium is often raised several milligrams per deciliter in a short period of time. Fatigue and lethargy are common side effects. Flushing, nausea, vomiting, and significant elevation in blood pressure may also occur and may last for several minutes. Particular caution must be observed in patients with cardiac arrhythmia and in subjects treated with digitalis glycosides. The **short calcium infusion test** is relatively free of side effects, and serum calcium levels generally are not increased more than 1 mg/dL.

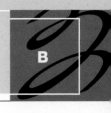

NORMAL REFERENCE LABORATORY VALUES FOR ENDOCRINE CHEMISTRY

B

Analyte	Fluid	MGH units	SI units	Method or instrument	Factor for conversion to SI units
Aldosterone					
Standing (normal-salt diet)	S, P	4–31 ng/dL	111–860 pmol/L	Immunoassay	27.74
Recumbent (normal-salt diet)	S, P	<16 ng/dL	<444 pmol/L	Immunoassay	27.74
Normal-salt diet (100–180 mEq of sodium)	U	6–25 μg/d	17–69 nmol/d	Immunoassay	2.774
Low-salt diet (10 mEq of sodium)	U	17–44 μg/d	47–122 nmol/d	Immunoassay	2.774
High-salt diet	U	0–6 μg/d	0–17 nmol/d	Immunoassay	2.774
Androstenedione	S	60–260 ng/dL	2.1–9.1 nmol/L	Immunoassay	0.0349
Antidiuretic hormone (arginine vasopressin)	P	1.0–13.3 pg/mL	1.0–13.3 ng/L	Immunoassay	1
Calcitonin	S			Immunoassay	
Female		0–20 pg/mL	0–20 ng/L		1
Male		0–28 pg/mL	0–28 ng/L		
Catecholamines					
Dopamine	U	65–400 μg/d	424–2 612 nmol/d	Liquid chromatography	6.53
	P	0–30 pg/mL	0–196 nmol/L	Liquid chromatography	6.53
Epinephrine	U	1.7–22.4 μg/d	9.3–122 nmol/d	Liquid chromatography	5.458
Supine	P	0–110 pg/mL	0–600 pmol/L	Liquid chromatography	5.458
Standing	P	0–140 pg/mL	0–764 pmol/L	Liquid chromatography	5.458
Norepinephrine	U	12.1–85.5 μg/d	72–505 nmol/d	Liquid chromatography	5.911
Supine	P	70–750 pg/mL	0.41–4.43 nmol/L	Liquid chromatography	0.005911
Standing	P	200–1 700 pg/mL	1.18–10.0 nmol/L	Liquid chromatography	0.005911
Chorionic gonadotropin (hCG) (nonpregnant)	S	<10 mIU/mL	<10 IU/L	Immunoassay	1
Corticotropin (ACTH)	P	6.0–76.0 pg/mL	1.3–16.7 pmol/L	Immunoassay	0.2202
Cortisol	P			Immunoassay	27.59
Fasting, 8 A.M.–12 noon		5.0–25.0 μg/dL	138–690 nmol/L		
12 noon–8 P.M.		5.0–15.0 μg/dL	138–410 nmol/L		
8 P.M.–8 A.M.		0.0–10.0 μg/dL	0–276 nmol/L		

(continued)

Analyte	Fluid	MGH units	SI units	Method or instrument	Factor for conversion to SI units
Cortisol, free	U	20–70 μg/d	55–193 nmol/d	Immunoassay	2.759
C-peptide	S	0.30–3.70 μg/L	0.10–1.22 nmol/L	Immunoassay	0.33
11-Deoxycortisol (after metyrapone)	P	>7.5 μg/dL	>216 nmol/L	Immunoassay	28.86
1,25-Dihydroxyvitamin D	S	16–42 pg/mL	38–101 pmol/L	Immunoassay	2.4
Erythropoietin	S	<19 mU/mL	≦19 U/L	Immunoassay	1
Estradiol	S, P			Immunoassay	3.671
Female					
Premenopausal adult		23–361 pg/mL	84–1 325 pmol/L		
Postmenopausal		<30 pg/mL	<110 pmol/L		
Prepubertal		<20 pg/mL	<73 pmol/L		
Male		<50 pg/mL	<184 pmol/L		
Gastrin	P	0–200 pg/mL	0–200 ng/L	Immunoassay	1
Growth hormone	P	2.0–6.0 ng/mL	2.0–6.0 μg/L	Immunoassay	1
Hemoglobin A$_{1c}$	P	3.8–6.4%	0.038–0.064%		0.01
Homovanillic acid	U	0.0–15.0 mg/d	0–82 μmol/d	Liquid chromatography	5.489
17-Hydroxycorticosteroids	U			Liquid chromatography	2.759
Female		2.0–6.0 mg/d	5.5–17 μmol/d	Colorimetry	
Male		3.0–10.0 mg/d	8–28 μmol/d		
5-Hydroxyindoleacetic acid (lower in women than in men)	U	2–9 mg/d	10–47 μmol/d	Colorimetry	5.23
17-Hydroxyprogesterone	S			Immunoassay	3.026
Female					
Prepubertal		0.20–0.54 μg/L	0.61–1.63 nmol/L		
Follicular		0.02–0.80 μg/L	0.61–2.42 nmol/L		
Luteal		0.90–3.04 μg/L	2.72–9.20 nmol/L		
Postmenopausal		<0.45 μg/L	<1.36 nmol/L		
Male					
Prepubertal		0.12–0.30 μg/L	0.36–0.91 nmol/L		
Adult		0.20–1.80 μg/L	0.61–5.45 nmol/L		

Analyte	Specimen	Conventional	SI	Method	Factor
25-Hydroxyvitamin D	S	8–55 ng/mL	20–137 nmol/L	Immunoassay	2.496
Insulin	S	0–29 µU/mL	0–208 pmol/L	Immunoassay	7.175
17-Ketogenic steroids	U			Colorimetry	3.467
Female		3.0–15.0 mg/d	10–52 µmol/d		
Male		5.0–23.0 mg/d	17–80 µmol/d		
17-Ketosteroids	U			Colorimetry	3.467
Female and male ≤10 y old		0.1–3.0 mg/d	0.4–10.4 µmol/d		
Female and male 11–14 y old		2.0–7.0 mg/d	6.9–24.2 µmol/d		
Female ≥15 y old		5.0–15.0 mg/d	17.3–52.0 µmol/d		
Male ≥15 y old		9.0–22.0 mg/d	31.2–76.3 µmol/d		
Metanephrines, total	U	0.0–0.90 mg/d	0.0–4.9 µmol/d	Spectrophotometry	5.458
Parathyroid hormone	P	10–60 pg/mL	10–60 ng/L	Immunoassay	1
Parathyroid-related protein	P	<1.5 pmol/L	<1.5 pmol/L	Immunoassay	1
Pregnanediol	U			Gas chromatography	3.12
Female					
Follicular phase		0.2–6.0 mg/d	0.6–18.7 µmol/d		
Luteal phase		0.1–1.3 mg/d	0.3–5.3 µmol/d		
Pregnancy		1.2–9.5 mg/d	3.7–29.6 µmol/d		
		Gestation-period dependent	Gestation-period dependent		
Male		0.2–1.2 mg/d	0.6–3.7 µmol/d		
Pregnanetriol	U	0.5–2.0 mg/d	1.5–6.0 µmol/d	Gas chromatography	2.972
Prolactin	S			Immunoassay	1
Female		0–15 ng/mL	0–15 µg/L		
Male		0–10 ng/mL	0–10 µg/L		
Renin activity	P			Immunoassay	0.2778
Normal salt intake					
Recumbent 6 h		0.5–1.6 ng/mL/h	0.14–0.44 ng/(L s)		
Upright 4 h		1.9–3.6 ng/mL/h	0.53–1.00 ng/(L s)		
Low salt intake					
Recumbent 6 h		2.2–4.4 ng/mL/h	0.61–1.22 ng/(L s)		
Upright 4 h		4.0–8.1 ng/mL/h	1.11–2.25 ng/(L s)		
Upright 4 h, with diuretic		6.8–15.0 ng/mL/h	1.89–4.17 ng/(L s)		

(continued)

Analyte	Fluid	MGH units	SI units	Method or instrument	Factor for conversion to SI units
Somatomedin C	P			Immunoassay	1
Female					
Preadolescent		60.8–724.5 ng/mL	60.8–724.5 μg/L		
Adolescent		112.5–450.0 ng/mL	112.5–450.0 μg/L		
Adult		141.8–389.3 ng/mL	141.8–389.3 μg/L		
Male					
Preadolescent		65.5–841.5 ng/mL	65.5–841.5 μg/L		
Adolescent		83.3–378.0 ng/mL	83.3–378.0 μg/L		
Adult		54.0–328.5 ng/mL	54.0–328.5 μg/L		
Testosterone, total, morning sample	P			Immunoassay	0.03467
Female		20–90 ng/dL	0.7–3.1 nmol/L		
Male, adult		300–1100 ng/dL	10.4–38.1 nmol/L		
Testosterone, unbound, morning sample	P			Equilibrium dialysis	34.67
Female, adult		0.09–1.29 ng/dL	3–45 pmol/L		
Male, adult		3.06–24.0 ng/dL	106–832 pmol/L		
Thyroglobulin	S	0–60 ng/mL	0–60 μg/L	Immunoassay	1
Thyroid hormone–binding index		0.83–1.17	0.83–1.17	Charcoal resin	1
Thyroid-stimulating hormone	S	0.5–5.0 μU/mL	0.5–5.0 mU/L	Immunoassay	1
Thyroxine, free	S	0.8–2.7 ng/dL	10–35 pmol/L	Direct equilibrium dialysis	12.87
Thyroxine-binding globulin	S	Age- and sex-dependent	Age- and sex-dependent	Immunoassay	
Thyroxine, free, index		4.6–11.2	4.6–11.2	Calculation	1
Thyroxine, total (T_4)	S	4–12 μg/dL	51–154 nmol/L	Immunoassay	12.87
Tri-iodothyronine, total (T_3)	S	75–195 ng/dL	1.2–3.0 nmol/L	Immunoassay	0.01536
Vanillylmandelic acid	U	1.4–6.5 mg/d	7.1–32.7 μmol/d	Liquid chromatography	5.046

S, serum; P, plasma; U, urine.
From Jordan CD, et al. Normal reference laboratory values. *N Engl J Med* 1992;327:718.

Note: Page numbers followed by f indicate figures; page numbers followed by t indicate tables.